Dermatology

Comprehensive Board Review and Practice Examinations

Caroline A. Nelson, MD

With

Hovik J. Ashchyan, MD
John S. Barbieri, MD, MBA
Jeff Gehlhausen, MD, PhD
Daniel M. Klufas, MD
Sherry H. Yu, MD

Editors

Paul L. Haun, MD: *Dermatopathology*
Nicole R. LeBoeuf, MD, MPH: *Medical Dermatology*
Arash Mostaghimi, MD, MPA, MPH: *Medical Dermatology*
Ivy I. Norris, MD: *Surgical Dermatology*
Misha Rosenbach, MD: *Medical Dermatology*
James Treat, MD: *Pediatric Dermatology*

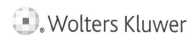
. Wolters Kluwer

Philadelphia · Baltimore · New York · London
Buenos Aires · Hong Kong · Sydney · Tokyo

Acquisitions Editor: James Sherman
Development Editor: Eric McDermott
Editorial Coordinator: Remya Divakaran, Varshaanaa SM
Editorial Assistant: Kristen Kardoley
Marketing Manager: Kirsten Watrud
Production Project Manager: Justin Wright
Manager, Graphic Arts & Design: Stephen Druding
Manufacturing Coordinator: Beth Welsh
Prepress Vendor: TNQ Technologies

1st edition

9 8 7 6 5 4 3 2 1

Printed in the United States of America.

Library of Congress Cataloging-in-Publication Data

ISBN-13: 978-1-975141-71-4

Cataloging in Publication data available on request from publisher.

shop.lww.com

Dedication

Caroline

To my husband for his unconditional love and support.

To my daughter for bringing sunshine into my life.

To my family, in particular my mother, my late father, my stepfather, and my brothers for showing me the joys of learning and giving back.

To my friends and colleagues for their encouragement.

To my mentors for teaching me to live and love dermatology.

To my residents, who teach me every day.

To my patients, who inspire me to be a better doctor.

Hovik

To my family for their unwavering support and unconditional love.

To my mentors and teachers, for being my confidants and helping me become the first college graduate and doctor in my family.

John

To my amazing wife, the love of my life.

To my family, for always being there for me.

To all my mentors, colleagues, and patients who push me to grow every day.

Jeff

A sincere thank you to my family and friends who offer support, understanding, and encouragement of my academic pursuits and the time and effort they require.

Dan

To my wife, the best and most steadfast partner one could imagine.

To my mother and father, whose unwavering support and love made me into the person I am today.

To my grandmother, who taught me the value of hard work and perseverance.

To my brothers, friends, classmates, teachers, mentors, coresidents, and patients, who have ridden alongside and guided me through this incredible journey of life—thank you.

Sherry

To my husband and our sons for their steadfast encouragement and support.

To my family, in particular my parents and sister, for encouraging me to do my best, as well as my friends and colleagues whose curiosity and drive constantly inspire me.

To my many mentors, past and present, for their continued guidance and friendship.

Authors

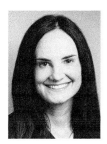

Caroline A. Nelson, MD
Director, Inpatient Dermatology
Assistant Professor of Dermatology
Yale New Haven Hospital
Yale University School of Medicine
New Haven, Connecticut

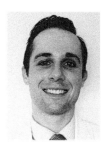

Jeff Gehlhausen, MD, PhD
Instructor of Dermatology
Yale New Haven Hospital
Yale University School of Medicine
New Haven, Connecticut

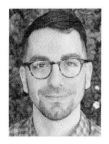

Hovik J. Ashchyan, MD
Fellow, Micrographic Surgery and
    Dermatologic Oncology
Memorial Sloan-Kettering Cancer
    Center
New York, New York

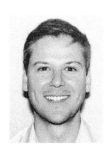

Daniel M. Klufas, MD
Assistant Professor of Dermatology
University of California San Francisco
San Francisco, California

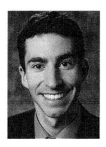

John S. Barbieri, MD, MBA
Director, Advanced Acne Therapeutics
    Clinic
Assistant Professor of Dermatology
Brigham and Women's Hospital
Harvard Medical School
Boston, Massachusetts

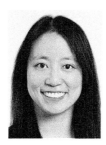

Sherry H. Yu, MD
Staff Physician
Department of Dermatology
Dermatology and Plastic Surgery
    Institute
Cleveland Clinic Foundation
Cleveland, Ohio

Editors

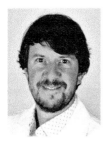

Paul L. Haun, MD: *Dermatopathology*
Assistant Professor of Dermatology and
  Dermatopathology
Assistant Professor of Anatomic
  Pathology and Laboratory Medicine
Hospital of the University of
  Pennsylvania
Perelman School of Medicine at the
  University of Pennsylvania
Philadelphia, Pennsylvania

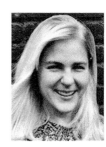

Ivy I. Norris, MD: *Surgical Dermatology*
Mohs Micrographic Surgeon
Valley View Dermatology
Salem, Oregon

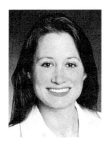

Nicole R. LeBoeuf, MD, MPH: *Medical
  Dermatology*
Director, Center for Cutaneous
  Oncology
Director, The Program in Skin Toxicities
  from Anticancer Therapies
Director, Cutaneous Oncology
  Fellowship Program
Co-Director, Complex Medical
  Dermatology Fellowship Program
Associate Professor of Dermatology
Brigham and Women's Hospital, Dana
  Farber Cancer Institute
Harvard Medical School, Boston,
  Massachusetts

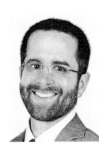

Misha Rosenbach, MD: *Medical
  Dermatology*
Program Director, Dermatology
  Residency
Vice Chair, Education and Training
Professor of Dermatology and Medicine
Hospital of the University of
  Pennsylvania
Perelman School of Medicine at the
  University of Pennsylvania
Philadelphia, Pennsylvania

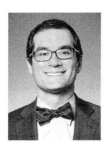

Arash Mostaghimi, MD, MPA, MPH:
  Medical Dermatology
Director, Dermatology Inpatient Service
Co-Director, Complex Medical
  Dermatology Fellowship Program
Assistant Professor of Dermatology
Brigham and Women's Hospital
Harvard Medical School
Boston, Massachusetts

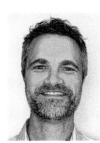

James Treat, MD: *Pediatric Dermatology*
Professor of Clinical Pediatrics and
  Dermatology
Education and Fellowship Directors for
  Pediatric Dermatology
Children's Hospital of Philadelphia
Perelman School of Medicine at the
  University of Pennsylvania
Philadelphia, Pennsylvania

Preface

Purpose of the Board Review and Practice Examinations

The American Board of Dermatology (ABD) has restructured its in-training and certification examinations to emphasize knowledge application over knowledge retention. The "Exam of the Future" is a staged evaluation consisting of multiple-choice questions as follows:

- *Basic* examination testing first-year residents on dermatology fundamentals (4 hours for approximately 200 questions);
- *Core* examination modules testing senior residents on advanced knowledge of medical dermatology, surgical dermatology, pediatric dermatology, and dermatopathology (2 hours for approximately 75-100 questions per module);
- *Applied* examination testing residency graduates on knowledge application to clinical scenarios (8 hours for approximately 240 questions).

This information is subject to change. Please check the ABD website for updates.

The Board Review and Practice Examinations are designed to help dermatology residents prepare for the "Exam of the Future." However, we hope that this presentation of the principles and practice of dermatology may be of benefit to learners around the world.

How to get the most out of the Board Review

The Board Review begins with an overview of science and research, progresses to review dermatologic diagnoses, and concludes with a summary of treatment techniques. It covers in-depth 100 diagnoses designated as "Group 1" or "Group 2" by the ABD Content Outline and Blueprint for the Basic Exam and 200 additional high-yield diagnoses. Other diagnoses selected by our editorial team are briefly summarized. Each section features a genodermatosis "spotlight." 200 "clinicopathological correlation," "side-by-side comparison," and "matching exercise" figures demonstrate high-yield histopathology.

To facilitate studying for the *basic* examination, diagnoses are labeled as "Group 1" or "Group 2". Online, the Board Review may be collapsed to view only these kodachromes or expanded to view all kodachromes.

To facilitate studying for the *core* examination modules, the Board Review is color-coded to indicate content most relevant to each module: medical dermatology in blue, surgical dermatology in red, pediatric dermatology in , and

dermatopathology in purple. The science and research chapter is divided according to the ABD as follows:

- Medical dermatology: epidemiology and statistics, immunology and inflammation, pharmacology.
- Surgical dermatology: carcinogenesis, photobiology, wound healing.
- Pediatric dermatology: embryology, genetics.
- Dermatopathology: structure and function, laboratory techniques.

Online, the Board Review may be collapsed to view only the content most relevant to each module. We used our best judgment; however, content overlap between modules is unavoidable.

To facilitate studying for the *applied* examination, the Board Review focuses on knowledge application to clinical practice. It reviews evidence-based recommendations for diagnosis and management, including relevant guidelines, with in-depth coverage of "Group 1" and "Group 2" diagnoses.

In the science and research chapter, clinical correlations boxes in orange highlight science and research applications to patient care. Summary tables are provided in the appendices: "Mucosal and Adnexal Disorders," "Dermatologic Signs of Internal Malignancy," and "Dermatologic Signs of Metabolic Disorders and Pregnancy." Dermoscopy, bedside diagnostics, and histopathology are reviewed in the "Dermatology Diagnostics" appendix. Finally, common codes and modifiers are reviewed in the "Billing" appendix. To facilitate learning, the Board Review includes memory aid boxes in and indicates high-yield content in the text with bold lettering.

Our understanding of what is high yield for the "Exam of the Future" will likely evolve over time. The optimal use of the Board Review is to refresh knowledge before each examination. It is NOT a substitute for reading textbooks or journal articles during residency.

How to get the most out of the Practice Examinations

The Practice Examinations contain 840 questions:

- One basic examination (200 questions);
- Four core examination modules: medical dermatology (100 questions), surgical dermatology (100 questions), pediatric dermatology (100 questions), and dermatopathology (100 questions);
- One applied examination (240 questions).

Answer choice rationales reference relevant sections of the Board Review for further reading.

Additional instructions on how to use the questions in the Practice Examinations may be found online at https://wolter-skluwer.vitalsource.com.

Additional Information

Comments from the readers for any omissions or errors are welcome. Please email Caroline.Nelson@yale.edu.

Acknowledgments

We are greatly indebted to Noel Turner, MD, MHS, Chief Resident in Dermatology and Christine J. Ko, MD, Professor in Dermatology and Dermatopathology at the Yale University School of Medicine for contributing histopathology images.

Many memory aids in the Board Review are of our own creation; however, for other memory aids, we are grateful for the creative effort of authors of other review books and dermatology learners past and present. We would like to specifically acknowledge the medical students, residents, fellows, faculty, and administrative staff at our respective institutions. They have been essential to our learning process and co-collaborators in bringing this project to life.

Finally, we appreciate the expertise of the editorial and publication team at Wolters Kluwer, without whom this project would not have been possible.

Contents

Authors   v
Editors   vii
Preface   ix
Acknowledgements   xi

1. Science and Research   1

    Structure and Function   1
    Embryology   15
    Genetics   15
    Carcinogenesis   19
    Photobiology   22
    Immunology and Inflammation   25
    Wound Healing   35
    Pharmacology   36
    Laboratory Techniques   38
    Epidemiology and Statistics   41

2. Nonneoplastic Disorders   49

Papulosquamous Disorders and Palmoplantar
Keratodermas   49
    Psoriasis: Group 1   49
    Reactive Arthritis   54
    Geographic Tongue: Group 2   55
    Parapsoriasis: Group 2   55
    Pityriasis Lichenoides   56
    Pityriasis Rosea: Group 1   56
    Pityriasis Rubra Pilaris: Group 2   58
    Spotlight on Hereditary Palmoplantar Keratodermas   59
    Granular Parakeratosis   62
    Acanthosis Nigricans: Group 1   62
    Confluent and Reticulated Papillomatosis   64

Eczematous Dermatoses and Related Disorders   64
    Atopic dermatitis: Group 1   65
    Asteatotic Dermatitis   67
    Dyshidrotic Eczema   67
    Nummular Dermatitis: Group 1   68
    Seborrheic Dermatitis Group 1   68
    Stasis Dermatitis: Group 1   69
    Contact Dermatitis: Group 1   70
    Ichthyosis Vulgaris: Group 2   78
    Spotlight on Hereditary Ichthyoses and
    Erythrokeratodermas   79
    Keratosis Pilaris   79

Pigmentary Disorders   83
    Vitiligo: Group 1   84
    Erythema Dyschromicum Perstans   85
    Pigmentary Demarcation Lines   87
    Prurigo Pigmentosa   88
    Spotlight on Incontinentia Pigmenti   88

Vesiculobullous Disorders   93
    Acute Generalized Exanthematous Pustulosis: Group 2 93
    Pemphigus Foliaceus   96
    Pemphigus Vulgaris: Group 2   96
    Immunoglobulin A Pemphigus   98
    Paraneoplastic Pemphigus   99
    Spotlight on Hailey-Hailey Disease and Darier Disease 100
    Grover Disease   102
    Bullous Pemphigoid: Group 2   102
    Linear Immunoglobulin A Bullous Dermatosis   105
    Mucous Membrane Pemphigoid   106
    Epidermolysis Bullosa Acquisita   107
    Dermatitis Herpetiformis: Group 2   107

Interface Dermatoses and Other Connective
Tissue Disorders   110
    Lichen Planus: Group 1   111
    Lichenoid Drug Eruption: Group 2   114
    Lichen Striatus: Group 2   114
    Lichen Nitidus   115
    Erythema Multiforme: Group 1   116
    Stevens-Johnson Syndrome/Toxic Epidermal
    Necrolysis: Group 1   117
    Fixed Drug Eruption: Group 2   119
    Toxic Erythema of Chemotherapy   120
    Graft-Versus-Host Disease   120
    Lupus Erythematosus: Group 1   121
    Dermatomyositis: Group 1   127
    Lichen Sclerosus: Group 2   129
    Morphea: Group 2   131
    Systemic Sclerosis: Group 2   134
    Eosinophilic Fasciitis   135
    Nephrogenic Systemic Fibrosis   136
    Relapsing Polychondritis   136
    Rheumatoid Arthritis   136
    Adult-Onset Still Disease   137
    Acquired Perforating Dermatosis   137
    Spotlight on Pseudoxanthoma Elasticum   141

Panniculitis and Lipodystrophy   144
    Erythema Nodosum: Group 2   144
    Lipodermatosclerosis: Group 2   147
    Spotlight on Hereditary Lipodystrophies   149

Urticaria and Other Erythemas   150
    Urticaria: Group 1   150
    Spotlight on Hereditary Angioedema   153
    Erythema Annulare Centrifugum   154
    Morbilliform Drug Eruption: Group 1   154
    Drug Reaction with Eosinophilia and Systemic
    Symptoms   155
    Polymorphic Eruption of Pregnancy   157
    Kawasaki Disease   158

Livedo Reticularis, Purpura, and Other Vascular
Disorders   158
    Livedo Reticularis: Group 1   161
    Livedoid Vasculopathy: Group 2   162

Spotlight on Neonatal Purpura Fulminans | 164
Malignant Atrophic Papulosis | 164
Cholesterol Emboli | 164
Calciphylaxis: Group 2 | 165
Pigmented Purpura: Group 2 | 168
Small Vessel Vasculitis: Group 1 | 169
Serum Sickness-Like Eruption | 170
Immunoglobulin A Vasculitis | 171
Urticarial Vasculitis | 171
Erythema Elevatum Diutinum | 172
Cryoglobulinemia | 172
Antineutrophil Cytoplasmic Antibody Vasculitis | 174
Polyarteritis Nodosa: Group 2 | 176
Giant Cell Arteritis | 177
Edema Blister | 177
Lymphedema | 178
Venous Ulcer | 178
Arterial Ulcer | 180
Diffuse Dermal Angiomatosis | 180
Erythromelalgia | 181

Neurocutaneous and Psychocutaneous Disorders | 181
Prurigo Nodularis: Group 1 | 181
Lichen Simplex Chronicus: Group 2 | 183
Complex Regional Pain Syndrome | 184
Spotlight on Familial Dysautonomia | 185
Delusions of Parasitosis | 186
Excoriation Disorder | 186
Factitial Dermatitis: Group 2 | 187

Disorders of Sebaceous, Apocrine, and Eccrine Glands | 188
Acne Vulgaris: Group 1 | 188
Hidradenitis Suppurativa: Group 2 | 193
Rosacea: Group 1 | 194
Periorificial Dermatitis: Group 1 | 196
Lupus Miliaris Disseminatus Faciei | 197
Hyperhidrosis | 197
Spotlight on Ectodermal Dysplasias | 198
Miliaria | 200

Disorders of the Hair and Nails | 200
Alopecia Areata: Group 1 | 200
Trichotillomania | 203
Androgenetic Alopecia | 204
Traction Alopecia | 205
Anagen Effluvium | 205
Telogen Effluvium | 205
Frontal Fibrosing Alopecia/Lichen Planopilaris | 206
Central Centrifugal Cicatricial Alopecia | 208
Acne Keloidalis | 208
Dissecting Cellulitis of the Scalp | 209
Hypertrichosis | 210
Beau Lines: Group 2 | 211
Spotlight on Pachyonychia Congenita | 213

Neutrophilic and Eosinophilic Dermatoses | 215
Sweet Syndrome: Group 2 | 215
Neutrophilic Eccrine Hidradenitis | 217
Recurrent Aphthous Stomatitis | 217
Behçet Disease | 219
Pyoderma Gangrenosum: Group 1 | 219
Spotlight on Syndromic Pyoderma Gangrenosum | 222
Bowel-Associated Dermatosis-Arthritis Syndrome | 222
Granuloma Faciale | 223
Eosinophilic Pustular Folliculitis | 223
Wells Syndrome | 224
Hypereosinophilic Syndrome | 225

Noninfectious Granulomas, Histiocytoses, and Xanthomas | 225
Sarcoidosis: Group 2 | 226
Spotlight on Blau syndrome | 230
Granuloma Annulare: Group 1 | 230
Necrobiosis Lipoidica: Group 2 | 232
Langerhans Cell Histiocytosis | 233
Necrobiotic Xanthogranuloma | 234
Xanthoma | 236

Depositional Disorders, Porphyrias, and Nutritional Deficiencies | 237
Scleromyxedema | 240
Scleredema | 240
Amyloidosis | 243
Gout | 245
Spotlight on Lipoid Proteinosis | 248
Porphyria Cutanea Tarda: Group 2 | 248
Zinc Deficiency | 252

3. Infections, Infestations, and Other Animal Kingdom Encounters | 265

Viral Diseases | 265
Herpes Simplex: Group 1 | 265
Eczema Herpeticum: Group 1 | 272
Varicella: Group 1 | 272
Herpes Zoster: Group 1 | 273
Infectious Mononucleosis | 274
Cytomegalovirus Infection | 275
Rubeola, Rubella, and Roseola | 277
Wart: Group 1 | 278
Spotlight on Epidermodysplasia Verruciformis | 280
Molluscum Contagiosum: Group 1 | 280
Erythema Infectiosum | 283
Coronavirus Disease 2019 | 283
Dengue | 284
Hand-Foot-Mouth Disease: Group 2 | 284

Bacterial Diseases | 285
Impetigo: Group 1 | 288
Staphylococcal Scalded Skin Syndrome | 289
Scarlet Fever | 290
Toxic Shock Syndrome | 291
Cellulitis: Group 1 | 291
Erysipelas | 292
Necrotizing Fasciitis | 292
Bacterial Abscess | 293
Spotlight on Chronic Granulomatous Disease | 294
Bacterial Folliculitis | 294
Paronychia | 295
Pitted Keratolysis: Group 2 | 295
Erythrasma | 296
Anthrax | 297
Actinomycosis | 298
Septic Vasculitis and Infective Endocarditis | 298
Ecthyma Gangrenosum | 300
Vibriosis | 301
Cat Scratch Disease | 303
Rocky Mountain Spotted Fever | 303
Lyme Disease | 304
Syphilis | 308
Tuberculosis | 309
Leprosy | 313

Fungal Diseases | 315
Tinea Versicolor: Group 1 | 315

Tinea Nigra 317
Piedra 318
Tinea: **Group 1** 318
Tinea Capitis 320
Onychomycosis: **Group 1** 321
Candidiasis: **Group 1** 322
Spotlight on Chronic Mucocutaneous Candidiasis 324
Blastomycosis, Chromoblastomycosis, and
Paracoccidioidomycosis 325
Coccidioidomycosis 327
Histoplasmosis and Talaromycosis 327
Cryptococcosis 329
Lobomycosis 329
Sporotrichosis: **Group 2** 330
Angioinvasive Fungal Infection 331
Mycetoma 333
Protothecosis 333

Parasitic Diseases and Other Animal Kingdom Encounters 334
Leishmaniasis 334
Cutaneous Larva Migrans: **Group 2** 336
Spotlight on Hyper-Immunoglobulin E Syndromes 343
Scabies and Lice: **Group 1** 343
Arthropod Bites: **Group 2** 347

4. Disorders Due to Physical Agents 353

Photodermatoses 353
Polymorphous Light Eruption: **Group 2** 353
Hydroa Vacciniforme 354
Chronic Actinic Dermatitis 355
Solar Urticaria 355
Spotlight on Xeroderma Pigmentosum 356
Photoallergic/Phototoxic Eruption: **Group 2** 358
Poikiloderma of Civatte: **Group 2** 359

Other Physical Agents 360
Erythema Ab Igne 363
Pernio 363
Spotlight on Sickle Cell Disease 364
Black Heel and Palm 364
Chondrodermatitis Nodularis Helicis: **Group 2** 365

5. Neoplasms and Cysts 367

Epidermal Neoplasms 367
Seborrheic Keratosis: **Group 1** 367
Epidermal Nevus 369
Clear Cell Acanthoma 370
Basal Cell Carcinoma: **Group 1** 370
Spotlight on Basal Cell Nevus Syndrome 374
Porokeratosis: **Group 2** 375
Actinic Keratosis: **Group 1** 376
Squamous Cell Carcinoma: **Group 1** 377
Keratoacanthoma 381
Mammary Paget Disease and
Extramammary Paget Disease 381

Melanocytic Neoplasms 382
Lentigo Simplex: **Group 1** 382
Dermal Melanocytosis 385
Blue Nevus: **Group 2** 386
Nevocellular Nevus and Atypical Nevus: **Group 1** 387
Congenital Melanocytic Nevus 389
Nevus Spilus: **Group 2** 390
Halo Nevus 390
Spitz Nevus: **Group 2** 391

Melanoma: **Group 1** 393
Spotlight on Familial Atypical Multiple
Mole Melanoma Syndrome 398

Fibrous Neoplasms 399
Keloid: **Group 1** 399
Angiofibroma: **Group 2** 401
Spotlight on Tuberous Sclerosis 402
Dermatofibroma: **Group 1** 403
Dermatofibrosarcoma Protuberans 406
Atypical Fibroxanthoma 406
Epithelioid Sarcoma 406

Adipose Neoplasms 407
Hibernoma 409
Lipoma 409
Spotlight on Cowden Syndrome 411

Vascular Malformations and Neoplasms 412
Angiokeratoma: **Group 2** 412
Capillary Malformation: **Group 2** 413
Venous Malformation 415
Lymphatic Malformation 417
Arteriovenous Malformation 418
Hemangioma: **Group 1** 419
Spotlight on PHACE(S) Syndrome and
LUMBAR Syndrome 422
Pyogenic Granuloma: **Group 2** 423
Cherry Angioma 424
Tufted Angioma and Kaposiform Hemangioendothelioma 424
Kaposi Sarcoma: **Group 2** 426
Angiosarcoma 428
Glomus Tumor and Glomuvenous Malformation 429

Neural Malformations and Neoplasms 430
Aplasia Cutis Congenita 431
Neurofibroma 432
Schwannoma 432
Spotlight on Neurofibromatosis: **Group 2** 434
Neuroma 435
Granular Cell Tumor 436
Merkel Cell Carcinoma 437

Neoplasms of Sebaceous, Apocrine, and Eccrine Glands 439
Nevus Sebaceous: **Group 2** 439
Sebaceous Gland Hyperplasia: **Group 1** 440
Sebaceous Adenoma and Sebaceoma 441
Sebaceous Carcinoma 442
Spotlight on Muir-Torre Syndrome 443
Cylindroma and Spiradenoma 443
Syringocystadenoma Papilliferum and Hidradenoma
Papilliferum 444
Hidradenoma 446
Poroma 446
Syringoma: **Group 2** 446
Microcystic Adnexal Carcinoma 448
Mucinous Carcinoma 450

Neoplasms of the Hair and Nails 450
Nevus Comedonicus 452
Trichoepithelioma 453
Spotlight on Birt-Hogg-Dubé Syndrome 455
Tricholemmoma 455
Pilomatricoma 457
Onychomatricoma 458

Other Malformations and Neoplasms 459
Accessory Tragus 459
Rudimentary Supernumerary Digit 460

■ Leiomyoma 461
Spotlight on Hereditary Leiomyomatosis and
Renal Cell Cancer 462
Becker Nevus: Group 2 462

Cysts and Pseudocysts 464
■ Epidermoid Cyst 464
Spotlight on Gardner Syndrome 467
■ Hidrocystoma 467
■ Digital Mucous Cyst 468

Hematolymphoid Neoplasms and Solid Organ
Metastases 470
■ Cutaneous T-Cell Lymphoma: Group 1 471
■ Lymphomatoid Papulosis 472
■ Cutaneous B-Cell Lymphoma 476
■ Cutaneous Lymphoid Hyperplasia 476
■ Leukemia Cutis 478
Spotlight on Mastocytosis 480
■ Solid Organ Metastasis 481

6. Medical Treatments 487

Immunosuppressants and Immunomodulators 487
Antihistamines and Related Drugs 497
Retinoids 497
Hormonal Drugs 500
Antimicrobials 501
Antineoplastics 511
Miscellaneous Drugs 523

7. Physical Treatments 529

Phototherapy 529
Photodynamic Therapy 529
Radiation Therapy 531
Cryosurgery 532
Electrocautery and Electrosurgery 533

8. Surgery 537

Surgical Anatomy 537
Preoperative Considerations 545
Anesthetics and Antiseptics 546
Surgical Instruments and Materials 549
Basic Surgical Procedures 557
Mohs Micrographic Surgery 558
Flaps and Grafts 561
Surgical Emergencies and Complications 566
Nail Unit Surgery 569

9. Cosmetics 573

Cosmetics and Cosmeceuticals 573
Chemical and Mechanical Skin Resurfacing 574
Lasers 576
Botulinum Neurotoxins 578
Soft-Tissue Dermal Fillers 580
Body Contouring 582
Sclerotherapy 583
Hair Restoration 583

Appendix 1: Mucosal and Adnexal Disorders 587

Appendix 2: Dermatologic Signs of Internal
Malignancy 605

Appendix 3: Dermatologic Signs of Metabolic
Disorders and Pregnancy 609

Appendix 4: Dermatology Diagnostics 613

Appendix 5: Billing 637

Abbreviations 641
Index 649

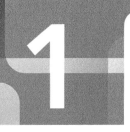

Science and Research

Caroline A. Nelson, MD

Structure and Function

Basic Concepts

- The skin consists of three layers: the epidermis, the dermis, and the subcutis.
- Key functions include maintenance of the skin barrier, prevention of infection, wound healing, nutrition, thermoregulation, and physical and interpersonal communication.

Skin (Figure 1.1)

Epidermis

Keratinocytes

- The cytoskeletal network of keratinocytes is made up of actin microfilaments and keratin (K) intermediate filaments.
- **Keratin intermediate filaments** are coexpressed as **heterodimers**:
  - **Type I**: low molecular weight, acidic, K9-28, K31-40, gene locus on chromosome 17.
  - **Type II**: high molecular weight, basic, K1-8, K71-86, gene locus on chromosome 12.
    - ◆ Table 1.1.
- Keratinocyte **stem cells** are located at the **base of rete ridges** in the interfollicular epithelium and the **bulge** region of hair follicles.

- Terminal keratinocyte **differentiation** (Figure 1.2) is mediated by p63 and NOTCH signaling along with an **increase in extracellular calcium. Phospholipids decrease and sphingolipids increase.** The lipid composition in the *stratum corneum* is **~45% to 50% ceramide, 25% cholesterol, 10% to 15% free fatty acids (FFAs), 5% cholesterol sulfate, and other lipids. Ceramide is the major lipid** component of the cornified lipid envelope, while **loricrin is the major protein** component of the cornified cell envelope.
  - Phospholipids are on the phloor.
  - ◆ Table 1.2.
- The total **transit time** of a keratinocyte through normal epidermis is **~28 days (14 days from *stratum basale* to *stratum corneum* and 14 days from *stratum corneum* to desquamation).**
  - ◆ Keratinocyte transit time decreases in hyperproliferative disease states such as psoriasis.

Langerhans Cells

- See Chapter 1: Immunology and Inflammation.

Melanocytes

- Melanocytes are derived from the **neural crest. KIT and KIT ligand signaling** is an important mediator of melanocyte migration.
  - ◆ Sporadic mutation of the gene encoding KIT disrupts melanocyte migration leading to piebaldism. Autosomal dominant (AD) gain-of-function mutation

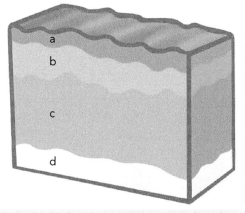
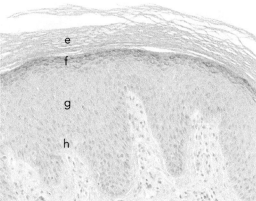

Figure 1.1. SKIN. a-epidermis, b-papillary dermis, c-reticular dermis, d-subcutis. Epidermal layers: e-*stratum corneum*, f-*stratum granulosum*, g-*stratum spinosum*, h-*stratum basale*.

(Illustration by Caroline A. Nelson, MD; Histology image courtesy of Noel Turner, MD, MHS and Christine J. Ko, MD.)

Table 1.1. DISORDERS OF KERATIN

Type II	Type I	Location of Expression	Associated Disorders[a]
1	10	Suprabasal layers	EI, ichthyosis with confetti, ichthyosis hystrix Curth-Macklin (K1)
1	9	Palmoplantar suprabasal layers	Vörner-Unna-Thost epidermolytic PPK, nonepidermolytic PPK (K1), striate PPK (K1)
2[b]	10	Upper spinous and granular layers	Superficial EI (K2)
3	12	Cornea	Meesmann corneal dystrophy
4	13	Mucosa	White sponge nevus
5	14	Basal layer	DDD (K5), EBS, EBS with mottled pigmentation (K5 > K14), NFJ syndrome/DPR (K14)
6a, 6b, 6c	16, 17	Hair follicle isthmus, nail bed	Hyperproliferative disease states such as psoriasis (increased K6 and K16), PC,[c] steatocystoma (K17), vellus hair cyst (K17)
81, 83, 86[d]		Hair cortex	Monilethrix

DDD, Dowling-Degos disease; DPR, dermatopathia pigmentosa reticularis; EBS, epidermolysis bullosa simplex; EI, epidermolytic ichthyosis; K, keratin; NFJ, Naegeli-Franceschetti-Jadassohn; PC, pachyonychia congenita; PPK, palmoplantar keratoderma.
[a]Illustrative examples provided for clinical correlation.
[b]Previous name K2e.
[c]Historical classification divided PC into type I (Jadassohn-Lewandowsky) due to mutations in K6a and K16 and type II (Jackson-Lawler) due to mutations in K6b and K17.
[d]Previous names Hb1, Hb3, Hb6; monilethrix is also due to mutations in desmoglein-4.

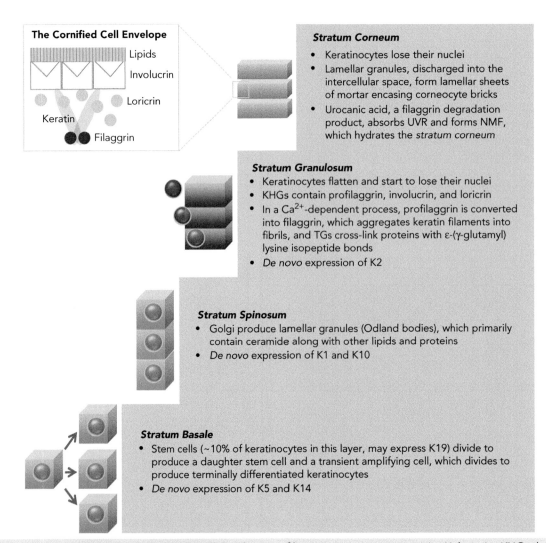

Figure 1.2. THE LIFE CYCLE OF KERATINOCYTES. Filaggrin, filament aggregating protein; K, keratin; KHGs, keratohyalin granules; NMF, natural moisturizing factor; TGs, transglutaminases; UVR, ultraviolet radiation.

in the gene encoding KIT ligand increases melanocyte migration, leading to familial progressive hyperpigmentation.

- Melanocytes are primarily located in the *stratum basale* in a ratio of **1 melanocyte to 10 keratinocytes**. Other sites include the **mucous membranes, hair, uveal tract of the eye (choroid, ciliary body, iris, retina), inner ear (*striae vascularis* of the cochlea), and leptomeninges.**
  - Congenital melanocytic nevi may be associated with increased melanocytes at other sites, such as neurocutaneous melanosis.
- Under the influence of **melanocyte-stimulating hormone (MSH), a product of the proopiomelanocortin (POMC) polypeptide**, melanocytes synthesize melanin pigment. POMC is also the **precursor of adrenocorticotropic hormone (ACTH).**
  - Stimulation of POMC is the mechanism of hyperpigmentation in Addison disease.
- Melanocytes synthesize melanin in **melanosomes (specialized lysosomes). Tyrosinase**, a product of the *TYR* gene, **is the copper-dependent rate-limiting enzyme** that catalyzes the conversion of tyrosine to dihydroxyphenylalanine (DOPA) and DOPA to dopaquinone.
  - Oculocutaneous albinism (OCA) may result from defective vesicle assembly, trafficking, or transport (eg, Chédiak-Higashi syndrome) or defective melanin synthesis (eg, *TYR* mutation in OCA, type I). Tyrosinase is also impaired in copper-deficient states such as Menkes kinky hair disease.
- Synthesis of pheomelanin versus eumelanin is primarily determined by the **melanocortin-1 receptor (MC1R):**
  - **Pheomelanin:** red-yellow, synthesized in spherical melanosomes with microvesicular structure.
  - **Eumelanin:** brown-black, synthesized in elliptical melanosomes with lamellar structure.
    - Dysfunction of the MC1R can lead to red hair, inability to tan following ultraviolet radiation (UVR) exposure, and increased risk of melanoma and nonmelanoma skin cancer.

- One melanocyte transfers melanin to ~30 to 40 keratinocytes via phagocytosis of melanocyte tips. This constitutes an epidermal melanin unit. Melanin absorbs UVR, thereby protecting against UVR-induced mutations. Melanocyte density is consistent across all skin phototypes (Table 1.3); however, melanosomes in darker skin are larger, darker, more stable, more numerous, and transferred as individual organelles as opposed to membrane-bound clusters, ultimately exhibiting a higher degree of dispersion within keratinocytes.

Merkel Cells

- Merkel cells are primarily located in the *stratum basale* in areas with **high tactile sensitivity** such as the hair follicle outer root sheath (ORS), lips, oral cavity, fingertips, and anogenital region.
- Merkel cells function as **mechanoreceptors** and contain **neuropeptides such as calcitonin gene–related peptide, chromogranin A, met-enkephalin, neuron-specific enolase, synaptophysin, and vasoactive intestinal peptide.**

Junctions

Intercellular Junctions (Figure 1.3)

- Keratinocytes are bound together by a variety of cell-cell junctions:
  - **Tight junctions (*zonula occludens*):** seal the intercellular space with claudins and occludins to prevent the free diffusion of macromolecules (eg, water loss in the granular layer).
  - **Adherens junctions (*zonula adherens*):** bind cells together with actin cytoskeleton linked to α-catenin linked to armadillo family proteins (β-catenin or plakoglobin) linked to transmembrane proteins (classic cadherins E and P).
  - **Desmosomes:** bind cells together with keratin cytoskeleton linked to plakin family protein (desmoplakin) linked to armadillo family proteins (plakoglobin or plakophilin) linked to calcium-dependent transmembrane proteins (cadherins desmocollin 1/2/3 and desmoglein 1/3). **Plakoglobin, also known as γ-catenin, is the only common protein between adherens junctions and desmosomes. Desmoglein 1 is 160 kDa and desmoglein 3 is 130 kDa.**

Table 1.2. DISORDERS OF CORNIFICATION

Target	Associated Disorders[a]
Lamellar granules	ARCI (decreased or absent), EI (increased but abnormal), Flegel disease (decreased or absent), steroid sulfatase deficiency
Filaggrin	AD, ichthyosis vulgaris, KP
Involucrin	Psoriasis (increased)
Loricrin	Loricrin keratoderma, psoriasis (decreased)
TG-1[b]	LI

AD, atopic dermatitis; ARCI, autosomal recessive congenital ichthyosis; DH, dermatitis herpetiformis; EI, epidermolytic ichthyosis; filaggrin, filament aggregating protein; KP, keratosis pilaris; LI, lamellar ichthyosis; TG, transglutaminase.
[a]Illustrative examples provided for clinical correlation.
[b]The auto-antigen in DH is TG-3.

Table 1.3. FITZPATRICK SCALE OF SKIN PHOTOTYPES

Skin Phototype	Response to UVR
I	Always burns, does not tan
II	Burns easily, tans with difficulty
III	Mild burns, tans gradually
IV	Rarely burns, tans easily
V	Very rarely burns, tans very easily
VI	Never burns, tans very easily

UVR, ultraviolet radiation.

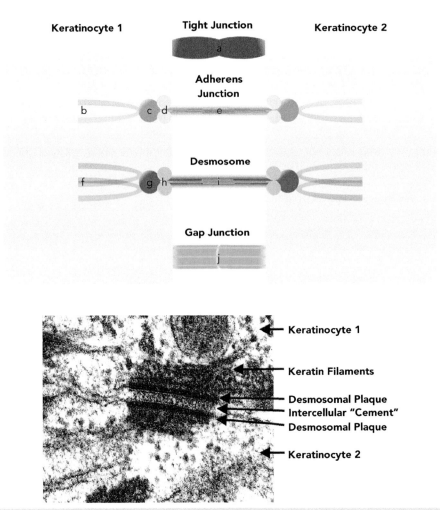

Figure 1.3. KERATINOCYTE INTERCELLULAR JUNCTIONS. a-claudins and occludins, b-actin monofilaments, c-α-catenin d-β-catenin and plakoglobin, e-classic cadherins E and P, f-keratin intermediate filaments, g-desmoplakin, h-plakoglobin and plakophilin, i-cadherins desmocollin 1/2/3 and desmoglein 1/3, j-6 connexins forming a connexon. Ultrastructure of a desmosome.

(Electron microscopy image reprinted with permission from Elder DE, Elenitsas R, Rosenbach M, et al. *Lever's Histopathology of the Skin.* 11th ed. Wolters Kluwer; 2015.)

◈ The name of a protein may provide a clue to its family. Armadillos are covered in plates (plakoglobin, plakophilin, plus β-catenin); plakins often end with plakin (desmoplakin, envoplakin, periplakin, plus bullous pemphigoid antigen 1 [BPAG1] and plectin). Cadherins are calcium-dependent.

○ **Gap junctions**: facilitate intercellular communication through connexons (six connexins).

Basement Membrane Zone (Figure 1.4)

● The basement membrane zone (BMZ) consists of dermo-epidermal junction (DEJ) and dermal blood vessels.
● The DEJ can be divided into four layers with the following key components:
  ○ **Basal keratinocyte hemidesmosomes**: keratin cytoskeleton linked to plakin family proteins (BPAG1 and plectin) linked to transmembrane proteins (bullous pemphigoid antigen 2 [BPAG2] and α6β4 integrin).

  ○ *Lamina lucida*: transmembrane proteins linked to anchoring filaments (eg, laminin 332).
  ○ *Lamina densa*: anchoring filaments linked to collagen IV linked to anchoring fibrils (collagen VII) along with heparin sulfate (provides a selective permeability barrier).
  ○ *Sublamina densa*: anchoring fibrils linked by anchoring plaques to collagen I and III along with elastic fibers.
● Based on molecular weight (kDa), BPAG1 is also known as BP230 and BPAG2 is also known as BP180. Another name for BPAG2 is collagen XVII. The amino terminus of BPAG2 is intracellular, the NC16A domain is the first extracellular segment, and the carboxy terminus extends into the *lamina lucida*.
  ◈ The risk of scarring associated with subepidermal blistering disorders increases with depth. For example, antibodies may preferentially target the carboxy terminus of BPAG2 in cicatricial pemphigoid (CP).
● In addition to their structural role, **integrins** transduce signals from keratinocytes to the extracellular matric (ECM) to control **cell proliferation, differentiation, and migration.**

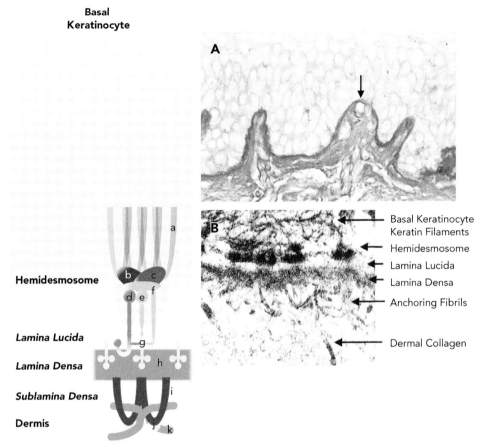

Basal
Keratinocyte

A

Hemidesmosome

Lamina Lucida

Lamina Densa

Sublamina Densa

Dermis

B — Basal Keratinocyte
Keratin Filaments
— Hemidesmosome
— Lamina Lucida
— Lamina Densa
— Anchoring Fibrils

— Dermal Collagen

Figure 1.4. THE BASEMENT MEMBRANE ZONE. a-keratin intermediate filaments, b-BPAG1, c-plectin, d-BPAG2, e-integrin subunit α6, f-integrin subunit β4, g-anchoring filaments (laminin 332), h-collagen IV, i-anchoring fibrils (collagen VII), j-anchoring plaques (collagen IV), k-collagens I and III. A, The BMZ stained with PAS separating the epidermis and the dermis. Solid arrow: basement membrane zone. B, Ultrastructure of the BMZ. BMZ basement membrane zone; BPAG1, bullous pemphigoid antigen 1; BPAG2, bullous pemphigoid antigen 2; PAS, periodic acid-Schiff.

(Histology and electron microscopy images reprinted with permission from Elder DE, Elenitsas R, Rosenbach M, et al. *Lever's Histopathology of the Skin.* 11th ed. Wolters Kluwer; 2015.)

- The *lamina lucida* is the weakest layer of the BMZ. Laminin 332 was previously known as epiligrin and laminin 5. Like integrins, **laminins** are also involved in **cell signaling.**
    - The *lamina lucida* is the cleavage plane in salt-split skin immunofluorescence testing for autoimmune blistering disorders.
- In focal adhesion complexes, the actin cytoskeleton is linked via intracellular proteins such as kindlins, talin, and vinculin to α3β1 integrin, which binds laminins 311 and 332.
    - Figure 1.5.

Dermis

- The dermis is divided into a superficial papillary layer and a deep reticular layer.
- **Fibroblasts** synthesize a variety of ECM components, primarily regulated by growth factors in the **transforming growth factor (TGF) β family:**
    - **Collagen (75% of dry weight)** is configured in a **triple helix** with each chain containing **Gly-X-Y repeats (glycine, X often proline, Y often hydroxylysine or hydroxy-**proline). It provides structural stability to the skin and other tissues.
        - Table 1.4.
    - **Elastin (4% of dry weight)** contains **desmosine and isodesmosine cross-links** and is surrounded by a **fibrillin scaffold. Oxytalan** fibers run **perpendicular** to the skin surface in the **papillary dermis,** while **elaunin** fibers run **parallel** to the skin surface in the **reticular dermis.** Elastin provides elasticity to the skin (capacity to resume its normal shape after deformation).
        - Oxytalan elastic fibers are like a "talon heel" (perpendicular); elaunin elastic fibers lay flat (parallel).
        - Elastin mutation causes cutis laxa.
        - Fibrillin mutations cause Marfan syndrome and congenital contractural arachnodactyly.
    - The **extrafibrillar matrix** (previously known as ground substance) consists of **glycosaminoglycans (GAGs).** GAGs can be *protein free* (eg, chondroitin sulfate, dermatan sulfate, heparin sulfate, and keratan sulfate). **Versican, a negatively charged proteoglycan bound to chondroitin/dermatan sulfate, forms aggregates with hyaluronic acid (HA)** in the dermis.

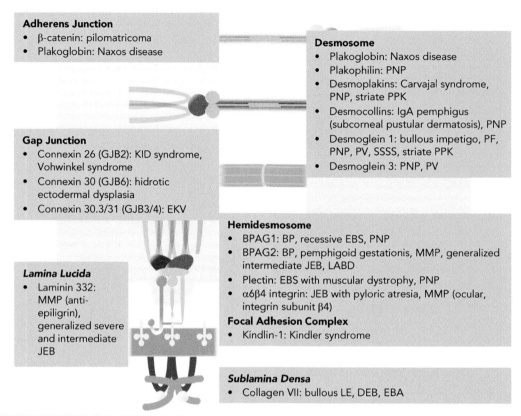

Adherens Junction
- β-catenin: pilomatricoma
- Plakoglobin: Naxos disease

Gap Junction
- Connexin 26 (GJB2): KID syndrome, Vohwinkel syndrome
- Connexin 30 (GJB6): hidrotic ectodermal dysplasia
- Connexin 30.3/31 (GJB3/4): EKV

Lamina Lucida
- Laminin 332: MMP (anti-epiligrin), generalized severe and intermediate JEB

Desmosome
- Plakoglobin: Naxos disease
- Plakophilin: PNP
- Desmoplakins: Carvajal syndrome, PNP, striate PPK
- Desmocollins: IgA pemphigus (subcorneal pustular dermatosis), PNP
- Desmoglein 1: bullous impetigo, PF, PNP, PV, SSSS, striate PPK
- Desmoglein 3: PNP, PV

Hemidesmosome
- BPAG1: BP, recessive EBS, PNP
- BPAG2: BP, pemphigoid gestationis, MMP, generalized intermediate JEB, LABD
- Plectin: EBS with muscular dystrophy, PNP
- α6β4 integrin: JEB with pyloric atresia, MMP (ocular, integrin subunit β4)

Focal Adhesion Complex
- Kindlin-1: Kindler syndrome

Sublamina Densa
- Collagen VII: bullous LE, DEB, EBA

Figure 1.5. DISORDERS OF JUNCTIONS. Illustrative Examples Provided For Clinical Correlation. BP, bullous pemphigoid; BPAG1, bullous pemphigoid antigen 1; DEB, dystrophic epidermolysis bullosa; EBA, epidermolysis bullosa acquisita; EBS, epidermolysis bullosa simplex; EKV, erythrokeratoderma variabilis; GJB2, gap junction beta-2; JEB; junctional epidermolysis bullosa; KID, keratitis-ichthyosis-deafness; LABD, linear IgA bullous dermatosis; LE, lupus erythematosus; MMP, mucous membrane pemphigoid; PF, pemphigus foliaceus; PNP, paraneoplastic pemphigus; PPK, palmoplantar keratoderma; PV, pemphigus vulgaris; SSSS, staphylococcal scalded skin syndrome.

Table 1.4. DISORDERS OF COLLAGEN

Collagen	Location	Associated Disorders[a]
I[b]	Bone, dermis, ligament, tendon, wound healing (remodeling phase)	EDS type VII (arthrochalasia), morphea/SSc, OI
II	Cartilage, vitreous humor	Morphea/SSc, relapsing polychondritis
III	Blood vessels, fetal skin, gastrointestinal tract, wound healing (proliferative phase)	EDS type III (vascular), keloid, morphea/SSc
IV	Basement membrane	Alport syndrome, Goodpasture disease
V	Dermis	EDS type I (classic)
VII[b]	Amnion, anchoring fibrils	Bullous SLE, DEB, EBA
XVII	Hemidesmosome	BP/pemphigoid gestationis, CP, generalized intermediate JEB, LABD

BP, bullous pemphigoid; CP, cicatricial pemphigoid; DEB, dystrophic epidermolysis bullosa; EBA, epidermolysis bullosa acquisita; EDS, Ehlers-Danlos syndrome; JEB, junctional epidermolysis bullosa; LABD, linear IgA bullous dermatosis; OI, osteogenesis imperfecta; SLE, systemic lupus erythematosus; SSc, systemic sclerosis.

[a]Illustrative examples provided for clinical correlation.

[b]Retinoids upregulate synthesis of collagen I and collagen VII.

GAGs on a proteoglycan are arranged like "bristles on a hairbrush."

- ◆ The mucopolysaccharidoses, such as Hunter syndrome and Hurler syndrome, are caused by mutations in enzymes that catabolize GAGs.
- **Prolyl hydroxylases are involved in collagen synthesis. Lysyl oxidase, a copper-dependent enzyme, is important for collagen and elastin cross-linking. Vitamin C is an essential cofactor for these enzymes.**
  - ◆ Lysyl hydroxylase is impaired in Ehlers-Danlos syndrome (EDS) type VI (kyphoscoliotic).
  - ◆ Lysyl oxidase is impaired in copper-deficient states such as Menkes kinky hair disease.
  - ◆ Figure 1.6.
- **Matrix metalloproteinases (MMPs)** are **zinc-dependent endopeptidases** that degrade ECM components.
- The ECM maintains the elasticity, resilience, and tautness of the skin. Both decreased production and increased degradation of ECM components contribute to normal skin aging.

Subcutis (Hypodermis)

- The subcutis contains lobules of adipose (fat) cells within loose connective tissue.
- The subcutis provides padding, insulation, and an energy reserve.

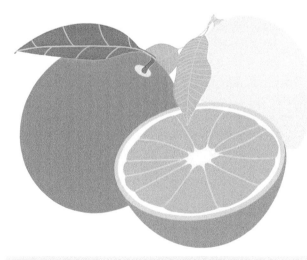

Figure 1.6. VITAMIN C. Scurvy was a feared complication of sailing, resulting in bleeding, impaired wound healing, "a strange dejection of the spirits," and death. In 1747, the Scottish surgeon James Lind conducted one of the first known controlled trials. He randomized 12 scorbutic sailors to receive a quart of cider daily, 25 drops of elixir of vitriol (sulfuric acid), six spoonfuls of vinegar, half a pint of seawater, two oranges and one lemon, or a spicy paste plus a drink of barley water. Vitamin C in the citrus fruit reversed the blood vessel fragility due to impaired collagen synthesis. Unfortunately, Lind's discovery was ignored for 42 y, but the admiralty eventually issued lemon juice to every sailor.
(Illustration by Caroline A. Nelson, MD.)

- Brown (immature) fat produces heat. It is more prominent in children.

Blood Vessels (Figure 1.7)

- Anatomy of blood vessels (arteries, veins, and lymphatics):
  - ○ Capillaries: supply the papillary dermis and adnexa.
  - ○ Superficial plexus: located in the upper part of the reticular dermis.
  - ○ Deep plexus: located in the lower part of the reticular dermis.
  - ○ Communicating blood vessels: connect the superficial and deep plexuses.
    - ◆ Cutaneous small vessel vasculitis (CSVV) is mediated by immune complex deposition in postcapillary venules, while cutaneous polyarteritis nodosa (PAN) primarily involves medium-sized arteries in the deep plexus.
- The walls of arteries have three layers: intima, media, and adventitia. The walls of veins are thinner and less clearly divided. Lymphatics do not have well-developed walls.
- **Vascular endothelial growth factor (VEGF)** is the primary mediator of **angiogenesis** (formation of new blood vessels).
  - ◆ Mutation of *FLT4*, which encodes VEGF receptor 3, causes hereditary lymphedema.
  - ◆ VEGF is the target of angiogenesis inhibitors such as bevacizumab.
- Blood vessels function to deliver oxygen, nutrients, and leukocytes to the skin and to regulate body temperature and blood pressure.
- Endothelial cells contain **Weibel-Palade bodies** that serve as storage organelles for the blood clotting protein **von Willebrand factor.**
- **Vimentin** is the intermediate filament **preferentially expressed over desmin in vascular smooth muscle**, which is under **adrenergic control.**
- **Glomus cells** are **modified smooth muscle cells** enriched on the distal extremities, particularly the **nail beds, palms, and soles.** They permit **shunting of blood from arterioles to venules**, bypassing capillaries. A glomus body consists of an afferent arteriole, **Sucquet-Hoyer canal**, efferent venule, and nerve fibers.
  - ◆ The subungual region of the finger is the leading site for glomus cell tumors. Temperature changes and pressure may provoke severe paroxysmal pain due to myofilament contraction.

Nerves (Figure 1.8)

Nonencapsulated (Free) Nerve Endings

- **Aβ-type fibers**: large diameter myelinated fibers that innervate dermal corpuscles and hair follicles. Aβ-type fibers detect light touch and moving stimuli.
- **Aδ-type fibers**: small diameter myelinated fibers that lose their myelin sheath as they terminate in the epidermis. Aδ-type fibers detect sharp pain, pruritus, temperature, and mechanical stimuli.

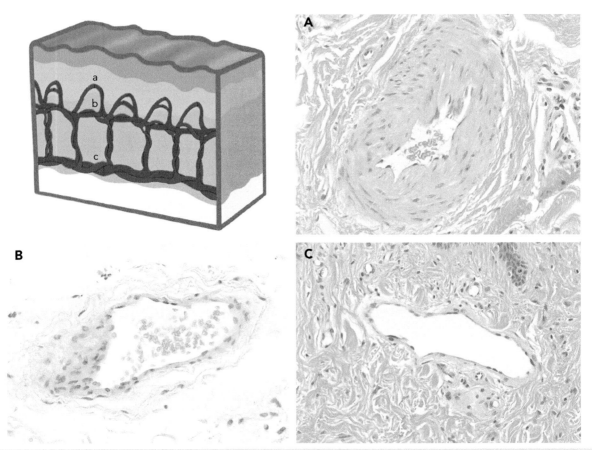

Figure 1.7. BLOOD VESSELS. a-capillary in the papillary dermis, b-superficial plexus, c-deep plexus. A, Artery. B, Vein. C, Lymphatic vessel.

(Illustration by Caroline A. Nelson, MD. A, Histology images courtesy of Noel Turner, MD, MHS and Christine J. Ko, MD.)

- **C-type fibers**: small diameter nonmyelinated fibers that terminate in the epidermis. C-type fibers detect dull pain, pruritus, temperature, and mechanical stimuli. They may be histaminergic or nonhistaminergic.
- **Merkel cells**: see above.
- **Primary mediators of pruritus** include **histamine,** tryptase, cathepsin S, and **interleukin (IL)-31**, while **secondary mediators of pruritus** include prostaglandin $E_{1,2}$, **substance P, μ-opioid receptor agonists,** nerve growth factor, and IL-2.
    - ◆ Opioids cause pruritus.
    - ◆ Antihistamines relieve pruritus.
    - ◆ Capsaicin, found in chili peppers and other nightshades (*Solanaceae*), releases and depletes substance P from C-type fibers. It initially causes erythema, edema, and burning but ultimately relieves pruritus.
    - ◆ Nemolizumab, a monoclonal antibody targeting IL-31, is under investigation for the treatment of pruritus associated with atopic dermatitis (AD).

Encapsulated Nerve Endings

- **Meissner corpuscles**: mechanoreceptors located in the dermal papillae. Meissner corpuscles detect light pressure and vibration and are enriched on sensitive areas such as the palms and soles.
    - ◆ Meissner corpuscles are shaped like "pine cones."

- **Ruffini corpuscles**: mechanoreceptors located in the deep dermis. Ruffini corpuscles detect sustained pressure or stretch and are concentrated around fingernails.
    - ◆ Ruffini corpuscles are shaped like "spindles."
- **Pacinian (lamellar) corpuscles**: mechanoreceptors located in the deep dermis and subcutis. Pacinian corpuscles detect deep pressure and vibration and are enriched on sensitive areas such as the palms and soles.
    - ◆ Pacinian corpuscles are shaped like "onions."
    - ◆ Pacinian Pressure.
- **Krause end bulbs (mucocutaneous end organs)**: mechanoreceptors located in the dermis. Krause end bulbs detect pressure and temperature and are enriched on the conjunctiva, mucosal lip, tongue, nipple, and anogenital region.

Glands (Figure 1.9)

Sebaceous Glands

- Sebaceous glands are present **nearly everywhere except the palms and soles,** but are **enriched on the scalp, face, chest, and upper back. Free** sebaceous glands (not associated with a hair follicle) are on the **superficial eyelid margin (glands of Zeis), eyelid tarsal plate (meibomian glands), buccal mucosa and vermillion border of the lips (Fordyce**

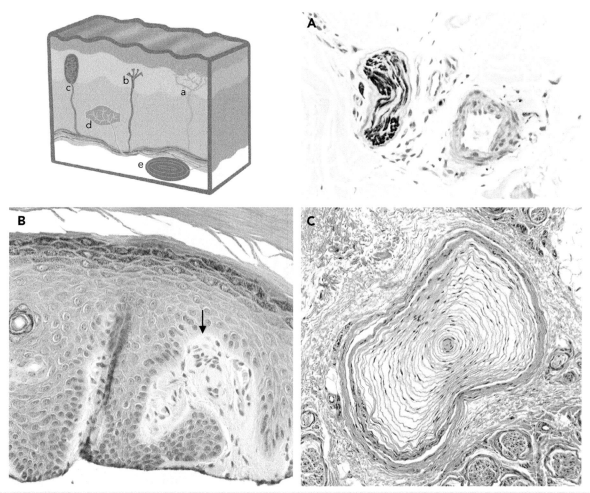

Figure 1.8. NERVES. a-free nerve endings, b-Merkel disks, c-Meissner corpuscle, d-Ruffini corpuscle, e-Pacinian corpuscle. A, Dermal nerve fibers demonstrated by S100 immunohistochemical staining. B, Meissner corpuscle within dermal papillae of human palm skin. Solid arrow: Meissner corpuscle. C, Pacinian corpuscle with characteristic concentric pattern.

(Illustration by Caroline A. Nelson, MD. A and C, Histology image reprinted with permission from Elder DE, Elenitsas R, Rosenbach M, et al. *Lever's Histopathology of the Skin.* 11th ed. Wolters Kluwer; 2015. B, Histology image courtesy of Noel Turner, MD, MHS and Christine J. Ko, MD.)

granules), **nipple and areola (Montgomery tubercles), and prepuce and labia minora (Tyson glands).**

◆ Zeis is on the zurface.

◆ Fordyce granules present as multiple asymptomatic yellow to white papules on the buccal mucosa/vermilion upper lip. They are considered a normal anatomic variant.

• Sebaceous glands are under **adrenergic hormonal control.** They are **transiently stimulated in infancy and mature under the influence of androgens during puberty.**

◆ Androgen stimulation explains the appearance of infantile acne between 2 and 12 months of age and the onset of acne vulgaris during adolescence.

• The primary functions of sebaceous glands are to promote skin barrier function and modulate inflammation. They exhibit **holocrine secretion.** Sebocytes in lobules shed into the lumen of the excretory duct, which opens into the hair follicle at the junction between the isthmus and infundibulum.

• **Sebum is roughly 57% triglycerides, 26% wax esters, 12% squalene, 3% cholesterol esters, and 1.5% cholesterol.**

◆ Do NOT get confused! Ceramide predominates in the cornified lipid envelope. Triglycerides predominate in sebum.

• Sebaceous follicles harbor **bacteria, for example, *Staphylococcus epidermidis* and *Cutibacterium acnes*** (formally *Propionibacterium acnes*), **fungi, for example, *Malassezia* species, and *Demodex* mites.**

◆ *C. acnes* contributes to the pathogenesis of acne.

◆ *Malassezia* species cause tinea versicolor (TV) and *Malassezia folliculitis* and have been implicated in confluent and reticulated papillomatosis (CARP), seborrheic dermatitis, and neonatal acne.

◆ *Demodex* mites cause folliculitis and have been implicated in the pathogenesis of rosacea.

Apocrine Glands

• Apocrine glands are present on the **vermillion border of the lip, axilla, nipple and areola, periumbilical region, and anogenital region.** Modified apocrine glands are present on the **superficial eyelid margin (Moll glands),**

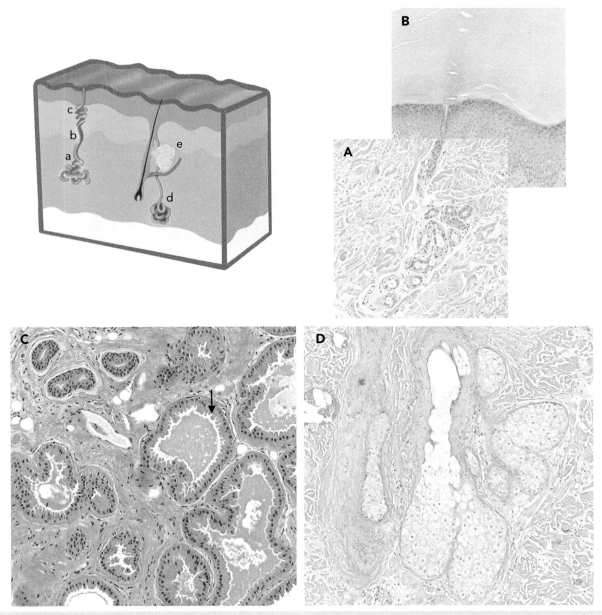

Figure 1.9. GLANDS. a-eccrine gland secretory coil, b-eccrine gland straight duct, c-eccrine gland acrosyringium, d-apocrine gland, e-sebaceous gland. A, Eccrine gland secretory coil and straight duct. B, Eccrine gland acrosyringium. C, Apocrine glands. Solid arrow: decapitation secretion. D, Sebaceous gland.

(Illustration by Caroline A. Nelson, MD. A, Histology image courtesy of Noel Turner, MD, MHS and Christine J. Ko, MD. B, Histology image courtesy of Noel Turner, MD, MHS and Christine J. Ko, MD. C, Histology image reprinted with permission from Elder DE, Elenitsas R, Rosenbach M, et al. *Lever's Histopathology of the Skin.* 11th ed. Wolters Kluwer; 2015. D, Histology image courtesy of Noel Turner, MD, MHS and Christine J. Ko, MD.)

external auditory canal (ceruminous glands), and areola (**mammary glands**).

- Apocrine glands are under **adrenergic control** (circulating catecholamines). They are **present at birth but become functional under the influence of androgens during puberty.**
- Apocrine glands are thought to play a role in olfactory communication. They exhibit **decapitation secretion.** Vesicles pinch off from secretory cells in the subcutis and degrade in the lumen of the excretory duct, which typically opens into the infundibulum of the hair follicle above the sebaceous duct. Fatty sweat, mixed with sebum, is **odorless until it reaches the skin surface and is degraded by bacteria.** Specialized apocrine glands open directly to the skin surface.

Eccrine Glands

- Eccrine glands are present **nearly everywhere except the external auditory canal, vermillion lip, nail bed, prepuce, glans penis, labia minora, and clitoris.**
- Eccrine glands are **functionally cholinergic** (acetylcholine neurotransmitter), but **anatomically adrenergic** (enervated by postganglionic sympathetic fibers).
    - Sympathectomy is a treatment for hyperhidrosis, but may cause compensatory hyperhidrosis.
- The primary function of eccrine glands is **thermoregulation.** They exhibit **merocrine secretion.** Sweat is secreted via exocytosis from the secretory coil in the subcutis or reticular dermis

and transported through the straight duct into the intraepidermal spiral acrosyringium. **Sweat is initially isotonic but becomes hypotonic due to sodium absorption.** When it reaches the skin surface, it cools the body by evaporation.

   ◆ Heat intolerance is a prominent feature of hypohidrotic ectodermal dysplasia. Decreased electrolyte reabsorption by the eccrine duct in cystic fibrosis (CF) results in electrolyte loss that poses a risk in hot environments.

Hair (Figure 1.10)

- Hair anatomy and histopathology (cross-sectional from inner to outer): **medulla, cortex, cuticle (hair shaft), cuticle of the inner root sheath (IRS), Huxley layer of the IRS, Henle layer of the IRS, ORS, vitreous or glassy layer, fibrous root sheath.**

   ○ Huxley layer overlying the cuticle is like the "husk on a corncob."

- Hair anatomy and histopathology (longitudinal from bulb to epidermal surface):

   ○ **Bulb**: base to Adamson fringe. The bulk of mitotic activity happens below the **critical line of Auber (widest diameter)** in the matrix, which receives its blood supply from the dermal papilla. Adamson fringe is the point above which the hair shaft is completely keratinized. The IRS keratinizes first and contains citrulline.

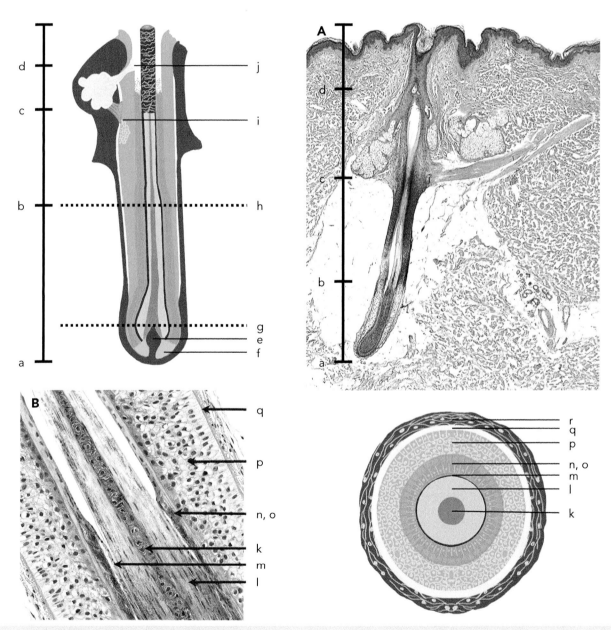

Figure 1.10. HAIR. A, Low-power view of a hair follicle: a-bulb, b-suprabulbar zone, c-isthmus, d-infundibulum, e-papillary mesenchymal body, f-matrix, g-critical line of Auber, h- Adamson fringe, i-arrector pili muscle insertion site (bulge), j-sebaceous gland ostium. B, High-power view of the suprabulbar zone: k-medulla, l-cortex, m-cuticle (hair shaft and IRS), n- Huxley layer of the IRS, o- Henle layer of the IRS, p- ORS, q-vitreous layer, r-fibrous root sheath. IRS, inner root sheath; ORS, outer root sheath.

(Illustration by Caroline A. Nelson, MD. Histology images reprinted with permission from Elder DE, Elenitsas R, Rosenbach M, et al. *Lever's Histopathology of the Skin.* 11th ed. Wolters Kluwer; 2015.)

○ **Suprabulbar zone (lower segment):** Adamson fringe to *arrector pili* muscle insertion site. The *arrector pili* muscle is under adrenergic control.

◆ Piloerection (eg, during the fight or flight response) causes goose bumps.

○ **Isthmus:** *arrector pili* muscle insertion site to sebaceous gland ostium. The IRS disappears. The ORS keratinizes without a granular layer (trichilemmal keratinization) and expresses K6, K16, and K17.

◆ The absence of a granular layer is a histopathological feature that distinguishes pilar cysts arising from the isthmus from epidermoid cysts arising from the infundibulum.

○ **Infundibulum:** sebaceous gland ostium to epidermal surface. The ORS keratinizes with a granular layer and is contiguous with the epidermis.

● Keratinocyte **stem cells** are primarily located at the **bulge** (*arrector pili* **muscle insertion site**) of hair follicles. Stem cells contribute to hair cycling, tissue regeneration, and wound healing. The enzyme **ornithine decarboxylase (ODC)** plays a role in **cellular growth and differentiation** and is a **marker of proliferative activity.**

◆ ODC is inhibited by eflornithine, a treatment for hypertrichosis.

● **Sonic hedgehog (SHH) and the Wnt, bone morphogenic protein (BMP), and fibroblast growth factor (FGF) families** are important mediators of **hair follicle development and cycling.**

◆ Gardner syndrome, caused by *APC* mutation in the Wnt/β-catenin signaling pathway, is associated with epidermoid cysts.

● There are ~**100,000 hairs on the scalp** and ~**100 to 200 are lost each day.** The hair cycle has three phases:

○ **Anagen (85%-90%):** growth phase. Hair grows at a rate of ~0.4 mm/d. The length of the anagen phase determines hair length (2-6 years on the scalp).

◆ Anagen effluvium (AE) occurs when a trigger such as cytotoxic chemotherapy leads to shedding of anagen hairs.

○ **Catagen (<1%):** regression phase. The bulb regresses, the IRS is lost, and melanocytes apoptose. This is the shortest phase (2-3 weeks on the scalp).

○ **Telogen (10%-15%):** rest phase. After the telogen phase (~3 months on the scalp), hairs are shed (exogen) leaving behind an empty follicle (kenogen).

◆ Unlike animals that molt, humans have asynchronous hair cycling to maintain a fairly uniform density of hair. Telogen effluvium (TE) occurs when triggers such as systemic diseases reset the hair follicle biological clock, leading to synchronous shedding.

● **Melanocytes,** enriched in the **matrix,** transfer melanin to hair keratinocytes during anagen (**ratio 1:5**). Follicular melanocyte stem cells contribute to **interfollicular repigmentation.** Hair graying is due to a decline in the number of melanocytes with aging.

◆ Perifollicular repigmentation is the predominant pattern in vitiligo vulgaris.

● The hair follicle represents a site of **immune privilege.**

◆ Collapse of immune privilege is implicated in alopecia areata (AA).

● The **cortex** contains the majority of **hair keratins**; while the **cuticle** maintains the **integrity of hair fibers.**

◆ Excessive heat and mechanical stress can damage the cuticle, leading to trichoptilosis (split ends).

● **Hair strength** is primarily proportional to the number of **disulfide bonds. Round follicles** produce **straight hair,** while **oval (elliptical) follicles** produce **curly hair.**

◆ Figure 1.11.

● There are **three types** of hair: **lanugo** (fine hairs shed in first wave during the third trimester and in a second wave 3-4 months after birth), **vellus** (fine hairs over face and body), and **terminal** hairs (long, thick, and dark-colored hairs on scalp, eyebrows, and eyelashes).

◆ Hypertrichosis lanuginosa may be congenital or acquired (paraneoplastic).

◆ Excess of lanugo-like hair may occur in nutritional deficiencies (eg, marasmus).

● During puberty, androgens cause vellus hair follicles to be replaced with terminal hair follicles in the axillae and anogenital region. Men and women with increased androgens will also develop terminal hairs on the face (moustache and beard), chest, back, arms, thighs, pubic and lower abdominal areas, and buttocks. Terminal hair follicles on the scalp exposed to the same androgens revert to vellus hair follicles in genetically susceptible individuals. 5α-reductase type 2 converts testosterone to its more potent metabolite dihydrotestosterone (DHT). Androgen signaling does not influence eyebrow and eyelash hair growth. Estrogen signaling prolongs anagen but reduces the hair growth rate.

◆ The paradoxical effect of androgens on body versus scalp hair explains the excess of terminal hairs in hirsutism and the miniaturization of terminal hairs in androgenetic alopecia (AGA). Finasteride blocks 5α-reductase type 2.

Nails (Figure 1.12)

● Nail anatomy and histopathology:

○ **Nail matrix:** wedge-shaped epithelium that synthesizes the nail plate. The proximal matrix synthesizes 80% of the nail plate. It begins at the mid-distal phalanx, while the

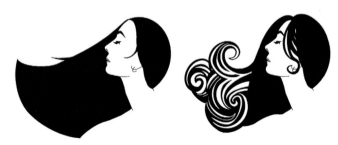

Figure 1.11. DISULFIDE BONDS. Ammonium thioglycolate and glyceryl thioglycolate are reducing agents used in permanent waves. They dissolve disulfide bonds, allowing keratin molecules to rearrange into curls, reformed by neutralizers. Unfortunately, they also cause contact dermatitis.
(Illustration by Caroline A. Nelson, MD.)

distal matrix may be visible under the nail plate (*lunula*). The matrix keratinizes without a granular layer.

> The *lunula* looks like a "crescent <u>moon</u>" under the thumbnail.

- ○ **Nail bed**: epithelium tightly apposed to the undersurface of the nail plate. The nail bed extends from the *lunula* to the onychodermal band. It keratinizes without a granular layer and expresses K6, K16, and K17. The dermis is contiguous with the periosteum of the distal phalanx (no subcutis). Capillaries in the dermis cause nails to be pink and to blanch with pressure. Glomus cells are enriched in the subungual region.
- ○ **Nail plate**: semitranslucent convex sheet of cornified onychocytes that express hair-type keratins.

- ○ **Nail folds**: epithelium that folds over the proximal and lateral edges of the nail plate. The nail folds keratinize with a granular layer.
- ○ **Eponychium (cuticle)**: cornified layer of the proximal nail fold that creates a seal between the nail plate and the proximal nail fold.
- ○ **Hyponychium**: anatomic region between the nail bed and the distal groove, where the nail plate detaches from the distal digit.
- Keratinocyte **stem cells** are primarily located in the basal layer of the nail **matrix. The proximal matrix synthesizes the dorsal aspect of the plate; the distal matrix synthesizes the ventral aspect of the plate.**

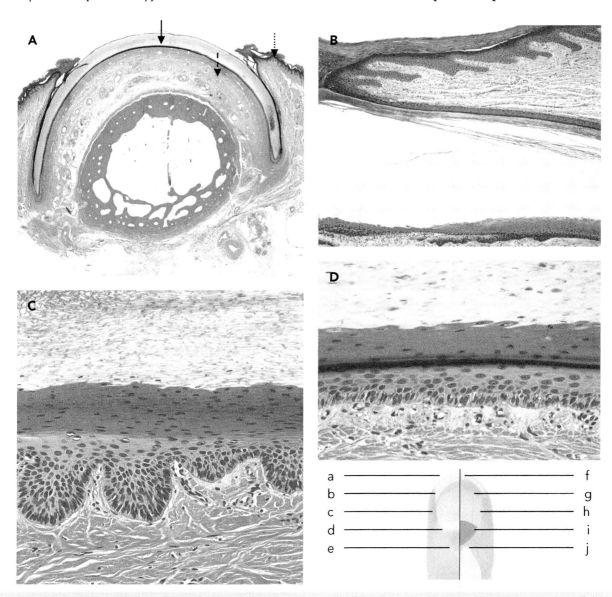

Figure 1.12. NAILS. a-nail plate, b-onychodermal band, c-lateral nail fold, d-eponychium (cuticle), e-proximal nail fold, f-hyponychium, g-distal phalanx, h-nail bed, i-nail matrix (lunula), j-extensor tendon. A, Low-power view of a transverse section of the distal portion of a finger including the nail unit. Solid arrow: nail plate. Dashed arrow: nail bed. Dotted arrow: lateral nail fold. B, Proximal nail fold forming the roof of the nail groove. C. Nail matrix. Note the lack of a granular layer and presence of multilayered germinative basal cells. D. Nail bed. Note the lack of a granular layer. The epithelium shows a paucity of germinative basal cells.

(Illustration by Caroline A. Nelson, MD. Histology images reprinted with permission from Elder DE, Elenitsas R, Rosenbach M, et al. *Lever's Histopathology of the Skin*. 11th ed. Wolters Kluwer; 2015.)

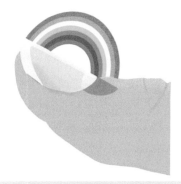

Figure 1.13. NAIL GROWTH.
(Illustration by Caroline A. Nelson, MD.)

The nail grows out like a "rainbow." The proximal matrix synthesizes the dorsal aspect of the plate. The distal matrix synthesizes the ventral aspect of the plate.

◆ Figure 1.13.
◆ Biopsy of the proximal matrix is more likely to result in visible nail dystrophy than biopsy of the distal matrix.
- **Fingernails** grow **2 to 3 mm/mo** and take approximately **6 months** to replace. **Toenails** grow **1 mm/mo** and take approximately **18 months** to replace.
- **Melanocytes**, enriched in the distal **matrix**, transfer melanin to nail keratinocytes.
- The nail unit represents a site of **relative immune privilege.**

Special Sites (Figure 1.14)

- **Areola**: histology shows epidermal acanthosis, basilar hyperpigmentation, central invagination leading to a follicle and sebaceous glands, smooth muscle bundles, and apocrine glands.

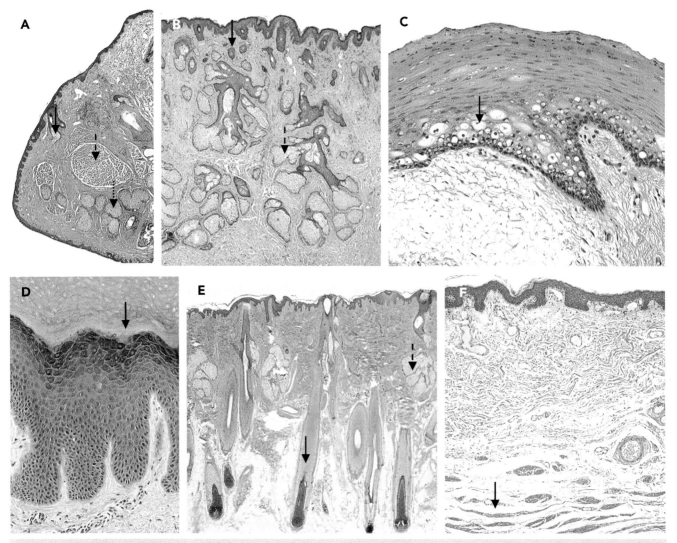

Figure 1.14. SPECIAL SITES. A, Eyelid skin (top) and transition to eyelid mucosa (bottom). Solid arrow: Zeis gland. Dashed arrow: skeletal muscle bundle. Dotted arrow: meibomian gland. B, Face. Solid arrow: vellus hair follicle. Dashed arrow: sebaceous gland. C, Oral cavity mucosa. Solid arrow: pale keratinocyte containing glycogen. Note the lack of well-formed granular or cornified layers. D, Palmoplantar skin. Solid arrow: *stratum lucidum*. Note the absence of hair follicles. E, Scalp. Solid arrow: terminal hair follicle extending to the subcutis. Dashed arrow: sebaceous gland. F, Scrotal skin. Solid arrow: smooth muscle bundle in the *dartos* layer.

◆ Polythelia (accessory nipples) are remnants of the embryologic mammary ridges (milk lines).
- **Ear**: histology shows cartilage and vellus hair follicles.
  ◆ Accessory tragi are remnants of the first branchial arch.
- **Eyelid**: histology shows a thin *stratum corneum* transitioning to a conjunctival surface with goblet cells, vellus hair follicles, superficial Zeis and Moll glands, Meibomian glands deep within the tarsal plate, and skeletal muscle bundles.
- **Face**: histology shows hair follicles, sebaceous glands, *Demodex* mites, and solar elastosis (deposition of degenerative elastotic material in the dermis).

Embryology

Basic Concepts

- **Gastrulation**: formation of three primary germ layers (ectoderm, mesoderm, and endoderm) at 3 weeks estimated gestational age (EGA).
  ◆ 3 layers at 3 weeks.
- Skin structures are derived from the following layers:
  ○ **Ectoderm**: epidermis, adnexal structures, melanocytes, Merkel cells, and nerves (neuroectoderm).
    ◆ Ecto- is derived from the Greek word *ektos* meaning "outside" (epidermis).
  ○ **Mesoderm**: fibroblasts, Langerhans cells (LCs), blood vessels, and inflammatory cells.
    ◆ Meso- is derived from the Greek word *mesos* meaning "middle" (dermis).

Development of the Skin, Hair, and Nails (Figure 1.15)

- Infants attain **full skin barrier function ~ 3 weeks after birth. Premature** infants, especially those born before 28 weeks' EGA, have an immature *stratum corneum* and **impaired skin barrier function.**
  ◆ Premature infants have an increased risk of infection, dehydration, and excessive absorption of topical medications or chemicals.

Genetics

Basic Concepts

- **Allele**: alternative forms of a particular gene.
- **Locus**: location on a chromosome.
- **Genotype**: alleles present at a specific locus.
- **Phenotype**: physical manifestation of a particular genotype.
- **Allelic heterogeneity**: mutations in a single gene causing more than one disorder.
  ◆ An example of allelic heterogeneity is *PTEN* gene mutation causing both Cowden syndrome and Bannayan-Riley-Ruvalcaba (BRR) syndrome.
- **Locus heterogeneity**: mutations in different genes causing the same disorder.

- **Mucosa**: (noncornified) histology shows pale keratinocytes containing glycogen and lacking well-formed granular or cornified layers.
- **Palmoplantar**: histology shows a *stratum lucidum* (lucent layer under the *stratum corneum*) and Meissner and Pacinian corpuscles with absence of hair follicles (glabrous). Palmoplantar skin is the thickest ~1.5 mm (compared to ~0.04 mm eyelid skin).
- **Scalp**: histology shows hair follicles extending to the subcutis associated with sebaceous glands and arrector pili muscles.
- **Scrotum**: histology shows smooth muscle bundles in the *dartos* layer.

◆ An example of locus heterogeneity is tuberous sclerosis complex (TSC) caused by mutations in either hamartin or tuberin.
- **Homozygous**: genotype with two identical alleles at a given locus.
- **Heterozygous**: genotype with two different alleles at a given locus.
- **Hemizygous**: genotype with only one allele at a given locus.
- **Nullizygous**: genotype with no alleles at a given locus.
- **Haploinsufficiency**: protein produced by one wild-type allele is not sufficient to sustain normal function.
  ◆ An example of haploinsufficiency is Hailey-Hailey disease, an AD disorder in which one wild-type allele of the *ATP2C1* gene is not sufficient to sustain normal function of a Golgi calcium pump.
- **Dominant negative effect**: mutated protein interferes with normal function of wild-type proteins.
  ◆ An example of the dominant negative effect is epidermolysis bullosa (EB) simplex, which is most commonly due to mutations in K5 or K14 that interfere with normal wild-type function.
- **Exon**: protein-coding region of a gene.
- **Intron**: non–protein-coding region of a gene.
- **Epigenetics**: heritable changes affecting gene expression that do not result from alterations in the deoxyribonucleic acid (DNA) sequence.
  ◆ An example of epigenetics is the alteration in DNA methylation, histone modifications, and micro-ribonucleic acid (RNA) profiling that have been found in patients with lupus erythematosus (LE).

Genetic Disorders

- **Monogenic (Mendelian)** disorders are caused by a defect in a **single gene** (Table 1.5).
  ◆ Table 1.6.
- Modifying factors to Mendelian inheritance patterns:
  ○ **Age-dependent penetrance**: in late-onset diseases, not all affected individuals are old enough to manifest the disease.
  ○ *De novo* **mutations**: new mutation in an individual with a negative family history.
  ○ **Imprinting**: epigenetic phenomenon in which the sex of the transmitting parent determines which allele is expressed in the children.

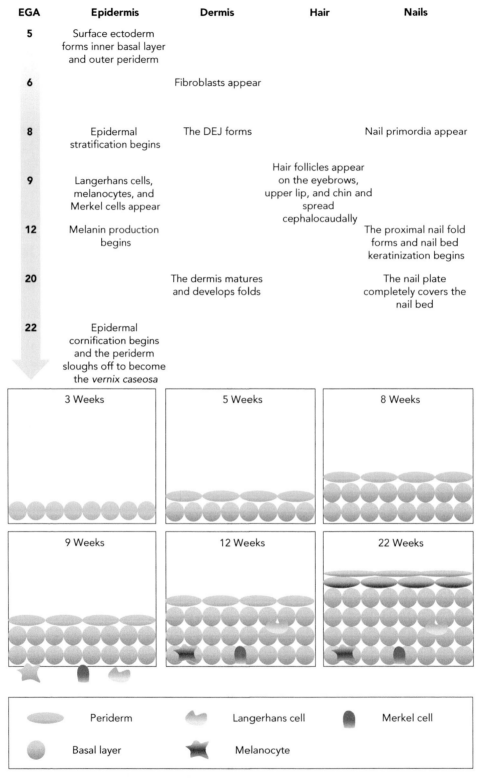

EGA	Epidermis	Dermis	Hair	Nails
5	Surface ectoderm forms inner basal layer and outer periderm			
6		Fibroblasts appear		
8	Epidermal stratification begins	The DEJ forms		Nail primordia appear
9	Langerhans cells, melanocytes, and Merkel cells appear		Hair follicles appear on the eyebrows, upper lip, and chin and spread cephalocaudally	
12	Melanin production begins			The proximal nail fold forms and nail bed keratinization begins
20		The dermis matures and develops folds		The nail plate completely covers the nail bed
22	Epidermal cornification begins and the periderm sloughs off to become the *vernix caseosa*			

Figure 1.15. DEVELOPMENT OF THE SKIN, HAIR, AND NAILS. Development of the skin, hair, and nails according to approximate EGA in weeks. DEJ, dermal-epidermal junction; EGA, estimated gestational age.

Table 1.5. MENDELIAN INHERITANCE PATTERNS

Pattern	Description	Punnet Square	Notes
AR	If both parents are carriers, children have a 25% risk of being affected.		Risk factors include consanguinity and isolated population.
AD	If one parent is affected, children have a 50% risk of being affected.		*De novo* mutations. Mechanisms include haploinsufficiency or a dominant negative effect.
XLR	If the mother is a carrier, male children have a 50% risk of being affected. If the father is affected, children have a 0% risk of being affected.		*De novo* mutations. May be mosaic in female carriers.
XLD	If the mother is affected, children have a 50% risk of being affected. If the father is affected, female children have a 100% risk of being affected.		*De novo* mutations. Often lethal in affected males and mosaic in affected females.

Punnett squares:

AR

	A	A^R
A	AA	$A^R A$
A^R	AA^R	$\mathbf{A^R A^R}$

AD

	A	A^D
A	AA	$\mathbf{A^D A}$
A	AA	$\mathbf{A^D A}$

XLR

	X	X^R		X	X
X	XX	$X^R X$	X^R	XX^R	XX^R
Y	XY	$\mathbf{X^R Y}$	Y	XY	XY

XLD

	X	X^D		X	X
X	XX	$\mathbf{X^D X}$	X^D	$\mathbf{XX^D}$	$\mathbf{XX^D}$
Y	XY	$\mathbf{X^D Y}$	Y	XY	XY

AD, autosomal dominant; AR, autosomal recessive; XLD, X-linked dominant; XLR, X-linked recessive.

Table 1.6. MNEMONICS FOR X-LINKED GENETIC DISORDERS

XLR: CHADS kinky WIFE CHANdra   **XLD: BIG CHOMP**

XLR: CHADS kinky WIFE CHANdra	XLD: BIG CHOMP
CGD[a]	Bazex syndrome
Hunter syndrome	IP
Anhidrotic/hypohidrotic ectodermal dysplasia[a]	Goltz syndrome
DKC[a]	CHILD syndrome
SCID[a]	Oro-facial-digital syndrome[a]
Menkes kinky hair disease	MIDAS syndrome
WAS	Chondrodysplasia punctata (Conradi-Hünermann)[a]
Ichthyosis[a]	
Fabry disease	
EDS (V, IX, X)[b]	
Chondrodysplasia punctata (not Conradi-Hünermann)[a]	
Anhidrotic/hypohidrotic ectodermal dysplasia with immune deficiency[a]	
Bruton agammaglobulinemia	
Lesch-Nyhan syndrome	

[a]Steroid sulfatase deficiency.
[b]Historical classification. Types V and X have unknown molecular basis. Type IX has been reclassified as cutis laxa (occipital horn syndrome).
CGD, chronic granulomatous disease; CHILD, congenital hemidysplasia with ichthyosiform erythroderma and limb defects; DKC, dyskeratosis congenita; EDS, Ehlers-Danlos syndrome; IP, incontinentia pigmenti; MIDAS, micrognathia, dermal aplasia, and sclerocornea; SCID, severe combined immunodeficiency; WAS, Wiskott-Aldrich syndrome; XLD, X-linked dominant; XLR, X-linked recessive.

○ **Incomplete penetrance**: not all affected individuals manifest the disease.
○ **Loss of heterozygosity (second hit)**: an individual with a heterozygous loss of function mutation in a tumor suppressor gene develops a cancer following mutation of the wild-type allele.
   ◆ An example of loss of heterozygosity is Muir-Torre syndrome, which is due to heterozygous germline mutations in DNA mismatch repair genes. Somatic inactivation of the wild-type allele results in microsatellite instability and mutations, leading to sebaceous neoplasms and other malignancies.
○ **Mitochondrial inheritance**: a mother transmits a disease, the severity of which is determined by the proportion of mutant versus normal mitochondrial proteins.
   Mothers pass on mitochondria.
○ **Mosaicism**: presence of two or more populations of cells with different genotypes in an individual who has developed from a single fertilized egg; often manifests as skin lesions following lines of Blaschko, but may take on a variety of patterns including blocklike, dermatomal, garment-like, patchy, phylloid, or segmental (Figure 1.16).
○ **Pseudodominant inheritance**: children of an individual homozygous for an autosomal recessive (AR) mutant allele and a carrier have a 50% risk of being affected.
○ **Variable expression**: not all affected individuals manifest the same severity of disease.

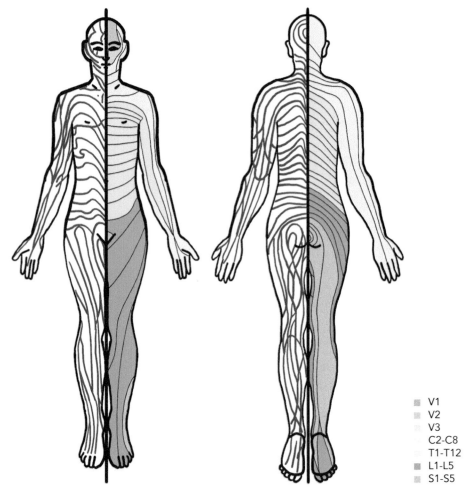

V1
V2
V3
C2-C8
T1-T12
L1-L5
S1-S5

Figure 1.16. LINES OF BLASCHKO AND DERMATOMES.
(Illustration by Caroline A. Nelson, MD.)

- Mosaicism may be divided into three subtypes:
  - **Genomic mosaicism**: due to either somatic postzygotic mutations (cannot be transmitted to children) or postzygotic mutations affecting the gonads (may be transmitted to children and result in generalized disease).
    - Mosaic epidermolytic ichthyosis (EI) is characterized by streaks of hyperkeratosis following lines of Blaschko. It is caused by a postzygotic mutation in *K1* or *K10* during embryogenesis. If the mutation involves gonadal cells, it can be transmitted to the patient's children, resulting in generalized EI.
  - **Functional mosaicism**: due to variable X-inactivation (lyonization) in females and males with Klinefelter syndrome.
    - In female patients with X-linked dominant male-lethal genetic disorders such as incontinentia pigmenti (IP), and in female carriers of X-linked recessive disorders, functional mosaicism can produce lesions following lines of Blaschko.
  - **Revertant mosaicism**: due to rescue of a mutation in a mosaic clone of cells that regain normal function.

  - In ichthyosis with confetti, due to *K10* mutation, revertant mosaicism is responsible for the appearance of small islands of normal skin on a background of ichthyosiform erythroderma.
    - Revertant mosaicism is called "natural gene therapy."
- **Polygenic** disorders are caused by defects in **more than one gene.**
- **Complex** genetic disorders are caused by **interaction of genetic and environmental factors.**
- **Chromosomal** genetic disorders are caused by abnormalities in the number, structure, or parental contribution of chromosomes.
  - **Number**: one chromosome (monosomy) or extra chromosomes (eg, trisomy) affecting one pair of homologous chromosomes (aneuploidy) or the whole genome (polyploidy).
  - **Structure**: inversion (reversal of part of a homologous chromosome) or translocation (rearrangement of parts between nonhomologous chromosomes).
  - **Parental contribution**: inheritance of both homologous chromosomes from one parent (uniparental disomy)

resulting in disease due to imprinting or transmission of two AR mutant alleles.

◆ Chromosome 15 provides a classic example of uniparental disomy. Inheritance of the maternal allele causes Prader-Willi syndrome, with features including insatiable appetite and intellectual disability. Inheritance of the paternal allele causes Angelman syndrome, with features including intellectual disability, seizures, and speech impairment.

- McKusick's Online Mendelian Inheritance in Man (OMIM) database provides access to current information on human genes and genetic diseases.

Carcinogenesis

Basic Concepts

- Carcinogenesis occurs in **four stages (initiation —> promotion —> progression —> malignant conversion).**
- **Telomeres**, maintained by the enzyme telomerase, **protect the ends of chromosomes.** Normal cells enter senescence (a nonproliferative but viable state) and ultimately undergo apoptosis as a consequence of accumulating genetic or epigenetic alterations and telomere shortening.
  - Telo- is derived from the Greek word *telos* meaning "end."
  - ◆ Defective telomere maintenance is a feature of dyskeratosis congenita (DKC).
- **Apoptosis** may be induced by stimuli including DNA damage, withdrawal of growth cytokines, and death-promoting agents. It is **mediated by caspases.**
  - "Casper the friendly ghost" (caspases mediate apoptosis).
- Cancer cells display a **mutator phenotype (higher degree of genomic instability)** in comparison to normal cells, often due to decreased efficiency in DNA repair systems.
- **Driver mutations** confer a **selective survival advantage** to cancer cells, while **passenger mutations** have **no effect on carcinogenesis.**
- Six hallmarks of cancer:
  - Sustaining proliferative signaling (eg, **gain-of-function mutations in oncogenes such as the *RAS* family,** which behave in a dominant fashion).
  - Evading growth suppressors (eg, **loss-of-function mutations in tumor suppressor genes such as RB,** which behave in a recessive fashion [two hits]).
  - Resisting cell death (eg, **mutations that upregulate antiapoptotic factors like B-cell lymphoma 2 [BCL2]**).
  - Enabling replicative immortality (eg, **mutations that upregulate telomerase**).
  - Inducing angiogenesis (eg, **mutations that upregulate growth factors such as VEGF**).
  - Activating invasion and metastasis (eg, **mutations that downregulate cell adhesion molecules, such as E-cadherin**).
- Predisposing factors for **skin cancer** include **age, anatomic site, chemical carcinogen exposure (eg, alcohol, arsenic, betel nut, tobacco), gender, genetic disorders, immunosuppression, oncogenic virus infection, scarring or chronic ulceration, skin phototype, and ultraviolet (UV) or ionizing radiation.**

◆ Arsenical keratoses on the palms and soles have premalignant potential for aggressive squamous cell carcinomas (SCCs).

The Cell Cycle (Figure 1.17)

- The cell cycle is the process of DNA replication and mitosis. It progresses through G_1 (gap 1 phase) to S (DNA synthesis phase) to G_2 (gap 2 phase) to M (mitosis phase), at which point the cell cycle may repeat or the cell may enter G_0 (resting phase).
  - ◆ Conventional antineoplastics may be cell cycle specific or cell cycle nonspecific.
- The cell cycle has **three primary checkpoints: G_1, G_2, and M,** which are regulated by cyclins, cyclin-dependent kinases (CDKs), and cyclin-dependent kinase inhibitors (CKIs).
- **P53 (encoded by the *TP53* gene on chromosome 17)** is the most common mutation in human cancer. It protects DNA integrity by regulating cell cycle progression, DNA repair, and apoptosis. **P53 activates P21, a CKI, leading to cell cycle arrest at G_1. P53 also activates P53 unregulated modulator of apoptosis (PUMA), which inhibits BCL2, leading to apoptosis.**
  - ◆ Germline *TP53* mutation causes Li-Fraumeni syndrome. Somatic *TP53* mutation is the leading gene mutation in SCC.
- **CDKN2A activates P16, a CKI, which leads to cell cycle arrest at G_1. CDKN2A also activates P14ARF (alternative reading frame), which inhibits mouse double minute 2 (MDM2), decreasing P53 degradation and leading to cell cycle arrest and apoptosis.**
  - ◆ *CDKN2A* mutation causes familial atypical multiple mole melanoma (FAMMM) syndrome.
- The G_1 checkpoint is controlled by CDK-cyclin complex-mediated phosphorylation of retinoblastoma (RB) protein. **Underphosphorylated RB arrests the cell cycle, while phosphorylated RB releases E2F, which promotes the transcription of cyclins, leading to cell cycle progression.**
  - ◆ Human papillomavirus (HPV) co-opts host cell machinery to replicate viral DNA. In high-risk types, the early (E) 6 oncoprotein destroys P53, while the E7 oncoprotein binds underphosphorylated RB, releasing E2F.

Molecular Signaling Pathways (Figure 1.18)

- **Mitogen-activated protein kinase (MAPK) signaling pathway**:
  - Growth factors (mitogens) bind to and activate receptor tyrosine kinases (RTKs) such as KIT.

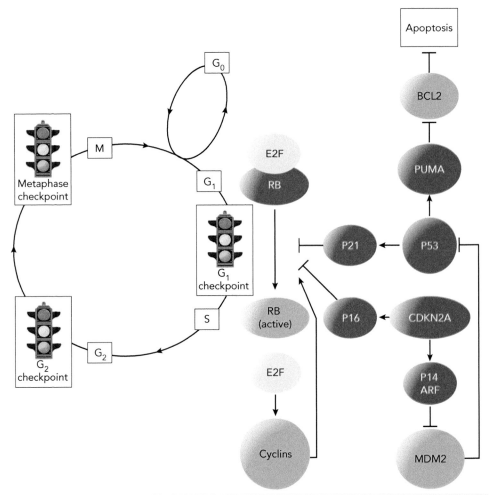

Figure 1.17. THE CELL CYCLE. ARF, alternative reading frame; BCL2, B-cell lymphoma 2; CDKN2A, cyclin-dependent kinase inhibitor 2A; G_0, resting phase; G_1, gap 1 phase; G_2, gap 2 phase; M, mitosis phase; MDM2, mouse double minute 2; PUMA, p53 upregulated modulator of apoptosis; RB, retinoblastoma protein; S, deoxyribonucleic acid synthesis phase. (Illustration by Caroline A. Nelson, MD.)

- ○ RTKs activate GTPases in the RAS family.
- ○ The RAS family activates kinases BRAF, MEK, and ERK/MAPK.
- ○ ERK/MAPK activates cyclin D1, thereby promoting cell proliferation, among other targets.
  - ◦ "Rebecca Brings Matzah Every Passover" (RAS, BRAF, MEK, ERK/MAPK proliferation).
- • **Phosphoinositide 3-kinase (PI3K) signaling pathway:**
  - ○ Growth factors (mitogens) bind to and activate RTKs such as KIT.
  - ○ RTKs activate PI3Ks.
  - ○ PI3Ks phosphorylate phosphatidylinositol 4,5-bisphosphate (PIP2) to active phosphatidylinositol (3,4,5)-trisphosphate (PIP3).
  - ○ PIP3 activates AKT.
  - ○ AKT activates the mammalian target of rapamycin (MTOR), thereby promoting cell growth, among other targets.
- • **SHH signaling pathway:**

- ○ SHH binds to the SHH receptor patched (encoded by *PTCH1* or *PTCH2*).
- ○ Patched releases smoothened (SMO).
- ○ SMO inhibits suppressor of fused (SUFU).
- ○ SUFU releases GLI.
- ○ GLI activates BCL2, thereby promoting cell survival, among other targets.
- • **Ubiquitin-proteasome pathway:**
  - ○ Enzymes link chains of ubiquitin on to proteins to tag them for degradation.
  - ○ Tagged proteins are recognized by the 26S proteasome that degrades them into peptides.
  - ○ Peptides are either degraded by peptidases in the cytoplasm into amino acids or used in antigen presentation.
  - ○ Proper function of the proteasome is important for protein recycling and therefore cell survival.
    - ◆ Table 1.7.
    - ◆ Targeted antineoplastics inhibit cellular membrane or intracellular molecular signaling pathways.

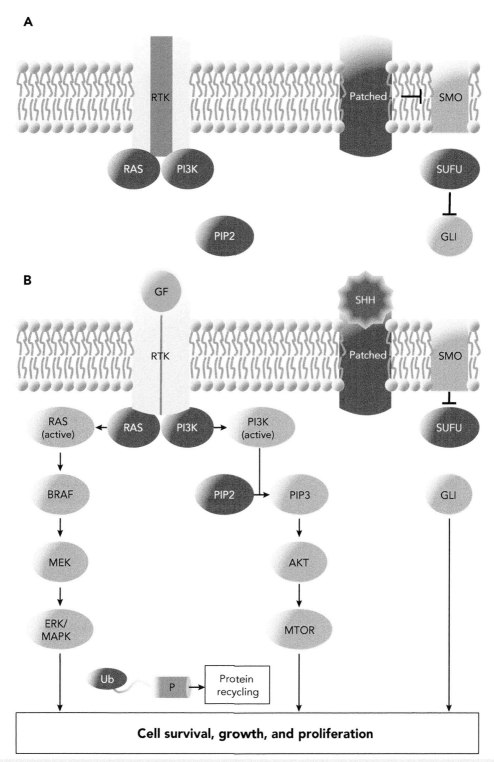

Figure 1.18. MOLECULAR SIGNALING PATHWAYS. A, Unbound state. B, Bound state. GF, growth factor; MAPK, mitogen-activated protein kinase; MTOR, mammalian target of rapamycin; P, proteasome; PI3K, phosphoinositide 3-kinase; PIP2, phosphatidylinositol 4,5-bisphosphate; PIP3, phosphatidylinositol (3,4,5)-trisphosphate; RTK, receptor tyrosine kinase; SHH, sonic hedgehog; SMO, smoothened; SUFU, suppressor of fused; Ub, ubiquitin.

Table 1.7. MOLECULAR SIGNALING PATHWAY MUTATIONS IN NEOPLASMS AND GENODERMATOSES

Pathway	Gene	Associated Neoplasms[a]	Associated Genodermatoses[a]
MAPK[b]	BRAF	LCH (Erdheim-Chester disease), common acquired nevocellular nevus, atypical epithelioid Spitz nevus, superficial spreading melanoma, lentigo maligna/lentigo maligna melanoma, acral lentiginous melanoma	Cardiofaciocutaneous syndrome
	HRAS, KRAS, NRAS	Epidermal nevus (HRAS > NRAS > KRAS), congenital melanocytic nevus, nevus spilus (HRAS), Spitz nevus (HRAS), superficial spreading melanoma (NRAS), lentigo maligna/lentigo maligna melanoma (NRAS), acral lentiginous melanoma (NRAS), nodular melanoma (NRAS), woolly hair nevus (HRAS), nevus sebaceous (HRAS > KRAS)	Costello syndrome (HRAS > KRAS), phakomatosis pigmentokeratotica (HRAS), Schimmelpenning syndrome (HRAS > KRAS)
	NF1	Neurofibroma	Neurofibromatosis type I
	PTPN11		Noonan (LEOPARD) syndrome
	RASA1		CM-AVM syndrome
	SPRED1		Legius syndrome
PI3K	AKT1		Proteus syndrome
	PIK3CA	Epidermal nevus, venous malformation, lymphatic malformation	PIK3CA-related segmental overgrowth spectrum
	PTEN		PTEN hamartoma syndrome spectrum[c]
	TSC1, TSC2		TSC
SHH	PTCH1, SMO	BCC	Basal cell nevus syndrome
Ubiquitin-proteasome	BAP1	Atypical epithelioid Spitz nevus, uveal melanoma	BAP1 tumor predisposition syndrome
	CTSC		Haim-Munk syndrome, Papillon-Lefèvre syndrome
	CYLD		Brooke-Spiegler syndrome
	PSMB8		Proteasome-associated autoinflammatory syndrome
	RHBDF2		Howel-Evans syndrome

BAP1, BRCA1-associated protein-1; BCC, basal cell carcinoma; CM-AVM, capillary malformation–arteriovenous malformation; LCH, Langerhans cell histiocytosis; LEOPARD, lentigines electrocardiographic conduction defects, ocular hypertelorism, pulmonary stenosis, abnormalities of the genitalia, retarded growth, and deafness; MAPK, mitogen-activated protein kinase; PI3K, phosphoinositide 3-kinase; SHH, sonic hedgehog; TSC, tuberous sclerosis complex.
[a]Illustrative examples provided for clinical correlation.
[b]RASopathies have significant allelic and locus heterogeneity.
[c]Historical classification divided PTEN hamartoma syndrome into Bannayan-Riley-Ruvalcaba syndrome and Cowden syndrome.

Photobiology

Basic Concepts

- Light has properties of both waves and photons. The electromagnetic spectrum (Figure 1.19) consists of radio waves, microwaves, infrared radiation, visible light, UVR, X-rays, and gamma rays. UVR is further subdivided into UVA I, UVA II, UVB, and UVC. X-rays and gamma rays are termed ionizing radiation.
- **Wavelength (nm) decreases while frequency (Hz) and energy (J) increase across the spectrum.**
- Formulas:
  - **Power** (J/s or Watts) = energy per unit time.
  - **Irradiance** ($J/s \cdot cm^2$) = power per unit area.
  - **Dose** (J/cm^2) = irradiance ($J/s \cdot cm^2$) · exposure time (s).
- The **absorption spectrum** is the portion of electromagnetic spectrum **absorbed by a particular molecule or chromophore.** The major chromophores in the skin are **hemoglobin, melanin, and water.** The **action spectrum** is the portion of electromagnetic spectrum **producing a particular biologic effect.**
  - The action of each laser depends on the absorption spectrum of the targeted chromophore. For example, the pulsed dye laser (PDL) emits light at 595 nm, corresponding with a hemoglobin absorption peak. As such, PDL is the treatment of choice for many cutaneous vascular lesions.

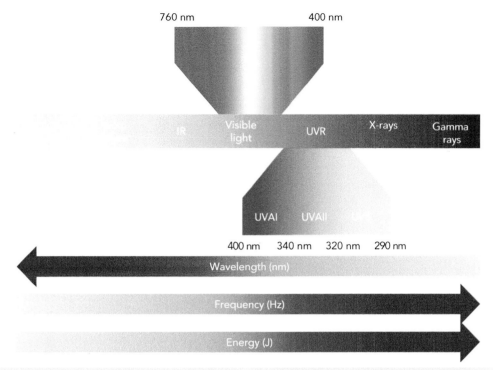

Figure 1.19. THE ELECTROMAGNETIC SPECTRUM. IR, infrared radiation; UVR, ultraviolet radiation.

Ultraviolet Radiation (Table 1.8)

- **Photoaging**:
  - Chronic and repetitive inflammatory responses to UVR upregulate ECM-degrading proteases and downregulate collagen synthesis.
    - Cutaneous signs of photoaging include acquired elastotic hemangioma, acrokeratoelastoidosis, colloid milium, elastoma of Dubreuilh, ephelides/solar lentigines, erosive pustular dermatosis, Favre-Racouchot syndrome, skin fragility, idiopathic guttate hypomelanosis (IGH), poikiloderma of Civatte, pseudoscars, solar elastosis (includes cutis rhomboidalis nuchae, solar elastotic bands of the forearm, elastotic nodules of the ear), solar purpura, and weathering nodules.
  - UVR induces mutations in mitochondrial DNA that lead to cellular senescence.
- **Photoallergy**: delayed-type, cell-mediated (type IV) reaction to an allergen activated or produced by the effect of light on a chemical or drug.
- **Phototoxicity**: dose-dependent reaction between light and a chemical or drug that generates reactive oxygen species (ROS) and cellular damage.
- **Immunomodulation**:
  - UVR **stimulates the immune system (innate > adaptive)** through induction of antimicrobial peptides, activation of endothelial cells, release of pro-inflammatory cytokines (eg, **type I IFNs**), and recruitment of inflammatory cells (eg, cluster of differentiation (**CD)4$^+$ and CD8$^+$ T cells, plasmacytoid dendritic cells [pDCs]**).
    - UVR exacerbates LE and other autoimmune connective tissue disorders (AI-CTDs).

- UVR **suppresses the immune system (adaptive > innate)** through release of anti-inflammatory cytokines (eg, **IL-10**) that **increase regulatory** T cells and **decrease the number and function of antigen-presenting cells (APCs)** such as LCs. This results in **decreased delayed-type, cell-mediated reactions.** UVR-induced immunosuppression is mediated by photoreceptors: DNA damage, **urocanic acid isomerization from *trans* to *cis***, and membrane lipids alteration of redox potential.
    - UV phototherapy is efficacious for the treatment of psoriasis and other inflammatory disorders.
  - UVR **induces mast cell degranulation and prostaglandin release.**
- **Photocarcinogenesis**:
  - UVR directly damages cellular DNA, most commonly through production of **cyclobutane pyrimidine dimers** (T-T > C-T, T-C). Photoproducts may induce apoptosis, DNA repair, or DNA mutation.
  - UVR (UVA) indirectly damages cellular DNA through production of **ROS.**
  - UVR **decreases immune surveillance** of cancer and cells infected with oncogenic viruses.
    - The DNA repair disorder xeroderma pigmentosum (XP) is associated with photosensitivity and an increased risk of actinic keratoses (AKs), basal cell carcinomas (BCCs), SCCs, and melanomas.
  - Protective mechanisms include pigmentation, epidermal hyperplasia, and antioxidant enzymes (controversial). **Tocopherol (vitamin E derivative) is the primary antioxidant in the epidermis.** Other antioxidants identified in mice include **silymarin, tea polyphenols, and vitamin C.**

Table 1.8. ULTRAVIOLET RADIATION

Characteristic	UVA	UVB	Notes
Wavelength	321-400 nm UVA I: 341-400 nm UVA II: 321-340 nm[a]	290-320 nm[a]	For UVB, UVA II, and UVA I wavelengths, dial the phone number 290-320-3440.
Solar radiation	Present from sunrise to sunset	Peaks at noon	Longer wavelength light penetrates more deeply. The atmosphere absorbs UVC.
			nbUVB phototherapy is a treatment for patch-stage CTCL. For thicker plaque stage CTCL, PUVA photochemotherapy is desirable.
Glass penetration	Yes	No	
Skin penetration	Epidermis to deep dermis	Epidermis	
Solar erythema	Immediate erythema and minor role in delayed erythema	Major role in delayed erythema (sunburn)	Delayed erythema occurs 6-24 h after exposure. UVB radiation is 1000× more erythemogenic than UVA radiation and produces apoptotic keratinocytes on histopathology, followed by epidermal hyperplasia.
Pigmentation	Immediate pigment darkening	Delayed pigmentation (tanning)	Immediate pigment darkening (also caused by visible light) occurs hours after exposure due to oxidation and redistribution of existing melanin and is transient. Delayed pigmentation occurs 48-72 h after exposure due to increased size and number of melanocytes, melanin synthesis, arborization of melanocytes, and transfer of melanosomes to keratinocytes.
Vitamin D_3 synthesis	No	Yes	UVB converts provitamin D_3 (7-dehydrocholesterol) to previtamin D_3, which isomerizes to vitamin D_3. Lumisterol and tachysterol are inert reservoirs of vitamin D_3 in the epidermis. Vitamin D_3 is converted to 25-OH-vitamin D_3 in the liver and 1,25-OH$_2$-vitamin D_3 (active form) in the kidneys. Vitamin D inhibits ODC.
Other major biologic effects	Photoaging, photoallergy, phototoxicity	Immunomodulation, photocarcinogenesis	

CTCL, cutaneous T-cell lymphoma; ODC, ornithine decarboxylase; nbUVB, narrowband UVB, OH, hydroxy; PUVA, psoralen-UVA; UV, ultraviolet.
[a]The defined boundary between UVA and UVB differs between the Food and Drug Administration (320 nm) and the International Commission on Illumination (315 nm).

Photoprotection

- **Minimal erythema dose (MED)**: minimal amount of a specific wavelength of light resulting in minimal erythema of the skin completely filling the test square after 24 hours of exposure.
- **Sun protection factor (SPF)**: MED of protected skin/MED of unprotected skin. SPF is measured following application of 2 mg/cm² of sunscreen (~1 ounce or a shot glass for an adult).
- **Water resistance**: ability of a sunscreen to persist on the skin following water immersion (substantivity). According to the Food and Drug Administration (FDA), sunscreens may be labeled as water resistant (40 minutes) or water resistant (80 minutes), but not waterproof.
- **The American Academy of Dermatology (AAD) recommends water-resistant sunscreens** (Table 1.9) **that provide broad-spectrum protection against UVA and UVB with an SPF of 30 or higher.**
- Potential side effects of sunscreen include minor skin irritation; **allergic contact dermatitis (ACD) and photoallergic contact dermatitis**; and impaired vitamin D synthesis. According to the 2010 Institute of Medicine consensus statement, the **recommended dietary allowance for vitamin D is 600 international units (IU) per day (800 IU/day for those over 70 years of age).**
- In February 2018, the FDA issued a proposed rule updating regulatory requirements for most sunscreen products in the United States (US). Under this rule, the FDA determined zinc oxide and titanium dioxide to be generally recognized as safe and effective in contrast to para-aminobenzoic acid (PABA) and trolamine salicylate. Other elements of the rule included raising the maximum proposed SPF value on sunscreen labels from 50 to 60 and requiring sunscreens with an SPF value of 15 or higher to provide broad-spectrum protection.
- Application of commercially available sunscreens under maximal use conditions has resulted in plasma concentrations of active ingredients exceeding the threshold established by the FDA for potentially waiving some nonclinical toxicology studies. This is an active area of investigation.
- UV filters have been identified in water sources worldwide and have been implicated in coral reef bleaching (controversial). The Hawaiian state legislature in 2018 was the first to ban sunscreens containing oxybenzone and octinoxate. The AAD issued a statement expressing concern that the public's

Table 1.9. PHYSICAL AND CHEMICAL SUNSCREENS

Sunscreen Type	Sunscreen Mechanism	Examples of UVA Blockers	Examples of UVB Blockers	Examples of UVA and UVB Blockers
Physical	Inert agents that reflect and scatter radiation			Titanium dioxide, zinc oxide
				Titanium dioxide and zinc oxide are white tattoo pigments.
Chemical	Organic agents that absorb and convert radiation into longer, lower-energy wavelengths	Avobenzone (Parsol 1789), ecamsule	PABA and its derivative padimate O, cinnamates, and salicylates	Benzophenones (eg, oxybenzone)
		Avobenzone blocks UV<u>A</u>.		Benzophenones are the leading cause of photoallergic contact dermatitis.

PABA, para-aminobenzoic acid; UV, ultraviolet.

- risk of developing skin cancer could increase and encouraging those who are concerned to use physical sunscreens.
- According to the AAD, other sun-safe practices include **limiting sun exposure, especially between the hours of 10 AM and 2 PM; seeking shade; and wearing sun-protective clothing, hats, and sunglasses.**

- Systemic photoprotective agents include the **natural fern leaf extract** *Polypodium leucotomos* **(Heliocare)**, the α-MSH analogue afamelanotide, carotenoids, polyphenols, and nonsteroidal anti-inflammatory drugs (NSAIDs) such as celecoxib.
- The active ingredient in most **sunless tanning** products is **dihydroxyacetone.**

Immunology and Inflammation

Basic Concepts

- **Innate immunity** is a **rapid** response in which **nonspecific** effectors recognize **non–self**-antigens, while **adaptive immunity** is a **delayed** initial response with subsequent rapid response due to **memory** in which **specific** effectors recognize **self and non–self-antigens** (Table 1.10).
  - **Humoral immunity**, mediated by **antibodies** also known as immunoglobulins (Igs) produced by **B cells**, primarily defends against **extracellular pathogens.**
  - **Cell-mediated immunity**, mediated by **CD4⁺ helper T cells and CD8⁺ cytotoxic T cells**, primarily defends against **intracellular pathogens.**
- Innate and adaptive immune responses are synergistic (eg, antibodies trigger the complement cascade).
- The **major histocompatibility complex (MHC)** is a large family of membrane-bound glycoproteins encoded by the **human leukocyte antigen (HLA) complex of genes on chromosome 6.**
  - Table 1.11.
- **HLA-A, HLA-B, HLA-C are MHC class I; HLA-DP, HLA-DQ, HLA-DR are MHC class II.**
  - ABCs are taught in class I; DP, DQ, DR each have II letters.

Table 1.10. INNATE AND ADAPTIVE IMMUNITY

	Innate Immunity	Adaptive Immunity
Molecular effectors	• Complement • TLRs • Inflammasomes • Antimicrobial peptides • Cytokines (eg, IFNα, IFNβ, IL-1α, IL-1β, IL-6, IL-8, IL-10, TNF-α)	• Cytokines (eg, IFNγ, IL-2, IL-4, IL-5, IL-12, IL-13, IL-17, IL-22, IL-23, IL-31, IL-36, TGF-β) • Antibodies
Cellular effectors	• Macrophages and neutrophils • Eosinophils • Basophils and mast cells • NK cells	• APCs • B cells • T cells

APCs, antigen presenting cells; IFN, interferon; IL, interleukin; NK, natural killer; TGF, transforming growth factor; TLR, toll-like receptor; TNF-α, tumor necrosis factor α.

Table 1.11. DISORDERS ASSOCIATED WITH HUMAN LEUKOCYTE ANTIGENS

HLA	Associated Disorders[a]	Notes
MHC Class I		
HLA-A3101	SCAR to carbamazepine in European populations	
HLA-B8	Oral LP, SCLE, Sjögren syndrome, MCTD	
HLA-B13	Early-onset psoriasis, SCAR to dapsone in Asian populations (HLA-B1301)	
HLA-B1502	SCAR to carbamazepine in Asian and East Indian populations, SCAR to lamotrigine in Han Chinese population, SCAR to phenytoin in Han Chinese population	
HLA-B17	Early onset and guttate psoriasis	
HLA-B27	Pustular psoriasis, psoriatic arthritis (spondylitis and sacroiliitis variant), reactive arthritis	
HLA-B35	Cutaneous LP	
HLA-B51	Behçet disease	
HLA-B57	SCAR to abacavir (HLA-B5701)	
HLA-B5801	SCAR to allopurinol in Han Chinese population	
HLA-Cw6	Early onset/guttate psoriasis	Strongest association with early onset psoriasis.
MHC Class II		
HLA-DR1	LP	
HLA-DR2	SLE	
HLA-DR3	Pemphigoid gestationis, SLE, SCLE, Sjögren syndrome	
HLA-DR4	PV, pemphigoid gestationis, MCTD, relapsing polychondritis, chronic urticaria, actinic prurigo	
HLA-DR6	PV	
HLA-DR7	Early onset psoriasis	
HLA-DQ2	DH	Strongest association with DH.
HLA-DQ7	LS	
HLA-DQ8	Chronic urticaria	

DH, dermatitis herpetiformis; HIV, human immunodeficiency virus; HLA, human leukocyte antigen; LP, lichen planus; LS, lichen sclerosus; MCTD, mixed connective tissue disease; PV, pemphigus vulgaris; SCAR, severe cutaneous adverse reaction; SCLE, subacute cutaneous lupus erythematosus; SLE, systemic lupus erythematosus.
[a]Illustrative examples provided for clinical correlation.

- **MHC class I** molecules, present on nucleated cells, process and express intracellular antigens degraded by proteasomes in the cytosol to CD8⁺ cytotoxic T cells; **MHC class II** molecules, present on APCs, process and express extracellular antigens that are internalized and degraded in endosomes to CD4⁺ helper T cells.
  - $1 \times 8 = 2 \times 4$ (MHC class I, CD8⁺ T cells; MHC class II, CD4⁺ T cells).

Molecular Effectors

Complement

- Complements are proteins in the blood or on the surface of cell membranes.

- There are **three complement pathways** (Figure 1.20) with different triggers:
  - **Alternative pathway**: interaction of polysaccharides derived from microbial cell walls (eg, lipopolysaccharide) with complement 3b (C3b) (may be activated by IgA).
  - **Classical pathway**: interaction of antigen with antibodies (IgM or IgG excepting IgG4).
  - **Lectin pathway**: interaction of microbial carbohydrates with mannose-binding lectin (MBL) (may be activated by IgA).
- Functions of the complement cascade include:
  - B-cell activation and tolerance.

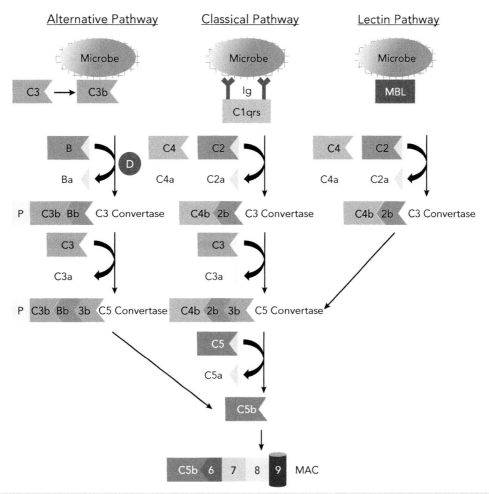

Figure 1.20. COMPLEMENT. In the classical complement pathway, C1qrs bound to the antigen-antibody complex converts C4 and C2 to form C4a, C2a, and C4b2b. C4b2b converts C3 to form C3a and C4b2b3b. C4b2b3b converts C5 to form C5a and C5b, which assembles C6, C7, C8, and C9 to form the membrane attack complex. In the alternative pathway, C3 is spontaneously converted into C3a and C3b, which binds the antigen. Factor D converts Factor B into Ba and C3bBb, which is stabilized by properdin. C3bBb converts C3 into C3a and C3bBb3b, which is stabilized by properdin. C3bBb3b converts C5 to form C5a and C5b, which assembles C6, C7, C8, and C9 to form the membrane attack complex. In the lectin pathway, mannose-binding lectin bound to the antigen converts C4 and C2 to form C4a, C2a, and C4b2b. C4b2b converts C3 to form C3a and C4b2b3b. C4b2b3b converts C5 to form C5a and C5b, which assembles C6, C7, C8, and C9 to form the membrane attack complex. B, factor B; D, factor D; Ig, immunoglobulin; MAC, membrane attack complex; MBL, mannose-binding lectin; P, properdin.

○ **Mast cell degranulation (C3a, C5a > C4a).**
　Anaphylatoxins (C3a, C5a > C4a).
○ **Microbe opsonization to enhance phagocytosis (C3b > C4b).**
　Goldilocks (phagocyte) ate the porridge (microbe) prepared by the 3 bears (C3b opsonization).
○ **Leukocyte chemotaxis (C5a).**
○ Osmotic lysis of microbes due to pores created by the **membrane attack complex (C5b-C9).**
○ Prevention and solubilization of immune complexes.
• Human cells express a variety of proteins such as **complement receptor type 1 (CR1)** that inhibit activation of the complement cascade. **C1-inhibitor (C1-inh)** is an acute-phase protein that circulates in blood and **inhibits activation of the complement cascade.**
　◈ Table 1.12.

Antimicrobial Peptides

• Human epithelia secrete antimicrobial peptides, which defend against bacteria and other microbes. The antimicrobial peptide cathelicidin (LL-37) is also secreted by granulocytes.
• Some antimicrobial peptides such as human β-defensins attract APCs and memory T cells, serving as a bridge between the innate and adaptive immune systems.
• While some antimicrobial peptides are **constitutively expressed** (eg, antileukoprotease, dermcidin, and lysozyme), the expression of others may be **stimulated by bacteria or pro-inflammatory cytokines (e.g., human β-defensins, cathelicidin,** psoriasin, and RNase 7).
　◈ Decreased expression of antimicrobial peptides contributes to *Staphylococcus aureus* colonization in AD.
　◈ Antimicrobial peptide expression is increased in psoriasis, LE, and acne.

Table 1.12. DISORDERS OF COMPLEMENT

Complement	Associated Disorders[a]
Early complement components (C1-C4)	• Hereditary deficiency resulting in susceptibility to pyogenic infections (encapsulated bacteria) and autoimmune disorders (eg, SLE) • Acquired deficiency in patients with autoimmune disorders (eg, SLE)
Late complement components (C5[b]-C9)	• Hereditary deficiency resulting in susceptibility to neisserial infections
C1-inh[c]	• Hereditary angioedema type I (deficiency) and type II (dysfunction) • Acquired angioedema type I (consumption) and type II (autoantibodies) in patients with B-cell lymphoproliferative disorders/ plasma cell dyscrasias and autoimmune disorders (eg, SLE)

C, complement; CH50, total hemolytic complement; inh, inhibitor; PNH, paroxysmal nocturnal hemoglobinuria; SLE, systemic lupus erythematosus.
[a]Illustrative examples provided for clinical correlation. A low CH50 level suggests deficiency of a classical or late complement component.
[b]Eculizumab is a monoclonal antibody targeting C5 approved for PNH.
[c]C1-inh protein and functional levels are normal in hereditary angioedema type III.

Toll-Like Receptors

- Toll-like receptors (TLRs) are a family of **10 receptors** expressed in immune cells such as **dendritic cells (DCs) and macrophages** and nonimmune cells such as **epithelial cells and fibroblasts.**
- **TLRs 1 to 9** recognize **pathogen-associated molecular patterns (PAMPs)** on pathogens as well as **damage-associated molecular patterns (DAMPs)** released by damaged host cells.
- Upon PAMP or DAMP recognition (Table 1.13):
  - TLRs 1 to 9 signal through adaptor proteins such as **myeloid differentiation factor 88 (MyD88)** that activate downstream transcription factors such as **nuclear factor κ-light-chain-enhancer of activated B-cells (NF-κB)** to upregulate release of proinflammatory cytokines.
  - APCs that express TLRs mature and migrate to lymph nodes, where they present pathogen-derived antigens to T cells, serving as a bridge between the innate and adaptive immune systems.
- **TLR10** exerts an **anti-inflammatory** effect. Both the ligand and signaling pathway are unknown.

Inflammasomes

- Inflammasomes are innate immune complexes that, like TLRs, sense **PAMPs and DAMPs.** Activation results in cleavage of pro-IL-1β into the inflammatory cytokine **IL-1β.**
- The most important inflammasome is **nucleotide-binding domain leucine-rich repeat-containing receptor 3 (NLRP3),** the gene that encodes **cryopyrin. Pyrin inhibits formation of the NLRP3 inflammasome. Proline-serine-threonine phosphatase-interacting protein 1 (PSTPIP1) binds pyrin.**
  - The cryopyrin-associated periodic syndromes (CAPS) include chronic infantile articular neurological periodic syndrome (CINCA)/neonatal-onset multisystem inflammatory disease (NOMID), familial cold autoinflammatory syndrome (FCAS), and Muckle-Wells syndrome (MWS).
  - Pyrin mutation causes familial Mediterranean fever (FMF).
  - PSTPIP 1 mutation may cause syndromic pyoderma gangrenosum (PG).
  - The NLRP3 inflammasome is stimulated in acquired inflammatory disorders (eg, acne).

Table 1.13. TOLL-LIKE RECEPTORS

TLR	PAMP
TLR2 (in association with TLR1 or TLR6)	Lipoproteins and peptidoglycans
	Inflammatory acne is associated with increased expression of TLR2 and TLR4 by keratinocytes. Tretinoin, which is approved for acne, regulates TLRs, especially TLR2.
TLR3	Viral dsRNA
TLR4	LPS on GN bacteria
TLR5	Flagellin in bacterial flagella
TLR7 and TLR8	Viral ssRNA
	Imiquimod is a TLR7 ± TLR8 agonist approved for condyloma acuminata, AKs, and superficial BCCs.
TLR9	Bacterial CpG DNA sequences

AKs, actinic keratoses; BCCs, basal cell carcinomas; DNA, deoxyribonucleic acid; ds, double-stranded; GN, gram-negative; LPS, lipopolysaccharide; PAMP, pathogen-associated molecular pattern; RNA, ribonucleic acid; ss, single-stranded; TLR, toll-like receptor.

Cytokines

- Cytokines are small proteins involved in cell signaling (Table 1.14).
  - Figure 1.21.
- Immune cells such as **macrophages, mast cells, and T cells** are important mediators of cytokine signaling.
- **Chemokines** are a subclass of cytokines that attract and direct **migration (chemotaxis)** of leukocytes. For example, **mast cells recruit neutrophils by secreting IL-8.**
- A wide variety of other cell types mediate cytokine signaling. For example, **adipocytes promote systemic inflammation through secretion of IL-6.**
- The **Janus kinase (JAK) enzymes**, JAK1, JAK2, JAK3, and tyrosine kinase 2 (TYK2), are involved in the **transduction of cytokine-mediated signals.**

- Table 1.15.
- Table 1.16.
- Table 1.17.

Antibodies

- Antibodies are secreted by a mature subset of B cells called **plasma cells.**
- Each Ig has a basic structure (Figure 1.22) consisting of **two identical heavy chains and two identical light chains (κ or λ)** connected by disulfide bonds.
- The **antigen-binding fragment (Fab)** has a variable domain containing **three hypervariable complementarity-determining regions (CDRs)** that are determined by gene arrangement during B-cell development and division after antigen stimulation (**somatic hypermutation**). The fragment crystallizable (Fc) also known as the **constant frag-**

Table 1.14. CYTOKINES

Cytokine	Category[a]	Function
G-CSF, GM-CSF	Hematopoiesis	↑granulocyte/macrophage marrow progenitors
Type I: IFNα, IFNβ Type II: IFNγ	Type I: innate immunity Type II: adaptive immunity	Type I: ↑MHC class I molecules, ↑NK cells, ↑Th1 response, ↓viral replication Type II: ↑B cells, ↑macrophages, ↑Th1 response, ↓viral replication
		Interferons interfere with viral replication.
IL-1α, IL-1β	Innate immunity	↑acute phase reactants, ↑chemokines, ↑endothelial cell adhesion molecules, fever
IL-2	Adaptive immunity	↑B cells, ↑NK cells, ↑Th1 response, ↑T cells and differentiation into memory T cells, pruritus
IL-3	Hematopoiesis	↑multilineage marrow progenitors
IL-4	Adaptive immunity	↑B cells, ↑B cell class switching to IgE, ↑Th2 response
IL-5	Adaptive immunity	↑B cells, ↑B cell class switching to IgA, ↑eosinophils
IL-6	Innate immunity	↑acute phase reactants, ↑B cells, ↑Th2 response
IL-8	Innate immunity	↑chemotaxis of neutrophils
IL-10	Innate immunity	↓macrophage activation, ↓Th1 response
IL-12	Adaptive immunity	↑Th1 response
IL-13	Adaptive immunity	↑B cell class switching to IgE, ↑Th2 response
IL-17	Adaptive immunity	↑chemokines
IL-22	Adaptive immunity	↑Th17 cells
IL-23	Adaptive immunity	↑Th17 response, ↑Th22 response
IL-31	Adaptive immunity	↑Th2 response, pruritus
IL-36	Adaptive immunity	↓T cells
TGF-β	Adaptive immunity	↓macrophage activation, ↓T cells but ↑T-regs
		β-ouncers calm down bar hoppers.
TNF-α	Innate immunity	↑endothelial cell adhesion molecules, ↑chemokines, ↑acute-phase reactants, fever, ↑Th1 response

G-CSF, granulocyte colony-stimulating factor; GM-CSF, granulocyte-monocyte colony-stimulating factor; IFN, interferon; Ig, immunoglobulin; IL, interleukin; MHC, major histocompatibility complex; NK, natural killer; TGF, transforming growth factor; Th, T helper cell type; TNF, tumor necrosis factor; Tregs, T regulatory cells.

[a]Cytokines are often involved in cross talk between the innate and adaptive immune systems and therefore categories are not mutually exclusive.

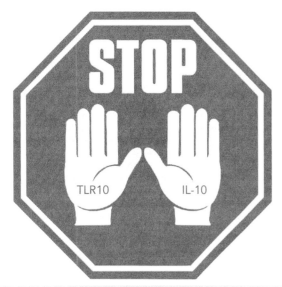

Figure 1.21. ANTI-INFLAMMATORY SIGNALS, 10 fingers up means STOP IL-10, interleukin 10; TLR10, toll-like receptor 10.

(Illustration by Caroline A. Nelson, MD.)

Table 1.15. CYTOKINE SIGNATURES

Cytokines	Associated Disorder[a]
↑Th2 cytokines such as IL-4, IL-13, and IL-31	AD (acute), morphea/SSc
↑IL-1	Contact dermatitis, DIRA, acne
↑IL-36	DITRA
↑Type I IFNs	LE
↑Th1 cytokines such as TNF-α and IL-12, IL-17, IL-22, and IL-23	Psoriasis, AD (chronic), acne
↑TGF-β	Morphea/SSc

AD, atopic dermatitis; DIRA, deficiency of the IL-1 receptor antagonist; DITRA, deficiency of the IL-36 receptor antagonist; G-CSF, granulocyte colony-stimulating factor; GM-CSF, granulocyte-monocyte colony-stimulating factor; IFNs, interferons; IL, interleukin; LE, lupus erythematosus; SSc, systemic sclerosis; TGF, transforming growth factor; Th, T helper cell type; TNF-α, tumor necrosis factor α
[a]Illustrative examples provided for clinical correlation.

Table 1.16. CYTOKINE TREATMENTS

Cytokines	FDA-Approved Dermatology Indications[a]
G-CSF, GM-CSF[b]	Melanoma (T-VEC)
IFNα, IFNβ	AIDS-associated Kaposi sarcoma, condyloma acuminata, melanoma
IFNγ	CGD
IL-2	Melanoma

AIDS, acquired immune deficiency syndrome; CGD, chronic granulomatous disease; FDA, Food and Drug Administration; G-CSF, granulocyte colony-stimulating factor; GM-CSF, granulocyte-monocyte colony-stimulating factor; IFN, interferon; T-VEC, talimogene laherparepvec.
[a]Illustrative examples provided for clinical correlation.
[b]CSF use in the supportive care of oncology patients may trigger neutrophilic dermatoses such as Sweet syndrome.

ment classifies the Ig into one of **five isotypes** (Table 1.18) and induces its effector functions.

- ◆ Intravenous immune globulin (IVIG), a sterile solution of globulins extracted from pooled plasma, is approved for Kawasaki disease, primary humoral immunodeficiency syndromes such as agammaglobulinemia and common variable immunodeficiency (CVID), and prophylaxis for viral infections such as measles, rubella, and varicella.

Cellular Effectors

- Cellular effectors of the immune system include macrophages and neutrophils, eosinophils, basophils and mast cells, natural killer (NK) cells, APCs, B cells, T cells, and keratinocytes.
  - ◆ Figure 1.23.

Macrophages and Neutrophils

- **Macrophages** are **mononuclear phagocytes** that exit the bloodstream to **reside in tissues.** They also function as **APCs and mediate cytokine signaling.**
- **Neutrophils** are the **most abundant leukocyte.** They are classified as **granulocytes** and function as **phagocytes.**
- In response to **chemokines (eg, C5a, IL-8),** neutrophils exit the bloodstream and enter the dermis through postcapillary venules. **Capture and rolling of leukocytes** is primarily mediated by **selectins** (eg, E-selectin and P-selectin on endothelial cells and L-selectin on leukocytes) and their ligands. **Firm adhesion and transmigration** is primarily mediated by **integrins.**
- Once in the tissue, macrophages and neutrophils identify microbes using antibody, complement, mannose, and other receptors and **ingest and destroy microbes with ROS (the respiratory burst) and lysosomal enzymes (eg, myeloperoxidase (MPO) and nicotinamide adenine dinucleotide phosphate hydrogen (NADPH) oxidase).** Neutrophils destroy microbes within primary (azurophilic) granules and release ectosomes and neutrophilic extracellular traps (NETs).
  - ◆ Chronic granulomatous disease (CGD), due to decreased NADPH oxidase activity, results in severe recurrent infections. Diagnosis is made with the nitro blue tetrazolium test, in which phagocytes are unable to reduce yellow dye to blue dye.

Eosinophils

- Eosinophils are **granulocytes** that primarily function to **defend against parasitic infections and mediate allergic reactions.**
- Eosinophils respond to **chemokines (eg, C5a, eotaxin).**
  - ◆ Increased expression of eotaxin is observed in Kimura disease, a chronic inflammatory disorder characterized by head and neck tumors, enlarged lymph nodes, increased eosinophil counts, and high serum IgE.
- Eosinophils express a **low affinity receptor for the Fc region of IgE (FcεRII).** Upon binding IgE, they become activated and release **major basic protein (MBP)** and other proteins from their granules. MBP is cytotoxic and induces basophil and mast cell degranulation.

Table 1.17. CYTOKINE INHIBITORS

Cytokine Pathway	Inhibitors	FDA-Approved Dermatology Indications[a]
GM-CSF	Namilumab	Psoriasis/psoriatic arthritis[b]
Type I IFN	Anifrolumab	SLE
IL-1	Anakinra, canakinumab, rilonacept	CAPS, FMF, HIDS, TRAPS
IL-2[c]	Basiliximab	
IL-4	Dupilumab	AD
IL-5	Mepolizumab, reslizumab	EGPA
IL-6	Sarilumab, siltuximab, tocilizumab	GCA
IL-12	Ustekinumab	Psoriasis/psoriatic arthritis
IL-13	Dupilumab	AD
IL-17	Brodalumab, ixekizumab, secukinumab	Psoriasis/psoriatic arthritis
IL-23	Guselkumab, risankizumab, tildrakizumab, ustekinumab	Psoriasis/psoriatic arthritis
IL-31	Nemolizumab	Pruritus associated with AD[b]
JAK	Baricitinib, ruxolitinib, tofacitinib	GVHD, psoriatic arthritis
TNF-α	Adalimumab, certolizumab, etanercept, golimumab, infliximab	HS, psoriasis/psoriatic arthritis

AD, atopic dermatitis; CAPS, cryopyrin-associated periodic syndromes; CTCL, cutaneous T-cell lymphoma; EGPA, eosinophilic granulomatosis with polyangiitis; FDA, Food and Drug Administration; FMF, familial Mediterranean fever; GCA, giant cell arteritis; GM-CSF, granulocyte-monocyte colony stimulating factor; GVHD, graft-versus-host disease; HIDS, hyperimmunoglobulinemia D syndrome; HS, hidradenitis suppurativa; IFN, interferon; IL, interleukin; JAK, Janus kinase; R, receptor; SLE, systemic lupus erythematosus; TNF-α, tumor necrosis factor α; TRAPS. TNF receptor–associated periodic syndrome.
[a]Illustrative examples provided for clinical correlation.
[b]Under investigation.
[c]IL-2 is also the primary downstream target of calcineurin inhibitors. Systemic cyclosporine is approved for psoriasis and topical tacrolimus is approved for AD. Denileukin diftitox (discontinued) was an IL-2 diphtheria toxin fusion protein targeting the IL-2 receptor (IL-2R) that was approved for CTCL.

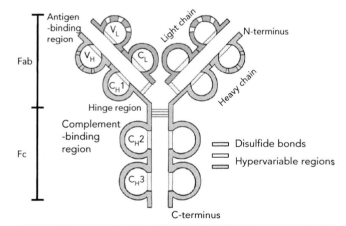

Figure 1.22. IMMUNOGLOBULIN. Basic Structure. C$_H$, constant region of the heavy chain; C$_L$, constant region of the light chain; Fab, fragment antigen binding; Fc, fragment crystallizable; V$_H$, variable region of the heavy chain; V$_L$, variable region of the light chain.

Basophils and Mast Cells

- Basophils and mast cells are **granulocytes** that **mediate allergic reactions.** Mast cells help to **defend mucosal surfaces from infection.** Basophils are located in the blood, while mast cells are primarily located in perivascular spaces within the **papillary dermis.**
- **Mast cells are derived from CD34/c-kit/CD13⁺ cells in the bone marrow.** They express the **kit** receptor and its ligand,

Table 1.18. ANTIBODIES

Ig	Notes
IgA	Predominant Ig in mucosal surfaces, activates the alternative and lectin complement pathways
	Open your mouth and say "A."
	Selective IgA deficiency is a hereditary immunodeficiency syndrome.
IgD	Unknown function
	MKD/HIDS is a hereditary periodic fever syndrome.
IgE	Allergic, atopic, and helminthic responses
	Hyper-IgE syndromes are hereditary immunodeficiency syndromes. Omalizumab is a monoclonal antibody targeting IgE approved for chronic idiopathic urticaria.
IgG	Predominant Ig in the circulation, activates the classical complement pathway (IgG3 > IgG1 > IgG2), crosses the placenta
	Neonatal pemphigus occurs when maternal IgG antibodies cross the placenta.
IgM	Pentamer, predominant Ig in the primary immune response, agglutinates antigens, activates the classical complement pathway
	Selective IgM deficiency and hyper-IgM syndrome are hereditary immunodeficiency syndromes.

HIDS, hyper-IgD syndrome; Ig, immunoglobulin; MKD, mevalonate kinase deficiency.

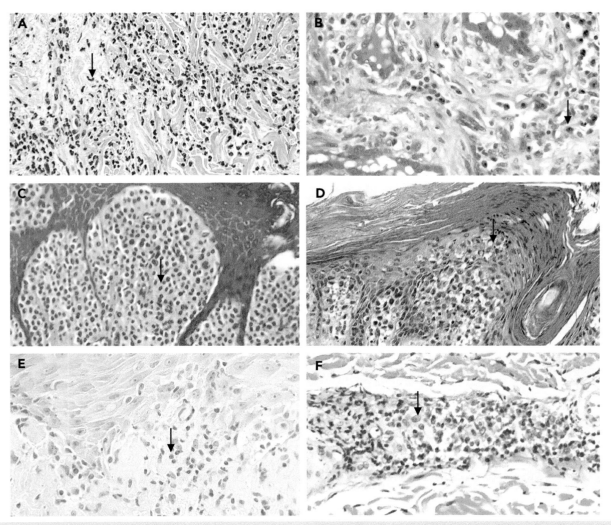

Figure 1.23. CELLULAR EFFECTORS. A, Solid arrow: neutrophil in Sweet syndrome. Note the multilobed nucleus. B, Solid arrow: eosinophil in an epithelioid hemangioma. Note the pink cytoplasm and bilobed nucleus resembling "sunglasses." C, Solid arrow: mast cell in urticaria pigmentosa. Note the "fried egg" appearance. D, Solid arrow: Langerhans cell in Langerhans cell histiocytosis. Note the reniform "kidney bean–shaped" nucleus. E, Solid arrow: lymphocyte in lichen planus. Note the nucleus is approximately the size of a normal erythrocyte. F, Solid arrow: plasma cell in secondary syphilis. Note the eccentric nucleus with heterochromatin in a "clockface" arrangement and the pale cytoplasmic hoff (Golgi).

(B, Histology image reprinted with permission from Elder DE, Elenitsas R, Rosenbach M,et al. *Lever's Histopathology of the Skin*. 11th ed. Wolters Kluwer; 2015. C, Histology image reprinted with permission from Elder DE, Elenitsas R, Rosenbach M, et al. *Lever's Histopathology of the Skin*. 11th ed. Wolters Kluwer; 2015. D, Histology image reprinted with permission from Elder DE, Elenitsas R, Rosenbach M, et al. *Lever's Histopathology of the Skin*. 11th ed. Wolters Kluwer; 2015. E, Histology image courtesy of Noel Turner, MD, MHS and Christine J. Ko, MD. F, Histology image reprinted with permission from Elder DE, Elenitsas R, Rosenbach M, et al. *Lever's Histopathology of the Skin*. 11th ed. Wolters Kluwer; 2015.)

stem cell factor, which are critical for their survival and proliferation.

  ◆ Activating mutations in *c-KIT* **proto-oncogene** are often implicated in mastocytosis.

• Basophils and mast cells express **receptors for complement and high-affinity FcεRI. Cross-linking of two bound IgE molecules by antigen, anti-IgE antibodies, or other substances induces degranulation.** Other triggers for mast cell degranulation include **anaphylatoxins** and **substance P.**

  ◆ Urticaria may be immunologic (eg, allergy to a β-lactam antibiotic) or nonimmunologic (eg, nettle stings).

• Prostaglandin E_2 inhibits mast cell degranulation.

• Degranulation results in release of preformed and newly formed mediators (Table 1.19). Effects include pruritus, vascular permeability, bronchoconstriction, and cytokine signaling to induce eosinophil and neutrophil chemotaxis.

Table 1.19. MAST CELL MEDIATORS

	Mast Cell Mediator
Preformed	Carboxypeptidase, cathepsin G, chymase, heparin, histamine, serotonin, tryptase
Newly formed	Leukotrienes, platelet activating factor, prostaglandin D_2

Natural Killer Cells

- NK cells are **lymphocytes** that **identify virally infected cells and cancer cells that have attempted to evade the immune system by downregulating expression of MHC class I molecules.** NK cells also **mediate antibody-dependent cellular cytotoxicity,** serving as a bridge between the innate and adaptive immune systems.
- NK cells secrete **interferon γ (IFNγ)** and other pro-inflammatory cytokines.
- NK cells destroy target cells using a variety of mechanisms:
  - **Perforins** produced by NK cells **form pores in the membranes** of target cells.
  - **Granzymes** injected by NK cells through pores **fragment DNA, leading to apoptosis** of target cells.
  - **Fas ligand on NK cells binds to Fas on target cells, leading to apoptosis.**
    - Fas is fastened to all cells; Fas ligand is a land mine.

Antigen-Presenting Cells

- APCs are cells that **present antigens on MHC class II molecules to CD4+ helper T cells.**
- **LCs are the most important APCs in the epidermis.** They are derived from a **CD34+ monocyte-macrophage lineage in the bone marrow.** They are primarily located in the *stratum spinosum* connected to keratinocytes via **E-cadherin receptors.** They are **poorly phagocytic** as compared to other APCs. Similar to basophils and mast cells, they **express high-affinity FcεRI.**
  - LCs are spies that hide among the spines.
- **DCs are APCs** located in the **dermis.** They are **highly phagocytic.**

B Cells

- B cells are **lymphocyte APCs;** however, their primary function is to **produce antibodies.**
- During early development, Igs function as antigen-specific B-cell receptors on the cell membrane.
- Upon activation, B cells divide and mature into plasma cells and memory B cells. **B lymphocyte stimulator (BLyS) is a B-cell activator. CD20 is a B-cell surface molecule that plays a role in the development and differentiation of B cells into plasma cells.**
  - Belimumab is a monoclonal antibody targeting BLyS approved for systemic lupus erythematosus (SLE). Rituximab is a monoclonal antibody targeting CD20 approved for granulomatosis with polyangiitis (GPA), microscopic polyangiitis (MPA), and pemphigus vulgaris (PV).
- B-cell activation to secrete IgM may be T cell independent; however, this response is short lived and has poor specificity due to lack of germinal center formation, affinity maturation, Ig class switching, and memory. Therefore, **most B-cell activation is T cell dependent.**

T Cells

- T cells are **lymphocytes** that **recognize antigens bound to MHC molecules** via the **T-cell receptor (TCR).**
- The diversity of TCRs results from gene rearrangement during T-cell development. T cells undergo **positive selection (ability to recognize MHC molecules)** and **negative selection (recognition of self-antigens)** within the **thymus.** The vast **majority** of T cells express the **α/β TCR;** however, a **subset** of T cells express the **γ/δ TCR,** such as dendritic epidermal T cells.
- **CD4+ helper T cells** recognize extracellular antigens bound to **MHC class II molecules on APCs** and are divided into the following subtypes:
  - **T helper type 1 (Th1) cells:** primarily secrete IFNγ to stimulate phagocyte-mediated defense.
  - **T helper type 2 (Th2) cells:** primarily secrete IL-4, IL-5, IL-6, IL-10, and IL-13 to stimulate IgE and eosinophil and mast cell–mediated defense.
    - The balance between Th1/Th2 responses influences disease evolution. For example, tuberculoid leprosy is characterized by a Th1 response, while lepromatous leprosy is characterized by a Th2 response.
  - **T helper type 17 (Th17) cells:** primarily secrete IL-17 to recruit neutrophils.
  - **T helper type 22 (Th22) cells:** primarily secrete IL-22 to amplify the Th17 response.
    - Chronic mucocutaneous candidiasis (CMC) results from impaired Th17 response. Th1, Th17, and Th22 cells have been implicated in psoriasis.
- T cell–dependent B-cell activation:
  - An antigen binds to IgM on the B-cell surface.
  - The antigen is internalized, processed, and reexpressed within the MHC class II molecule on the B-cell surface and presented to a CD4+ helper T cell.
  - Primed CD4+ helper T cells secrete B-cell growth factor cytokines (IFNγ, IL-2, IL-4, IL-5, and IL-6) that induce proliferation, isotype switching, and differentiation into plasma cells.
    - *IL-2RG* mutation causes X-linked severe combined immunodeficiency (SCID).
  - **Interaction of CD40 with CD40 ligand (CD154) on T cells leads to B cell class switching from IgM to IgG and formation of memory B cells.**
  - Upon antigen reexposure, follicular DCs in the germinal centers of lymph nodes trap antigen-antibody complexes and stimulate T cell–dependent B-cell activation.
- **CD8+ cytotoxic T cells** recognize intracellular antigens bound to **MHC class I molecules on nucleated cells** and destroy virally infected cells and cancer cells with **perforin, granzymes, and Fas ligand.** Along with **NK T cells,** which share properties of NK cells and T cells, they secrete **IFNγ** and other pro-inflammatory cytokines.
  - γ looks like a gun in a holster (natural killer cells, Th1 cells, CD8+ cytotoxic T cells).
- **Resident memory T cells** in the skin **defend against previously encountered antigens.**
- **CD4/CD25+ regulatory T cells (T-regs),** under the influence of the transcription factor **FOXP3,** function to **downregulate the immune response (e.g., via IL-10 and TGF-β).**
  - *AIRE* mutation in autoimmune regulator causes autoimmune polyendocrinopathy-candidiasis-ectodermal dys-

Table 1.20. T-CELL SURFACE MOLECULES

T-Cell Surface Molecule	Binding Site	T-Cell Function
CD2	LFA3 on APCs and endothelial cells	Adhesion of naïve T cells, costimulatory signal
		Alefacept (discontinued) was an LFA-3/Fc-IgG1 fusion protein targeting CD2 that was approved for psoriasis.
CD3	MHC	Activation of T cells
CD4	MHC II on APCs	Activation of helper T cells
CD8	MHC I	Activation of cytotoxic T cells
CD28	B7-1/2 (CD80/86) on APCs	Costimulatory signal
CD40L (CD154)	CD40 on APC	Upregulation of B7, B cell class switching from IgM to IgG, formation of memory B cells
CD30	CD30L	Costimulatory signal
		Brentuximab vedotin is a monoclonal antibody drug conjugate targeting CD30 approved for CTCL.
CD52	Anchored to GPI	Costimulatory signal
		Alemtuzumab is a monoclonal antibody targeting CD52 approved for ATLL and CTCL.
CLA	E-selectin on endothelial cells	Adhesion of memory T cells
CTLA4	B7-1/2 (CD80/86) on APCs	Anergy or apoptosis of T cells
		Abatacept is a CTLA-4/Fc-IgG1 fusion protein targeting B7-1 approved for psoriatic arthritis. CTLA-4 is an ICI target.
LFA1 (CD11a)	ICAM1 on APCs and endothelial cells	Tight adhesion leading to transmigration of T cells, costimulatory signal
		LFA1-ICAM-1 interaction is disrupted in LAD. Efalizumab (discontinued due to risk of PML) was a monoclonal antibody targeting CD11a that was approved for psoriasis.
PD-1	PD-L1 on cancer cells	Anergy or apoptosis of T cells
		PD-1 and PD-L1 are ICI targets.

APC, antigen-presenting cell; ATLL, T-cell leukemia/lymphoma; CD, cluster of differentiation; CLA, cutaneous lymphocyte antigen; CTCL, cutaneous T-cell lymphoma; CTLA, cytotoxic T lymphocyte–associated protein; Fc, fragment crystallizable; GPI, glycosylphosphatidylinositol; ICAM, intercellular adhesion molecule; ICI, immune checkpoint inhibitor; Ig, immunoglobulin; L, ligand; LAD, leukocyte adhesion deficiency; LFA, lymphocyte function–associated antigen; MHC, major histocompatibility complex; PD, programmed death; PML, progressive multifocal leukoencephalopathy; TNF-α, tumor necrosis factor α

trophy (APECED) syndrome. *FOXP3* mutation causes immune dysregulation, polyendocrinopathy, enteropathy, X-linked (IPEX) syndrome.

- **A costimulatory signal is required to form effector and memory T cells** (Table 1.20).
- **Immune checkpoints** are regulators of the immune system that are **crucial for self-tolerance, but may be exploited by cancer cells** (Figure 1.24).
  - Immune checkpoint inhibitors (ICIs) activate the antitumor immune response.

Keratinocytes

- Keratinocytes are both effectors and targets of immune reactions.
- Keratinocytes **express pattern recognition receptors such as TLRs and secrete antimicrobial peptides and both pro- and anti-inflammatory cytokines (eg, IL-1 and IL-10, respectively).**
- Keratinocytes express MHC class I molecules and can be **induced to express MHC class II molecules by cytokines (e.g., IFNγ)** and thereby induce proliferation of allogeneic CD4⁺ T-cell lines.

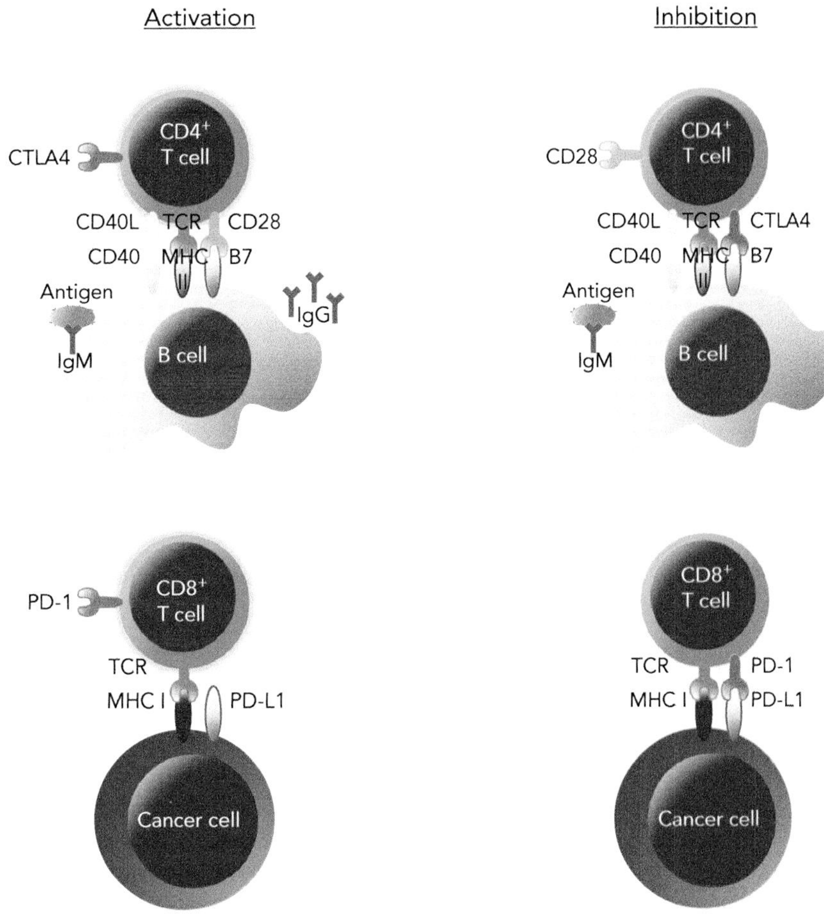

Activation   Inhibition

Figure 1.24. IMMUNE CHECKPOINTS Interaction of B7 on B cells with cluster of differentiation 28 (CD28) on CD4$^+$ T cells serves as a costimulatory signal for T-cell activation. Interaction of CD40 on B cells and CD40 ligand (CD40L) on T cells upregulates B-cell expression of B7 and leads to class switching from immunoglobulin M (IgM) to IgG and formation of memory B cells. In contrast, interaction of B7 with CTLA4 on T cells causes T-cell anergy (nonreactivity) or apoptosis. Programmed death-ligand 1 (PD-L1) is expressed by some cancer cells. Interaction of PD-L1 with PD-1 on CD8$^+$ T cells inhibits T-cell activation, thereby circumventing cytotoxic T cell–mediated destruction. CD, cluster of differentiation; CTLA4, cytotoxic T lymphocyte–associated protein 4; Ig, immunoglobulin; L, ligand; MHC, major histocompatibility complex; PD, programmed death; TCR, T-cell receptor.

Wound Healing

Basic Concepts

- **Regeneration**: wound healing process during the first third of gestation that occurs without scarring.
- **Scarring**: wound healing process that tackles pathogens quickly, walls off foreign bodies, and seals off injured areas from the environment.
- **Erosion**: defect that affects only the epidermis (heals without scarring).
- **Ulceration**: defect that affects the dermis (heals with scarring):
  - **Partial thickness**: ulcer extends to the mid-dermis (reepithelialization occurs from preserved adnexal structures [if preserved] and intact wound edges).

  - **Full thickness**: ulcer extends to the subcutis (reepithelialization occurs from the intact wound edges only with relatively increased contraction).

    Do NOT get confused! Wounds and grafts are opposites. Split-thickness skin grafts lack adnexal structures and have poor cosmesis and relatively increased contraction compared to full-thickness skin grafts.

The Three Phases of Wound Healing (Table 1.21)

Table 1.21. THE THREE PHASES OF WOUND HEALING

Phase	Description
Inflammatory (days 1-3)	Fibrin is the first ECM component deposited.
	Platelets initiate clot formation and release chemotactic factors for other platelets, fibroblasts, and immune cells such as fibrinogen, fibronectin, PDGF, TGF-α, and TGF-β. <ul><li>PDGF, TGF-β_1, TGF-β_2, IL-6, and IL-8 augment scarring;</li><li>TGF-β_3 and IL-10 reduce scarring.</li></ul>
	TGF-β upregulation has been implicated in keloid formation.
	Fibronectin, required for granulation tissue formation, acts as a reservoir for growth factor signaling, a matrix for fibroblast migration, and a template for collagen deposition.
	Fibroblasts and neutrophils arrive after ~48 hours.
	Macrophages ultimately outnumber neutrophils. They are crucial because they not only debride tissue and kill pathogens but also secrete growth factors that simulate fibroblasts.
Proliferative (days 4-21)	Reepithelialization begins within 24 hours as keratinocytes, aided by collagenase, leapfrog over each other from the wound edges.
	After ~4 days, fibroblasts deposit granulation tissue with type III collagen into the wound.
	During weeks 1-2, angiogenesis occurs and myofibroblasts contract the wound.
	Angiogenesis inhibitors such as bevacizumab disturb wound healing, leading to ulcers that characteristically localize to *striae distensae*.
Remodeling (day 21 to year 1)	Fibroblasts gradually remodel the scar, replacing type III collagen with type I collagen to increase tensile strength.
	Scar strength is ~5% at 1 week, ~20% at 3 weeks, ~50% at 3 months, and ~80% at 1 year.

ECM, extracellular matrix; IL, interleukin; PDGF, platelet-derived growth factor; TGF, transforming growth factor.

Pharmacology

Basic Concepts

- **Pharmacodynamics**: study of the relationship between the concentration of a drug at its site of action and the magnitude of the pharmacological response.
  - Pharmacodynamics is "what the drug does to the body."
- **Pharmacokinetics**: study of the time course of absorption, distribution, metabolism, and excretion of a drug after its administration.
  - Pharmacokinetics is "what the body does to the drug."
- **Bioavailability** is the proportion of a drug that enters the circulation and is able to exert an effect.
- **Half-life** is the time it takes for the drug concentration in the plasma or the body to decrease by 50%.
- **Absorption** of a drug may be enteral (eg, oral or rectal) or parenteral (eg, topical, intradermal, intralesional, intramuscular [IM], subcutaneous [SC], or intravenous [IV]).
  - Drug interactions may affect bioavailability of a drug by altering its absorption.
    - For example, antacids, particularly those containing aluminum hydroxide, magnesium hydroxide, and/or calcium carbonate, impair absorption of fluoroquinolones.
  - Efflux pumps such as P-glycoprotein may also impair drug absorption.
    - For example, efflux of certain aminoglycoside antibiotics by brush border cells of the small intestine limits efficacy of oral administration.
- **Distribution** is the reversible transfer of a drug from one location to another within the body.
  - Drug interactions may affect bioavailability of a drug by altering its distribution.
    - For example, NSAIDs displace methotrexate from plasma protein–binding sites, increasing free concentration.
- **Metabolism** of a drug may occur in the liver, intestine (enterocytes and microbiome), kidney, lung, plasma, red blood cells, placenta, skin, and brain. In general, enzymatic processes transform a lipophilic substrate into a more hydrophilic metabolite in order to facilitate drug excretion. **Cytochrome p-450 (CYP) enzymes** are primarily located in the **endoplasmic reticulum of hepatocytes** (Table 1.22). **CYP2D6** accounts for ~25% of drug metabolism. **CYP3A4** accounts for ~50% of drug metabolism.
  - Drug interactions may affect bioavailability of a drug by altering its metabolism. Mechanisms include inhibition or induction of CYP enzymes and microbiome alteration.
    - For example, rifampin decreases the efficacy of oral contraceptive pills (OCPs) by inducing CYP3A4, thereby accelerating metabolism, and by reducing the bacterial population of the small intestine,

thereby interfering with enterohepatic cycling of ethinylestradiol.

○ Individuals with certain genotypes may reach increased blood concentrations of a drug and have an increased risk of a drug reaction.

◆ For example, epoxide hydroxylase deficiency has been linked to anticonvulsant hypersensitivity syndrome.

▫ In the setting of e̲p̲oxide hydroxylase deficiency, an anticonvulsant may start the e̲p̲ocalypse.

▫ Figure 1.25.

- Drug **excretion** occurs primarily through biliary and renal routes. Skin, hair, and sweat are among the secondary excretion processes.

○ Drug interactions may affect bioavailability of a drug by altering its excretion. For example, **probenecid decreases renal tubular excretion of β-lactams.**

Skin Absorption and Penetration

- Absorption: amount of drug that builds up in the skin over a certain period of time.
- Penetration: amount of drug that crosses the skin per unit area per unit time.

- The extracellular, lipid-enriched matrix of the *stratum corneum* serves as a reservoir for the absorption and release of lipid-soluble drugs and limits penetration of hydrophilic drugs.

- Topical drugs consist of an active ingredient in a nonactive base:

○ **Cream:** emulsion of oil and water.

○ **Foam:** liquid or solid in gas.

○ **Gel:** transparent semisolid emulsion (aqueous or alcohol base).

○ **Lotion:** oil mixed with a liquid (aqueous or alcohol base).

○ **Ointment:** semisolid oil.

○ **Paste:** mixture of oil, water, and powder.

○ **Solution:** powder dissolved in liquid (aqueous or alcohol base).

- Factors that affect absorption:

○ Characteristics of the skin: skin barrier immaturity, disruption, hydration, and/or occlusion increase absorption while *stratum corneum* thickness decreases absorption. The **mucous membranes and scrotum are the sites of highest absorption**, while the palms, soles, and nails are the sites of lowest absorption.

Table 1.22. CYTOCHROME P450 ENZYMES: SUBSTRATES, INHIBITORS, AND INDUCERS

CYP Enzyme	CYP1A2	CYP2C9	CYP2D6	CYP3A4
Example substrates	Warfarin	Phenytoin, warfarin	Doxepin, pimozide, propranolol	Nifedipine, OCP, pimozide, simvastatin, terfenadine, warfarin
Example inhibitors	Ciprofloxacin, tobacco	Fluconazole	Sertraline, terbinafine	Azoles, cyclosporine, gemfibrozil, grapefruit juice, macrolides, protease inhibitors
				CYP3A4 inhibitors –> bleeding, rhabdomyolysis, and *torsades de pointes*.
Example inducers				Bexarotene, carbamazepine, griseofulvin, rifampin, St. John's wort
				CYP3A4 inducers –> clotting and unintended pregnancy.

CYP, cytochrome P450; HMG-CoA, 3-hydroxy-3-methylglutaryl-coenzyme A; OCPs, oral contraceptive pills.

Coadministration of warfarin with a CYP3A4 inhibitor increases risk of bleeding

Azoles
Cyclosporine
Gemfibrozil
Grapefruit juice
Macrolides
Protease inhibitors

Coadministration of warfarin with a CYP3A4 inducer increases risk of clotting

Bexarotene
Carbamazepine
Griseofulvin
Rifampin
St. John's wort

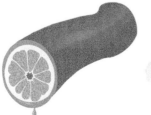

Figure 1.25. CYP3A4 INTERACTIONS. CYP, cytochrome P450.

(Illustration by Caroline A. Nelson, MD.)

Table 1.23. IMMUNOLOGIC DRUG REACTIONS

Drug Reaction	Gell-Coombs Classification	Mechanism	Example(s)
IgE-dependent	Type I	Mast cell degranulation	Urticaria, angioedema, anaphylaxis
Cytotoxic	Type II	Antigen-antibody interactions	Petechiae secondary to drug-induced thrombocytopenia
Immune complex–dependent	Type III	Antigen-antibody interactions in the blood	CSVV, leprosy type 2 reaction (ENL), leprosy type 3 (Lucio) reaction
Delayed-type, cell-mediated	Type IV	Activation of CD4[+] and CD8[+] T cells	ACD, AGEP,[a] EN, lichenoid drug eruption, SJS/TEN,[a] FDE, morbilliform drug eruption/DRESS,[a] leprosy type 1 (reversal) reaction, PMLE, CAD, photoallergic eruption

[a]Alternatively classified as idiosyncratic drug reactions.
ACD, allergic contact dermatitis; AGEP, acute generalized exanthematous pustulosis; CAD, chronic actinic dermatitis; CSVV, cutaneous small-vessel vasculitis; DRESS, drug reaction with eosinophilia and systemic symptoms; EN, erythema nodosum; ENL, erythema nodosum leprosum; FDE, fixed drug eruption; Ig, immunoglobulin; PMLE, polymorphous light eruption; SJS/TEN, Stevens-Johnson syndrome/toxic epidermal necrolysis.

○ Characteristics of the drug: small molecular size and/or low frictional coefficient, lipophilicity, and high concentration and/or solubility increase absorption.
○ Characteristics of the vehicle: occlusive vehicles (eg, ointments) increase absorption.
• One fingertip unit is ~0.5 g. The appropriate amount to treat the entire body of an adult man is ~20 g (~250 g/wk if applied twice daily).

Pregnancy, Lactation, and Reproduction

• FDA pregnancy risk categories (1979-2015):
  ○ **A**: Controlled studies show no risk. Adequate well-controlled studies in pregnant women have failed to demonstrate risk to the fetus.
  ○ **B**: No evidence of risk in humans. Either animal studies show risk, but human studies do not, or if no adequate human studies have been done, animal findings are negative.
  ○ **C**: Risk cannot be ruled out. Human studies are lacking, and animal studies are either positive for fetal risk or lacking as well. However, potential benefits may justify the potential risk.

○ **D**: Positive evidence for risk. Human studies, or investigational or postmarketing data, show risk to fetus. Nevertheless, potential benefits may outweigh potential risk.
○ **X**: Contraindicated in pregnancy. Studies in animals or humans, or investigational or postmarketing reports, have shown fetal risk, which clearly outweighs any possible benefit to the patient.
• In 2015, the FDA Pregnancy and Lactation Labeling Rule replaced pregnancy risk categories with narrative sections on pregnancy, lactation, and females and males of reproductive potential.

Drug Reactions

• The mechanism of a drug reaction may be:
  ○ **Immunologic**: drug or its metabolites act as haptens to induce a specific immune response.
    ◆ Table 1.23.
  ○ **Nonimmunologic**: overdose, pharmacologic side effects, cumulative toxicity, delayed toxicity, drug-drug interactions, alterations in metabolism, and/or exacerbation of disease.
  ○ **Idiosyncratic**: possible interplay between an immunologic mechanism and genetic predisposition.

Laboratory Techniques

Basic Concepts

• The cell theory holds that all living things are made of cells, which are the basic units of life.

Cell Extraction (Table 1.24)

Measurement of Cellular Components (Table 1.25)

• Cellular components include DNA, RNA, and protein.
  ◇ Figure 1.26.

Genetic Modification (Table 1.26)

Table 1.24. CELL EXTRACTION

Technique	Description
Laser capture microdissection	A specific population of cells is dissected from a tissue section with a laser while the slide is viewed under a microscope.
Flow cytometry	Cells in suspension are sorted according to expression of specific markers.
	An example use of flow cytometry is testing the blood of CTCL patients for circulating lymphoma cells.

CTCL, cutaneous T-cell lymphoma.

Table 1.25. MEASUREMENT OF CELLULAR COMPONENTS

Technique	Description
DNA	
Southern blot	A DNA sample is separated by size with electrophoresis and then a hybridization probe is used to detect a specific DNA sequence by radiographic, chemiluminescent, or chromogenic detection.
PCR	A specific DNA sequence is amplified from a DNA sample in four steps: (1) denaturation of dsDNA to ssDNA, (2) hybridization of primers,[a] (3) primer extension by DNA polymerase, and (4) repeat. Quantitative PCR measures the amount of PCR product formed after each cycle. Array CHG can detect changes in copy number and SNP arrays can be analyzed in GWAS to determine the genetic architecture of complex diseases.
	An example use of PCR is detecting HSV infection.
DNA FISH	A fluorescently labeled probe hybridizes to a specific DNA sequence on a tissue section. Fluorescence microscopy is used to visualize its cellular location.
	An example use of FISH is detecting DNA deletions or amplifications in cancer cells.
DNA sequencing	A primer hybridizes to the DNA of interest and is extended by DNA polymerase. Chain termination occurs when DNA polymerase incorporates a nucleotide analogue instead of a normal nucleotide. Each nucleotide analogue (A, G, C, T) is labeled with a different color fluorochrome. Electrophoresis through a fluorochrome detector sequences the DNA. Next-generation sequencing is high throughput. Whole exome sequencing sequences exons, while whole genome sequencing sequences exons and introns.
	An example use of next-generation sequencing is identifying genetic mutations.
RNA	
Northern blot	Analogous procedure to Southern blot for RNA.
RT-PCR	Analogous procedure to PCR for mRNA, which is first converted into cDNA by reverse transcriptase. RNA arrays can profile the expression of thousands of genes simultaneously.
RNA FISH	Analogous procedure to DNA FISH for RNA.
RNA sequencing (RNA-seq)	Analogous procedure to DNA sequencing for RNA, which is first converted into cDNA by reverse transcriptase.
Protein	
Western blot	Analogous procedure to Southern blot for protein, which can also determine molecular weight.
	An example use of Western blot is confirmatory testing for Lyme disease.
Immunoprecipitation	Analogous procedure to Western blot, except that the antibody is added to the protein mixture prior to electrophoresis.
	An example use of immunoprecipitation is detecting circulating autoantibodies in autoimmune blistering disorders.
Immunoblotting	Analogous procedure to Western blot, except that the antibody is added to the denatured protein mixture prior to electrophoresis.
	An example use of immunoblotting is detecting circulating autoantibodies in autoimmune blistering disorders.

(Continued)

Table 1.25. MEASUREMENT OF CELLULAR COMPONENTS (CONTINUED)

Technique	Description
ELISA	An antibody to a specific protein is applied to a plate coated with the sample. The antibody is detected using a secondary antibody coupled to an enzyme that reacts with a substrate to produce a colored precipitate.
	An example use of ELISA is detecting circulating autoantibodies in autoimmune blistering disorders.
IHC	Analogous procedure to ELISA to visualize the cellular location of a specific protein on a tissue section.
	An example use of IHC is differentiating MCC from SCLC metastasis by demonstrating a negative reaction for TTF-1.
DIF	A fluorescent antibody is used to visualize the cellular location of a specific protein on a tissue section.
	An example use of DIF is detecting autoantibodies in perilesional skin or mucosa in autoimmune blistering disorders.
IIF	An antibody to a specific protein is applied to a tissue section. The antibody is detected using a secondary fluorescent antibody.
	An example use of IIF is detecting circulating autoantibodies in autoimmune blistering disorders.
Proteomics with mass spectrometry	Proteins are ionized and the time of flight is measured to determine which proteins are present in a specific cell population based on their mass/charge ratio.

A, adenosine; c, complementary; C, cytosine; CGH, comparative genomic hybridization; DIF, direct immunofluorescence; DNA, deoxyribonucleic acid; ds, double-stranded; ELISA, enzyme-linked immunosorbent assay; FISH, fluorescence in situ hybridization; G, guanine; GWAS, genome-wide association studies; HSV, herpes simplex virus; IHC, immunohistochemistry; IIF, indirect immunofluorescence; m, messenger; MCC, Merkel cell carcinoma; PCR, polymerase chain reaction; RNA, ribonucleic acid; RT-PCR, reverse transcription polymerase chain reaction; SCLC, small-cell lung carcinoma; SNP, single nucleotide polymorphism; ss, single-stranded; T, thymidine; TTF-1, thyroid transcription factor 1.
aPrimers are short ssDNA strands designed to hybridize at each end of the specific DNA sequence.

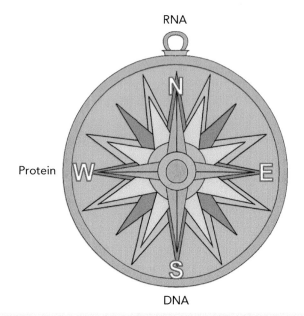

Figure 1.26. BLOT COMPASS. The Southern blot for DNA was named after its inventor Edwin Southern. As a joke, the analogous procedures for RNA and protein were later called Northern blot and Western blot. #nerdhumor (Illustration by Caroline A. Nelson, MD.)

Table 1.26. GENETIC MODIFICATION

Technique	Description
Transgenic mice	A transgene is injected into a fertilized mouse egg or single-cell embryo and randomly integrates into the genome. It is expressed in tissues where the promoter/enhancer regulatory region is active. Genes can also be knocked out in specific tissues or at a specific time point in development. Transgenic mice can be used to study the in vivo biologic effects of genetic modifications.
Gene therapy	Genes can be introduced, corrected, or knocked down. In the in vivo approach, the desired gene is introduced into the skin by a viral or nonviral vector. In the ex vivo approach, keratinocytes are removed from the donor, genetically modified in culture, and grafted back onto the donor. Alternatively, fibroblasts may be reprogramed into iPS cells and then differentiated into keratinocytes. To avoid the risk of insertional mutagenesis, genes may be corrected with nucleases (ZFNs, TALENs, and CRISPR-Cas9). Finally, specific mRNAs may be targeted for degradation, eg, with vectors delivering siRNA or miRNA.
	An example of gene therapy is correcting LAMB3-deficient skin in JEB by transplantation of stem cell–enriched epidermal grafts transduced ex vivo with a retroviral vector encoding LAMB3 cDNA.

c, complementary; CRISPR-Cas9, clustered regularly interspaced short palindromic repeats and CRISPR-associated protein 9; DNA, deoxyribonucleic acid; iPS, induced pluripotent stem; JEB, junctional epidermolysis bullosa; LAMB3, laminin subunit β3; m, messenger; mi, micro; RNA, ribonucleic acid; si, short interfering; TALENS, transcription activator–like effector nucleases; ZFNs, zinc finger nucleases.

Epidemiology and Statistics

Basic Concepts

- For a sample:
  - **Mean (average)**: sum of values divided by the sample size.
  - **Median**: middle value (odd sample) or mean of the two middle values (even sample) ordered from smallest to largest.
  - **Mode**: most frequent value.
  - **Standard deviation (SD)**: measure of variability of the data distribution.
  - **Standard error (SE) of the mean**: measure of how well the sample mean approximates the population mean (mean ± SD divided by the square root of the sample size).
  - **95% confidence interval (CI)**: range of values 95% certain to contain the population mean (mean ± 1.96 × SE for a normal distribution).
- In statistics:
  - **Association**: relationship between variables.
  - **Causation**: cause and effect relationship between variables.
  - **Null hypothesis: no relationship between variables.**
  - **Probability value (*P*-value)**: probability under the null hypothesis of obtaining a result equal or more extreme than what was observed.
  - **Type I error (α, false positive)**: incorrect rejection of the null hypothesis (α is often set at 0.05 equivalent to a 5% false positive rate).
  - **When the *P*-value is less than or equal to α, than the null hypothesis is rejected and the relationship between variables is considered statistically significant.**
  - **When 95% CIs for two independent populations do not overlap, there is a statistically significant difference between the means (α = 0.05).**
  - **Type II error (β, false negative)**: incorrect acceptance of the null hypothesis.
  - **Power (1 − β)**: probability of avoiding a type II error; **increases with sample size.**
    - "The power rests with the people."

Clinical Studies

Observational Studies

- **Case reports or series are descriptive.** These studies provide the **lowest level of evidence** for or against an intervention, but can be valuable for reporting **rare or first (sentinel) observations.**
- **Case-control studies analyze a study group with an outcome (eg, a disease) and a control group by retrospectively comparing the frequency of an exposure (eg, a risk factor).** These studies cannot establish causation, but can yield an **odds ratio (OR)**, which approximates the relative risk (RR) for rare diseases.
- **Cross-sectional surveys analyze a study group with an exposure (eg, a risk factor) and a control group by comparing the frequency of an outcome (eg, a disease) at a point in time.** These studies cannot establish causation, but can yield the **prevalence** of the exposure and the disease (**total number of cases divided by the total at risk population**) and the relative prevalence of the disease in exposed versus unexposed groups.
- **Cohort studies analyze a study group with an exposure (eg, a risk factor) and a control group by prospectively or retrospectively comparing the frequency of an outcome (eg, a disease) over time.** These studies **infer causation** and yield the **incidence** of the disease (**number of new cases divided by the total at risk population**) and a **RR.**
- The Strengthening the Reporting of Observational studies in Epidemiology (STROBE) guidelines are generally accepted for the proper reporting of observational studies.

Experimental Studies

- **Randomized controlled trials (RCTs) analyze an exposure (eg, a treatment) by comparing the frequency of an outcome (eg, mortality) in participants randomly assigned to an intervention group or a control group.** These studies **establish causation** and yield a variety of outcome measures, such as **RR.** An RCT is the standard for single-study designs. **A double-blind RCT conceals the intervention from participants and observers to minimize bias.**
- **Meta-analyses of RCTs pool data.** These studies provide the **highest level of evidence** for or against an intervention.
- The Consolidated Standards of Reporting Trials (CONSORT) guidelines are generally accepted for the proper reporting of RCTs.

Calculations (Table 1.27)

- The **OR** (eg, case-control study) is the ratio of the odds of the outcome in exposed versus unexposed groups (**odds$_{exposed}$/odds$_{unexposed}$ = a/b/c/d**).
- The **RR** (eg, cohort study) is the ratio of the probability of the outcome in exposed versus unexposed groups (**risk$_{exposed}$/risk$_{unexposed}$ = a/(a + b)/c/(c + d)**).
- For both OR and RR:
  - **95% CI < 1** suggests that exposure **decreases risk** of the outcome,
  - **95% CI including 1** suggests that exposure **does not impact risk** of the outcome,
  - **95% CI > 1** suggests that exposure **increases risk** of the outcome.
- If exposure (eg, a risk factor) increases risk of the outcome (eg, a disease):
  - **Absolute risk increase (ARI)** is the difference in the probability of disease in exposed versus unexposed groups (**risk$_{exposed}$ − risk$_{unexposed}$ = a/(a + b) − c/(c + d)**),
  - **Number needed to harm (NNH)** is the average number of individuals who need to be exposed to the risk factor over a specific time period to cause disease in an average of one additional individual (**1/ARI**).

- If exposure (eg, a treatment) decreases risk of the outcome (eg, mortality):
  - **Absolute risk reduction (ARR)** is the difference in the probability of mortality in unexposed versus exposed groups ($\mathbf{risk_{unexposed} - risk_{exposed}} = \mathbf{c/(c + d) - a/(a+b)}$),
  - **Number needed to treat (NNT)** is the average number of individuals who need to be treated over a specific time period to prevent mortality in an average of one additional individual (**1/ARR**).

Bias, Confounding, and Effect Modification

- **Bias (systematic sources of error)** examples include:
  - **Ascertainment bias**: not all of those who are supposed to be represented in a population are represented.
  - **Selection bias**: participants are selected differently across exposure or disease categories.
  - **Misclassification bias**: participants are wrongfully thought to belong to one category of exposure or disease, when they actually belong to another.
  - **Information bias**: inaccuracies in the collection of data on the exposure or disease (eg, recall bias, in which groups of participants have a different accuracy or completeness of recall to memory of the exposure).
- **Confounding**: variable associated with both the exposure and the outcome (outside the causal pathway) accounts for a part or all of the relationship between the exposure and the outcome (Figure 1.27).
- **Effect modification**: variable that differentially modifies the effect of the exposure on the outcome for different subgroups of the population.

Clinical Tests

- **Precision** indicates the **reproducibility** of the result, while **accuracy (validity)** indicates how **close the result comes to the truth.**
  - Figure 1.28.
- **Sensitivity** is the proportion of correctly identified positive test results ($\mathbf{a/(a + c)}$). High sensitivity indicates **few false negatives.**
- **Specificity** is the proportion of correctly identified negative test results ($\mathbf{d/(b + d)}$). High specificity indicates **few false positives.**

Table 1.27. CALCULATIONS

2 × 2 Table		Outcome	
		Present	Absent
Exposure	**Present**	a	b
	Absent	c	d

Example Applications

- The exposure is a risk factor and the outcome is a disease
- The exposure is a treatment and the outcome is mortality
- The exposure is a test result and the outcome is true presence or absence of the disease

2 × 2 Table Formula Summary

OR	a/b/c/d
RR	a/(a + b)/c/(c + d)
ARI	a/(a + b) − c/(c + d)
NNH	1/ARI
ARR	c/(c + d) − a/(a + b)
NNT	1/ARR
Sensitivity	a/(a + c)
Specificity	d/(b + d)
PPV	a/(a + b)
NPV	d/(c + d)

ARI, absolute risk increase; ARR, absolute risk reduction; NNH, number needed to harm; NNT, number needed to treat; NPV, negative predictive value; OR, odds ratio; PPV, positive predictive value; RR, relative risk.

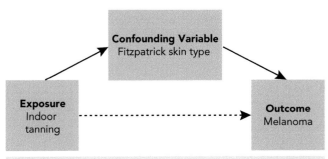

Figure 1.27. CONFOUNDING.

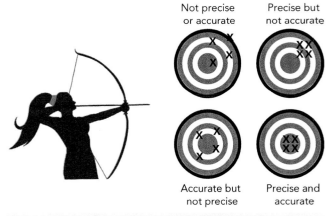

Figure 1.28. PRECISION VERSUS ACCURACY
(Illustration by Caroline A. Nelson, MD.)

- **Positive predictive value (PPV)** is the likelihood that a patient with a positive test result does have the disease ($a/(a + b)$). PPV **increases with increasing prevalence.**
- **Negative predictive value (NPV)** is the likelihood that a patient with a negative test result does not have the disease ($d/(c + d)$). NPV **decreases with increasing prevalence.**
  - ◆ Table 1.28.
  - ◆ Table 1.29.
  - ◆ Table 1.30.

Principles of Patient-Centered Care

- Communication:
  - Review the chart and prepare to pay attention before entering the examination room.
  - Sit instead of stand to convey full attention to the patient.
  - Elicit patient concerns at the beginning of the visit without interrupting.
  - Tactfully ask for permission to interrupt if the patient will not stop talking.
  - If the patient brings in a long list of concerns, invite the patient to cooperate in setting the agenda for the current visit.
  - Use reflective listening to verify information and to show active listening.
    - ◆ <u>NURS</u> = <u>N</u>ame, <u>U</u>nderstand, <u>R</u>espect, <u>S</u>upport.
  - Show empathy for the patient's thoughts and emotions.
  - Check that all concerns have been addressed before reaching a mutual decision with the patient to end the visit.

Table 1.28. SAMPLE CALCULATION WHAT IS THE RR, ARI, AND NNH IN THIS HYPOTHETICAL COHORT STUDY FOR WHICH THE EXPOSURE IS CARPET AND THE OUTCOME IS CARPET BEETLE INFESTATION?

2 × 2 Table		Carpet Beetle Infestation	
		Present	Absent
Carpet	**Present**	50	75
	Absent	50	200

Calculations

- RR = risk$_{exposed}$/risk$_{unexposed}$ = a/(a + b)/c/(c + d) = 0.4/0.2 = 2
- ARI = risk$_{exposed}$ – risk$_{unexposed}$ = a/(a + b) – c/(c + d)) = 0.4 – 0.2 = 0.2
- NNH = 1/ARI = 5

ARI, absolute risk increase; NNH, number needed to harm; RR, relative risk.

Table 1.29. SAMPLE CALCULATION WHAT IS THE RR, ARR, AND NNT IN THIS HYPOTHETICAL RANDOMIZED CONTROLLED TRIAL FOR WHICH THE EXPOSURE IS IPILIMUMAB AND THE OUTCOME IS MELANOMA-SPECIFIC MORTALITY?

2 × 2 Table		Melanoma-Specific Mortality	
		Present	Absent
Ipilimumab	**Present**	50	200
	Absent	50	75

Calculations

- RR = risk$_{exposed}$/risk$_{unexposed}$ = a/(a + b)/c/(c + d) = 0.2/0.4 = 0.5
- ARR = risk$_{unexposed}$ – risk$_{exposed}$ = c/(c + d) – a/(a + b) = 0.4 – 0.2 = 0.2
- NNT = 1/ARR = 5

ARR, absolute risk increase; NNT, number needed to harm; RR, relative risk.

Table 1.30. SAMPLE CALCULATION WHAT IS THE SENSITIVITY, SPECIFICITY, PPV, AND NPV FOR THIS HYPOTHETICAL TEST FOR SARCOIDOSIS?

2 × 2 Table		Sarcoidosis	
		Present	Absent
Test	**Positive**	200	25
	Negative	50	75

Calculations

- Sensitivity = a/(a + c) = 0.8 (80%)
- Specificity = d/(b + d) = 0.75 (75%)
- PPV = a/(a + b) = 0.89 (89%)
- NPV = d/(c + d) = 0.6 (60%)

NPV, negative predictive value; PPV, positive predictive value.

- Communication in special situations:
  - Acknowledge patient anger and explore its causes prior to explanation or defense.
  - In the face of patient disappointment, form a therapeutic alliance.
  - Educate the patient to set realistic expectations of treatment outcomes.
  - Engage the patient while interfacing with health information technology (eg, maintain eye contact and verbalize actions).
- Education:
  - Assess the patient's needs and goals, health beliefs, and health literacy.
  - Gain the patient's attention, provide clear and memorable explanations, and assess understanding.
  - Use teaching aids (eg, handouts, visual aids, audiovisual media, and Internet websites).

Principles of Quality Improvement

- Physicians are under increasing pressure from purchasers of insurance, government, the media, and patients to measure quality of care and develop systems to reduce errors and improve quality.
- **Major patent safety issues** in dermatology established by the AAD Association Ad Hoc Task Force:
  - **Misdiagnosis and delayed diagnosis.**
  - **Medication errors.**
  - **Pathology specimen processing.**
  - **Timely and accurate communication of biopsy and laboratory results.**
  - **Wrong-site procedures.**
  - **Patient identification.**
  - **Supervision and competency assessment of ancillary staff.**
- **A culture of patient safety is based on learned behaviors** (eg, systems-based approach to error reduction, communication skills, and root cause analysis).
- The Accreditation Council for Graduate Medical Education (ACGME) has incorporated patient safety into its requirements for all residency programs and the American Board of Dermatology (ABD) has incorporated patient

Table 1.31. MAINTENANCE OF CERTIFICATION

Component[a]	Description
License attestation	Attest active license to practice medicine or osteopathy in the US or Canada and no adverse actions against these licenses every year
CME attestation	Attest 25 hours of Category 1 Credit every year (eg, AMA PRA Category 1 Credit™)
Periodic self-assessment	Complete 100 self-assessment credits in years 1-3, 4-6, and 7-10 of the 10-year cycle for a total of 300 credits every 10 years
Practice improvement	Complete 1 QI activity every 5 years
CertLink	52 questions every year
MOC fee	Pay a fee to the ABD every year

ABD, American Board of Dermatology; AMA PRA, American Medical Association Physician's Recognition Award; CME, continuing medical education; MOC, maintenance of certification; QI, quality improvement; US, United States.
[a]This information is subject to change. Please check the ABD website for updates.

Table 1.32. SAMPLE PATIENT SAFETY PROGRAM TO REDUCE WRONG-SITE PROCEDURES

- Gather data on wrong-site procedures in the practice
- Establish a nonpunitive culture of patient safety that encourages error reporting
- Identify best practices, in this case, biopsy-site photography
- Establish the goal to take a high-quality photograph at the time of biopsy within 3 months
- Create a system to train medical personnel in high-quality biopsy-site photography (at least one visible anatomic landmark) and for ongoing assessment and certification
- Establish reasonable limits on work hours and volume to ensure that medical personnel are well-rested and able to allocate time during the visit to biopsy-site photography
- Establish accountability and incentives, for example, that each each provider who achieves over a 90% rate of biopsy-site photography is able to fulfill the 5-year MOC practice improvement component

MOC, maintenance of certification.

safety into its requirements for maintenance of certification (MOC) (Table 1.31).

- **Performance measures**:
  - **Outcome**: end results of care.
  - **Process**: performance at different steps within the care pathway.
  - **Structural**: system-level adjuncts to multiple care processes.
- Steps to a successful patient safety program:
  - Gather data on adverse events in the practice or similar practices.
  - Establish a nonpunitive culture of patient safety that encourages error reporting.
  - Identify best practices appropriate to the practice.
  - Establish achievable goals and a timeline.
  - Create a system for the assessment and certification of procedural skills for medical personnel.
  - Establish reasonable limits on work hours and volume.
  - Establish accountability and incentives based on measurable targets.
    - ◈ Table 1.32.

FURTHER READING

Abbas AKL, Andrew H. *Basic Immunology: Functions and Disorders of the Immune System.* 3rd ed. Elsevier Saunders; 2009.

Aebersold R, Mann M. Mass-spectrometric exploration of proteome structure and function. *Nature.* 2016;537(7620):347-355.

Amatya N, Garg AV, Gaffen SL. IL-17 signaling: the yin and the yang. *Trends Immunol.* 2017;38(5):310-322.

American Academy of Dermatology Spot Skin Cancer. How to select a sunscreen. Accessed January 13, 2019. https://www.aad.org/public/spot-skin-cancer/learn-about-skin-cancer/prevent/how-to-select-a-sunscreen

American Board of Dermatology. Maintenance of certification requirements. Accessed January 19, 2019. https://www.abderm.org/diplomates/fulfilling-moc-requirements/moc-requirements.aspx

Anbunathan H, Bowcock AM. The molecular revolution in cutaneous biology: the era of genome-wide association studies and statistical, big data, and computational topics. *J Invest Dermatol.* 2017;137(5):e113-e118.

Online Mendelian Inheritance in Man: An Online Catalog of Human Genes and Genetic Disorders. Accessed January 20, 2019. https://www.omim.org/

FDA advances new proposed regulation to make sure that sunscreens are safe and effective. Accessed March 10, 2019. https://www.fda.gov/NewsEvents/Newsroom/PressAnnouncements/ucm631736.htm

American Academy of Dermatology Association statement on sunscreen access. Accessed March 22, 2019. https://www.aad.org/media/news-releases/aada-statement-on-sunscreen-access

Pregnancy and Lactation Labeling (Drugs) Final Rule. Accessed January 20, 2019. https://www.fda.gov/drugs/developmentapprovalprocess/developmentresources/labeling/ucm093307.htm

AMA PRA credit system. Accessed January 19, 2019. https://www.ama-assn.org/education/cme/ama-pra-credit-system

Arthur G, Bradding P. New developments in mast cell biology: clinical implications. *Chest.* 2016;150(3):680-693.

Bagci IS, Ruzicka T. IL-31: a new key player in dermatology and beyond. *J Allergy Clin Immunol.* 2018;141(3):858-866.

Baker RE, Murray PJ. Understanding hair follicle cycling: a systems approach. *Curr Opin Genet Dev.* 2012;22(6):607-612.

Bauer J. The molecular revolution in cutaneous biology: era of cytogenetics and copy number analysis. *J Invest Dermatol.* 2017;137(5):e57-e59.

Bohan KH, Mansuri TF, Wilson NM. Anticonvulsant hypersensitivity syndrome: implications for pharmaceutical care. *Pharmacotherapy.* 2007;27(10):1425-1439.

Bolognia JL, Schaffer JV, Cerroni L. *Dermatology.* 4th ed. Elsevier Saunders; 2018.

Borradori L, Sonnenberg A. Structure and function of hemidesmosomes: more than simple adhesion complexes. *J Invest Dermatol.* 1999;112(4):411-418.

Butler DC, Heller MM, Murase JE. Safety of dermatologic medications in pregnancy and lactation: part II. Lactation. *J Am Acad Dermatol.* 2014;70(3):417.e1-10. quiz 427.

Califf RM, Shinkai K. Filling in the evidence about sunscreen. *JAMA.* 2019;321(21):2077-2079.

Carroll MC. The role of complement in B cell activation and tolerance. *Adv Immunol.* 2000;74:61-88.

de Torre-Minguela C, Mesa Del Castillo P, Pelegrin P. The NLRP3 and pyrin inflammasomes: implications in the pathophysiology of autoinflammatory diseases. *Front Immunol.* 2017;8:43.

Diercks GF, Pas HH, Jonkman MF. Immunofluorescence of autoimmune bullous diseases. *Surg Pathol Clin.* 2017;10(2):505-512.

Elder DE, et al. *Lever's Histopathology of the Skin.* 11th ed. Wolters Kluwer; 2015.

Elston DM, Ferringer T. *Dermatopathology.* 2nd ed. Elsevier Saunders; 2014.

Elston DM, Stratman E, Johnson-Jahangir H, Watson A, Swiggum S, Hanke CW. Patient safety: part II. Opportunities for improvement in patient safety. *J Am Acad Dermatol.* 2009;61(2):193-205. quiz 206.

Elston DM, Taylor JS, Coldiron B, et al. Patient safety: Part I. Patient safety and the dermatologist. *J Am Acad Dermatol.* 2009;61(2):179-190. quiz 191.

Emri G, Paragh G, Tosaki A, et al. Ultraviolet radiation-mediated development of cutaneous melanoma: an update. *J Photochem Photobiol B.* 2018;185:169-175.

Fan J, de Lannoy IAM. Pharmacokinetics. *Biochem Pharmacol.* 2014;87(1):93-120.

Fuchs E. Scratching the surface of skin development. *Nature.* 2007;445(7130):834-842.

Ghadially R. 25 years of epidermal stem cell research. *J Invest Dermatol.* 2012;132(3 pt 2):797-810.

Guitart JR, Jr. Johnson JL, Chien WW. Research techniques made simple: the application of CRISPR-Cas9 and genome editing in investigative dermatology. *J Invest Dermatol.* 2016;136(9):e87-e93.

Hafner C, Groesser L. Mosaic RASopathies. *Cell cycle (Georgetown, Tex).* 2013;12(1):43-50.

Hanahan D, Weinberg RA. Hallmarks of cancer: the next generation. *Cell.* 2011;144(5):646-674.

Happle R. The molecular revolution in cutaneous biology: era of mosaicism. *J Invest Dermatol.* 2017;137(5):e73-e77.

Hawkes JE, Yan BY, Chan TC, Krueger JG. Discovery of the IL-23/IL-17 signaling pathway and the treatment of psoriasis. *J Immunol.* 2018;201(6):1605-1613.

Heineke MH, Ballering AV, Jamin A, Ben Mkaddem S, Monteiro RC, Van Egmond M. New insights in the pathogenesis of immunoglobulin A vasculitis (Henoch-Schonlein purpura). *Autoimmun Rev.* 2017;16(12):1246-1253.

Hess NJ, Felicelli C, Grage J, Tapping RI. TLR10 suppresses the activation and differentiation of monocytes with effects on DC-mediated adaptive immune responses. *J Leukoc Biol.* 2017;101(5):1245-1252.

Hirsch T, Rothoeft T, Teig N, et al. Regeneration of the entire human epidermis using transgenic stem cells. *Nature.* 2017;551(7680):327-332.

Hoath SB, Leahy DG. The organization of human epidermis: functional epidermal units and phi proportionality. *J Invest Dermatol.* 2003;121(6):1440-1446.

Hong J, Nguyen TV, Prose NS. Compassionate care—enhancing physician-patient communication and education in dermatology—Part II: patient education. *J Am Acad Dermatol.* 2013;68(3):364.e1-364.10.

James WD, Elston DM, Treat JR, Rosenbach MA, Neuhaus IM. *Andrews' Diseases of the Skin: Clinical Dermatology.* 13th ed. Elsevier; 2020.

Jansen R, Osterwalder U, Wang SQ, Burnett M, Lim HW. Photoprotection: part II. Sunscreen—development, efficacy, and controversies. *J Am Acad Dermatol.* 2013;69(6):867.e1-14. quiz 881-862.

Jansen R, Wang SQ, Burnett M, Osterwalder U, Lim HW. Photoprotection: part I. Photoprotection by naturally occurring, physical, and systemic agents. *J Am Acad Dermatol.* 2013;69(6):853.e1-12. quiz 865-856.

Jhaj R, Sivagnanam G. Concomitant prescription of oral fluoroquinolones with an antacid preparation. *J Pharmacol Pharmacother.* 2013;4(2):140-142.

Johnston A, Sarkar MK, Vrana A, Tsoi LC, Gudjonsson JE. The molecular revolution in cutaneous biology: the era of global transcriptional analysis. *J Invest Dermatol.* 2017;137(5):e87-e91.

Kawakami A, Fisher DE. Key discoveries in melanocyte development. *J Invest Dermatol.* 2011;131(E1):E2-E4.

Kawasaki T, Kawai T. Toll-like receptor signaling pathways. *Front Immunol.* 2014;5:461.

Kim N, Fischer AH, Dyring-Andersen B, Rosner B, Okoye GA. Research techniques made simple: choosing appropriate statistical methods for clinical research. *J Invest Dermatol.* 2017;137(10):e173-e178.

Lambert AW, Pattabiraman DR, Weinberg RA. Emerging biological principles of metastasis. *Cell.* 2017;168(4):670-691.

Lecker SH, Goldberg AL, Mitch WE. Protein degradation by the ubiquitin-proteasome pathway in normal and disease states. *J Am Soc Nephrol.* 2006;17(7):1807-1819.

Madison KC. Barrier function of the skin: "la raison d'etre" of the epidermis. *J Invest Dermatol.* 2003;121(2):231-241.

Matta MK, Zusterzeel R, Pilli NR, et al. Effect of sunscreen application under maximal use conditions on plasma concentration of sunscreen active ingredients: a randomized clinical trial. *JAMA.* 2019;321(21):2082-2091.

Meroni PL, Penatti AE. Epigenetics and systemic lupus erythematosus: unmet needs. *Clin Rev Allergy Immunol.* 2016;50(3):367-376.

Michel M, Torok N, Godbout MJ, et al. Keratin 19 as a biochemical marker of skin stem cells in vivo and in vitro: keratin 19 expressing cells are differ-

entially localized in function of anatomic sites, and their number varies with donor age and culture stage. *J Cell Sci.* 1996;109(pt 5):1017-1028.

Millar SE. Molecular mechanisms regulating hair follicle development. *J Invest Dermatol.* 2002;118(2):216-225.

Monk D, Mackay DJG, Eggermann T, Maher ER, Riccio A. Genomic imprinting disorders: lessons on how genome, epigenome and environment interact. *Nat Rev Genet.* 2019;20(4):235-248.

Mukaida N. Interleukin-8: an expanding universe beyond neutrophil chemotaxis and activation. *Int J Hematol.* 2000;72(4):391-398.

Murase JE, Heller MM, Butler DC. Safety of dermatologic medications in pregnancy and lactation: part I. Pregnancy. *J Am Acad Dermatol.* 2014;70(3):401.e1-14. quiz 415.

Nguyen TV, Hong J, Prose NS. Compassionate care—enhancing physician-patient communication and education in dermatology—part I: patient-centered communication. *J Am Acad Dermatol.* 2013;68(3):353.e1-353.e8.

Overbosch D, Van Gulpen C, Hermans J, Mattie H. The effect of probenecid on the renal tubular excretion of benzylpenicillin. *Br J Clin Pharmacol.* 1988;25(1):51-58.

Profyris C, Tziotzios C, Do Vale I. Cutaneous scarring: pathophysiology, molecular mechanisms, and scar reduction therapeutics Part I. The molecular basis of scar formation. *J Am Acad Dermatol.* 2012;66(1):1-10. quiz 11-12.

Ronacher K, Sinha R, Cestari M. IL-22: an underestimated player in natural resistance to tuberculosis? *Front Immunol.* 2018;9:2209.

Saito M, Ohyama M, Amagai M. Exploring the biology of the nail: an intriguing but less-investigated skin appendage. *J Dermatol Sci.* 2015;79(3):187-193.

Salo T, Lyons JG, Rahemtulla F, Birkedal-Hansen H, Larjava H. Transforming growth factor-beta 1 up-regulates type IV collagenase expression in cultured human keratinocytes. *J Biol Chem.* 1991;266(18):11436-11441.

Sarig O, Sprecher E. The molecular revolution in cutaneous biology: era of next-generation sequencing. *J Invest Dermatol.* 2017;137(5):e79-e82.

Scales SJ, de Sauvage FJ. Mechanisms of Hedgehog pathway activation in cancer and implications for therapy. *Trends Pharmacol Sci.* 2009;30(6):303-312.

Schacherer J. Beyond the simplicity of Mendelian inheritance. *C R Biol.* 2016;339(7-8):284-288.

Schmieder S, Patel P, Krishnamurthy K. Research techniques made simple – drug delivery techniques, Part 1: concepts in transepidermal penetration and absorption. *J Invest Dermatol.* 2015;135(11):1-5.

Schneider SL, Lim HW. Review of environmental effects of oxybenzone and other sunscreen active ingredients. *J Am Acad Dermatol.* 2019;80(1):266-271.

Schutte RJ, Sun Y, Li D, Zhang F, Ostrov DA. Human leukocyte antigen associations in drug hypersensitivity reactions. *Clin Lab Med.* 2018;38(4):669-677.

Shendure J, Balasubramanian S, Church GM, et al. DNA sequencing at 40: past, present and future. *Nature.* 2017;550(7676):345-353.

Silverberg JI. Study designs in dermatology: practical applications of study designs and their statistics in dermatology. *J Am Acad Dermatol.* 2015;73(5):733-740. quiz 741-732.

Silverberg JI. Study designs in dermatology: a review for the clinical dermatologist. *J Am Acad Dermatol.* 2015;73(5):721-731. quiz 731-722.

Smack DP, Korge BP, James WD. Keratin and keratinization. *J Am Acad Dermatol.* 1994;30(1):85-102.

Stratman E, Kirsner RS, Horn TD. Maintenance of Certification in dermatology: requirements for diplomates. *J Am Acad Dermatol.* 2013;69(1):13.e11-14. quiz 17-18.

Stratman E, Kirsner RS, Horn TD. Maintenance of Certification in dermatology: what we know, what we don't. *J Am Acad Dermatol.* 2013;69(1):1.e1-11. quiz 12.

Tang JY, Fu T, Lau C, Oh DH, Bikle DD, Asgari MM. Vitamin D in cutaneous carcinogenesis: part II. *J Am Acad Dermatol.* 2012;67(5):817.e1-11. quiz 827-818.

Tang JY, Fu T, Lau C, Oh DH, Bikle DD, Asgari MM. Vitamin D in cutaneous carcinogenesis: part I. *J Am Acad Dermatol.* 2012;67(5):803.e1-12. quiz 815-806.

Titeux M, Izmiryan A, Hovnanian A. The molecular revolution in cutaneous biology: emerging landscape in genomic dermatology—new mechanistic ideas, gene editing, and therapeutic breakthroughs. *J Invest Dermatol.* 2017;137(5):e123-e129.

Tsao H, Fukunaga-Kalabis M, Herlyn M. Recent advances in melanoma and melanocyte biology. *J Invest Dermatol.* 2017;137(3):557-560.

Visscher MO, Taylor T, Narendran V. Neonatal intensive care practices and the influence on skin condition. *J Eur Acad Dermatol Venereol.* 2013;27(4):486-493.

Wei SC, Duffy CR, Allison JP. Fundamental mechanisms of immune checkpoint blockade therapy. *Cancer Discov.* 2018;8(9):1069-1086.

Werner S, Krieg T, Smola H. Keratinocyte-fibroblast interactions in wound healing. *J Invest Dermatol.* 2007;127(5):998-1008.

Zhanel GG, Siemens S, Slayter K, Mandell L. Antibiotic and oral contraceptive drug interactions: is there a need for concern? *Can J Infect Dis.* 1999;10(6):429-433.

Zhang J, Rosen A, Orenstein L, et al. Factors associated with biopsy site identification, postponement of surgery, and patient confidence in a dermatologic surgery practice. *J Am Acad Dermatol.* 2016;74(6):1185-1193.

Zhu J, Clark RAF. Fibronectin at select sites binds multiple growth factors and enhances their activity: expansion of the collaborative ECM-GF paradigm. *J Invest Dermatol.* 2014;134(4):895-901.

Nonneoplastic Disorders

Caroline A. Nelson, MD

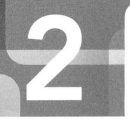

Papulosquamous Disorders and Palmoplantar Keratodermas

Basic Concepts

- **Papulosquamous disorders** are characterized by **scaling papules and plaques.**
- **Palmoplantar keratodermas (PPKs)** are disorders of cornification characterized by **hyperkeratosis of the palms and soles.**

PSORIASIS
→ Diagnosis Group 1

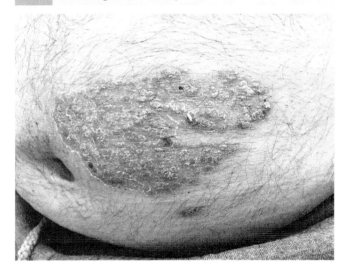

Epidemiology

- Psoriasis is a papulosquamous disorder caused by a complex interplay of genetic and environmental factors. The **pathogenesis of psoriasis** (Figure 2.1) is primarily mediated by **T cells.**
- Psoriasis affects ~2% of the world's population. The age of onset is bimodal, occurring in peaks from 20 to 30 years and 50 to 60 years.
- Associations include **cardiovascular disease, inflammatory bowel disease (IBD), metabolic syndrome, psoriatic arthritis, and depression/anxiety.**
- Drug associations include **tumor necrosis factor alpha (TNFα) inhibitors, dupilumab, IFNs, ICIs, imiquimod, β-blockers, and lithium. Rapid tapering of systemic corticosteroids** may trigger **generalized pustular psoriasis (GPP).**

- Dupilumab can swing the pendulum from eczema to psoriasis ("Th2 to Th1 shift").
- The leading HLA association is **-Cw6 within psoriasis susceptibility region 1 (PSORS1),** which accounts for ~50% of psoriasis risk. Specific HLA associations include:
  - **Early-onset psoriasis: -B13, -B17, -Cw6, -DR7.**
  - **Guttate psoriasis: -B17, -Cw6.**
  - **Psoriatic arthritis (spondylitis and sacroiliitis variant): -B27.**
  - **Pustular psoriasis: -B27.**
    - PSORS1 is #1. HLA-B17 association is easy to recall because psoriasis is a Th17 disease.

Clinicopathological Features

- Psoriasis vulgaris classically presents with **sharply demarcated, scaly, erythematous plaques favoring the scalp, intergluteal fold, elbows, and knees.** Pruritus is common.
  - In infants, psoriasis is in the differential diagnosis for **diaper dermatitis.** In contrast to contact dermatitis, psoriasis classically presents with **sharply demarcated psoriasiform plaques involving the inguinal creases,** and often involves the umbilicus.
  - Diaper-area psoriasis is also known as "napkin psoriasis."
- The **Auspitz sign** refers to **pinpoint bleeding after scraping psoriatic lesions.**
  - Thin suprapapillary plates and tortuous blood vessels in dermal papillae on histopathology are responsible for the Auspitz sign.
- **Woronoff ring** refers to **blanching around psoriatic lesions due to decreased prostaglandin E2.**
- **Psoriasiform alopecia** classically presents with **nonscarring circumscribed** hair loss. Involvement of the **nail unit** occurs in **10% to 80%** of patients and may be the sole manifestation of psoriasis. Nail psoriasis is a strong predictor of psoriatic arthritis.
- **Psoriasis variants** are summarized in Table 2.1.
  - **Guttate psoriasis** is the most common variant in **children and adolescents.**
  - Figure 2.2.
- The **Koebner phenomenon (isomorphic response)** describes the appearance of **new psoriatic lesions at sites of cutaneous trauma.**
  - Psoriasis Vulgaris Honestly Loves Koebnerizing like Vitiligo, Halo nevus, Lichen planus (LP), Kyrle disease, and Keratoacanthoma (KA), while warts and molluscum contagiosum pseudo-Koebnerize.

Table 2.1. PSORIASIS VARIANTS

Variant[a]	Subvariant	Classic Description	Notes
Guttate	N/A	Numerous, small, widely disseminated psoriasiform papules and plaques.	Associations include streptococcal pharyngitis. Tonsillectomy may help prevent recurrence. Drug associations include β-blockers.
		The appearance of guttate psoriasis is often compared to "rain drops."	
Erythrodermic	N/A	Erythema and scaling > 80%-90% BSA ± PPK and ectropion; alopecia; onychodystrophy. Lymphadenopathy is the leading systemic feature.	Erythroderma may by complicated by hypothermia, peripheral edema, and fluid/electrolyte/albumin loss leading to tachycardia and high-output cardiac failure.
Location-specific	Scalp	Psoriatic lesions on the scalp ± periphery of the face, retroauricular areas, and posterior upper neck.	Scalp psoriasis is the leading cause of pityriasis amiantacea.
	Inverse	Psoriatic lesions on flexural sites and/or genitalia.	
	Palmoplantar	Psoriatic lesions on palms and/or soles.	
Nail	N/A	Irregular pitting, the "oil drop" sign (salmon patch), and onycholysis with an erythematous border > onychauxis, paronychia, splinter hemorrhages (distal), and subungual hyperkeratosis.	Nail psoriasis is a strong predictor of psoriatic arthritis.
		Figure 2.2.	
Pustular	GPP (von Zumbusch)	Primary, relapsing (>1 episode) or persistent (>3 months), sterile pustules on nonacral skin ± psoriasis vulgaris. Patterns include annular and exanthematic. Annulus migrans resembling geographic tongue may occur. Patients may exhibit fever and other constitutional symptoms.	Triggers include rapid tapering of systemic corticosteroids, hypocalcemia, and infection.
	PPP	Primary, persistent (>3 months), sterile pustules on palms and/or soles ± psoriasis vulgaris.	Associations include SAPHO syndrome. Triggers include stress, local infections, and smoking.
	Acrodermatitis continua of Hallopeau	Primary, persistent (>3 months), sterile pustules affecting the nail apparatus. Annulus migrans may occur. Nail bed involvement may result in onycholysis.	
		Acrodermatitis continua of Hallopeau is often described as "lakes of pus."	
	Pustular psoriasis of pregnancy (impetigo herpetiformis)	Presents in late pregnancy or postpartum with GPP favoring flexural sites.	Increases risk of maternal hypocalcemia and placental insufficiency leading to stillbirth and neonatal demise.
			Pustular psoriasis of pregnancy harms the placenta.

BSA, body surface area; GPP, generalized pustular psoriasis; N/A, not applicable; PPK, palmoplantar keratoderma; PPP, palmoplantar pustulosis; SAPHO, synovitis, acne, pustulosis, hyperostosis, and osteitis.
[a]Illustrative examples provided. Since pustular psoriasis of pregnancy is a GPP variant, some authors do not classify it as a pregnancy dermatosis.

- The **Renbök phenomenon** (reverse Koebner phenomenon) describes one skin condition inhibiting another (eg, regression of a psoriatic plaque on the scalp coinciding with appearance of a patch of AA).
  - In German, _Renbök_ is a reversal of the letters of _Köbner._
- Other psoriasis triggers relate to infection (eg, **human immunodeficiency virus [HIV], streptococcal pharyngitis**), stress, weight gain, alcohol consumption, smoking, and associated drugs.
- **Psoriatic arthritis** occurs in **5% to 30%** of patients and may be the initial manifestation of psoriasis. Clinical features include **tendonitis** (inflammation of juxta-articular tendons), **enthesitis** (inflammation of sites where tendons insert into bones), and **dactylitis** (swelling of the fingers). **Morning stiffness** is common. **Psoriatic arthritis variants** are summarized in Table 2.2.
- Psoriasis may overlap with **seborrheic dermatitis (sebopsoriasis).**
- Psoriasis may overlap with **lichen simplex chronicus (LSC).**
  - Figure 2.3.

Table 2.2. PSORIATIC ARTHRITIS VARIANTS

Variant[a]	Classic Description	Notes
Mono- and asymmetric oligoarthritis	Involvement of PIP and DIP ± larger joints may result in dactylitis.	Most common variant. Spares MCP joints (in contrast to RA).
	Dactylitis is also called "sausage digit."	
Arthritis of the DIPs	Exclusive involvement of DIP joints may result in permanent flexion.	
Symmetric polyarthritis	Involvement of small- and medium-sized joints (eg, elbow, wrist, ankle, MCP, PIP).	Resembles RA.
Arthritis mutilans	Severe and rapidly progressive joint involvement with osteolysis.	Least common variant.
	Osteolysis results in a "telescoping" joint deformity.	
Spondylitis and sacroiliitis	Involvement of axial, sacroiliac, and knee ± peripheral joints.	Resembles ankylosing spondylitis. Associations include IBD and uveitis.

DIP, distal interphalangeal; IBD, inflammatory bowel disease; MCP, metacarpal phalangeal; PIP, proximal interphalangeal; RA, rheumatoid arthritis; RF, rheumatoid factor.
[a]Illustrative examples provided.

1 Stressed keratinocytes release self DNA and RNA, which complex with cathelicidin and induce IFN-α release from pDCs, thereby activating dDCs.

2 Keratinocytes release IL-1β, IL-6, and TNF-α, which further activate dDCs.

3 dDCs migrate to regional lymph nodes to present an as-yet-unknown antigen to naïve T cells.

4 Activation of T cells via IL-12 and IL-23 released from dDCs generates Th1, Th17, and Th22 cells that migrate to the skin.

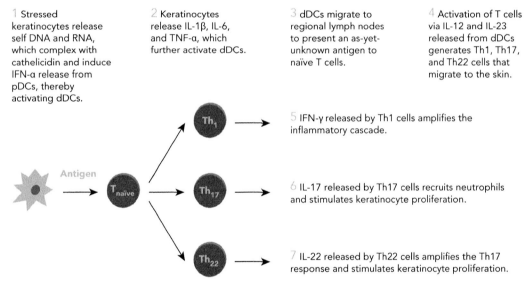

5 IFN-γ released by Th1 cells amplifies the inflammatory cascade.

6 IL-17 released by Th17 cells recruits neutrophils and stimulates keratinocyte proliferation.

7 IL-22 released by Th22 cells amplifies the Th17 response and stimulates keratinocyte proliferation.

8 Memory CD8+ T cells at the DEJ release Th1 and Th17 cytokines, and neutrophils enter the epidermis.

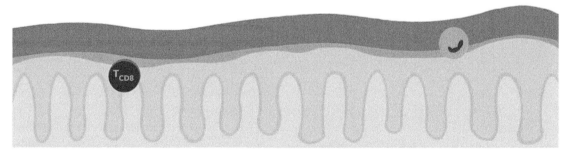

9 Keratinocyte proliferation, driven by the transcription factor STAT3, results in increased K6 and K16 expression, increased involucrin and decreased loricrin expression, and decreased keratinocyte transit time.

10 Increased expression of antimicrobial peptides (eg, cathelicidin, human β-defensin, SKALP/elafin, SLPI) decreases the risk of secondary infection.

Figure 2.1. PATHOGENESIS OF PSORIASIS. CD, cluster of differentiation; dDCs, dermal dendritic cells; DEJ, dermal-epidermal junction; DNA, deoxyribonucleic acid; IFN, interferon; IL, interleukin; K, keratin; pDCs, plasmacytoid dendritic cells; RNA, ribonucleic acid; SKALP, skin-derived antileukoproteinase; SLPI, secretory leukocyte protease inhibitor; STAT, signal transducer and activator of transcription; Th, T helper; TNFα, tumor necrosis factor α.

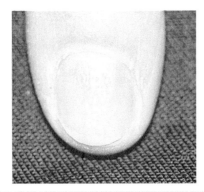

Figure 2.2. PITTING. (Psoriatic pitting image reprinted with permission from Goodheart HP. *Goodheart's Photoguide of Common Skin Disorders: Diagnosis and Management.* 2nd ed. Lippincott Williams & Wilkins; 2003.) AA, alopecia areata.

Psoriasis and AA are associated with punctate depressions in the nail plate surface; however, these pits have subtle distinguishing features.
- Pits in psoriasis are large and irregularly distributed within the nail plate.
- Pits in AA are small and geometrically distributed within the nail plate. Pits derive from the proximal matrix, while the "oil drop" sign (salmon patches) and onycholysis in psoriasis derive from the nail bed.

Evaluation

- The differential diagnosis of psoriasis includes other papulosquamous disorders, eczematous dermatoses, lichenoid dermatoses, dermatomyositis (DM), secondary syphilis, dermatophytosis, and cutaneous T-cell lymphoma (CTCL). Lichenoid keratosis (LK), superficial BCC, and squamous cell carcinoma in situ (SCCis) are important mimickers of isolated plaque psoriasis. **Acrokeratosis paraneoplastica (Bazex sign) is characterized by psoriasiform lesions on the nose, ear helices, palms, and soles ± onychodystrophy** in association with **malignancy of the upper aerodigestive tract.**
  - Do NOT confuse <u>Bazex</u> sign with <u>Bazex</u>-Dupré-Christol syndrome.
- The differential diagnosis of erythroderma includes erythrodermic psoriasis, pityriasis rubra pilaris (PRP), eczematous dermatoses (especially AD, seborrheic dermatitis, contact dermatitis, and chronic actinic dermatitis [CAD]), morbilliform drug eruption/drug reaction with eosinophilia and systemic symptoms (DRESS), papuloerythroderma of Ofuji, CTCL, and paraneoplastic erythroderma (eg, lymphoma). **Preexisting dermatoses are the leading cause of erythrod-**

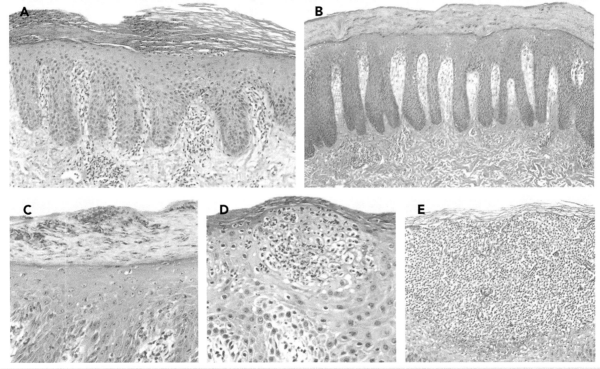

Figure 2.3. CLINICOPATHOLOGICAL CORRELATION: PSORIASIS. Characteristic features are alternating neutrophils and parakeratosis, hypogranulosis, regular acanthosis with thin suprapapillary plates, neutrophilic spongiform pustules in the *stratum corneum* (Munro microabscesses) and *stratum spinosum* (spongiform pustules of Kogoj) with variable spongiosis, and tortuous vessels in the dermal papillae. A, Early psoriasis. B, Late psoriasis. C, Munro microabscess. D, Spongiform pustule of Kogoj. E, Pustular psoriasis. PR, pityriasis rosea.

(Histology images reprinted with permission from Elder DE, Elenitsas R, Rosenbach M, et al. *Lever's Histopathology of the Skin.* 11th ed. Wolters Kluwer; 2015.)

- **Guttate variant:** neutrophils above mounded parakeratosis.
- **Pustular variant:** exaggerated neutrophilic spongiform pustules in the *stratum corneum* (Munro microabscesses) and *stratum spinosum* (spongiform pustules of Kogoj).

Regular acanthosis may be described as "club shaped." Remember <u>Munro</u> microabscesses are in the *stratum corneum* because Marilyn <u>Monro</u> was on top of Hollywood, while spongiform pustules of Kogoj are deeper in the *stratum spinosum*. Mounded parakeratosis is a shared feature between guttate psoriasis and PR. On high-power, psoriasis can NOT be distinguished from clear cell acanthoma on histopathology.

erma overall, while drug eruption (eg, allopurinol) is the leading cause of erythroderma in HIV-infected patients. Idiopathic erythroderma ("red man syndrome") occurs in ~25% of patients.

 ◦ Do NOT get confused! "Red man syndrome" is used to refer to idiopathic erythroderma OR a rate-dependent infusion reaction to vancomycin.

 In infants, the differential diagnosis of erythroderma additionally includes ichthyoses (eg, epidermolytic ichthyosis [EI]), immunodeficiencies (eg, SCID [Omenn syndrome]), and infections (eg, staphylococcal scalded skin syndrome [SSSS]).

- The differential diagnosis of pustulosis includes pustular psoriasis, acute generalized exanthematous pustulosis (AGEP), pemphigus foliaceus (PF)/pemphigus erythematosus, IgA pemphigus (subcorneal pustular dermatosis [SPD] type), SPD (Sneddon-Wilkinson disease), amicrobial pustulosis of the folds, impetigo, superficial folliculitis, superficial candidiasis, and dermatophytosis.

 In infants, the differential diagnosis of pustulosis additionally includes transient neonatal pustular melanosis, erythema toxicum neonatorum, autoinflammatory syndromes (eg, deficiency of the interleukin-1 receptor antagonist [DIRA], deficiency of the interleukin-36 receptor antagonist [DITRA], *CARD14*-mediated pustular psoriasis, *ADAM17* deletion), and acropustulosis of infancy.

- **Dermoscopy** features include **white superficial scales and dotted vessels in a uniform distribution against a light red background ± red globular rings.**
- Psoriasis is primarily a clinical diagnosis, but skin scraping and/or biopsy may be helpful.
- In patients with guttate psoriasis, antistreptolysin O (ASO) and anti-DNase B or streptozyme titer may be considered to identify streptococcal pharyngitis.
- In patients with erythroderma, longitudinal evaluation (eg, repeated skin biopsies, peripheral blood flow cytometry, and high-throughput sequencing [HTS]) may be required to rule out CTCL.
- There is no specific serologic test that establishes the diagnosis of psoriatic arthritis, and most patients are **seronegative for rheumatoid factor (RF)**. Radiographic changes include joint erosions, joint-space narrowing, bony proliferation, osteolysis, ankylosis, spur formation, and spondylitis.

 Osteolysis results in a "pencil in cup deformity."

Management

- Psoriasis is a chronic relapsing disorder that requires a long-term treatment strategy (clearing phase followed by maintenance phase).
- Recommendations from the **Joint AAD/NPF (National Psoriasis Foundation) Guidelines of Care for the Management of Psoriasis** include:
 ◦ Awareness and attention to comorbidities: Patients should receive screening and education regarding cardiovascular disease, IBD, metabolic syndrome, psoriatic arthritis, and depression/anxiety, including advice on how to practice a healthy lifestyle.

 ◦ Topical therapies: **Corticosteroids** play a key role, especially for localized disease. Steroid-sparing agents include **vitamin D analogues (eg, calcipotriene), retinoids (eg, tazarotene), and calcineurin inhibitors (eg, pimecrolimus, tacrolimus).** "Proactive treatment" to reduce frequency of flares typically involves twice-weekly treatment of clinically quiescent at-risk areas. Other recommended topical therapies are **emollients, salicylic acid, anthralin, and coal tar preparations. Roflumilast** was subsequently approved.
 ◦ Phototherapy: Narrowband ultraviolet B (nbUVB) is recommended over broadband ultraviolet B (bbUVB) for generalized plaque psoriasis. Options for localized psoriasis include **targeted UVB (eg, excimer laser)** and **topical psoralen ultraviolet A (PUVA)**, especially for palmoplantar disease. Bath and oral PUVA are also available. Though less effective, nbUVB is preferred to PUVA because of enhanced safety, convenience, and cost savings. **Goeckerman therapy** involves application of **coal tar followed by nbUVB.**
 ◦ Systemic nonbiological therapies: **Acitretin** is recommended for **plaque, erythrodermic, and pustular** psoriasis. **Apremilast and methotrexate** are recommended for **moderate to severe** psoriasis, while **cyclosporine** is recommended for **severe, recalcitrant** psoriasis.
 ◦ Biologics: **TNFα inhibitors (adalimumab, certolizumab, etanercept, golimumab, infliximab), the IL-12/IL-23 inhibitor (ustekinumab), IL-17 inhibitors (brodalumab, ixekizumab, secukinumab), and IL-23 inhibitors (guselkumab, risankizumab, tildrakizumab)** are recommended for **moderate to severe** psoriasis.

 The **TNFα inhibitor etanercept (age ≥ 4 years) and the IL-12/IL-23 inhibitor ustekinumab (age ≥ 6 years)** are recommended for **moderate to severe** psoriasis in **pediatric patients.**

- **Body surface area (BSA)** of involved skin is an important measure of psoriasis severity **to risk stratify patients for future comorbidities and to assess response to treatment** (Figure 2.4). The **Psoriasis Area and Severity Index (PASI)** measures average erythema, induration, and scaling of psoriatic lesions on a scale of 0 to 4 and is weighted by area of involvement. A common outcome measure in clinical trials, the PASI is seldom used in clinical practice.

"Real World" Advice

- It is important to recognize the **negative impact of psoriasis on quality of life and psychosocial well-being**, which is **comparable to** other chronic diseases such as **type 2 diabetes mellitus.**
- **Cost-effectiveness** is an important consideration when treating patients. In a prior study, **methotrexate** was found to be the least costly systemic psoriasis therapy.
- **Acitretin** is not immunosuppressive and is therefore beneficial for immunosuppressed patients (eg, **HIV**).
- **Early diagnosis of psoriatic arthritis** is critical to prevent disease progression resulting in irreversible joint destruction and loss of function. In these patients, remember to select a therapy efficacious for both skin and joint disease (eg, **biologics are preferred to phototherapy**).

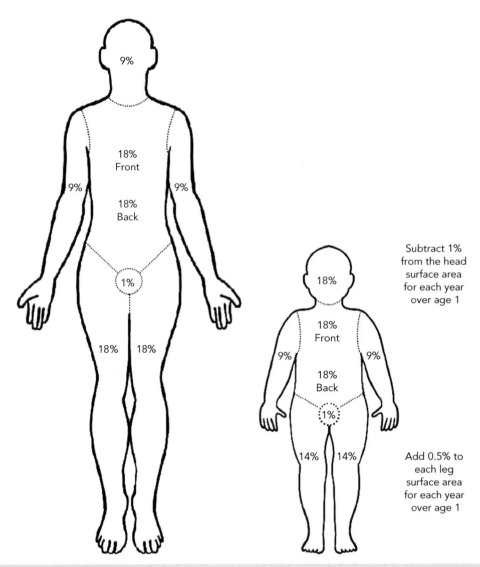

Figure 2.4. BODY SURFACE AREA.
(Illustration by Caroline A. Nelson, MD.)

REACTIVE ARTHRITIS

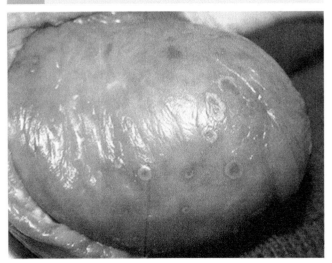

Balanitis circinata reprinted with permission from Reprinted with permission from Edwards L, Lynch P. *Genital Dermatology Atlas and Manual*. 3rd ed. Wolters Kluwer; 2017.

- Reactive arthritis is a psoriasiform disorder. It occurs most often in **men**. The leading association is **urethritis (eg, *Chlamydia trachomatis*)** followed by **enteritis (eg, *Shigella flexneri*)**. **HIV**-infected patients may develop **severe** disease. The leading HLA association is **-B27.**
  - The historical name for reactive arthritis, Reiter disease, is no longer in use due to Reiter's activities during the German Nazi regime.
- Reactive arthritis presents in ~5% of patients with **psoriasiform skin lesions favoring the scalp, genitalia, and acral areas. Balanitis circinata** refers to involvement of the **penis**, while **keratoderma blennorrhagicum** refers to involvement of the **palms and soles**, often with pustules. Other mucocutaneous findings include **oral ulcers and psoriasiform onychodystrophy**. Patients may exhibit fever and other constitutional symptoms. **Arthritis (polyarthritis/sacroiliitis ≥ 1 month)** occurs in ~**20%** of patients. **Morning stiffness** is common. Other systemic features include **ocular findings (eg, conjunctivitis)** and **urethritis** (±cystitis, cervicitis, salpingitis).

The "classic triad" of reactive arthritis—conjunctivitis, urethritis, arthritis—may be remembered with the popular saying, "can't see, can't pee, can't climb a tree."
 ◈ Reactive arthritis exhibits psoriasiform dermatitis.
- NSAIDs are first line for acute disease, which typically self-resolves within 6 to 12 months but may flare. For ~25% of patients who develop chronic disease, **biologics (eg, TNFα inhibitors)** are increasingly popular.

GEOGRAPHIC TONGUE
→ **Diagnosis Group 2**
Synonym: benign migratory glossitis

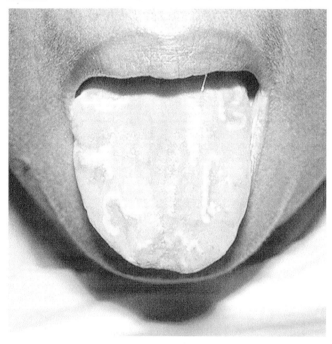

Reprinted with permission from Goodheart HP. *Goodheart's Photoguide of Common Skin Disorders: Diagnosis and Management.* 2nd ed. Lippincott Williams & Wilkins; 2003.

Epidemiology

- Geographic tongue is a common psoriasiform disorder (1%-3% of the general population).
- The incidence of geographic tongue may be increased in patients with **psoriasis.**

Clinicopathological Features

- Geographic tongue classically presents with **asymptomatic sharply demarcated erythematous patches with yellow-white serpiginous borders favoring the lateral and dorsal tongue.**
 ◈ Geographic tongue exhibits psoriasiform mucositis and atrophy of filiform papillae.

Evaluation

- The differential diagnosis of geographic tongue includes LP, candidiasis, and leukoplakia.
- No evaluation is typically indicated for geographic tongue.

Management

- No treatment is typically indicated for geographic tongue. A topical corticosteroid gel may be helpful in some patients with burning or sensitivity to hot or spicy foods.

"Real World" Advice

- Given the striking appearance of geographic tongue, reassurance regarding its benign nature is important.

PARAPSORIASIS
→ **Diagnosis Group 2**

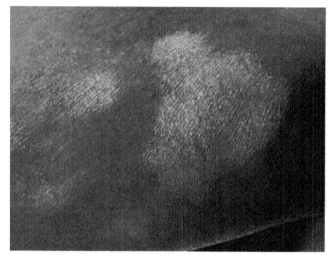

Reprinted with permission from Shaw KN, Bachur RG, Chamberlain JM, et al. *Fleisher & Ludwig's Textbook of Pediatric Emergency Medicine.* 7th ed. Wolters Kluwer; 2015.

Epidemiology

- Parapsoriasis is an umbrella term for two distinct papulosquamous disorders: **small plaque parapsoriasis and large plaque parapsoriasis.**
- Parapsoriasis, pityriasis lichenoides (PL), and lymphomatoid papulosis (LyP) are overlapping **clonal T cell–related dermatoses associated with CTCL.**

Clinicopathological Features

- Parapsoriasis classically presents with **asymptomatic round-oval scaly erythematous patches. Small plaque parapsoriasis lesions are <5 cm, while large plaque parapsoriasis lesions are >5 cm.** Lesions may wax and wane but ultimately become **persistent.**
 ◈ Beware the misnomer! Lesions of small and large "plaque" parapsoriasis are patches.
- The **digitate dermatosis** variant of small plaque parapsoriasis is characterized by **elongated patches symmetrically distributed on the flanks.**
 ◈ Digitate dermatosis lesions are elongated like <u>fingers</u>.
 ◈ Parapsoriasis exhibits parakeratosis and spongiotic dermatitis. Large plaque parapsoriasis may exhibit a lichenoid interface dermatitis. There is a predominance of CD4+ T cells. TCR gene rearrangement may detect T-cell clonality. For discussion of risk of progression to CTCL, see below.

Evaluation

- The differential diagnosis of parapsoriasis includes other papulosquamous disorders and mycosis fungoides (MF). Nummular dermatitis and secondary syphilis are important mimickers of small plaque parapsoriasis, while poikiloderma and chronic radiation dermatitis are important mimickers of large plaque parapsoriasis.

Management

- Treatments for parapsoriasis include topical corticosteroids, coal tar preparations, and **phototherapy.**

"Real World" Advice

- The risk of progression from large plaque parapsoriasis to CTCL is well established (10%-35% over 6-10 years), leading some to consider it the earliest stage of MF. In contrast, the risk of progression from small plaque parapsoriasis to CTCL remains controversial. Some consider small plaque parapsoriasis a *forme fruste* of MF, while others recommend reassurance.
- Topical calcineurin inhibitors carry a boxed warning for lymphoma and other malignancies. Although a causal relationship has not been established, exercise caution in parapsoriasis.

PITYRIASIS LICHENOIDES

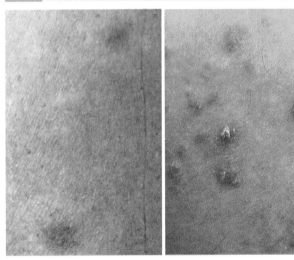

Pityriasis lichenoides et varioliformis acuta (left) courtesy of Sa Rang Kim, MD. Pityriasis lichenoides chronica (right).

- PL is a papulosquamous disorder. **Pityriasis lichenoides et varioliformis acuta (PLEVA)** is at the acute end of the spectrum, while **pityriasis lichenoides chronica (PLC)** is at the chronic end of the spectrum. Parapsoriasis, PL, and LyP are overlapping **clonal T cell–related dermatoses associated with CTCL.**
- PL classically presents with **recurrent crops of asymptomatic erythematous papules that involve spontaneously.**

PLEVA lesions are crusty or vesiculopustular and heal with varioliform scars, while PLC lesions are scaly and heal with hypopigmentation. Patients with the **febrile ulceronecrotic Mucha-Habermann disease** variant of PLEVA may exhibit mucosal involvement, fever, and other constitutional symptoms, along with gastrointestinal and pulmonary involvement.

    ◆ Figure 2.5.

- Varicella is an important mimicker of PLEVA, while secondary syphilis is an important mimicker of PLC.
- The prognosis of PL depends on its distribution, as **patients with diffuse lesions have the shortest average disease course** (11 vs 33 months). Treatments for PL are similar to parapsoriasis with the addition of systemic antiinflammatory antibacterials (eg, doxycycline, erythromycin) and immunosuppressants (eg, methotrexate).

PITYRIASIS ROSEA
→ Diagnosis Group 1

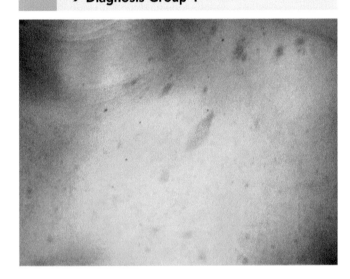

Epidemiology

- Pityriasis rosea (PR) is a papulosquamous disorder. A role for **human herpes virus (HHV)-7 > HHV-6** in PR has been hypothesized but remains unproven.

    ◆ HHV-6 and HHV-7 have been implicated in PR, DRESS, and roseola infantum.

- PR most commonly occurs in healthy young adults with a seasonal predilection for **spring and fall.**

    The peak incidence of PR is during adolescence.

- PR may increase the risk of **spontaneous abortion,** particularly during the **first 15 weeks** of pregnancy (controversial).

Clinicopathological Features

- PR classically presents with a **scaling erythematous plaque on the trunk.** Within hours to days, **scaly erythematous**

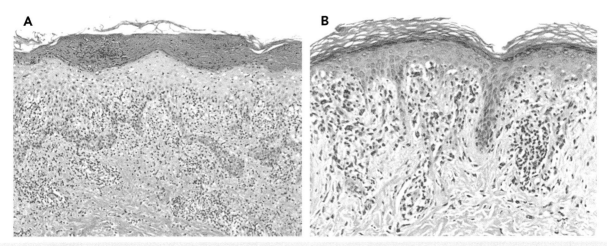

Figure 2.5. CLINICOPATHOLOGICAL CORRELATION: PITYRIASIS LICHENOIDES. Characteristic features are a perivascular interface dermatitis and erythrocyte extravasation extending to the epidermis. There is a predominance of CD8+ T cells in PLEVA versus CD4+ T cells in PLC. TCR gene rearrangement may detect T-cell clonality. CD, cluster of differentiation; PLC, pityriasis lichenoides chronica; PLEVA, pityriasis lichenoides et varioliformis acuta; TCR, T-cell receptor. A, PLEVA. B, PLC. (Histology images reprinted with permission from Husain AN. *Biopsy Interpretation of Pediatric Lesions.* Wolters Kluwer; 2014.)

The histopathology of PLC is more subtle than PLEVA, the latter of which has a denser "V-shaped" infiltrate and variable epidermal changes (eg, parakeratosis, crust, ulceration, necrotic keratinocytes).

papules with long axes along Langer lines erupt on the trunk and proximal extremities. Lesions are characterized by a subtle advancing border and collarette of scale. Follicular prominence and hyperpigmentation are often observed in darkly pigmented skin. Pruritus is common.

- Pityriasis is derived from the Greek word *pítouro* meaning "bran." Collectively, the pityriases are characterized by fine "branlike" scale.
- In PR, the initial lesion is known as the "herald patch." On the posterior trunk, lesions with long axes along Langer lines may create a "Christmas tree" pattern.
- Patients may exhibit fever and other constitutional symptoms.
- Rare variants include **vesicular, pustular, erythema multiforme (EM)-like, purpuric, and inverse PR.**
    - Figure 2.6.

Evaluation

- The differential diagnosis of PR includes other papulosquamous disorders, nummular dermatitis, and secondary syphilis. The pityriases include:
    - **Pityriasis amiantacea** refers to **thick scales, often adhering to hair shafts in clumps.** It is not a specific disease, but rather a clinical finding associated with multiple dermatoses. Scalp psoriasis is the leading cause, followed by seborrheic dermatitis and Darier disease.
        - Amiantacea is derived from the French word *amiante* meaning "asbestos."
    - **PL** (see above).
    - **PR** (see above).
    - **Pityriasis rotunda** refers to **large sharply demarcated circular and polycyclic scaly hyperpigmented patches favoring the trunk and extremities.** This disorder is hypothesized to arise from malnutrition in genetically

susceptible individuals (eg, Far East, Mediterranean basin, African descent) with an underlying disorder (eg, gastric or hepatocellular carcinoma, hepatic cirrhosis, plasma cell dyscrasia, mycobacterial infection).

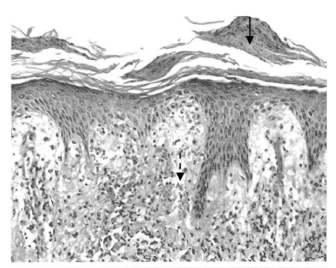

Figure 2.6. CLINICOPATHOLOGICAL CORRELATION: PITYRIASIS ROSEA. Characteristic features are mounded parakeratosis, spongiosis, a superficial perivascular and interstitial lymphohistiocytic infiltrate, and erythrocyte extravasation extending to the epidermis. Dashed arrow: erythrocyte extravasation. Solid arrow: mounded parakeratosis. PR, pityriasis rosea.

(Histology image reprinted with permission from Husain AN, Stocker JT, Dehner LP. *Stocker and Dehner's Pediatric Pathology.* 5th ed. Wolters Kluwer; 2021.)

Mounded parakeratosis is a shared feature between guttate psoriasis and PR.

○ **PRP** (see below).
○ **Drug-induced PR-like eruption** such as **angiotensin-converting enzyme inhibitors (ACEIs), β-blockers, and gold.**
- **Serologic testing** may be considered to rule out syphilis.

Management

- PR typically self-resolves within 6 to 8 weeks; therefore, **observation** is satisfactory.
- Optional treatments for PR include topical corticosteroids, oral antihistamines, and phototherapy. Small studies have additionally reported the efficacy of **oral acyclovir and erythromycin.**

"Real World" Advice

- Classic time course is helpful to distinguish PR from PLC and small plaque parapsoriasis. PR self-resolves more rapidly than PLC (6-8 weeks vs 11-33 months), while small plaque parapsoriasis is chronic.

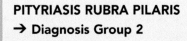

PITYRIASIS RUBRA PILARIS
→ Diagnosis Group 2

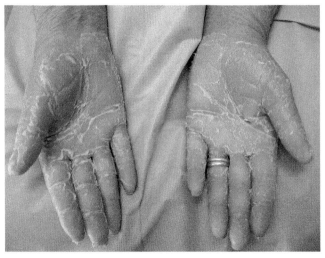

Courtesy of Victoria Werth, MD.

Epidemiology

- PRP is a disorder of follicular keratinization.

Clinicopathological Features

- PRP classically presents with **follicular hyperkeratosis on an erythematous base with follicular plugging. Lesions coalesce into orange-red (salmon) patches sparing discrete areas of skin. ± Waxy orange-red PPK.** Psoriasiform onychodystrophy may occur (without pitting).
    ◆ PRP, like lichen spinulosus, has a "nutmeg grater" texture. "Islands of sparing" is an important clue. The PPK is "sandal-like."
- PRP morphology and distribution vary based on type. **PRP types in adults** are summarized in Table 2.3.
    PRP types in children are summarized in Table 2.4.

- Generalization of PRP may lead to **erythroderma.**
    ◆ Figure 2.7.

Evaluation

- The differential diagnosis of PRP includes other papulosquamous disorders, seborrheic dermatitis, PRP-like (Wong) type DM, and CTCL.

Management

- PRP prognosis varies based on type. Types I and III PRP typically self-resolve within 3 to 5 years, while types II and V have a chronic course. Types IV and VI have a variable course.
- Treatments for PRP include **systemic retinoids (eg, acitretin, isotretinoin)**, methotrexate, and biologics (eg, TNFα inhibitors, IL-17 inhibitors). PRP type VI may improve with antiretroviral therapy.

"Real World" Advice

- Biologics carry a boxed warning for lymphoma and other malignancies. Since CTCL may clinically mimic PRP, exercise caution.

Table 2.3. PITYRIASIS RUBRA PILARIS TYPES IN ADULTS

Type[a]	Classic Description	Notes
I (classic adult)	Classic PRP. Spreads caudally.	55% (most common type in adults).
II (atypical adult)	Eczematous dermatitis, ichthyosiform scale on the legs, PPK with course, lamellated scale ± alopecia.	5%.
VI (HIV-associated)	Classic PRP ± acne conglobata and HS.	<1%.

[a]Illustrative examples provided.
HIV, human immunodeficiency virus; HS, hidradenitis suppurativa; PPK, palmoplantar keratoderma; PRP, pityriasis rubra pilaris.

Table 2.4. PITYRIASIS RUBRA PILARIS TYPES IN CHILDREN

Type[a]	Classic Description	Notes
III (classic juvenile)	Classic PRP. Spreads caudally.	10%.
IV (circumscribed juvenile)	Classic PRP localized to elbows and knees.	25% of patients (most common subtype in children).
V (atypical juvenile)	Scleroderma-like changes of the hands and feet.	5%. Associated with *CARD14* mutation.

PRP, pityriasis rubra pilaris.
[a]Illustrative examples provided.

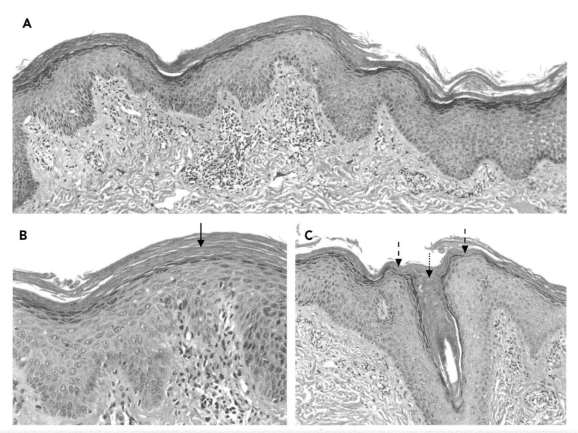

Figure 2.7. CLINICOPATHOLOGICAL CORRELATION: PITYRIASIS RUBRA PILARIS. Characteristic features are alternating vertical and horizontal ortho- and parakeratosis, parakeratosis adjacent to follicles, follicular plugging, acanthosis, and acantholysis with thick suprapapillary plates. A, Low-power view. B, High-power view. Solid arrow: "checkerboard parakeratosis." C, High-power view. Dashed arrows: "shoulder parakeratosis." Dotted arrow: follicular plugging. DLE, discoid lupus erythematosus; LS, lichen sclerosus; PRP, pityriasis rubra pilaris.

Alternating vertical and horizontal ortho- and parakeratosis is often called "checkerboard parakeratosis." Parakeratosis adjacent to follicles is often called "shoulder parakeratosis." "Shoulder parakeratosis" is a shared feature between PRP and seborrheic dermatitis. Follicular plugging is a shared feature between PRP, DLE, and LS.

SPOTLIGHT ON HEREDITARY PALMO-PLANTAR KERATODERMAS

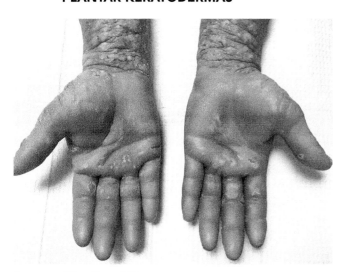

Courtesy of Sara Berg, MD.

- Hereditary PPKs are disorders of cornification that may be **nonsyndromic or syndromic.** PPK classification is based on pattern:
  - **Diffuse:** involvement of the entire palmoplantar surface.
  - **Focal:** oval lesions over pressure points (**areata**) or linear lesions over flexor tendons (**striate**).
  - **Punctate:** multiple small keratotic papules or pits.
- Hereditary PPKs are summarized in Table 2.5. **Transgrediens** refers to **extension beyond volar skin. Pseudoainhum** refers to **keratotic constriction bands around digits** that may lead to **autoamputation.**
  - Histopathological features depend on the hereditary PPK. Note that Vörner-Unna-Thost epidermolytic PPK demonstrates epidermolytic hyperkeratosis (EHK) (Figure 2.8).
  - **Keratoderma climacterum**, a **focal PPK favoring pressure points of the soles of women > 45 years**, is the most common acquired PPK. Other acquired PPKs include aquagenic PPK and circumscribed palmar or plantar hyperkeratosis.

Table 2.5. HEREDITARY PALMOPLANTAR KERATODERMAS

Diagnosis[a]	Inheritance pattern	Gene(s)	Classic Description	Notes
Nonsyndromic Diffuse PPKs				
Vörner-Unna-Thost epidermolytic PPK	AD	*K1* encoding K1 and *K9* encoding K9 Remember *K1* mutation in Vörner-Unna-Thost epidermolytic PPK by the card game UNO.	Diffuse PPK with a smooth surface, sharply demarcated erythematous border, and pseudoainhum.	
Nonepidermolytic PPK	AD, AR	Variable	Diffuse PPK similar to epidermolytic PPK with a less erythematous border.	
Mal de Meleda nonepidermolytic PPK	AR	*SLURP1* encoding SLURP1	Diffuse PPK, mutilating and transgradient, with pseudoainhum; angular cheilitis; hyperhidrosis with malodor; onychodystrophy (eg, koilonychia). Mal de Meleda is malodorous.	Increased risk of skin infections.
Loricrin keratoderma	AD	*LOR* encoding loricrin	Diffuse PPK (Vohwinkel-like) and ichthyosis.	Variant Vohwinkel syndrome.
Nonsyndromic Focal PPKs				
Striate PPK	AD	*DSG1* encoding desmoglein 1, *DSP* encoding desmoplakin, and *K1* encoding K1	Focal PPK (striate on the palms and areata on the soles).	
Nonsyndromic Punctate PPKs				
Punctate PPK	AD	Variable	Punctate PPK. Spiny keratoderma variant: numerous tiny keratotic spines. Marginal papular keratoderma variant: small, keratotic yellow (acrokeratoelastoidosis) or skin-colored (FAH) papules along the margins of the palms, soles, and digits.	Punctate PPK favors palmar creases in adults with African ancestry. Pits on palms and soles may also be identified in reticulate acropigmentation of Kitamura, Darier disease, PAON/PEODDN/ porokeratosis punctata palmaris et plantaris, Gorlin syndrome, and Cowden syndrome.
Syndromic PPKs				
Vohwinkel syndrome	AD	*GJB2* encoding connexin 26	Diffuse PPK, mutilating, with pseudoainhum and stellate knuckle keratoses; alopecia; onycholysis; and subungual hyperkeratosis. Systemic features include congenital sensorineural hearing impairment. PPK is "honeycomb-like," knuckle keratoses are "starfish-like."	Classic Vohwinkel syndrome.
Bart-Pumphrey syndrome	AD	*GJB2* encoding connexin 26	Diffuse PPK (Vohwinkel-like) with knuckle pads; leukonychia (true). Extracutaneous features include congenital sensorineural hearing impairment.	

Table 2.5. HEREDITARY PALMOPLANTAR KERATODERMAS (CONTINUED)

Diagnosis[a]	Inheritance pattern	Gene(s)	Classic Description	Notes
Olmstead syndrome	AD > AR	*TRPV3* encoding TRPV3	Diffuse PPK, mutilating, with pseudoainhum and periorificial and intertriginous keratotic plaques. Systemic features include visual and hearing impairment.	
	XLR	*MBTPS2* encoding MBTPS2		
Papillon-Lefèvre syndrome/Haim-Munk syndrome	AR	*CTSC* encoding cathepsin C	Diffuse PPK, mutilating and transgradient, with pseudoainhum and hyperkeratotic psoriasiform plaques on elbows and knees; periodontitis. Haim-Munk syndrome features onychodystrophy (eg, onychogryphosis).	Intracranial calcification of choroid plexus and tentorium on radiographic examination. Increased risk of skin infections. *Papillon* is the French word for butterfly. The "butterfly-shaped" choroid plexus is calcified in Papillon-Lefèvre syndrome.
Naxos disease	AR	*JUP* encoding junction plakoglobin	Diffuse PPK. The characteristic hair shaft abnormality without increased fragility is woolly hair. Systemic features include right ventricular cardiomyopathy with arrhythmias.	Perform cardiac evaluation.
Carvajal syndrome	AR > AD	*DSP* encoding desmoplakin	Focal (areata and striate) PPK. The characteristic hair shaft abnormality without increased fragility is woolly hair. Systemic features include dilated, often left-sided, cardiomyopathy. To remember left- vs right-sided cardiomyopathy, align the "plaks": desmoplakin-plakoglobin. Carvajal is on the left and Naxos is on the right.	Perform cardiac evaluation.
Richner-Hanhart syndrome (oculocutaneous tyrosinemia)	AR	*TAT* encoding hepatic TAT	Focal (areata) PPK, painful. Systemic features include dendritic keratitis with corneal ulcers and intellectual disability.	Treat with a tyrosine and phenylalanine-restricted diet. In Richner-Hanhart syndrome, tyrosine- and phenylalanine-rich foods make hands hurt.
Howel-Evans syndrome (TOC)	AD	*RHBDF2* encoding RhBDF2	Focal (areata) PPK; premalignant leukoplakia. Systemic features include esophageal leukokeratosis.	Increased risk of esophageal cancer. Perform serial endoscopy.
Miscellaneous				
Aquagenic PPK	AD, AR	Variable	Transient translucent to white papules on the palms shortly after water immersion. Aquagenic PPK has a "pebbly" appearance.	Associations include CF and marasmus. Drug associations include COX-2 inhibitors.

AD, autosomal dominant; AR, autosomal recessive; CF, cystic fibrosis; COX, cyclooxygenase; EB, epidermolysis bullosa; FAH, focal acral hyperkeratosis; K, keratin; MBTPS2, membrane-bound transcription factor peptidase, site 2; PAON, porokeratotic adnexal ostial nevus; PC, pachyonychia congenita; PEODDN, porokeratotic eccrine ostial and dermal duct nevus; PPK, palmoplantar keratoderma; RHBDF2, rhomboid 5 homolog 2; SLURP1, secreted LY6/PLAUR domain containing 1; TAT, tyrosine aminotransferase; TOC, tylosis with esophageal cancer; TRPV3, transient receptor potential vanilloid 3; XLR, X-linked recessive.

[a]Illustrative examples provided. Other hereditary disorders that feature PPK (eg, selected ichthyoses, erythrokeratodermas, EB, ectodermal dysplasias, PC) are discussed elsewhere.

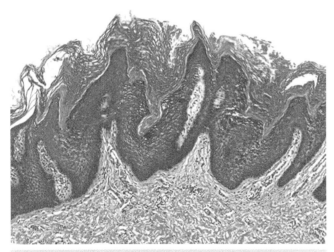

Figure 2.8. CLINICOPATHOLOGICAL CORRELATION: EPIDERMOLYTIC HYPERKERATOSIS. Characteristic features are dense orthohyperkeratosis, acanthosis, hypergranulosis, vacuolar degeneration of the granular and suprabasal layers, and clumped keratin intermediate filaments. EHK, epidermolytic hyperkeratosis; EI, epidermolytic ichthyosis; PPK, palmoplantar keratoderma.

(Reprinted with permission from Elder DE, Elenitsas R, Rubin AI, et al. *Atlas of Dermatopathology: Synopsis and Atlas of Lever's Histopathology of the Skin.* 4th ed. Wolters Kluwer; 2020.)

EHK may be identified in Vörner-Unna-Thost epidermolytic PPK, EI, epidermolytic acanthoma, and epidermolytic epidermal nevus. The granular layer appears "chewed up."

- Screen with **hearing and sweat tests.** Skin biopsy may be helpful to establish the diagnosis, along with **genetic testing.** Other diagnostic tests are highlighted in the table.
- Topical therapies to reduce hyperkeratosis include emollients, humectants, and keratolytics. **Oral retinoids** may have a role in treatment of severe PPKs.

GRANULAR PARAKERATOSIS

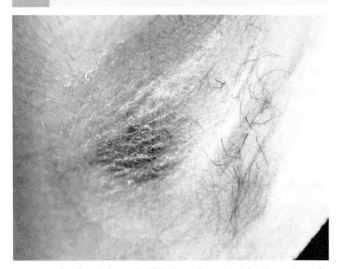

Courtesy of Seth J. Orlow, MD, PhD. From Gru AA, Wick MR, Mir A, et al. *Pediatric Dermatopathology and Dermatology.* Wolters Kluwer; 2018.

- Granular parakeratosis is a papulosquamous disorder. The hypothesized pathogenesis is a defect in processing profilaggrin to filaggrin.
- Granular parakeratosis classically presents with **brownish-red keratotic papules coalescing into plaques favoring flexural sites (especially the axillae).** Pruritus is common.
  In infants, granular parakeratosis is in the differential diagnosis for **diaper dermatitis.**

◆ Figure 2.9.
- Treatments for granular parakeratosis include topical corticosteroids, vitamin D analogues, retinoids, ammonium lactate, and antifungals.

ACANTHOSIS NIGRICANS
→ Diagnosis Group 1

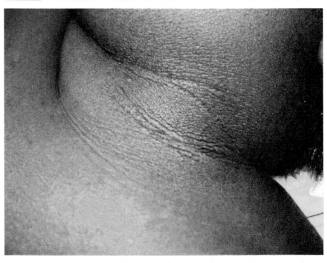

Reprinted with permission from Berek JS. *Berek & Novak's Gynecology.* 16th ed. Wolters Kluwer; 2019.

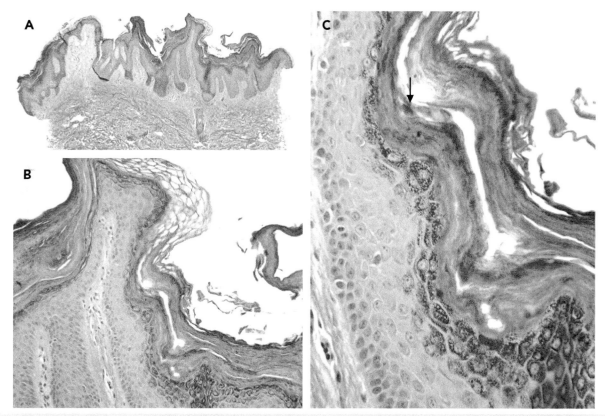

Figure 2.9. CLINICOPATHOLOGICAL CORRELATION: GRANULAR PARAKERATOSIS. Characteristic features are compact orthohyperkeratosis, parakeratosis, basophilic KHGs in the *stratum corneum*, acanthosis, and papillomatosis. A, Low-power view. B, Medium-power view. C, High-power view. Solid arrow: granules in the *stratum corneum*. KHGs, keratohyalin granules.

Epidemiology

- Acanthosis nigricans (AN) is an epidermal proliferation.
- The leading association is **insulin resistance (eg, diabetes mellitus, hyperandrogenism, insulin resistance, AN (HAIR-AN) syndrome).** Malignancy-associated AN is most often due to **gastric carcinoma**, and this holds true when AN is accompanied by **florid cutaneous papillomatosis and/or tripe palms syndrome.** However, **tripe palms syndrome in isolation** is most often due to **lung carcinoma.**

    Beare-Stevenson cutis gyrata syndrome, due to **AD *FGFR2*** gene mutation encoding fibroblast growth factor receptor 2 (FGFR2), leads to **cutis gyrata, AN,** furrowed palms and soles, craniosynostosis, and anogenital anomalies.
- Drug associations include corticosteroids, OCPs, and human growth hormone (HGH).

Clinicopathological Features

- **AN** is characterized by **velvety hyperpigmentation favoring flexural sites (eg, neck, axillae, groin).**
- **Florid cutaneous papillomatosis** is characterized by **verrucous skin lesions favoring the dorsal wrists and hands.**
- **Tripe palms syndrome** is characterized by **rigid velvety hyperpigmentation of the palms with pronounced dermatoglyphs.**
    - Figure 2.10.

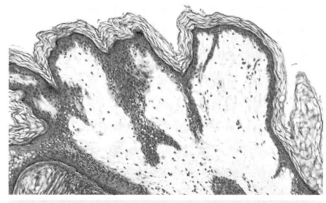

Figure 2.10. CLINICOPATHOLOGICAL CORRELATION: ACANTHOSIS NIGRICANS. Characteristic features are loose orthohyperkeratosis, acanthosis, papillomatosis, and pigment at the base of bulbous rete ridges. AN, acanthosis nigricans; CARP, confluent and reticulated papillomatosis.

(Reprinted with permission from Elder DE, Elenitsas R, Rubin AI, et al. *Atlas of Dermatopathology: Synopsis and Atlas of Lever's Histopathology of the Skin.* 4th ed. Wolters Kluwer; 2020.)

Pigment at the base of bulbous rete ridges may give AN the appearance of "dirty feet." AN can NOT be distinguished from CARP on histopathology.

Evaluation

- The differential diagnosis of AN includes CARP and pseudoatrophoderma colli (PC).
- Evaluation for insulin resistance is appropriate for patients who are overweight or obese.
- Evaluation for hyperandrogenism is appropriate for patients with AGA, hirsutism, and/or hormonal acne.
- Evaluation for malignancy is appropriate for patients with rapid onset AN, widespread distribution (eg, lips, oral mucosa, palms), weight loss, and/or other dermatologic signs (eg, florid cutaneous papillomatosis, tripe palms syndrome, sign of Leser-Trélat).

Management

- Treatment of AN should be directed at the underlying disorder.

"Real World" Advice

- Classic morphology is helpful to distinguish AN from CARP and PC. In contrast to the velvety hyperpigmentation of AN, CARP demonstrates brown verrucous papules and plaques, while PC demonstrates brown atrophic macules. Some consider PC to be a variant of CARP.

CONFLUENT AND RETICULATED PAPILLOMATOSIS

Synonym: confluent and reticulated papillomatosis of Gougerot and Carteaud

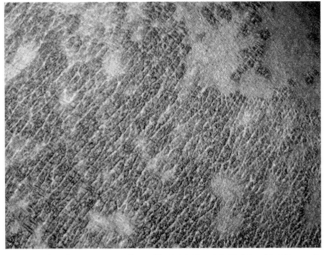

Reprinted with permission from Craft N, Fox LP, Goldsmith LA, et al. *VisualDx: Essential Adult Dermatology.* Wolters Kluwer Health/ Lippincott Williams & Wilkins; 2010

- CARP is an epidermal proliferation. Onset is most common in individuals of color during puberty.
- CARP classically presents with **brown verrucous papules and plaques (confluent centrally, reticulated peripherally) that spread from the inframammary area** to the upper trunk and other flexural sites.
  - ◆ CARP can NOT be distinguished from AN on histopathology.
- **Minocycline** is first line.

Eczematous Dermatoses and Related Disorders

Basic Concepts

- **Eczematous dermatoses** arise due to a combination of **skin barrier dysfunction** leading to increased transepidermal water loss (TEWL) and **immune dysregulation.**
- Related disorders include:
  - **Ichthyoses**: disorders of cornification characterized by **generalized scaling ± erythema.**
  - **Erythrokeratodermas**: disorders of cornification characterized by **circumscribed erythema and hyperkeratosis.**
  - **Keratosis pilaris (KP)**: disorder of follicular keratinization characterized by **prominent keratin plugs within follicular orifices.**

ATOPIC DERMATITIS
→ Diagnosis Group 1

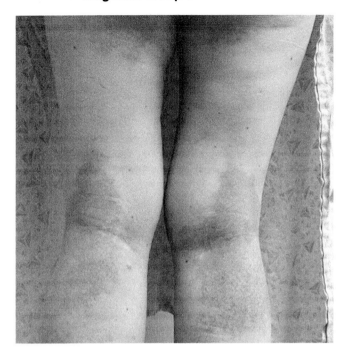

Epidemiology

- AD is an eczematous dermatosis due to a complex interplay of genetic factors (eg, **filaggrin deficiency**) and environmental factors (eg, **high income, urban areas**). **Acute AD** involves upregulation of **Th2 cytokines (eg, IL-4, IL-13, IL-31) and basophils.** Over time, **chronic AD** reflects a "**Th2 to Th1 shift.**" **Decreased expression of antimicrobial peptides (eg, cathelicidin, human β-defensins)** contributes to *Staphylococcus aureus* **colonization.**
- AD affects up to 20% to 30% of children. It typically presents during **infancy or early childhood** and follows a **chronic or relapsing course.**
  - While AD is more common in children, it affects 2% to 10% of adults. Age-associated skin barrier dysfunction may lead to **senile-onset AD** (>60 years).
- Associations include **allergic rhinoconjunctivitis, asthma, food allergies, and eosinophilic esophagitis.** The "**atopic march**" refers to progression from AD and food allergies (infancy or early childhood) to asthma (late childhood) to allergic rhinoconjunctivitis (adolescence).
  - The "allergic salute" refers to nasal creases in patients with AD and allergic rhinoconjunctivitis caused by habitual upward rubbing to relieve congestion.

Clinicopathological Features

- **Stages of eczematous dermatitis:**
  - **Acute:** papules and plaques with erythema and edema ± vesiculation, oozing, and crust.
  - **Subacute:** variably thick plaques with scale and subtle erythema and edema ± crust.

- **Chronic:** thick plaques with scale.
- Eczematous dermatitis often heals with **pigmentary changes.**
- In AD, the classic morphology and distribution pattern shift with age:
  - **Infants: acute** eczematous dermatitis on the **scalp, cheeks, and extensor extremities.** The **diaper area is typically spared**; however, AD is in the differential diagnosis for **diaper dermatitis.**
  - **Children: chronic** eczematous dermatitis on **flexural sites** (eg, neck, antecubital/popliteal fossae, wrists/ankles).
    - **Adults: chronic** eczematous dermatitis on **eyelids, flexural sites, and hands.**
- **Papular eczema with a follicular predilection** is more common in **African** and **Asian** populations.
- Other mucocutaneous findings include madarosis (Hertoghe sign) and onychodystrophy (eg, large and irregular pitting, Beau lines).
- Atypical vascular responses include **delayed blanching, midface pallor, and white dermatographism** (blanching due to capillary vasoconstriction after stroking the skin).
- AD may be associated with **peripheral hypereosinophilia and elevated IgE.**
- Ocular findings include **infraorbital darkening and pleats, recurrent conjunctivitis, keratoconus (progressive corneal thinning), and anterior subcapsular cataracts.**
  - "Allergic shiners" refer to infraorbital darkening, while "Dennie-Morgan lines" refer to infraorbital pleats. Anterior neck creases are also characteristic.
- Regional AD variants affect specific sites (eg, head/neck, eyelids, lips, ears, nipples, anogenital area).
- Generalization of AD may lead to **erythroderma.**
- AD is accompanied by **intense pruritus** that is often worse in the evening. Unfortunately, rubbing or scratching can trigger or exacerbate AD.
  - AD is the "itch that rashes."
Other AD triggers relate to **climate** (eg, extreme temperatures, low humidity, sunlight), **environmental allergies** (eg, contact allergens, dust mites, pollen), **food allergies** (eg, egg > milk, peanuts/tree nuts, shellfish/fish, soy, wheat), **irritants** (eg, wool), **infections** (eg, eczema herpeticum [Kaposi varicelliform eruption], molluscum contagiosum, eczema coxsackium, *S. aureus*).
- AD may overlap with **LSC.** Other dermatologic disorders associated with AD include:
  - **AA:** see Chapter 2: Disorders of the Hair and Nails.
  - Atopic eruption of pregnancy (AEP): classically presents in **early pregnancy** in women with atopy and recurs in subsequent pregnancies.
  - **Disseminate and recurrent infundibulofolliculitis:** superficial folliculitis (more common in **adults with darkly pigmented skin**) characterized by numerous pruritic, uniform, skin-colored papules favoring the neck, trunk, and upper extremities.
    - Disseminate and recurrent infundibulofolliculitis resembles "goose bumps."

○ **Follicular mucinosis (secondary):** see Chapter 2: Depositional Disorders, Porphyrias, and Nutritional Deficiencies.

○ **Frictional lichenoid eruption:** multiple small, flat-topped, pink to skin-colored papules on the elbows > knees and dorsal hands.

○ **Ichthyosis vulgaris:** see below.

○ **Immunologic contact urticaria:** see Chapter 2: Urticaria and Other Erythemas.

○ **Juvenile plantar dermatosis: shiny red plaques with scale on the balls of the feet and toepads** in prepubertal children due to friction.

◈ The colloquial name for juvenile plantar dermatosis is "sweaty sock syndrome."

○ **KP:** see below.

○ **Periorificial dermatitis:** see Chapter 2: Disorders of Sebaceous, Apocrine, and Eccrine Glands.

○ **Pityriasis alba:** hypopigmented patches with minimal scale.

○ **Xerosis:** see below.

◈ The histopathological correlate to eczematous dermatitis is spongiotic dermatitis (Figure 2.11).

Evaluation

• The differential diagnosis of eczematous dermatitis includes:

○ Nonneoplastic disorders such as eczematous dermatoses and related disorders, psoriasis, and nutritional deficiencies.

○ Hyper-IgE syndromes, Wiskott-Aldrich syndrome (WAS), and infections/infestations such as human T-lymphotropic virus (HTLV)-associated infective dermatitis, dermatophytosis, and scabies.

○ Neoplastic disorders such as CTCL.

○ Eczematous drug eruptions (eg, **TNFα inhibitors, ICIs, calcium channel blockers [CCBs]**).

LK, superficial BCC, and SCCis are important mimickers of isolated eczematous dermatitis.

• Evaluation of eczematous dermatitis may include skin scraping and/or biopsy, patch testing, blood and skin prick testing for allergen-specific IgE.

• The differential diagnosis of peripheral hypereosinophilia includes:

○ Nonneoplastic disorders such as atopy, bullous pemphigoid (BP), eosinophilic fasciitis (EF), urticaria, cholesterol emboli, eosinophilic granulomatosis with polyangiitis (EGPA), and eosinophilic dermatoses.

○ Hyper-IgE syndromes and infections/infestations such as parasites.

○ Neoplastic disorders such as systemic mastocytosis.

○ Drug eruptions such as morbilliform drug eruption/DRESS.

• Evaluation of peripheral hypereosinophilia may include skin biopsy, complete blood count (CBC), peripheral smear, IgE, C-reactive protein (CRP)/erythrocyte sedimentation rate (ESR), antinuclear antibody (ANA), antineutrophil cytoplasmic antibody (ANCA), vitamin B_{12}, HIV, stool ova and parasites, *Strongyloides* serology, flow cytometry, and tryptase.

Management

• **AD remits in ~60% of infants and children by 12 years of age.** However, appropriate management is critical not only to provide symptomatic relief but also to prevent epicutaneous sensitization and cutaneous inflammation that drive the "atopic march."

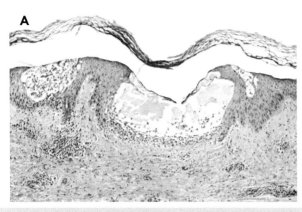
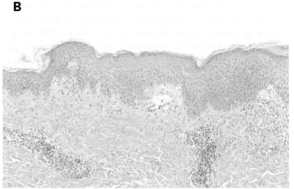

Figure 2.11. CLINICOPATHOLOGICAL CORRELATION: SPONGIOTIC DERMATITIS. Spongiosis refers to intercellular edema in the epidermis with stretching of cell-cell junctions. A, Acute spongiotic dermatitis. B, Subacute spongiotic dermatitis. LSC, lichen simplex chronicus.

(A, Histology image reprinted with permission from Elder DE, Elenitsas R, Rosenbach M, et al. *Lever's Histopathology of the Skin.* 11th ed. Wolters Kluwer; 2015. B, Histology image courtesy of Noel Turner, MD, MHS and Christine J. Ko, MD.)

Stages of Spongiotic Dermatitis:
• **Acute:** spongiosis and exocytosis of inflammatory cells.
• **Subacute:** parakeratosis, acanthosis, spongiosis, and exocytosis of inflammatory cells.
• **Chronic:** hyperkeratosis, hypergranulosis, irregular acanthosis, and papillary dermal fibrosis with capillary proliferation (angiofibroplasia) and vertically oriented collagen.

In acute and subacute spongiotic dermatitis, fluid accumulates in the epidermis like a "sponge." Chronic spongiotic dermatitis can NOT be distinguished from LSC on histopathology.

- Strategies for the primary prevention of AD may involve **emollient therapy from birth, exclusive breastfeeding for 3 to 4 months, and probiotics/prebiotics.**
- In general, patients with AD should **bathe or shower for 5 to 10 minutes in warm (not hot) water daily, use a gentle fragrance-free cleanser, and apply an emollient shortly after.**
- AAD Guidelines of Care for the Management of AD include:
  - **Topical corticosteroids and calcineurin inhibitors** (first line). Techniques to enhance penetration are **"soak and smear"** (soaking in plain water for 20 minutes followed by application) and **"wet wraps"** (application followed by an inner wet layer and an outer dry layer of cotton gauze or garments, 8-24 hours/day, <2 weeks). **Crisaborole** was subsequently approved (age ≥ 3 months).
  - **Phototherapy** (second line).
  - Systemic immunomodulatory agents including cyclosporine, azathioprine, methotrexate, mycophenolate mofetil, and IFN-γ (third line). Short-term corticosteroids may be used to control an acute flare as a bridge to steroid-sparing therapy. **Dupilumab** was subsequently approved.
- Trigger avoidance involves:
  - Short-term sedating antihistamines to reduce itch and sleep disturbance during an acute flare.
  - Climate control.
  - Allergen and irritant avoidance.
  - Strategies to reduce *S. aureus* colonization (eg, "bleach baths" with intranasal mupirocin). Bacteriotherapy (topical coagulase negative *Staphylococcus* strains with antimicrobial activity) is being explored as a potential strategy. Short-term antimicrobials may be necessary for superinfection.

"Real World" Advice

- It is important to recognize the **negative impact of AD on quality of life and psychosocial well-being.**
- Patch testing should be considered in case of refractory disease or an unusual distribution. Blood and skin prick testing for allergen-specific IgE has high NPV but low PPV. Clinical history ± provocation testing is required to conclude that an allergen is triggering AD. Food allergy testing should only be considered in case of refractory disease or immediate reliable reaction after ingestion of a specific food. Nutritional deficiencies may result from unnecessarily restrictive diets.
- Patients often state that topical corticosteroids "do not work" for them. Before reaching that conclusion, it is important to assess for **poor adherence** and corticosteroid contact dermatitis.
- Given the risk of adverse events (eg, skin atrophy, cataracts/glaucoma), **low-potency topical corticosteroids or calcineurin inhibitors are preferred on the face, axillae, and groin.**
- Long-term systemic corticosteroids, antihistamines, and antimicrobials are not indicated for AD.

ASTEATOTIC DERMATITIS

Synonyms: desiccation dermatitis, eczema craquelé, winter eczema, winter itch

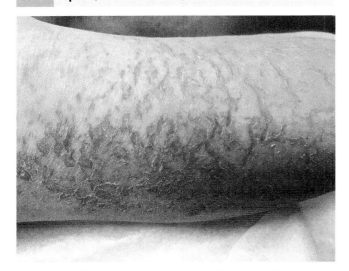

- Asteatotic dermatitis is an eczematous dermatosis due to **xerosis.** *Stratum corneum* dysfunction including **decreased natural moisturizing factor (NMF)** occurs with **aging.** Other associations include nutritional deficiencies and metabolic disorders (eg, **hypothyroidism**). Drug associations include **retinoids, epidermal growth factor receptor (EGFR) inhibitors, mitogen-activated protein kinase (MEK) 1/2 inhibitors, and statins.**
- Asteatotic dermatitis classically presents with **skin scaling, erythema, and cracking favoring the shins.**
  - Skin cracks in asteatotic dermatitis may resemble a "dried riverbed."

◈ Asteatotic dermatitis exhibits spongiotic dermatitis.

- Topical corticosteroids are first line, followed by emollient application to prevent relapse.

DYSHIDROTIC ECZEMA

Synonym: pompholyx

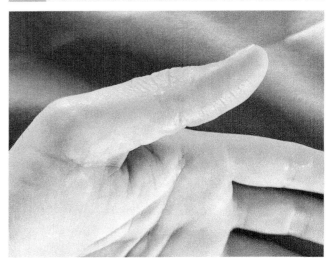

- Dyshidrotic eczema is an eczematous dermatosis associated with AD > contact dermatitis. Drug associations include **IVIG.**
- Dyshidrotic eczema is characterized by **symmetric, firm, deep-seated vesicles on the palms and lateral/medial fingers** > soles and toes. The mildest variant of dyshidrotic eczema is *dyshidrosis lamellosa sicca* (keratolysis

exfoliativa) with small annular collarettes of white scale in place of vesicles. Dyshidrotic eczema is accompanied by **intense pruritus.** Triggers include stress and hot climates.

- ◈ Vesicles in dyshidrotic eczema may resemble "tapioca pudding."
- ◆ Dyshidrotic eczema exhibits spongiotic dermatitis with vesicles on palmoplantar skin.
- Management of dyshidrotic eczema is similar to AD (see above).

NUMMULAR DERMATITIS
→ **Diagnosis Group 1**

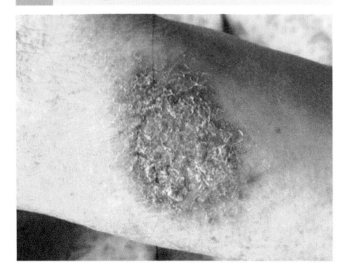

Epidemiology

- Nummular dermatitis is an uncommon eczematous dermatosis.

Clinicopathological Features

- Nummular dermatitis is characterized by **round eczematous lesions favoring the extremities.**
  - ◈ Nummular is derived from the Latin word *nummus* meaning "coin."
  - ◆ Nummular dermatitis exhibits spongiotic dermatitis.

Evaluation

- For the differential diagnosis of eczematous dermatitis, see above. SCCis is an important mimicker of isolated nummular dermatitis.

Management

- Management of nummular dermatitis is similar to AD (see above).

"Real World" Advice

- Round eczematous lesions may occur in other eczematous dermatoses; therefore, the existence of nummular dermatitis as an independent clinical entity is controversial.

SEBORRHEIC DERMATITIS
→ **Diagnosis Group 1**

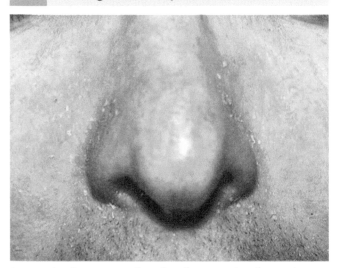

Reprinted with permission from Goodheart HP. *Goodheart's Same-Site Differential Diagnosis: A Rapid Method of Diagnosing and Treating Common Skin Disorders.* Wolters Kluwer Health/Lippincott Williams & Wilkins; 2011.

Epidemiology

- Seborrheic dermatitis is an eczematous dermatosis due to colonization with ***Malassezia* species** (yeasts that are part of normal resident skin flora) in areas with **active sebaceous glands.**
- In **adults,** seborrheic dermatitis peaks in the fourth to sixth decades and follows a **chronic** course.
  - In **infants,** seborrheic dermatitis typically **presents ~1 week after birth and self-resolves within 3 months.**
- Associations include **seborrhea, acne, hirsutism, and androgenetic alopecia (SAHA) syndrome.** Severe seborrheic dermatitis may signal **HIV infection** or a neuropsychiatric disorder (eg, **Parkinson disease**).
- A seborrheic dermatitis-like reaction has been reported to **BRAF inhibitors.**

Clinicopathological Features

- Seborrheic dermatitis is characterized by **pink-yellow to red-brown patches or thin plaques with scale in a seborrheic distribution** (scalp, face, ears, presternal > flexural sites, anogenital area).
  - ◈ The scale in seborrheic dermatitis is often described as "greasy." Chest lesions may have a "petaloid" appearance. In **infants,** seborrheic dermatitis typically involves the **scalp (cradle cap) ± diaper area.** As such, seborrheic dermatitis is in the differential diagnosis for **diaper dermatitis.**
- The mildest variant of seborrheic dermatitis is **pityriasis simplex capillitii (dandruff).** Thick scaling may result in pityriasis amiantacea.
- Generalization of seborrheic dermatitis may lead to **erythroderma.**
- Seborrheic dermatitis may **overlap with psoriasis (sebopsoriasis).**
  - ◈ Figure 2.12.

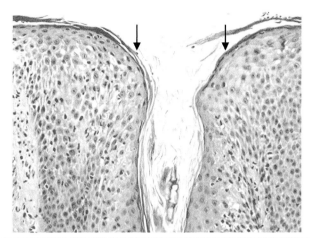

Figure 2.12. CLINICOPATHOLOGICAL CORRELATION: SEBORRHEIC DERMATITIS. Chronic seborrheic dermatitis. Acute seborrheic dermatitis exhibits spongiotic dermatitis. Chronic seborrheic dermatitis exhibits psoriasiform dermatitis with neutrophilic parakeratosis adjacent to follicles. Solid arrows: "shoulder parakeratosis." PRP, pityriasis rubra pilaris.

(Histology image reprinted with permission from Husain AN. *Biopsy Interpretation of Pediatric Lesions.* Wolters Kluwer; 2014.)

"Shoulder parakeratosis" is a shared feature between PRP and seborrheic dermatitis.

Evaluation

- For the differential diagnosis of eczematous dermatitis, see above. Langerhans cell histiocytosis (LCH) is a rare but important mimicker of seborrheic dermatitis in flexural sites.

Management

- In adults, antifungal therapy with **topical ketoconazole** or ciclopirox (cream or shampoo) ± short-term low-potency topical corticosteroid therapy is first line. Second-line therapies include tar, selenium sulfide, or zinc pyrithione shampoos and topical calcineurin inhibitors.

    In **infants**, bathing followed by **emollient application (eg, mineral oil)** is typically sufficient to control seborrheic dermatitis. Topical antifungal ± short-term low-potency topical corticosteroid therapy can be considered for refractory disease.

"Real World" Advice

- Understanding differing hair care practices between racial and ethnic groups is important. For example, a study assessing hair care practices among African American girls determined that hair extensions, chemical relaxers, and use of hair oil every 2 weeks versus daily were significantly associated with seborrheic dermatitis, while hair washing every 1 to 2 weeks was not. A recommendation to shampoo with ketoconazole or ciclopirox twice weekly may not be feasible in this patient population.

STASIS DERMATITIS
→ Diagnosis Group 1

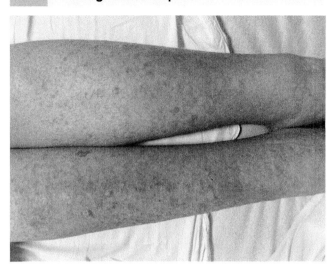

Epidemiology

- Stasis dermatitis is an eczematous dermatosis due to **venous insufficiency/hypertension.**
- Risk factors include age, family history, female gender, height, obesity, pregnancy, and prolonged standing.

Clinicopathological Features

- Stasis dermatitis is characterized by **scaling and erythema of the distal lower extremities.**
- Contact dermatitis is often present. **Disseminated eczema (autoeczematization, autosensitization, id reaction)** refers to development of secondary lesions distant from the primary site. This phenomenon occurs most often in **ACD and stasis dermatitis**, along with other eczematous disorders and tinea pedis.
    - Figure 2.13.

Evaluation

- For the differential diagnosis of eczematous dermatitis, see above.

Management

- Treatment should be directed at the underlying venous insufficiency/hypertension including **leg elevation and compression.**
- Topical corticosteroids and emollients are first line.

"Real World" Advice

- Other cutaneous signs of venous insufficiency/hypertension may provide helpful clues to the diagnosis of stasis dermatitis: **acroangiodermatitis, edema, lipodermatosclerosis, livedoid vasculopathy, petechiae superimposed on yellow-brown discoloration (hemosiderin), varicosities, venous ulcers.**

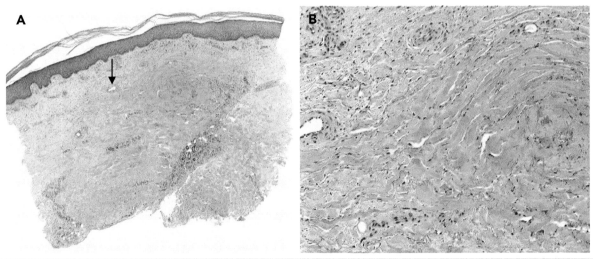

Figure 2.13. CLINICOPATHOLOGICAL CORRELATION: STASIS DERMATITIS. Stasis dermatitis demonstrates spongiotic dermatitis with superficial vascular ectasia, nodular angioplasia, erythrocyte extravasation, and hemosiderin deposition in the superficial dermis. A, Low-power view. Solid arrow: nodular "cannonball-like" angioplasia. B, High-power view.

Nodular angioplasia is "cannonball-like." Hemosiderin is refractile, while melanin is not.

CONTACT DERMATITIS
→ Diagnosis Group 1

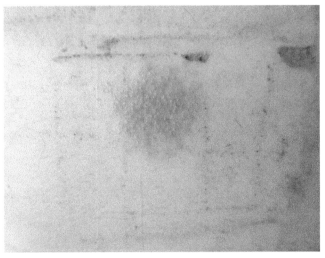

Courtesy of Ari Goldminz, MD.

Epidemiology

- Contact dermatitis is an eczematous dermatosis that occurs in two forms: **ACD (20%) and irritant contact dermatitis (ICD) (80%).** The **pathogenesis** is illustrated in Figure 2.14.
- In ACD, polysensitization is subcategorized into **co-reactivity** (concurrent, immunologically distinct chemicals) and **cross-reactivity** (immunologically indistinct chemicals).
- Common **contact allergens and irritants** are summarized in Tables 2.6 and 2.7, respectively.

- Common **plant allergens and irritants** are summarized in Tables 2.8 and 2.9, respectively.
  - Plant recognition skills, while of uncertain relevance to examinations, may prevent a raging case of poison ivy dermatitis (Figure 2.15).

Clinicopathological Features

- Contact dermatitis classically presents with **eczematous dermatitis localized to the site of allergen or irritant exposure. Linear configuration** is common when a plant brushes against the skin. ACD occurs within **hours to days** after exposure, while ICD occurs within **minutes to hours** after exposure.
  - Clinical features can NOT distinguish ACD from ICD; however, timing and pruritus in ACD versus burning, pain, and stinging in ICD are clues.
- In contact dermatitis, the distribution pattern depends on allergen or irritant exposure. Patterns include:
  - **Airborne:** ACD due to an aerosolized allergen (eg, **sesquiterpene lactones, usnic acid**) or ICD due to an aerosolized irritant (eg, **fiberglass, solvents**).
  - **Photoinduced:** photoallergic contact dermatitis (eg, **benzophenones, musk ambrette**) or phototoxic contact dermatitis (eg, **furocoumarins**).
  - **Symmetrical drug-related intertriginous and flexural exanthema (SDRIFE):** see Chapter 2: Interface Dermatoses and Other Connective Tissue Disorders.
  - **Systemic:** widespread ACD due to systemic exposure to an allergen. In addition to foods/plants, triggers include medications (eg, **ethylenediamine in IV aminophylline or oral cetirizine/hydroxyzine, thiuram in disulfiram**) and metals (eg, **nickel**).

ACD

1 Allergen penetrates the skin and couples with host proteins to form a hapten.

2 Hapten induces keratinocytes to release cytokines (IL-1β) that activate APCs.

3 APCs migrate to regional lymph nodes to present hapten to naïve T cells.

4 Activation of T cells generates CD8⁺ T cells and Tregs that migrate to the skin.

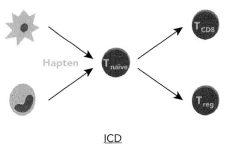

ICD

1 Irritant penetrates the skin, causing direct cytotoxic damage to keratinocytes.

2 Keratinocytes release cytokines (IL-1α, TNFα) that activate T cells.

Figure 2.14. PATHOGENESIS OF CONTACT DERMATITIS. ACD is a delayed-type, cell-mediated (type IV) reaction. Sensitization versus tolerance is determined by the balance of CD8⁺ T cells and Tregs. Similar reactions may not occur in other exposed individuals. ICD is dose dependent. Sensitization is not required. Similar reactions occur in other exposed individuals. ACD, allergic contact dermatitis; APCs, antigen-presenting cells; CD, cluster of differentiation; ICD, irritant contact dermatitis; IL, interleukin; TNF, tumor necrosis factor; Tregs, T-regulatory cells.

Table 2.6. CONTACT ALLERGENS

Allergen	Exposure(s)[a]	TRUE TEST[b]	Notes
Adhesives			
p-tert-Butylphenol formaldehyde resin	Glues (eg, leather), resins	X	
Colophony (rosin)	Dental lacquers/varnishes, glues, mascaras, resins (eg, string instruments)	X	Colophony is derived from the pine tree.
Cyanoacrylates	Commercial "super glues," tissue adhesives		
Epoxy resin (bisphenol A)	Glues, resins	X	
Ethyl acrylate	Nail glue		
Methacrylates	Artificial nails, bone and dental cements		Methacrylate may diffuse through intact gloves to cause paresthesia of the fingers (eg, nail technicians, orthopedic surgeons, dentists). Common cause of contact stomatitis.
Propolis	Beeswax-containing lip balms		Propolis is also known as "bee glue."
Shellac	Food coating, resin, varnishes		
Fragrances			
Balsam of Peru	Cosmetics, flavorings, perfumes	X	Balsam of Peru is derived from the *Myroxylon balsamum pereirae* tree.

(Continued)

Table 2.6. CONTACT ALLERGENS (CONTINUED)

Allergen	Exposure(s)[a]	TRUE TEST[b]	Notes
Fragrance mix I	Cosmetics, flavorings, perfumes	X	Together, Balsam of Peru and fragrance mix I detect ~75% of fragrance ACD.
Fragrance mix II	Cosmetics, flavorings, perfumes		
Musk ambrette	After shave, perfumes		Musk ambrette causes both ACD and photoallergic contact dermatitis.
Hair and Nail Products			
Ammonium persulfate	Flour bleach, hair bleach		Ammonium persulfate also causes contact urticaria.
Ammonium thioglycolate, glyceryl thioglycolate	Permanent waves		
PPD	Black henna, black rubber products, hair dyes, photographic developer, temporary tattoos	X	Cross-reactivity: azo dyes, ester anesthetics, PABA, parabens, PAS, PPD, sulfonamides.
Tosylamide formaldehyde resin	Nail polish		Tosylamide formaldehyde resin in nail polish is a common cause of eyelid dermatitis in women.
Medications			
Bacitracin	Antibacterial	X	Bacitracin is a common cause of ACD around venous stasis ulcers. Co-reactivity: bacitracin, neomycin. Bacitracin also causes contact urticaria.
Budesonide	Corticosteroid	X	Delayed reaction to patch testing is common. Cross-reactivity: group 1 corticosteroids.
Caine mix	Anesthetics	X	Cross-reactivity: see PPD. Benzocaine is a common cause of contact stomatitis.
Hydrocortisone 17-butyrate	Corticosteroid	X	Delayed reaction to patch testing is common. Cross-reactivity: see budesonide.
Mechlorethamine (aqueous > ointment)	Antineoplastic		
Neomycin	Antibacterial	X	Neomycin is a common cause of ACD around venous stasis ulcers. Delayed reaction to patch testing is common. Co-reactivity: see bacitracin. Neomycin also causes contact urticaria.
Quinoline mix	Antibacterial	X	
Retapamulin	Antibacterial		
Tixocortol-21-pivalate	Corticosteroid	X	Delayed reaction to patch testing is common. Cross-reactivity: see budesonide.
Metals			
Cobalt	Cement, ceramics, hair dyes, metal objects	X	Poral reaction: erythematous to violaceous dots due to cobalt residing in acrosyringia after patch testing. Co-reactivity: other metals.
Gold	Dental fillings, metal objects	X	Delayed reaction to patch testing is common. Co-reactivity: other metals.
Nickel	Metal objects	X	Nickel is the most common cause of ACD worldwide. Nickel may cause systemic ACD. The dimethylglyoxime test uses a pink color indicator to detect nickel. Co-reactivity: other metals.

Table 2.6. CONTACT ALLERGENS (CONTINUED)

Allergen	Exposure(s)[a]	TRUE TEST[b]	Notes
Potassium dichromate (metal salt derived from chromium)	Cement, green dyes (eg, pool table felt), leather, metal objects	X	Co-reactivity: other metals.
Silver	Amalgam dental fillings		Common cause of contact stomatitis. Co-reactivity: other metals.

Preservatives (Formaldehyde Releasing)

2-Bromo-2-nitropropane-1,3-diol (bronopol)	Cosmetics	X	Formaldehyde and quaternium-15 are the second most common preservatives to cause cosmetic ACD.
Diazolidinyl urea (Germall II)	Cosmetics	X	
DMDM hydantoin	Cosmetics		
Imidazolidinyl urea (Germall 115)	Cosmetics	X	Cosmetics with formaldehyde-releasing preservatives are typically applied "QD to BID": quaternium-15, diazolidinyl urea, tris(hydroxymethyl)nitromethane, 2-bromo-2-nitropropane-1,3-diol, imidazolidinyl urea, DMDM hydantoin.
Quaternium-15 (Dowicil 200)	Cosmetics	X	
Tris(hydroxymethyl) nitromethane	Cosmetics		

Preservatives (Non-Formaldehyde-Releasing)

MCI/MI (Kathon CG)[c]	Cosmetics, wipes	X	MI is the most common preservative to cause cosmetic ACD and is a common cause of contact dermatitis in the anogenital area.
Ethylenediamine	Medications	X	Ethylenediamine in IV aminophylline or oral cetirizine/hydroxyzine may cause systemic ACD.
Methyldibromoglutaronitrile (Euxyl K400)	Cosmetics	X	
Parabens	Cosmetics	X	Parabens have a relatively low sensitization potential. Cross-reactivity: see PPD.
Thimerosal	Contact lens solution, cosmetics, eye/nose/ear drops, vaccines	X	Thimerosal is a mercury-based preservative. Cross-reactivity: piroxicam (photosensitizer), thimerosal.

Rubber Products

Black rubber mix	Black rubber products	X	
Carba mix	Rubber accelerator (eg, elastics, gloves)	X	Repeated washing of elastics with bleach increases availability of carbamates implicated in elastic dermatitis, termed "bleached rubber syndrome."
MBT	Rubber accelerator (eg, gloves, shoes)	X	MBT is a common cause of shoe ACD. Shoe ACD spares the toewebs.
Mercapto mix	Rubber accelerator (eg, gloves)	X	
Mixed dialkyl thioureas	Rubber accelerator neoprene, photocopying, photography		
Thiuram	Rubber accelerator (eg, gloves)	X	Thiuram is a common cause of ACD in healthcare workers. Thiuram in disulfiram may cause systemic ACD.

Sunscreen Components

Benzophenones (eg, oxybenzone)	Chemical sunscreens		Oxybenzone is the leading cause of photoallergic contact dermatitis. Photoallergic contact dermatitis spares the upper eyelids, philtrum, and submental region.

(Continued)

Table 2.6. CONTACT ALLERGENS (CONTINUED)

Allergen	Exposure(s)[a]	TRUE TEST[b]	Notes
PABA and its derivative padimate O	Chemical sunscreens		Cross-reactivity: see PPD.
Textiles			
Disperse blue 106 and 124	Blue textiles	X	Textile ACD may be purpuric.
			Textile ACD spares the axillary vault.
Formaldehyde	Permanent press textiles (wrinkle resistant)	X	Formaldehyde is ubiquitous. 100% polyester contains less formaldehyde than other textiles.
Miscellaneous			
Cinnamon	Flavoring		Common cause of contact stomatitis.
Cocamidopropyl betaine/oleamidopropyl dimethylamine	Cosmetics, shampoos		
Dimethyl fumarate	Antimold sachets inside leather products		
Essential oils	Clove, lemon, orange		Common cause of contact stomatitis.
Glutaraldehyde	Cold sterilization (eg, dental/medical equipment)		
Parthenolide	Supplements	X	Parthenolide is a sesquiterpene lactone derived from the *Asteraceae* family.
Plants	See below.		
Propylene glycol	Antifreeze, cosmetics, lubricants, medications		Propylene glycol in medications (eg, minoxidil) may cause ACD.
Tocopherol (vitamin E derivative)	Antioxidant		
Wool alcohols (lanolin)	Emollients	X	Lanolin is a common cause of ACD around venous stasis ulcers.

ACD, allergic contact dermatitis; DMDM, dimethylol dimethyl; MBT, mercaptobenzothiazole; MCI, methylchloroisothiazolinone; MI, methylisothiazolinone; PABA, para-aminobenzoic acid; PAS, para-aminosalicylic acid; PPD, p-phenylenediamine; TRUE, thin-layer rapid use epicutaneous patch test.
[a]Illustrative examples provided.
[b]The TRUE TEST evaluates sensitivity to 35 allergens. There are 36 patches but patch 9 is a negative control.
[c]MCI/MI (Kathon CG) should be tested at twice the TRUE TEST concentration for improved sensitivity.

Table 2.7. CONTACT IRRITANTS

Irritant	Exposure(s)[a]	Notes[b]
Acids	Cosmetics, medications	Medications include azelaic acid and retinoids. The most severe injury results from hydrofluoric acid (antidote 2.5% calcium gluconate gel) or sulfuric acid. Aspirin is a common cause of contact stomatitis.
Alcohols/glycols	Antiseptics, medications, solvents	Propylene glycol in medications (eg, minoxidil) may cause ICD.
Alkalis	Construction (eg, cement work), soap	Alkalis cause more severe injury than acids (except hydrofluoric acid).
Body fluids	Saliva (lip licker's dermatitis), urine/feces (diaper dermatitis)	
Detergents and cleansers	Antiseptics, cosmetics	
Disinfectants	Antiseptics, medications	Medications include benzoyl peroxide.

Table 2.7. CONTACT IRRITANTS (CONTINUED)

Irritant	Exposure(s)[a]	Notes[b]
Fibers	Fiberglass	Aerosolized fiberglass may cause airborne ICD.
Foods and food additives	Food work	
Metal salts	Metal work	
Plants	See below.	
Plastics	Plastics work	
Solvents	Dry cleaning, medications	Medications include coal tar. Aerosolized solvents may cause airborne ICD.
Water	Wet work	

ICD, irritant contact dermatitis.
[a]Illustrative examples provided.
[b]Other medications causing ICD include sulfa antimicrobials (dapsone, mafenide, silver sulfadiazine, sulfacetamide, sulfur, and sulfacetamide), calcipotriene, and antipruritics (camphor, doxepin, menthol, phenol).

Table 2.8. PLANT ALLERGENS

Allergen	Family[a]	Plant(s)[a]	Notes
Plants			
Balsam of Peru	*Fabaceae*	*Myroxylon balsamum pereirae* tree	Balsam of Peru is a fragrance (see above).
Colophony (rosin), terpenes (eg, 3-carene)	*Pinaceae*	Pine tree (oleoresin)	Colophony is an adhesive (see above). Abietic acid is a major sensitizer.
Diallyl disulfide, allicin	*Alliaceae*	Garlic > chives, onion	Diallyl disulfide and allicin cause ACD on fingertips of the nondominant hand.
Musk ambrette			Musk ambrette is a fragrance (see above).
Primin	*Primulaceae*	Primrose	
Sesquiterpene lactones (eg, parthenolide)	*Asteraceae* (*Compositae*)	Chrysanthemum, dandelion, ragweed, sunflower, wild feverfew	Aerosolized sesquiterpene lactones may cause airborne ACD. Pyrethrin is an insecticide derived from chrysanthemums. Cross-reactivity: permethrin, pyrethrin.
Tea tree oil	*Myrtaceae*	Tea tree (oil)	Limonene is a major sensitizer.
			Limonene in <u>tea</u> tree oil; <u>lemon</u> in tea.
Tuliposide	*Alstroemeriaceae*	Peruvian lily	Tuliposide A > B is a common cause of ACD in florists.
	Liliaceae	Tulip	
Urushiol	*Anacardiaceae* genus *Toxicodendron* (*Rhus*)	Poison ivy, poison oak, poison sumac (oleoresin)	Urushiol is the most common cause of ACD in the United States. Catechols > resorcinols are major sensitizers. Cross-reactivity: Brazilian pepper tree (sap), cashew tree (oil and nut shells), gingko (seed pulp), Indian marking nut (black juice), Japanese lacquer tree (sap), mango (rinds), poison ivy, poison oak, poison sumac (oleoresin). Urushiol oxidation is responsible for "black spot" poison ivy.
Usnic acid	N/A	Lichen (fungal component)	Usnic acid and other lichen acids may cause airborne ACD and are included in fragrance mix I ("oak moss absolute").
		Technically speaking, lichen is not a plant!	In lichen, fungi live with algae ("<u>us</u>") and produce <u>usn</u>ic acid.

ACD, allergic contact dermatitis; N/A, not applicable.
[a]Illustrative examples provided.

Table 2.9. PLANT IRRITANTS

Irritant(s)	Family[a]	Plant(s)[a]	Notes
ICD			
Bromelain	*Bromelia*	Pineapple	In pineapple ICD, calcium oxalate–induced microabrasions allow bromelain to exert its proteolytic effect.
Calcium oxalate	*Amaryllidaceae* genus *Narcissus*	Daffodil	Calcium oxalate in daffodils is the leading cause of dermatitis in florists.
	Araceae	Dumb cane	
	Bromelia	Pineapple	
	Liliaceae	Tulip	
Capsaicin	*Solanaceae*	Hot pepper	Capsaicin, a topical antipruritic therapy, causes erythema, edema, and burning (not dermatitis).
Glochids	*Cactaceae*	Prickly pear	Glochids cause mechanical ICD (eg, Sabra dermatitis).
Phorbol esters	*Euphorbiaceae*	Poinsettia	
Protoanemonin	*Ranunculaceae*	Buttercup	Protoanemonin causes linear vesiculation that heals without hyperpigmentation.
Thiocyanates	*Alliaceae*	Garlic > chives, onion	Thiocyanates cause ICD on fingertips of the nondominant hand.
	Brassicaceae	Black mustard, radish	
Phototoxic Contact Dermatitis			
Furocoumarins (psoralens and angelicins)	*Apiaceae* (*Umbelliferae*)	Celery, hogweed	Phytophotodermatitis refers to linear erythema ± vesiculation that heals with hyperpigmentation. Celery is the leading cause, followed by limes and rue.
	Moraceae	Fig tree (sap)	Strimmer dermatitis (weed-whacker dermatitis) develops when weeds (eg, hogweed) splatter onto the body.
	Rutaceae (Citrus and Ruta species)	Burning bush, grapefruit, lemon, lime, mokihana (Hawaiian lei flowers), orange, rue	5-MOP in bergamot oil colognes causes berloque dermatitis. 8-MOP is utilized in PUVA phototherapy.
Hypericin	*Hypericaceae*	St. John's wort	St. John's wort is a CYP3A4 inducer.

ACD, allergic contact dermatitis; CYP, cytochrome P450; ICD, irritant contact dermatitis; MOP, methoxsalen; PUVA, psoralen ultraviolet A.
[a]Illustrative examples provided.

- Generalization of contact dermatitis may lead to **erythroderma.**
- Disseminated eczema may occur in ACD, most often in the setting of stasis dermatitis.
- Other mucocutaneous findings include cheilitis, stomatitis, and balanitis/vulvovaginitis; onychodystrophy (eg, chronic paronychia, hapalonychia, onycholysis).

  In **infants**, contact dermatitis (ICD > ACD) is in the differential diagnosis for **diaper dermatitis.** In contrast to psoriasis, contact dermatitis classically presents with **poorly demarcated eczematous patches sparing the inguinal creases.** Severe anogenital ICD is called **Jacquet erosive diaper dermatitis. Granuloma gluteale infantum/adultorum** is a reactive condition that exists on a spectrum with **perianal pseudoverrucous papules/nodules.** In addition to chronic irritation (eg, diarrhea), predisposing factors include topical corticosteroid use, occlusion, and candidal infection.

  ◆ Contact dermatitis exhibits spongiotic dermatitis. ACD is characterized by a mixed dermal infiltrate with variable eosinophils. ICD is characterized by keratinocyte necrosis and a neutrophil-rich dermal infiltrate. Contact stomatitis is characterized by lichenoid mucositis.

Evaluation

- For the differential diagnosis of eczematous dermatitis, see above. Other rare but important mimickers of contact dermatitis include:
  ○ **Autoimmune progesterone dermatitis:** progesterone sensitization (eg, during pregnancy or postpartum) leads to cyclic eczematous dermatitis during the **luteal phase of the menstrual cycle (ovulation to menses).** A majority of patients react to **intradermal injection of progesterone. Combined OCPs** are first line.
  ○ **Contact urticaria/protein contact dermatitis**: see Chapter 2: Urticaria and Other Erythemas.
  ○ **Infectious eczematous dermatitis**: sensitization to bacterial antigens (eg, *Staphylococcus* or *Streptococcus* species).
- **Patch testing** is often required to differentiate ACD from ICD. Patients should avoid corticosteroids for ≥1 week

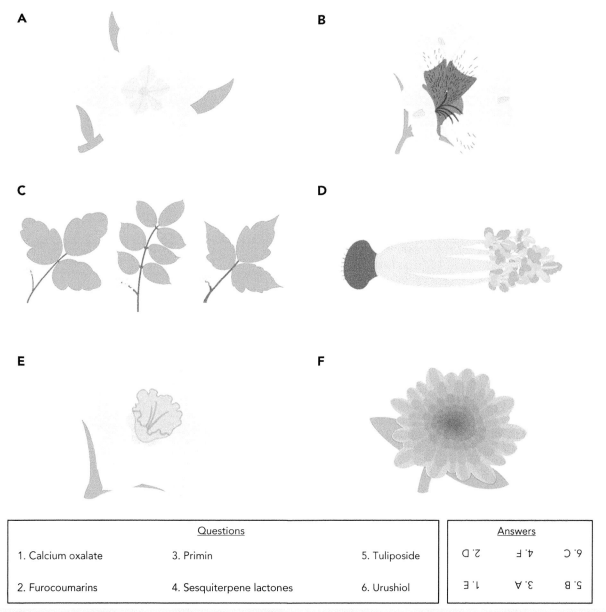

Figure 2.15. MATCHING EXERCISE: PLANT ALLERGENS AND IRRITANTS. A, Primrose. Family *Primulaceae*. Allergen: primin. B, Peruvian lily. Family *Alstroemeriaceae*. Allergen: tuliposide. C, Poison oak (left), poison sumac (center), poison ivy (right). Family *Anacardiaceae* genus *Toxicodendron* (*Rhus*). Allergen: urushiol. D, Celery. Family *Apiaceae* (*Umbelliferae*). Photoirritant: furocoumarins. E, Daffodil. Family *Amaryllidaceae* genus *Narcissus*. Irritant: calcium oxalate. F, Chrysanthemum. Family *Asteraceae* (*Compositae*). Allergen: sesquiterpene lactone.

(Illustration by Caroline A. Nelson, MD.)

beforehand (<20 mg prednisone equivalent daily if necessary) but may continue antihistamines. The upper back is the most common site of patch application. While the TRUE TEST is convenient, expanded testing improves diagnostic accuracy. Testing unknown personal care products is dangerous due to risk of "chemical burn." As a general rule of thumb, "leave-on" products can be tested, while "rinse-off" products require dilution. The first reading occurs at **48 hours** (when patches are removed) and the second reading occurs between **72 hours and 1 week.** The second reading is required to detect **delayed reactions (eg, corticosteroids, gold, neomycin).** The **International Grading System for Patch Tests** is:

○ ± doubtful reaction, faint macular erythema.

○ + weak, nonvesicular reaction with erythema, infiltration, and papules.

○ ++ strong, vesicular reaction with erythema, infiltration, and papules.

○ +++ spreading bullous reaction.

○ − negative reaction.

○ IR irritant reaction.

Ultimately, the diagnosis of ACD relies on finding a reaction of current relevance.

• The **open use test** can be helpful to evaluate sensitivity to a product when patch testing is unavailable or to confirm a patch test reaction. The product is applied to a predetermined location (eg, antecubital fossa, flexor forearm) twice daily for 1 to 2 weeks to determine whether dermatitis develops.

◆ The open use test is sometimes called "the poor man's patch test."

Management

- **Allergen avoidance** is essential for the prevention of ACD (≥6 weeks may be required). **Irritant avoidance** is essential for the prevention of ICD. Barriers include emollient, clear nail polish over nickel, and personal protective equipment. In some patients, ICD may resolve spontaneously with continued exposure; however, this phenomenon (accommodation or hardening) is unpredictable.
- **Topical corticosteroids** are first line. If corticosteroid contact dermatitis is suspected, prescribe ointment (to avoid preservatives) and switch to a **Group 3 topical corticosteroid.**
  ◆ Group 1 corticosteroids are the #1 cause of corticosteroid contact dermatitis.
- Severe ACD (eg, poison ivy dermatitis) may require **prednisone 1 to 2 mg/kg/d tapered over 2 to 3 weeks.**

"Real World" Advice

- It is important to counsel patients that the terms "clean beauty" or "natural skin care" do not mean "safe." In fact, companies "greenwashing" products have often substituted low-risk chemicals for ACD (eg, parabens) for high-risk chemicals (eg, methylchloroisothiazolinone/methylisothiazolinone [MCI/MI]).
  ◆ Poison ivy is "natural," but that does not mean it should be included in a skin care line.
- Patients with poison ivy dermatitis often state that prednisone "did not work" for them when, in fact, the duration was not sufficient.
- In case of poison ivy reexposure, patients should immediately wash with water (soap may enhance oleoresin permeability).

ICHTHYOSIS VULGARIS
→ Diagnosis Group 2

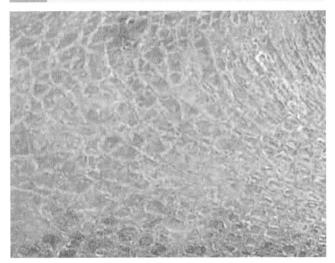

Reprinted with permission from Elder DE, Elenitsas R, Rubin AI, et al. *Atlas of Dermatopathology: Synopsis and Atlas of Lever's Histopathology of the Skin.* 4th ed. Wolters Kluwer; 2020.

Epidemiology

- Ichthyosis vulgaris is a disorder of cornification.
  For hereditary ichthyosis vulgaris, see below.
- Associations with acquired ichthyosis vulgaris include inflammatory disorders (eg, **sarcoidosis**), nutritional deficiencies (eg, **marasmus, vitamin A deficiency**), metabolic disorders (eg, **hypothyroidism, end-stage renal disease [ESRD] ± uremic frost**), infections (eg, **HIV, HTLV-I/II**), and malignancies (eg, **Hodgkin lymphoma**).
- Drug associations with acquired ichthyosis vulgaris include cimetidine, clofazimine, and statins.

Clinicopathological Features

- Ichthyosis vulgaris classically presents with **fine, adherent scales on the trunk and extremities with flexural sparing, hyperlinear palms/soles, and furrowed heels.**
  ◆ Ichthyosis is derived from the Greek root *ichthy* in reference to "fish scales."
  ◆ Figure 2.16.

Evaluation

- The differential diagnosis of acquired ichthyosis vulgaris includes late-onset hereditary ichthyosis vulgaris and xerosis.
  Terra firma-forme dermatosis is a disorder of cornification in **children and adolescents.** It classically presents with **brown patches and plaques favoring the neck.**

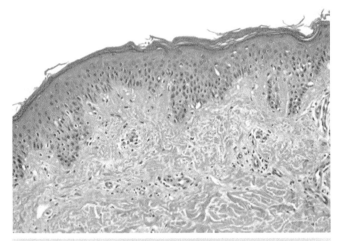

Figure 2.16. CLINICOPATHOLOGICAL CORRELATION: ICHTHYLOSIS VULGARIS. Characteristic features are compact orthohyperkeratosis and hypogranulosis. KP, keratosis pilaris; PXE, pseudoxanthoma elasticum.

(Histology image reprinted with permission from Elder DE, Elenitsas R, Rosenbach M, et al. *Lever's Histopathology of the Skin.* 11th ed. Wolters Kluwer; 2015.)

At scanning power, the "normal skin" differential diagnosis includes guttate psoriasis, seborrheic dermatitis, ichthyosis vulgaris, KP atrophicans faciei, vitiligo, chrysiasis, argyria, PXE, urticaria, scleredema, macular amyloidosis, tinea, candidiasis, onchocerciasis, and mastocytosis. Diagnosis relies on systematic evaluation and clinicopathological correlation. Do NOT forget to search for organisms in the *stratum corneum*.

Although terra firma-forme does not relate to poor hygiene, the Latin words *terra firma* meaning "dry land" reference its "dirty" appearance.

Management

- If possible, treatment of acquired ichthyosis vulgaris should be directed at the underlying cause.
- Topical therapies to reduce hyperkeratosis include emollients, humectants, and keratolytics. Topical retinoids cause skin irritation and oral retinoids are rarely indicated.

"Real World" Advice

- Patients with ichthyosis vulgaris should be carefully monitored for skin infection.
- Application of salicylic acid over a large BSA may lead to salicylism.

SPOTLIGHT ON HEREDITARY ICHTHYOSES AND ERYTHROKERATODERMAS

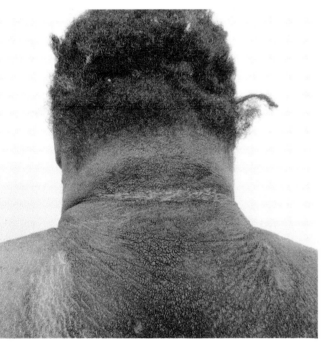

Epidermolytic ichthyosis courtesy of Leslie Castelo-Soccio, MD, PhD and Douglas Pugliese, MD, MPH.

- Hereditary ichthyoses and erythrokeratodermas are disorders of cornification that may be **nonsyndromic or syndromic.** Ichthyosis classification is based on absence or presence of a **collodion membrane** at birth.
  - The collodion membrane is a taut, shiny, transparent membrane comprised of thickened *stratum corneum* that appears to wrap the neonate in "cellophane."
- **Hereditary ichthyoses and erythrokeratodermas** are summarized in Table 2.10.
  - Histopathological features depend on the hereditary ichthyosis or erythrokeratoderma. Note that epidermolytic ichthyosis (EI) demonstrates EHK. Note that neutral lipid storage disease with ichthyosis demonstrates oil stain positivity (eg, Oil Red O, Sudan Black) on frozen skin biopsy specimens.
- Skin biopsy may be helpful to establish the diagnosis, along with **genetic testing.** Specific diagnostic tests are highlighted in the table.

- Treatment of hereditary ichthyoses is similar to acquired ichthyosis vulgaris. **Oral retinoids** are indicated for some severe ichthyoses (eg, **acitretin 1 mg/kg/d in Harlequin ichthyosis**) but **may enhance blistering in EI.**
  - Harlequin ichthyosis was historically considered universally fatal; however, due to advances in postnatal care and oral retinoid therapy, that is no longer true.

KERATOSIS PILARIS

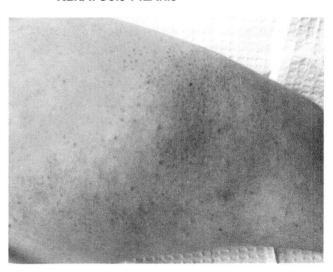

- KP is a disorder of follicular keratinization. **Filaggrin deficiency** may be present. Associations include **atopy, ichthyosis vulgaris, and Down syndrome.** A KP-like reaction may occur in association with **BRAF inhibitors.**
- KP classically presents with **keratotic papules with a rim of erythema favoring the lateral cheeks, upper arms, and thighs.** Background erythema is prominent in the **widespread keratosis pilaris rubra (KPR) variant.** The characteristic hair shaft abnormality without increased fragility is **rolled hairs.**
  - Figure 2.17.
- Beyond KP, other disorders of follicular keratinization include:
  - **Erythromelanosis follicularis faciei et colli:** multiple pinpoint follicular papules superimposed on a red-brown patch favoring the lateral cheeks/neck. May co-occur with KP.
  - FFA/LPP: see Chapter 2: Disorders of the Hair and Nails.

Table 2.10. HEREDITARY ICHTHYOSES AND ERYTHROKERATODERMAS

Diagnosis[a]	Inheritance Pattern	Gene(s)	Classic Description	Notes
Nonsyndromic Ichthyoses Without Collodion Membrane				
Ichthyosis vulgaris	AD	*FLG* encoding filaggrin	See above.	Associations include atopy, KP, and multiple eruptive clear cell acanthoma.
Steroid sulfatase deficiency (XLR ichthyosis)	XLR	*STS* encoding steroid sulfatase	Fine to large dark adherent scales on lateral face, neck, trunk, and extremities with sparing of the skin folds. Systemic features include corneal opacities and cryptorchidism. / Scales in steroid sulfatase deficiency have a "dirty" appearance.	Increased plasma (hydroxy)cholesterol sulfate and decreased steroid sulfatase activity (eg, in leukocytes). Increased risk of hypogonadism and testicular cancer. Female carriers may have corneal opacities and prolonged labor.
EI (bullous CIE)	AD > AR	*K1* encoding K1 and *K10* encoding K10	Erythroderma, blistering, and erosions at birth evolving into hyperkeratosis overlying joints and flexural ridging. ± PPK with pseudoainhum (K1). Malodor. Systemic features include gait and posture abnormalities. EI is the leading cause of the ichthyosis hystrix phenotype (massive hyperkeratosis). / Scales in EI have a "cobblestone" appearance. Flexural ridging may resemble "corrugated cardboard." Ichthyosis hystrix may resemble a "porcupine."	K1 is expressed in the suprabasal layers. K10 is expressed in the suprabasal layers excepting palms/soles. Lamellar granules are increased but abnormal. Monitor for sepsis and fluid and electrolyte imbalances. Mosaic EI, caused by a postzygotic mutation in *K1* or *K10* during embryogenesis, follows lines of Blaschko. If the mutation involves gonadal cells, it can be transmitted to the patient's children, resulting in generalized EI.
Superficial EI (ichthyosis bullosa of Siemens)	AD	*K2* encoding K2	Similar to EI (without erythroderma or PPK). Skin molting. / In ichthyosis bullosa of Siemens, the skin molts like the plumage of a seabird.	K2 is expressed in the upper spinous and granular layers.
Ichthyosis with confetti	AD	*K10* encoding K10 > *K1* encoding K1	Ichthyosiform erythroderma with development of small islands of normal skin.	Revertant mosaicism.
Ichthyosis hystrix, Curth-Macklin	AD	*K1* encoding K1	Similar to EI (without skin fragility). Severe mutilating PPK with digital contractures and pseudoainhum.	
Nonsyndromic Ichthyoses With Collodion Membrane				
LI/CIE (nonbullous CIE)	AR	LI: *TGM1* encoding TG-1, *ABCA12* encoding ABC lipid transporter CIE: *ALOXE3/ALOXI2B* encoding lipoxygenases[a,b]	Desquamation of the collodion membrane that evolves into large, thick, dark scales ± erythroderma (LI) or erythroderma and fine white scales (CIE). ± PPK with pseudoainhum. Ectropion > eclabium; scarring alopecia.	Collectively categorized as ARCI. Lamellar granules are decreased or absent. Premature delivery. Monitor for sepsis, fluid and electrolyte imbalances (eg, hypernatremic dehydration), and thermoinstability. Sepsis and respiratory insufficiency are the leading causes of mortality in Harlequin ichthyosis. To facilitate gradual desquamation of the collodion membrane, place the neonate in a humidified incubator and treat with wet compresses and emollients. Avoid manual removal (except if concern for autoamputation due to constricting skin bands) and topical keratolytics. Topical NAC has shown benefit.
		Do NOT confuse TG-1 with TG-3, the targeted antigen in DH.	Scales in LI have a "plate-like" appearance. Scales in CIE have a "powdery" appearance.	
Harlequin ichthyosis	AR	*ABCA12* encoding ABC lipid transporter	Desquamation of large, very thick, dark scales with red fissuring leaves erythroderma in the neonate that evolves into a severe CIE phenotype. / Scales in Harlequin ichthyosis have an "armor-like" appearance. The hands and feet resemble "mittens."	
Self-improving collodion ichthyosis	AR	Variable	Desquamation of the collodion membrane may leave normal skin.	

Table 2.10. HEREDITARY ICHTHYOSES AND ERYTHROKERATODERMAS

Diagnosis[a]	Inheritance Pattern	Gene(s)	Classic Description	Notes
Syndromic Ichthyoses				
Netherton syndrome	AR	*SPINK5* encoding serine-protease inhibitor LEKT1	Eczematous dermatitis, ichthyosis (ichthyosis linearis circumflexa with double-edged scale or CIE-like), and pruritus. Characteristic hair shaft abnormalities with increased fragility are trichorrhexis invaginata (most specific, eyebrow) and trichorrhexis nodosa (most common).	Elevated IgE. Monitor for sepsis, fluid and electrolyte imbalances (eg, hypernatremic dehydration), and thermoinstability. Increased risk of skin infection and allergies. Exercise caution with topical corticosteroids and calcineurin inhibitors due to increased absorption.
Sjögren-Larsson syndrome	AR	*ALDH3A2* encoding FALDH	Ichthyosis and pruritus. ± PPK. Systemic features include spastic di- and tetraplegia, intellectual disability, and perifoveal glistening white dots. Spastic di- and tetraplegia leads to a "scissor gate."	Accumulation of leukotriene B$_4$ is implicated in pruritus. Treat with 5-lipoxygenase inhibitors.
Neutral lipid storage disease with ichthyosis (Chanarin-Dorfman syndrome)	AR	*ABHD5* encoding an activator ATGL	Ichthyosis (CIE-like). Systemic features include hepatomegaly.	Lipid vacuoles in circulating leukocytes on peripheral smear.
Trichothiodystrophy with ichthyosis	See Chapter 4: Photodermatoses.			
Refsum disease (hereditary sensory motor neuropathy type IV)	AR	*PHYH* encoding phytanoyl-CoA hydroxylase and *PEX7* encoding peroxisomal type 2 targeting signal receptor	Ichthyosis (ichthyosis vulgaris–like). Systemic features include cerebellar dysfunction, peripheral neuropathy, retinitis pigmentosa, and sensorineural hearing impairment. *Refsum disease leads to retinitis pigmentosa.*	Elevated plasma phytanic acid. Treat with dietary restriction of phytanic acid in dairy products and animal fats. *Refsum disease patients should refuse the dairy products and fat of ruminants.*
Erythrokeratodermas				
EKV (Mendes da Costa disease)	AD > AR	*GJB3* encoding connexin 31 and *GJB4* encoding connexin 30.3[a]	Transient erythematous patches and stable hyperkeratotic plaques. ± PPK with pseudoainhum.	
PSEK	AD, AR	Variable	Progressive erythematous hyperkeratotic plaques. ± PPK with pseudoainhum.	
KID syndrome	AD	*GJB2* encoding connexin 26	Erythematous hyperkeratotic plaques. PPK (Vohwinkel-like). Systemic features include keratitis and congenital sensorineural hearing impairment. *KID syndrome in a kid is summarized by the name: keratitis-ichthyosis-deafness.*	Erythrokeratoderma. Increased risk of skin infections and skin cancer.

(Continued)

Table 2.10. HEREDITARY ICHTHYOSES AND ERYTHROKERATODERMAS (CONTINUED)

Diagnosis[a]	Inheritance Pattern	Gene(s)	Classic Description	Notes
XLD Ichthyosiform Disorders				
CHILD syndrome	XLD	*NSDHL* encoding 3β-hydroxysteroid dehydrogenase	Unilateral ichthyosiform erythroderma sparing the face at birth that evolves into verrucous hyperkeratosis. Verruciform xanthoma. Systemic features include ipsilateral organ hypoplasia and skeletal hemidysplasia.	XR demonstrates stippled epiphyses (chondrodysplasia punctata) during infancy. Treat with topical 2% lovastatin or simvastatin/2% cholesterol.
			CHILD syndrome in a *child* is summarized by the name: congenital *hemidysplasia* with *ichthyosiform erythroderma* and *limb defects*.	
Conradi-Hünermann-Happle syndrome (XLD chondrodysplasia punctata)[c]	XLD	*EBP* encoding EBP	Ichthyosiform erythroderma along lines of Blaschko that evolves into follicular atrophoderma and scarring alopecia. Systemic features include asymmetric skeletal abnormalities (eg, rhizomelia).	Accumulation of plasma 8(9) cholesterol. XR demonstrates stippled epiphyses (chondrodysplasia punctata) during infancy.
Miscellaneous				
Flegel disease (hyperkeratosis lenticularis perstans)	AD		Symmetric keratotic papules favoring the distal extremities and dorsal feet.	Lamellar granules are decreased or absent.
			Keratotic papules in Flegel disease have a "disc-like" appearance.	

AD, autosomal dominant; AR, autosomal recessive; ARCI, autosomal recessive congenital ichthyoses; ATGL, adipose triglyceride lipase; CIE, congenital ichthyosiform erythroderma; CHILD, congenital hemidysplasia with ichthyosiform erythroderma and limb defects; CoA, coenzyme A; DH, dermatitis herpetiformis; EBP, emopamil-binding protein; EI, epidermolytic ichthyosis; EKV, erythrokeratoderma variabilis; FALDH, fatty aldehyde dehydrogenase; Ig, immunoglobulin; K, keratin; KID, keratitis-ichthyosis-deafness; LEKT1, lymphoepithelial Kazal-type-related inhibitor; LI, lamellar ichthyosis; NAC, N-acetylcysteine; PPK, palmoplantar keratoderma; PSEK, progressive symmetric erythrokeratoderma; TG, transglutaminase; XLD, X-linked dominant; XLR, X-linked recessive; XR, x-ray.

[a]Illustrative examples provided.

[b]LI and CIE exist on a spectrum. Eleven genes that favor one phenotype have been identified.

[c]An AR variant (rhizomelic chondrodysplasia punctata) due to *PEX7* mutation has been described.

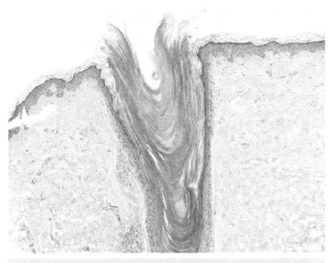

Figure 2.17. CLINICOPATHOLOGICAL CORRELATION: KERATOSIS PILARIS. Characteristic features are an orthokeratotic keratin plug that dilates the follicular orifice, rolled hairs, and a mild perivascular lymphocytic infiltrate.

(Histology image reprinted with permission from Gru AA, Wick MR, Mir A, et al. *Pediatric Dermatopathology and Dermatology.* Wolters Kluwer; 2018.)

- ○ **KP atrophicans**: KP with atrophy and scarring alopecia (Table 2.11).
- ○ **Lichen spinulosus**: multiple skin-colored papules with keratotic spines.
    - Lichen spinulosus, like PRP, has a "nutmeg grater" texture.
- ○ Phrynoderma: see Chapter 2: Depositional Disorders, Porphyrias, and Nutritional Deficiencies.
- ○ PRP: see Chapter 2: Papulosquamous Disorders and Palmoplantar Keratodermas.
- KP may improve after puberty. Keratolytics are first line. Topical retinoids cause skin irritation. Strategies to reduce erythema include topical corticosteroids and PDL.

Table 2.11. KERATOSIS PILARIS ATROPHICANS

Diagnosis[a]	Inheritance Pattern	Onset	Classic Description	Notes
Atrophoderma vermiculatum	Sporadic > AD	Childhood	KP atrophicans favoring the cheeks in a reticulated pattern.	Associations include Nicolau-Balus syndrome and Rombo syndrome.
			Vermiculatum means "worm eaten," referring to the reticulated pattern.	Do NOT confuse atrophoderma vermiculatum with follicular atrophoderma: follicular "dimple-like" or "ice pick" depressions favoring the cheeks and dorsal hands/feet associated with chondrodysplasia punctata and Bazex-Dupré-Christol syndrome.
Keratosis follicularis spinulosa decalvans	XLR	Childhood	KP atrophicans.	
	AD	Puberty	Follicular pustules.	
KP atrophicans faciei (ulerythema ophryogenes)	AD	Infancy	KP atrophicans favoring the lateral one third of the eyebrows.	Associations include cardiofaciocutaneous syndrome and Noonan syndrome.

AD, autosomal dominant; KP, keratosis pilaris; XLR, X-linked recessive.
[a]Illustrative examples provided.

Pigmentary Disorders

Basic Concepts

- **Hypopigmentation** (leukoderma) results either from **hypomelanosis or decreased cutaneous blood supply.** Hypomelanosis is further classified into melanocytopenic (decreased melanocyte number) or melanopenic (decreased melanin synthesis or transfer to keratinocytes). **Depigmentation** results from **amelanosis.** The distribution pattern of hypopigmentation/depigmentation may be **circumscribed, diffuse, guttate, or linear. Hair** hypopigmentation/depigmentation may present as **circumscribed poliosis** (leukotrichia) or **diffuse canities. Pigmentary dilution** refers to **diffuse hypopigmentation/depigmentation** of the skin and hair ± eyes.
- **Hyperpigmentation** may result from **hypermelanosis or dermal deposition of exogenous substances.** The distribution pattern of hyperpigmentation may be **circumscribed, diffuse, linear, or reticulated.**
- **Dyschromatoses** are disorders characterized by **both hypopigmentation and hyperpigmentation.**

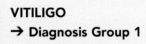

VITILIGO
→ Diagnosis Group 1

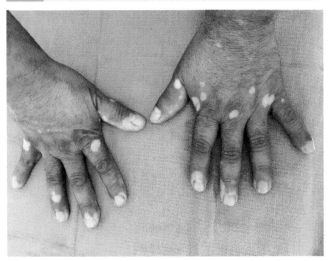

Courtesy of Zelma Chiesa-Fuxench, MD, MSCE.

Epidemiology

- Vitiligo results from **autoimmune destruction of functional melanocytes.**
- Associations include **AA**, LE, lichen sclerosus (LS), **halo nevi/melanoma**, Addison disease, adult-onset insulin-dependent diabetes mellitus, **autoimmune thyroid disease**, pernicious anemia, and rheumatoid arthritis (RA).

  Vitiligo is a characteristic feature of **APECED/IPEX syndromes.**
- Drug associations include **ICIs.**

Clinicopathological Features

- **Generalized vitiligo** may be classified as **vulgaris, acrofacial, mixed, or universal. Localized vitiligo** may be classified as **focal, segmental, or mucosal.**

  While vitiligo vulgaris is the most common type in children, **segmental vitiligo is relatively more common in children than adults.**
- Vitiligo vulgaris classically presents with **circumscribed depigmented macules and patches favoring the face (periorificial)**, nipples, axillae, umbilical/sacral/inguinal/anogenital regions, and dorsal hands.
- **Poliosis** may be observed.
- Onset is typically insidious. **Koebnerization** is a known trigger.
- Vitiligo variants include blue vitiligo (areas of postinflammatory hyperpigmentation), hypochromic vitiligo (hypopigmented macules in a seborrheic distribution), inflammatory vitiligo (erythematous border), trichrome/quadrichrome/pentachrome vitiligo (hypopigmented zone between normal and depigmented skin), and vitiligo ponctué (multiple discrete macules).

  Vitiligo ponctué is also called "confetti-like" vitiligo.
- Vitiligo syndromes include:
  - **Alezzandrini syndrome:** unilateral facial vitiligo and poliosis, ipsilateral ocular involvement (retinal pigment epithelial degeneration), and otic involvement (hypoacusis).
  - **Kabuki syndrome:** vitiligo, congenital heart defects, hemolytic anemia, idiopathic thrombocytopenic purpura, and thyroiditis.
  - **Vogt-Koyanagi-Harada (VHK) syndrome:** vitiligo and poliosis, alopecia, aseptic meningitis, ocular involvement (**uveitis**), and otic involvement (**dysacusis/tinnitus**).

    Figure 2.18.

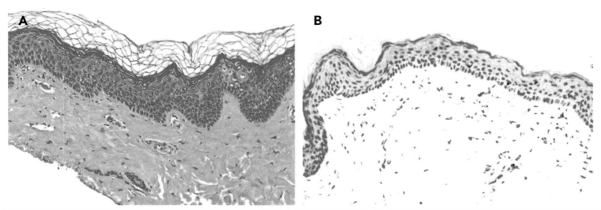

Figure 2.18. CLINICOPATHOLOGICAL CORRELATION: VITILIGO. Vitiligo is characterized by absent or decreased melanocytes. Melanocyte stains include HMB-45, melan A (MART-1), MITF, S100, SOX10, while melanin stains include Fontana-Masson. A, H&E demonstrates total loss of melanocytes. B, S100 protein immunoperoxidase staining confirms the loss of melanocytes. H&E, hematoxylin and eosin; HMB, human melanoma black; MART, melanoma antigen recognized by T cells; MITF, microphthalmia-associated transcription factor; SOX10, sry-related HMg-Box gene 10.

(Histology images reprinted with permission from Mills SE. *Histology for Pathologists.* 5th ed. Wolters Kluwer; 2019.)

Evaluation

- The differential diagnosis of vitiligo includes:
  - **Circumscribed** (eg, vitiligo vulgaris): pityriasis alba, hypopigmented lesions of LS, sarcoidosis, halo nevi/melanoma-associated leukoderma, CTCL.
  - **Diffuse** (universal vitiligo): nutritional deficiencies (eg, copper deficiency/Menkes kinky hair disease, selenium deficiency).
  - **Guttate** (vitiligo ponctué): IGH characterized by **guttate hypopigmentation favoring extensor forearms and shins**, progressive macular hypomelanosis (PMH) characterized by **guttate hypopigmentation in young women with darkly pigmented skin from the tropics**, **arsenic poisoning** (see below).
  - **Linear** (segmental vitiligo): intralesional corticosteroids.
  - Hypopigmentation/depigmentation in **multiple distribution patterns**: postinflammatory (eg, LE), postinfectious (eg, treponematoses, leprosy, TV, onchocerciasis), posttraumatic (eg, cryotherapy), **chemical (eg, phenols/catechols, sulfhydryls),** and drug-induced (eg, topical corticosteroids, topical retinoids, kinase receptor/breakpoint cluster region-Abelson platelet-derived growth factor receptor [BCR-ABL/Kit/PDGFR] inhibitors, topical imiquimod).
- The **Wood's lamp (nickel oxide–doped glass, peaks as 365 nm)** can aid in the diagnosis of vitiligo by **enhancing contrast between hypomelanosis and amelanosis.**
- Skin biopsies comparing melanocyte density in affected and unaffected skin may be helpful.

Management

- **Mucosal involvement** is associated with a **poor prognosis.**
- Treatment options for vitiligo (in addition to psychological support) have differing goals:
  - **Repigmentation: Topical corticosteroids, topical calcineurin inhibitors, and light devices (eg, phototherapy, excimer laser and lamp, helium-neon laser)** are first line. Surgical options (eg, minigrafting of small punch biopsies from unaffected to affected skin) may be considered; however, risks include Koebnerization and keloiding. Emerging treatment options include afamelanotide and JAK inhibitors.
  - **Camouflage:** Permanent dermal **micropigmentation** utilizes a nonallergenic iron oxide pigment.
  - **Depigmentation:** Depigmentation (eg, with **20% monobenzyl ether of hydroquinone**) may be considered for patients with **widespread vitiligo** who understand the significant impact depigmentation will have on their appearance and the need for lifelong strict photoprotection.

"Real World" Advice

- Vitiligo depigmentation and repigmentation each progress in a characteristic pattern. Peripheral hypopigmentation and poorly defined borders predict vitiligo activity. **Repigmentation initially appears in a perifollicular pattern** and/or at the periphery of vitiligo lesions.
- Treatment options for vitiligo repigmentation are **more effective in combination** than as monotherapy.

ERYTHEMA DYSCHROMICUM PERSTANS
Synonyms: ashy dermatosis, dermatosis cenicienta

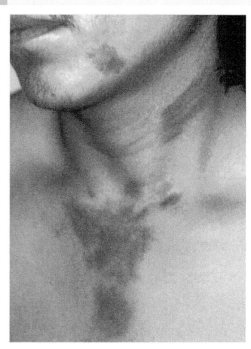

Reprinted with permission from Craft N, Fox LP, Goldsmith LA, et al. *VisualDx: Essential Adult Dermatology.* Wolters Kluwer Health/Lippincott Williams & Wilkins; 2010.

- Erythema dyschromicum perstans (EDP) is an idiopathic disorder that most often occurs in **adults from Latin America with skin phototypes III-IV.**
- EDP classically presents with **symmetric gray-brown to blue-gray macules and patches favoring the neck, trunk, and proximal extremities.**
  - The gray color of EDP lesions is reflected in its alternative names: ashy dermatosis and dermatosis cenicienta (Cinderella in Spanish).
  - Figure 2.19.
- Beyond EDP, disorders with **circumscribed and diffuse hyperpigmentation** include:
  - **Melasma (circumscribed hyperpigmentation favoring the face and forearms**, 90% in women with triggering factors including **sun exposure, pregnancy, and OCPs**).
  - Interface dermatoses and other CTDs (eg, LP pigmentosus, lichenoid drug eruption, fixed drug eruption [FDE], sclerodermoid disorders).
  - Metabolic disorders (eg, **Addison disease, hyperthyroidism, primary biliary cirrhosis [PBC], and hemochromatosis), carotenemia (eg, diabetes mellitus, hypothyroidism), ectopic ACTH syndrome** (eg, small-cell lung cancer).
    - Hemochromatosis is called "bronze diabetes" due to its association with diffuse hyperpigmentation and diabetes mellitus.
  - Depositional disorders, porphyrias, and nutritional deficiencies (eg, macular/lichen amyloidosis, porphyria cutanea tarda [PCT], vitamin B_9 deficiency).
  - Postinflammatory hyperpigmentation (eg, acne vulgaris).

- ○ Postinfectious hyperpigmentation (eg, TV).
- ○ Posttraumatic hyperpigmentation (eg, cryotherapy).
- ○ **Heavy metal and drug-induced hyperpigmentation or discoloration** (Table 2.12).
- ○ **Pregnancy** (areolar hyperpigmentation, linea nigra, longitudinal melanonychia, melasma, darkening of preexisting nevi).
- • There is no consistently effective treatment for EDP. Treatments for hyperpigmentation include:
  - ○ **Photoprotection and camouflage facial foundations.**
  - ○ **Topical hydroquinone** (2%-4%, more effective if pigmentation is limited to the epidermis and in combination with a topical corticosteroid and a topical retinoid than as monotherapy).
  - ○ **Topical azelaic acid, α-hydroxy acids, β-hydroxy acids, kojic acid, and vitamin C.**
  - ○ **Chemical peels** (eg, glycolic acid, salicylic acid).
  - ○ **Lasers** (eg, Q-switched ruby, alexandrite, and neodymium-doped yttrium aluminum garnet [Nd:YAG]) and **intense pulsed light (IPL).**

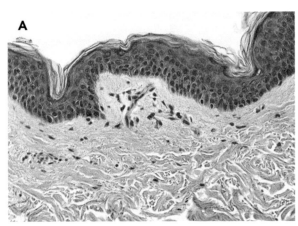
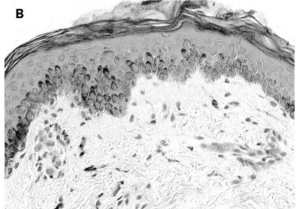

Figure 2.19. CLINICOPATHOLOGICAL CORRELATION: ERYTHEMA DYSCHROMICUM PERSTANS. Active EDP is characterized by increased epidermal melanin, vacuolar degeneration of the basal cell layer, and a sparse perivascular lymphocytic infiltrate with melanophages. A, H&E. B, Fontana-Masson. EDP, erythema dyschromicum perstans; H&E, hematoxylin and eosin.

Table 2.12. HEAVY METAL AND DRUG-INDUCED HYPERPIGMENTATION OR DISCOLORATION

Heavy metal or Drug[a]	Classic Description
Heavy Metals	
Arsenic	Guttate hypopigmentation superimposed on hyperpigmentation.
	Arsenic poisoning resembles "raindrops on a dusty road."
Bismuth	Generalized blue-gray discoloration ± mucosal involvement.
Gold (chrysiasis)	Blue-gray discoloration in a sun-exposed distribution.
Iron	Brown decorative tattoo or tattoo following application of ferric subsulfate (Monsel solution) for hemostasis.
Lead	"Lead line" in gingival margin and nail discoloration.
Mercury	Slate gray discoloration favoring skin folds.
Silver (argyria)	Localized or diffuse slate-gray discoloration ± sclerae, blue lunulae.
Antineoplastics	
Alkylating agents	Hyperpigmentation at sites of occlusion (eg, cyclophosphamide, ifosfamide, thiotepa) or pressure (eg, cisplatin).
Antibiotics	Flagellate hyperpigmentation (eg, bleomycin), longitudinal melanonychia (eg, doxorubicin).
Antimetabolites	Sun-exposed hyperpigmentation (eg, 5-FU, methotrexate) and serpentine supravenous hyperpigmentation (eg, 5-FU).
Miscellaneous Drugs	
Antimalarials	Blue-gray pigmentation (chloroquine, hydroxychloroquine) and yellow pigmentation (quinacrine).
TCAs	Blue-gray pigmentation.

(Continued)

Table 2.12. HEAVY METAL AND DRUG-INDUCED HYPERPIGMENTATION OR DISCOLORATION (CONTINUED)

Heavy metal or Drug[a]	Classic Description
OCPs	Melasma.
Zidovudine	Mucocutaneous hyperpigmentation and blue lunulae/longitudinal melanonychia.
Clofazimine	Red-brown hyperpigmentation.
Minocycline	Type 1: focal blue-black pigmentation in areas of previous inflammation or scarring. Type 2: blue-gray pigmentation favoring the legs. Type 3: diffuse brown pigmentation favoring the sun-exposed skin. Blue lunulae/longitudinal melanonychia.
ACEIs	Acquired brachial cutaneous dyschromatosis.
Afamelanotide	Hyperpigmentation, darkening of preexisting nevi.
Amiodarone	Slate-gray to violaceous discoloration in a sun-exposed distribution.
Chlorpromazine	Slate-gray pigmentation.
Diltiazem	Slate-gray to gray-brown discoloration in a sun-exposed distribution (skin phototypes IV-VI).
Hydroquinone	Exogenous ochronosis.
PUVA	Hyperpigmentation and lentigines.
Tobacco	Oral hyperpigmentation (smoker's melanosis), often in association with nicotinic stomatitis, periodontal disease, and oral cancer.

ACEIs, angiotensin-converting enzyme inhibitors; CCBs, calcium channel blockers; 5-FU, 5-fluorouracil; OCPs, oral contraceptive pills; PUVA, psoralen and ultraviolet A; TCA, tricyclic antidepressants.
[a]Illustrative examples provided.

PIGMENTARY DEMARCATION LINES

Synonyms: Ito lines, Futcher lines, Voight lines

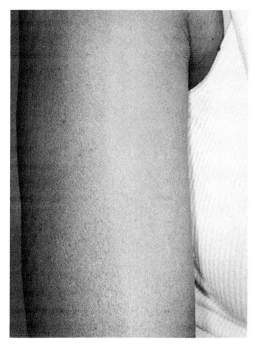

Reprinted with permission from Lugo-Somolinos A, McKinley-Grant L, Goldsmith LA, et al. *VisualDx: Essential Dermatology in Pigmented Skin.* Wolters Kluwer Health/Lippincott Williams & Wilkins; 2011

- **Pigmentary demarcation lines separate relatively hyperpigmented dorsal surfaces from ventral surfaces.** They are more readily apparent in individuals with **darkly pigmented skin.**
- Pigmentary demarcation lines may be classified into eight types:
  - **A: Vertical line along anterolateral upper arm.**
  - **B: Curved line on the posteromedial thigh.**
  - C: Vertical or curved hypopigmented band on the midchest.
  - D: Vertical pre- or paraspinal line.
  - E: Bilateral chest markings.
  - F, G: "V-" or "W"-shaped lines between lateral temple and malar prominence.
  - H: Diagonal line from oral commissure to lateral chin.
    - Pigmentary demarcation lines have normal histopathology.
- Beyond pigmentary demarcation lines, other acquired disorders with **linear hyperpigmentation** include **linea nigra (linear hyperpigmentation extending from the umbilicus to the pubis in pregnant women)**, linear postinflammatory hyperpigmentation (eg, linear LP, phytophotodermatitis), flagellate hyperpigmentation (eg, bleomycin, **Shiitake mushrooms**), and serpentine supravenous hyperpigmentation (eg, 5-fluorouracil [5-FU]). **Wallace lines** separate **dorsal (hair bearing) skin from palmoplantar (glabrous) skin.**
- Pigmentary demarcation lines are normal. No treatment is indicated.

PRURIGO PIGMENTOSA

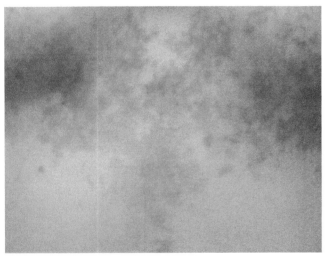

Courtesy of William James, MD.

- Prurigo pigmentosa is an idiopathic disorder that most often occurs in **young adults from Japan.** Prurigo pigmentosa is associated with nutrition (eg, **strict ketogenic diet**).
- Prurigo pigmentosa classically presents with **recurrent crops of pruritic erythematous papules and papulovesicles favoring the neck, chest, and back.** Lesions involve within a week, leaving behind **macular reticulated hyperpigmentation.**
  - ◈ Prurigo pigmentosa has three histopathologic stages: (1) neutrophilic exocytosis, spongiosis, papillary dermal edema, and a superficial perivascular neutrophilic infiltrate; (2) intra-/subepidermal vesiculation, necrotic keratinocytes, and a patchy lichenoid infiltrate of lymphocytes > eosinophils; and (3) variable parakeratosis, acanthosis, and hyperpigmentation of the epidermis with dermal melanophages.
- Beyond prurigo pigmentosa, other acquired disorders with **reticulated hyperpigmentation** include CARP, atopic "dirty neck," reticulated postinflammatory hyperpigmentation, erythema ab igne (EAI), and reticulated drug-induced hyperpigmentation.
- Treatment options for prurigo pigmentosa include minocycline, doxycycline, and dapsone.

SPOTLIGHT ON INCONTINENTIA PIGMENTI
Synonym: Bloch-Sulzberger syndrome

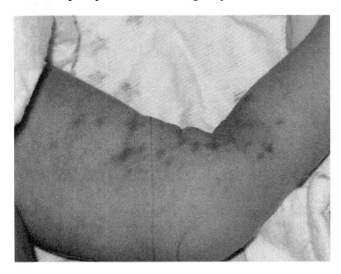

- IP is a neurocutaneous disorder due to **XLD** mutation in **NEMO**, also known as *IKBKG* (inhibitor of κ light polypeptide gene enhancer in B cells, kinase γ). The gene product, **NF-κB essential modulator**, protects against apoptosis induced by the TNF cytokine family. IP is **lethal in males (unless XXY or mosaic)** and has a **variable phenotype**

in females due to lyonization. Female carriers of hypohidrotic ectodermal dysplasia with immune deficiency due to X-linked recessive (XLR) *NEMO* mutation may have mild IP.
- Skin lesions of IP **follow lines of Blaschko** and evolve through four classic stages: **vesicular (birth-2 weeks), verrucous (2-6 weeks), hyperpigmented (3-6 months), and hypopigmented/atrophic (2nd-3rd decade).** There is overlap (eg, older children can still have areas of blistering while developing hyperpigmentation). Patients may also develop **periungual/subungual keratotic tumors** and adnexal involvement (eg, anhidrosis, patchy scarring alopecia, onychodystrophy). Systemic features include dental (eg, **hypodontia, conical teeth**), neurologic (eg, **seizures**), and/or ophthalmologic (eg, **retinal vascular abnormalities**).
  - ◈ Remember that X-linked dominant (XLD) <u>NEMO</u> mutation in IP leads to <u>striped</u> skin lesions along lines of Blaschko by remembering that <u>Nemo</u> has become a popular name for <u>striped</u> clown fish.
  - ◈ Figure 2.20.
- IP must be distinguished from other **hereditary pigmentary disorders** (Table 2.13). Skin biopsy may be helpful to establish the diagnosis, along with **genetic testing.**
- While skin lesions of IP do not require treatment, patients should be referred for dental, neurologic, and ophthalmologic evaluation.

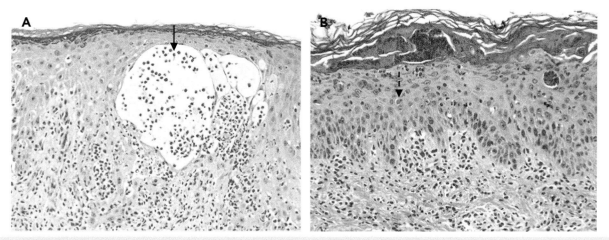

Figure 2.20. CLINICOPATHOLOGICAL CORRELATION: INCONTINENTIA PIGMENTI. The four classic stages of IP may overlap. Each of the four classic stages of IP is characterized by apoptotic keratinocytes. A, Vesicular stage. Solid arrow: eosinophilic spongiosis and vesiculation with eosinophils. B, Verrucous stage. Dashed arrow: dyskeratosis. IP, incontinentia pigmenti.

(Histology images reprinted with permission from Husain AN. *Biopsy Interpretation of Pediatric Lesions.* Wolters Kluwer; 2014.)

Stages:
- **Vesicular**: eosinophilic spongiosis.
- **Verrucous**: hyperkeratosis and papillomatosis with prominent dyskeratosis in whorls and clusters.
- **Hyperpigmented**: pigment incontinence.
- **Hypopigmented**: normal to decreased melanocytes ± dermal fibrosis.

Table 2.13. HEREDITARY PIGMENTARY DISORDERS

Category	Diagnosis[a]	Type	Inheritance pattern	Gene(s)	Classic Description	Notes
Hypopigmentation/Depigmentation						
Circumscribed	Piebaldism	N/A	AD	*KIT > SNAI2*	Congenital stable depigmentation/poliosis favoring the midscalp (white forelock), mid-forehead ± eyebrows/eyelashes, midtrunk, or mid-extremities.	*KIT* mutation disrupts melanocyte migration.
	WS	1	AD > AR	*PAX3*	Depigmentation of the skin and/or hair, congenital deafness, heterochromia iridis, synophrys, broad nasal root, dystopia canthorum.	To remember common gene(s) implicated in each WS type, remember the phrase, "*Pack* (*PAX3*) your *mittens* (*MITF*), *pack* (*PAX3*) your *socks* (*SOX10*)."
		2		*MITF, SNAI2, SOX10*	Similar to WS1 without dystopia canthorum and increased rate of deafness.	
		3		*PAX3*	Similar to WS1 with upper limb abnormalities.	
		4		*EDN3, EDNRB, SOX10*	Similar to WS1 with Hirschsprung disease.	

(Continued)

Table 2.13. HEREDITARY PIGMENTARY DISORDERS (CONTINUED)

Category	Diagnosis[a]	Type	Inheritance pattern	Gene(s)	Classic Description	Notes
Diffuse	OCA	1A	AR	*TYR* encoding tyrosinase	White skin and hair, blue-gray eyes, amelanotic nevi, photosensitivity, and ocular manifestations (eg, photophobia, reduced visual acuity, strabismus, nystagmus, lack of binocular vision).	OCA has normal melanocyte number but reduced or absent melanin. OCA1A corresponds to tyrosinase-negative albinism (absent melanin). Increased risk of skin cancer (eg, SCC).
		1B		*TYR* encoding tyrosinase	Little to no pigment at birth, some pigmentation in first and second decades (may be temperature sensitive), amelanotic or pigmented nevi.	OCA1B corresponds to yellow albinism. Temperature-sensitive tyrosinase activity in OCA1B (active only in colder areas of the body) is akin to the Siamese cat phenotype.
		2		*P* gene	Minimal to moderate pigmentary dilution, pigmented nevi.	OCA2 corresponds to tyrosinase-positive albinism. Most common in individuals of African descent. Responsible for hypopigmentation in Prader-Willi syndrome or Angelman syndrome.
		3		*TYRP1* encoding tyrosinase-related protein 1	Red-bronze skin color, ginger-red hair, blue or brown irides.	OCA3 corresponds to rufous > brown albinism.
		4		*SLC45A2* encoding solute carrier family 45 member 2	Variable pigmentary dilution.	Most common in Japan.
	HPS	10 types	AR	*BLOC1/2/3* encoding biogenesis of lysosome-related organelles complexes 1-3 except for *AP3B1* in HPS2 and *AP3D1* in HPS10, which encode AP-3 complex β3A and δ1 subunits	Pigmentary dilution (skin/hair/eyes), bleeding diathesis, IPF (premature death), granulomatous cheilitis ± renal failure, cardiomyopathy. Immunodeficiency (HPS2, HPS10). Neurologic dysfunction (HPS10).	HPS is a ceroid lysosomal storage disease characterized by absence of dense bodies within platelets. Most common in Puerto Rico. HPS is most common in Puerto Rico.
	CHS	N/A	AR	*LYST* encoding lysosomal trafficking regulator	Pigmentary dilution (skin/silvery hair/eyes), bleeding diathesis, immunodeficiency, neurologic dysfunction. 85% develop HLH (accelerated phase).	CHS is characterized by giant lysosome-related organelles (melanosomes—evenly distributed, neutrophil granules, platelet dense granules). Consider HSCT.

Table 2.13. HEREDITARY PIGMENTARY DISORDERS (CONTINUED)

Category	Diagnosis[a]	Type	Inheritance pattern	Gene(s)	Classic Description	Notes
	GS	1	AR	*MYO5A* encoding myosin 5A	Pigmentary dilution (skin/silvery hair), neurologic dysfunction.	GS is characterized by pigment clumping within melanocytes. To distinguish CHS from GS, perform hair shaft microscopy and a peripheral smear. Elejalde syndrome is a GS1 variant. Consider HSCT for GS2.
		2		*RAB27A* encoding a small Ras-like GTPase	Pigmentary dilution (skin/silvery hair), immunodeficiency. HLH (accelerated phase) may occur.	
		3		*MLPH* encoding melanophilin	Pigmentary dilution (skin/silvery hair).	
Guttate	TSC	See Chapter 5: Fibrous Neoplasms.				
Linear	Linear nevoid hypopigmentation/ hypomelanosis of Ito	N/A	Sporadic	N/A	Unilateral or bilateral hypopigmented streaks and whorls along lines of Blaschko. Hypomelanosis of Ito is associated with CNS, eye (eg, strabismus, hypertelorism), tooth, and/or musculoskeletal abnormalities.	Pigmentary mosaicism.
	IP (stage 4)	See above.				
	Goltz syndrome (focal dermal hypoplasia)	N/A	XLD	*PORCN* (porcupine gene family, Wnt pathway)	Cribriform linear atrophy along lines of Blaschko with fat herniation/ telangiectasias/hypopigmentation/ hyperpigmentation, perioral/ anogenital papillomas, and bone (eg, osteopathia striata), eye (eg, coloboma), face, hair, limb (eg, ectrodactyly), nail, and tooth abnormalities.	Lethal in males (unless mosaic); variable phenotype in females due to lyonization. To distinguish IP from Goltz syndrome, look for vesicles. Note that vestibular papillomatosis is a normal finding.
					Papillomas in Goltz syndrome are "raspberry-like."	
	Nevus depigmentosus	N/A	Sporadic	N/A	Hypopigmented patch that may or may not follow lines of Blaschko.	The block-like variant of nevus depigmentosus is synonymous with the hypopigmented form of segmental pigmentation disorder.

Hyperpigmentation

Category	Diagnosis[a]	Type	Inheritance pattern	Gene(s)	Classic Description	Notes
Circumscribed	Segmental pigmentation disorder	N/A	Sporadic	N/A	Block-like pattern of hyperpigmentation > hypopigmentation.	Pigmentary mosaicism.
Diffuse	Familial progressive hyperpigmentation	N/A	AD	*KITLG* encoding KIT ligand	Hyperpigmented patches develop during infancy and increase in size, number, and confluence with age.	Gain-of-function mutation.
	FA	See Chapter 4: Photodermatoses.				
Linear	Linear and whorled nevoid hypermelanosis	N/A	Sporadic	N/A	Unilateral or bilateral hyperpigmented streaks and whorls along lines of Blaschko. 10%-25% associated with CNS, musculoskeletal, and/or cardiac abnormalities.	Pigmentary mosaicism.
	IP (stage 3)	See above.				

(Continued)

Table 2.13. HEREDITARY PIGMENTARY DISORDERS (CONTINUED)

Category	Diagnosis[a]	Type	Inheritance pattern	Gene(s)	Classic Description	Notes
Reticulated	DKC	See Chapter 4: Photodermatoses.				
	NFJ syndrome	N/A	AD	*KRT14* encoding K14	Reticulated hyperpigmentation, ectodermal dysplasia with hypohidrosis and dental anomalies, and PPK.	Ectodermal dysplasias. Reticulated hyperpigmentation improves during adolescence in patients with NFJ syndrome but persists in patients with DPR. Both conditions can lead to hypoplastic or absent dermatoglyphs.
	DPR	N/A	AD		Reticulated hyperpigmentation, nonscarring alopecia, nail hypoplasia, and punctate PPK.	
	X-linked reticulate pigmentary disorder	N/A	XLD	*POLA1* encoding DNA polymerase α catalytic subunit	Reticulated hyperpigmentation, recurrent infections (males), dermal amyloid deposits.	Reticulated hyperpigmentation is generalized in males and follows lines of Blaschko in females.
	DDD	N/A	AD	*KRT5* encoding K5 (most common)	Reticulated hyperpigmentation favoring flexural sites, pitted scars on face, and comedone-like lesions on neck and back.	Galli-Galli disease is a DDD variant with prominent suprabasal non-dyskeratotic acantholysis on histopathology. Haber syndrome is a DDD variant with comedones and rosacea-like facial erythema.

Dyschromatosis

Category	Diagnosis[a]	Type	Inheritance pattern	Gene(s)	Classic Description	Notes
N/A	DSH (acropigmentation of Dohi)	N/A	AD	*ADAR (DSRAD)* encoding dsRNA adenosine deaminase	Hypo- and hyperpigmented macules favoring dorsal distal extremities.	
	DUH	N/A	AD > AR	*ABCB6* encoding ATP-binding cassette transporter protein (most common)	Generalized hypo- and hyperpigmented macules.	

AD, autosomal dominant; AP-3, activator protein-3; AR, autosomal recessive; CHS, Chédiak-Higashi syndrome; CNS, central nervous system; DDD, Dowling-Degos disease; DKC, dyskeratosis congenita; DNA, deoxyribonucleic acid; DPR, dermatopathia pigmentosa reticularis; ds, double-stranded; DSH, dyschromatosis symmetrica hereditaria; DUH, dyschromatosis universalis hereditaria; EBS, epidermolysis bullosa simplex; FA, Fanconi anemia; GS, Griscelli syndrome; HLH, hemophagocytic lymphohistiocytosis; HPS, Hermansky-Pudlak syndrome; HSCT, hematopoietic stem cell transplantation; IP, incontinentia pigmenti; IPF, interstitial pulmonary fibrosis; K, keratin; N/A, not applicable; NFJ, Naegeli-Franceschetti-Jadassohn; OCA, oculocutaneous albinism; PPK, palmoplantar keratoderma; RNA, ribonucleic acid; SCC, squamous cell carcinoma; TSC, tuberous sclerosis complex; WS, Waardenburg syndrome; XLD, X-linked dominant.
[a]Illustrative examples provided.

Vesiculobullous Disorders

Basic Concepts

- **Vesiculobullous disorders** are often categorized according to the level at which the split occurs in the skin: **subcorneal, intraepidermal, and/or subepidermal.**
- Pathogenetic mechanisms include autoimmune, drug-induced, and genetic disorders. Edema (see Chapter 2: Livedo Reticularis, Purpura, and Other Vascular Disorders) and physical agents (see Chapter 4: Other Physical Agents) may also lead to blister formation.
- A variety of techniques are available for the diagnosis of autoimmune blistering disorders. The optimal approach for obtaining biopsy specimens is as follows:
  - **Biopsy a fresh vesicle or edematous papule.** Otherwise, **biopsy the edge of a fresh vesicle or bulla including the inflammatory rim.** In pemphigus, a Tzanck smear may be helpful to reveal acantholytic epidermal cells within the blister cavity but cannot substitute for a biopsy.
  - **Direct immunofluorescence (DIF) is the most reliable and sensitive diagnostic test.** To avoid negative staining due to secondary degeneration of target antigens and immunoreactants, **biopsy for DIF should be perilesional in pemphigus and pemphigoid and should sample adjacent normal skin in dermatitis herpetiformis (DH).**

ACUTE GENERALIZED EXANTHEMATOUS PUSTULOSIS

→ Diagnosis Group 2

Synonym: pustular drug eruption

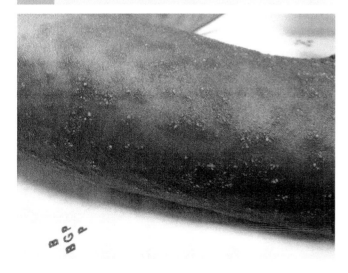

Epidemiology

- AGEP may be classified as a **delayed-type, cell-mediated (type IV) severe cutaneous adverse reaction (SCAR).** The hypothesized mechanism is neutrophil and T-cell activation leading to release of chemokines such as CXC chemokine ligand 8 (CXCL8) and cytokines such as granulocyte-monocyte colony stimulating factor (GM-CSF).
- Drug associations include **β-lactams, macrolides, ICIs, and CCBs (eg, diltiazem).** Other triggers include **iodinated radiocontrast media, mercury,** peritoneal dialysate, and enteroviral infection.
  - Urticaria after iodinated radiocontrast media is immediate, while reactions delayed 1 hour to 1 week include AGEP, SDRIFE, morbilliform drug eruption/DRESS, and iododerma.

Clinicopathological Features

- AGEP characteristically presents with **erythema studded with numerous, nonfollicular, sterile pustules** that starts on the **face and/or intertriginous zones. Edema of the face and hands** may be present, and patients may exhibit **fever, neutrophilia, and hypocalcemia.** Pustules resolve with pinpoint desquamation.
- The timing of AGEP relative to initial drug exposure is typically **<4 days.**
  - Acute generalized exanthematous pustulosis.
- AGEP may present with multiorgan involvement (liver > kidney > lung) in a minority of patients.
  - Figure 2.21.

Evaluation

- The differential diagnosis for the pustules of AGEP is similar to pustular psoriasis.
  - In neonates, the differential diagnosis for sterile pustules includes transient neonatal pustular melanosis and erythema toxicum neonatorum (Table 2.14).
  - Transient neonatal pustular melanosis is characterized by subcorneal pustules with neutrophils > eosinophils.
  - Erythema toxicum neonatorum is characterized by intrafollicular, subcorneal, or intraepidermal pustules with eosinophils > neutrophils.
- The differential diagnosis for the confluent erythema of AGEP includes other drug reactions, acute graft-versus-host disease (GVHD), Kawasaki disease, and infections (eg, toxic shock syndrome).
  - Table 2.15.
- The EuroSCAR validation score categorizes cases as definite, probable, possible, or no AGEP.

Management

- AGEP has a 1% to 2% reported mortality rate (controversial).
- **Discontinuation of the suspected drug** along with all nonessential drugs is the first step. *In-vitro* assays to establish the culprit drug are under investigation. However, given uncertain sensitivity and specificity, their utility remains limited in clinical practice. **50% to 60% of patients are patch test positive.** While AGEP is drug associated in 70% to 90% of cases, it is important to consider alternative etiologies.
- **Topical corticosteroids** are first line.

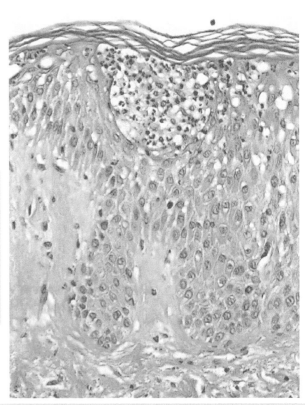

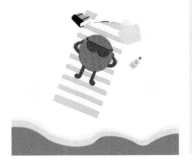

The presence of eosinophils with bilobed nuclei resembling "sunglasses" helps distinguish AGEP from pustular psoriasis.

Figure 2.21. CLINICOPATHOLOGICAL CORRELATION: ACUTE GENERALIZED EXANTHEMATOUS PUSTULOSIS. Characteristic features are subcorneal or superficial epidermal pustules, mild spongiosis, papillary dermal edema, and a superficial mixed infiltrate with neutrophils and eosinophils. AGEP, acute generalized exanthematous pustulosis.

(Histology image reprinted with permission from Elder DE, Elenitsas R, Rosenbach M, et al. *Lever's Histopathology of the Skin.* 11th ed. Wolters Kluwer; 2015.) (Illustration by Caroline A. Nelson, MD.)

Table 2.14. TRANSIENT NEONATAL PUSTULAR MELANOSIS AND ERYTHEMA TOXICUM NEONATORUM

Characteristic	Transient Neonatal Pustular Melanosis	Erythema Toxicum Neonatorum
Epidemiology	Term infants (favors infants with darkly pigmented skin, ~5%). Onset at birth.	Term infants (~50%). Onset typically 24-48 hours after birth.
Classic description	Pustules without erythema, collarettes of scale, hyperpigmented macules.	Blotchy erythematous macules, papules, pustules > vesicles, wheals sparing the palms and soles.
Smear (Wright stain)	Neutrophils > eosinophils.	Eosinophils > neutrophils.
		The pustules in E tox are riddled with eosinophils on Wright stain.
Management	Observation.	

Table 2.15. DIFFERENTIATING SELECTED DRUG REACTIONS

Drug Reaction	Morphology and Distribution	Timing (Relative to Initial Drug Exposure)	Systemic Involvement	Drugs[a]
AGEP	Erythema studded with numerous, nonfollicular, sterile pustules that starts on the face and/or intertriginous zones, edema	<4 days	Fever, neutrophilia, hypocalcemia, and liver > kidney > lung involvement (minority)	β-lactams, macrolides, ICIs, CCBs
SJS/TEN	Dusky and/or dusky-red macules with epidermal detachment and erosions, macular atypical targets, and bullous lesions favoring the face and trunk; + Nikolsky sign; + Asboe-Hansen sign	7-21 days	Fever, lymphadenopathy, cytopenias, hepatitis, and cholestasis TFN: nephritis	Dapsone, rituximab, NNRTIs, sulfonamides, bortezomib,[b] ICIs,[b] allopurinol, aromatic anticonvulsants including lamotrigine, NSAIDs
FDE	Round to oval, sharply demarcated, erythematous and edematous plaques with variable duskiness and blister formation favoring the face, genitalia, hands and feet, lips, anogenital mucosa	7-14 days (reexposure < 24 hours)	Rare	Dapsone, sulfonamides, tetracyclines, antimicrotubule taxanes (bullous), NSAIDs, pseudoephedrine (nonpigmenting)
Urticaria	Transient, often pruritic, erythematous edematous wheals	Minutes to hours	*Anaphylaxis*: swelling of the oropharynx, larynx, epiglottis, and intestinal wall; tachycardia; hypotension	*Immunologic*: monoclonal antibodies, IVIG, β-lactams, platinum alkylating agents *Nonimmunologic*: polymyxin B, atracurium/mivacurium, opiates, thiopental, NSAIDs, ACEIs
Morbilliform drug eruption	Symmetrically distributed, often pruritic, erythematous macules, papules and/or urticarial lesions that start on the trunk and upper extremities	4-14 days	Low grade fever, peripheral hypereosinophilia	Antimalarials, NRTIs/NtRTIs, NNRTIs, β-lactams, sulfonamides, minocycline, BCR-ABL/Kit/PDGFR inhibitors, BRAF inhibitors, MEK 1/2 inhibitors, ICIs, allopurinol, aromatic anticonvulsants
DRESS	Morbilliform drug eruption, edema	15-40 days	Fever, lymphadenopathy, atypical lymphocytosis, peripheral hypereosinophilia, and muscle/heart, liver, pancreas, kidney, lung, and other organ involvement	Azathioprine, dapsone, NRTIs/NtRTIs, NNRTIs, sulfonamides, minocycline, vancomycin, ICIs, allopurinol, aromatic anticonvulsants including lamotrigine

ACEIs, angiotensin-converting enzyme inhibitors; AGEP, acute generalized exanthematous pustulosis; CCBs, calcium channel blockers; DRESS, drug reaction with eosinophilia and systemic symptoms; FDE, fixed drug eruption; Kit/BCR-ABL, kinase receptor/breakpoint cluster region-Abelson; ICIs, immune checkpoint inhibitors; IVIG, intravenous immunoglobulin; MEK, mitogen-activated protein kinase; NNRTIs, nonnucleoside reverse transcriptase inhibitors; NRTIs, nucleoside reverse transcriptase inhibitors; NSAIDs, nonsteroidal anti-inflammatory drugs; NtRTIs, nucleotide reverse transcriptase inhibitors; PDGFR, platelet-derived growth factor receptor; SJS/TEN, Stevens-Johnson syndrome/toxic epidermal necrolysis

[a]Illustrative examples provided.
[b]SJS/TEN-like eruptions.

"Real World" Advice

- The presence of confluent pustules mimicking Nikolsky sign (see below) and desquamation in AGEP often prompts dermatology consultation to "rule out Stevens-Johnson syndrome (SJS)/toxic epidermal necrolysis (TEN)." The key distinguishing feature is the superficial split in AGEP, which can be demonstrated by skin biopsy, if necessary.
- Facial edema is a helpful diagnostic clue in both AGEP and DRESS.

PEMPHIGUS FOLIACEUS

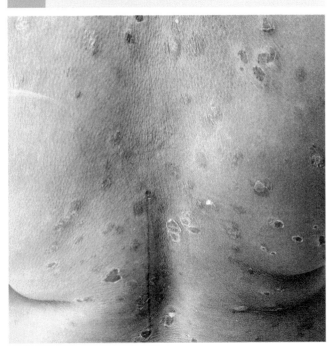

- PF is characterized by circulating autoantibodies to **desmoglein 1. Jewish ancestry** is a risk factor. Drug associations include **ACEIs and D-penicillamine (PF > PV). Fogo selvagem** is an **endemic** form of PF in **rural Brazil** that may be transmitted by the **black fly (genus *Simulium*).**
  - ◈ Fogo selvagem <u>simul</u>ates PF (transmitted by <u>Simul</u>*ium*). Mutation of desmoglein 1 leads to striate PPK and toxin-mediated cleavage of desmoglein 1 occurs in bullous impetigo and SSSS.
- The classic presentation of PF is **scaly crusted erosions favoring a seborrheic distribution.** The lack of mucosal involvement in PF may be explained by the **desmoglein compensation theory** (Figure 2.22). **Pemphigus erythematosus (Senear-Usher syndrome)** is a **localized** PF variant, most notably on the **malar region of the face** that may **overlap with LE. Pemphigus herpetiformis** is a PF variant that classically presents with **herpetiform erythematous urticarial plaques and tense vesicles.**
  - ◈ The scaly crusted erosions of PF have been described as "corn flakes" pasted to the skin.
  - ◈ Figure 2.23.
- Obtain **biopsies for hematoxylin and eosin (H&E) and perilesional DIF.** To optimize sensitivity, **indirect immunofluorescence (IIF)** may be performed on human skin and **guinea pig esophagus. Enzyme-linked immunosorbent assay (ELISA)** can detect circulating autoantibodies to **desmoglein 1.**
- Untreated PF rarely results in death with the exception of **fogo selvagem, which has a 40% mortality rate within 2 years. Topical corticosteroids** are first line for localized PF. Management of generalized PF is similar to PV.

PEMPHIGUS VULGARIS
→ Diagnosis Group 2

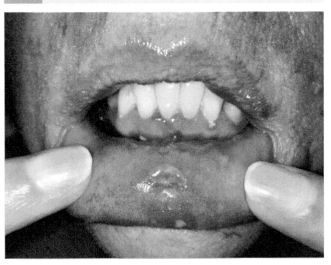

Courtesy of Erin Wei, MD.

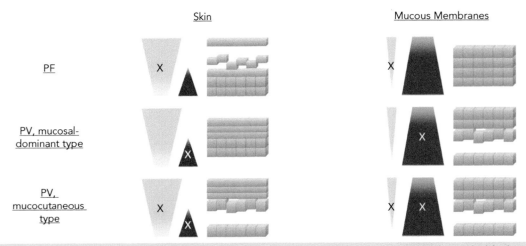

Figure 2.22. THE DESMOGLEIN COMPENSATION THEORY. The desmoglein compensation theory holds that desmoglein 1 and 3 compensate for each other when coexpressed in the same cell. The distribution of desmoglein 1 (light blue) and desmoglein 3 (dark blue) in the skin and mucous membranes explains the distribution of pemphigus lesions. PF, pemphigus foliaceus; PV, pemphigus vulgaris.

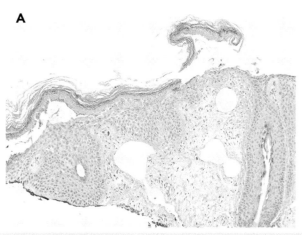
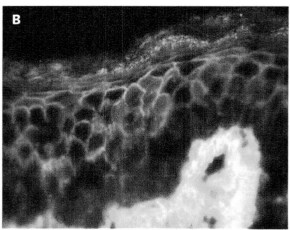

Figure 2.23. CLINICOPATHOLOGICAL CORRELATION: PEMPHIGUS FOLIACEUS. Characteristic features are a subcorneal split with acantholysis. Dyskeratosis may be present in the granular layer. Neutrophils and occasional eosinophils may be present in the blister cavity. DIF classically demonstrates intercellular deposition of IgG and C3 between keratinocytes in the upper epidermis. A, H&E. B, DIF (IgG). C, complement; DEJ, dermal-epidermal junction; DIF, direct immunofluorescence; GPCs, Gram-positive cocci; Ig, immunoglobulin; LE, lupus erythematosus; PF, pemphigus foliaceous; SSSS, staphylococcal scalded skin syndrome.

(Histology image courtesy of Noel Turner, MD, MHS and Christine J. Ko, MD.) B, DIF (IgG) (Histology image reprinted with permission from Elder DE, Elenitsas R, Rosenbach M, et al. *Lever's Histopathology of the Skin*. 11th ed. Wolters Kluwer; 2015.)

> Acantholytic cells on the blister roof ("cling ons") provide a helpful diagnostic clue.
> The DIF pattern has been described as "chicken wire," "lace-like," or "net-like."

- **Pemphigus erythematosus variant**: resembles PF. When pemphigus erythematosus overlaps with LE, DIF classically demonstrates granular deposition of IgM, IgG, IgA, and C3 along the DEJ.
- **Pemphigus herpetiformis variant**: eosinophilic spongiosis and subcorneal pustules with minimal to no acantholysis.

> PF can NOT be distinguished from bullous impetigo or SSSS on histopathology. GPCs may be evident in bullous impetigo. DIF is positive in PF and negative in bullous impetigo and SSSS.

Epidemiology

- PV is characterized by circulating autoantibodies to **desmoglein 3 (mucosal dominant type, ~50% of cases) or desmogleins 1 and 3 (mucocutaneous type, ~50% of cases).**

  > The desmoglein compensation theory explains why neonates manifest PV (30%-45%) but rarely manifest PF. Maternal IgG autoantibodies cross the placenta in both disorders; however, desmoglein 3 is distributed throughout neonatal skin (similar to the mucous membranes), compensating for desmoglein 1.

- **Jewish ancestry** is a risk factor.
- Drug associations include **ACEIs and D-penicillamine (PF > PV).**
- **HLA** associations include -DR4 and -DR6.

Clinicopathological Features

- PV presents on the **oral mucosa in 70% to 90%** of patients, with **painful erosions that favor the buccal and palatine mucosa.** When the gingiva is involved, patients present with **desquamative gingivitis.** The lack of skin involvement in mucosal-dominant PV may be explained by the **desmoglein compensation theory.**

- PV on the skin is characterized by **flaccid blisters that rupture to form painful crusted erosions that ooze and bleed.** PV heals with pigmentary changes but **not scarring.**
- Lack of cohesion within the epidermis may be demonstrated by the **Nikolsky sign (lateral movement of the upper epidermis with slight pressure or rubbing)** and the **Asboe-Hansen sign (spread of fluid under the skin with gentle pressure on an intact bulla).**
- **Pemphigus herpetiformis** may rarely present as a PV variant.
- **Pemphigus vegetans** is a PV variant that classically presents with flaccid pustules that become erosions and then form **vegetating papillomatous plaques favoring intertriginous areas,** the scalp, and the face. It is divided into the **Neumann type (severe)** and the **Hallopeau type (mild).**
  - Figure 2.24.

Evaluation

- The differential diagnosis for mucosal PV includes mucous membrane pemphigoid (MMP), LP, EM or SJS/TEN, SLE, aphthous stomatitis, and acute herpetic stomatitis. Desquamative gingivitis must be distinguished from necrotizing ulcerative gingivitis caused by bacteria belonging to the normal oral flora.
- The differential diagnosis for cutaneous PV includes other forms of pemphigus, Hailey-Hailey disease, BP, linear IgA bullous dermatosis (LABD), EM or SJS/TEN, and Grover disease (GD).

A

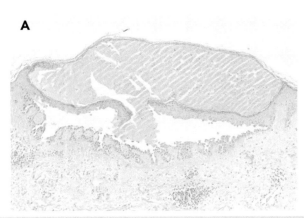

B

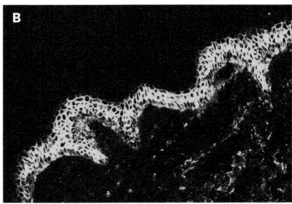

Figure 2.24. CLINICOPATHOLOGICAL CORRELATION: PEMPHIGUS VULGARIS. Characteristic features are a suprabasal split with acantholysis tracking down adnexal structures. Eosinophils may be present in the blister cavity and the dermis alongside lymphocytes. DIF classically demonstrates intercellular deposition of IgG and C3 between keratinocytes in the lower epidermis. A, H&E. B, DIF (IgG). C, complement; DIF, direct immunofluorescence; H&E, hematoxylin & eosin; Ig, immunoglobulin; PEH, pseudoepitheliomatous hyperplasia.

(A, Histology image courtesy of Noel Turner, MD, MHS and Christine J. Ko, MD. B, Histology image courtesy of Kim B. Yancey, MD. From Gru AA, Wick MR, Mir A, et al. *Pediatric Dermatopathology and Dermatology*. Wolters Kluwer; 2018.)

> The row of cells ("tombstones") covering dermal papillae ("villi") provides a helpful diagnostic clue.
> The DIF pattern has been described as "chicken wire," "lace-like," or "net-like."

- **Pemphigus herpetiformis variant**: eosinophilic spongiosis and subcorneal pustules with minimal to no acantholysis.
- **Pemphigus vegetans variant**: suprabasal acantholysis, acanthosis, papillomatosis, PEH with intraepidermal pustules, and an eosinophil-rich inflammatory infiltrate.

- Obtain **biopsies for H&E and perilesional DIF.** To optimize sensitivity, **IIF** may be performed on **monkey esophagus. ELISA** can detect circulating autoantibodies to **desmogleins 1 and 3.**
  - The monkey is vulgar (IIF on monkey esophagus in pemphigus vulgaris).

Management

- Untreated PV has a **poor prognosis,** resulting in death within 2 to 5 years due to loss of body fluids or to secondary bacterial infections.
- **Systemic corticosteroids** are first line. **Rituximab** may be given 375 mg/m^2 once weekly for 4 weeks ("lymphoma dosing") or 1 g initially then at 2 weeks ("rheumatoid arthritis dosing"). Other steroid-sparing therapies include azathioprine, IVIG, methotrexate, mycophenolate mofetil, and plasmapheresis or extracorporeal photopheresis (ECP).
- Pemphigus Disease Area Index (PDAI) and Autoimmune Bullous Skin Disorder Intensity Score (ABSIS) are commonly used indices for disease activity. **Autoantibody levels often correlate with disease activity** and are therefore useful for **assessing response to treatment and predicting flares or relapses** before they are clinically evident.

"Real World" Advice

- Rituximab resistance can develop due to genetic polymorphisms (*FCGR3A*) or human antichimeric antibodies against its murine fragment that prevent binding to B cells. There are no commercially available tests; however, "lymphoma dosing" optimizes B-cell depletion by increasing serum levels.

- Look out for novel therapies coming down the pipeline for PV, such as the use of chimeric autoantibody receptor (CAR) T cells to eliminate desmoglein-specific B cells.

IMMUNOGLOBULIN A PEMPHIGUS

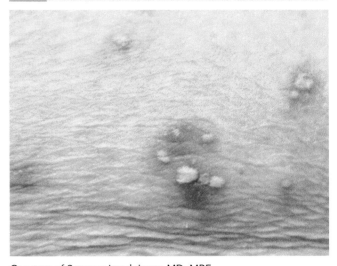

Courtesy of Sotonye Imadojemu, MD, MBE.

- IgA pemphigus typically occurs in **middle-age or elderly** persons. It may be divided into the **SPD type** and the **intraepidermal neutrophilic (IEN) type.** The SPD type is characterized by circulating autoantibodies to **desmocollin 1**, while the antigen in the IEN type has not been fully characterized. Associations include **ulcerative colitis and IgA monoclonal gammopathy.**

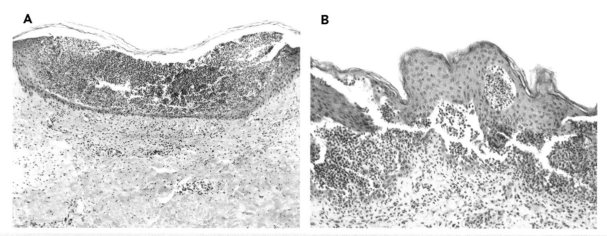

Figure 2.25. CLINICOPATHOLOGICAL CORRELATION: IgA PEMPHIGUS. IgA pemphigus is characterized by the formation of intraepidermal pustules. Acantholysis is rarely present. DIF classically demonstrates intercellular deposition of IgA between keratinocytes. A, Subcorneal pustular dermatosis subtype. B, Intraepidermal neutrophilic subtype. DIF, direct immunofluorescence; Ig, immunoglobulin.

(A, Histology image reprinted with permission from Elder DE, Elenitsas R, Rosenbach M, et al. *Lever's Histopathology of the Skin*. 11th ed. Wolters Kluwer; 2015. B, Histology image reprinted with permission from Gru AA, Wick MR, Mir A, et al. *Pediatric Dermatopathology and Dermatology*. Wolters Kluwer; 2018.)

- **Subcorneal pustular dermatosis variant**: pustules in the upper epidermis.
- **Intraepidermal neutrophilic variant**: pustules in the lower epidermis.

- The classic presentation of IgA pemphigus is **flaccid blisters or pustules in an annular or circinate pattern favoring intertriginous areas.**
  - The configuration of the IEN type has been likened to a "sunflower."
  - Figure 2.25.
- Immunofluorescence studies are required to distinguish the SPD type from classic SPD (Sneddon-Wilkinson disease).
- **Dapsone** is first line.

PARANEOPLASTIC PEMPHIGUS

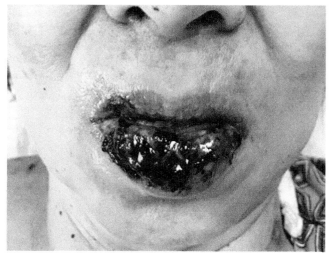

Courtesy of Sotonye Imadojemu, MD, MBE.

- Paraneoplastic pemphigus (PNP) is characterized by circulating autoantibodies to **desmoglein 1 and 3** along with a diverse array of antigens including **desmocollins,** members of the **plakin family** (BPAG1, desmoplakins I and II, envoplakin, epiplakin, periplakin, plectin), **plakophilin,** and the protease inhibitor **alpha-2-macroglobulin-like 1.** The pathogenesis of PNP involves **both humoral autoimmunity and cell-mediated cytotoxicity,** explaining its polymorphic and refractory presentation. In adults, the most common association is **non-Hodgkin lymphoma (NHL).** Other associations include **Castleman disease, chronic lymphocytic leukemia (CLL), and thymoma.** Drug associations include **rituximab, bendamustine, and fludarabine.**
  - Castleman disease is the most common association with PNP in children and adolescents.
- The classic presentation of PNP is **intractable stomatitis, often involving the entire oropharynx and extending on to the vermillion lip. Pseudomembranous conjunctivitis may lead to blindness,** and all mucosal surfaces may be affected. Skin lesions are **polymorphic** (erythematous macules, flaccid blisters and erosions, tense blisters, EM-like lesions, and **lichenoid eruptions). Bronchiolitis obliterans may lead to respiratory failure.**
  - Figure 2.26.
- Obtain biopsies for H&E and perilesional DIF. To optimize sensitivity, **IIF** may be performed on guinea pig esophagus, monkey esophagus, and **rat bladder** (antiplakin). **ELISA** can detect circulating autoantibodies to **desmogleins 1 and 3, BPAG1, envoplakin, and periplakin.** To evaluate for bronchiolitis obliterans, it is important to obtain **pulmonary function tests (PFTs),** as chest x-ray (CXR) and computed tomography (CT) chest may be normal.
- PNP has a **90% mortality rate.** Unfortunately, PNP is often **refractory** to treatment of the associated neoplasm. **Benign neoplasms such as localized Castleman disease or thymomas should be excised.** Management of PNP is similar to PV with the addition of therapies directed against cell-mediated cytotoxicity such as alemtuzumab.

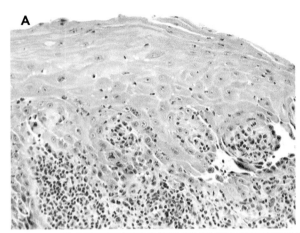

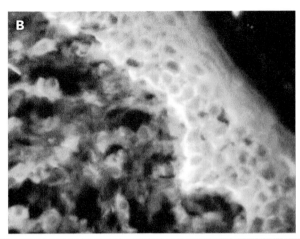

Figure 2.26. CLINICOPATHOLOGICAL CORRELATION: PARANEOPLASTIC PEMPHIGUS. PNP exhibits a combination of PV-like, LP-like, or EM-like patterns. DIF classically demonstrates intercellular deposition of IgG and C3 between keratinocytes, primarily in the lower epidermis, and linear deposition of IgG and C3 along the DEJ. A, H&E (lichen planus–like pattern). B, DIF (IgG). C, complement; DEJ, dermal-epidermal junction; DIF, direct immunofluorescence; EM, erythema multiforme; H&E, hematoxylin and eosin; Ig, immunoglobulin; LP, lichen planus; PNP, paraneoplastic pemphigus; PV, pemphigus vulgaris.

(Histology images reprinted with permission from Elder DE, Elenitsas R, Rosenbach M, et al. *Lever's Histopathology of the Skin*. 11th ed. Wolters Kluwer; 2015.)

SPOTLIGHT ON HAILEY-HAILEY DISEASE AND DARIER DISEASE

Hailey-Hailey disease synonym: familial benign chronic pemphigus

Darier disease synonym: keratosis follicularis

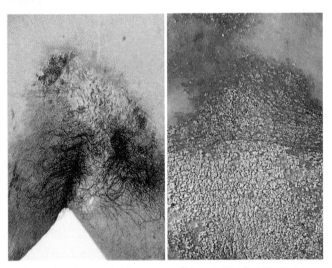

Hailey-Hailey disease (left) courtesy of Victoria Werth, MD. Darier disease (right).

- Hailey-Hailey disease and Darier disease are **AD** genetic disorders due to mutations in genes encoding **Ca²⁺ ATPase pumps.** Abnormal intracellular Ca²⁺ signaling leads to **impaired processing of junctional proteins**, resulting in **acantholytic dyskeratosis.**
  - Do NOT confuse <u>Darier</u> disease with the "<u>Darier</u> sign" of mastocytosis.
- **Hailey-Hailey disease and Darier disease** are compared and contrasted in Table 2.16.
  - Figure 2.27.
  - Figure 2.28.
- **Acrokeratosis verruciformis of Hopf** may clinically mimic Darier disease, with **warty papules favoring the dorsal hands and feet.**
- Common treatments include antimicrobial washes and ablative or surgical therapies. Additional treatments for Hailey-Hailey disease include local corticosteroids, naltrexone, and botulinum toxin, while additional treatments for Darier disease include keratolytic emollients and retinoids.

Table 2.16. HAILEY-HAILEY DISEASE AND DARIER DISEASE

Characteristic	Hailey-Hailey Disease	Darier Disease
Pathogenesis	*ATP2C1* mutation on 3q22.1 results in dysfunction of a Golgi-associated Ca^{2+} ATPase hSPCA1. It is important to see one Halley's Comet in a lifetime. Gene: *ATP2C1*.	*ATP2A2* mutation on 12q23 results in dysfunction of an endoplasmic reticulum Ca^{2+} ATPase SERCA2.
Epidemiology	Age of onset varies widely, but peaks in the second and third decades. Triggers include friction, heat, sweating, and UVR. Complications include secondary infections (eg, Kaposi varicelliform eruption) and SCC. Segmental variant.	Age of onset peaks during puberty. Triggers include friction, heat, sweating, and UVR. Associations include neuropsychiatric disorders (eg, epilepsy, intellectual impairment, mood disorders). Drug associations include lithium. Complications include secondary infections (eg, Kaposi varicelliform eruption) and SCC. Segmental variant.
Classic description	Malodorous pruritic flaccid blisters favoring intertriginous areas that rupture to form painful macerated or crusted erosions and heal without scarring; rare involvement of the mucosa; longitudinal leukonychia.	Malodorous pruritic keratotic and crusted red to brown papules favoring seborrheic (pityriasis amiantacea) and intertriginous areas, warty papules favoring the dorsal hands and feet, and pits on palms and soles; cobblestoning of the oral and anogenital mucosa; longitudinal erythronychia and longitudinal leukonychia with "V-shaped" nicking of the distal nail plate. Figure 2.27.

hSPCA, human secretory pathway Ca^{2+}/Mn^{2+} ATPase; SCC, squamous cell carcinoma; SERCA, sarco(endo)plasmic reticulum Ca^{2+} ATPase; UVR, ultraviolet radiation.

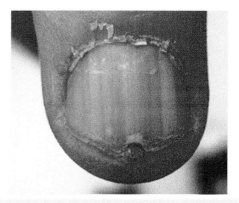

Figure 2.27. CANDY CANE NAILS. Darier disease is characterized by longitudinal erythronychia and longitudinal leukonychia. These red and white bands are often referred to as "candy cane nails." "V-shaped" nicking of the distal nail plate is pathognomonic.

(Darier disease image reprinted with permission from Gru AA, Wick MR, Mir A, et al. *Pediatric Dermatopathology and Dermatology.* Wolters Kluwer; 2018.)

A

B

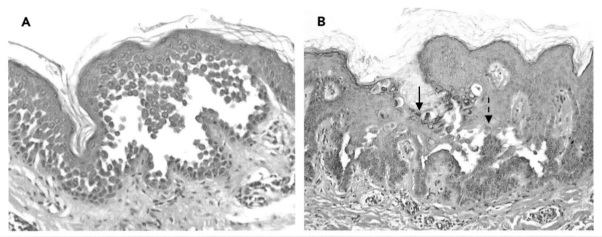

Figure 2.28. SIDE-BY-SIDE COMPARISON: HAILEY-HAILEY DISEASE AND DARIER DISEASE. Both Hailey-Hailey disease and Darier disease* are characterized by acantholytic dyskeratosis and a superficial perivascular lymphocytic infiltrate. Hailey-Hailey disease demonstrates acanthosis and acantholysis at all levels of the epidermis. Acantholysis in Darier disease is accentuated in the lower epidermis, forming suprabasal clefts. There is papillomatosis and hyperkeratosis. Grains classically occur in the *stratum corneum* and corps ronds classically occur in the *stratum spinosum*. A, Hailey-Hailey disease. B, Darier disease. Solid arrow: grain. Dashed arrow: *corps rond.*

(Histology image A reprinted with permission from Husain AN, Stocker JT, Dehner LP. *Stocker and Dehner's Pediatric Pathology.* 5th ed. Wolters Kluwer; 2021.)

Acantholysis in Hailey-Hailey disease resembles a "dilapidated brick wall."
Acrokeratosis verruciformis of Hopf is warty due to "church spire" hyperkeratosis, papillomatosis, and acanthosis.

GROVER DISEASE
Synonym: transient acantholytic dermatosis

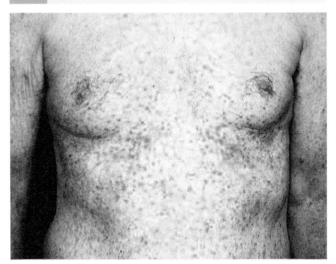

Reprinted with permission from Schalock PC, Hsu JTS, Arndt KA. *Lippincott's Primary Care Dermatology.* Wolters Kluwer Health/ Lippincott Williams & Wilkins; 2010.

- GD most often affects **older White men** with a peak onset in the **winter.** Triggers include heat, occlusion, sweating, UVR, and xerosis.
  - President <u>Grover</u> Cleveland was an <u>older White man.</u>
- GD classically presents with an **intensely pruritic papulovesicular eruption favoring the trunk.**

- Grover disease may exhibit a variety of patterns including PV-like, Hailey-Hailey disease–like, Darier disease–like, or spongiotic with minimal acantholysis.
- GD is typically **self-limited** over weeks to months but may persist for years. First-line therapies include emollients, topical corticosteroids, topical vitamin D analogues, and oral antihistamines.
  - <u>Transient</u> acantholytic dermatosis.

BULLOUS PEMPHIGOID
→ Diagnosis Group 2

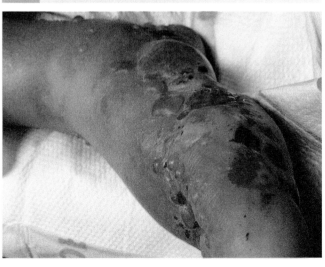

Epidemiology

- BP is characterized by circulating autoantibodies to **BPAG1 and BPAG2 (NC16A domain)**.
- **Advanced age (>60 years old) and male sex** are risk factors: **the relative risk of BP in patients over 90 years old is ~300-fold higher than in patients 60 years old or younger.**
- BP is commonly associated with **neurological disorders (eg, Parkinson disease)**.
- While reported drug associations include β-lactams, ACEIs, and diuretics (eg, furosemide), the most compelling evidence exists for **ICIs and dipeptidyl peptidase-4 (DPP-4) inhibitors.**

Clinicopathological Features

- BP is characterized by **tense blisters on apparently normal or erythematous skin** and annular or figurate urticarial and infiltrated papules and plaques favoring the flexural extremities and lower trunk. **10% to 30% of patients exhibit oral mucosal involvement.** BP heals with pigmentary changes and occasionally milia.

   Infantile and childhood BP classically presents with **acral bullae.**

- BP may be associated with **peripheral hypereosinophilia (~50%) and elevated IgE.**

- **Nonbullous** BP is a BP variant that classically presents with **intractable pruritus ± eczematous and/or fixed urticarial lesions** and often precedes the development of blisters (prodrome).
- **Pemphigoid vegetans** is a BP variant that classically presents with blisters that form **vegetating plaques favoring intertriginous areas.**
- Other clinical variants include dyshidrosiform pemphigoid, eczematous pemphigoid, erythrodermic pemphigoid, large erosive TEN-like lesions, papular pemphigoid, pemphigoid nodularis, and vesicular pemphigoid. Localized BP may also occur (eg, distal end of amputated limb, paralyzed limb, peristomal, pretibial, radiation therapy sites, umbilical, vulvar).
- BP may **overlap with LP in LP pemphigoides** (reactivity against **BPAG2**).
   ❖ Figure 2.29.

Evaluation

- The differential diagnosis for nonbullous BP includes eczematous dermatoses, urticarial dermatoses, prurigo nodularis, arthropod assault, and drug reactions.
- The differential diagnosis for bullous BP includes other **subepidermal autoimmune blistering disorders** (Table 2.17),

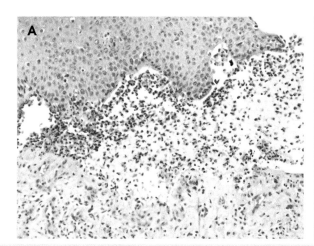 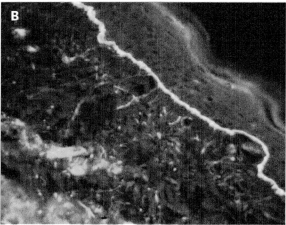

Figure 2.29. CLINICOPATHOLOGICAL CORRELATION: BULLOUS PEMPHIGOID. Characteristic features are a subepidermal split and a predominantly eosinophilic infiltrate. DIF classically demonstrates linear deposition of IgG and C3 along the DEJ in an *n-serrated* pattern. A, H&E. B, DIF (IgG). BP, bullous pemphigoid; C, complement; DEJ, dermal-epidermal junction; DH, dermatitis herpetiformis; DIF, direct immunofluorescence; EBA, epidermolysis bullosa acquisita; H&E, hematoxylin and eosin; Ig, immunoglobulin; LABD, linear IgA bullous dermatosis; MMP, mucous membrane pemphigoid; PCT, porphyria cutanea tarda; SJS/TEN, Stevens-Johnson syndrome/toxic epidermal necrolysis; SLE, systemic lupus erythematosus.

(Histology images reprinted with permission from Elder DE, Elenitsas R, Rosenbach M, et al. *Lever's Histopathology of the Skin.* 11th ed. Wolters Kluwer; 2015.)

- **Nonbullous variant**: eosinophilic spongiosis and/or dermal infiltrates.
- **Pemphigoid vegetans variant**: subepidermal split, epidermal hyperplasia, and an eosinophil-rich inflammatory infiltrate.

The intensity of inflammation can be a helpful clue to differentiate subepidermal blisters:
- Inflammatory: BP, LABD, MMP (variable), EBA (inflammatory variant), bullous SLE, DH
- Pauci-inflammatory: EBA (noninflammatory variant), SJS/TEN, PCT, pseudoporphyria
   In urticarial nonbullous BP, look for eosinophils "lined up" along the DEJ.

bullous eczematous dermatoses, SJS/TEN, PCT, pseudopor-phyria, bullous diabeticorum (tense acral blisters), and bul-lous arthropod assault.

- Obtain **biopsies for H&E and perilesional DIF.** To optimize sensitivity, **IIF** should be performed on **salt-split human skin** (epidermal ± dermal). **ELISA** can detect circulating autoantibodies to **BPAG1 and BPAG2.**
  - ◆ Figure 2.30.

Management

- **Systemic corticosteroids** are first line. **Potent topical corticosteroids have been shown to have equivalent efficacy, fewer adverse events, and reduced mortality.** The next step on the therapeutic ladder for mild and/or localized BP is the combination of **nicotinamide** (500-2000 mg/d) **with doxy-**cycline, minocycline, or tetracycline. Steroid-sparing therapies are similar to PV, with additions including **dapsone, dupilumab, and omalizumab.**

- The BP Disease Area Index (BPDAI) and daily blister count are commonly used indices for disease activity. **Autoantibody levels may correlate with disease activity**; however, this is not well established.

"Real World" Advice

- It is important to maintain a high level of suspicion for BP in older adults with unexplained generalized pruritus.
- Pemphigoid incipiens refers to the presence of circulating autoantibodies to BPAG1 and/or BPAG2 without a confirmatory DIF or IIF. A subset of these patients will eventually develop BP.

Table 2.17. SUBEPIDERMAL AUTOIMMUNE BLISTERING DISORDERS

Diagnosis[a]	Classic Description	Notes
BP[b]	See above	
Pemphigoid gestationis	Presents in late pregnancy or postpartum with BP-like skin lesions involving the umbilicus. Commonly recurs with menstruation, OCPs, and subsequent pregnancies.	Characterized by circulating autoantibodies to BPAG2 (NC16A domain) (epidermal staining on IIF of salt-split human skin). Associations in addition to pregnancy include trophoblastic tumors (eg, choriocarcinoma). HLA associations include -DR3 and -DR4. Increased risk of maternal Graves disease. Increased risk of prematurity, SGA, and mild and transient skin lesions (~10%) in neonates. While antihistamines and topical corticosteroids are preferred, systemic corticosteroids (prednisolone) are often required.
Anti-p105 pemphigoid	Presents with extensive TEN or PV-like skin and mucosal lesions.	The antigen has not been fully characterized (dermal staining on IIF of salt-split human skin).
Anti-p200 pemphigoid	Presents with BP-like skin lesions but in a younger age group with significant acral and cephalic distribution and mucosal involvement.	Characterized by circulating autoantibodies to laminin γ1 (dermal staining on IIF of salt-split human skin).
LABD	See below.	
MMP	See below.	
EBA	See below.	
Bullous SLE	See Chapter 2: Interface Dermatoses and Other Connective Tissue Disorders.	

BP, bullous pemphigoid; BPAG2, bullous pemphigoid antigen 2; EBA, epidermolysis bullosa acquisita; HLA, human leukocyte antigen; IIF, indirect immunofluorescence; LABD, linear IgA bullous dermatosis; MMP; mucous membrane pemphigoid; OCP, oral contraceptive pill; PV, pemphigus vulgaris; SGA, small for gestational age; SLE, systemic lupus erythematosus; TEN, toxic epidermal necrolysis
[a]Illustrative examples provided.
[b]Four clinical criteria were reported to indicate a diagnosis of BP over other subepidermal autoimmune blistering disorders: (1) absence of skin atrophy; (2) absence of mucosal involvement; (3) absence of head and neck involvement; and (4) age greater than 70 years.

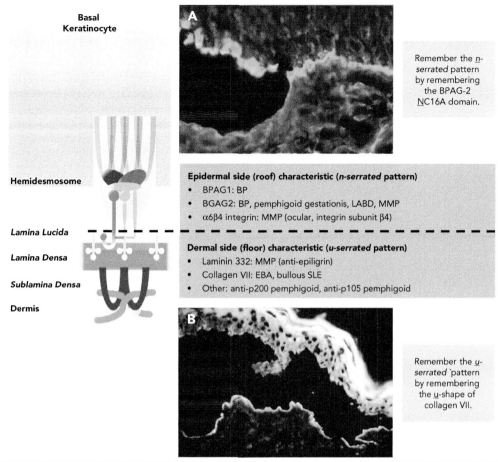

Basal
Keratinocyte

Remember the *n-serrated* pattern by remembering the BPAG-2 NC16A domain.

Hemidesmosome

Epidermal side (roof) characteristic (*n-serrated* pattern)
- BPAG1: BP
- BGAG2: BP, pemphigoid gestationis, LABD, MMP
- α6β4 integrin: MMP (ocular, integrin subunit β4)

Lamina Lucida

Lamina Densa

Dermal side (floor) characteristic (*u-serrated* pattern)
- Laminin 332: MMP (anti-epiligrin)
- Collagen VII: EBA, bullous SLE
- Other: anti-p200 pemphigoid, anti-p105 pemphigoid

Sublamina Densa

Dermis

Remember the *u-serrated* `pattern by remembering the *u*-shape of collagen VII.

Figure 2.30. THE SALT SPLIT-SKIN TECHNIQUE FOR DIFFERENTIATING SUBEPIDERMAL AUTOIMMUNE BLISTERING DISORDERS. Normal human skin is incubated in 1 M NaCl, resulting in a split in the lower portion of the *lamina lucida*. Using immunofluorescence to determine whether autoantibodies are bound to the epidermal side (roof) or dermal side (floor) helps to differentiate subepidermal autoimmune blistering disorders. A, Salt-split DIF of BP reveals IgG deposition on the epidermal side. B, Salt-split DIF of EBA reveals IgG deposition on the dermal side. BP, bullous pemphigoid; BPAG1, bullous pemphigoid antigen 1; BPAG2, bullous pemphigoid antigen 2; EBA, epidermolysis bullosa acquisita; Ig, immunoglobulin; LABD, linear IgA bullous dermatosis; MMP, mucous membrane pemphigoid; SLE, systemic lupus erythematosus.

(Histology images reprinted with permission from Elder DE, Elenitsas R, Rosenbach M, et al. *Lever's Histopathology of the Skin.* 11th ed. Wolters Kluwer; 2015.)

LINEAR IMMUNOGLOBULIN A BULLOUS DERMATOSIS

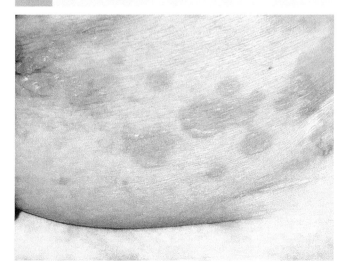

- LABD may be divided into a *lamina lucida* type (majority) and a *sublamina densa* type. The *lamina lucida* type is characterized by circulating IgA autoantibodies to BPAG1 and BPAG2, specifically a **120 kDa LAD antigen that corresponds to the cleaved shed extracellular domain of BPAG2 and a 97 kDa LAD antigen that results from further proteolytic degradation.** The antigen in the *sublamina densa* type has not been fully characterized. Drug associations include **vancomycin >>> β**-lactams, ACEIs, NSAIDs, and vaccinations (eg, influenza).
- LABD classically presents with **herpetiform tense blisters** with variable mucosal involvement.
    - The configuration of LABD is often described as a "crown of jewels."
    - Pediatric LABD, **chronic bullous disease of childhood,** typically presents in **preschool age children in flexural areas** (eg, the lower trunk, thigh, groin) and remits in 2 to 4 years.
    - Figure 2.31.

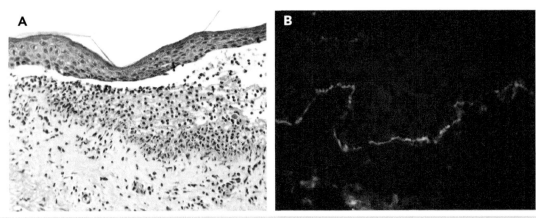

Figure 2.31. CLINICOPATHOLOGICAL CORRELATION: LINEAR IgA BULLOUS DERMATOSIS. Characteristic features are a subepidermal split and a predominantly neutrophilic infiltrate. DIF classically demonstrates linear deposition of IgA along the DEJ. A, H&E. B, DIF (IgA). DEJ, dermal-epidermal junction; DIF, direct immunofluorescence; H&E, hematoxylin and eosin; Ig, immunoglobulin.

(Histology images reprinted with permission from Elder DE, Elenitsas R, Rosenbach M, et al. *Lever's Histopathology of the Skin.* 11th ed. Wolters Kluwer; 2015.)

- Obtain **biopsies for H&E and perilesional DIF.** To optimize sensitivity, IIF should be performed on **salt-split human skin (epidermal).**
- After **discontinuation of the suspected drug, dapsone** is first line.

MUCOUS MEMBRANE PEMPHIGOID
Synonym: cicatricial pemphigoid

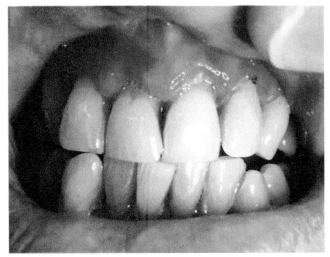

Courtesy of Erin Wei, MD.

- MMP constitutes a disease phenotype. The first subgroup is **anti-laminin-332 MMP (anti-epiligrin MMP),** associated with solid > liquid tumors (eg, **gastrointestinal, lung**). The second subgroup is **ocular MMP** in which **integrin subunit β4** is the characteristic target antigen. The third subgroup is **anti-BP antigen MMP** in which **BPAG2 (c-terminus)** is the characteristic target antigen. The fourth subgroup is heterogeneous. **Advanced age and female sex** are risk factors for MMP.
   - To remember that integrin subunit β4 is a target antigen in ocular MMP, rotate β 90° clockwise to form eyeglasses.

- The C-terminus extends into the *lamina densa*, which explains why the inflammation is cicatricial.
- MMP classically presents with **desquamative gingivitis. Conjunctival involvement in ~40%** of patients may lead to progressive scar tissue formation (eg, **symblepharon, ankyloblepharon, trichiasis, entropion**) and ultimately **blindness. Cutaneous involvement in 25% to 40%** of patients is characterized by erythematous plaques ± blisters that heal with **scarring. Brunsting-Perry pemphigoid** is a clinical MMP variant with **skin lesions favoring the head and neck and minimal to absent mucosal involvement.** Complications include **scarring alopecia and dorsal pterygium.**
   - Figure 2.32.

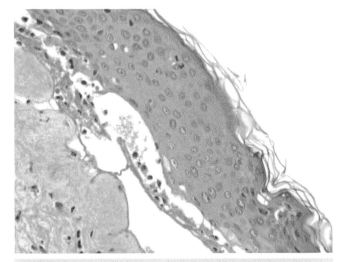

Figure 2.32. CLINICOPATHOLOGICAL CORRELATION: MUCOUS MEMBRANE PEMPHIGOID. Characteristic features are a subepidermal split, a predominantly neutrophilic infiltrate, and scarring in the upper dermis. DIF classically demonstrates linear deposition of IgG and C3 along the DEJ. C, complement; DEJ, dermal-epidermal junction; DIF, direct immunofluorescence; H&E, hematoxylin and eosin; Ig, immunoglobulin.

(Histology image reprinted with permission from Stelow EB, Mills S. *Biopsy Interpretation of the Head and Neck.* 3rd ed. Wolters Kluwer; 2020.)

- Obtain **biopsies for H&E and perilesional DIF (ideally mucosal).** To optimize sensitivity, **IIF** should be performed on **salt-split human skin (epidermal with the exception of anti-laminin-332 MMP)** and normal oral or genital mucosa or conjunctiva. **ELISA** can detect circulating auto-antibodies to **desmogleins 1 and 3, BPAG1, envoplakin, and periplakin.**
- **Topical corticosteroids and dapsone** are first line. **Cyclophosphamide and rituximab** are the treatments of choice for **rapidly progressive or severe ocular MMP.**

EPIDERMOLYSIS BULLOSA ACQUISITA

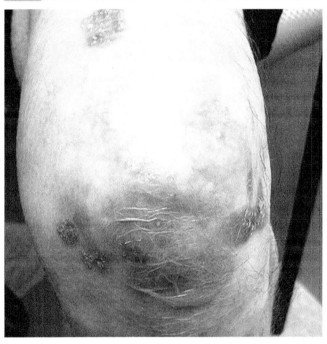

Reprinted with permission from Krakowski AC, Shumaker PR. *The Scar Book: Formation, Mitigation, Rehabilitation and Prevention.* Wolters Kluwer; 2017.

- Epidermolysis bullosa acquisita (EBA) is characterized by circulating autoantibodies to **collagen VII.** The most common association is **IBD.**
  > **Hereditary EB** (Table 2.18) leads to mechanical fragility of the skin and other epithelial surfaces with formation of **blisters** that often heal with **scarring** and may result in **alopecia and onychoatrophy. ± PPK with pseudoainhum.** Since there is considerable overlap in clinical features, types can be distinguished based on immunofluorescence antigenic mapping, transmission electron microscopy, or genetic analysis. Current management primarily focuses on blister prevention, wound care, and treatment of systemic complications; however, gene therapy holds promise for the future.
- EBA classically presents with **acral blisters** that heal with **dyspigmentation, milia, and atrophic scarring** that may result in **alopecia and onychoatrophy,** as well as **pseudosyndactyly.** EBA may be associated with **verruciform xanthoma.** Inflammatory EBA has also been described.

  > Pseudosyndactyly has been described as a "mitten" hand deformity.
  * Figure 2.33.
- Obtain **biopsies for H&E and perilesional DIF.** To optimize sensitivity, **IIF** should be performed on **salt-split human skin (dermal). ELISA** can detect circulating autoantibodies to **collagen VII.**
- EBA is notoriously **refractory** to treatment. Management of EBA is similar to BP.

DERMATITIS HERPETIFORMIS
→ **Diagnosis Group 2**
Synonym: Duhring disease

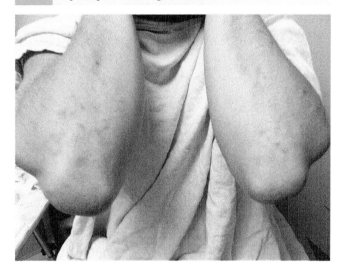

Epidemiology

- DH is a cutaneous manifestation of **gluten sensitivity** characterized by circulating **IgA** autoantibodies to **epidermal transglutaminase-3 (TG-3).**
  > Do NOT confuse TG-3 with TG-1, an abnormal gene product in lamellar ichthyosis.
- The mean age of onset is in the **fourth decade.** Male sex and **Northern European ancestry** are risk factors.
- DH is associated with several autoimmune disorders, most commonly **thyroid disease (eg, Hashimoto thyroiditis), insulin-dependent diabetes mellitus, and pernicious anemia.** While only ~20% of DH patients have intestinal symptoms of celiac disease, >90% have **gluten-sensitive enteropathy.** Long-standing enteropathy may lead to **enteropathy-associated T-cell lymphoma.**
- Drug associations include **ICIs.**
- The **strongest HLA** association is **-DQ2.** The pathogenesis of DH involves **epitope spreading. Gluten** digestion forms **gliadin,** which is absorbed via the *lamina propria* and deamidated by TG-2. Deamidated gliadin binds to HLA-DQ2 on APCs and is presented to sensitized helper T cells, which stimulate B cells. Differentiated plasma cells produce IgA antibodies to gliadin, gliadin–TG-2, TG-2, and epidermal TG-3. Deposition of IgA anti–TG-3 antibodies

Table 2.18. EPIDERMOLYSIS BULLOSA VARIANTS

Variant[a]	Inheritance Pattern	Gene Product(s)	Distinctive Clinical Features	Notes
EBS (Split: Intraepidermal)				
EBS, generalized	AD	K5 and K14	Grouped or herpetiform blisters, sometimes in a figurate array, confluent palmoplantar keratoderma.	Formerly known as Dowling-Meara type. Keratin filaments coalesce into electron-dense clumps.
EBS, generalized intermediate				Formerly known as Koebner type.
EBS, localized			Primary palm and sole involvement.	Formerly known as Weber-Cockayne type.
EBS with mottled pigmentation	AD	K5 > K14	Reticulated hyperpigmented macules.	
EBS with muscular dystrophy	AR	Plectin	Associated with muscular dystrophy.	Plectin is expressed in skeletal muscle.
JEB (Split: *intralamina lucida*)				
JEB, generalized severe	AR	Laminin 332	Symmetric excessive granulation tissue favoring the periorificial area, nape of the neck, upper back, intertriginous areas, and periungual areas. Systemic complications in a majority of patients include oral[b] (enamel hypoplasia, excessive carries and premature loss of teeth, tracheolaryngeal stenosis), gastrointestinal (malnutrition/FTT), and hematologic (anemia).	Formerly known as Herlitz type. Often due to premature truncating mutations. May develop benign EB nevi that clinically resemble melanoma.
JEB, generalized intermediate	AR	Laminin 332, BPAG2		Formerly known as non-Herlitz type or GABEB.
JEB, localized	AR	BPAG2, α6β4 integrin	Primarily acral involvement.	
JEB with pyloric atresia	AR	α6β4 integrin	Associated with pyloric atresia.	
DEB (Split: *sublamina densa*)				
DDEB, generalized	AD	Collagen VII		Formerly known as non–Hallopeau-Siemens type. DDEB Cockayne-Touraine (primarily acral involvement). DDEB Pasini (albopapuloid lesions).
RDEB, generalized severe	AR		Systemic complications in a majority of patients include ocular (corneal scarring), oral (enamel hypoplasia, excessive carries and premature loss of teeth, microstomia), gastrointestinal[c] (eg, esophageal strictures, GERD, malnutrition/FTT, severe constipation), musculoskeletal (eg, osteoporosis/osteopenia, pseudosyndactyly), and hematologic (eg, anemia).	Formerly known as Hallopeau-Siemens type. Often due to premature truncating mutations resulting in undetectable anchoring fibrils. SCC is a leading cause of death. Consider a systemic retinoid for prevention.
RDEB, generalized intermediate				
RDEB, inversa			Primary axillae and groin involvement.	

Table 2.18. EPIDERMOLYSIS BULLOSA VARIANTS (CONTINUED)

Variant[a]	Inheritance Pattern	Gene Product(s)	Distinctive Clinical Features	Notes
Kindler Syndrome (Split: Mixed)				
Kindler syndrome	AR	Kindlin-1	Atrophy, photosensitivity/poikiloderma. Kindle a match—photosensitivity.	Disruption of actin assembly due to *FERMT1* mutation results in basement membrane reduplication.

AD, autosomal dominant; AR, autosomal recessive; DEB, dystrophic EB; DDEB, dominant dystrophic EB; EB, epidermolysis bullosa; EBS, EB simplex; FTT, failure to thrive; GABEB, generalized atrophic benign EB; GERD, gastroesophageal reflux disease; JEB; junctional EB; K, keratin; RDEB, recessive dystrophic EB; SCC, squamous cell carcinoma.

[a]Illustrative examples provided.

[b]Enamel hypoplasia occurs in a majority of patients with all JEB subtypes.

[c]Esophageal strictures also occur in a majority of patients with RDEB inversa and GERD occurs in a majority of patients with all RDEB subtypes.

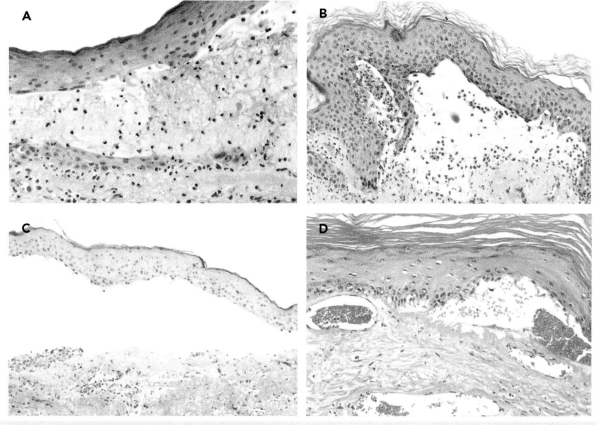

Figure 2.33. SIDE-BY-SIDE COMPARISON: EPIDERMOLYSIS BULLOSA ACQUISITA AND BULLOUS SYSTEMIC LUPUS ERYTHEMATOSUS. Both EBA and bullous SLE are characterized by a subepidermal split with a variable inflammatory infiltrate. DIF classically demonstrates linear deposition along the DEJ in a *u-serrated* pattern: IgG in EBA and IgM, IgG, IgA, and C3 in bullous SLE. A and C, EBA (inflammatory type and noninflammatory type, respectively). B and D, Bullous SLE (neutrophilic type and mononuclear type, respectively). C, complement; DEJ, dermal-epidermal junction; DIF, direct immunofluorescence; EBA, epidermolysis bullosa acquisita; Ig, immunoglobulin; SLE, systemic lupus erythematosus.

(Histology images reprinted with permission from Elder DE, Elenitsas R, Rosenbach M, et al. *Lever's Histopathology of the Skin*. 11th ed. Wolters Kluwer; 2015.)

EBA:
• **Inflammatory variant:** predominantly neutrophilic infiltrate.
• **Noninflammatory variant:** minimal to absent inflammatory infiltrate.

Bullous SLE:
• **Noninflammatory variant:** predominantly neutrophilic infiltrate.
• **Mononuclear variant:** predominantly mononuclear infiltrate.

within dermal papillae leads to neutrophil recruitment and degranulation.

◇ HLA-<u>DQ</u>2 carriers should avoid the cones at <u>D</u>airy Queen.

Clinicopathological Features

- DH classically presents with **urticarial plaques, papules, and vesicles symmetrically distributed on the back, buttocks, elbows, extensor forearms, and knees.**
- DH is associated with **intense pruritus.**
  ◆ Figure 2.34.

Evaluation

- The differential diagnosis of DH includes subepidermal autoimmune blistering disorders, EM, arthropod assault, and drug reactions.
- Obtain **biopsies for H&E and sample adjacent normal skin for DIF.** Test for IgA anti–TG-3 antibody (if available). Test total IgA and IgA anti–TG-2 antibodies. If positive, test for IgA antiendomysial antibody. If IgA is low, test for IgG anti–TG-2 antibody. If positive, test for IgG antiendomysial antibody.

Management

- **Gluten avoidance** is first line. **IgA anti–TG-3 antibody** may be helpful to **assess compliance.**

- **Dapsone** is highly efficacious for DH, **relieving pruritus in 48 to 72 hours.** Unfortunately, it has **no effect on gluten-sensitive enteropathy.**

"Real World" Advice

- Even though the hallmark lesion in DH is a papulovesicle, patients in practice often present with secondary changes from scratching. A high index of suspicion is required for diagnosis.
- Gluten is found in **wheat, rye, barley,** and hybrids of these grains (eg, Kamut). **Safe grains** for patients with DH include **corn, oats, and rice.**

Interface Dermatoses and Other Connective Tissue Disorders

Basic Concepts

- **Connective tissue disorders (CTDs)** affect tissues that **support, ensheath, and bind tissues together.**
- **Interface dermatoses** are characterized by a **predominantly lymphocytic infiltrate that abuts or obscures the DEJ** on histopathology.
  ◆ Interface dermatitis may be divided into lichenoid and vacuolar patterns (Figure 2.35).

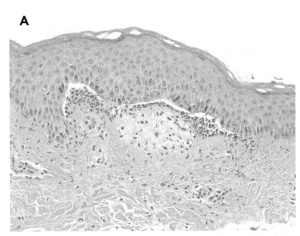
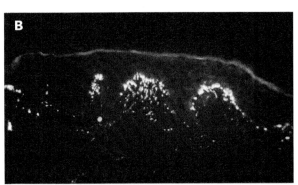

Figure 2.34. CLINICOPATHOLOGICAL CORRELATION: DERMATITIS HERPETIFORMIS. Characteristic features are a subepidermal split and dermal papillary neutrophilic microabscesses. DIF classically demonstrates granular deposition of IgA at the tips of the dermal papillae. A, H&E. B, DIF (IgA). DIF, direct immunofluorescence; H&E, hematoxylin and eosin; Ig, immunoglobulin.

(A, Histology image courtesy of Noel Turner, MD, MHS and Christine J. Ko, MD. B, Histology image reprinted with permission from Elder DE, Elenitsas R, Rosenbach M, et al. *Lever's Histopathology of the Skin.* 11th ed. Wolters Kluwer; 2015.)

The DIF pattern has been described as a "picket fence" due to the granules.

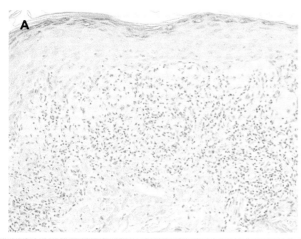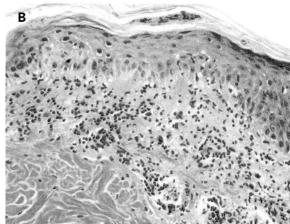

Figure 2.35. SIDE-BY-SIDE COMPARISON: LICHENOID AND VACUOLAR INTERFACE DERMATITIS. Both lichenoid and vacuolar interface dermatitis are characterized by a predominantly lymphocytic infiltrate that abuts or obscures the DEJ. Lichenoid interface dermatitis demonstrates destruction of the basal layer with apoptotic keratinocytes (colloid bodies) (PAS positive, diastase resistant) and conical rete. Vacuolar interface dermatitis demonstrates preservation of the basal layer with vacuoles and rounded rete. A, Lichenoid interface dermatitis: LP. B, Vacuolar interface dermatitis: SCLE. Colloid bodies are alternatively known as Civatte, cytoid, or hyaline bodies. DEJ, dermal-epidermal junction; LP, lichen planus; PAS, periodic acid-Schiff; SCLE, subacute cutaneous lupus erythematosus.

(A, Histology image courtesy of Noel Turner, MD, MHS and Christine J. Ko, MD.)

> Lymphocytes in lichenoid interface dermatitis are often described as "band-like."
> Lymphocytes in vacuolar interface dermatitis tend to aggregate.

LICHEN PLANUS
→ Diagnosis Group 1

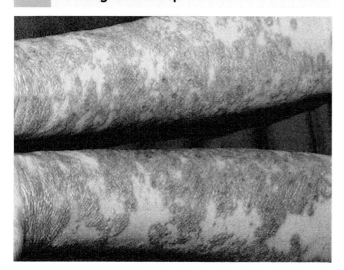

Reprinted with permission from Craft N, Fox LP, Goldsmith LA, et al. *VisualDx: Essential Adult Dermatology.* Wolters Kluwer Health/ Lippincott Williams & Wilkins; 2010.

Epidemiology

- LP is a T cell–mediated autoimmune reaction against keratinocyte epitopes modified by viral/drug antigens. IFN-γ is central to the pathogenesis.
- The mean age of onset is **50 years.**

- Associations include **viral infection (eg, hepatitis C virus [HCV] infection, especially oral LP), vaccinations (eg, influenza, hepatitis B virus [HBV]), drugs (see below), and dental restorative materials (eg, amalgam [mercury], copper, and gold).**
- HLA associations include **-B8 (oral LP), -B35 (cutaneous LP), and -DR1 (cutaneous and oral LP).**
  > Beatrice eight with her mouth open (HLA-B8 is associated with oral LP).

Clinicopathological Features

- **Cutaneous LP** classically presents with **pruritic, flat-topped, polygonal, violaceous papules that favor the wrists, forearms, distal lower extremities, and presacral area.**
  > Lichen is derived from the Greek word *leichen* meaning "tree moss." In dermatology, "lichen" is used to describe an eruption of flat papules.
  > The five Ps of cutaneous LP: pruritic planar, polygonal, purple papules.
- LP may involve the **oral cavity** and **nail unit.**
- **Koebnerization** is common.
- **LP variants** are summarized in Table 2.19.
  > 20-nail dystrophy is more common in children than adults.
  > Figure 2.36.
- Some experts consider **keratosis lichenoides chronica,** which classically presents with **symmetric keratotic**

Table 2.19. LICHEN PLANUS VARIANTS

Variant[a]	Classic Description	Notes
Actinic LP	Photodistribution of LP.	Majority of reported patients are from the Middle East.
Acute (exanthematous) LP	Rapid onset of LP over a wide distribution.	
Annular LP	Annular LP favoring the axillae > penis, groin, and extremities.	
Atrophic LP	LP with central atrophy and hyperpigmentation.	
Bullous LP	Blisters within existing LP lesions.	Blisters in bullous LP are due to cytotoxic keratinocyte damage (expanded Max-Joseph spaces).
	In contrast, blisters in LP pemphigoides may arise within existing LP lesions or on previously unaffected skin.	
Hypertrophic LP	Hyperkeratotic LP favoring the lower extremities.	Increased risk of SCC.
Inverse LP	LP favoring flexural zones (especially the axillae).	
LP pigmentosus	Gray-brown macules in sun-exposed areas > intertriginous zones.	Majority of reported patients are from South Asia, Latin America, and the Middle East.
Lichen planopilaris	See Chapter 2: Disorders of the Hair and Nails.	
Linear LP	LP following the lines of Blaschko.	
Nail LP	Onychoatrophy, onychorrhexis/trachyonychia, and onychoschizia may lead to scarring and dorsal pterygium formation. Red lunulae may also occur.	
	Trachyonychia is also referred to as "sandpapered nails." Figure 2.36.	
Oral LP	Desquamative gingivitis. Reticular (most common) oral LP classically presents with symmetric raised white linear lines or rings with short radiating spines favoring the buccal and gingival mucosa (Wickham striae).	Oral LP is present in 75% of patients, 10%-20% of whom develop cutaneous lesions. Increased risk of esophageal LP and SCC.
	Reticular oral LP has been described as a "lace-like" pattern.	
Ulcerative LP	Ulcerative LP favoring the palms/soles.	Increased risk of SCC.
Vulvovaginal LP	Erosive LP that may lead to scarring with dyspareunia and postcoital bleeding.	Often overlaps with oral LP (vulvovaginal-digital syndrome). Increased risk of SCC.

LP, lichen planus; SCC, squamous cell carcinoma.
[a]Illustrative examples provided.

lichenoid papules arranged in a linear and reticulated pattern on the trunk and extremities and dorsal hands and feet, to be an LP variant.
- LP may **overlap with BP in LP pemphigoides** (reactivity against **BPAG2**).
- LP may **overlap with LE.**
  - Figure 2.37.

Evaluation

- The differential diagnosis of cutaneous LP includes other lichenoid dermatoses and GVHD, papulosquamous dermatoses, CTDs, and secondary syphilis. LP pigmentosus should be differentiated from EDP and vulvovaginal LP should be differentiated from LS.

- **Dermoscopy** features include **white crossing streaks (Wickham striae) and dotted or linear vessels at the periphery.**
- There is no established guideline for the evaluation of LP. A skin biopsy may be helpful in case of diagnostic uncertainty, and some experts recommend **HCV screening.**
- Patients with oral LP in apposition to dental restorative materials should undergo **patch testing.** Even if negative, removal may lead to improvement by reducing Koebnerization due to irritation.
- **Early detection of esophageal LP with endoscopy is important to avoid scarring stenosis.**
- It is important to **monitor for the development of SCC** in patients with LP, particularly in high-risk variants (**hypertrophic, oral, ulcerative, and vulvovaginal**).

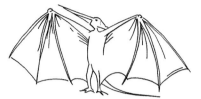

Pterygium, like pterodactal, is derived from the Greek word *pteron* meaning wing.

Dorsal pterygium results from adhesion of the proximal nail fold to the nail matrix and bed, creating a winglike appearance. Associations include MMP and LP.

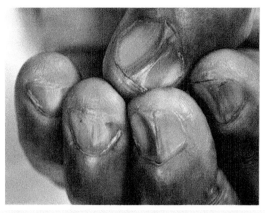

Figure 2.36. PTERYGIUM. By contrast, ventral pterygium (pterygium inversus unguis) results from adhesion of the distal nail plate to the hyponychium. It is associated with impaired peripheral perfusion in SSc. LP, lichen planus; MMP, mucous membrane pemphigoid; SSc, systemic sclerosis.

(Dorsal pterygium image reprinted with permission from Craft N, Fox LP, Goldsmith LA, et al. *VisualDx: Essential Adult Dermatology.* Wolters Kluwer Health/Lippincott Williams & Wilkins; 2010. Illustration by Misha Rosenbach, MD.)

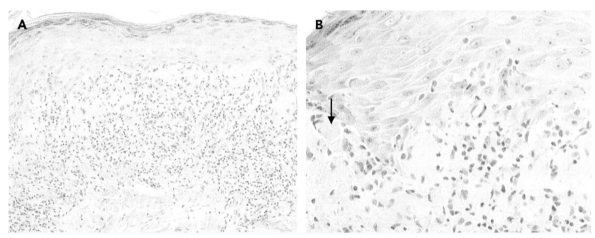

Figure 2.37. CLINICOPATHOLOGICAL CORRELATION: LICHEN PLANUS. Characteristic features are orthohyperkeratosis, "wedge-shaped" hypergranulosis, acanthosis, a lichenoid interface dermatitis, and dermal melanophages. Artifactual clefts between the epidermis and the dermis are called Max-Joseph spaces. DIF classically demonstrates shaggy deposition of fibrin and granular deposition of IgM, IgG, IgA, and C3 staining apoptotic keratinocytes at the DEJ. Oral LP is characterized by parakeratosis (not hyperkeratosis) and epidermal atrophy (not acanthosis). A, Low-power view. B, High-power view. Solid arrow: apoptotic keratinocyte (colloid body). C, complement; DEJ, dermal-epidermal junction; DIF, direct immunofluorescence; Ig, immunoglobulin; LP, lichen planus.

(Histology images courtesy of Noel Turner, MD, MHS and Christine J. Ko, MD.)

Management

- LP may **resolve spontaneously (~ 1 year for cutaneous LP vs ~5 years for oral LP)** or with treatment of an associated disease or discontinuation of an associated trigger; however, disease-targeted therapy is often required.
  - Oral LP is sustained, leading to strictures and squames.
- **High-potency topical corticosteroids** are first line, but **systemic corticosteroids** may be required. Diverse steroid-sparing therapies have been reported, including **topical calcineurin inhibitors, antimalarials, phototherapy,** and **retinoids.**

"Real World" Advice

- **Beware of pseudoepitheliomatous hyperplasia in hypertrophic LP masquerading as multiple SCCs.**

LICHENOID DRUG ERUPTION
→ Diagnosis Group 2

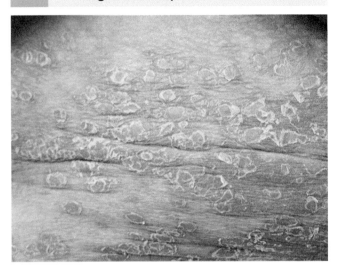

Epidemiology

- Lichenoid drug eruption may be classified as a **delayed-type, cell-mediated (type IV) reaction.** The mean age of onset is **65 years.**
- Drug associations include **antimalarials,** TNFα inhibitors, **ICIs,** anticonvulsants, anxiolytics, antidepressants, antipsychotics, **anti-hypertensives (eg, ACEIs, diuretics),** hypoglycemic agents, **metals (eg, gold salts),** NSAIDs, and D-penicillamine.

Clinicopathological Features

- Clinical clues to differentiate lichenoid drug eruption from LP include **older age at presentation, generalized or photodistributed lesions, and mucous membrane sparing.**
  - ◆ Histopathological clues to differentiate lichenoid drug eruption from LP include parakeratosis and eosinophils.
- The timing of lichenoid drug eruption relative to initial drug exposure ranges from months to years (~**12 months**).

Evaluation

- The differential diagnosis of lichenoid drug eruptions is similar to LP.

Management

- **Discontinuation of the suspected drug** along with all non-essential drugs is the first step. *In vitro* assays to establish the culprit drug are under investigation. However, given uncertain sensitivity and specificity, their utility remains limited in clinical practice. Patch testing has high false negative rates.
- Treatment strategies for lichenoid drug eruptions mirror those for LP.
- Lichenoid drug eruptions often resolve within weeks to months but may persist.

"Real World" Advice

- Beware of the long latency period. In a patient with a lichenoid eruption, it is important to perform a detailed medication history and not to disregard chronic medications.

LICHEN STRIATUS
→ Diagnosis Group 2

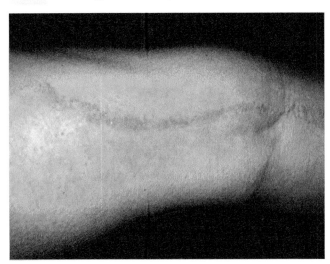

Reprinted with permission from Schalock PC, Hsu JTS, Arndt KA. *Lippincott's Primary Care Dermatology.* Wolters Kluwer Health/ Lippincott Williams & Wilkins; 2010.

Epidemiology

- Lichen striatus is a linear dermatosis that primarily affects **preschool-age children.**

Clinicopathological Features

- Lichen striatus classically presents with **flat-topped papules extending in a continuous or interrupted band along the lines of Blaschko down an extremity.** Lichen striatus typically resolves with **hypopigmentation.** While lichen striatus is typically asymptomatic, intense pruritus may occur.
- **Nail involvement** is common.
  - ◆ Figure 2.38.

Evaluation

- The differential diagnosis of lichen striatus includes other linear dermatoses (eg, blaschkitis, linear LP, GVHD, pigmented purpura) and neoplasms (eg, inflammatory linear verrucous epidermal nevus [ILVEN]).
  - ◆ Blaschkitis and linear LP are linear dermatoses that primarily affect adults. In contrast to lichen striatus, blaschkitis classically presents with multiple recurrent

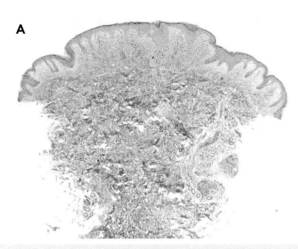

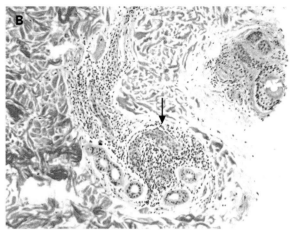

Figure 2.38. CLINICOPATHOLOGICAL CORRELATION: LICHEN STRIATUS. Lichen striatus is characterized by lichenoid interface dermatitis with variable adnexal involvement. A, Low-power view. B, High-power view. Solid arrow: lymphoid aggregates in the eccrine coil. H&E, hematoxylin & eosin.

A striation is a line. Lichen striatus follows the lines of Blaschko. Under the microscope, lymphocytes follow adnexal structures, forming blue lines on H&E staining.

lesions on the trunk with eczematous features and linear LP resolves with hyperpigmentation.
- There is no established guideline for the evaluation of lichen striatus. Skin biopsy may be helpful.

Management

- Lichen striatus **resolves spontaneously in a few months to a few years.**
- High-potency topical corticosteroids are first line; however, the efficacy of topical calcineurin inhibitors has also been reported.

"Real World" Advice

- Lichen striatus is self-limited; therefore, treatment is usually not needed.

LICHEN NITIDUS

- Lichen nitidus is a rare disorder that is more prevalent in **children and adolescents.**
- Lichen nitidus classically presents with **multiple clusters of tiny, discrete, shiny papules that favor the anterior trunk, genitalia, and flexor aspects of the upper extremities.**
  - Figure 2.39.
- Treatment includes topical corticosteroids and antihistamines.

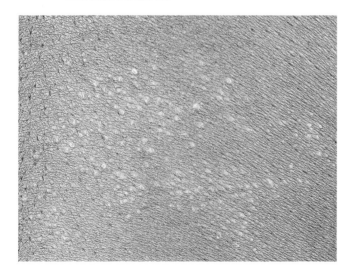

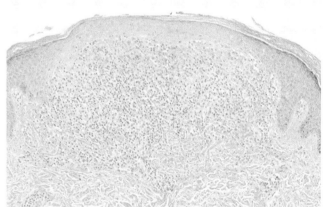

Figure 2.39. CLINICOPATHOLOGICAL CORRELATION: LICHEN NITIDUS. Characteristic features are parakeratosis, hypogranulosis, and epidermal atrophy with hyperplastic rete ridges surrounding a well-circumscribed lichenoid infiltrate. The infiltrate, spanning < 2-3 dermal papillae, is typically composed of lymphocytes, epithelioid cells, and occasionally Langhans giant cells.

(Histology image courtesy of Noel Turner, MD, MHS and Christine J. Ko, MD.)

The well-circumscribed infiltrate with surrounding hyperplastic rete ridges has been described as the "ball and claw" configuration.

ERYTHEMA MULTIFORME
→ **Diagnosis Group 1**

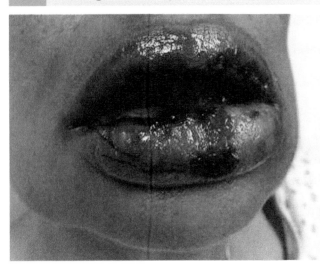

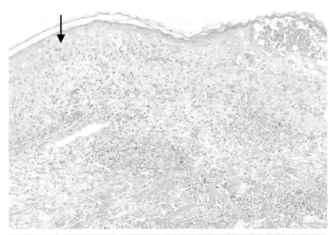

Figure 2.40. CLINICOPATHOLOGICAL CORRELATION: ERYTHEMA MULTIFORME. Characteristic features are an acute *stratum corneum*, individual necrotic keratinocytes that may progress to confluent epidermal necrosis, papillary dermal edema, and a dermal lymphocytic infiltrate. DIF may demonstrate granular deposition of IgM and C3 focally along the DEJ. Solid arrow: necrotic keratinocyte (present at all levels of the epidermis).

(Histology image courtesy of Noel Turner, MD, MHS and Christine J. Ko, MD.)

Cell death occurs out of proportion to inflammation.

Epidemiology

- EM is an acute inflammatory disorder.
- The EM spectrum is categorized into:
  - **EM minor** (EM von Hebra): absent or mild mucosal involvement.
  - **EM major:** severe mucosal involvement and **systemic features.**
- The leading association is infection (~**90%** of patients), most often **herpes simplex virus (HSV).** EM major may be associated with *Mycoplasma pneumoniae* (***Mycoplasma pneumoniae*-induced rash and mucositis [MIRM]**). Less common associations include other infections (eg, *Histoplasma capsulatum*, particularly in patients with concomitant **erythema nodosum [EN]**) and exposures (eg, poison ivy).
- Drugs associations (eg, NSAIDs) are rare.

Clinicopathological Features

- Skin involvement in EM is characterized by **abrupt onset of papular target lesions favoring the face and extremities** (elbows, wrists, hands, knees). Target lesions may be **typical (at least three different zones)** or **atypical (papular, only two different zones and/or a poorly defined border).** Bullous lesions are occasionally present in EM major.
  - Target lesions may resemble a "bull's eye."
- Mucosal involvement in EM major is characterized by **vesiculobullous lesions that rapidly evolve into painful crusted erosions on the buccal mucosa and lips > ocular and anogenital mucosae.**
- Systemic features in EM major include **fever and arthralgias.**
- EM may **overlap with LE (Rowell syndrome).**
  - Figure 2.40.

Evaluation

- The differential diagnosis of EM includes SJS/TEN, generalized bullous fixed drug eruption (GBFDE), subacute cutaneous lupus erythematosus (SCLE), erythema annulare centrifugum (EAC), and CSVV.

  In the pediatric population, urticaria multiforme and Kawasaki disease are often misdiagnosed as EM.

Management

- EM is self-limited. There is no risk of progression to TEN.
- Oral corticosteroids and other systemic immunosuppressive therapies may be required.
- For patients with **HSV-associated EM with frequent recurrences, consider prophylaxis (eg, valacyclovir 500-1000 mg/d)** for at least 6 months.

"Real World" Advice

- Distinguishing EM from SJS/TEN is challenging. Four clinical criteria are (1) type of elementary skin lesion, (2) distribution of skin lesions, (3) presence or absence of overt mucosal lesions, and (4) presence or absence of systemic symptoms.
  - Histopathological features that suggest EM over SJS/TEN are decreased cell death and increased inflammation.
- Use of systemic corticosteroids is controversial in EM given concern for increased risk of infection.

STEVENS-JOHNSON SYNDROME/TOXIC EPIDERMAL NECROLYSIS
→ Diagnosis Group 1

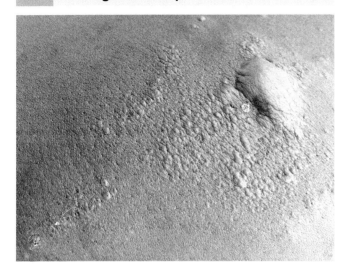

Epidemiology

- SJS/TEN may be classified as a **delayed-type, cell-mediated (type IV) SCAR.** The hypothesized mechanism is activation of **CD4⁺ and CD8⁺ T cells** leading to release of cytokines (eg, IFN-γ). Mediators of apoptosis include **Fas-FasL interactions and granulysin.**
- The SJS/TEN spectrum is **categorized according to BSA of detached (and detachable) epidermis** into:
  - **SJS: < 10% BSA.**
  - **SJS/TEN overlap: 10% to 30% BSA.**
  - **TEN** (Lyell syndrome): **>30% BSA.**
- Drug associations include **dapsone, rituximab, nonnucleoside reverse transcriptase inhibitors (NNRTIs; eg, nevirapine), sulfonamides (eg, trimethoprim-sulfamethoxazole [TMP-SMX]), allopurinol, aromatic anticonvulsants (eg, carbamazepine, phenobarbital, phenytoin), lamotrigine, and NSAIDs.** Additionally, **SJS/TEN-like reactions** have been reported to antineoplastics such as **bortezomib and ICIs.** Other SJS triggers include infection or vaccination.
- **HLA** associations include **-A3101 (carbamazepine in European populations), -B1502 (carbamazepine in Asian and East Indian populations; lamotrigine in Han Chinese population; phenytoin in Han Chinese population), and -B5801 (allopurinol in Han Chinese population).** Other risk factors include **slow acetylator genotype (eg, sulfonamides), immunosuppression (eg, HIV),** and concomitant anticonvulsants or radiation therapy.

Clinicopathological Features

- SJS/TEN classically presents with a **prodrome of upper respiratory infection (URI) symptoms, fever, and skin pain.**
- **Mucosal involvement (>90% of patients)** is characterized by **erythema and erosions of the buccal, ocular, and anogenital mucosae.** TEN may involve the respiratory and gastrointestinal mucosa.

- **Skin involvement** is characterized by **dusky and/or dusky-red macules with epidermal detachment and erosions, macular atypical targets, and bullous lesions favoring the face and trunk.**
  - Epidermal detachment may resemble "wet cigarette paper" peeling away from "scalded skin."
- The **Nikolsky sign** and the **Asboe-Hansen sign** are positive in SJS/TEN.
- Systemic features include **fever, lymphadenopathy, cytopenias, hepatitis, and cholestasis.** TEN may be further complicated by **nephritis.**
- The timing of SJS/TEN relative to initial drug exposure is typically **7 to 21 days** (earlier in case of rechallenge).
- Sequalae may be cutaneous (eg, scarring, dyspigmentation, eruptive melanocytic nevi), mucosal (eg, **symblepharon**), or adnexal (eg, alopecia, onychodystrophy).
  - ◈ Figure 2.41.

Evaluation

- The differential diagnosis of SJS/TEN includes AGEP, autoimmune blistering disorders, EM, GBFDE, toxic erythema of chemotherapy (TEC), GVHD (stage IV), Rowell syndrome/acute syndrome of apoptotic pan-epidermolysis (ASAP), morbilliform drug eruption/DRESS, and disseminated intravascular coagulation (DIC).
  - In the pediatric population, Kawasaki disease, SSSS, and invasive fungal dermatitis (eg, candidal) are often misdiagnosed as SJS/TEN.
- **Skin biopsy,** often with an additional **frozen section** for rapid evaluation, is helpful. Obtaining a frozen section of the blister roof to evaluate for a subepidermal split is termed the **"jelly roll" preparation.**
  - ◈ The "jelly roll" preparation can help to distinguish SJS/TEN from SSSS.

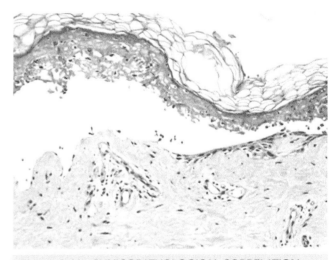

Figure 2.41. CLINICOPATHOLOGICAL CORRELATION: STEVENS-JOHNSON SYNDROME/TOXIC EPIDERMAL NECROLYSIS. Characteristic features are an acute *stratum corneum,* a subepidermal blister with overlying confluent epidermal necrosis, and a sparse dermal lymphocytic infiltrate.

(Histology image reprinted with permission from Husain AN. *Biopsy Interpretation of Pediatric Lesions.* Wolters Kluwer; 2014.)

Cell death occurs out of proportion to inflammation.

Table 2.20. SCORTEN		
SCORTEN[a]		
Prognostic Factors		**Points**
TAMEBUG = Tachycardia, Age, Malignancy, Epidermal loss, Bicarbonate, Urea, Glucose.		
Tachycardia (>120 bpm)		1
Age (>40 years)		1
Malignancy		1
Initial percentage of epidermal detachment (>10%)		1
Serum bicarbonate level (<20 mmol/L)		1
Serum urea level (>10 mmol/L)		1
Serum glucose level (>14 mmol/L)		1
SCORTEN		**Mortality Rate (%)**
0-1		3.2
2		12.1
3		35.8
4		58.3
≥5		90

BSA, body surface area; SJS/TEN, Stevens-Johnson syndrome/toxic epidermal necrolysis
[a]Age, Bicarbonate, Cancer, Dialysis, 10% BSA (ABCD-10) is an alternative severity-of-illness score for SJS/TEN.

Management

- SJS may progress to TEN. While the **average mortality rate for SJS is ~5%**, the **average mortality rate for TEN is ~30%**. The primary cause of death is **infection (eg, *S. aureus*, *Pseudomonas aeruginosa*)**. SCORTEN is a TEN-specific severity-of-illness score (Table 2.20). Among these, **low serum bicarbonate level** was associated with the **greatest risk of death**.

  - TEN: >30% BSA; ~30% average mortality rate.
- **Discontinuation of the suspected drug** along with all nonessential drugs is the first step. *In vitro* assays to establish the culprit drug are under investigation. However, given uncertain sensitivity and specificity, their utility remains limited in clinical practice. Prick and intradermal tests are contraindicated. 10% to 25% of patients are patch test positive. While SJS/TEN is **drug-associated in 70% to 90%** of cases, it is important to consider alternative etiologies.

- **Supportive care** (eg, admission to a skilled nursing unit, daily wound care with emollients and/or topical antibiotics) is first line. A **multidisciplinary team** (eg, ophthalmology, urology) is preferred. While no therapy has demonstrated efficacy in prospective controlled clinical studies, limited data support **cyclosporine** (3-5 mg/kg/d × 7 days), **IVIG** (>2 g/kg total over 3-4 days), **systemic corticosteroids** (eg, dexamethasone 1.5 mg/kg/d × 3 days), and **TNFα inhibitors** (eg, etanercept 25-50 mg SC twice weekly).

"Real World" Advice

- If the suspected drug is an **aromatic anticonvulsant**, alternatives for seizure prophylaxis include **benzodiazepines, levetiracetam, and valproic acid.**
- Use of systemic corticosteroids is controversial in SJS/TEN given concern for delayed wound healing and increased risk of infection.

FIXED DRUG ERUPTION
→ Diagnosis Group 2

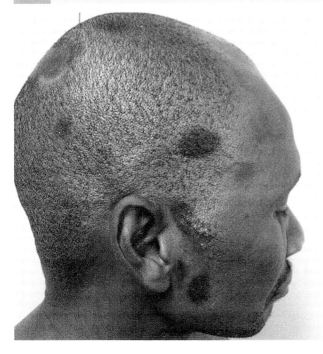

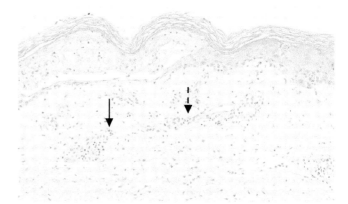

Figure 2.42. CLINICOPATHOLOGICAL CORRELATION: FIXED DRUG ERUPTION. Characteristic features are an acute *stratum corneum*, a vacuolar interface dermatitis, variable keratinocyte necrosis, a dermal mixed infiltrate with eosinophils, and perivascular melanin pigment incontinence. Solid arrow: melanin pigment incontinence. Bullous FDE. Solid arrow: eosinophil. Dashed arrow: perivascular melanin pigment incontinence. FDE, fixed drug eruption.

(Histology image courtesy of Noel Turner, MD, MHS and Christine J. Ko, MD.)

The mismatch between the *stratum corneum* (acute changes) and the dermis (chronic changes) is due to the episodic nature of FDE: perivascular melanin pigment incontinence tells the story of prior episodes.

Epidemiology

- FDE may be classified as a **delayed-type, cell-mediated (type IV) reaction.** GBFDE may be classified as a **SCAR.** The hypothesized mechanism is activation of **CD8⁺ resident memory T cells** leading to release of cytokines (eg, IFN-γ).
    - Fixed drug eruption is mediated by residents NOT transients.
- Drug associations include **dapsone, sulfonamides (eg, TMP-SMX), tetracyclines, antimicrotubule taxanes (bullous), NSAIDs, and pseudoephedrine (nonpigmenting).**

Clinicopathological Features

- FDE characteristically presents with **round to oval, sharply demarcated, erythematous and edematous plaques with variable duskiness and blister formation favoring the face and hands and feet.** Involvement of the **lips and anogenital mucosa** is common. Lesions resolve with postinflammatory hyperpigmentation. Upon reexposure, the number of sites may remain constant or increase.
- The timing of FDE relative to initial drug exposure is typically **7 to 14 days.** The timing of FDE relative to drug reexposure is typically **<24 hours.**
    - Figure 2.42.

Evaluation

- The differential diagnosis for FDE includes infection and arthropod assault.
- The differential diagnosis for GBFDE includes EM and SJS/TEN.

Management

- FDE has a 0% reported mortality rate; however, GBFDE may be lethal.
- **Discontinuation of the suspected drug** along with all nonessential drugs is the first step. *In vitro* assays to establish the culprit drug are under investigation. However, given uncertain sensitivity and specificity, their utility remains limited in clinical practice. An in situ **patch test (at the site of a previous lesion) is recommended** (>40% of patients are positive), and topical provocation or rechallenge may be considered.
- **Topical corticosteroids** are first line. **Systemic corticosteroids** are first line for GBFDE.

"Real World" Advice

- Recurrent FDE on the lips and genitalia is often misdiagnosed as HSV.
- Distinguishing GBFDE from SJS/TEN is challenging. Clinical features that suggest GBFDE include more rapid onset (<24 hours) and absent or mild mucosal and systemic involvement.
    - Histopathological features that suggest GBFDE over SJS/TEN are eosinophils and perivascular melanin pigment incontinence.

TOXIC ERYTHEMA OF CHEMOTHERAPY

Synonyms: acral erythema, "Ara-C" (cytarabine arabinoside) ears, chemotherapy-induced eccrine squamous syringometaplasia, epidermal dysmaturation, hand-foot syndrome, intertriginous eruption associated with chemotherapy, palmoplantar erythrodysesthesia

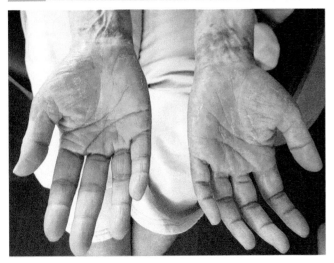

Courtesy of Robert Micheletti, MD.

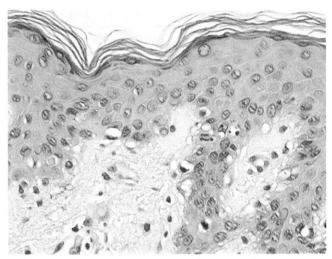

Figure 2.43. CLINICOPATHOLOGICAL CORRELATION: TOXIC ERYTHEMA OF CHEMOTHERAPY. Characteristic features are epidermal dysmaturation exemplified by keratinocyte loss of polarity and disorganization, keratinocyte necrosis, vacuolar degeneration of basilar keratinocytes with cleft formation, and perivascular lymphocytic infiltrate in the dermis with scattered eosinophils.

(Histology image reprinted with permission from Elder DE, Elenitsas R, Rosenbach M, et al. *Lever's Histopathology of the Skin.* 11th ed. Wolters Kluwer; 2015.)

- TEC is associated with multiple antineoplastics including **alkylating agents, antimetabolites, antimicrotubule taxanes, and antitumor antibiotics.**
- TEC is characterized by **symmetric erythematous to dusky patches** that can develop edema, erosions, desquamation, or purpura. The distribution favors **intertriginous zones,** elbows, knees, and **acral sites. Hand-foot syndrome (HFS)** typically favors the **palms and soles;** however, **HFS due to antimicrotubule taxanes** favors the **dorsal hands and feet,** Achilles tendon, and malleoli. TEC may disproportionately impact skin warmed with **heating devices.**
    - Figure 2.43.
- Given its intertriginous distribution, TEC must be differentiated from **SDRIFE** (historically called baboon syndrome), by history of antineoplastic exposure as opposed to other drugs (eg, **β-lactams**) or triggers (eg, **iodinated radiocontrast media**).
- Preventative measures for HFS include pretreatment with systemic corticosteroids and **cooling** before, during, and after chemotherapy infusions. NSAIDs may be efficacious for HFS due to capecitabine (eg, celecoxib 200 mg twice daily).

GRAFT-VERSUS-HOST DISEASE

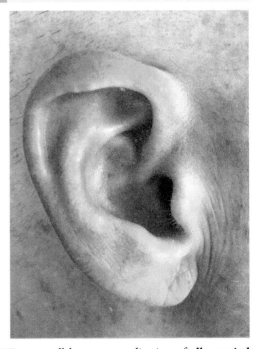

- GVHD is a well-known complication of **allogeneic hematopoietic stem cell transplantation (HSCT).** Risk factors may relate to the donor (eg, **HLA incompatibility with recipient, unrelated to recipient, female sex**), the recipient (eg, **older age**), the stem cell source (eg, **peripheral blood**), and other (eg, **myeloablative conditioning regimen**). **HLA incompatibility is the most important.** Historically, GVHD was classified into acute (first 100 days post-HSCT) and chronic subtypes. The traditional timeline has been altered by trends such as the use of donor lymphocyte infusions to augment the graft-versus-tumor effect post-HSCT, prompting the National Institutes of Health (NIH) Consensus Project to propose a new classification of chronic GVHD using organ-specific criteria. GVHD may also occur following transfusion of nonirradiated blood products (to immunocompromised hosts), by maternal-fetal transmission, or in the setting of solid organ transplantation, particularly the small bowel.

- Among solid organ transplants, it stands to reason that the small bowel carries the highest risk of GVHD due to the large number of lymphoid cells.
- Maternofetal GVHD may lead to seborrheic dermatitis–like or morbilliform eruptions in infants with SCID.

- **Acute GVHD (peak 4-6 weeks post-HSCT)** is characterized by a **morbilliform eruption with a follicular predilection that favors the upper trunk and acral areas (including the ear pinna)** ± bullae formation (stage IV). Acute GVHD may involve multiple organs, with the classic triad involving the skin, liver (eg, **bilirubin elevation**), and gut (eg, **diarrhea**). **Chronic GVHD** may resemble a variety of skin disorders both **nonsclerotic such as LP** and **sclerotic such as LS, morphea, systemic sclerosis (SSc), and EF. Limited range-of-motion (ROM)** most often affects the **wrists and fingers.**
  - A positive "prayer sign" indicates limited ROM of the wrists.
  - Figure 2.44.
- In chronic sclerotic GVHD, **magnetic resonance imaging (MRI)** may be helpful to evaluate for fascial involvement.
- **Systemic corticosteroids** are first line for both acute and chronic GVHD. Phototherapy is a common treatment. **Patients with steroid refractory acute GVHD have a poor prognosis.**

LUPUS ERYTHEMATOSUS
→ **Diagnosis Group 1**

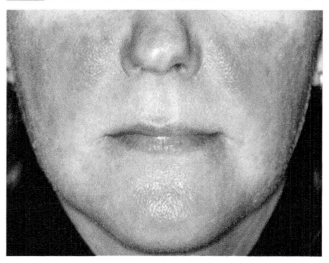

Acute cutaneous lupus erythematosus reprinted with permission from Craft N, Fox LP, Goldsmith LA, et al. *VisualDx: Essential Adult Dermatology.* Wolters Kluwer Health/Lippincott Williams & Wilkins; 2010.

Epidemiology

- LE is an AI-CTD that leads to **inflammation of multiple organ systems, primarily the skin.**
  - Do NOT confuse <u>lupus</u> erythematosus with <u>lupus</u> miliaris disseminatus faciei, <u>lupus</u> pernio, or <u>lupus</u> vulgaris. The distribution of each of these disorders favors the face, but lupus miliaris disseminatus faciei (LMDF) is related to rosacea, lupus pernio is a sarcoidosis variant, and lupus vulgaris is a tuberculosis (TB) variant.

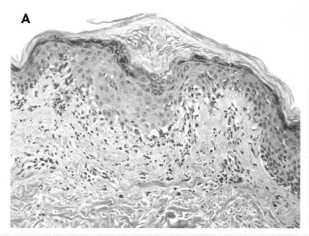
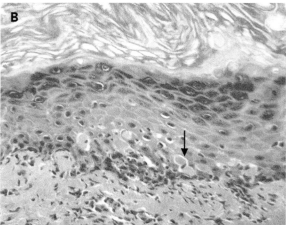

Figure 2.44. CLINICOPATHOLOGICAL CORRELATION: GRAFT-VERSUS-HOST DISEASE. Acute GVHD is characterized by a vacuolar interface dermatitis, keratinocyte necrosis, and a dermal lymphocytic infiltrate. The histopathological features of chronic GVHD may resemble a variety of skin disorders both nonsclerotic such as LP and sclerotic such as LS, morphea, SSc, and EF. A, Low-power view. B, High-power view. Solid arrow: "satellite cell necrosis." EF, eosinophilic fasciitis; GVHD, graft-versus-host disease; LP, lichen planus; LS, lichen sclerosis; SSc, systemic sclerosis.

"Satellite cell necrosis" refers to the presence of necrotic keratinocytes surrounded by lymphocytes.

- The pathogenesis of LE involves a complex interplay of genetic and environmental factors. **UVR induces apoptosis** with translocation of cellular and nuclear antigens and **activates the immune system** through induction of antimicrobial peptides, activation of endothelial cells, release of pro-inflammatory cytokines (eg, **type I IFNs**), and recruitment of inflammatory cells (eg, **$CD4^+$ and $CD8^+$ T cells, pDCs**). Type I IFN release from pDCs creates an amplification loop that culminates in **cytotoxic keratinocyte damage.**
- LE peaks in women during child-bearing years. Approximately 50% of patients have isolated cutaneous disease (female:male ratio 3:1) and ~50% of patients have **SLE (female:male ratio 6:1). African American women have a fourfold higher prevalence of SLE than Caucasian American women**, in addition to earlier disease onset and a higher mortality rate.
- LE may occur as part of an overlapping AI-CTD. Other associations depend on subtype.

Clinicopathological Features

- **LE subtypes and related disorders** are summarized in Table 2.21.
    - Figure 2.45.
      Neonatal LE primarily occurs in infants whose mothers have **anti-ro/la > anti-U1-ribonucleoprotein (RNP) autoantibodies.** The incidence is ~2%, with a **recurrence rate of ~20%** in subsequent pregnancies. While some mothers have identified LE or Sjögren syndrome, **the majority of mothers are asymptomatic.** Neonatal LE classically presents with **SCLE lesions favoring the scalp and periorbital face.** Lesions **heal 6 to 8 months after birth with dyspigmentation ± telangiectasias. Photosensitivity** is common. **Patients with anti-ro/la autoantibodies may develop congenital heart block (15%-30%).** Other systemic features include **hepatobiliary disease** and cytopenias, especially **thrombocytopenia.**
    - Periorbital neonatal LE may have a "raccoon eye" appearance.
      Children and adolescents with SLE have higher mortality rates and more disease damage (eg, LE nephritis) than adults.
- LE may **overlap with pemphigus erythematosus (Senear-Usher syndrome).**
- LE may **overlap with LP.**
- LE may **overlap with EM (Rowell syndrome).**
- **Classification criteria for SLE** are presented in Table 2.22.
    - Figure 2.46.

Evaluation

- The differential diagnosis of LE is extensive and depends on the subtype.
- In discoid lupus erythematosus (DLE), trichoscopy demonstrates **follicular red dots and hair casts.**

- **Lesional skin biopsy ± lesional DIF** (when skin biopsy is not definitive) is recommended to diagnose cutaneous LE. **In nonlesional skin, a true positive "lupus band" test correlates with SLE.** However, this test is often superfluous in the setting of clinical evaluation and serologic testing.
- Laboratory evaluation for SLE includes comprehensive metabolic panel (CMP), CBC, C3/C4, CRP/ESR, urinalysis (UA), ANA with profile, and antiphospholipid antibodies.
      In neonatal LE, serial monitoring with CBC, liver function tests (LFTs), and electrocardiogram (ECG) is recommended.
- ANAs are autoantibodies that target primarily nuclear components (eg, DNA). ANAs are conventionally detected using IIF, but ELISA assays may have similar clinical utility. When detected using IIF, positive ANAs are reported with both **pattern** (Figure 2.47) and **titer ≥ 1:40** (last dilution at which the pattern is detectable). Positive ANA titer is nonspecific and may be present in **apparently normal individuals** (~**one third at 1:40, ~13% at 1:80, ~5% at 1:160** ages 20-60 years). **ANA titer ≥ 1:160 is often clinically significant.**
- **Autoantibodies in LE and related disorders** are summarized in Table 2.23.

Management

- For cutaneous LE, topical therapies include **photoprotection**, corticosteroids, calcineurin inhibitors, and retinoids. **Hydroxychloroquine** is the first-line systemic antimalarial therapy, with chloroquine and quinacrine as alternatives. For antimalarial-resistant cutaneous disease, consider other systemic immunosuppressives (eg, corticosteroids), thalidomide/lenalidomide, and retinoids. Tobacco use is associated with refractory cutaneous LE; therefore, smoking cessation is an adjunctive therapy.
    - DLE is a rare exception when the use of high-potency topical corticosteroids on the face is appropriate to PREVENT atrophy.
      When **neonatal LE with congenital heart block** is identified, consider preemptive treatment with **hydroxychloroquine during subsequent pregnancies.**
- For mild SLE, NSAIDs are first line. For moderate to severe SLE, consider systemic immunosuppressives including **anifrolumab, belimumab, and rituximab.** Severe SLE may warrant **pulse cyclophosphamide ± pulse corticosteroids.** For bullous SLE, **dapsone** is first line.

"Real World" Advice

- Clinical clues to differentiate LE from PMLE include absence of pruritus and longer duration (weeks to months as compared to days to weeks).
- Remember to advise patients that the response to antimalarials is slow (~2-3 months). The retinotoxic effect of chloroquine and hydroxychloroquine is additive; therefore, using quinacrine in combination is preferred. Unfortunately, quinacrine is not currently marketed in the United States.

Table 2.21. LUPUS ERYTHEMATOSUS SUBTYPES AND RELATED DISORDERS

Diagnosis[a]	Classic Description	Notes
Acute Cutaneous		
ACLE	Malar erythema sparing the nasolabial folds. Photosensitivity is common Figure 2.45.	ACLE is typically associated with SLE.
Subacute Cutaneous		
SCLE	Erythematous scaling thin papules and plaques favoring the lateral face, upper trunk, and extensor upper extremities. The configuration may be annular or papulosquamous. Lesions heal with dyspigmentation ± telangiectasias. Photosensitivity is common.	Drug associations include TNFα inhibitors, terbinafine, antimicrotubule taxanes, antiepileptics, CCBs, HCTZ, PPIs, and thrombocyte inhibitors. HLA associations include -B8 and -DR3. Up to 50% of patients have SLE.
Chronic Cutaneous		
DLE	Erythematous scaling indurated papules and plaques favoring the scalp, face, and ears. Lesions heal with dyspigmentation, atrophy, and scarring. Scarring circumscribed hair loss may occur. DLE variants are localized, widespread, or hypertrophic. Hypertrophic DLE resembles hypertrophic LP but favors the extensor upper extremities > face and trunk. If the scale from a follicular area is lifted, conical projections may extend downward. This correlates with follicular plugging on histopathology and is the "carpet tack sign."	A lupus-like syndrome, in particular DLE, may be observed in both XLR CGD patients and female carriers. SCC may develop within long-standing DLE lesions. ~10%-20% of patients have SLE (higher risk in widespread variant).
LE tumidus	Erythematous plaques favoring the face and trunk without DLE surface changes. The configuration may be annular. Photosensitivity is common.	May overlap with reticular erythematous mucinosis and lymphocytic infiltrate of Jessner.
LE panniculitis	Tender erythematous subcutaneous nodules and plaques favoring the scalp, face, upper trunk, breasts, buttocks, upper arms, and thighs ± overlying features of DLE. Lesions heal with significant atrophy. The skin overlying LE panniculitis may have a "tethered" appearance.	Similar to LE panniculitis, a predominantly lobular panniculitis may occur in DM and RA.
Chilblain lupus	Red-to-purple papules and plaques favoring the fingers and toes > nose, elbows, knees, and lower legs. Chilblain lupus resembles pernio but may evolve to resemble DLE over time.	Triggered by cold wet exposure.
Systemic		
SLE	Cutaneous features depend on LE subtype. Nonspecific cutaneous lesions include Raynaud phenomenon, palmar erythema, APLS/Degos-like lesions, vasculitis (eg, CSVV, hypocomplementemic urticarial vasculitis, cryoglobulinemic vasculitis), Sweet syndrome–like neutrophilic dermatosis, PNGD, papulonodular mucinosis, and multiple DFs. Diffuse nonscarring alopecia may occur, as well as proximal nail fold dilated capillaries with normal density and red lunulae. The diagnostic criteria (see below) summarize systemic features of SLE, which also include fever and nonbacterial thrombotic endocarditis. Short, broken hairs along the frontal scalp line are called "lupus hairs."	Associations include hereditary and acquired deficiency of early complement components (C1-C4) and C1-inh (acquired angioedema, MAS resulting in HLH) and solar urticaria. HLA associations include -DR2 and -DR3. Drug associations include TNFα inhibitors IFNs, ICIs, and D-penicillamine.
Bullous SLE	Tense blisters mimicking BP, LABD, or inflammatory EBA.	Acquired autoimmune blistering disorder characterized by circulating autoantibodies to collagen VII.
ASAP	Large erosions mimicking TEN.	Blisters due to cytotoxic keratinocyte damage.
Drug-induced LE	Arthralgias, myalgias, serositis, and fever. Rare cutaneous involvement mimicking ACLE.	Drug associations include INH, minocycline, chlorpromazine, hydralazine, methyldopa, procainamide, and quinidine. Slow acetylation is associated with hydralazine- and procainamide-induced LE.

(Continued)

Table 2.21. LUPUS ERYTHEMATOSUS SUBTYPES AND RELATED DISORDERS (CONTINUED)

Diagnosis[a]	Classic Description	Notes
Related Disorders		
Sjögren syndrome	Xerostomia, xerophthalmia, and arthritis. Nonspecific cutaneous features include xerosis, Raynaud phenomenon, and vasculitis (CSVV, hypocomplementemic urticarial vasculitis, cryoglobulinemic vasculitis). Complications include ILD, peripheral neuropathy, and B-cell lymphomas, in particular extranodal marginal zone lymphomas of the MALT type.	AI-CTD that involves inflammation of secretory glands. Associations include other autoimmune disorders (eg, RA, SLE). HLA associations include -B8 and -DR3. Vasculitis, hypocomplementemia, cryoglobulinemia, and parotid enlargement are poor prognostic factors. 50% of salivary glands must be destroyed before sicca symptoms arise. In the Schirmer test, lacrimal gland dysfunction is indicated by ≤ 5 mm migration of the aqueous component of the tear film on a piece of Whatman paper wick folded over the lower eyelid for 5 minutes. Consider biopsy of the minor salivary glands.
MCTD	Raynaud phenomenon, swollen hands or sclerodactyly, PAH > ILD, esophageal dysmotility, myositis, and arthritis.	AI-CTD with overlapping features of SLE, PM, SSc, and RA. HLA associations include -B8 and -DR4. PAH is the leading cause of death.

ACLE, acute cutaneous lupus erythematosus; AI-CTD, autoimmune connective tissue disorder; APLS, antiphospholipid antibody syndrome; ASAP, acute syndrome of apoptotic pan epidermolysis; BP, bullous pemphigoid; C, complement; CCBs, calcium channel blockers; CGD, chronic granulomatous disease; CSVV, cutaneous small-vessel vasculitis; DFs, dermatofibromas; DLE, discoid lupus erythematosus; EBA, epidermolysis bullosa acquisita; 5-FU, 5-fluorouracil; HCTZ, hydrochlorothiazide; HLA, human leukocyte antigen; HLH, hemophagocytic lymphohistiocytosis; ICIs, immune checkpoint inhibitors; IFNs, interferons; ILD, interstitial lung disease; inh, inhibitor; INH, isoniazid; LABD, linear IgA bullous dermatosis; LE, lupus erythematosus; LP, lichen planus; MALT, mucosa-associated lymphoid tissue; MAS, macrophage activation syndrome; MCTD, mixed connective tissue disease; PAH, pulmonary arterial hypertension; PM, polymyositis; PNGD, palisaded neutrophilic granulomatous dermatitis; PPIs, proton pump inhibitors; RA, rheumatoid arthritis; SCC, squamous cell carcinoma; SCLE, subacute cutaneous lupus erythematosus; SLE, systemic lupus erythematosus; SSc, systemic sclerosis; TEN, toxic epidermal necrolysis; XLR, X-linked recessive.
[a]Illustrative examples provided. LE subtypes may overlap in the same patient.

Table 2.22. CLASSIFICATION CRITERIA FOR SYSTEMIC LUPUS ERYTHEMATOSUS

1997 Update of the 1982 ACR revised criteria for classification of SLE[a,b]

1. Malar rash
2. Discoid rash
3. Photosensitivity
4. Oral ulcers (oral or nasopharyngeal, usually painless, observed by physician)
5. Nonerosive arthritis (involving ≥2 peripheral joints)
6. Pleuritis OR pericarditis
7. Renal disorder (persistent proteinuria OR cellular casts)
8. Neurologic disorder (seizures OR psychosis in the absence of offending drugs or known metabolic derangements)
9. Hematologic disorder (hemolytic anemia with reticulocytosis OR leukopenia on ≥ 2 occasions OR lymphopenia on ≥ 2 occasions OR thrombocytopenia in the absence of offending drugs)
10. Immunologic disorder (autoantibodies: anti-dsDNA OR anti-Sm OR antiphospholipid)
11. ANA (in the absence of drugs)

ACR, American College of Rheumatology; ANA, antinuclear antibody; DNA, deoxyribonucleic acid; ds, double-stranded; EULAR, European League Against Rheumatism; SLE, systemic lupus erythematosus; SLICC, Systemic Lupus International Collaborating Clinics; Sm, Smith.
[a]Four criteria, serially or simultaneously, are required for diagnosis.
[b]Alternative classification criteria include the 2012 SLICC criteria and the 2019 EULAR/ACR criteria.

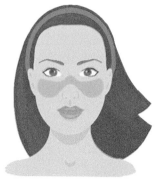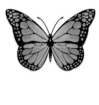

Figure 2.45. THE BUTTERFLY RASH. Malar erythema sparing the nasolabial folds in ACLE is commonly called the "butterfly rash." Do NOT confuse the "butterfly rash" with the "butterfly sign" of self-induced skin findings. ACLE, acute cutaneous lupus erythematosus.

(Illustration by Caroline A. Nelson, MD.)

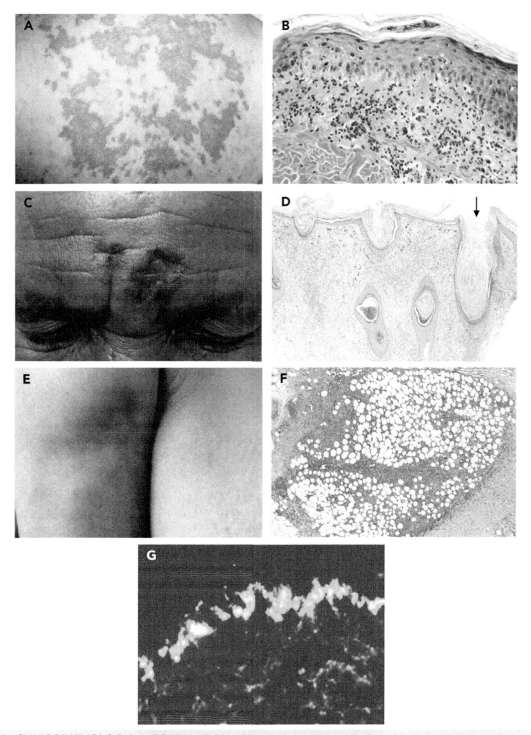

Figure 2.46. CLINICOPATHOLOGICAL CORRELATION: LUPUS ERYTHEMATOSUS. A, SCLE. B, SCLE. C, DLE. D, DLE. Solid arrow: follicular plugging. E, LE panniculitis. F, LE panniculitis. G, DIF (IgG). ACLE, acute cutaneous LE; BMZ, basement membrane thickening; C, complement; CD, cluster of differentiation; DEJ, dermal-epidermal junction; DIF, direct immuno-fluorescence; DLE, discoid LE; FFA, frontal fibrosing alopecia; GAG, glycosaminoglycan; H&E, hematoxylin and eosin; Ig, immunoglobulin; LE, lupus erythematosus; LPP, lichen planopilaris; LS, lichen sclerosus; pDCs, plasmacytoid dendritic cells; PRP, pityriasis rubra pilaris; SCLE, subacute cutaneous LE; SLE, systemic lupus erythematosus; SPTCL, subacute panniculitis–like T-cell lymphoma; SSA, anti–Sjögren syndrome-related antigen A; SSB, anti–Sjögren syndrome-related antigen B; TCR. T-cell receptor.

(A, Image courtesy of Victoria Werth, MD. D, Histology image courtesy of Noel Turner, MD, MHS and Christine J. Ko, MD. G, Histology image reprinted with permission from Elder DE, Elenitsas R, Rosenbach M, et al. *Lever's Histopathology of the Skin.* 11th ed. Wolters Kluwer; 2015.)

Figure 2.46. Continued

- **ACLE:** vacuolar interface dermatitis.
- **SCLE/Neonatal Lupus:** vacuolar interface dermatitis and lymphohistiocytic infiltrates in the dermis.
- **DLE:** vacuolar interface dermatitis and perivascular and periadnexal lymphohistiocytic infiltrates in the dermis. Perifollicular infiltrates are concentrated at the isthmus and lower infundibulum. DLE > SCLE may demonstrate hyperkeratosis, follicular plugging, BMZ thickening, and melanin pigment incontinence. Hypertrophic DLE is characterized by lichenoid interface dermatitis.
- **LE tumidus:** perivascular and periadnexal lymphohistiocytic infiltrates in the dermis. Vacuolar interface dermatitis is absent.
- **LE panniculitis:** lymphoplasmacytic infiltrates with nodular lymphocytic aggregates (lymphoid follicles) and hyaline fat necrosis ± overlying features of DLE.
- **Chilblain lupus:** vacuolar interface dermatitis, lymphohistiocytic infiltrates, and papillary dermal edema.
- **Bullous SLE:** see Chapter 2: Vesiculobullous Disorders.

CD123 is a marker of pDCs. Though not specific, the pattern and intensity of CD-123 staining may help diagnose LE. Mucin, an amorphous mixture of acid GAGs, is variably present (most prominent in tumid LE). Mucin appears blue on H&E with stains including Alcian blue, colloidal iron, crystal violet, and toluidine blue. DIF in LE classically demonstrates continuous granular deposition of IgM, IgG, IgA, and C3 along the DEJ.*

The depth of interface dermatitis helps distinguish DLE (isthmus > infundibulum) from FFA/LPP (infundibulum > isthmus). Follicular plugging is a shared feature between PRP, DLE, and LS.
TCR gene rearrangement is more likely to detect T-cell clonality in SPTCL than LE panniculitis.
The "full house" DIF pattern in LE is also known as the "lupus band."

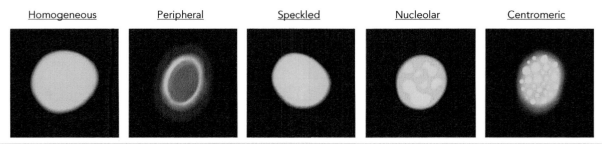

| Homogeneous | Peripheral | Speckled | Nucleolar | Centromeric |

Figure 2.47. ANTINUCLEAR ANTIBODY PATTERNS. The homogenous pattern is also called diffuse, the peripheral pattern is also called rim, the specked pattern is also called particulate, and the centromeric pattern is also called discrete speckled. (Illustration by Caroline A. Nelson, MD.)

Table 2.23. AUTOANTIBODIES IN LUPUS ERYTHEMATOSUS AND RELATED DISORDERS

Autoantibody[a]	Association(s)[a]
ANA	SLE (99%).
Anti-collagen VII	Bullous SLE.
Anti-C1q	SLE (severe).
Anti-dsDNA (peripheral ANA pattern)	SLE (highly specific) with LE nephritis (correlates with disease activity).
Anti-α-fodrin	Sjögren syndrome.
Anti-histones	Drug-induced LE.
Anti-Ku	SLE overlap with DM/PM or SSc.
Antiphospholipid.	SLE overlap with APLS.
Anti-ro (SSA)/la (SSB) (speckled ANA pattern)	Neonatal LE with congenital heart block. SCLE. Sjögren syndrome.
Anti-rRNP	SLE (highly specific) with neuropsychiatric LE.
Anti-Sm (speckled ANA pattern)	SLE (highly specific).
Anti-ssDNA	SLE (possible risk for SLE in DLE patients).
Anti-U1RNP (speckled ANA pattern)	MCTD (100%). Neonatal LE without congenital heart block. SLE (as part of an overlapping AI-CTD).
p-ANCA	Drug-induced LE due to minocycline.

AI-CTD, autoimmune connective tissue disorder; ANA, antinuclear antibody; APLS, antiphospholipid antibody syndrome. C, complement; DLE, discoid lupus erythematosus; DM, dermatomyositis; DNA, deoxyribonucleic acid; ds, double-stranded; LE, lupus erythematosus; MCTD, mixed connective tissue disease; p-ANCA, perinuclear antineutrophil cytoplasmic antibody; PM, polymyositis; r, ribosomal; RNP, ribonucleoprotein; SCLE, subacute cutaneous lupus erythematosus; SLE, systemic lupus erythematosus; Sm, Smith; ss, single-stranded; SSA, anti–Sjögren syndrome-related antigen A; SSB, anti–Sjögren syndrome-related antigen B; SSc, systemic sclerosis.
[a]Illustrative examples provided.

DERMATOMYOSITIS
→ Diagnosis Group 1

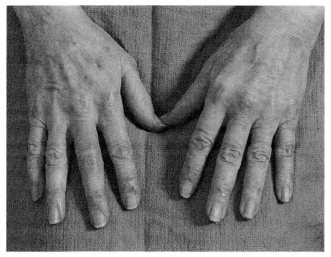

Courtesy of Victoria Werth, MD.

Epidemiology

- DM is an AI-CTD classified, along with polymyositis (PM) and inclusion body myositis, as an idiopathic inflammatory myopathy.
- DM has a **bimodal age distribution** with the first peak occurring from **5 to 14 years (juvenile-onset DM)** and the second peak occurring from **45 to 64 years (adult-onset DM)**. The female:male ratio ranges from 2:1 to 3:1. DM may be **classic, hypomyopathic, or amyopathic.**
- DM may occur as part of an overlapping AI-CTD. **Adult-onset DM is associated with malignancy in up to 25% of patients**, with the **risk of malignancy returning to a relative baseline after 3 years.** The most common malignancy is **ovarian**, with others include breast, colorectal, gastric, lung, NHL, pancreatic, and nasopharyngeal (in some Southeast Asian populations).
    Juvenile-onset DM is not associated with malignancy.
- Drug associations include **cyclophosphamide, TNFα inhibitors, hydroxyurea, ICIs, NSAIDs, D-penicillamine, and statins.** Other triggers include the **bacille Calmette-Guérin (BCG) vaccine.**

Clinicopathological Features

- **Skin findings in DM** are presented in Figure 2.48.
    Dystrophic calcification and vascular occlusion are more common in juvenile-onset DM than adult-onset DM. In patients with the **TNFα 308A allele,** vascular occlusion may relate to increased circulating concentrations of the potent anti-angiogenic factor **thrombospondin 1.**
- DM may cause significant morbidity due to **pruritus.**
- DM is a **symmetric, proximal, extensor inflammatory myopathy (triceps/quadriceps).** Patients may be unable to comb their hair or rise to their feet from a sitting position. Other systemic features include **arrhythmias, dysphagia/gastroesophageal reflux disease (GERD), inflammatory polyarthritis, and interstitial lung disease (ILD).**

- **PRP-like (Wong) type DM** primarily occurs in **Asian** populations.
    ❖ Figure 2.49.

Evaluation

- The differential diagnosis of DM is extensive and depends on the variant.
- **Lesional skin biopsy** is recommended to diagnose DM.
- Laboratory evaluation includes CMP, fasting lipid panel, CBC, and direct autoantibody panel.
- All patients should also undergo evaluation for:
    o Overlapping AI-CTDs.
    o Myositis (at baseline and at 2-3-month intervals for at least 2 years): **examination for proximal extensor muscle weakness, creatine kinase (CK)/aldolase ± electromyography (EMG), MRI, and/or US of proximal muscles, muscle biopsy (triceps).**
        Ignore outdated dogma regarding the deltoid! In patients with suspected myositis, biopsy of the triceps is preferred as the deltoid is often spared until late in the disease.
    o ILD: **high-resolution CT chest, PFTs with diffusing capacity for carbon monoxide (DLCO).**
    o Malignancy (at baseline and annually for at least 3 years): UA, fecal occult blood test (FOBT), cancer antigen (CA)19-9, CA125 (women), prostate-specific antigen (PSA) (men), CT chest/abdomen/pelvis, mammogram (women), **transvaginal pelvic US (women),** Papanicolaou smear (women) ± colonoscopy/upper endoscopy.
- Patients with myositis should also undergo ECG ± transthoracic echocardiogram (TTE) and/or Holter monitor (if symptoms) and esophageal barium swallow or manometry (if symptoms).
- **Autoantibodies in DM** are summarized in Table 2.24.

Management

- Malignancy is a poor prognostic factor in adult-onset DM.
    Juvenile-onset DM has a more favorable prognosis than adult-onset DM.
- For cutaneous DM, topical therapies are similar to cutaneous LE. **Hydroxychloroquine** is the first-line systemic antimalarial therapy; however, there is an **increased risk of a cutaneous drug reaction to hydroxychloroquine in patients with DM** as compared to LE. Antimalarial-resistant cutaneous disease is often treated with methotrexate, mycophenolate mofetil, and finally **IVIG.** Therapies for dystrophic calcification include diltiazem and surgical excision.
    IVIG is first line for severe or refractory juvenile-onset DM.
- For myositis, **systemic corticosteroids** are first line. **Physical therapy** is important to preserve muscle strength and endurance.
- The Dermatomyositis Skin Severity Index (DSSI) and the updated Cutaneous Dermatomyositis Disease Area and Severity Index (CDASI) are validated instruments to measure the severity of cutaneous DM and assess response to treatment in clinical trials.

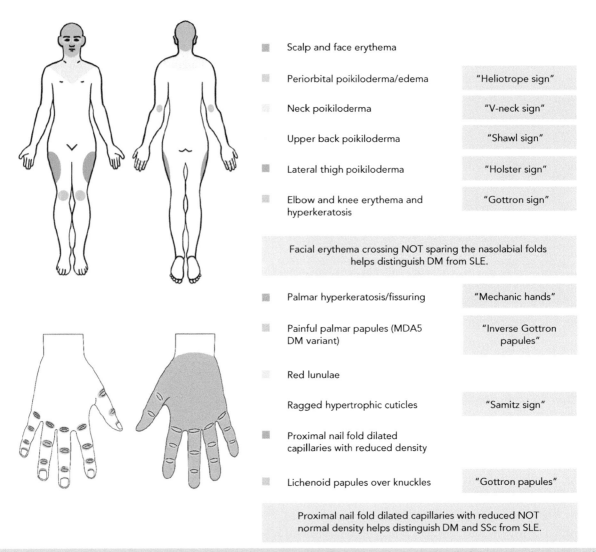

Scalp and face erythema		
Periorbital poikiloderma/edema	"Heliotrope sign"	
Neck poikiloderma	"V-neck sign"	
Upper back poikiloderma	"Shawl sign"	
Lateral thigh poikiloderma	"Holster sign"	
Elbow and knee erythema and hyperkeratosis	"Gottron sign"	

Facial erythema crossing NOT sparing the nasolabial folds helps distinguish DM from SLE.

Palmar hyperkeratosis/fissuring	"Mechanic hands"
Painful palmar papules (MDA5 DM variant)	"Inverse Gottron papules"
Red lunulae	
Ragged hypertrophic cuticles	"Samitz sign"
Proximal nail fold dilated capillaries with reduced density	
Lichenoid papules over knuckles	"Gottron papules"

Proximal nail fold dilated capillaries with reduced NOT normal density helps distinguish DM and SSc from SLE.

Figure 2.48. SKIN FINDINGS IN DERMATOMYOSITIS. Other skin findings include Raynaud phenomenon, centripetal flagellate erythema, dystrophic calcification, necrosis/ulceration, diffuse nonscarring alopecia, and papulonodular mucinosis. Illustrative examples provided. DM, dermatomyositis; MCP, metacarpophalangeal; MDA5, melanoma differentiation–associated protein 5; SLE, systemic lupus erythematosus; SSc, systemic sclerosis.
(Illustration by Caroline A. Nelson, MD.)

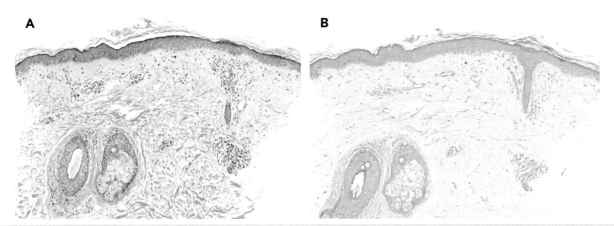

Figure 2.49. CLINICOPATHOLOGICAL CORRELATION: DERMATOMYOSITIS. The histopathology of DM resembles LE but is often more subtle. Epidermal atrophy is characteristic except in "Gottron papules," which demonstrate hyperkeratosis and acanthosis. A, H&E. B, Alcian blue stain. DM, dermatomyositis; H&E, hematoxylin and eosin; LE, lupus erythematosus.

Table 2.24. AUTOANTIBODIES IN DERMATOMYOSITIS

Autoantibody[a]	Association(s)[a]
ANA	DM/PM (40%).
Anti-Ku	DM/PM overlap with SLE or SSc.
	Anti-Ku suggests muscular involvement in SLE or SSc.
Anti-MDA5 (CADM-140)	MDA5 DM (highly specific): amyopathic DM with cutaneous and oral ulcerations, painful palmar papules, and diffuse nonscarring alopecia; rapidly progressive ILD; arthritis.
Anti-Mi2	Classic DM (highly specific, good prognosis).
Anti-NXP-2 (p140)	DM/PM (highly specific) with dystrophic calcification and subcutaneous edema. Malignancy-associated adult-onset DM.
Anti-PM-Scl	DM/PM overlap with SSc.
Anti-SAE	Adult-onset DM.
Anti-SRP	Fulminant DM/PM (highly specific) with cardiac involvement (poor prognosis).
Anti-TIF1γ (p155)	Amyopathic > classic DM (highly specific) with extensive cutaneous disease. Malignancy-associated adult-onset DM.
Anti-aminoacyl-tRNA synthetases (eg, anti-Jo-1, anti-PL-7, anti-PL-12 > anti-EJ, anti-OJ)	Antisynthetase syndrome (highly specific): Raynaud phenomenon, palmar hyperkeratosis and fissuring, fever, ILD, erosive polyarthritis.

ANA, antinuclear antibody; CADM, clinically amyopathic dermatomyositis; DM, dermatomyositis; ILD, interstitial lung disease; MDA5, melanoma differentiation-associated protein 5; NXP, nuclear matrix protein; PM, polymyositis; SAE, small ubiquitin-like modifier activating enzyme; SLE, systemic lupus erythematosus; SRP, signal recognition particle; SSc, systemic sclerosis; TIF, transcription intermediary factor; tRNA, transfer ribonucleoprotein.
[a]Illustrative examples provided.

"Real World" Advice

- Some clinicians perform MRI and/or US before or instead of EMG and muscle biopsy.
- **Older age and extensive cutaneous disease with necrosis/ulceration** are among the characteristics of adult-onset DM reported in **association with malignancy.**
- Cutaneous DM is often refractory to systemic corticosteroids, which are the mainstay of treatment for myositis. As a result, **systemic corticosteroids** are first line in **classic but not amyopathic DM.**

LICHEN SCLEROSUS
→ Diagnosis Group 2
Synonym: lichen sclerosus et atrophicus

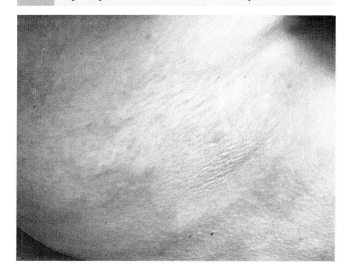

Epidemiology

- LS is an AI-CTD that leads to **cutaneous sclerosis, primarily of the epidermis and dermis.** There is no internal organ involvement.
- LS peaks in the fifth and sixth decades. The female:male ratio ranges from 1:1 to 10:1.
- In women, LS is associated with **other autoimmune disorders (eg, thyroid).**
- The leading HLA association is -**DQ7.**

Clinicopathological Features

- LS classically presents with **sclerotic, white, flat papules and plaques with epidermal atrophy favoring the anogenital area.** Involvement of the **penis (balanitis xerotica obliterans)** may be complicated by **phimosis,** paraphimosis, or recurrent balanitis. Involvement of the **perivulvar area** may be complicated by burying of the clitoris, fusion of the labia minora to the labia majora, and **scarring of the vaginal introitus.** DEJ fragility causes **subepidermal hemorrhagic bullae. Extragenital LS (~15%)** classically presents with **follicular plugging and telangiectasias favoring the trunk and proximal extremities.**
    - LS lesions may be described as "ivory white" and "parchment-like." The perivulvar and perianal configuration in women may resemble a "figure of eight."
- Involvement of the oral cavity is rare.

- **Anogenital LS** may cause significant morbidity due to **pruritus and pain leading to dysuria, dyspareunia, and dyschezia.** LS may induce eruptive melanocytic nevi. Increased risk of **SCC and vulvar intraepithelial neoplasia (VIN)** remains controversial. **Extragenital LS** is often **asymptomatic.**
- LS **may overlap with morphea.**
    - Figure 2.50.

Evaluation

- The differential diagnosis of LS in adults includes morphea, erosive LP, and SCCis.
- Autoantibodies in LS include **ECM-1.**

Management

- **High-potency topical corticosteroids** are first line. Other topical therapies include calcineurin inhibitors and calcipotriene.

- LS is a rare exception when the use of high-potency topical corticosteroids in the anogenital area is appropriate to PREVENT atrophy.
- **Phototherapy (PUVA, UVA1)** may be helpful for **extragenital LS.**
- Systemic therapies for severe LS include corticosteroids, cyclosporine, **methotrexate**, and retinoids.
- **Circumcision** is first line for **balanitis xerotica obliterans** complicated by phimosis or paraphimosis.

"Real World" Advice

- The absence of vaginal mucosal involvement helps distinguish LS from LP.

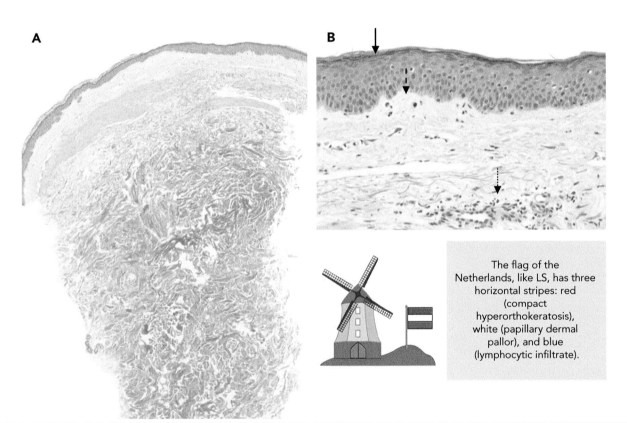

The flag of the Netherlands, like LS, has three horizontal stripes: red (compact hyperorthokeratosis), white (papillary dermal pallor), and blue (lymphocytic infiltrate).

Figure 2.50. CLINICOPATHOLOGICAL CORRELATION: LICHEN SCLEROSUS. LS is characterized by compact hyperorthokeratosis ± epidermal atrophy, papillary dermal pallor, and a vacuolar lymphocytic dermal infiltrate. Other features include follicular plugging, pigment incontinence, and subepidermal hemorrhagic bullae. A, Low-power view. B, High-power view. Solid arrow: compact hyperorthokeratosis (red). Dashed arrow: papillary dermal pallor (white). Dotted arrow: lymphocytic infiltrate (blue). LS may overlap with morphea on histopathology. DLE, discoid lupus erythematosus; LS, lichen sclerosus; PRP, pityriasis rubra pilaris.

(Illustration by Caroline A. Nelson, MD.)

Follicular plugging is a shared feature between PRP, DLE, and LS.

MORPHEA
→ Diagnosis Group 2
Synonym: localized scleroderma

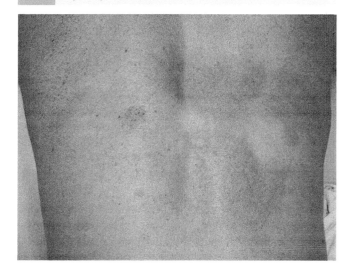

Epidemiology

- Morphea is an AI-CTD that leads to **cutaneous sclerosis, primarily of the dermis ± subcutis.** There is no internal organ involvement. The pathogenesis of sclerosis involves hypoxia resulting from vascular injury followed by T-cell infiltration. **Upregulation of Th2 cytokines (eg, IL-4, IL-13, IL-31) and TGF-β activates dermal fibroblasts** to enhance production of collagen (I, II, III) and other ECM proteins. **CXCL4,** secreted by pDCs, is anti-angiogenic and promotes the Th2 response.
- A hypothesized role for **Borrelia burgdorferi** infection in triggering morphea remains controversial.

Clinicopathological Features

- **Plaque-type** morphea classically presents with **asymmetric 2 to 15 cm indurated plaques favoring the trunk. Active lesions** are characterized by a **lilac border and central hypo- or dyspigmentation,** while **inactive lesions** are characterized by hyperpigmentation.
- **Scarring circumscribed hair loss** may occur.
- Morphea can cause significant morbidity due to **pain, skin tightness, and joint contractures.**
- Less common **morphea variants** are summarized in Table 2.25.

   Linear morphea is the most common variant in **children.** Disabling pansclerotic morphea of children is similar to generalized morphea of the adult.
- Morphea may **overlap with LS.**
   ◆ Figure 2.51.

Table 2.25. MORPHEA VARIANTS

Variant[a]	Classic Description	Notes
Bullous	Indurated plaques associated with bullae.	Bullous morphea develops when cutaneous sclerosis is accompanied by diffuse, rapidly progressive edema with lymphoceles resulting from stasis of lymphatic fluid.
Deep (morphea profunda)	Few deeply indurated plaques ± dystrophic calcification.	Similar to deep morphea, a predominantly septal panniculitis may occur in SSc.
Generalized	Multiple indurated plaques rapidly coalesce, most often on the trunk extending to the extremities.	Aggressive therapy is important to prevent difficulty breathing due to impaired thorax mobility and intercostal muscle inflammation.
Guttate	Multiple nummular indurated plaques.	
Linear	Deeply indurated linear plaque, most often on an extremity. Hemifacial atrophy (Parry-Romberg syndrome) refers to progressive loss of subcutaneous fat with little or no sclerosis in the distribution of the trigeminal nerve. Ocular or neurologic symptoms may rarely occur in linear morphea of the head or hemifacial atrophy.	Linear morphea may be associated with linear melorheostosis. Aggressive therapy is important to prevent joint contractures and growth retardation (eg, micromelia).
	En coup de sabre, meaning a stroke or blow with a single-edged sword, refers to linear morphea of the scalp and forehead.	The radiographic finding in linear melorheostosis is linear hyperostosis, which resembles "tallow drippings on the side of a burning candle."
Nodular (keloidal)	Thick keloid-like nodules or bands.	

SSc, systemic sclerosis.
[a]Illustrative examples provided. For atrophoderma of Pasini and Pierini/linear atrophoderma of Moulin, which some consider a very superficial variant of plaque-type morphea, see Chapter 5: Fibrous Neoplasms.

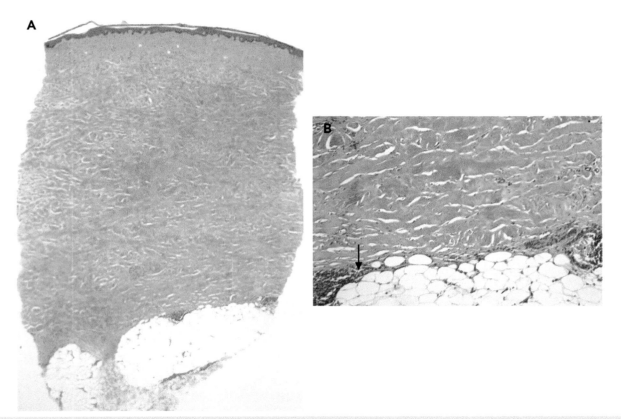

Figure 2.51. CLINICOPATHOLOGICAL CORRELATION: MORPHEA. Early morphea is characterized by an interstitial lymphoplasmacytic infiltrate separating dermal collagen bundles. Collagen bundles become thick, hypocellular, and swollen over time, resulting in a square punch. The infiltrate surrounds eccrine coils in the deep dermis, and there is loss of adventitial fat and CD34$^+$ DCs. Late morphea is characterized by absent appendages and sparse inflammation localized at the dermal–subcutaneous junction. Elastic fibers separated by collagen fibers are brightly eosinophilic and stain black on VVG stain in a parallel array. Morphea may overlap with LS on histopathology. Late morphea. A, Low-power view. B, High-power view. Solid arrow: lymphoplasmacytic infiltrate at the dermal-subcutaneous junction. CD, cluster of differentiation; DCs, dendritic cells; LS, lichen sclerosis; SSc, systemic sclerosis; VVG, Verhoeff-van Gieson.

(Histology images reprinted with permission from Elder DE, Elenitsas R, Rosenbach M, et al. *Lever's Histopathology of the Skin.* 11th ed. Wolters Kluwer; 2015.)

• **Deep morphea**: lymphoplasmacytic infiltrates with nodular lymphocytic aggregates (lymphoid follicles) and subcutaneous septal thickening with involvement of the underlying fascia ± muscle/bone.

Loss of adventitial fat gives eccrine glands a "trapped" appearance.
Morphea can NOT be distinguished from SSc on histopathology, although early morphea tends to have a more robust inflammatory infiltrate.

Evaluation

• The differential diagnosis of morphea includes other sclerosing disorders. **Sclerosing disorders induced by exogenous substances** are summarized in Table 2.26.

   Stiff skin syndrome is a hereditary disorder due to **AD mutation of *FBN1* encoding fibrillin-1** that classically presents with **thick skin favoring the buttocks and thighs with joint contractures.** Other hereditary disorders with sclerosis include PRP type V, pachydermoperiostosis, phenylketonuria, porphyrias, progeria, adult progeria, and ataxia-telangiectasia (A-T).

   Thick skin in stiff skin syndrome may be "rock hard."

• **Biopsy should include the subcutis (eg, telescoping [double] punch, incisional, or excisional biopsy).**

• **Autoantibodies in morphea and SSc** are summarized in Table 2.27.

Management

• Morphea typically progresses over 3 to 5 years, then regresses spontaneously. The exception is linear morphea, which typically persists.

• Management of morphea is similar to LS. **Physical therapy** is important to preserve joint mobility.

"Real World" Advice

• Distinguishing morphea from SSc is challenging. Clinical features that suggest morphea include:
   ○ Localized asymmetric sclerosis (except generalized morphea) without sclerodactyly.
   ○ Absent Raynaud phenomenon.
   ○ Absent internal organ involvement (except rare ocular and/or neurologic symptoms in linear morphea of the head or hemifacial atrophy).

Table 2.26. SCLEROSING DISORDERS INDUCED BY EXOGENOUS SUBSTANCES

Diagnosis[a]	Classic Description	Exogenous Substance(s)[a]
Eosinophilia-myalgia syndrome	Morbilliform eruption with possible evolution into a sclerodermoid reaction (with acral sparing). Systemic features include fever, peripheral hypereosinophilia, and myalgias.	Contaminated L-tryptophan (historical).
Radiation-induced morphea	Resembles morphea at sites of radiation therapy.	Radiation therapy.
Sclerodermoid reaction	Resembles SSc.	Drugs: bleomycin, taxanes. Chemicals: epoxy resins, organic solvents, pesticides, vinyl chloride. Miscellaneous: silica.
Sclerosis at injection sites	Resembles morphea at injection sites. Texier disease (due to vitamin K injections) favors the buttocks and thighs.	Bleomycin, IFNs, paraffin or silicone, vaccinations, vitamin B_{12}, and vitamin K.
	The configuration of Texier disease resembles a "cowboy gun belt and holster."	
Toxic oil syndrome	Morbilliform eruption with possible evolution into an LP-like, morpheaform, or sclerodermoid reaction. Systemic features include fever and peripheral hypereosinophilia.	Adulterated rapeseed oil (historical).

IFNs, interferons; LP, lichen planus; SSc, systemic sclerosis.
[a]Illustrative examples provided.

Table 2.27. AUTOANTIBODIES IN MORPHEA AND SYSTEMIC SCLEROSIS

Autoantibody[a]	Association(s)[a]
ANA	Morphea (40% most often generalized or linear variants). SSc (95%).
Anti-CENP-B (centromeric ANA pattern)	Limited cutaneous SSc with PAH.
Anti-fibrillarin (U3RNP) (nucleolar ANA pattern)	Diffuse cutaneous SSc with internal organ involvement.
Anti-Ku	SSc overlap with SLE or DM/PM.
Anti-PM-Scl	SSc overlap with DM/PM.
Anti-RNA polymerase III (speckled ANA pattern)	Diffuse cutaneous SSc (correlates with extent of cutaneous and renal involvement). Malignancy-associated diffuse cutaneous SSc (eg, breast cancer).
	Anti-RNA polymerase III correlates with renal involvement.
Anti-DNA topoisomerase I (scl70) (speckled ANA pattern)	Diffuse cutaneous SSc with ILD (poor prognosis).
Anti-ssDNA	Morphea (most often linear variant, correlates with disease activity). SSc.
	Anti-ssDNA is a single strand resembling *en coup de sabre*.
Anti-topoisomerase IIα	Morphea.

ANA, antinuclear antibody; CENP, centromere protein; DM, dermatomyositis; DNA, deoxyribonucleic acid; ILD, interstitial lung disease; PAH, pulmonary arterial hypertension; PM, polymyositis; RNA, ribonucleic acid; RNP, ribonucleoprotein; ss, single-stranded; SSc, systemic sclerosis; SLE, systemic lupus erythematosus.
[a]Illustrative examples provided.

SYSTEMIC SCLEROSIS
→ Diagnosis Group 2
Synonym: scleroderma

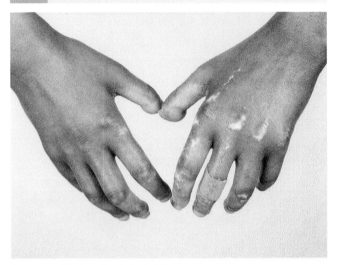

Courtesy of Robert Micheletti, MD.

Epidemiology

- SSc is an AI-CTD that leads to **cutaneous sclerosis, primarily of the dermis ± subcutis, in addition to Raynaud phenomenon and internal organ involvement (heart, lungs, gastrointestinal tract, and kidneys)**. The pathogenesis of cutaneous sclerosis is similar to morphea.
- SSc peaks between the ages of 35 and 50 years. The female:-male ratio ranges from 3:1 to 4:1.
- **Raynaud phenomenon** refers to **episodic vasospasm of digital arteries secondary to cold stimulus** resulting in **white, blue, and red finger discoloration.**
  - **Primary:** Raynaud disease **(onset at puberty, <5 attacks per day, precipitated by cold and emotional stress, absent ischemic injury, normal capillaroscopy, absent autoantibodies)** occurs in 3% to 5% of the population with a 20:1 female:male ratio.
  - **Secondary:** Associations include structural vasculopathies (eg, SLE, Sjögren syndrome, mixed connective tissue disease [MCTD]), DM (especially antisynthetase syndrome), SSc, physical agents (eg, cold injury, vibration injury), abnormal blood elements (eg, cryoglobulinemia), or abnormal vasomotion (eg, pheochromocytoma). Drug associations include **bleomycin (periungual wart treatment) and β-blockers.**

Clinicopathological Features

- SSc classically presents with **Raynaud phenomenon and hand/finger edema** that evolves into **sclerodactyly.** Involvement of the face may lead to a **beaked nose, microstomia, and a more youthful appearance.** Other mucocutaneous features of SSc include **leukoderma sparing perifollicular skin, elastosis perforans serpiginosa (EPS), dystrophic calcification, papulonodular mucinosis, and mat telangiectasias.** Raynaud phenomenon and dystrophic calcification may result in **ulcers or pitted scars.**
  - Leukoderma sparing perifollicular skin in SSc is known as the "salt and pepper sign."

- **Proximal nail fold dilated capillaries with reduced density and ventral pterygium** may occur.
  - Proximal nail fold dilated capillaries with reduced NOT normal density help distinguish DM and SSc from SLE.
  - Ventral NOT dorsal pterygium helps distinguish SSc from MMP and LP.
- SSc can cause significant morbidity due to **pain, skin tightness, and joint contractures.**
- Cutaneous involvement is **symmetric** and depends on subtype:
  - **Limited cutaneous SSc: face, hands/fingers.**
  - **Diffuse cutaneous SSc: hands/fingers** with progression to **face, trunk, and extremities.**
- Internal organ involvement depends on subtype:
  - **Limited cutaneous SSc** (later, after 10-15 years): **restrictive cardiomyopathy, esophageal dysmotility, pulmonary arterial hypertension (PAH) > ILD.**
    - Limited cutaneous SSc was formerly called <u>CREST</u> syndrome: <u>C</u>alcification, <u>R</u>aynaud phenomenon, <u>E</u>sophageal dysmotility, <u>S</u>clerodactyly, <u>T</u>elangiectasia.
  - **Diffuse cutaneous SSc** (earlier, after ~5 years): **restrictive cardiomyopathy, esophageal dysmotility, renal involvement, ILD > PAH.**
    - SSc can NOT be distinguished from morphea on histopathology, although early morphea tends to have a more robust inflammatory infiltrate.

Evaluation

- The differential diagnosis of SSc includes other sclerosing disorders.
- **Biopsy should include the subcutis.**
- Patients with SSc should be monitored for internal organ involvement including:
  - Kidney disease: **blood urea nitrogen (BUN)/creatinine (Cr), UA, blood pressure.**
  - PAH: **serum N-terminal prohormone of brain natriuretic peptide (NT-pro-BNP), TTE.**
  - ILD: **high-resolution CT chest, PFTs with DLCO.**
- **CXCL4** has been proposed as a **novel biomarker for pulmonary involvement.**
- For autoantibodies in SSc, see above.

Management

- Limited cutaneous SSc has a better prognosis than diffuse cutaneous SSc. **PAH is the leading cause of death in limited cutaneous SSc, while ILD is the leading cause of death in diffuse cutaneous SSc.**
- Management of cutaneous SSc is similar to LS. **Physical therapy** is important to preserve joint mobility.
- For **Raynaud phenomenon,** cold avoidance, hand and feet warming packets, and tobacco avoidance are first line. **CCBs (eg, nifedipine)** are second line. **PDE5 inhibitors (eg, sildenafil)** are third line.
- Management of internal organ involvement is beyond the scope of this chapter, except to note that **ACEIs** are helpful for the **treatment (but not prevention) of kidney disease.**

"Real World" Advice

- Cold avoidance to prevent Raynaud phenomenon requires attention to the core, not just the extremities.

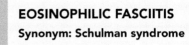

EOSINOPHILIC FASCIITIS
Synonym: Schulman syndrome

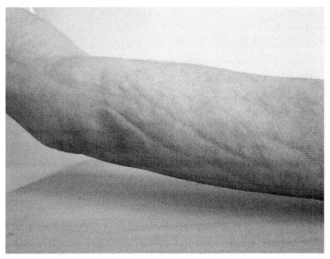

Courtesy of Robert Micheletti, MD.

- EF is an AI-CTD that leads to **cutaneous sclerosis, primarily of the subcutis and fascia ± muscle/bone. A history of strenuous physical activity** precedes EF in ~30% of patients. Associations include malignancy (eg, **myeloproliferative disorders**).
- EF classically presents with **edema and pain of the involved extremities, which rapidly progresses to symmetric cutaneous sclerosis sparing the face, hands, and feet.** EF can cause significant morbidity due to **pain, skin tightness, and joint contractures.**
  - EF has a "dimpled" or "pseudocellulite" appearance. The "dry river bed" sign or "groove" sign refers to linear depressions where veins appear to be sunken within the indurated skin.
  - Figure 2.52.
- **Biopsy including the fascia and/or MRI** are required for diagnosis. Laboratory findings include **peripheral hypereosinophilia,** elevated ESR, and hypergammaglobulinemia.
- **Systemic corticosteroids** are first line. Steroid-sparing therapies include methotrexate and mycophenolate. **Physical therapy** is important to preserve joint mobility.

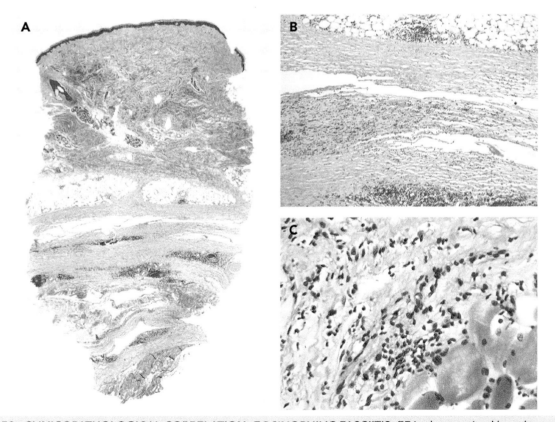

Figure 2.52. CLINICOPATHOLOGICAL CORRELATION: EOSINOPHILIC FASCIITIS. EF is characterized by subcutaneous septal thickening with involvement of the underlying fascia ± muscle/bone. A lymphoplasmacytic infiltrate ± eosinophils is variably present. A, Low-power view. B, Medium-power view. C, High-power view. EF, eosinophilic fasciitis.

Do NOT get confused! EF is named for its association with peripheral hypereosinophilia. Eosinophils are NOT required and are often NOT identified on histopathology.

NEPHROGENIC SYSTEMIC FIBROSIS
Synonym: nephrogenic fibrosing dermopathy

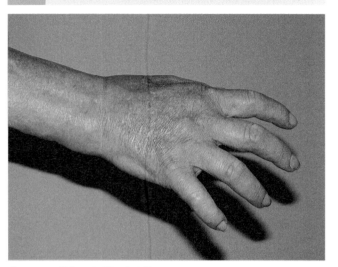

Courtesy of Victoria Werth, MD.

- Nephrogenic systemic fibrosis (NSF) is a CTD related to **gadolinium-based contrast exposure in patients with acute kidney injury (AKI) or severe chronic kidney disease (CKD).**
- NSF classically presents with **symmetric patterned indurated plaques on the trunk and extremities.** Systemic features include **heart/skeletal muscle/lung fibrosis** and **yellow scleral plaques.** NSF can cause significant morbidity due to **pain, skin tightness, and joint contractures.**
  - Indurated plaques in NSF are often described as "band-like" and "woody."
  - NSF can NOT be distinguished from scleromyxedema on histopathology. Unlike scleromyxedema, however, NSF tends to involve the subcutis.
- **Improvement in renal function after renal transplantation** may be beneficial. **Physical therapy** is important to preserve joint mobility.

RELAPSING POLYCHONDRITIS

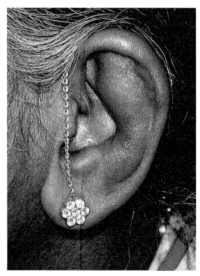

Reprinted with permission from Garg SJ. *Uveitis*. 2nd ed. Wolters Kluwer; 2018

- Relapsing polychondritis is an AI-CTD that involves **inflammation of cartilage.** Relapsing polychondritis peaks between 20 and 60 years of age. **Men and women are equally affected.** Associations include other autoimmune disorders and **myelodysplastic syndrome (MDS).** The leading HLA association is **-DR4.**
- Relapsing polychondritis classically presents with **painful erythema and edema of the cartilaginous portion of the ears (sparing the earlobes) with destruction of cartilage over time.** Audiovestibular damage may lead to **hearing loss and vestibular dysfunction.** Other sites of involvement include the **nose, costochondral joints, and respiratory tract (larynx, trachea, bronchi).** Systemic features include cardiovascular/renal/neurologic involvement, **seronegative inflammatory arthritis**, and **ocular inflammation (eg, conjunctivitis).** Relapsing polychondritis may **overlap with Behçet disease in mouth and genital ulcers with inflamed cartilage (MAGIC) syndrome.**
  - Destruction of auricular cartilage results in "cauliflower ears." Destruction of nasal cartilage results in a "saddle nose."
  - Relapsing polychondritis is characterized by early neutrophilic infiltrates and late lymphoplasmacytic infiltrates, with breakdown of the normal lacunar structure of cartilage and replacement by granulation tissue and fibrosis. DIF classically demonstrates a continuous granular band of IgG, IgA, IgM, and C3 in the perichondrium.
- Autoantibodies in relapsing polychondritis include **anticollagen II (<50%, not required for diagnosis)** and **anti-matrilin-1 (a cartilage ECM protein).**
- **Pneumonia is the leading causes of death. Systemic corticosteroids** are first line.

RHEUMATOID ARTHRITIS

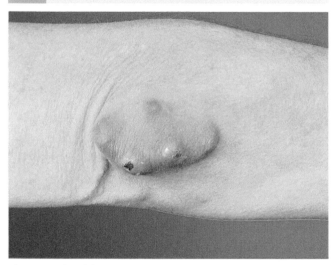

Rheumatoid nodule.

- RA is an AI-CTD that involves **inflammation of the joints.**
- RA classically presents with **deforming arthritis favoring the metacarpophalangeal (MCP) joints** (in contrast to the most common variant of psoriatic arthritis). Extra-articular manifestations include:

- Rheumatoid nodules: firm, semimobile papulonodules on periarticular and extensor surfaces, especially the hands. Accelerated rheumatoid nodulosis refers to the sudden appearance of multiple rheumatoid nodules associated with methotrexate or TNFα inhibitors.
- Felty syndrome: seropositive RA with leg ulcers, granulocytopenia, and splenomegaly.
    - Felty syndrome has a <u>faulty</u> spleen.
- Neutrophilic lobular panniculitis.
- Vasculitis (CSVV, hypocomplementemic urticarial vasculitis, EED, cryoglobulinemic vasculitis): see Chapter 2: Livedo Reticularis, Purpura, and Other Vascular Disorders. The term "Bywaters lesions" refers to nailfold thromboses and purpuric papules on the distal digits (especially the digital pulp) with CSVV on histopathology. The term "rheumatoid vasculitis" refers to small- and medium-vessel vasculitis in long-standing RA.
- Intravascular/intralymphatic histiocytosis: dilated vessels filled with histiocytes, leading to reticular erythema, induration, and papules overlying joints, especially the elbows.
- Red lunulae.
- Neutrophilic dermatoses (eg, Sweet syndrome, rheumatoid neutrophilic dermatosis [RND], PG): see Chapter 2: Neutrophilic and Eosinophilic Dermatoses.
- Granulomatous dermatoses (eg, interstitial granulomatous dermatitis [IGD], palisaded neutrophilic granulomatous dermatitis [PNGD]): see Chapter 2: Noninfectious Granulomas, Histiocytoses, and Xanthomas.
    - ◆ For the histopathology of a rheumatoid nodule, see Figure 2.102.
- Autoantibodies in RA include RF and cyclic citrullinated peptide (CCP).
- Treatment options include NSAIDs, systemic corticosteroids, disease-modifying antirheumatic drugs (DMARDs) (eg, methotrexate), and biologics (eg, TNFα inhibitors).

ADULT-ONSET STILL DISEASE

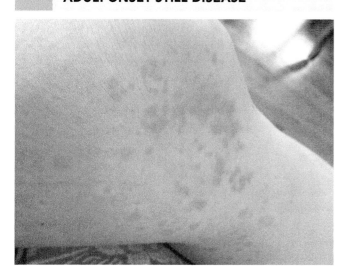

Courtesy of Robert Micheletti, MD.

- Adult-onset Still disease (AoSD) is an autoinflammatory syndrome characterized by increased IL-1.
- AoSD classically presents with evanescent salmon-colored macules in the setting of periodic fever and arthritis with carpal ankylosis. Persistent papules and plaques may also occur.
    - Periodic fever and other autoinflammatory syndromes are summarized in Table 2.28.
    - ◆ AoSD is characterized by an interstitial and perivascular neutrophil-dominant infiltrate.
- Laboratory abnormalities include elevated CRP/ESR and elevated ferritin (sometimes >4000 mg/mL), which correlates with disease activity.
- NSAIDs and/or systemic corticosteroids are first line. For refractory disease, anakinra and tocilizumab are often preferred when systemic inflammation is predominant, while methotrexate and TNFα inhibitors are often preferred when arthritis is predominant.

ACQUIRED PERFORATING DERMATOSIS

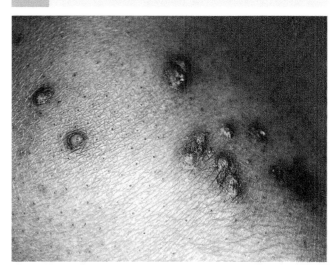

- Acquired perforating dermatosis (APD) arises due to transepidermal elimination of connective tissue or other materials. Associations depend on the variant (see below).
- APD variants are summarized in Table 2.29.
    - Children with hereditary reactive perforating dermatosis (RPD) and EPS develop pruritic papulonodules with keratotic plugs similar to adults.
    - ◆ Figure 2.53.
- bbUVB or nbUVB are first line.

Table 2.28. AUTOINFLAMMATORY SYNDROMES

Diagnosis[a]	Inheritance Pattern	Gene(s)	Classic Description	Notes
Inflammasomopathies				
FMF	AR	*FEFV* encoding pyrin	Periodic fever, erysipelas-like eruption on the lower extremities, pleuritis, arthritis, and myalgia.	Associated with secondary systemic amyloidosis. Colchicine is first line.
MKD/HIDS	AR	*MVK* encoding mevalonate kinase	Periodic fever, recurrent aphthous stomatitis, arthralgia, and myalgia.	
TRAPS	AD	*TNFRSF1A* encoding TNF receptor superfamily member 1 A	Periodic prolonged fever, pseudocellulitic eruption, periorbital edema, pleurisy, arthralgia, and myalgia.	Associated with secondary systemic amyloidosis. Etanercept is first line.
CINCA/NOMID	AD	*NLRP3* encoding cryopyrin	Early-onset persistent urticaria-like eruption, conjunctivitis, hypertrophic arthropathy of long bones, and chronic arthritis. Facial dysmorphia.	Classified under CAPS. Associated with secondary systemic amyloidosis. Anakinra or canakinumab are first line.
FCAS			Cold-induced fever, urticaria-like eruption, conjunctivitis, and arthralgia.	
MWS			Fever, urticaria-like eruption, conjunctivitis, and arthralgia without specific trigger. Sensorineural hearing loss.	
			Loud sounds are muffled well for patients with Muckle-Wells.	
Syndromic PG	See Chapter 2: Neutrophilic and Eosinophilic Dermatoses.			
NF-kβ–Related Autoinflammatory Syndromes				
Blau syndrome	See Chapter 2: Noninfectious Granulomas, Histiocytoses, and Xanthomas.			
Familial PRP	See Chapter 2: Noninfectious Granulomas, Histiocytoses, and Xanthomas.			
Interferonopathies				
CANDLE syndrome	AD	*PSMB8* encoding a proteasome ring protein.	Periodic fever and Sweet syndrome and pernio-like skin lesions. Facial dysmorphia, FTT, progressive lipodystrophy.	Classified under PRAAS. Emerging role for JAK inhibitors.
			Remember that CANDLE syndrome is a periodic fever syndrome because candles are periodically hot.	
SAVI	AD	*TMEM173* encoding STING	Fever, livedo reticularis, pernio-like skin lesions, ILD, anemia, and FTT.	Emerging role for JAK inhibitors.

Table 2.28. AUTOINFLAMMATORY SYNDROMES (CONTINUED)

Diagnosis[a]	Inheritance Pattern	Gene(s)	Classic Description	Notes
Miscellaneous				
ADA2 deficiency	See Chapter 2: Livedo Reticularis, Purpura, and Other Vascular Disorders.			
Cherubism	AD	*SH3BP2* encoding SH3 binding protein 2	Osteolytic lesions of mandibles followed by fibrotic dysplastic soft-tissue overgrowth. Overgrowth leads to puffy cheeks resembling a "cherub."	
CRMO	N/A	Polygenic	Pediatric counterpart to SAPHO syndrome (see Chapter 2: Disorders of Sebaceous, Apocrine, and Eccrine Glands).	
DIRA	AR	*IL1RN* encoding IL-1 receptor antagonist	Periodic fever, generalized pustulosis, and osteitis/periostitis.	Anakinra is first line.
DITRA	AR	*IL36RN* encoding IL-36 receptor antagonist	Periodic fever and generalized pustulosis.	
SoJIA (Still disease)	N/A	Polygenic	Pediatric counterpart to adult Still disease (see above).	

AD, autosomal dominant; AR, autosomal recessive; CANDLE, chronic atypical neutrophilic dermatosis with lipodystrophy and elevated temperature; CAPS, cryopyrin-associated periodic syndromes; CINCA, chronic infantile articular neurological periodic syndrome; CRMO, chronic recurrent multifocal osteomyelitis; DIRA, deficiency of the IL-1 receptor antagonist; DITRA, deficiency of IL-36 receptor antagonist; FCAS, familial cold autoinflammatory syndrome; FMF, familial Mediterranean fever; FTT, failure to thrive; HIDS, hyper-IgD syndrome; Ig, immunoglobulin; IL, interleukin; ILD, interstitial lung disease; JAK, Janus kinase; MKD, mevalonate kinase deficiency; MWS, Muckle-Wells syndrome; N/A, not applicable; NF-κβ, nuclear factor κβ; NOMID, neonatal onset multisystem inflammatory disease; PG, pyoderma gangrenosum; PRAAS, proteasome-associated autoinflammatory syndromes; PRP, pityriasis rubra pilaris; SAPHO, synovitis, acne, pustulosis, hyperostosis, and osteitis; SAVI, STING-associated vasculopathy with onset in infancy; SoJIA, juvenile idiopathic arthritis; STING, stimulator of interferon genes; TRAPS, TNF receptor-associated periodic syndrome; TNF, tumor necrosis factor.
[a]Illustrative examples provided.

Table 2.29. ACQUIRED PERFORATING DERMATOSIS VARIANTS

Variant[a]	Classic Description	Notes
RPD Kyrle disease	Pruritic papulonodules with keratotic plugs favoring the lower extremities in a linear configuration due to Koebnerization.	Collagen fibers (RPD) and nonspecific connective tissue (Kyrle disease) are the primary extruded materials. Associations include diabetes mellitus and stage 3-4 CKD.
EPS	Pruritic papulonodules with keratotic plugs favoring flexural sites (eg, the neck) in an annular configuration.	Elastic fibers are the primary extruded material. For associations, see below.
		MADD PORES: Marfan syndrome, acrogeria, Down syndrome, D-penicillamine, PXE, OI, Rothmund-Thompson syndrome, EDS, SSc.
Perforating periumbilical calcific elastosis	Periumbilical plaque with peripheral keratotic papules.	Elastic fibers are clumped, distorted, and calcified similar to PXE. Most commonly affects middle-aged, obese, hypertensive, multiparous Black women.

APD, acquired perforating dermatosis; CKD, chronic kidney disease; EDS, Ehlers-Danlos syndrome; EPS, elastosis perforans serpiginosa; OI, osteogenesis imperfecta; PXE, pseudoxanthoma elasticum; RPD, reactive perforating dermatosis; SSc, systemic sclerosis.
[a]Illustrative examples provided. Perforating folliculitis refers to hair follicle rupture in the setting of folliculitis. It is variably classified as an APD variant.

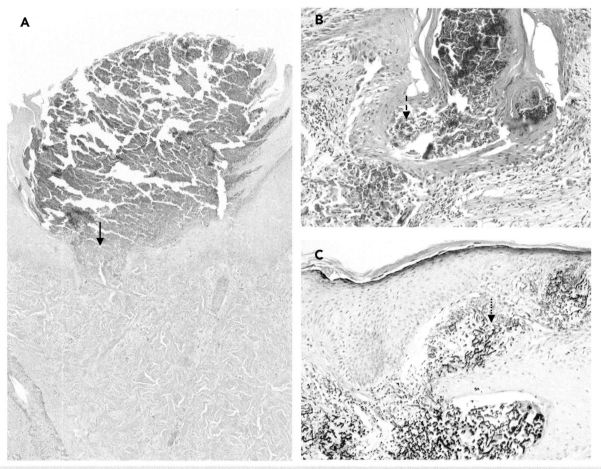

Figure 2.53. SIDE-BY-SIDE COMPARISON: REACTIVE PERFORATING DERMATOSIS AND ELASTOSIS PERFORANS SERPIGINOSA. Both RPD and EPS are characterized by a tortuous channel through an acanthotic epidermis. RPD demonstrates perforating collagen fibers that are basophilic and stain blue-green on Masson trichrome stain. EPS demonstrates perforating elastic fibers that are brightly eosinophilic and stain black on VVG stain. A, RPD. Solid arrow: perforating collagen fibers. B, EPS. Dashed arrow: perforating elastic fibers. C, EPS. VVG stain. Dotted arrow: perforating elastic fibers. EPS, elastosis perforans serpiginosa; RPD, reactive perforating dermatosis; VVG, Verhoeff-van Gieson.

(A, Histology image courtesy of Noel Turner, MD, MHS and Christine J. Ko, MD.)

SPOTLIGHT ON PSEUDOXANTHOMA ELASTICUM

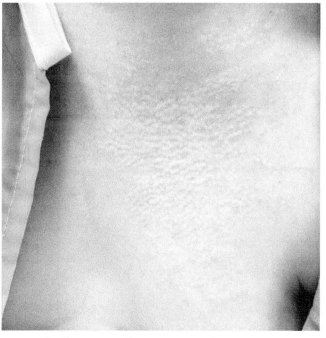

Reprinted with permission from Gru AA, Wick MR, Mir A, et al. *Pediatric Dermatopathology and Dermatology.* Wolters Kluwer; 2018.

- Pseudoxanthoma elasticum (PXE) is a **hereditary CTD** (Table 2.30) due to **AR** mutation in **ABCC6** encoding a transmembrane transporter. The pathogenesis involves decreased antimineralization activity resulting in **calcification of elastic fibers in the reticular dermis, the walls of medium-sized arteries, and Bruch membrane of the eye.**
  - To remember <u>ABCC6</u> mutation in <u>PXE</u>, sing, "<u>ABCCPXE</u>."
- PXE classically presents with **yellow papules** in flexural areas (eg, **lateral neck**), **EPS**, secondary cutis laxa, and **dystrophic calcification**. Cardiovascular complications include **atherosclerosis (eg, myocardial infarction [MI]), hemorrhage (eg, gastric), and mitral valve prolapse (MVP). Angioid streaks reflect breaks in the calcified elastic lamina of Bruch membrane. Loss of visual acuity** may result from choroidal neovascularization and hemorrhage.
  - Yellow papules in PXE resemble "cobblestones" or the skin of a "plucked chicken."
  - Figure 2.54.
- PXE is associated with **early death** and an increased risk of **first trimester miscarriage.** Skin-directed therapies are limited; multidisciplinary care should involve cardiology and ophthalmology.

Table 2.30. HEREDITARY CONNECTIVE TISSUE DISORDERS

Diagnosis[a]	Type	Inheritance Pattern	Gene(s)	Classic Description	Notes
OI	Multiple	AD	*COL1A1/COL1A2* encoding collagen I[b]	Cutaneous features include thin skin and EPS. Systemic features include blue sclerae, hearing loss, cardiac valvular regurgitation, and bone fragility with decreased pulmonary function associated with early death.	OI is unified by bone fragility and deformity.
EDS[c]	Classic	AD	*COL5A1/COL5A2* encoding collagen V[b]	Cutaneous features include hyperextensible and fragile skin with atrophic scars, dystrophic calcification, ecchymoses, EPS, molluscoid pseudotumors, and piezogenic pedal papules. Systemic features include MVP, skeletal abnormalities (pes planus, scoliosis), and joint hypermobility. Gorlin sign refers to the ability to touch the tongue to the nasal tip. Atrophic scars have a "cigarette paper" appearance and gape like a "fish mouth."	EDS is unified by defective function of collagens, the collagen-associated protein tenascin-X, or ECM-processing enzymes.
	Classic-like	AR	*TNXB* encoding tenascin-X	Systemic features include CAH.	
	Hypermobile	AD	*TNXB* encoding tenascin-X (10%)	Systemic features include pronounced joint hypermobility.	

(Continued)

Table 2.30. HEREDITARY CONNECTIVE TISSUE DISORDERS (CONTINUED)

Diagnosis[a]	Type	Inheritance Pattern	Gene(s)	Classic Description	Notes
	Vascular	AD	*COL3A1* encoding collagen III	Cutaneous features include thin translucent skin and pronounced ecchymoses. Systemic features include arterial/gastrointestinal/uterine rupture associated with early death.	
	Kyphoscoliotic	AR	*PLOD1* encoding lysyl hydroxylase[b]	Systemic features include marfanoid body habitus with pronounced scoliosis and blue sclerae/ocular fragility.	
	Arthrochalasia	AD	*COL1A1/COL1A2* encoding collagen I	Systemic features include pronounced joint hypermobility (congenital bilateral hip dislocation).	
	Dermatosparaxis	AR	*ADAMTS2* encoding procollagen I N-peptidase	Cutaneous features include pronounced skin fragility and laxity. Systemic features include hernias.	
	Spondylodysplastic	AR	*B4GALT7* encoding galactosyl transferase 1, *B3GALT6* encoding galactosyltransferase II, and *SLC39A13* encoding the zinc transporter ZIP13	Cutaneous features include progeroid facies. Systemic features include joint hypermobility.	
Cutis laxa[d]	AD cutis laxa	AD	*ELN* encoding elastin, *FBLN5* encoding fibulin 5	Cutaneous features include loose sagging skin with decreased elasticity and resilience. Systemic features include craniofacial anomalies, emphysema, hernias, and diverticula.	Cutis laxa is unified by sparse and fragmented elastic fibers.
	AR cutis laxa	AR	*FBLN4/FBLN5* encoding fibulins 4/5[b]		
	Occipital horn syndrome	XLR	*ATP7A*, encodes copper-transporting ATPase	Loose sagging facial skin in cutis laxa is sometimes called "bloodhound facies."	
Costello syndrome	N/A	AR	*HRAS* encoding HRAS	Cutaneous features include acral cutis laxa. Systemic features include cardiac malformations.	Increased risk of malignancy (eg, rhabdomyosarcoma).
Nonsyndromic "Michelin tire baby"	N/A	AD	Unknown	Multiple circumferential creases/folds of excess skin ± fat, smooth muscle, and hypertrichosis favoring the extremities.	May spontaneously resolve.
Marfan syndrome	N/A	AD	*FBN1* encoding fibrillin 1	Cutaneous features include EPS and *striae distensae;* dolichonychia. Systemic features include lens subluxations (upward), high-arched palate, MVP and dilation/dissection of ascending aorta, spontaneous pneumothorax, and skeletal abnormalities (arachnodactyly, pectus excavatum, scoliosis, tall stature). Arachnodactyly refers to "spider-like" digits.	Upward lens subluxations differentiate Marfan syndrome from homocystinuria. Strategies to prevent aortic dissection include ARBs and β-blockers.
Loeys-Dietz syndrome	Type I	AD	*TGFBR1* encoding TGF-β receptor	Overlap between vascular EDS and Marfan syndrome.	
	Type II		*TGFBR2* encoding TGF-β receptor 2		
Congenital contractural arachnodactyly (Beals syndrome)	N/A	AD	*FBN2* encoding fibrillin 2	Similar to Marfan syndrome without ocular involvement and with joint contractures. "Crumpled ears" are a diagnostic clue.	

Table 2.30. HEREDITARY CONNECTIVE TISSUE DISORDERS (CONTINUED)

Diagnosis[a]	Type	Inheritance Pattern	Gene(s)	Classic Description	Notes
Homocystinuria	N/A	AR	*CBS* encoding CBS[b]	Cutaneous features include pigmentary dilution, atrophic scars, malar flush, and livedo reticularis. Systemic features include lens subluxations (downward), venous and arterial thrombosis, intellectual disability, and marfanoid habitus.	Downward lens subluxations differentiate homocystinuria from Marfan syndrome.
PXE	See above.				
Buschke-Ollendorff syndrome	N/A	AD	*LEMD3* encoding LEM domain–containing 3	Cutaneous features include connective tissue nevi (dermatofibrosis lenticularis disseminata). Systemic features include osteopoikilosis.	LEM domain–containing 3 is an antagonist of BMP and TGF-β signaling.

AD, autosomal dominant; AR, autosomal recessive; ARBs, angiotensin receptor blockers; BMP, bone morphogenic protein; CAH, congenital adrenal hyperplasia; CBS, cystathionine β synthase; ECM, extracellular matrix; EDS, Ehlers-Danlos syndrome; EPS, elastosis perforans serpiginosa; MVP, mitral valve prolapse; N/A, not applicable; OI, osteogenesis imperfecta; PXE, pseudoxanthoma elasticum; TGF, transforming growth factor; XLR, X-linked recessive.
[a]Illustrative examples provided.
[b]Selected genes provided.
[c]EDS is currently classified on a molecular basis into 13 types. Cardiac valvular, musculocontractural, periodontal, brittle cornea syndrome, and myopathic types are omitted from this table. Historically, EDS was classified on a clinical basis into 11 types. Types IX and XI have been reclassified as occipital horn syndrome (XLR cutis laxa) and familial joint hypermobility syndrome, respectively.
[d]Cutis laxa may also be acquired in the setting of an inflammatory disorder (eg, Marshall syndrome), monoclonal gammopathy/plasma cell dyscrasia, or long-term exposure to D-penicillamine.

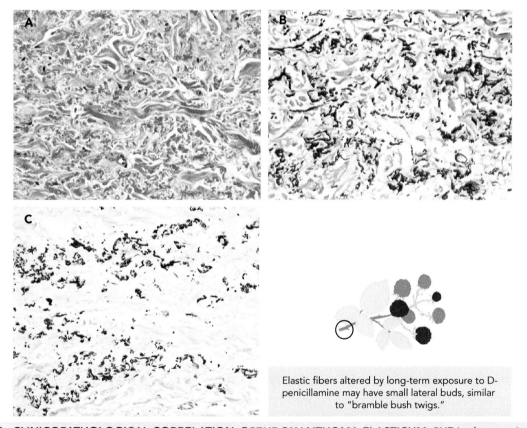

Elastic fibers altered by long-term exposure to D-penicillamine may have small lateral buds, similar to "bramble bush twigs."

Figure 2.54. CLINICOPATHOLOGICAL CORRELATION: PSEUDOXANTHOMA ELASTICUM. PXE is characterized by clumped, distorted, and calcified elastic fibers in the reticular dermis. VVG and Von Kossa stain elastic fibers and calcium, respectively. D-penicillamine interferes with elastin cross-linking. On histopathology, long-term exposure may induce cutis laxa-like changes, EPS, or PXE-like changes without calcification. A, H&E. B, VVG stain. C, von Kossa stain. PXE, pseudoxanthoma elasticum; VVG, Verhoeff-van Gieson.

(Histology images reprinted with permission from Elder DE, Elenitsas R, Rosenbach M, et al. *Lever's Histopathology of the Skin.* 11th ed. Wolters Kluwer; 2015. Illustration by Caroline A. Nelson, MD.)

Panniculitis and Lipodystrophy

Basic Concepts

- **Panniculitis** refers to **inflammation of the subcutaneous fat.**
  - ◆ Panniculitis may be divided into predominantly septal and lobular patterns (Figure 2.55).
- **Lipodystrophy** refers to **selective lipoatrophy (fat loss) ± lipohypertrophy (fat accumulation).**

ERYTHEMA NODOSUM
→ Diagnosis Group 2

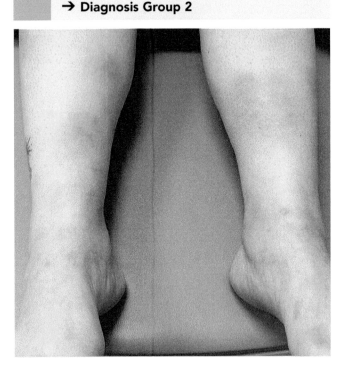

Epidemiology

- EN is a predominantly septal panniculitis due to a **delayed-type, cell-mediated (type IV) reaction.** It is the **most common panniculitis.**
  - ◆ Do NOT confuse erythema nodosum with erythema nodosum leprosum.
- EN is **idiopathic in 30% to 50%** of cases. The most common associations are **sarcoidosis, IBD (Crohn disease > ulcerative colitis), infections (eg, streptococcal, coccidioidomycosis), and drugs.** In **sarcoidosis and coccidioidomycosis,** EN is a **positive prognostic factor.**
  - **Streptococcal infection** is the leading cause of EN in **children.**
- Drug associations include **TNFα inhibitors, OCPs, sulfonamides (eg, TMP-SMX), tetracyclines, BRAF inhibitors, ICIs, and NSAIDs.**
- Panniculitides in adults are summarized in Table 2.31.
  - Panniculitides in children are summarized in Table 2.32.

Clinicopathological Features

- EN classically presents with **symmetric tender, erythematous, subcutaneous nodules favoring the shins.** Late lesions may resemble ecchymoses and gradually involute **without scarring.**
- Patients may exhibit fever and other constitutional symptoms.
- **Subacute nodular migratory panniculitis (EN migrans)** is characterized by chronic unilateral nodules favoring the lower extremities that migrate or undergo centrifugal spread with central clearing.
  - ◆ Figure 2.56.

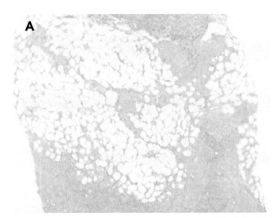
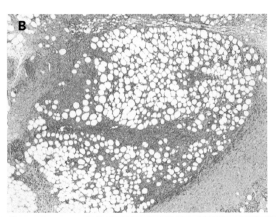

Figure 2.55. SIDE-BY-SIDE COMPARISON: SEPTAL AND LOBULAR PANNICULITIS. Both septal and lobular panniculitis are characterized by inflammation within the subcutaneous fat. Septal panniculitis demonstrates intact lobules of adipocytes that are similar in size and shape. Lobular panniculitis demonstrates necrotic lobules of adipocytes, lipophages, and free lipid accumulation in pools that vary in size and shape. A, Septal panniculitis: EN. B, Lobular panniculitis: LE panniculitis. EN, erythema nodosum; LE, lupus erythematosus.

(A, Histology image courtesy of Noel Turner, MD, MHS and Christine J. Ko, MD.)

In septal panniculitis, inflammation "spills over" into the lobule. In lobular panniculitis, inflammation "spills over" into the septum. Therefore, lobule architecture is the most reliable means of differentiation.

Table 2.31. PANNICULITIDES IN ADULTS

Diagnosis[a]	Classic Description	Notes
Predominantly Septal		
EN	See below.	
Connective tissue panniculitis	For deep morphea and SSc panniculitis, see Chapter 2: Interface Dermatoses and Other Connective Tissue Disorders.	
Predominantly Lobular		
Cold panniculitis—equestrian panniculitis	Tender, erythematous, subcutaneous nodules and plaques favoring the thighs.	Associated with cold injury—typically in young women horse riding in the cold wearing tight-fitting clothing. Self-limited.
Connective tissue panniculitis	For LE, DM, and RA panniculitis, see Chapter 2: Interface Dermatoses and Other Connective Tissue Disorders.	
Cytophagic histiocytic panniculitis	Tender, erythematous, subcutaneous nodules.	Associated with lymphoma, most often extranodal NK/T-cell lymphoma, nasal type or PCGD-TCL.
Factitial panniculitis	See Chapter 2: Neurocutaneous and Psychocutaneous Disorders.	
Infection-induced panniculitis	See Chapter 3: Bacterial Diseases.	
Lipodermatosclerosis	See below.	
Malignancy-related panniculitis-like infiltrates	For SPTCL, see Chapter 5: Hematolymphoid Neoplasms and Solid Organ Metastases.	
Nodular vasculitis/EI of Bazin	Tender, erythematous, subcutaneous nodules ± ulceration favoring the calves.	Some authorities use the term nodular vasculitis when patients are PPD/IFN-γ release assay negative and EI of Bazin when patients are PPD/IFN-γ release assay positive. In EI of Bazin, other tuberculids may be present. PCR has been used to identify mycobacterial DNA within lesional tissue.
Pancreatic panniculitis	Tender, erythematous, subcutaneous nodules ± ulceration with oily discharge. Lesions heal with scarring. Patients may exhibit fever, ascites, pleural effusions, abdominal pain, and arthritis.	Amylase, lipase, and trypsin are involved in the pathogenesis of pancreatic panniculitis. Associations include pancreatitis and pancreatic carcinoma. Schmidt's triad (subcutaneous nodules, eosinophilia, polyarthritis) is associated with a poor prognosis.
Panniculitis due to blunt trauma	Tender, ecchymotic, subcutaneous nodules and plaques favoring the extremities.	Associated with blunt trauma.
Sclerosing lipogranuloma	See Chapter 2: Noninfectious Granulomas, Histiocytoses, and Xanthomas.	

DNA, deoxyribonucleic acid; EI, erythema induratum; EN, erythema nodosum; IFN, interferon; LE, lupus erythematosus; PCGD-TCL, primary cutaneous γ/δ T-cell lymphoma; PCR, polymerase chain reaction; PPD, purified protein derivative; NK, natural killer; RA, rheumatoid arthritis; SPTCL, subacute panniculitis–like T-cell lymphoma; SSc, systemic sclerosis.
[a]Illustrative examples provided.

Table 2.32. PANNICULITIDES IN CHILDREN

Diagnosis[a]	Classic Description	Notes
Predominantly Lobular		
α1AT deficiency panniculitis	Tender, erythematous, subcutaneous nodules, or plaques ± ulceration with oily discharge. Lesions heal with scarring. Patients may exhibit fever, pleural effusions, and pulmonary emboli. Systemic features of α1AT deficiency include chronic liver disease with cirrhosis and emphysema.	Classification of α1AT deficiency panniculitis as predominantly lobular vs septal is controversial. Age of onset ranges from infancy to the eighth decade. Homozygotes for the Z allele of the *SERPINA1* gene have the most severe disease. α1AT replacement is first line.
Cold panniculitis—popsicle panniculitis	Tender, erythematous, subcutaneous nodules, and plaques favoring the cheeks.	Associated with cold injury—typically in infants and children. Self-limited.
Sclerema neonatorum	Diffuse skin induration.	Onset typically occurs in the first week of life of severely ill premature neonates. Associations include hypothermia and perinatal asphyxia. Complications include hypothermia and early death due to sepsis.
	Infants with sclerema neonatorum are "stiff as a board."	

(Continued)

Table 2.32. PANNICULITIDES IN CHILDREN (CONTINUED)

Diagnosis[a]	Classic Description	Notes
Subcutaneous fat necrosis of the newborn	Erythematous subcutaneous nodules favoring the cheeks, shoulders, back, buttocks, and thighs.	Onset typically occurs in the first 2-3 weeks of life of healthy full-term neonates. Associations include hypoglycemia, hypothermia, and perinatal hypoxemia. Complications include hypercalcemia. Serial monitoring of calcium levels for at least 4 months is recommended.
Poststeroid panniculitis	Erythematous subcutaneous nodules favoring the cheeks, trunk, and upper extremities.	Triggered by rapid tapering of systemic corticosteroids, most often in children.

α1AT, α1-antitrypsin.
[a]Illustrative examples provided.

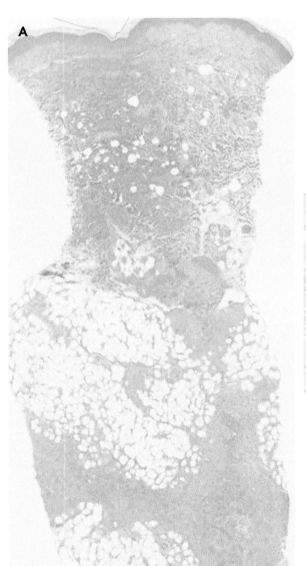
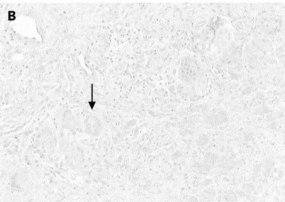

Figure 2.56. CLINICOPATHOLOGICAL CORRELATION: ERYTHEMA NODOSUM. EN is a septal panniculitis. The acute phase of EN is characterized by neutrophilic inflammation. The chronic phase of EN is characterized by lymphohistiocytic inflammation. Miescher radial granulomas contain central extracellular clefts. A, Low-power view. B, High-power view. Solid arrow: Miescher radial granuloma with central "slit-like" extracellular cleft. EN, erythema nodosum.

(Histology images courtesy of Noel Turner, MD, MHS and Christine J. Ko, MD.)

Extracellular clefts in Miescher radial granulomas may be radial or "slit-like."

Evaluation

- The differential diagnosis of EN includes other panniculitides.
- At a minimum, initial testing should include **CBC, CRP/ESR, UA, ASO, purified protein derivative (PPD) or IFN-γ release assay, throat culture, and CXR.**
- EN is primarily a clinical diagnosis; however, **a biopsy that includes the subcutis** may be helpful.

Management

- EN is typically **self-limited** over 3 to 4 weeks but may recur in up to one third of cases.
- Treatment should be directed at the underlying disorder.
- **Bed rest, leg elevation, and compression** provide symptomatic relief. **NSAIDs and saturated solution of potassium iodide (SSKI)** are first line. Other therapies include **colchicine** and **TNFα inhibitors.**

"Real World" Advice

- Distribution is a helpful clue to distinguish **EN**, which favors the **shins**, from **nodular vasculitis/erythema induratum (EI) of Bazin**, which favors the **calves.**

LIPODERMATO SCLEROSIS
→ Diagnosis Group 2
Synonym: sclerosing panniculitis

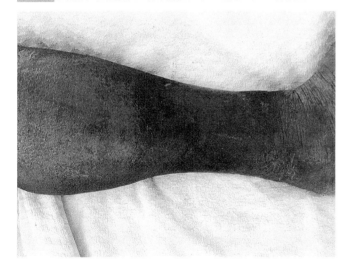

Epidemiology

- Lipodermatosclerosis is a predominantly lobular and septal panniculitis due to **venous insufficiency/hypertension.**

Clinicopathological Features

- **Acute** lipodermatosclerosis is characterized by **warmth (calor), pain (dolor), erythema (rubor), and swelling (tumor)**, while **chronic** lipodermatosclerosis is characterized by **induration and hyperpigmentation**. The distribution favors the **medial lower extremities above the malleolus.**
  - Chronic lipodermatosclerosis has an "inverted wine bottle" appearance.
  - Figure 2.57.

Evaluation

- The differential diagnosis of lipodermatosclerosis includes other panniculitides and cellulitis (acute).
- Lipodermatosclerosis is primarily a clinical diagnosis and biopsy should be reserved for atypical cases given the risk of poor wound healing and ulceration.

Management

- Treatment should be directed at the underlying venous insufficiency/hypertension including **leg elevation and compression.**
- Other treatment options include **androgens (eg, danazol) and pentoxifylline.**

"Real World" Advice

- Distinguishing acute lipodermatosclerosis from cellulitis is challenging. Clinical features that suggest acute lipodermatosclerosis include bilateral distribution and associated venous stasis changes.

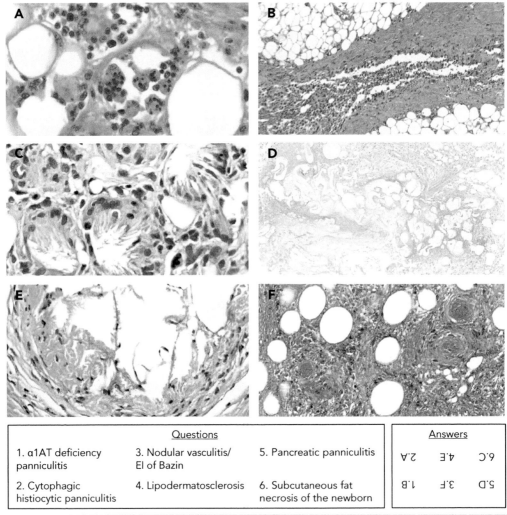

Questions		
1. α1AT deficiency panniculitis	3. Nodular vasculitis/EI of Bazin	5. Pancreatic panniculitis
2. Cytophagic histiocytic panniculitis	4. Lipodermatosclerosis	6. Subcutaneous fat necrosis of the newborn

Answers		
2.A	4.E	6.C
1.B	3.F	5.D

Figure 2.57. MATCHING EXERCISE: LOBULAR PANNICULITIS. A, Cytophagic histiocytic panniculitis. Note the cytophagic histiocytes ("bean bag cells") that have engulfed erythrocytes, lymphocytes, and/or karyorrhectic debris. B, α1AT deficiency panniculitis. Note the neutrophilic inflammation. α1AT deficiency panniculitis is characterized by liquefactive fat necrosis. C, Subcutaneous fat necrosis of the newborn. Note the "needle-shaped" clefts within adipocytes and multinucleated histiocytes. "Needle-shaped" clefts are also present in sclerema neonatorum and poststeroid panniculitis. In sclerema neonatorum, the clefts are only present in adipocytes, inflammation is sparse, and septal thickening is prominent. In poststeroid panniculitis, the clefts are present in adipocytes and multinucleated histiocytes. D, Pancreatic panniculitis. Note the necrotic adipocytes with thick walls and absent nuclei ("ghost cells") and deposition of basophilic material due to saponification of fat by calcium salts. Neutrophilic inflammation may be present. E, Lipodermatosclerosis. Note the fat necrosis with lipomembranous change (eosinophilic lining of cystic adipocytes resembling "frost on the windowpane"). Other features of lipodermatosclerosis include septal thickening, septal PXE-like elastosis with calcification, pericapillary fibrin, and overlying stasis change. F, Nodular vasculitis. Note the vasculitis. Inflammation may be neutrophilic, lymphocytic, or granulomatous. Caseation necrosis is associated with PCR positivity for mycobacterial DNA. For the histopathology of LE panniculitis, see Figure 2.46. α1AT, α1-antitrypsin; DNA, deoxyribonucleic acid; EI, erythema induratum; LE, lupus erythematosus; PCR, polymerase chain reaction; PXE, pseudoxanthoma elasticum.

(A, Histology image reprinted with permission from Elder DE, Elenitsas R, Rosenbach M, et al. *Lever's Histopathology of the Skin*. 11th ed. Wolters Kluwer; 2015. B, Histology image reprinted with permission from Elder DE, Elenitsas R, Rosenbach M, et al. *Lever's Histopathology of the Skin*. 11th ed. Wolters Kluwer; 2015. C, Histology image reprinted with permission from Elder DE, Elenitsas R, Rosenbach M, et al. *Lever's Histopathology of the Skin*. 11th ed. Wolters Kluwer; 2015. D, Histology image courtesy of Noel Turner, MD, MHS and Christine J. Ko, MD. E, Histology image reprinted with permission from Elder DE, Elenitsas R, Rosenbach M, et al. *Lever's Histopathology of the Skin*. 11th ed. Wolters Kluwer; 2015. F, Histology image reprinted with permission from Elder DE, Elenitsas R, Rosenbach M, et al. *Lever's Histopathology of the Skin*. 11th ed. Wolters Kluwer; 2015.)

SPOTLIGHT ON HEREDITARY LIPODYS-TROPHIES

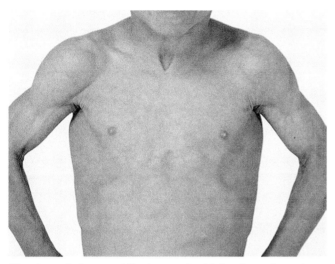

Chronic atypical neutrophilic dermatosis with lipodystrophy and elevated temperature syndrome reprinted with permission from Gru AA, Wick MR, Mir A, et al. *Pediatric Dermatopathology and Dermatology*. Wolters Kluwer; 2018.

- Lipodystrophy classification is based on distribution: **generalized, partial, or localized.**
- **Hereditary lipodystrophies** are summarized in Table 2.33.
    - Hereditary lipodystrophies demonstrate lipoatrophy ± lipohypertrophy.
    - **Acquired lipodystrophies** are summarized in Table 2.34.
- Lipodystrophy management focuses on cosmesis (eg, soft tissue dermal fillers) and treatment directed at **metabolic syndrome** (eg, cardiovascular disease, hepatic steatosis, insulin resistant diabetes mellitus, dyslipidemia) and other systemic features.

Table 2.33. HEREDITARY LIPODYSTROPHIES

Diagnosis[a]	Inheritance pattern	Gene(s)	Classic Description
CGL (Berardinelli-Seip syndrome)	AR	*AGPAT2* encoding AGPAT2 (type 1) *BSCL2* encoding seipin (type 2)[a]	Generalized lipoatrophy with cadaveric facies and a muscular-appearing body habitus at birth. Other cutaneous features include AN, hirsutism, and tuberous/tuberoeruptive xanthomas. Systemic features may be anabolic (eg, increased basal metabolic rate), metabolic (eg, metabolic syndrome), and gynecologic (eg, female infertility) along with organomegaly/organ dysfunction. Type 2 has more severe intellectual disability, hypertrophic cardiomyopathy, and premature death.
FPLD2 (Dunnigan type)	AD	*LMNA* encoding lamins A and C	Onset after puberty of lipoatrophy favoring the extremities with compensatory lipohypertrophy of the head and neck. Other features are similar to CGL.
CANDLE syndrome	See Chapter 2: Interface Dermatoses and Other Connective Tissue Disorders.		

AD, autosomal dominant; AGPAT2, 1-acylglycerol-3-phosphate O-acyltransferase 2; AN, acanthosis nigricans; AR, autosomal recessive; CGL, congenital generalized lipodystrophy; CANDLE, Chronic Atypical Neutrophilic Dermatosis with Lipodystrophy and Elevated temperature; FPLD2, familial partial lipodystrophy 2.
[a]Illustrative examples provided.

Table 2.34. ACQUIRED LIPODYSTROPHIES

Diagnosis[a]	Classic Description	Notes
AGL (Lawrence syndrome)	Onset in childhood or after puberty of panniculitis that evolves into generalized lipoatrophy (may affect palms and soles). Other features are similar to CGL but less severe.	Associations include antecedent autoimmune disease or infection. Preservation of bone marrow fat helps distinguish AGL from CGL.
APL (Barraquer-Simons syndrome)	Onset in childhood of lipodystrophy with a cephalocaudal progression. Three patterns: (1) upper body lipoatrophy, (2) upper body lipoatrophy with lower body lipohypertrophy, or (3) hemilipodystrophy. Other features are similar to CGL but less severe. ~1/5 patients have MPGN II.	Associations include antecedent autoimmune disease or infection. AD mutations in *LMNB2* encoding lamin B2 have been detected. Low C3 and C3 nephritic factor may result in unopposed activation of the alternative complement pathway and adipocyte lysis.
HIV/ART-associated lipodystrophy syndrome	See Chapter 6: Antimicrobials.	
Acquired localized lipodystrophy	Localized lipoatrophy or lipohypertrophy.	Associations with lipoatrophy include panniculitis, antecedent autoimmune disease, pressure, and drug (eg, corticosteroids, nonhuman insulin) or vaccine injections. Associations with lipohypertrophy include insulin therapy.

AD, autosomal dominant; AGL, acquired generalized lipodystrophy; APL, acquired partial lipodystrophy; ART, antiretroviral therapy; C, complement; CGL, congenital generalized lipodystrophy; HIV, human immunodeficiency virus; MPGN II, mesangiocapillary glomerulonephritis type II.
[a]Illustrative examples provided.

Urticaria and Other Erythemas

Basic Concepts

- **Erythema** describes a **pink > red or violaceous color change** of the skin due to **blood vessel dilation.** Given the underlying pathophysiology, **erythema blanches (turns white) with pressure.**
- **Urticaria** results from blood vessel dilation and transient edema within the **dermis.**

> **URTICARIA**
> **→ Diagnosis Group 1**
> **Synonym: hives**

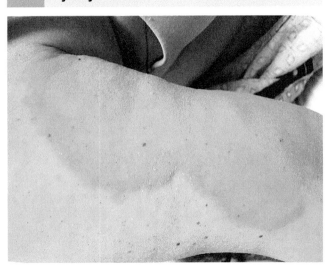

Epidemiology

- Urticaria is common (8%-22% lifetime prevalence) and most types are **female predominant.**
- Urticaria may be divided into **acute** versus **chronic (>6 weeks) subtypes** and **spontaneous** versus **inducible** (Table 2.35) subtypes. Chronic urticaria develops in 20% to 45% of patients with acute urticaria.
- Chronic urticaria may be associated with autoimmune disorders (eg, Graves disease) and infections (eg, *Helicobacter pylori* gastritis, *Strongyloides*).
- **HLA** associations with chronic urticaria include **-DR4 and -DQ8.**
- Mechanistically, urticaria may be:
  - **Immunologic:**
    - **Autoimmune:** Autoantibodies against **FcεRI or IgE.**
    - **IgE-dependent (type I) reaction:** contactants (eg, **latex**), drugs (eg, **monoclonal antibodies, IVIG, β-lactams, platinum alkylating agents**), foods (eg, **nuts, fish, and fruit**), and UVR (solar urticaria).
    - **Immune complex–dependent (type III) reaction:** urticarial vasculitis.
    - **Kinin and complement dependent:** angioedema.
  - **Nonimmunologic:**
    - **Direct mast cell–releasing agents** (eg, **polymyxin B, atracurium/mivacurium, opiates, thiopental, iodinated radiocontrast media, tartrazine**).
    - **Vasoactive stimuli** (eg, **stinging nettles in the *Urticaceae* family coated with sharp hairs containing acetylcholine, histamine, and serotonin**).
    - **NSAIDs (eg, aspirin [ASA]),** dietary pseudoallergens.
    - **ACEIs.**

Table 2.35. INDUCIBLE URTICARIAS

Type[a]	Classic Description	Notes
Urticaria Due to Mechanical Stimuli		
Dermatographism	Linear wheals at sites of scratching or friction.	
Delayed pressure	Deep erythematous swellings at sites of sustained pressure.	Delay may be 30 minutes to 12 hours.
Vibratory angioedema	Erythematous swellings at sites of vibration.	Hereditary or acquired.
Urticaria Due to Temperature Changes		
Heat	Wheals at sites of heat contact.	
Cold	Wheals at sites of cold exposure after rewarming.	May be secondary to reflex cold urticaria, familial cold urticaria, or cryoglobulinemia. Cold baths and swimming may cause anaphylaxis; therefore, patients should not swim alone.
Urticaria Due to Sweating or Stress		
Adrenergic	Pink wheals surrounded by blanched (vasoconstricted) skin after sudden stress.	
Cholinergic	Pale wheals surrounded by a pink halo after sweat-inducing stimuli (eg, physical exertion, hot baths, sudden emotional stress).	
Exercise induced	Pale wheals surrounded by a pink halo after physical exertion only.	
Contact Urticaria		
Immunologic	Wheals after contact with an allergen (eg, bacitracin/neomycin/polymyxin B, latex, potatoes).	Atopy is a risk factor. Latex is derived from *Hevea brasiliensis* (rubber tree). Repeated mucosal contact (eg, urinary catheterization in spina bifida patients) may cause anaphylaxis. Allergic patients should wear a medical alert bracelet. Measures to reduce sensitization include use of powder-free gloves and nonlatex alternatives (eg, nitrile, vinyl). Oral allergy syndrome describes immunologic mucosal contact urticaria due to antigens similar to allergenic pollen. Protein contact dermatitis is an eczematous eruption due to repeated urticarial reactions.
	A person with a latex allergy will "<u>BACK</u> away" from certain fruits (eg, <u>B</u>ananas, <u>A</u>vocados, <u>C</u>hestnuts, and <u>K</u>iwis).	
Nonimmunologic	Wheals after contact with a vasoactive stimulus (eg, plants, caterpillars, jellyfish).	The *Urticaceae* (nettle family), *Euphorbiaceae* (spurge family), and *Hydrophyllaceae* (water-leaf family) have sharp hairs that contain histamine, acetylcholine, and serotonin. Nonimmunologic contact urticaria has a low risk of anaphylactoid reaction.
Unknown mechanism	Wheals after contact (eg, ammonium persulfate).	Contact urticaria to ammonium persulfate is most common in bakers and hairdressers.
Other Inducible Urticarias		
Aquagenic	Wheals after contact with water of any temperature.	
Solar	See Chapter 4: Photodermatoses.	

[a]Illustrative examples provided.

- Urticaria may present with **angioedema** and/or **anaphylaxis,** which may be **life threatening.** Drug associations with anaphylaxis include **omalizumab, rituximab, and IVIG (IgA deficiency).** The distinction between anaphylaxis and an anaphylactoid reaction is mechanistically analogous to the distinction between immunologic and nonimmunologic urticaria.

Clinicopathological Features

- **Urticaria** characteristically presents with **transient (<24 hours), often pruritic, erythematous, and edematous wheals.**
- **Anaphylaxis** characteristically presents with **swelling of the oropharynx, larynx, epiglottis, and intestinal wall** that can result in impaired swallowing, stridor, abdominal pain, nausea, vomiting, and diarrhea. Patients may exhibit **tachycardia and hypotension.**
- Urticaria may be associated with **peripheral hypereosinophilia and elevated IgE.**
- The timing of urticaria relative to initial drug exposure is typically **minutes to hours.**
    - ◆ Figure 2.58.

Evaluation

- The differential diagnosis for urticaria includes papular urticaria and distinctive urticarial syndromes, urticarial pemphigoid, urticarial vasculitis, and Sweet syndrome. **Schnitzler syndrome is characterized by recurrent, nonpruritic wheals with intermittent fevers, bone pain, arthralgia or arthritis, an increased ESR, and an IgM monoclonal gammopathy.** For Still disease and CAPS, see Chapter 2: Interface Dermatoses and Other Connective Tissue Disorders.
- **Skin biopsy is indicated if lesions persist >24 hours to rule out urticarial vasculitis.**
- Consider **LFTs, CBC, CRP/ESR, and thyroid-stimulating hormone (TSH)** on a case-by-case basis. Other tests may include complement activity tests, thyroid/FcɛRI/IgE autoantibodies, ANA, RF/anti-CCP, cryoglobulins, HBV/HCV, stool ova and parasites, serologic or skin testing for immediate hypersensitivity, imaging studies, and physical challenge tests (US practice parameters).

Management

- While urticaria has a 0% reported mortality rate, the reported mortality rate for anaphylaxis is 5%.
- **The first step is treating with second-generation histamine-1 (H₁) antihistamines and avoiding triggers.**

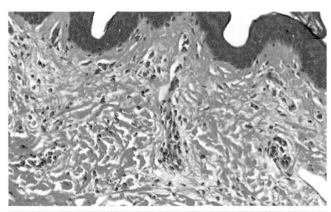

Figure 2.58. CLINICOPATHOLOGICAL CORRELATION: URTICARIA. Early lesions demonstrate superficial dermal vessels filled with neutrophils. Late lesions demonstrate a sparse superficial perivascular and interstitial neutrophilic, eosinophilic, and lymphocytic infiltrate.

(Histology image reprinted with permission from Elder DE, Elenitsas R, Rubin AI, et al. *Atlas and Synopsis of Lever's Histopathology of the Skin.* 3rd ed. Wolters Kluwer Health/Lippincott Williams & Wilkins; 2012.)

Do NOT get confused! Mast cell degranulation induces urticaria; however, neutrophils fill the superficial dermal vessels of early lesions on histopathology.

Only 10% of urticaria and 30% of anaphylaxis are drug-associated, so it is important to consider alternative etiologies. **Radioallergosorbent tests (RASTs) that detect specific IgE autoantibodies and prick tests** (performed under medical supervision due to the risk of anaphylaxis) can be helpful. Additional therapeutic options include first-generation antihistamines, H₂ receptor antagonists, leukotriene receptor antagonists, immunosuppressives, and/or omalizumab. **Use of oral corticosteroids should be limited to ≤1 to 3 weeks** (US practice parameters). Consider allergy and immunology consultation for **desensitization.**

Viral infection is the leading cause of urticaria in children.

"Real World" Advice

- Patients often state that antihistamines "do not work" for them. Before reaching that conclusion, it is important to ensure that a preventative regimen has been trialed at an appropriate dose (eg, cetirizine may be increased twofold to fourfold).

SPOTLIGHT ON HEREDITARY ANGIOEDEMA

Synonym(s): angioneurotic edema, Quincke edema

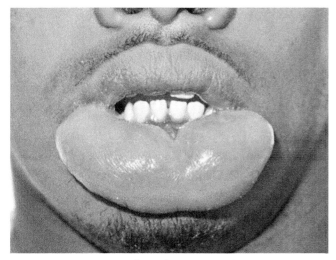

Reprinted with permission from Plantz SH, Huecker M. *Step-Up to Emergency Medicine*. Wolters Kluwer Health; 2015.

- **Angioedema** results from edema within **deep dermal, subcutaneous, and submucosal tissues. Hereditary angioedema due to C1-inh deficiency** typically presents in the first or second decade and may be divided into **type I (reduced level) and type II (reduced function)**. A third type, likely due to activation of factor XII (the Hageman factor), is now recognized. All forms result from **bradykinin accumulation.**
  - ◆ **Acquired C1-inh deficiency** typically presents after the fourth decade and may be divided into **type I (consumption) and type II (autoantibodies) in patients with autoimmune disorders (eg, SLE) or B-cell lymphoproliferative disorders/plasma cell dyscrasias.** Acquired angioedema may also be induced by **NSAIDs and ACEIs (more prevalent in African Americans).**
- The classic presentation of angioedema is **asymmetric, often painful, subcutaneous swelling favoring the face,** which may also involve the oropharynx and intestinal wall.
  - ◆ Hereditary angioedema is characterized by subcutaneous and submucosal edema without infiltrating inflammatory cells.
  - ◆ **Ascher syndrome** is a distinct disorder with a **classic triad of blepharochalasis (from recurrent eyelid edema), double lip, and nontoxic thyroid enlargement.**
- **Laboratory findings in hereditary C1-inh deficiency** are summarized in Table 2.36.
  - ◆ **Laboratory findings in acquired C1-inh deficiency** are summarized in Table 2.37.
  C4 is the optimal screening test.
- Angioedema may be **life threatening. C1-inh concentrate** is first line for an **acute attack** and may be given as **prophylaxis 1 hour prior to elective surgery.** Alternatives include **danazol or stanozolol.**

Table 2.36. LABORATORY FINDINGS IN HEREDITARY C1 INHIBITOR DEFICIENCY

Type	C1-inh Level	C1-inh Function	C4	C1q
HAE, type I	Low	Low	Low	Normal
HAE, type II	Normal	Low	Low	Normal

C1-inh, complement 1 inhibitor; HAE, hereditary angioedema.

Table 2.37. LABORATORY FINDINGS IN ACQUIRED C1 INHIBITOR DEFICIENCY

Type	C1-inh level	C1-inh function	C4	C1q Acquired = low C1q
AAE, type I	Low	Low	Low	Low
AAE, type II	Low	Low	Low	Low

AAE, acquired angioedema; C1-inh, C1 inhibitor.

ERYTHEMA ANNULARE CENTRIFUGUM

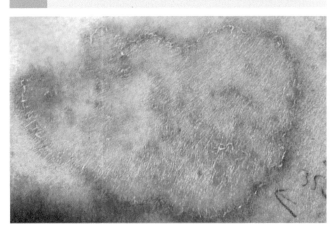

Reprinted with permission from Elder DE, Elenitsas R, Rubin AI, et al. *Atlas of Dermatopathology: Synopsis and Atlas of Lever's Histopathology of the Skin.* 4th ed. Wolters Kluwer; 2020.

- EAC is classified as a **figurate (annular, arciform, or polycyclic) erythema** that may be idiopathic or secondary to an identifiable trigger, most commonly **tinea.**
- EAC classically presents with **pink papules that expand centrifugally and then develop central clearing. Trailing scale** is a feature of **superficial** EAC.
    - ◈ Figure 2.59.
- Other **erythemas** are summarized in Table 2.38.
- Treat the underlying disorder. Topical corticosteroids may be considered, if needed.

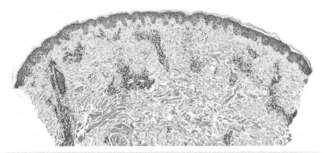

Figure 2.59. CLINICOPATHOLOGICAL CORRELATION: ERYTHEMA ANNULARE CENTRIFUGUM. Characteristic features are intact vessels with a dense perivascular lymphoid infiltrate. Spongiosis and parakeratosis are present in superficial EAC. EAC, erythema annulare centrifugum.

(Histology image reprinted with permission from Elder DE, Elenitsas R, Rubin AI, et al. *Atlas of Dermatopathology: Synopsis and Atlas of Lever's Histopathology of the Skin.* 4th ed. Wolters Kluwer; 2020.)

> The dense perivascular lymphoid infiltrate has been described as "coat sleeving." Clinically, the infiltrate corresponds to the erythematous rim of the lesion, while parakeratosis corresponds to the trailing scale of superficial EAC.

MORBILLIFORM DRUG ERUPTION
→ **Diagnosis Group 1**
Synonyms: exanthematous drug eruption, maculopapular drug eruption

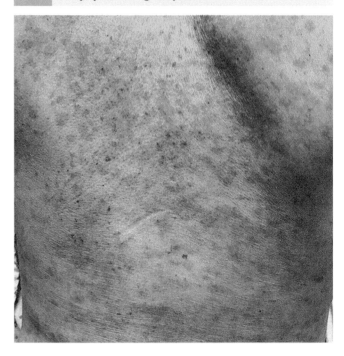

Epidemiology

- Morbilliform drug eruption may be classified as a **delayed-type, cell-mediated (type IV) reaction.**
- Drug associations include **antimalarials, nucleoside reverse transcriptase inhibitors (NRTIs)/nucleotide reverse transcriptase inhibitors (NtRTIs) (eg, abacavir), NNRTIs (eg, nevirapine), β-lactams, sulfonamides, minocycline, BCR-ABL/Kit/PDGFR inhibitors, BRAF inhibitors, MEK 1/2 inhibitors, ICIs, allopurinol, and aromatic anticonvulsants.** Other triggers include **iodinated radiocontrast media.**
    > **Infectious mononucleosis increases the risk of aminopenicillin-induced morbilliform drug eruption** (33%-100% of patients).

Clinicopathological Features

- Morbilliform drug eruptions classically present with **symmetrically distributed, pruritic, erythematous macules, papules, and/or urticarial lesions that start on the trunk and upper extremities.** Over time, lesions can become confluent and extend distally. Patients may exhibit **low-grade fever and peripheral hypereosinophilia.** The eruption typically self-resolves but may progress to **erythroderma.**
- The timing of morbilliform drug eruptions relative to initial drug exposure is typically **4 to 14 days** (earlier in case of rechallenge).
    - ◈ Morbilliform = "measles-like."
    - ◈ Morbilliform drug eruption has nonspecific histopathology. Superficial infiltrates composed of lymphocytes, neutrophils, and/or eosinophils are often present ± interface changes.

Table 2.38. ERYTHEMAS

Diagnosis[a]	Classic Description	Notes
EAC	See above.	
Erythema gyratum repens	Migratory concentric erythematous rings with scale. Erythema gyratum repens has a "woodgrain" appearance.	The leading association is lung cancer.
Erythema marginatum	Migratory, annular and polycyclic, erythematous eruption.	Major criterion of acute rheumatic fever due to antecedent group A streptococcal infection (major Jones criteria: carditis, erythema marginatum, migratory polyarthritis, Sydenham chorea, subcutaneous nodules).
Erythema migrans	Annular erythema at the site of the bite of a *Borrelia*-infected tick.	Initial manifestation of Lyme disease.
Necrolytic acral erythema	Acral pink to violet-brown plaques with hyperkeratosis, blisters, and/or erosions.	Associations include zinc deficiency and HCV.
Necrolytic migratory erythema	Similar to necrolytic acral erythema but distribution favors the face (especially perioral), intertriginous areas, and distal extremities.	Glucagonoma syndrome (necrolytic migratory erythema, angular cheilitis, glossitis) is associated with diabetes mellitus and weight loss.
Palmar erythema	Erythema of the palms.	Associations include TEC, SLE, cirrhosis, Crohn disease, diabetes mellitus, and pregnancy.

HCV, hepatitis C virus; SLE, systemic lupus erythematosus; TEC, toxic erythema of chemotherapy.
[a]Illustrative examples provided.

Evaluation

- The primary mimicker of morbilliform drug eruption is **viral exanthem.** The differential diagnosis includes other drug reactions, acute GVHD, urticaria, Kawasaki disease, and infections (eg, toxic shock syndrome). **Unilateral laterothoracic exanthem** is a morbilliform eruption in the **axilla and lateral trunk.**
  - **Only 10% to 20% of pediatric morbilliform eruptions are drug associated** (favor viral exanthem).
  - The "statue of liberty" sign refers to the visualization of unilateral laterothoracic exanthem when the patient raises the affected upper extremity.

Management

- Morbilliform drug eruptions have a 0% reported mortality rate.
- **Discontinuation of the suspected drug** along with all nonessential drugs is the first step. *In vitro* assays to establish the culprit drug are under investigation. However, given uncertain sensitivity and specificity, their utility remains limited in clinical practice. 10% to 40% of patients are patch test positive, and prick testing may be considered if patch testing is negative. While morbilliform eruptions are drug associated in 50% to 70% of cases, it is important to consider alternative etiologies.
- **Topical corticosteroids** are first line. Consider allergy and immunology consultation for **desensitization.**

"Real World" Advice

- "Treating through" a morbilliform drug eruption may be considered, especially when the suspected drug is of paramount importance to the patient's health and there is no satisfactory substitute.

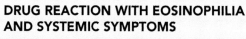

DRUG REACTION WITH EOSINOPHILIA AND SYSTEMIC SYMPTOMS
Synonym: drug-induced hypersensitivity syndrome

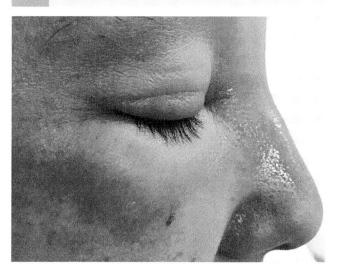

- Drug reaction with eosinophilia and systemic symptoms (DRESS) may be classified as a **delayed-type, cell-mediated (type IV) SCAR.** The pathogenesis involves a complex interplay between drugs, viruses, and the immune system primarily mediated by T-cells. In a subset of patients, recruitment and activation of eosinophils involves cytokine signaling (eg, IL-4, IL-5, IL-13, and eotaxin). Drug associations include **azathioprine, dapsone, NRTIs/NtRTIs (eg, abacavir), NNRTIs (eg, nevirapine), sulfonamides, minocycline, vancomycin, ICIs, allopurinol, aromatic anticonvulsants including lamotrigine.** Other triggers include **iodinated radiocontrast media. Inability to detoxify arene oxide metabolites** plays a role in aromatic anticonvulsant hypersensitivity syndrome. DRESS may also be associated with **viral reactivation (cytomegalovirus [CMV], Epstein-Barr virus [EBV], HHV-6, and HHV-7).** HLA associations include **-B1301 (dapsone in Asian populations), -B5701 (abacavir), and -B5801 (allopurinol in Asian populations).**
  - HHV-6 and HHV-7 have been implicated in PR, DRESS, and roseola infantum.
- The **European Registry of Severe Cutaneous Adverse [Drug] Reactions (RegiSCAR) scoring system** (Table 2.39) summarizes DRESS. The classic cutaneous eruption is **morbilliform** with **facial edema** that may progress to **erythroderma.** The timing of DRESS relative to initial drug exposure is typically **15 to 40 days** (earlier in case of rechallenge).
  - In practice, a morbilliform drug eruption with systemic features that does not exceed the diagnostic threshold for DRESS is often called "mini-DRESS" or "skirt syndrome".
  - DRESS may mimic a variety of disorders ranging from spongiotic dermatitis to AGEP to interface dermatitis.
- At a minimum, evaluation for systemic involvement should include **BUN/Cr, UA, spot urine for protein:Cr ratio, LFTs, CBC, and peripheral smear** with additional testing depending on the patient. Autoimmune complications such as **type I diabetes mellitus** and **Graves disease** may be delayed (**check TSH and free thyroxin (T4) at 3 months, 1 year, and 2 years).**
- DRESS has a **5% to 10%** reported mortality rate (**hepatic necrosis is the leading cause of death). Discontinuation of the suspected drug** along with all nonessential drugs is the first step. *In vitro* assays to establish the culprit drug are under investigation. However, given uncertain sensitivity and

---

Table 2.39. THE EUROPEAN REGISTRY OF SEVERE CUTANEOUS ADVERSE [DRUG] REACTIONS (REGISCAR) SCORING SYSTEM FOR DRUG REACTION WITH EOSINOPHILIA AND SYSTEMIC SYMPTOMS

RegiSCAR scoring System for DRESS[a,b]

Criteria[a]	No	Yes	Unknown/Unclassifiable
Fever (≥38.5 °C)	−1	0	−1
Lymphadenopathy (≥2 sites; >1 cm)	0	1	0
Circulating atypical lymphocytes	0	1	0
Peripheral hypereosinophilia • 700-1499/μL or 10%-19.9%[c] • ≥1500/μL *or* ≥20%[c]	0	1 2	0
It is possible to exceed the diagnostic threshold for DRESS without the "E" (eosinophilia).			
Skin involvement • Extent of cutaneous eruption >50% BSA • Cutaneous eruption suggestive of DRESS[d] • Biopsy suggests DRESS	0 −1 −1	1 1 0	0 0 0
Internal organs involved[e] • One • Two or more	0	1 2	0
Resolution in ≥15 days	−1	0	−1
Laboratory results negative for at least three of the following (and none positive): (1) ANA; (2) blood cultures; (3) HAV/HBV/HCV serology; and (4) *Chlamydia* and *Mycoplasma* serology	0	1	0

ANA, antinuclear antibody; BSA, body surface area; DRESS, drug reaction with eosinophilia and systemic symptoms; HAV, hepatitis A virus; HBV, hepatitis B virus; HCV, hepatitis C virus.

[a]Final score: <2, no case; 2 to 3, possible case; 4 to 5, probable case; >5, definite case.

[b]This scoring system has been validated. The Japanese Research Committee on Severe Cutaneous Adverse [Drug] Reactions (J-SCAR) provides an alternative diagnostic criteria to RegiSCAR.

[c]If leukocytes <4000/μL.

[d]At least two of the following: edema, infiltration, purpura, scaling.

[e]Liver, kidney, lung, muscle/heart, pancreas, or other organ and after exclusion of other explanations.

specificity, their utility remains limited in clinical practice. Thirty percent to 60% of patients are patch test positive; however, **patch testing should be delayed until at least 6 months after clinical resolution.** While DRESS is drug-associated in 70% to 90% of cases, it is important to consider alternative etiologies. **Systemic corticosteroids** are first line, with a **slow taper** over weeks to months. Emerging data support the use of cyclosporine as a steroid-sparing therapy for DRESS.

POLYMORPHIC ERUPTION OF PREGNANCY
Synonym: pruritic urticarial papules and plaques of pregnancy

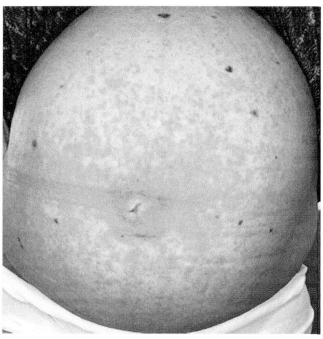

Courtesy of Sotonye Imadojemu, MD, MBE

- Polymorphic eruption of pregnancy (PEP) is the most common pregnancy-related dermatosis. Risk factors include **primiparous, multiple-gestation pregnancy, and increased maternal weight gain.**
- PEP classically presents in **late pregnancy or postpartum** with **urticarial papules and plaques arising in** *striae distensae* **with periumbilical sparing.** Other morphologies (eg, eczematous lesions, vesicles, target lesions, erythema) may develop with disease progression.
    Figure 2.60.
    Polymorphic eruption of pregnancy (PEP) is more accurate than pruritic urticarial papules and plaques of pregnancy (PUPPP) because lesions are polymorphic.
    PEP has nonspecific histopathology. A perivascular lymphocytic or mixed infiltrate is often present ± epidermal spongiosis or acanthosis and dermal edema.
- PEP typically self-resolves 7 to 10 days after delivery and does not recur. Topical corticosteroids and oral antihistamines are first line.

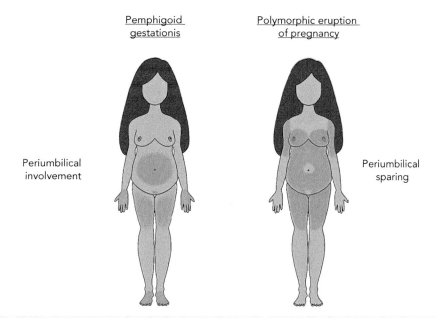

Figure 2.60. DISTRIBUTION: A HELPFUL DIAGNOSTIC CLUE IN PREGNANCY DERMATOSES.
(Illustration by Caroline A. Nelson, MD.)

KAWASAKI DISEASE

Synonym: mucocutaneous lymph node syndrome

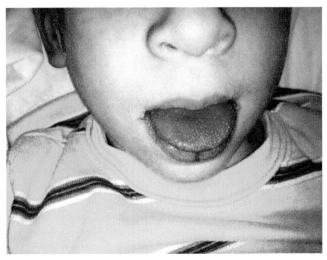

Reprinted with permission from Shaw KN, Bachur RG, Chamberlain JM, et al. *Fleisher & Ludwig's Textbook of Pediatric Emergency Medicine.* 7th ed. Wolters Kluwer; 2015.

- Kawasaki disease most commonly affects children **6 months to 5 years of age**; however, infants <6 months of age are at high risk of complications due to delayed or missed diagnosis. The incidence is highest in **Asian populations (eg, Japan)**.
- The classic findings of Kawasaki disease are summarized in the **diagnostic criteria** (Table 2.40). In **infants**, Kawasaki disease is in the differential diagnosis for **diaper dermatitis**. Kawasaki disease is the **leading cause of acquired pediatric heart disease in the United States and other developed countries. Coronary artery lesions are the most common complication,** leading to ectasia and aneurysms in **15% to 25%** of untreated patients. Associated laboratory abnormalities include **elevated cardiac troponin 1, endothelin 1,**

Table 2.40. DIAGNOSTIC CRITERIA FOR KAWASAKI DISEASE

Diagnostic criteria for Kawasaki Disease[a]

Fever CREAM = Fever, Conjunctivitis, Rash, Extremity changes, Adenopathy, Mucosal changes.

Criteria	Classic Description
Fever	Present ≥ 5 days
Conjunctivitis	Bilateral
Rash	Polymorphous (maculopapular > psoriasiform, erythrodermic, EM-like, urticarial) ± early perineal desquamation
Extremity changes	Erythema and induration of hands and/or feet (acute phase); periungual desquamation (subacute phase)
Adenopathy	Cervical lymphadenopathy (single node >1.5 cm or several smaller, firm, nonfluctuant nodes bilaterally)
Mucosal changes	• Erythema, cracking, peeling of lips • Strawberry tongue • Diffuse erythema of oral mucosa

EM, erythema multiforme.
[a]Fever must be present ≥5 days, with 4/5 other criteria met OR ≥ 4 days with 5/5 other criteria met.

neutrophil count, platelet count, ESR, low albumin, and hemoglobin (Hb).
- ◆ Kawasaki disease has nonspecific histopathology. A perivascular lymphocytic infiltrate and dermal edema are often present.
- **TTE** should be obtained early in the disease course.
- **ASA and IVIG** are first line. Treat within 10 days of symptom onset to reduce complications. Infliximab is used in refractory disease.

Livedo Reticularis, Purpura, and Other Vascular Disorders

Basic Concepts

- **Vascular disorders** affect **blood vessels.**
- **Livedo reticularis** describes a **mottled, reticulated vascular pattern** due to **alterations in blood flow** through the cutaneous microvasculature.
  - ◆ Reticularis means "net-like."
- **Purpura** describes a **violaceous color change** due to **visible hemorrhage** in the skin. Given the underlying pathophysiology, **purpura does not blanch with pressure.**

- In **primary purpura** (Table 2.41), hemorrhage is an integral part of lesion formation. The differential diagnosis varies based on morphology: **macular, palpable, or retiform.**
  - ◆ Figure 2.61.
- In **secondary purpura,** hemorrhage occurs within established lesions.
- **Vasculopathy** is an umbrella term that encompasses **vascular occlusion and vasculitis.**
- **Cutaneous vasculitis** (Table 2.42) is a specific pattern of **inflammation of the blood vessel wall** that may be (1) a skin-limited disease, (2) a primary cutaneous vasculitis with secondary systemic involvement, or (3) a cutaneous manifestation of systemic vasculitis.

Table 2.41. PRIMARY PURPURA					
Category	**Pathogenesis**	**Etiologies[a]**	**Classic Description**	**Notes**	

Category	Pathogenesis	Etiologies[a]	Classic Description	Notes
Macular Purpura				
Petechiae	Thrombocytopenia (<10,000-20,000/mm³)	Decreased platelet production (eg, bone marrow disorder, chemotherapy), increased platelet destruction (eg, early DIC, HIT, ITP, TTP/HUS/other thrombotic microangiopathy, quinine, quinidine), and platelet sequestration (eg, splenomegaly)	Purpuric macules favoring the lower extremities	Immune-mediated HIT is due to antibodies to the heparin-PF4 complex.
	Abnormal platelet function	Hereditary platelet function defects (eg, VWD), acquired platelet function defects (eg, renal insufficiency, monoclonal gammopathy, NSAIDs), and thrombocytosis secondary to myeloproliferative neoplasms		Myeloproliferative neoplasms include essential thrombocytosis, PV, primary myelofibrosis, and CML. ~95% of PV patients have activating *JAK2* mutations.
	Miscellaneous	Inflammatory disorders (eg, pigmented purpura, hypergammaglobulinemic purpura of Waldenström), vitamin C deficiency, increased external pressure (eg, the Rumpel-Leede sign of a blood pressure cuff), increased intravascular venous pressure (eg, vomiting), trauma		
Ecchymoses	Platelet disorders plus minor trauma	See above	Purpuric patches favoring the forearms	Solar purpura is also known as actinic or senile purpura.
	Procoagulant defects plus minor trauma	Vitamin E excess, vitamin K deficiency, hepatic insufficiency, anticoagulant use		
	Weak blood vessels plus minor trauma	EDS, solar purpura, primary systemic amyloidosis, vitamin C deficiency, hypothyroidism, corticosteroid therapy		
	Miscellaneous	Papular purpuric gloves and socks syndrome due to parvovirus infection		
Palpable Purpura				
Palpable purpura	Vascular inflammation	Vasculitis	Palpable purpura with peripheral erythema	Palpable purpura is the hallmark lesion of CSVV.
	Miscellaneous	PLEVA, EM, pigmented purpura, hypergamma-globulinemic purpura of Waldenström		
Retiform Purpura				
Noninflammatory retiform purpura	Vascular occlusion by emboli	Cholesterol emboli, oxalate emboli, HES, cardiac vegetations (eg, infective endocarditis, nonbacterial thrombotic endocarditis), aortic or cardiac tumor (eg, atrial myxoma), Nicolau syndrome (embolia cutis medicamentosa)	Angulated purpura	Nonbacterial thrombotic endocarditis is also known as Libman-Sacks or marantic endocarditis.
	Vascular occlusion by organisms	Bacteria (eg, ecthyma gangrenosum, Lucio phenomenon of leprosy, RMSF), angioinvasive fungi, and parasites (eg, disseminated *Strongyloides*)		
	Vascular occlusion by thrombi	Platelet-related thrombopathy (eg, HIT, TTP/HUS/other thrombotic microangiopathy PNH, thrombocytosis secondary to myeloproliferative neoplasms), systemic coagulopathy (eg, APLS), DIC (eg, Trousseau syndrome), protein C or S deficiency or dysfunction), or vascular coagulopathy (eg, livedoid vasculopathy, malignant atrophic papulosis, Sneddon syndrome, COVID-19).		PNH is a Coombs-negative intravascular hemolytic anemia due to *PIG-A* mutations.

(Continued)

Table 2.41. PRIMARY PURPURA (CONTINUED)

Category	Pathogenesis	Etiologies[a]	Classic Description	Notes
	Vascular occlusion due to abnormal circulating blood	Cryoglobulinemia, cryofibrinogenemia, cold agglutinins, crystalglobulin vasculopathy, malaria, sickle cell disease		
	Miscellaneous	Calciphylaxis, *Loxosceles* (brown recluse) spider bite, intravascular large B cell lymphoma, hydroxyurea		
Inflammatory retiform purpura	Vascular inflammation	Cutaneous vasculitis	Angulated purpura with peripheral erythema	Inflammatory retiform purpura is the hallmark lesion of PAN.
	Miscellaneous	Livedoid vasculopathy, PG, septic vasculitis, pernio		

APLS, antiphospholipid antibody syndrome; CML, chronic myelogenous leukemia; COVID-19, coronavirus disease 2019; CSVV, cutaneous small-vessel vasculitis; DIC, disseminated intravascular coagulation; EDS, Ehlers-Danlos syndrome; EM, erythema multiforme; HES, hypereosinophilic syndrome; HIT, heparin-induced thrombocytopenia; HUS, hemolytic uremic syndrome; ITP, idiopathic thrombocytopenic purpura; NSAIDs, nonsteroidal anti-inflammatory drugs; PAN, polyarteritis nodosa; PF4, platelet factor 4; PG, pyoderma gangrenosum; PLEVA, pityriasis lichenoides et varioliformis acuta; PNH, paroxysmal nocturnal hemoglobinuria; PV, polycythemia vera; RMSF, Rocky Mountain spotted fever; TTP, thrombotic thrombocytopenic purpura; VWD, von Willebrand disease.
[a]Illustrative examples provided.

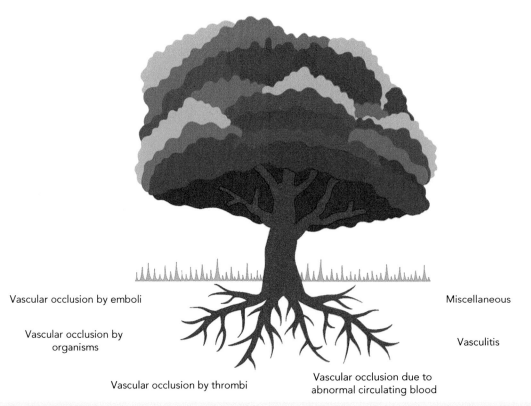

Figure 2.61. RETIFORM PURPURA: THE ROOT CAUSES. The cutaneous microvasculature is analogous to the rainforest canopy: a dense ceiling formed by the interlocking branches of closely spaced trees. Occlusion deprives the skin supplied by the affected vessel of oxygen and nutrients, resulting in retiform purpura.

(Illustration by Caroline A. Nelson, MD.)

Retiform means "net-like."

Table 2.42. CUTANEOUS VASCULITIS

Predominant Caliber of Inflamed Blood Vessel[a]	Classification[b]	Subclassification or Etiologies
Small	CSVV	IgA vasculitis (Henoch-Schönlein purpura) Acute hemorrhagic edema of infancy Urticarial vasculitis EED Mixed cryoglobulinemia (types II and III)
	Secondary causes	See below
Small and medium	ANCA-associated vasculitis	MPA GPA EGPA Drug-induced
	Secondary causes	Inflammatory disorders (eg, SLE, Sjögren syndrome, rheumatoid vasculitis), infections, neoplasms
Medium	PAN	Classic (systemic) PAN Cutaneous PAN
Large	Temporal arteritis	
	Takayasu arteritis	

ANCA, antineutrophil cytoplasmic antibody; CSVV, cutaneous small-vessel vasculitis; EED, erythema elevatum diutinum; EGPA, eosinophilic granulomatosis with polyangiitis; GPA, granulomatosis with polyangiitis; Ig, immunoglobulin; MPA, microscopic polyangiitis; PAN, polyarteritis nodosa; SLE, systemic lupus erythematosus.
[a]Small vessels include arterioles, capillaries, and postcapillary venules in the superficial and mid dermis. Medium vessels include arteries and veins in the deep dermis and subcutis. Large vessels include the aorta and named arteries.
[b]The American College of Rheumatology 1990 criteria and the 2012 revised International Chapel Hill Consensus Conference Nomenclature system are alternative classification schemes.

LIVEDO RETICULARIS
→ Diagnosis Group 1

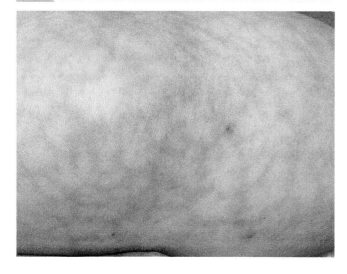

Epidemiology

- **Physiologic** livedo reticularis is a **vasospastic response to cold exposure.**
    - **Physiologic livedo reticularis**, also known as **cutis marmorata**, is common in **neonates, infants, and children.**

- Livedo reticularis may also be **primary or secondary** to an underlying disorder (eg, **vasospasm, vessel wall pathology, intraluminal pathology**).
    - **Cutis marmorata telangiectatica congenita (CMTC)** results in **congenital livedo reticularis often limited to one extremity.** Associations include **vascular malformations and limb asymmetry.** Livedo reticularis is a cutaneous feature of **STING-associated vasculopathy with onset in infancy (SAVI) and homocystinuria.**
- Drug associations include **amantadine and norepinephrine.**

Clinicopathological Features

- Livedo reticularis classically presents with a **mottled, reticulated vascular pattern favoring the extremities.** It often **co-occurs with acrocyanosis (painless red-to-purple hand/foot discoloration).**
- **Livedo racemosa** is a **livedo reticularis variant** with a **larger, branching, and more irregular pattern favoring both the trunk and extremities.** It is typically associated with **blood vessel occlusion.**
    - Physiologic and primary livedo reticularis do not demonstrate histopathological abnormalities. The histopathology of secondary livedo reticularis depends on the etiology.

Evaluation

- The differential diagnosis of livedo reticularis includes other reticulated skin disorders (eg, EAI).
- To diagnose an underlying disorder, it is often necessary to perform **serial elliptical biopsies from the pale center of the reticular pattern.**

Management

- Livedo reticularis does not require treatment. Physiologic livedo reticularis will typically disappear with warming. Treatment of secondary livedo reticularis should be directed at the underlying disorder.

"Real World" Advice

- The pattern of livedo reticularis may provide a clue to the etiology. A **complete network** is indicative of alterations in blood flow due to **vasospasm or abnormal circulating blood,** while a **patchy network** is indicative of **blood vessel inflammation or occlusion.**
- Hyperpigmentation distinguishes the reticulated pattern of EAI from livedo reticularis.

LIVEDOID VASCULOPATHY
→ **Diagnosis Group 2**
Synonym: atrophie blanche

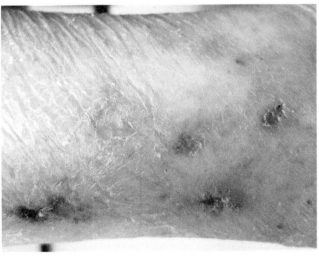

Courtesy of Robert Micheletti, MD.

Epidemiology

- Livedoid vasculopathy is a vascular coagulopathy of unknown etiology. It may be primary or secondary with an associated **prothrombotic abnormality** in ~50% of patients.
- Livedoid vasculopathy is **female predominant.**

Clinicopathological Features

- Livedoid vasculopathy classically presents with **painful well-demarcated ulcers favoring the distal lower extremities ± livedo reticularis and retiform purpura.** Lesions tend to heal as **white atrophic scars with peripheral telangiectasias.**
  - Well-demarcated ulcers in livedoid vasculopathy may be described as "punched out" and may be surrounded by prominent livedo reticularis.
  - Figure 2.62.

Evaluation

- The differential diagnosis of livedoid vasculopathy includes other causes of retiform purpura including **coagulopathies with cutaneous manifestations** (Table 2.43).
  - **Hereditary thrombophilias include factor V Leiden mutation (most common),** prothrombin mutation, protein C or S deficiency, antithrombin deficiency, and hyperhomocysteinemia.
  - Consider the AR autoinflammatory syndrome **adenosine deaminase 2 (ADA2) deficiency in children** who present with **Sneddon syndrome and PAN-like lesions.**
- **A biopsy that includes the subcutis** should be performed.
- **BUN/Cr, LFTs, CBC, blood smear, partial thromboplastin time (PTT), and ANCAs should be obtained in all patients with suspected vascular occlusion. Cryoglobulins ± cryofibrinogen ± cold agglutinins** should be obtained in patients with suspected cold-induced vascular occlusion.

Management

- Treatment options include **anticoagulants,** anabolic steroids, IVIG, and **antiplatelet agents.**

"Real World" Advice

- Beware of atrophie blanche–like lesions in antiphospholipid antibody syndrome (APLS) masquerading as livedoid vasculopathy.

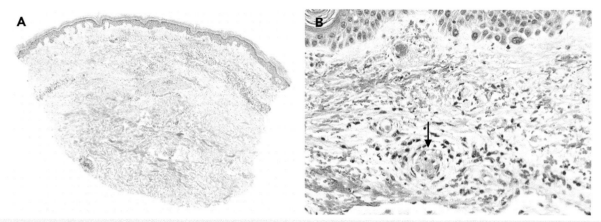

Figure 2.62. CLINICOPATHOLOGICAL CORRELATION: LIVEDOID VASCULOPATHY. Characteristic features are superficial dermal vessels with hyalinized walls and luminal fibrin deposition, a perivascular lymphocytic infiltrate, and erythrocyte extravasation. A, Low-power view. B, High-power view. Solid arrow: hyalinized vessel wall and intraluminal fibrin deposition.

Hyalinized vessel walls appear to be "outlined with a pink crayon."

Table 2.43. COAGULOPATHIES WITH CUTANEOUS MANIFESTATIONS

Diagnosis[a]	Classic Description	Notes
Systemic Coagulopathies		
APLS	Livedo reticularis/racemosa, bland necrosis, retiform purpura, atrophie blanche or Degos-like lesions, and splinter hemorrhages (proximal).	F > M. The leading association is SLE. Other triggers include levamisole-adulterated cocaine. CAPS may be fatal. To confirm the diagnosis of APLS in a patient with vascular thrombosis and/or pregnancy morbidity (eg, spontaneous abortion), anticardiolipin antibodies (IgG or IgM), lupus anticoagulant, and/or anti-β2 glycoprotein 1 antibodies (IgG or IgM) must be present on ≥ 2 occasions ≥12 weeks apart.
Protein C or S deficiency or dysfunction	Retiform purpura. Warfarin necrosis is characterized by symmetric retiform purpura favoring sites with abundant adipose tissue.	Protein C deficiency may occur in sepsis associated DIC. Warfarin necrosis, classified as a SCAR, is due to protein C dysfunction, while postinfectious purpura fulminans is due to protein S dysfunction.
Trousseau syndrome	Recurrent (migratory) superficial thrombophlebitis.	Chronic DIC associated with cancer (eg, pancreatic, lung). The differential diagnosis includes Mondor syndrome of superficial thrombophlebitis, which affects the anterolateral thoracoabdominal wall and is associated with infection, breast cancer, trauma, and surgical procedures.
Vascular Coagulopathies		
Livedoid vasculopathy	See above	
Malignant atrophic papulosis	See below	
Sneddon syndrome	Persistent livedo reticularis/racemosa.	F > M. Systemic features include labile hypertension and CNS disease (eg, strokes, dementia). Check antiphospholipid antibodies.

APLS, antiphospholipid antibody syndrome; CAPS, catastrophic antiphospholipid antibody syndrome; CNS, central nervous system; DIC, disseminated intravascular coagulation; F, female; M, male; SCAR, severe cutaneous adverse reaction; SLE, systemic lupus erythematosus.
[a]Illustrative examples provided.

SPOTLIGHT ON NEONATAL PURPURA FULMINANS

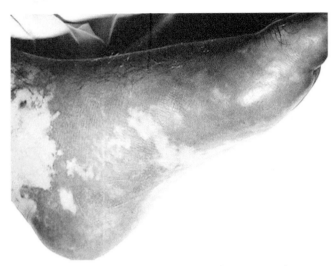

Homozygous protein C deficiency courtesy of Steven Manders, MD. From Graessle WR. Nonblanching rashes. In: Chung EK, Atkinson-McEvoy LR, Lai LN, et al, eds. *Visual Diagnosis and Treatment in Pediatrics*. 3rd ed. Wolters Kluwer; 2015:564-572.

- Proteins C and S are vitamin K–dependent anticoagulant proteins. **Homozygous (or compound heterozygous) deficiency or severe dysfunction in protein C or S** leads to neonatal purpura fulminans.
- Neonatal purpura fulminans classically presents **hours to 5 days after birth with noninflammatory retiform purpura and large-scale cutaneous and limb necrosis.** It is associated with visceral organ involvement (eg, cerebral thrombosis, retinal vein occlusion).
  - Neonatal purpura fulminans is characterized by bland thrombi ± hemorrhagic infarcts, epidermal and dermal necrosis, or subepidermal bullae formation.
  - In common parlance, the term "purpura fulminans" is used to describe any patient with cutaneous vascular occlusion and bland thrombi on histopathology.
- Neonatal purpura fulminans is fatal without treatment. Protein C deficiency may be treated with IV protein C concentrate or fresh frozen plasma (FFP), ultimately transitioned to lifelong anticoagulation.

MALIGNANT ATROPHIC PAPULOSIS
Synonym: Degos disease

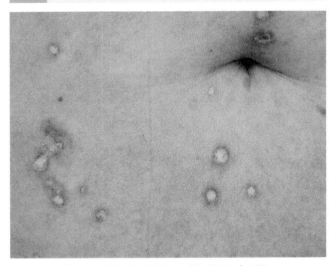

Courtesy of Robert Micheletti, MD and Badri Modi, MD.

- Malignant atrophic papulosis is a small-vessel vasculopathy. It may be divided into **systemic and benign (skin-limited)** subtypes.
- Malignant atrophic papulosis classically presents with **crops of small erythematous papules favoring the trunk and extremities.** Each lesion develops a **central depression** over 2 to 4 weeks and ultimately evolves into a **white scar with a rim of telangiectasias.** Gastrointestinal (eg, **bowel perforation**) and central nervous system (CNS) (eg, **stroke**) involvement are the leading causes of death.
  - White scars in malignant atrophic papulosis are often likened to "porcelain."

  - Figure 2.63.
- Degos-like lesions have been reported in **APLS, SLE, and DM.**
- Systemic malignant atrophic papulosis has a **poor prognosis.** Treatments include ASA, dipyridamole, **eculizumab,** and treprostinil.

CHOLESTEROL EMBOLI

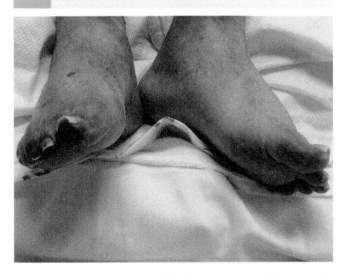

- Cholesterol emboli are caused by fragmentation of ulcerated atheromatous plaques typically in patients with **severe atherosclerotic disease.** Three clinical settings known to prompt embolization are **(1) arterial or coronary catheterization, (2) prolonged anticoagulation,** and **(3) acute thrombolytic therapy.**
- Cholesterol emboli classically present with **livedo reticularis and cyanosis,** with rarer findings including ulcer-

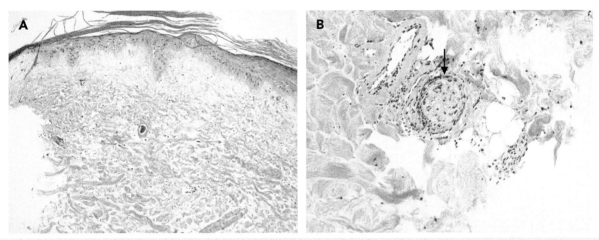

Figure 2.63. CLINICOPATHOLOGICAL CORRELATION: MALIGNANT ATROPHIC PAPULOSIS. Characteristic features are a wedge-shaped superficial and deep perivascular lymphoid infiltrate with vascular damage. Chronic lesions demonstrate central epidermal atrophy, avascular necrosis of dermal structures, and marked dermal mucinosis. A, Low-power view (superficial dermis). B, High-power view (subcutis). Solid arrow: thrombosed arteriole.

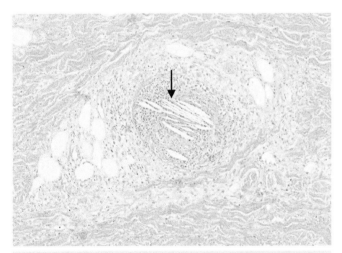

Figure 2.64. CLINICOPATHOLOGICAL CORRELATION: CHOLESTEROL EMBOLI. Cholesterol emboli form elongated clefts ± thrombi in arterioles at the dermal-subcutaneous junction. Peripheral hypereosinophilia is common. Solid arrow: cholesterol emboli that result from the release of material from atherosclerotic plaques in a submucosal artery.

(Histology image courtesy of Noel Turner, MD, MHS and Christine J. Ko, MD.)

Cholesterol emboli may resemble "potato chips" on histopathology.

CALCIPHYLAXIS
→ Diagnosis Group 2
Synonym: calcific uremic arteriolopathy

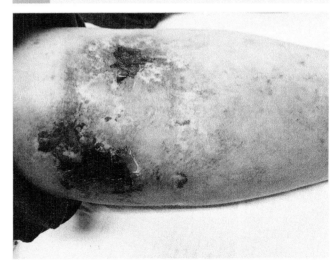

Epidemiology

ation, necrosis, nodules, and retiform purpura. Multisystem embolic complications may be fatal.

　　Figure 2.64.

- Patients may exhibit **peripheral hypereosinophilia.**
- Supportive care is first line unless surgical bypass or endovascular stent grafting can eliminate the source of embolism. Other treatments include antiplatelet agents (eg, ASA) and statins.

- Calciphylaxis is a **mixed calcifying disorder of the skin** (Table 2.44). The **first hit is medial calcification** resulting in vessel lumen narrowing and endothelial cell damage. The **second hit is thrombotic occlusion** leading to downstream cutaneous necrosis.

　　Calciphylaxis is analogous to a "heart attack of the skin."

　　Genetic disorders with **dystrophic calcification** of the skin include **EDS and PXE. Heel sticks** may result in dystrophic calcification of the skin in neonates.

　　Genetic disorders with **ossification** of the skin include **fibrodysplasia ossificans progressiva (FOP)**

Table 2.44. CALCIFYING AND OSSIFYING DISORDERS OF THE SKIN

Classification	Etiologies[a]
Dystrophic calcification (secondary to preexisting damage to the skin)	AI-CTD (eg, DM, deep morphea, SSc), panniculitis, infections (eg, parasitic), cutaneous tumors or cysts (eg, pilomatricomas), trauma
Metastatic calcification (secondary to calcium dysregulation)	Sarcoidosis, hypervitaminosis D, milk-alkali syndrome, renal disease, hyperparathyroidism, tumoral calcinosis (familial), neoplasms
Mixed calcification (dystrophic and metastatic)	Calciphylaxis
Idiopathic calcification	Idiopathic calcified nodules of the scrotum, subepidermal calcified nodule, tumoral calcinosis (sporadic), milia-like calcinosis
Iatrogenic calcification	Extravasation of IV solutions containing calcium or phosphate (most common)
Ossification (calcium combines with phosphorus and deposits as hydroxyapatite crystals in a proteinaceous matrix)[b]	Miliary osteomas of the face (associated with chronic acne vulgaris)

AI-CTD, autoimmune connective tissue disease; CKD, chronic kidney disease; DM, dermatomyositis; IV, intravenous; SSc, systemic sclerosis.
[a]Illustrative examples provided.
[b]Secondary ossification may also occur, often preceded by calcification.

characterized by **malformed great toes**, progressive osseous heteroplasia, plate-like osteoma cutis, and **Albright hereditary osteodystrophy (pseudohypoparathyroidism, pseudo-pseudohypoparathyroidism, obesity, brachydactyly, short stature)**.

◈ Do NOT confuse <u>Albright</u> hereditary osteodystrophy with McCune-<u>Albright</u> syndrome.
- Calciphylaxis is **female predominant.**
- The leading association with calciphylaxis is **end-stage renal disease (ESRD)**. For **nonuremic calciphylaxis**, however, associations include **obesity, cirrhosis, diabetes mellitus, and chronic corticosteroid use. Calcium and vitamin D intake** also increase risk of calciphylaxis. In converse, **vitamin K deficiency or antagonism (eg, warfarin)** increases risk of calciphylaxis due to the vitamin K–dependent vascular factor matrix Gla protein, a powerful local calcification inhibitor in the arterial wall.

Clinicopathological Features

- Calciphylaxis classically presents with **subcutaneous plaques or nodules favoring sites with abundant adipose tissue or sites of trauma** that progress to **retiform purpura with bullae and central ulceration.**
  ◈ Black eschars overlying calciphylaxis ulcers have been described as "leathery."
- Calciphylaxis may be **fatal**, most often due to secondary infection leading to **sepsis.**
  ◈ Figure 2.65.

Evaluation

- The differential diagnosis of calciphylaxis includes other causes of retiform purpura.
- **Biopsy should include the subcutis. Imaging (plain x-ray (XR), nuclear bone scan)** revealing **"net-like" soft-tissue calcifications** has been proposed as an alter-

native method of diagnosis; however, biopsy remains the gold standard.
- In addition to the common vascular occlusion work-up, evaluation of calciphylaxis should include **parathyroid hormone (PTH).**

Management

- Calciphylaxis has a reported **1-year mortality rate ranging from 45% to 80%. Proximal lesion location and ulceration** have been associated with a **poor prognosis**, while **nonuremic calciphylaxis** has been associated with a **better prognosis.**
- Measures to correct mineral imbalance include **increased frequency and duration of dialysis, elimination of high-calcium dialysate, and non-calcium phosphate binders** (eg, sevelamer, lanthanum).
- In patients with **hyperparathyroidism, cinacalcet or etelcalcetide** are first line, with **parathyroidectomy and kidney transplant** reserved for refractory cases.
- **Sodium thiosulfate (STS)**, hypothesized to increase calcium solubility, may be used IV (with dialysis sessions at 5-25 g doses) or intralesionally for localized disease.
- **Bisphosphonates** may be effective, particularly in nonuremic calciphylaxis, but should be used with caution in ESRD to avoid adynamic bone disease.
- In patients with ulcerations, **wound care ± hyperbaric oxygen therapy** is critical. Data on **surgical debridement** are conflicting.

"Real World" Advice

- **The optimal site for biopsy is the most active margin** not the central necrotic area of a lesion.
- It is important to counsel patients receiving STS about **nausea and vomiting** and to **monitor for metabolic acidosis (anion gap) and QT prolongation (ECG).**

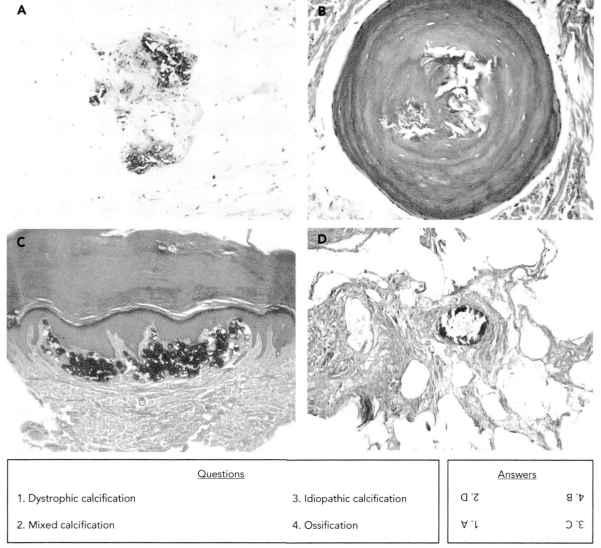

Questions

1. Dystrophic calcification

2. Mixed calcification

3. Idiopathic calcification

4. Ossification

Answers

2. D   4. B

1. A   3. C

Figure 2.65. MATCHING EXERCISE: CALCIFYING AND OSSIFYING DISORDERS. Calcium is basophilic on H&E and stains with alizarin red (more specific) and von Kossa. A, Dystrophic calcification. Note the granules and globules of calcium beneath the epidermis in this patient with DM. B, Ossification. Note the resident osteocytes in oval lacunae of the laminations about a central nidus of mature keratin flakes that were likely extruded from a follicle or cyst in this patient with osteoma cutis. C, Idiopathic calcification. Note the large deposit of calcium in the dermis distorting the overlying epidermis in this patient with a subepidermal calcified nodule. D, Mixed calcification. Note the calcification of the media of a small vessel in the panniculus, with delicate fibroplasia of the intima in this patient with calciphylaxis. There may be interstitial deposition of calcium as well. DM, dermatomyositis; H&E, hematoxylin and eosin.

(Histology images reprinted with permission from Elder DE, Elenitsas R, Rosenbach M, et al. *Lever's Histopathology of the Skin*. 11th ed. Wolters Kluwer; 2015.)

PIGMENTED PURPURA
→ **Diagnosis Group 2**
Synonyms: capillaritis, pigmented purpuric dermatoses, pigmented purpuric eruptions

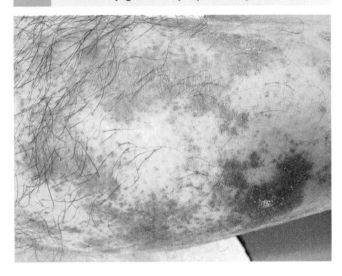

Epidemiology

- Pigmented purpura is due to **capillaritis.** There is no systemic alteration in control of coagulation.

Clinicopathological Features

- Pigmented purpura classically presents with **petechial hemorrhage favoring the lower extremities.**
- Pigmented purpura variants are summarized in Table 2.45.
  ◈ Figure 2.66.

Evaluation

- The differential diagnosis of pigmented purpura includes other causes of macular and palpable purpura, angioma serpiginosum, and early-stage CTCL.
- While pigmented purpura is a clinical diagnosis, biopsy may be required to exclude CSVV and CTCL.
- As a rule, **laboratory investigations are unremarkable.**

Management

- Topical corticosteroids may be helpful, particularly in cases associated with erythema and pruritus. Other treatments include phototherapy and ascorbic acid plus rutoside.

"Real World" Advice

- Beware the golfer. Golfer vasculitis is a CSVV variant induced by prolonged exercise in hot weather that closely resembles pigmented purpura.

Table 2.45. PIGMENTED PURPURA VARIANTS		
Variant[a]	**Classic Description**	**Notes**
Schamberg disease	Successive crops of pinpoint petechiae within yellow-brown patches	Most common variant
	Pinpoint petechiae share the color of "cayenne pepper."	
Purpura annularis telangiectodes of Majocchi	Punctate telangiectasias and petechiae within the border of 1-3 cm annular plaques that may slowly expand	
Pigmented purpuric lichenoid dermatosis of Gougerot and Blum	Schamberg-like lesions admixed with purpuric red-brown lichenoid papules	
Eczematid-like purpura of Doucas and Kapetanakis	Purpura within pruritic eczematous lesions	
Lichen aureus	Solitary golden to rust to purple-brown patch	
	The Latin word *aureus* means "golden."	
Linear pigmented purpura	Schamberg or lichen aureus–like lesions in a linear configuration often on a single extremity	
Granulomatous pigmented purpura	Hemorrhagic papules superimposed on brown patches	

[a]Illustrative examples provided.

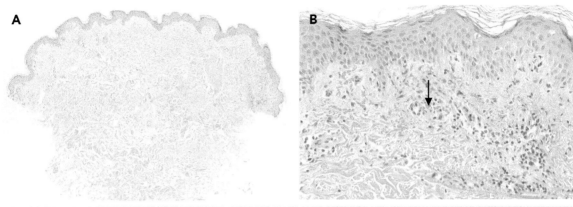

Figure 2.66. CLINICOPATHOLOGICAL CORRELATION: PIGMENTED PURPURA. Characteristic features are endothelial cell swelling, a perivascular lymphocytic infiltrate, erythrocyte extravasation, and hemosiderin-containing macrophages that stain with Perls Prussian blue. A, Low-power view. B, High-power view. Solid arrow: erythrocyte extravasation. (Histology images courtesy of Noel Turner, MD, MHS and Christine J. Ko, MD.)

SMALL VESSEL VASCULITIS
→ **Diagnosis Group 1**
Synonym: leukocytoclastic vasculitis

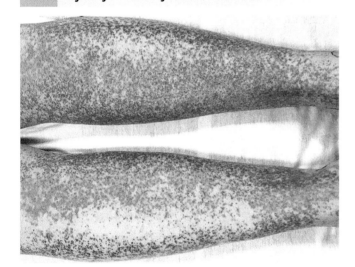

Courtesy of Robert Micheletti, MD.

Epidemiology

- CSVV is mediated by **deposition of immune complexes within postcapillary venules**, inducing complement-mediated chemotaxis of neutrophils. CSVV may be classified as an **immune complex–dependent (type III) drug reaction.**
- CSVV is **idiopathic in 50%** of patients. Associations include:
  - **Inflammatory disorders** (15%-20%): **SLE, Sjögren syndrome, RA.**
  - **Infections** (15%-20%): bacterial (eg, **group A β-hemolytic Streptococcus [GAS]**) and viral (eg, **HCV, HIV**).
  - **Neoplasms** (2%-5%): plasma cell dyscrasias, MDS, myeloproliferative disorders, lymphoproliferative disorders, hairy cell leukemia.
  - **Drug exposures** (10%-15%): TNFα inhibitors, ß-lactams, sulfonamides, quinolones, ICIs, allopurinol, hydrochlo-

rothiazide (HCTZ), NSAIDs. Nonhuman proteins (eg, antithymocyte globulin) may cause **serum sickness.**

Clinicopathological Features

- CSVV classically presents with **palpable and macular purpura favoring areas that are dependent or under tight-fitting clothing.** Urticarial papules, vesicles, pustules, and targetoid lesions may occur, along with burning, pain, or pruritus.
  - "Sock line purpura" illustrates the role of hydrostatic pressure and stasis in the pathophysiology of CSVV.
- **Proximal splinter hemorrhages** may be observed.
- CSVV can present as a **multisystem** disease in 5% to 25% of patients (**arthralgias and arthritis > gastrointestinal and/or genitourinary involvement**).
- The timing of CSVV relative to the triggering event is typically **7 to 10 days.**
  - Figure 2.67.

Evaluation

- The differential diagnosis of CSVV includes other causes of macular and palpable purpura.
- **Punch biopsies for H&E and DIF (lesional)** should be performed **within 24 to 48 hours.**
- **BUN/CR, LFTs, CBC, CRP/ESR, UA, and FOBT should be obtained in all patients** to evaluate for systemic involvement. Additional evaluation for associated triggers and other vasculitides may include:
  - Inflammatory disorders: **total hemolytic complement (CH50)/C3/C4 (and C1q if low C4), ANA with profile, ANCAs, cryoglobulins, RF.**
  - Infections: **ASO and anti-DNase B or streptozyme titer, HBV/HCV/HIV, blood, urine, and/or throat cultures.**
  - Neoplasms: **blood smear, age-appropriate malignancy screening ± sign/symptom-directed evaluation for malignancies, serum protein electrophoresis with immunofixation (SPEP/IFE), urine protein electrophoresis with immunofixation (UPEP/IFE).**

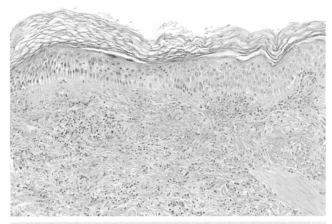

Figure 2.67. CLINICOPATHOLOGICAL CORRELATION: CUTANEOUS SMALL-VESSEL VASCULITIS. Characteristic features are a predominantly neutrophilic transmural infiltrate of small vessel walls with karyorrhexis, fibrinoid necrosis of vessel walls, leukocytoclasia, and erythrocyte extravasation. DIF classically demonstrates granular deposition of C3, IgM, IgA, and IgG in vessels. C, complement; DIF, direct immunofluorescence, Ig, immunoglobulin.
(Histology image courtesy of Noel Turner, MD, MHS and Christine J. Ko, MD.)

Palpable = infiltrating neutrophils.
Purpura = extravasating erythrocytes.

Management

- **The prognosis of CSVV depends on the severity of systemic involvement.** Skin lesions **resolve spontaneously in ~90%** of patients within weeks to months.
- Treatment should be directed at the underlying disorder. **Supportive care, NSAIDs, and antihistamines** are first line. Chronic or severe CSVV may be treated with **colchicine** and/or **dapsone. Systemic corticosteroids** may be considered for severe, ulcerating, or progressive CSVV.

"Real World" Advice

- Remember that the optimal site for DIF is **lesional for CSVV** as opposed to **perilesional for pemphigus and pemphigoid and adjacent normal skin for DH.** While the timing of a CSVV lesion (≤24 hours) takes precedence, it is preferable to select the most proximal lesions in order to avoid nonspecific vascular fluorescence due to hydrostatic pressure.

SERUM SICKNESS–LIKE ERUPTION

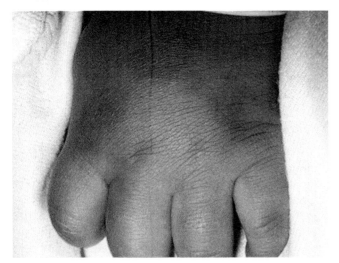

Reprinted with permission from Lugo-Somolinos A, McKinley-Grant L, Goldsmith LA, et al. *VisualDx: Essential Dermatology in Pigmented Skin.* Wolters Kluwer Health/Lippincott Williams & Wilkins; 2011.

- Serum sickness–like eruption resembles serum sickness but occurs in the absence of exposure to nonhuman proteins. It is **not a vasculitis.** It is more common in **children** than adults. Drug associations include biologics (eg, TNFα inhibitors, dupilumab, omalizumab, rituximab), **ß-lactams (eg, cefaclor),** minocycline, sulfonamides, bupropion, NSAIDs, phenytoin, propranolol, and vaccinations (eg, influenza).
- Serum sickness–like eruption classically presents with an **urticarial or morbilliform eruption.** Systemic features include **fever, lymphadenopathy, and arthralgias/arthritis.** The timing of serum sickness–like eruption relative to initial drug exposure is typically **1 to 3 weeks.**
    - ◆ Unlike serum sickness, serum sickness–like eruption lacks vasculitis on histopathology.
- **Discontinuation of the suspected drug** along with all nonessential drugs is the first step, followed by symptomatic treatment (eg, antihistamines, NSAIDs, systemic corticosteroids).

IMMUNOGLOBULIN A VASCULITIS
Synonym: Henoch-Schönlein purpura

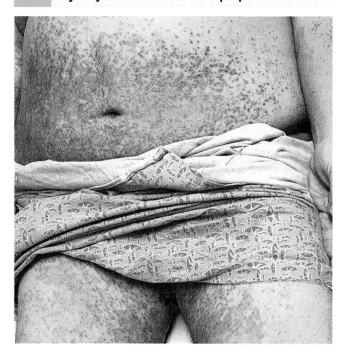

- IgA vasculitis is a vasculitis of predominantly small vessels. In contrast to CSVV, it is more commonly associated with solid organ neoplasms (eg, lung).
- IgA vasculitis classically presents with **intermittent palpable purpura favoring the extensor extremities and buttocks.** Patients may exhibit fever. Other systemic features include **gastrointestinal involvement, arthralgias/arthritis, and renal involvement. Colicky abdominal pain**, bleeding, and vomiting are common, while intussusception and bowel perfora-

tion are rare. **Nephritis (microscopic hematuria ± proteinuria evident in 40%-50% of patients within 3 months of the appearance of cutaneous lesions) may progress to chronic renal insufficiency (in up to 30% of patients). Spread of purpura above the waist has been reported to predict the risk of renal involvement**; however, data are conflicting.

   - Palpable purpura, abdominal pain, arthritis, and hematuria are often called the tetrad of IgA vasculitis.
   - Figure 2.68.
   - In children, **acute hemorrhagic edema of infancy (AHEI)** may clinically mimic IgA vasculitis (Table 2.46).
- **Supportive care** is first line. While systemic corticosteroids do not prevent renal disease, they may be used to treat severe nephritis (controversial).

URTICARIAL VASCULITIS

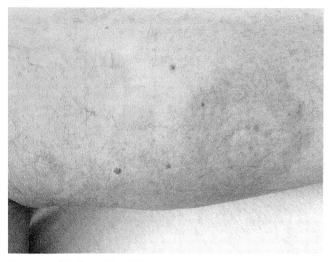

Courtesy of Sa Rang Kim, MD.

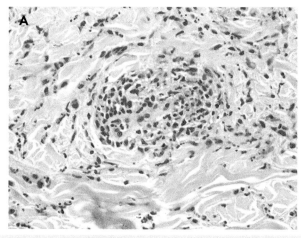
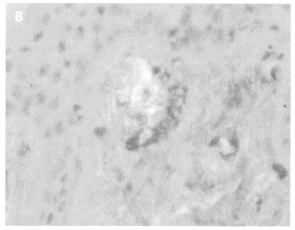

Figure 2.68. CLINICOPATHOLOGICAL CORRELATION: IMMUNOGLOBULIN A VASCULITIS. IgA vasculitis demonstrates CSVV on H&E. DIF classically demonstrates granular IgA (out of proportion to IgM and IgG) and C3 deposition in vessels. A, H&E. B, DIF (IgA). C, complement; CSVV, cutaneous small-vessel vasculitis; DIF, direct immunofluorescence; H&E, hematoxylin and eosin; Ig, immunoglobulin.

(Histology image reprinted with permission from Elder DE, Elenitsas R, Rosenbach M, et al. *Lever's Histopathology of the Skin.* 11th ed. Wolters Kluwer; 2015.)

Table 2.46. IGA VASCULITIS AND ACUTE HEMORRHAGIC EDEMA OF INFANCY

Characteristic	Immunoglobulin A vasculitis (Henoch-Schönlein purpura)	AHEI (Finkelstein Disease)
Epidemiology	Most common vasculitis in children (90% < 10 years of age). M > F. Associated with infections (eg, streptococcal URI).	Distinct vasculitis in children (<2 years of age). M > F. Associated with infections (eg, URI), drugs, and vaccines.
Classic description	See above. Children are less likely than adults to develop chronic renal insufficiency (1%-3%).	Annular, circular, or targetoid purpuric plaques favoring the face and extremities and tender, nonpitting edema of the face, ears, extremities, and scrotum. Patients may exhibit fever but are well appearing. Systemic involvement is rare.
		Lesions may resemble a "cockade," which is an ornament (eg, a rosette) usually worn on a hat as a badge.
Management	See above.	Supportive care is first line (resolves spontaneously in 1-3 weeks).

AHEI, acute hemorrhagic edema of infancy; F, female; M, male; URI, upper respiratory infection.

- Urticarial vasculitis is a vasculitis of predominantly small vessels. Associations include inflammatory disorders (eg, **SLE, Sjögren syndrome, RA**) and viral infections. Incidence peaks in the **fifth decade** and 60% to 80% of patients are **female.** Urticarial vasculitis is classically divided into **normocomplementemic (70%-80%) and hypocomplementemic** subtypes. It occurs in hypocomplementemic urticarial vasculitis syndrome (HUVS) and variably in Schnitzler syndrome.
- Urticarial vasculitis is characterized by **urticarial lesions ± angioedema.** Lesions **persist > 24 hours, present with burning and pain as opposed to pruritus, and resolve with postinflammatory hyperpigmentation. Hypocomplementemia is associated with systemic involvement. Diagnostic criteria** for HUVS are presented in Table 2.47.
  - ◆ Figure 2.69.
- Treatment options include antihistamines, indomethacin, dapsone ± pentoxifylline, and corticosteroids.

- Erythema elevatum diutinum (EED) is a vasculitis of predominantly small vessels. Associations include inflammatory disorders (eg, **RA**), infections (eg, **group A beta hemolytic streptococcal, HIV**), and hematologic disorders (eg, **IgA monoclonal gammopathy**).
- EED classically presents with **asymptomatic symmetric red-brown papules, plaques, and nodules favoring extensor surfaces.**
  - ◆ Apart from the nonfacial location, EED can NOT be distinguished from granuloma faciale on histopathology.
- NSAIDs, intralesional corticosteroids, and **dapsone** are first line.

CRYOGLOBULINEMIA

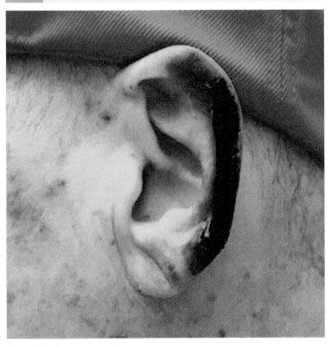

Cryoglobulinemia type I.

ERYTHEMA ELEVATUM DIUTINUM

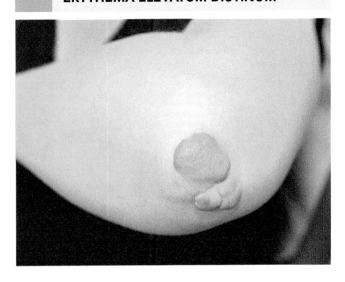

Table 2.47. DIAGNOSTIC CRITERIA FOR HYPOCOMPLEMENTEMIC URTICARIAL VASCULITIS SYNDROME

Diagnostic criteria for HUVS[a]

Major Criteria

1. Urticaria for 6 months
2. Hypocomplementemia

Minor Criteria

1. Vasculitis on skin biopsy
2. Arthralgia or arthritis
3. Uveitis or episcleritis
4. Glomerulonephritis
5. Recurrent abdominal pain
6. Positive C1q precipitin test with a low C1q level

HUVS, hypocomplementemic urticarial vasculitis syndrome.
[a]Both of the major and two minor criteria are required for diagnosis.

- **Cryoglobulins are cold-precipitable immunoglobulins detectable in both serum and plasma.** Cryoglobulinemia can be divided into **three subtypes**:
  - **Type I cryoglobulinemia (monoclonal IgM > IgG > IgA):** associations include **plasma cell dyscrasias and lymphoproliferative disorders.**
  - **Type II mixed cryoglobulinemia (monoclonal IgM > IgG against polyclonal IgG):** associations include inflammatory disorders (eg, **SLE, Sjögren syndrome, RA**), infections (eg, **HCV > HBV, HIV**), and lymphoproliferative disorders (eg, **NHL, CLL**).
  - **Type III mixed cryoglobulinemia (polyclonal IgM against polyclonal IgG):** same associations as type II mixed cryoglobulinemia.

Cryoglobulinemic vasculitis in ~15% of patients with mixed cryoglobulinemia is a vasculitis of predominantly small vessels.

  - Do NOT confuse cryoglobulins with cryofibrinogens (cold-precipitable fibrinogens detectable only in plasma) and cold agglutinins (antibodies that promote erythrocyte agglutination on exposure to cold), which are only rarely responsible for cold-related blood vessel occlusion.

- **Type I cryoglobulinemia** classically presents with **cold-induced retiform purpura and necrosis**, with rarer findings including **Raynaud phenomenon, livedo reticularis, and acrocyanosis. Cryoglobulinemic vasculitis** classically presents with **palpable purpura**, with rarer findings including **livedo reticularis and leg ulcers.** Systemic features of cryoglobulinemic vasculitis include **gastrointestinal disease or hepatitis, arthralgias and arthritis, mononeuritis multiplex and peripheral neuropathy**, and **membranoproliferative glomerulonephritis.**
  - Figure 2.70.

- **Cryoglobulins** can be falsely negative and need to be transported to the laboratory at 37 °C. Other laboratory findings include **hypocomplementemia**, positive RF (70%), positive **ANA** (20%), and **monoclonal gammopathy** (15%).
  - RF is sometimes called "the poor man's cryo."

- Treatment of cryoglobulinemia should be directed at the underlying disorder. Patients with type I cryoglobulinemia should **minimize cold exposure. Systemic corticosteroids** are first line for cryoglobulinemic vasculitis. Patients with HCV-associated mixed cryoglobulinemia should receive antiviral therapy. Historically, IFN-α plus ribavirin was the preferred regimen; although **IFN-α may trigger or worsen peripheral neuropathy.** More recent data support the use of newer regimens such as **sofosbuvir/velpatasvir plus ribavirin or sofosbuvir/ledipasvir.**

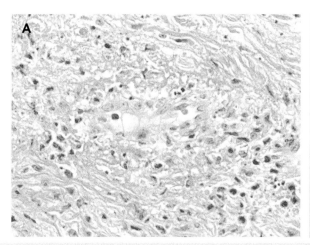
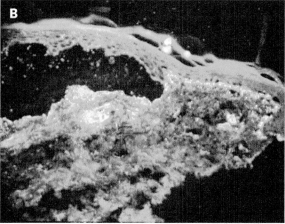

Figure 2.69. CLINICOPATHOLOGICAL CORRELATION: URTICARIAL VASCULITIS. Urticarial vasculitis demonstrates CSVV (vessel wall necrosis and leukocytoclasia at a minimum) on H&E. DIF classically demonstrates granular deposition of IgG, C3, and fibrinogen in vessels and the DEJ. A, H&E. B, DIF (IgG). C, complement; CSVV, cutaneous small-vessel vasculitis; DEJ, dermo-epidermal junction; DIF, direct immunofluorescence; H&E, hematoxylin and eosin; Ig, immunoglobulin.

(A, Histology image courtesy of Noel Turner, MD, MHS and Christine J. Ko, MD. B, Histology image reprinted with permission from Elder DE, Elenitsas R, Rosenbach M, et al. *Lever's Histopathology of the Skin.* 11th ed. Wolters Kluwer; 2015.)

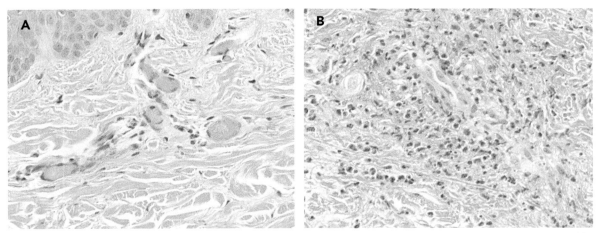

Figure 2.70. SIDE-BY-SIDE COMPARISON: TYPE I CRYOGLOBULINEMIA AND CRYOGLOBULINEMIC VASCULITIS.
Both type I and mixed cryoglobulinemia may demonstrate eosinophilic intramural and intravascular cryoprecipitates (PAS positive, diastase resistant). Type I cryoglobulinemia demonstrates prominent cryoprecipitates without inflammation. Cryoglobulinemic vasculitis demonstrates CSVV. DIF classically demonstrates granular deposition of IgM and C3 in vessels. A, Type I cryoglobulinemia. B, Cryoglobulinemic vasculitis. C, complement; CSVV, cutaneous small-vessel vasculitis; DIF, direct immunofluorescence; Ig, immunoglobulin; PAS, periodic acid-Schiff.

(Histology images courtesy of Noel Turner, MD, MHS and Christine J. Ko, MD.)

ANTINEUTROPHIL CYTOPLASMIC ANTI-BODY VASCULITIS

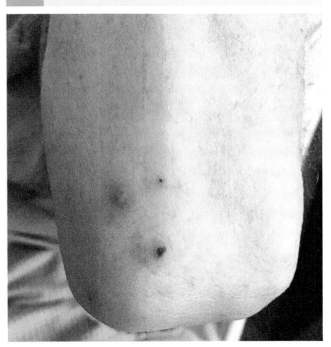

Granulomatosis with polyangiitis courtesy of Robert Micheletti, MD.

- ANCA vasculitis is a **pauci-immune** vasculitis of predominantly small and medium vessels (vessel wall damage is directly mediated by neutrophils). ANCAs are predominantly IgG autoantibodies to components of both **primary granules of neutrophils and monocyte**

lysosomes. **Cytoplasmic (c)-ANCAs to proteinase-3 (PR3)** and **perinuclear (p)-ANCAs to MPO** are implicated in vasculitis:
- **Anti-MPO** > anti-PR3 in **MPA.**
- **Anti-PR3** > anti-MPO in **GPA.**
  - The historical name for GPA, Wegener granulomatosis, is no longer in use due to Wegener's participation in the German Nazi Party.
- **Anti-MPO** > anti-PR3 in **EGPA.** Drug associations include **dupilumab, omalizumab, and leukotriene inhibitors.**
  - The historical name for EGPA is Churg-Strauss syndrome.
- **Anti-MPO** > anti-PR3 in **drug-induced ANCA vasculitis.** Drug associations include **minocycline and propylthiouracil.** Other triggers include **levamisole-adulterated cocaine.**
  - Propylthiouracil is associated with p-ANCA vasculitis. ANCAs may also be detected in inflammatory disorders (eg, **IBD**) and infections.
- ANCA vasculitis classically presents with **palpable purpura.** Other cutaneous and systemic features depend on the disease:
  - MPA: other cutaneous features include **acral erythematous macules.** Systemic features include neurologic involvement (eg, **mononeuritis multiplex and peripheral neuropathy**), renal involvement (**pauci-immune crescentic necrotizing glomerulonephritis**), and pulmonary involvement (**diffuse alveolar hemorrhage**).
  - GPA: other cutaneous manifestations include **subcutaneous nodules, PG-like lesions, and papulonecrotic**

lesions favoring the extremities; **oral ulcers and gingival hyperplasia.** Systemic features include renal involvement (**pauci-immune crescentic necrotizing glomerulonephritis**), upper respiratory tract involvement (eg, **recurrent epistaxis, nasal septal perforation, saddle nose deformity**), and lower respiratory tract involvement (eg, **pulmonary infiltrates and nodules**).

 Gingival hyperplasia in GPA is often called "strawberry gums."

o EGPA: other cutaneous manifestations include **subcutaneous nodules and papulonecrotic lesions favoring the extremities.** Systemic features include **peripheral hypereosinophilia and elevated IgE,** cardiac involvement (eg, **cardiomyopathy and pericarditis**), neurologic involvement (eg, **mononeuritis multiplex and peripheral neuropathy**), and respiratory tract involvement (eg, **allergic rhinitis, nasal polyps, asthma**).

 Figure 2.71.

- **Screen for ANCAs with IIF followed by confirmation with antigen-specific ELISAs for PR3 and MPO.** Consider a **urine toxicology screen.** Evaluation for systemic involvement depends on the disease and clinical findings. Beyond GPA, **gingival hyperplasia** is further associated with **vitamin C deficiency, hyaline fibromatosis syndrome, and drugs (eg, cyclosporine, CCBs, phenytoin).**
- Systemic corticosteroids are first line. Other recommendations for remission induction for active disease from the 2021 American College of Rheumatology/Vasculitis Foundation Guideline include:
  o MPA: **rituximab** (severe).
  o GPA: **methotrexate** (nonsevere); **rituximab** (severe).
  o EGPA: **mepolizumab** (nonsevere); **cyclophosphamide or rituximab** (severe).

ANCA levels often correlate with disease activity and are therefore useful for **monitoring response to therapy and predicting relapse.**

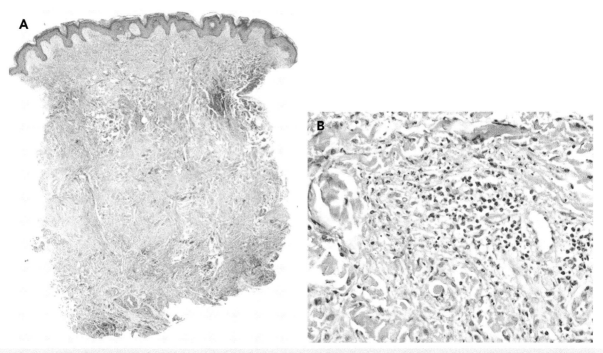

Figure 2.71. CLINICOPATHOLOGICAL CORRELATION: ANTINEUTROPHIL CYTOPLASMIC ANTIBODY VASCULITIS. Characteristic features are vasculitis of small and medium caliber vessels with endothelial necrosis. A, High-power view (EGPA). B, Low-power view (EGPA). ANCA, antineutrophil cytoplasmic antibody; EGPA, eosinophilic granulomatosis with polyangiitis; GPA, granulomatosis with polyangiitis; MPA, microscopic polyangiitis; RA, rheumatoid arthritis.

(Histology images reprinted with permission from Elder DE, Elenitsas R, Rosenbach M, et al. *Lever's Histopathology of the Skin.* 11th ed. Wolters Kluwer; 2015.)

ANCA Vasculitides
- **MPA**: No granuloma formation.
- **GPA**: Multinucleated giant cells palisade around stellate neutrophilic abscesses.
- **EGPA**: Epithelioid cells palisade around stellate eosinophilic abscesses.

GPA is a "blue granuloma." EGPA is a "red granuloma."
Despite its historic name, the "Churg-Strauss granuloma" occurs not only in EGPA but also in other vasculitides (eg, GPA), other inflammatory disorders (eg, RA), infections (eg, endocarditis), and lymphoproliferative disorders.

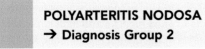

POLYARTERITIS NODOSA
→ Diagnosis Group 2

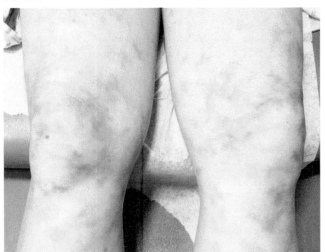

Courtesy of Robert Micheletti, MD.

Epidemiology

- PAN is a medium vessel vasculitis. It may be divided into **classic (systemic) PAN** and **cutaneous PAN** (~10%). It is unclear whether progression from cutaneous to classic PAN can occur.
- Associations include inflammatory disorders, infections (eg, **HBV** > HCV, streptococcal infection), vaccinations (eg, HBV), and neoplasms (eg, **hairy cell leukemia**).

◇ HCV = mixed cryoglobulinemia. HBV = PAN.
- Drug associations include **minocycline.**

Clinicopathological Features

- PAN classically presents with **livedo racemosa, palpable purpura, inflammatory retiform purpura, and well-demarcated ulcers. Subcutaneous nodules and digital infarcts** may occur.
- Patients may exhibit **fever, arthralgias and arthritis, and peripheral neuropathy.** Classic PAN is associated with cardiac (eg, congestive heart failure [CHF]), gastrointestinal (eg, mesenteric ischemia), neurologic (eg, stroke, mononeuritis multiplex), renal (eg, **renal hypertension and renal failure**), and testicular (eg, orchitis) involvement.
  ◇ Skin morphology provides a window into the body. In the kidneys, vasculitis of small vessels affects the glomerulus (a tuft of capillaries), while vasculitis of medium vessels affects the interlobar renal arteries.
  ◆ Figure 2.72.

Evaluation

- The differential diagnosis of PAN includes other causes of retiform purpura.
- **Biopsy should include the subcutis.**
- In addition to the common vasculitis work-up, evaluation for systemic involvement in classic PAN may include **mesenteric/renal/celiac angiogram to detect microaneurysms** and consideration of **muscle, nerve, kidney, and/or testicle biopsy.**

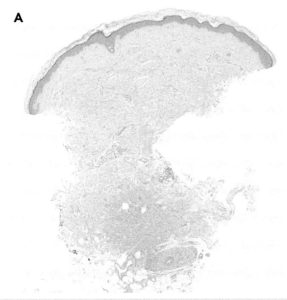

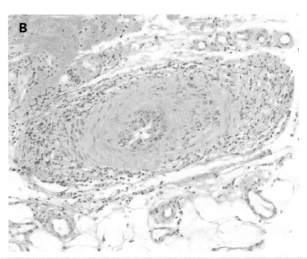

Figure 2.72. CLINICOPATHOLOGICAL CORRELATION: POLYARTERITIS NODOSA. Characteristic features are vasculitis of medium caliber vessels in the subcutaneous fat with fat necrosis. DIF classically demonstrates granular deposition of C3, IgM, and fibrin in vessels. A, Low-power view. B, High-power view. C, complement; DIF, direct immunofluorescence; Ig, immunoglobulin.
(Histology images courtesy of Noel Turner, MD, MHS and Christine J. Ko, MD.)

The media of a medium caliber vessel may resemble a "wreath."

Management

- Treatment should be directed at the underlying trigger. According to the 2021 American College of Rheumatology/Vasculitis Foundation Guideline, **systemic corticosteroids** are first line for classic PAN in addition to another immunosuppressant (eg, methotrexate, azathioprine) if nonsevere or cyclophosphamide if severe. Patients with HBV-associated classic PAN should receive **plasma exchange and antiviral therapy with IFN-α plus lamivudine. NSAIDs and topical, intralesional, and/or systemic corticosteroids** are first line for cutaneous PAN.

"Real World" Advice

- In contrast to ANCA vasculitis, PAN **often spares the lungs.**
- **The optimal site for biopsy is a subcutaneous nodule > retiform purpura > ulcer edge** including the peripheral rim of inflammation (if present). Incidental vasculitis underlying an ulcer is nondiagnostic.

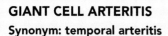

GIANT CELL ARTERITIS
Synonym: temporal arteritis

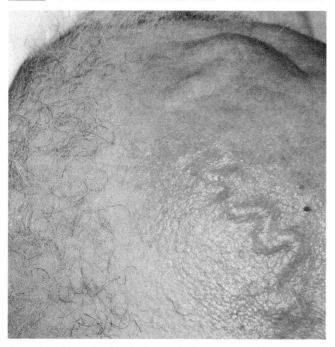

Reproduced from Mackie SL, Pease CT. Diagnosis and management of giant cell arteritis and polymyalgia rheumatica: challenges, controversies and practical tips. *Postgrad Med J.* 2013;89(1051):284-292; with permission from BMJ Publishing Group Ltd.

- Giant cell arteritis (GCA), like Takayasu arteritis, is a large vessel vasculitis. The former affects the temporal artery, while the latter affects the aorta and named arteries. GCA is associated with **polymyalgia rheumatica (PMR).**
- **Early** GCA is characterized by **erythematous or cyanotic skin, purpura, and tender nodules on the frontotemporal** scalp. **Late** GCA is characterized by **ulceration and/or gangrene of the frontotemporal scalp or tongue.** In contrast, cutaneous manifestations in Takayasu arteritis (eg, subcutaneous nodules and PG-like lesions) are rare. Systemic features of GCA include **new-onset headache, visual disturbances, and jaw claudication.** One or both temporal arteries may demonstrate **absent pulsation.**
  - Figure 2.73.
- Laboratory abnormalities include **elevated CRP/ESR.** Definitive diagnosis should then be made by **temporal artery biopsy.**
- Treatment should never be delayed for the purpose of diagnosis. According to the 2021 American College of Rheumatology/Vasculitis Foundation Guideline, **systemic corticosteroids ± tocilizumab** are first line.

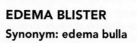

EDEMA BLISTER
Synonym: edema bulla

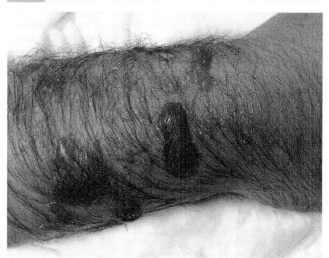

Courtesy of Robert G. Micheletti, MD.

- Edema results from an imbalance between capillary filtration and lymphatic drainage. Associations include **CHF, venous occlusion, hepatic cirrhosis, hypoalbuminemia, and renal disease.** Drug associations include **CCBs. Edema blisters** form in the setting of **acute exacerbation of chronic edema or anasarca.**
- An edema blister is characteristically **noninflammatory and tense, located on a lower extremity.** The surrounding skin is **edematous.**
  - An edema blister is characterized by marked epidermal spongiosis and dermal edema with widely spaced collagen bundles, dilated blood vessels, and a mild inflammatory infiltrate. A subepidermal split may be present.
- Treatment should be directed at the underlying edema including **diuretics and leg elevation and compression** (eg, gradient support stockings, pneumatic pumps, massage).

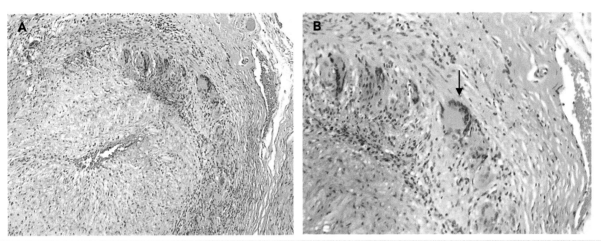

Figure 2.73. CLINICOPATHOLOGICAL CORRELATION: GIANT CELL ARTERITIS. Characteristic features are vasculitis of a large caliber vessel with subendothelial granulomatous inflammation and media disruption. A, Low-power view. B, High-power view. Solid arrow: Giant cell.

(Histology images reprinted with permission from Elder DE, Elenitsas R, Rosenbach M, et al. *Lever's Histopathology of the Skin.* 11th ed. Wolters Kluwer; 2015.)

The media of a large caliber vessel may resemble a "wreath."

LYMPHEDEMA

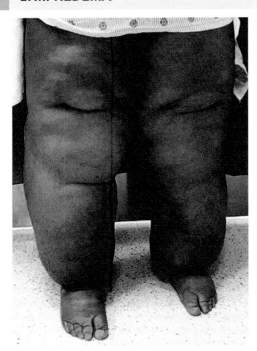

Reprinted with permission from Chung KC. *Grabb and Smith's Plastic Surgery.* 8th ed. Wolters Kluwer; 2019.

- Lymphedema results from a reduction in lymphatic drainage in the presence of normal capillary filtration, leading to accumulation of lymphatic fluid within the interstitium. It **may be primary or secondary.** Associations include inflammatory disorders (eg, acne/rosacea, granulomatous disorders), podoconiosis (exposure to mineral microparticles in volcanic soils), nephrotic syndrome, obesity, infections (eg, **filariasis, recurrent cellulitis/lymphangitis**), **malignant obstruction**, and procedures (eg, **lymph node dissection, radiation therapy**, surgical excisions).

Primary lymphedema is summarized in Table 2.48.
- Lymphedema begins with edema of the dorsal foot and progresses proximally. Complications include fibrosis, ulceration, **elephantiasis nostras verrucosa, verruciform xanthoma,** and secondary infection. **Yellow nail syndrome** may be present.
  - The appearance of elephantiasis nostras verrucosa has been likened to "cobblestones" or "moss."
  - Figure 2.74.
  - Lymphedema has nonspecific histopathology.
- **Leg elevation and compression are first line.** Diuretics have no role in lymphedema therapy. Topical keratolytics (eg, salicylic acid, urea) and retinoids may be helpful for elephantiasis nostras verrucosa.

VENOUS ULCER

Synonym: ulcer due to venous insufficiency/ venous hypertension

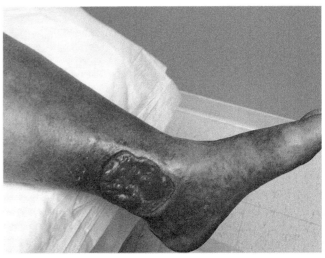

Courtesy of Douglas Pugliese, MD, MPH.

Table 2.48. PRIMARY LYMPHEDEMA

Classification	Diagnosis[a]	Inheritance pattern	Gene	Notes
Congenital lymphedema (onset 0-2 years)	Milroy disease (type 1A)	AD	*VEGFR3 (FLT4)*	
	Noonan syndrome	See Chapter 5: Vascular Malformations and Neoplasms.		
	Turner syndrome	See Chapter 5: Vascular Malformations and Neoplasms.		
Lymphedema praecox (onset peripubertal)	Meige disease (type II)	AD	*LMPH2*	Most common cause of primary lymphedema. Female predominance.
	Lymphedema-Distichiasis syndrome	AD	*FOXC2*	Distichiasis is abnormal growth of eyelashes from the orifices of meibomian glands, leading to a double row of eyelashes.
				Patients with lymphedema-distichiasis syndrome due to AD mutation of FOXC2 have "foxy" eyelashes.
	Yellow nail syndrome	See above.		
Lymphedema tarda (onset after age 35)	Due to an environmental trigger (eg, infection, trauma) superimposed on inherently weakened lymphatics.			

AD, autosomal dominant.
[a]Illustrative examples provided.

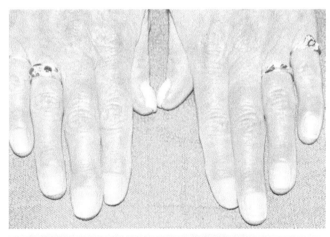

Figure 2.74. YELLOW NAIL SYNDROME. Yellow nail syndrome is characterized by arrested or reduced linear nail growth. Typically, the lunula and eponychium are absent and the nail plate is thick and yellow. It may be associated with lymphedema and respiratory tract involvement (eg, chronic bronchitis, bronchiectasis, sinusitis, pleural effusions). Remember the association between lymphedema and <u>yellow</u> nail syndrome by remembering that lymphatic fluid is <u>yellow</u> ("yeah, they were all yellow").

(Yellow nail syndrome image reprinted with permission from Goodheart HP. *Goodheart's Photoguide of Common Skin Disorders: Diagnosis and Management.* 2nd ed. Lippincott Williams & Wilkins; 2003.)

- **Venous insufficiency/hypertension is the leading cause of chronic leg ulceration.**
  - An ulcer may be the presenting sign of a genetic disorder. Patients with **Klinefelter syndrome (47, XXY)** are **tall** and often present with **multifactorial ulcers along with other features such as infertility due to primary testicular insufficiency.**
- A venous ulcer is characteristically **shallow with a yellow fibrinous base and irregular borders, located above the medial malleolus** (similar to a hydroxyurea ulcer). The skin surrounding a venous ulcer may be **yellow-brown due to hemosiderin deposits with pinpoint petechiae and lipodermatosclerosis.** Other findings include stasis dermatitis, varicosities, edema, and lymphedema.
  - A venous ulcer is characterized by ulceration with stasis change in the surrounding skin.
- Evaluate with **duplex ultrasonography, ankle-brachial index (ABI)** to exclude arterial insufficiency, and **nylon monofilament testing** to exclude neuropathy.
- Treatment should be directed at the underlying venous insufficiency/hypertension including **leg elevation and compression. Local wound care** involves dressings, debridement, treatment of surrounding stasis dermatitis (if present), antimicrobial therapy (if needed), vacuum-assisted closure (VAC) therapy (if needed), and tetanus booster vaccination. Venous surgery, skin constructs, and pinch grafts may be appropriate for nonhealing venous ulcers; however, the diagnosis should be carefully reconsidered (eg, skin biopsy and tissue culture to exclude a neoplastic or infectious process).

ARTERIAL ULCER
Synonym: ulcer due to atherosclerosis

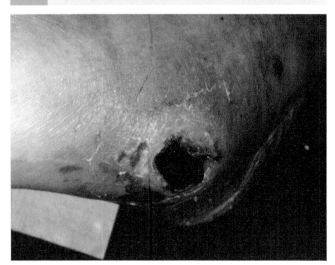

Courtesy of Douglas Pugliese, MD, MPH.

- **Peripheral arterial disease (PAD)** is a form of **arterial insufficiency** that may result in skin necrosis and impaired wound healing. Risk factors include **diabetes mellitus (acral dry gangrene) and cigarette smoking.**
- An arterial ulcer is characteristically **dry and well demarcated with a necrotic base, located around the lateral malleolus or on a distal point** (eg, a toe). The surrounding skin may be **shiny and atrophic with hair loss. Intermittent claudication** (leg pain induced by ambulation and relieved by resting) is the most common presenting symptom of PAD, progressing to rest pain. Other findings include weak or absent peripheral pulses, cool feet, prolonged capillary refill time (>3-4 seconds), pallor on leg elevation (45° for 1 min), and dependent rubor.
   ◆ An arterial ulcer has nonspecific histopathology.
- Evaluate arterial ulcer with **ABI** with additional tests including computed tomography angiogram (CTA) and magnetic resonance angiogram (MRA). While **Martorell hypertensive ischemic ulcer** may clinically mimic arterial ulcer, the location is **lateral** but typically more **posterior** overlying the Achilles tendon. **Buerger disease** is **distal** but often involves both the upper and lower extremities.

- Treatment should be directed at the underlying arterial insufficiency including **endovascular intervention or surgical reconstruction. Local wound care** is similar to venous ulcers except for **limiting sharp debridement** and **avoiding VAC therapy.**

DIFFUSE DERMAL ANGIOMATOSIS

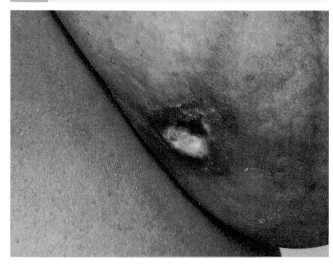

Courtesy of Alaina James, MD, PhD and Inbal Sander, MD.

- Diffuse dermal angiomatosis (DDA) is classified as a reactive angioendotheliomatosis along with intravascular reactive angioendotheliomatosis. DDA is associated with **atherosclerosis, large pendulous breasts, and cigarette smoking.**
- DDA classically presents with **rapid development of painful reticulated violaceous plaques with central ulceration favoring the breasts and extremities.**
   ◆ DDA is characterized by a diffuse interstitial proliferation of CD31-positive endothelial cells within the papillary and reticular dermis with focal formation of small vascular channels.
- Intravascular papillary endothelial hyperplasia (IPEH) is a distinct reactive vascular disorder that refers to recanalization of a thrombus within a vascular space.
- Treatment should be directed at the underlying disorder.

ERYTHROMELALGIA

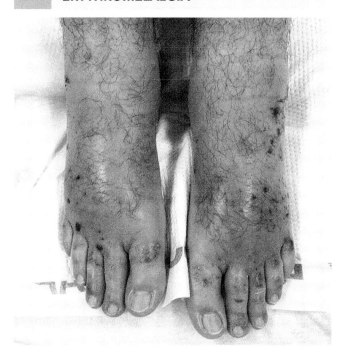

- Erythromelalgia is classically divided into three subtypes. **Type 1** is associated with **thrombocythemia. Type 2** is **primary or idiopathic. Type 3** is associated with other underlying disorders (eg, **myeloproliferative disorders, small fiber neuropathy**).
    - Gain-of-function missense mutations in *SCN9A*, which encodes the voltage-gated sodium channel alpha subunit Nav1.7, have been associated with **primary erythromelalgia.**
    - S<u>C</u>N9<u>A</u>: <u>s</u>odium (<u>Na</u>) channel.
- Erythromelalgia is characterized by **burning, erythema, and warmth of acral sites** (lower > upper).
    - Erythromelalgia has nonspecific histopathology with the exception of type 1, which shows intimal proliferation and occlusive thrombosis of affected arterioles, followed by complete fibrosis.
- **Cooling and limb elevation** generally reduce symptoms; however, it is important to exercise caution as prolonged water immersion contributes to maceration and ulceration. Therapy combines analgesia with treatments directed at any underlying disorder (eg, **ASA for type 1**).

Neurocutaneous and Psychocutaneous Disorders

Basic Concepts

- **Neurocutaneous disorders** primarily result from **pruritus**, an unpleasant sensation that elicits a desire to scratch. Pruritus may be categorized into **three groups: (1) affecting diseased (inflamed) skin, (2) affecting nondiseased (noninflamed) skin, and (3) presenting with chronic secondary scratch-induced lesions, such as prurigo nodularis.** Etiologies may be **dermatologic, systemic, neurologic, psychogenic**, mixed, or other/unknown (Table 2.49). Neurologic and psychogenic pruritus frequently manifest with **dysesthesia**, an unpleasant sensation of burning, numbness, pruritus, and/or tingling. Pruritus variants include **aquagenic pruritus**, pruritus in scars, postthermal burn pruritus, and fiberglass dermatitis.
- **Psychocutaneous disorders** primarily result from **four underlying psychopathologies: anxiety, depression, psychosis, and obsession-compulsion.** Psychocutaneous disorders include **primary psychiatric disorders** (self-induced skin findings), **secondary psychiatric disorders** (psychiatric findings induced by a skin disorder), **psychogenic pruritus and dysesthesia** (purely sensory complaints), and **psychophysiologic disorders** (skin disorder exacerbated by emotional factors).

PRURIGO NODULARIS
→ **Diagnosis Group 1**

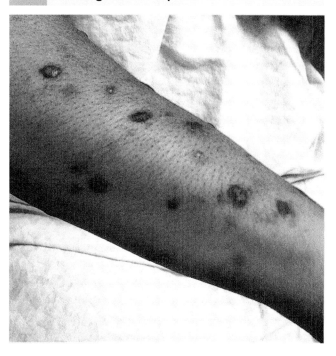

Epidemiology

- Prurigo nodularis is a **secondary skin disorder** associated with **pruritus.**

Clinicopathological Features

- Prurigo nodularis classically presents with **skin-colored to erythematous firm, dome-shaped papulonodules favoring the back (sparing the mid upper back), lumbosacral area, buttocks, and extensor extremities.** Central scale, crust, erosion, and ulceration are variably present. **Hyperpigmentation** is common.
    - Figure 2.75.
    - Figure 2.76.

Table 2.49. PRURITUS

Category	Subcategory	Diagnoses[a]	Notes
Dermatologic	Inflammatory dermatoses	Psoriasis, AD, AEP, LP, urticaria, PUVA phototherapy	AD is the leading cause of dermatologic pruritus (100% of patients). AEP is the leading cause of pruritus during pregnancy.
	Infectious dermatoses	Scabies, pediculosis	
	Neoplasms	CTCL	
Systemic	Endocrine and metabolic diseases	Chronic renal failure, cirrhosis, PBC, ICP, hyperthyroidism > hypothyroidism (xerosis), diabetes mellitus	ESRD on HD is the leading cause of systemic pruritus (25%-30% of patients). It peaks in the evening after 2 days without dialysis, is relatively high during dialysis, and is lowest the following day. Gabapentin, pregabalin, and phototherapy are first-line systemic therapies for moderate to severe renal pruritus. Renal transplant leads to resolution. Cholestyramine is first line for PBC. ICP classically presents in late pregnancy with elevated serum bile acid levels. Increased fetal risk of prematurity, intrapartum distress, and stillbirth. Ursodeoxycholic acid is first line. Recurs in 45%-70% of subsequent pregnancies.
	Infectious diseases	Viral (eg, VZV, HCV, HIV/AIDS) and parasitic	Thalidomide is first line for HIV/AIDS-associated pruritus.
	Hematological and lymphoproliferative diseases	Iron deficiency, PV, Hodgkin disease > NHL, CLL, HES	PV associated with aquagenic pruritus (starts within 30 minutes of water contact and lasts for up to 2 hours) often presents with a ruddy complexion.
	Visceral neoplasms	Solid tumors of the cervix, prostate, or colon, carcinoid syndrome	
	Pregnancy	AEP, pemphigoid gestationis, PEP, ICP	
	Drug-induced pruritus	OCPs, IL-2, ICIs, ACEIs, opioids	
Neurologic	Neurogenic origin (without neuronal damage)	Hepatic itch with increased endogenous μ-opioids (disinhibition of itch)	
	Neuropathic diseases (neuronal damage causes itch)	Cerebral or spinal infarcts, postherpetic neuralgia, neoplasms, MS, regional dysesthesias, small fiber neuropathy	
Psychogenic	Somatoform pruritus	Anxiety, depression, psychosis, obsession-compulsion	Pruritus in specific locations (eg, scalp pruritus, pruritus ani, pruritus scroti, pruritus vulvae) may be primary (psychogenic) or secondary.

ACEI, angiotensin-converting enzyme inhibitor; AD, atopic dermatitis; AEP, atopic eruption of pregnancy; AIDS, acquired immune deficiency syndrome; CLL, chronic lymphocytic leukemia; CTCL, cutaneous T-cell lymphoma; ESRD, end-stage renal disease; HCV, hepatitis C virus; HD, hemodialysis; HES, hypereosinophilic syndrome; HIV, human immunodeficiency virus; ICI, immune checkpoint inhibitor; ICP, intrahepatic cholestasis of pregnancy; Ig, immunoglobulin; IL, interleukin; LP, lichen planus; NHL, non-Hodgkin lymphoma; MS, multiple sclerosis; OCPs, oral contraceptive pills; PBC, primary biliary cholangitis; PEP, polymorphic eruption of pregnancy; PUVA, psoralen ultraviolet A; PV, polycythemia vera.
[a]Illustrative examples provided.

Evaluation

- The differential diagnosis of prurigo nodularis includes inflammatory disorders (eg, pemphigoid nodularis, hypertrophic LP, hypertrophic LE, perforating disorders), infestations (eg, scabies), and neoplasms (eg, keratoacanthomas, keratoacanthoma-type SCCs).

- Initial laboratory testing for patients with pruritus either affecting nondiseased skin or presenting with chronic secondary scratch-induced lesions includes **electrolytes, BUN/Cr, fasting glucose, LFTs, CBC, CRP/ESR, TSH ± FT4, and lactate dehydrogenase (LDH).** Additional evaluation depends on the suspected underlying disorder(s).

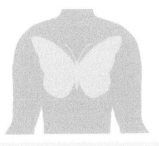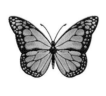

Figure 2.75. THE BUTTERFLY SIGN. Self-induced skin findings classically spare a "butterfly-shaped" area on the mid upper back where the patient cannot easily reach. This clinical feature is common in neurocutaneous disorders such as prurigo nodularis and psychocutaneous disorders such as delusions of parasitosis and excoriation disorder. Do NOT confuse the "butterfly" sign with the "butterfly" rash of ACLE. ACLE, acute cutaneous lupus erythematosus.

(Illustration by Caroline A. Nelson, MD.)

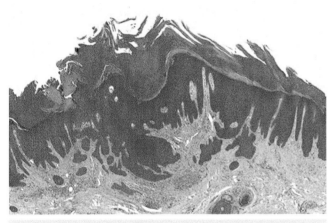

Figure 2.76. CLINICOPATHOLOGICAL CORRELATION: PRURIGO NODULARIS. Characteristic features are hyperkeratosis, hypergranulosis, acanthosis, and papillary dermal fibrosis with capillary proliferation (angiofibroplasia) and vertically oriented collagen.

(Histology image reprinted with permission from Elder DE, Elenitsas R, Rubin AI, et al. *Atlas of Dermatopathology: Synopsis and Atlas of Lever's Histopathology of the Skin*. 4th ed. Wolters Kluwer; 2020.)

Management

- Treatment of prurigo nodularis should be directed at pruritus along with any underlying disorders and obsessions and compulsions, if present.
- **Skin care** is the foundation of antipruritic therapy, and patients should **keep nails cut short.**
- Topical antipruritic agents include **cooling agents/counterirritants (eg, menthol, camphor, capsaicin), anesthetics (eg, pramoxine, lidocaine, prilocaine), and anti-inflammatory agents (eg, corticosteroids, calcineurin inhibitors).**
- Systemic antipruritic agents include **antihistamines, antidepressants, neuromodulators (eg, gabapentin, pregabalin), opioid antagonists/agonists (eg, difelikefalin, naltrexone), thalidomide, and aprepitant.**
- Physical antipruritic agents include **phototherapy** and **acupuncture.**
- Psychological approaches (eg, **behavior modification therapy**) may be beneficial.

"Real World" Advice

- The spontaneous pruritus of prurigo nodules leads to an **itch-scratch cycle.**
- Beyond pharmacodynamics, application of topical antipruritic agents may help break the itch-scratch cycle by replacing the actions of picking, rubbing, or scratching.
- **Doxepin can treat both pruritus (antihistamine effect) and obsessions and compulsions (tricyclic antidepressant [TCA] effect). Start at a low dose (eg, 10 mg/d) to avoid oversedation,** especially in the elderly.
    - Doxepin is a "double-hitter."
- The clinical resemblance between prurigo nodules, keratoacanthomas, and keratoacanthoma-type SCCs presents a challenge for oncologic surveillance. This is especially problematic in elderly patients with extensive actinic damage who may be predisposed to developing these lesions concurrently. Antipruritic therapy may improve prurigo nodules, reducing the need for diagnostic procedures.

LICHEN SIMPLEX CHRONICUS
→ **Diagnosis Group 2**

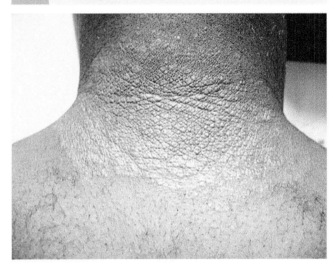

Reprinted with permission from Goodheart HP. *Goodheart's Same-Site Differential Diagnosis: A Rapid Method of Diagnosing and Treating Common Skin Disorders*. Wolters Kluwer Health/Lippincott Williams & Wilkins; 2011.

Epidemiology

- LSC is a **secondary skin disorder** associated with **pruritus.**

Clinicopathological Features

- LSC classically presents with **skin-colored to erythematous plaques with exaggerated skin lines favoring the occipital scalp, posterolateral neck, anogenital area, and extensor extremities. Hyperpigmentation** is common.
    - LSC is often said to have a "leathery" appearance. Clinical lesions are broader and thinner than prurigo nodules.
    - LSC resembles prurigo nodularis on histopathology.

Evaluation

- The differential diagnosis of LSC includes hypertrophic LE and lichen amyloidosis.
- Evaluation of LSC is similar to prurigo nodularis.

Management

- Management of LSC is similar to prurigo nodularis.

"Real World" Advice

- "Real world" advice for LSC is similar to that for prurigo nodularis.

COMPLEX REGIONAL PAIN SYNDROME

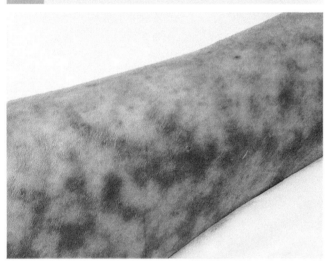

Courtesy of Douglas Pugliese, MD, MPH.

- Complex regional pain syndrome (CPRS) is a **regional dysesthesia** (Table 2.50, Figure 2.77) with **pain disproportionate to an inciting event (eg, distal radius or Colles fracture).** It is classically divided into two types based on whether damage to the peripheral nervous system is absent (CRPS type 1, formerly known as reflex sympathetic dystrophy) or present (CPRS type 2, formerly known as causalgia).
- CPRS classically presents in two phases. The **acute (warm) phase** is characterized by **inflammation** (*calor, dolor, rubor, tumor*). The **chronic (cold) phase** is characterized by **trophic changes** of the soft tissues and even bone. Clinical features include **burning pain, hyperalgesia, allodynia, vasomotor dysfunction** (eg, erythema, livedo reticularis, cyanosis, edema), **motor dysfunction, hyperhidrosis, hypertrichosis, onychodystrophy, and eventually atrophy.** CPRS favors the **upper > lower extremities.**
  - ◆ CPRS has nonspecific histopathology.
- Patients with suspected CPRS should be referred to neurology.

Table 2.50. REGIONAL DYSESTHESIAS

Diagnosis[a]	Classic Description	Notes
Sensory neuropathies	Secondary skin lesions localized to the receptive field of one or more sensory nerve branches. Trigeminal trophic syndrome (eg, after surgical trigeminal ablation by rhizotomy or alcohol injection into the Gasserian ganglion), is characterized by a crescentic ulcer on the nasal ala sparing the nasal tip due to recurrent self-inflicted trauma.	In addition to antipruritic therapy, consider MRI, orthopedic or neurology referral and treatment of the underlying cause (eg, physical therapy, nerve blocks, surgical decompression). Carbamazepine is first line for classic trigeminal neuralgia, while protective barriers at night and surgery are first line for trigeminal trophic syndrome. Patients with brachioradial pruritus may benefit from photoprotection. Notalgia paresthetica is associated with MEN type 2A.
Burning mouth syndrome	Burning mucosal pain of the anterior two-thirds of the tongue, palate, and lower lip without objective findings.	Exclude secondary causes including inflammatory disorders (eg, contact dermatitis), nutritional deficiencies, xerostomia, infections, trauma (eg, ill-fitting dentures), neoplasms (eg, SCC), systemic disorders (eg, diabetes mellitus, hypothyroidism), menopause, and psychiatric disorders (eg, depression, anxiety).
Burning scalp syndrome	Burning scalp pain without objective findings.	Exclude secondary causes including inflammatory disorders (eg, seborrheic dermatitis) and psychiatric disorders (eg, depression, anxiety).
Dysesthetic anogenital pain syndromes	Burning anogenital pain without objective findings.	Exclude secondary causes including vascular disorders (eg, hemorrhoids), infections, trauma (eg, fissures), neoplasms, and psychiatric disorders (eg, depression, anxiety).
CPRS	See above.	

CPRS, complex regional pain syndrome; MEN, multiple endocrine neoplasia; MRI, magnetic resonance imaging; SCC, squamous cell carcinoma.
[a]Illustrative examples provided.

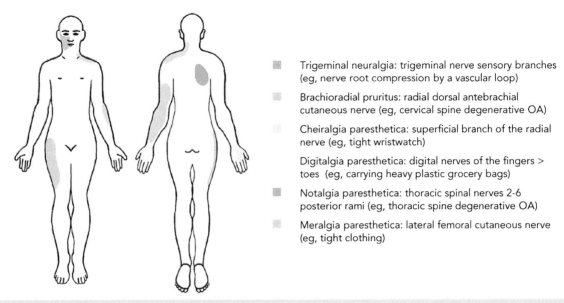

Trigeminal neuralgia: trigeminal nerve sensory branches (eg, nerve root compression by a vascular loop)

Brachioradial pruritus: radial dorsal antebrachial cutaneous nerve (eg, cervical spine degenerative OA)

Cheiralgia paresthetica: superficial branch of the radial nerve (eg, tight wristwatch)

Digitalgia paresthetica: digital nerves of the fingers > toes (eg, carrying heavy plastic grocery bags)

Notalgia paresthetica: thoracic spinal nerves 2-6 posterior rami (eg, thoracic spine degenerative OA)

Meralgia paresthetica: lateral femoral cutaneous nerve (eg, tight clothing)

Figure 2.77. DYSESTHESIA IN SENSORY NEUROPATHIES. OA, osteoarthritis.
(Illustration by Caroline A. Nelson, MD.)

SPOTLIGHT ON FAMILIAL DYSAUTONOMIA

Synonyms: hereditary sensory and autonomic neuropathy type III, Riley-Day syndrome

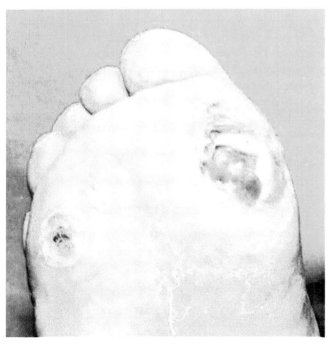

Neuropathic ulcers reprinted with permission from Pellico LH. *Focus on Adult Health: Medical-Surgical Nursing.* Wolters Kluwer Health/ Lippincott Williams & Wilkins; 2012.

- Familial dysautonomia is a hereditary sensory and autonomic neuropathy due to **AR mutation in** *IKBKAP*.
  - Familial dysautonomia causes vomiting. *IKBKAP* sounds like ipecac.
- Familial dysautonomia classically presents with **reduced sensitivity to pain and temperature, hyporeflexia,** hypotonia, ataxia, **lacrimation impairment, reduced lingual fungiform papillae,** cardiovascular instability, and gastrointestinal dysfunction. Reduced sensitivity to pain may lead to **neuropathic ulcers,** including **Riga-Fede disease.** Dysautonomic crises present with **erythematous skin rashes,** hypersalivation, hyperhidrosis, tachycardia, hypertension, **nausea, and vomiting.**
  - The most common association with **neuropathic ulcers** is **diabetes mellitus.** A neuropathic ulcer (mal perforans) is characteristically **well demarcated, located on a pressure site.** The surrounding skin may reveal a **thick callous.** Other findings include **peripheral neuropathy** with decreased sensation and foot deformities. Evaluate with nylon monofilament testing ± nerve conduction studies and electromyography.
  - Familial dysautonomia has nonspecific histopathology.
- Aspiration pneumonia is a leading cause of death.

DELUSIONS OF PARASITOSIS
Synonym: Ekbom disease

"Matchbox sign".

- Delusions of parasitosis is a primary psychiatric disorder that may be classified under **schizophrenia spectrum and other psychotic disorders** in the *Diagnostic and Statistical Manual of Mental Disorders, Fifth Edition* (DSM-5). Patients have an **encapsulated fixed false belief that the skin is infested with parasites. Morgellons disease** describes a subset of patients who **claim to observe fibers exuding from their skin.** Delusions may be shared by two or more people (*folie à deux* translates to "madness for two").
- Delusions of parasitosis classically presents with **scratch-induced skin lesions such as prurigo nodularis occurring in the setting of biting, crawling, or stinging sensations.**
  - The "matchbox sign" refers to a patient who brings in bits of skin, lint, and other samples they believe to be parasites. Remember to look before you label.

- Delusions of parasitosis have nonspecific histopathology.
- **Substance-induced formication** (sensation of ants crawling on the skin) is a diagnostic consideration.
- Antipsychotics are first line. **Psychiatry referral** is indicated; however, patients often **lack insight** and refuse.

EXCORIATION DISORDER
Synonyms: dermatillomania, neurotic excoriations, psychogenic excoriations, skin-picking disorder

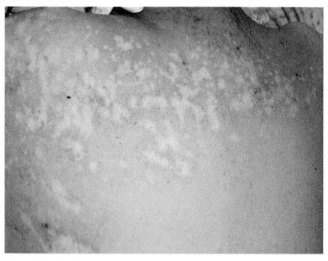

"Butterfly sign".

- Excoriation disorder is a primary psychiatric disorder that may be classified under **obsessive-compulsive and related disorders** in the DSM-5 (Table 2.51). Patients have a **conscious repetitive uncontrollable urge to pick, rub, or scratch.** Onset is typically **peripubertal** with a **3:1 female:-male ratio.**
- Excoriation disorder classically presents with **self-induced erosions, ulcerations, and/or scars.** Excoriations may be created **de novo or at preexisting skin lesions** (eg, **acne excoriée**).
  - Excoriation disorder has nonspecific histopathology.

Table 2.51. OBSESSIVE-COMPULSIVE AND RELATED PSYCHOCUTANEOUS DISORDERS

Diagnosis[a]	Classic Description	Notes
Body dysmorphic disorder[b]	Preoccupation with a nonexistent or slight defect in appearance. Commonly affected sites include the skin, nose, breasts, and genitalia.	It is important for cosmetic surgeons to be aware of body dysmorphic disorder, estimated to affect 10%-15% of dermatology patients, to avoid performing unnecessary procedures.
Body-focused repetitive behavior disorder	Repetitive behaviors include biting, chewing, licking, picking, pulling, rubbing, scratching, and sucking. Commonly affected sites include the lips, cheeks, nose, fingers, hair, and nails. Sequelae include lip licker's dermatitis, bite fibroma/*morsicatio buccarum*, and habit-tic deformity.	Excoriation disorder is called derma*tillo*mania; hair pulling is called tricho*tillo*mania; nail pulling is called onycho*tillo*mania. To remember that nail <u>biting</u> is called onycho<u>phagia</u>, think of a <u>biting phago</u>cyte.

[a]Illustrative examples provided.
[b]Body dysmorphic disorder may also include delusions that fall under schizophrenia and other psychotic disorders.

- Treatment of excoriation disorder should be directed at relieving pruritus. Alongside therapy sessions, drugs that treat obsessions and compulsions include **selective serotonin reuptake inhibitors (SSRIs) (eg, fluoxetine), serotonin -norepinephrine reuptake inhibitors (SNRIs) (eg, venlafaxine), TCAs (eg, doxepin), and N-acetylcysteine.** Patients may be receptive to **psychiatry referral.**

FACTITIAL DERMATITIS
→ Diagnosis Group 2
Synonym: dermatitis artefacta

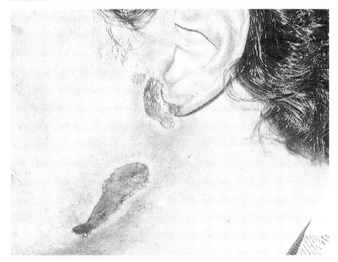

Reprinted with permission from Goodheart HP. *Goodheart's Photoguide of Common Skin Disorders: Diagnosis and Management.* 2nd ed. Lippincott Williams & Wilkins; 2003.

Epidemiology

- Factitial dermatitis is a primary psychiatric disorder that may be classified under **somatic symptom and related disorders** in the DSM-5. Patients have a **subconscious motive to self-inflict injury**, while patients with factitial disorder imposed on another (Munchausen syndrome by proxy) have a subconscious motive to inflict injury on another.
- Mechanisms of cutaneous injury include **burning (chemical, thermal, salt and ice challenge), carving with sharp instruments, and injecting foreign substances (eg, factitial panniculitis).** If asked, patients will **deny** any role in creating the skin lesions.
- Onset is typically in **adolescence and young adulthood** with an **8:1 female:male ratio.**
- Associations include **borderline personality disorder** and working or having a close family member working in health care.
- Other psychocutaneous disorders are summarized in Table 2.52.

Clinicopathological Features

- Factitial dermatitis presents with protean skin lesions including vesicles, bullae, erosions, and ulcerations. Clues to the diagnosis include **bizarre shapes with angulated edges and location within reach of the hands.**
  - Factitial dermatitis has nonspecific histopathology. A central nidus of inflammation may provide a clue to the diagnosis of factitial panniculitis. Look for evidence of a needlestick injury and vacuoles or foreign bodies.
- **Gardner-Diamond syndrome** is a factitial disorder that presents with **painful swollen ecchymoses at sites of trauma.**
  - On the Mohs scale of mineral hardness, <u>diamond</u>s are hard; therefore, trauma leads to <u>ecchymosis</u>. Gardner-<u>Diamond</u> syndrome presents with <u>ecchymoses</u>.

Evaluation

- The differential diagnosis of factitial dermatitis includes primary dermatologic disorders, other psychocutaneous disorders (eg, nonsuicidal self-injury) and **malingering,** in which patients have a **conscious motive to self-inflict cutaneous injury.**

Table 2.52. OTHER PSYCHOCUTANEOUS DISORDERS

Diagnosis[a]	Classic Description	Notes
Primary Psychiatric Disorders		
Nonsuicidal self-injury	Repetitive cutaneous injuries include burning, cutting, and stabbing. If asked, patients will admit to creating the skin lesions.	Classically associated with borderline personality disorder.
Excessive tanning behavior	Repetitive tanning despite potentially serious or fatal consequences.	Tanning can represent an addictive behavior.
Secondary Psychiatric Disorders		
Somatic symptom disorder	Somatic symptoms that cause significant distress or disrupt daily life.	Encompasses 75% of patients previously diagnosed with hypochondriasis.
Illness anxiety disorder	Preoccupation with the idea of having or acquiring a serious illness.	Encompasses 25% of patients previously diagnosis with hypochondriasis.

[a]Illustrative examples provided.

Management

- **Wound care** is first line.
- Treatment of factitial dermatitis should be directed at any underlying psychiatric disorder.

"Real World" Advice

- Confronting a patient with factitial dermatitis is controversial. It may be prudent to focus on creating a supportive doctor-patient relationship prior to addressing the psychological aspects of the disorder.

Disorders of Sebaceous, Apocrine, and Eccrine Glands

Basic Concepts

- **Gland disorders** arise from sebaceous, apocrine, and/or eccrine glands.
- Although the seborrheic pathogenesis of rosacea is no longer accepted, rosacea is included in this section along with related disorders and flushing.

ACNE VULGARIS
→ **Diagnosis Group 1**

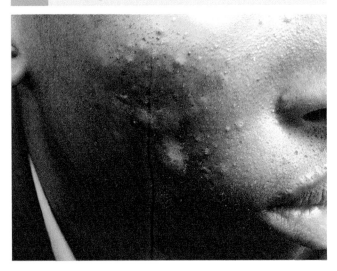

Epidemiology

- Acne vulgaris is a common inflammatory disorder with a multifactorial **pathogenesis** (Figure 2.78).
- Acne vulgaris is most common in **adolescents** but may also affect children and adults.
- Associations depend on the acne variant (see below).

Clinicopathological Features

- Noninflammatory acne vulgaris is characterized by **closed and open comedones**. Inflammatory acne is character-ized by **papules, pustules, nodules, and pseudocysts.** The distribution favors sites rich in sebaceous glands including the **face, upper chest, and back.** Acne lesions often heal with erythema and postinflammatory hypo- or hyperpig-mentation. **Atrophic and/or hypertrophic scarring** may result in lasting cosmetic disfigurement.
  - Atrophic scars are further characterized as "ice pick" (deep and narrow), "boxcar" (broad with sharply defined edges), or "rolling" (broad with sloping edges).
- **Acne variants and acneiform eruptions in adults** are sum-marized in Table 2.53.
  - **Acne variants and acneiform eruptions in children** are summarized in Table 2.54.
  - Figure 2.79.

Evaluation

- The differential diagnosis of acne includes rosacea and related disorders and gram-negative (GN) folliculitis. The follicular disorder **trichostasis spinulosa** is often clinically mistaken for open comedones; however, hair follicles con-tain keratin and **vellus hair shafts. Trichodysplasia spinu-losa** is an infection due to **trichodysplasia spinulosa–asso-ciated polyomavirus** that occurs in solid organ transplant recipients on immunosuppressive therapy and leukemia/lymphoma patients on chemotherapy. **Follicular hyperker-atotic spicules** on the face may alternatively occur in asso-ciation with **multiple myeloma.**
  - Do NOT confuse trichostasis spinulosa with tricho-dysplasia spinulosa.
- Routine microbiologic testing is not recommended except in cases suspicious for GN folliculitis.
- Women with hormonal acne and **irregular menses** or other signs of hyperandrogenism should undergo further evalua-tion. Initial laboratory studies are **dehydroepiandrosterone sulfate (DHEA-S), 17-hydroxyprogesterone (17-OHP), and total and free testosterone.** TSH, follicle-stimulating hormone (FSH), luteinizing hormone (LH), prolactin, and pelvic US may be considered. These studies should not be performed while the patient is taking an OCP.
  - **Elevated DHEA-S or 17-OHP** indicates **adrenal** hyperandrogenism.
  - **Elevated testosterone (100-200 ng/dL)** indicates **ovar-ian** hyperandrogenism. The most common etiology is **polycystic ovarian syndrome (PCOS),** further charac-terized by **LH:FSH > 2 to 3.** The diagnosis of PCOS is based on two or more **Rotterdam criteria: (1) oligo- or anovulatory cycles, (2) clinical or biochemical signs of hyperandrogenism, and (3) US evidence of polycystic ovaries.** PCOS is associated with **insulin resistance and obesity.**
  - **Elevated testosterone (>200 ng/dL) ± signs of viriliza-tion** (eg, amenorrhea, clitoromegaly, coarsening of the voice, increased muscle mass, male pattern alopecia, sud-den onset/rapid progression of hirsutism) may indicate an **adrenal or ovarian tumor, ovarian hyperthecosis, or HAIR-AN syndrome.**

1 Increased infundibular keratinization with obstruction of the pilosebaceous unit (microcomedo) may lead to:

- Infundibular dilation with keratin and sebum (closed comedone)
- Widening of the follicular orifice with sebum oxidation (open comedone)
- Follicular rupture with suppurative and granulomatous inflammation (superficial pustule or deep nodule)

2 Androgens*, especially DHT, act on the pilosebaceous unit to:

- Increase sebocyte proliferation/differentiation
- Increase lipid synthesis

3 Proliferation of *Cutibacterium acnes* in the pilosebaceous unit:

- Upregulates pro-inflammatory cytokines (eg, IL-1β, IL-17) via activation of TLR2 and the NLRP3 inflammasome
- Stimulates expression of antimicrobial peptides (eg, human β-defensins, cathelicidin)
- Converts triglycerides into FFAs^ via the activity of lipases, thereby increasing infundibular keratinization

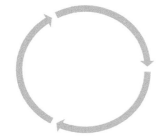

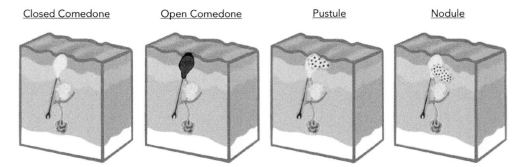

Closed Comedone   Open Comedone   Pustule   Nodule

Figure 2.78. PATHOGENESIS OF ACNE VULGARIS. * Other hormones implicated in the pathogenesis of acne include CRH, α-MSH, and HGH/IGF-1. ^ The sebum of individuals with acne has higher levels of pro-inflammatory lipids (eg, squalene MUFAs) and lower levels of linoleic acid. CRH, corticotropin-releasing hormone; DHT, dihydrotestosterone; FFAs, free fatty acids; HGH, human growth hormone; IGF-1, insulin-like growth factor 1; IL, interleukin; MSH, melanocyte-stimulating hormone; MUFAs, monounsaturated fatty acids; NLRP3, nucleotide-binding domain leucine-rich repeat-containing receptor 3; TLR, toll-like receptor.
(Illustration by Caroline A. Nelson, MD.)

Table 2.53. ACNE VARIANTS AND ACNEIFORM ERUPTIONS IN ADULTS

Acne Variant or Acneiform Eruption[a]	Classic Description	Notes
Acne Variants		
Acne conglobata	Severe inflammatory acne.	Associations include the follicular occlusion tetrad (acne conglobata, dissecting cellulitis of the scalp, HS, pilonidal sinus), syndromic PG, and IBD.
Acne excoriée	Acne vulgaris ritualistically excoriated into crusted erosions that heal with scarring.	Acne excoriée is under the umbrella of excoriation disorder. It occurs most often in young women (*acne excoriée des jeunes filles*).
Acne fulminans	Severe inflammatory acne with systemic manifestations (eg, fever). Osteolytic bone lesions favor the clavicle and sternum.	Associations include SAPHO syndrome.

(Continued)

Table 2.53. ACNE VARIANTS AND ACNEIFORM ERUPTIONS IN ADULTS (CONTINUED)

Acne Variant or Acneiform Eruption[a]	Classic Description	Notes
Hormonal acne (postadolescent acne in women)	Noninflammatory and inflammatory acne favoring the jawline. Premenstrual flares are common.	Hormonal acne is either caused by increased end-organ sensitivity to androgens or hyperandrogenemia: • Constitutional (normal or slightly elevated testosterone): familial; adrenal, ovarian, or hyperprolactinemic SAHA syndrome.[b] • Pituitary: Cushing disease, prolactinoma. • Adrenal (DHEA-S, 17-OHP): CAH (eg, 21-hydroxylase deficiency, 11-hydroxylase deficiency), Cushing syndrome (eg, primary nodular hyperplasia, adrenal adenoma, adrenal carcinoma). • Ovarian (Δ^4-androstenedione, testosterone[c]): PCOS, hyperthecosis, tumor (eg, arrhenoblastoma), late pregnancy. • Ectopic hormone production: ACTH (eg, small-cell lung cancer), HCG (eg, choriocarcinoma).

Acneiform Eruptions

Acne mechanica	Comedones.	Associated with recurrent mechanical obstruction of the pilosebaceous unit (eg, helmet/chin strap, mask, violin).
		During the COVID-19 pandemic, the term "mascne" was popularized to refer to acne mechanica occurring in the "O-zone" under a face mask.
Occupational acne, acne cosmetica, pomade acne	Comedones.	Associated with exposure to follicle-occluding substances: coal tar derivatives, chlorinated aromatic hydrocarbons, cutting oils, and petroleum; cosmetics; hair products.
Chloracne	Comedo-like papules and cysts favoring the malar cheeks, retroauricular region, axillae, and scrotum.	Associated with exposure to halogenated aromatic hydrocarbons (eg, 2,3,7,8-TCDD, a contaminant created in the herbicide Agent Orange used during the Vietnam War).
Tropical acne	Nodules and cysts favoring the trunk and buttocks.	Associated with exposure to extreme heat.
Drug-induced acne	Monomorphous eruption of papules and pustules (no comedones).	Drug associations include corticosteroids, androgens, INH, lithium, and phenytoin. Halogenoderma (eg, iododerma due to SSKI or iodinated radiocontrast media) may induce an acneiform eruption. Targeted antineoplastics (eg, EGFR inhibitors, MEK 1/2 inhibitors, mTOR inhibitors) may induce a papulopustular eruption.
Radiation acne	Comedo-like papules.	Associated with radiation therapy.

ACTH, adrenocorticotropic hormone; CAH, congenital adrenal hyperplasia; COVID-19, coronavirus disease of 2019; DHEA-S, dehydroepiandrosterone sulfate; DHT, dihydrotestosterone; EGFR, epidermal growth factor receptor; HAIR-AN, hyperandrogenemia, insulin resistance, and acanthosis nigricans; HCG, human chorionic gonadotropin; HS, hidradenitis suppurativa; IBD, inflammatory bowel disease; INH, isoniazid; MEK, mitogen-activated protein kinase; mTOR, mammalian target of rapamycin; 17-OHP, 17-hydroxyprogesterone; PCOS, polycystic ovary syndrome; PG, pyoderma gangrenosum; SAHA, seborrhea, acne, hirsutism, and androgenetic alopecia; SAPHO, synovitis, acne, pustulosis, hyperostosis, and osteitis; SSKI, saturated solution of potassium iodide; TCDD, tetrachlorodibenzo-P-dioxin.

[a]Illustrative examples provided.
[b]Ovarian SAHA syndrome may overlap with HAIR-AN syndrome.
[c]5α-reductase type 2 converts testosterone to its more potent metabolite DHT.

Table 2.54. ACNE VARIANTS AND ACNEIFORM ERUPTIONS IN CHILDREN

Acne Variant or Acneiform Eruption[a]	Classic Description	Notes
Acne Variants		
Neonatal acne (neonatal cephalic pustulosis)	Small papulopustules (not comedones) favoring the face > neck and upper trunk.	Presents in 20% of newborns between 2 weeks and 3 months of age possibly due to an inflammatory response to *Malassezia* species. Reassurance ± topical imidazole is first line.
Infantile acne	Acne vulgaris.	Presents between 2 and 12 months of age due to transient androgen production from the fetal adrenal gland. Topical retinoids and benzoyl peroxide are first line.
Midchildhood acne	Acne vulgaris.	Presents between 1 and 7 years of age due to aberrant androgen production (eg, hyperandrogenism, precocious puberty, XYY karyotype). In case of accelerated growth, obtain a hand/wrist x-ray to evaluate bone age ± endocrinology evaluation. Topical retinoids and benzoyl peroxide are first line.
Preadolescent acne	Comedones favoring the forehead and central face. Preadolescent acne favors the "T-zone."	Presents between 7 and 11 years of age due to adrenarche. Treatment is similar to acne vulgaris.
Apert syndrome	Severe inflammatory acne.	Early onset due to AD mutation in *FGFR2*. Nevus comedonicus may represent mosaic Apert syndrome.
Acneiform Eruptions		
Pseudoacne of the nasal crease	Comedones and milia along the transverse nasal crease.	Presents prior to onset of puberty. Mechanical expression or topical retinoids and benzoyl peroxide are first line.
Childhood flexural comedones	Discrete, double-orifice comedones favoring axillae > groin.	No association with acne vulgaris or HS.

AD, autosomal dominant; FGFR2, fibroblast growth factor receptor 2; HS, hidradenitis suppurativa.
[a]Illustrative examples provided.

Management

- The **AAD guidelines for the management of acne vulgaris** include the following first-line treatment algorithm based on severity:
  - **Mild: benzoyl peroxide OR topical retinoid OR topical combination therapy** (benzoyl peroxide with antibiotic and/or retinoid).
  - **Moderate: topical combination therapy OR topical combination therapy and oral antibiotic.**
  - **Severe: topical combination therapy and oral antibiotic OR oral isotretinoin.**
  Topical antibiotics include **clindamycin, erythromycin, and minocycline.** Oral antibiotics include **tetracyclines (doxycycline, minocycline) and macrolides (azithromycin, erythromycin).**
    Macrolides are preferred over tetracyclines in children <8 years of age.
- Other medical treatments for acne include topical **azelaic acid** (may reduce postinflammatory hyperpigmentation, **preferred in pregnancy**), topical **dapsone** (helpful for inflammatory acne), topical sulfacetamide or sulfur and sulfacetamide (limited evidence), **exfoliant cleansers**, topical cosmeceuticals (eg, **α-hydroxy acids, β-hydroxy acids**), and **ILK** (individual acne nodules).
- There is limited evidence to recommend the use of physical treatments for acne (eg, chemical peels, blue or red light, PDL). Treatments for **acne scarring** include the **trichloroacetic acid chemical reconstruction of skin scars (TCA-CROSS) technique, long-pulsed Nd:YAG laser, and soft-tissue dermal fillers (eg, Bellafill).**
- **Combined OCPs** and **antiandrogens** such as topical clascoterone and **spironolactone** are efficacious for the treatment of **hormonal acne** in women. Combined OCPs containing **progestins with greater intrinsic antiandrogen activity (eg, drospirenone)** may have greater efficacy. Low-dose oral corticosteroids are recommended in patients with adrenal hyperandrogenism.

"Real World" Advice

- It is important to recognize the **negative impact of acne on quality of life and psychosocial well-being.**
- The contribution of diet to the pathogenesis of acne remains controversial. The most compelling data exist for **skim**

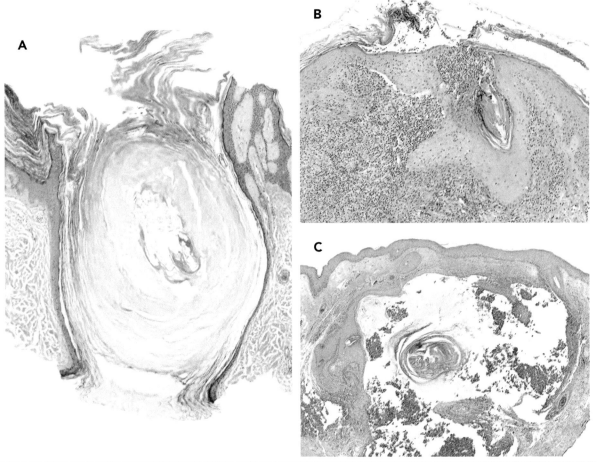

Figure 2.79. CLINICOPATHOLOGICAL CORRELATION: ACNE VULGARIS. The histopathology of acne vulgaris correlates with the clinical lesion. A, Open comedone. B, Pustule. C, Nodule.

(Histology images reprinted with permission from Elder DE, Elenitsas R, Rosenbach M, et al. *Lever's Histopathology of the Skin.* 11th ed. Wolters Kluwer; 2015.)

- **Comedone**: infundibular dilation with keratin and sebum ± widened follicular orifice.
- **Pustule**: superficial follicular rupture with suppurative and granulomatous inflammation.
- **Nodule**: deep follicular rupture with suppurative and granulomatous inflammation.

milk, whey protein, high glycemic-load diet, and vitamin B$_{12}$ supplementation.

- **No antibiotic resistance has been reported to benzoyl peroxide. To minimize antibiotic resistance:**
  - **Combine topical benzoyl peroxide with topical or oral antibiotics.**
  - **Limit oral antibiotics to the shortest possible duration (~3-4 months).**
  - Consider pulse dosing or submicrobial dosing.
- Discussion of the risks and benefits of isotretinoin should address the risks of IBD and psychiatric effects including suicidal ideation (SI); however, it is important to note that:
  - Inflammatory acne is associated with IBD; therefore, isotretinoin may be a confounding variable.
  - Data suggest that the incidence of depression and SI on isotretinoin may be no greater than the background incidence. Moreover, isotretinoin may attenuate the psychiatric burden of acne.
- **Acne fulminans** requires **systemic corticosteroids** prior to or concurrent with the initiation of **low-dose isotretinoin** to decrease risk of severe scarring.

HIDRADENITIS SUPPURATIVA
→ **Diagnosis Group 2**
Synonym: acne inversa

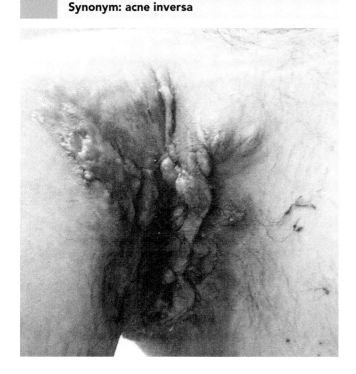

Epidemiology

- Hidradenitis suppurativa (HS) is an inflammatory disorder within the **follicular occlusion tetrad.** Similar to acne, the inciting event is **obstruction of the pilosebaceous unit.** Follicular rupture with release of keratin, sebum, and bacteria triggers subsequent **apocrine gland inflammation.**
- The most common demographic affected by HS is **young African American women.**
- Associations include **syndromic PG, obesity, and smoking.**

Clinicopathological Features

- HS classically presents with **boggy, fluctuant, interconnected nodules with purulent drainage favoring the axillae, inframammary area, and anogenital area.** HS may heal with **hypertrophic scarring** and is associated with an increased risk of SCC.
  - HS is characterized by perifollicular lymphocytic (early) to neutrophilic (late) inflammation extending from the dermis to the subcutaneous fat. Vascular proliferation, sinus tract formation, and fibrosis may occur.
  - Inflammation in HS "spills over" to involve apocrine glands.

Evaluation

- The differential diagnosis of HS includes staphylococcal furunculosis and cutaneous Crohn disease.

Management

- All patients with HS should be counseled regarding antiseptic soaps and avoidance of friction and moisture. If applicable, **weight loss and smoking cessation** should be encouraged.
- The **HS therapeutic ladder** (Table 2.55) may be categorized according to the **Hurley staging system.**

"Real World" Advice

- It is important to recognize the **negative impact of HS on quality of life and psychosocial well-being.**
- The **double-headed pseudocomedone** is a helpful clue to the presence of a sinus tract in HS.

Table 2.55. HIDRADENITIS SUPPURATIVA THERAPEUTIC LADDER

Hurley Stage[a]	Classic Description	Therapies
I	Single or multiple abscesses.	Topical: clindamycin, mupirocin (*Staphylococcus aureus* decolonization). Intralesional: corticosteroids. Oral: antibiotics, antiandrogens.
II	Single or multiple, widely separated, recurrent abscesses with sinus tracts and scarring.	Hurley stage I plus: Oral: acitretin, cyclosporine. SC: adalimumab.[b] IV: infliximab. Physical: local excision, CO_2 laser, Nd:YAG laser.
III	Diffuse or near-diffuse abscesses with multiple interconnected sinus tracts and scarring.	Hurley stage I and II plus: Physical: wide local excision.

CO_2, carbon dioxide; IL, interleukin; IV, intravenous; Nd:YAG, neodymium-doped yttrium aluminum garnet; SC, subcutaneous.
[a]Illustrative examples provided.
[b]IL-17 inhibitors and IL-12/23 inhibitors are under investigation.

ROSACEA
→ Diagnosis Group 1

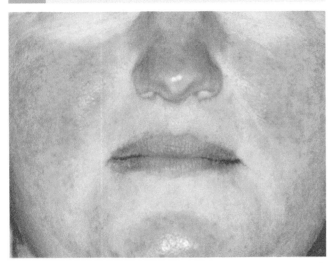

Erythematotelangiectatic rosacea reprinted with permission from Craft N, Fox LP, Goldsmith LA, et al. *VisualDx: Essential Adult Dermatology.* Wolters Kluwer Health/Lippincott Williams & Wilkins; 2010.

Epidemiology

- Rosacea is a common chronic facial dermatosis. The pathogenesis is incompletely understood; however, it appears to involve a complex interplay of genetic factors, environmental factors (eg, **alcohol, heat**), microbes (eg, *Demodex folliculorum* **mites**), skin barrier dysfunction, and **UVR** that result in neurovascular dysregulation and aberrant innate immunity (eg, **cathelicidin upregulation**).
- Rosacea most commonly occurs during middle age in individuals with skin phototypes I and II.

Clinicopathological Features

- Rosacea is divided into four subtypes:
  - **Erythematotelangiectatic rosacea (ETTR), type 1:** flushing on a background of persistent facial erythema ± telangiectasias.
  - **Papulopustular rosacea (PPR), type 2:** centrofacial eruption of erythematous papules and pustules that heal without scarring.
  - **Phymatous rosacea, type 3:** sebaceous gland hyperplasia and fibrosis initially manifesting with patulous follicles (dilated pores) and favoring the nose (rhinophyma).
  - **Ocular rosacea, type 4:** constellation of findings culminating in a **"red eye,"** most commonly a dry gritty sensation, blepharitis, conjunctivitis, chalazia, and hordeola.
- **Rosacea variants and related disorders** are summarized in Table 2.56.

  Idiopathic facial aseptic granuloma (IFAG) is characterized by a **solitary erythematous nodule on the cheek of a child** that **self-resolves** within months.
  - Figure 2.80.

Table 2.56. ROSACIA VARIANTS AND RELATED DISORDERS

Rosacea variant or related Disorder[a]	Classic Description	Notes
Rosacea Variants		
Granulomatous rosacea	Centrofacial skin-colored to red-brown papules that heal with scarring.	Some consider IFAG and LMDF to be variants of granulomatous rosacea.
Rosacea conglobata	Eruption of inflammatory cystic lesions that heal with scarring.	
Rosacea fulminans (pyoderma faciale)	Eruption of inflammatory papules and pustules that heal with scarring.	Most common in young women. Associated with pregnancy.
Related Disorders		
Haber syndrome	See Chapter 2: Pigmentary Disorders.	
Morbihan disease (solid facial edema)	Progressive persistent nonpitting centrofacial edema.	Often misdiagnosed as cellulitis.
Perioral dermatitis	See below.	
Pityriasis folliculorum	Roughened whitish scaling skin surface overlying erythema with papules/pustules not limited to the central face.	Most common in women who use facial creams in lieu of washing with water. KOH preparation reveals *Demodex folliculorum* mites.
Steroid-induced rosacea	Facial erythema and papules/pustules ± atrophy.	Associated with mid- to high-potency topical and systemic corticosteroids. KOH preparation reveals *D. folliculorum* mites.

IFAG, idiopathic facial aseptic granuloma; KOH, potassium hydroxide; LMDF, lupus miliaris disseminatus faciei.
[a]Illustrative examples provided.

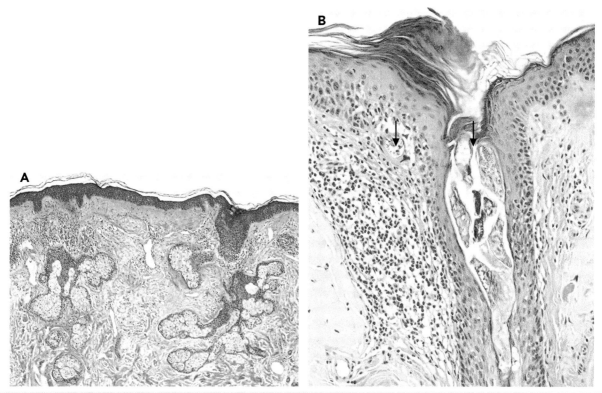

Figure 2.80. CLINICOPATHOLOGICAL CORRELATION: ROSACEA. Characteristic features are vascular dilation of upper and mid-dermal vessels with dermal edema and perivascular and perifollicular lymphohistiocytic inflammation. A, Perivascular and perifollicular lymphocytic inflammation with telangiectasias and solar elastosis. B, Demodicidosis with perifollicular lymphohistiocytic inflammation. Solid arrows: *Demodex folliculorum* mites. IFAG, idiopathic facial aseptic granuloma; PPR, papulopustular rosacea.

(Histology images reprinted with permission from Elder DE, Elenitsas R, Rosenbach M, et al. *Lever's Histopathology of the Skin.* 11th ed. Wolters Kluwer; 2015.)

- **PPR subtype**: suppurative inflammation.
- **Phymatous subtype**: dilated hair follicles, sebaceous gland hyperplasia.
- **Granulomatous variant/IFAG**: noncaseating granulomas.

The role of *Demodex folliculorum* mites in the pathogenesis of <u>rosacea</u> is a "<u>red-hot</u>" debate.

Evaluation

- The differential diagnosis of rosacea, in addition to the related disorders above, depends on the subtype:
  - ○ ETTR: physiologic or secondary flushing, seborrheic dermatitis, SLE, actinic damage.
  - ○ PPR: acne, follicular mucinosis, demodicosis/candida/ tinea incognito.
  - ○ Phymatous rosacea: discoid lupus erythematosus (DLE), lupus pernio, lupus vulgaris, neoplasms (eg, angiosarcoma).
  - ○ Ocular rosacea: drug-induced ocular rosacea, seborrheic dermatitis.
- Common triggers of physiologic flushing include **emotion, exercise, and heat.** Associations with **secondary flushing** include **menopause,** systemic diseases (eg, **diabetes mellitus [rubeosis], thyrotoxicosis, carcinoid syndrome, mastocytosis, pheochromocytoma**), **alcohol, spoiled scombroid fish,** food additives (eg, nitrites, sulfites, spicy foods), and neurologic disorders (eg, anxiety). **Alcohol-induced flushing** is exacerbated in the setting of

alcohol dehydrogenase deficiency (prevalent in **Asian** populations). Drug associations include the **disulfiram reaction (eg, metronidazole)** and vasoactive agents (eg, **L-asparaginase**).

    Malar flush is a cutaneous feature of homocystinuria. "Wet flush" (sweating) indicates vasodilation mediated by the autonomic nervous system. "Dry flush" indicates direct vasodilation mediated by vasoactive agents.

- The evaluation of sudden, severe, or symptomatic flushing may include:
  - ○ Blood: CBC, thyroid function tests (TFTs), estrogen/FSH/ LH, **tryptase**/chromogranin A/free metanephrines.
  - ○ Urine: **5-hydroxyindole acetic acid (5-HIAA), fractionated metanephrines,** methylimidazole acetic acid.
  - ○ Imaging: CT or MRI abdomen/pelvis, octreotide/somatostatin receptor scintigraphy.
- Bedside diagnostics to detect *D. folliculorum* mites include potassium hydroxide (KOH), mineral oil preparation, and Tzanck smear.

Management

- All patients with rosacea should be counseled regarding the avoidance of sun, irritants, and common triggers of flushing, as well as the utility of **green undercover foundation** to camouflage redness.
  - Remember that green is opposite red on the color wheel.
- Based on subtype, additional treatment options for rosacea include:
  - ETTR: α-adrenergic agonists **brimonidine and oxymetazoline, PDL.**
  - PPR: topical antimicrobials (eg, **azelaic acid, ivermectin, metronidazole, sulfur, and sulfacetamide**), oral antibiotics (eg, **doxycycline**), and oral retinoids (eg, isotretinoin). A meta-analysis showed a **higher efficacy and psychological benefit for topical ivermectin** as compared to azelaic acid, metronidazole, and placebo.
  - Phymatous rosacea: oral retinoids (eg, isotretinoin), physical treatments (eg, **carbon dioxide [CO_2] laser**).
  - Ocular rosacea: eyelid hygiene and artificial tears, topical cyclosporine, **doxycycline.**
- Treatment options for flushing include nonselective β-blockers (eg, propranolol) and clonidine. For **menopausal flushing**, consider **clonidine**, hormone replacement therapy, and/or SSRIs. Transthoracic endoscopic sympathectomy is a treatment of last resort.

"Real World" Advice

- While a skin biopsy is rarely indicated for the diagnosis of rosacea, it should be considered in refractory cases to exclude **angiosarcoma**, which is known as one of the **"great mimickers."**
- **Rebound redness** is an important limitation of **α-adrenergic agonists** for the treatment of ETTR.
- **Rosacea conglobata and rosacea fulminans** require **systemic corticosteroids** prior to or concurrent with the initiation of **low-dose isotretinoin** to decrease risk of severe scarring.

PERIORIFICIAL DERMATITIS
→ Diagnosis Group 1
Synonym: perioral dermatitis

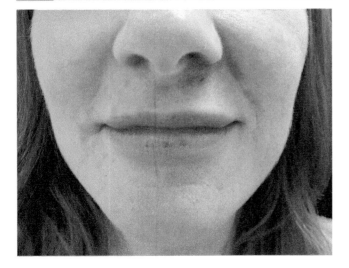

Epidemiology

- Periorificial dermatitis is a common facial dermatosis.
- Associations include **atopy.**
- Drugs associations include **topical, intranasal, and inhaled corticosteroids.**

Clinicopathological Features

- Periorificial dermatitis classically presents with **periocular, perinasal, and/or perioral monomorphous superficial pinpoint papules and pustules.**
  - Given the potential for perinasal and periocular involvement, the term "periorificial dermatitis" is preferred over "perioral dermatitis."
- Intolerance of sunlight and hot water are common symptoms.
  - Perioral dermatitis resembles rosacea but lacks vascular dilatation and dermal edema. The granulomatous variant demonstrates noncaseating granulomas.

Evaluation

- The differential diagnosis of periorificial dermatitis is similar to PPR.

Management

- Topical antimicrobial treatment options similar to PPR are first line.
- A 4- to 8-week course of oral antibiotic (eg, **doxycycline**) is second line.

"Real World" Advice

- Asthma is a "double hit" leading to periorificial dermatitis: (1) association with atopy and (2) association with inhaled corticosteroids. **Switching from a mask to a spacer** can help avoid inhaled corticosteroid contact with the skin.
- If corticosteroids are implicated in periorificial dermatitis, a gradual taper in strength and frequency is preferred over abrupt discontinuation to mitigate the risk of rebound flare.
- Periorificial dermatitis is differentiated from PPR by its monomorphous morphology and periorificial rather than centrofacial distribution. **Clearing around the vermillion border of the lips** may be a helpful clue.

LUPUS MILIARIS DISSEMINATUS FACIEI

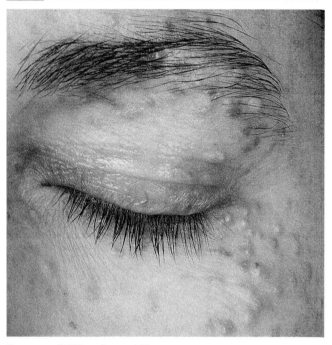

Courtesy of William James, MD.

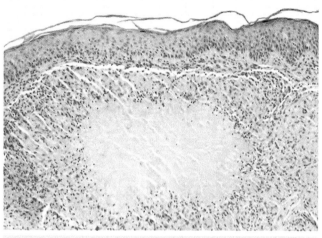

Figure 2.81. CLINICOPATHOLOGICAL CORRELATION: LUPUS MILIARIS DISSEMINATUS FACIEI. LMDF is characterized by tuberculoid granulomas: histiocytes with a peripheral lymphocytic infiltrate and central caseous necrosis. AFB, acid-fast bacilli; LMDF, lupus miliaris disseminatus faciei; TB, tuberculosis.

(Histology image reprinted with permission from Elder DE, Elenitsas R, Rosenbach M, et al. *Lever's Histopathology of the Skin.* 11th ed. Wolters Kluwer; 2015.)

Lupus <u>miliaris</u> disseminatus faciei and <u>miliary</u> TB are so named because the tiny tubercles are the size of "<u>millet</u> grains" (the main ingredient in bird seed). Absence of AFB distinguishes LMDF from miliary TB.

- LMDF is a rare, self-resolving granulomatous disorder. Some consider LMDF to be a variant of granulomatous rosacea.
  - Do NOT confuse <u>lupus</u> miliaris disseminatus faciei with <u>lupus</u> erythematosus, <u>lupus</u> pernio, or <u>lupus</u> vulgaris.
- LMDF classically presents with **symmetrical, monomorphic, reddish-brown papules on the face clustering around the forehead, eyelids, mouth, and cheeks** that heal with **scarring.**
  - Figure 2.81.
- Upon **diascopy**, LMDF lesions have the color of **apple jelly.**
- Topical calcineurin inhibitors are first line. Systemic corticosteroids may be required for extensive LMDF.

HYPERHIDROSIS

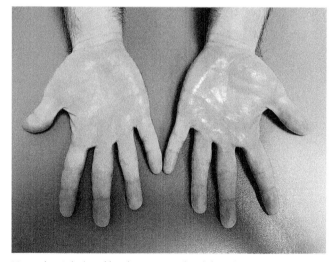

Note: the right hand has been treated with botulinum neurotoxin.
Courtesy of Juliana Choi, MD, PhD.

- Hyperhidrosis is defined as **excessive sweating.** 60% to 80% of patients with **primary focal hyperhidrosis** have a positive family history. The cause of **secondary hyperhidrosis** may be an underlying condition or a drug (eg, acetylcholine). **Frey syndrome** is a rare cause of **gustatory hyperhidrosis** after trauma to the **ipsilateral auriculotemporal branch of the trigeminal nerve (V3)** with haphazard nerve regeneration. It classically occurs after **parotid surgery.**
  - **Frey syndrome** may occur in neonates due to **forceps** assistance during delivery.
  - Granulosis rubra nasi is an AD genetic disorder leading to hyperhidrosis of the nose during the first decade of life that typically resolves by puberty.
- Primary focal hyperhidrosis is most often localized to the **axillae, palms, and/or soles.** Secondary hyperhidrosis may be localized or generalized.
  - Hyperhidrosis has nonspecific histopathology.
- Other sweat gland disorders include:
  - **Bromhidrosis**: defined as **exaggeration of body odor. Apocrine** bromhidrosis is caused by bacterial degradation of apocrine sweat. **Eccrine** bromhidrosis is caused by maceration of the *stratum corneum* and bacterial degradation of keratin but may be metabolic (eg, the **musty odor of phenylketonuria**) or exogenous (eg, **garlic**).
    - The smell of garlic wards off vampires and humans.
  - **Chromhidrosis**: defined as **colored sweating. Apocrine** chromhidrosis is caused by intrinsic excretion of **lipofuscin. Eccrine** chromhidrosis is caused by exogenous chemicals that color the sweat (eg, **red sweating induced by clofazimine or rifampin**).
  - **Hypohidrosis/anhidrosis**: defined as **decreased/absent sweating.** The cause may be central/neuropathic (eg, leprosy), peripheral (eg, hypohidrotic ectodermal dysplasia), or a drug (eg, glycopyrrolate).
- **Topical aluminum chloride and topical glycopyrronium** are first line. Other treatment options for hyperhidrosis include biofeedback therapy, iontophoresis, botulinum neurotoxin (BoNT), oral drugs (eg, glycopyrrolate), and surgery. The **starch-iodine technique** is a colorimetric technique to localize the most active sweat glands in order to **guide BoNT injections.** After application of iodine solution brushed with starch powder, sites with sweating turn blue-black.

SPOTLIGHT ON ECTODERMAL DYSPLASIAS

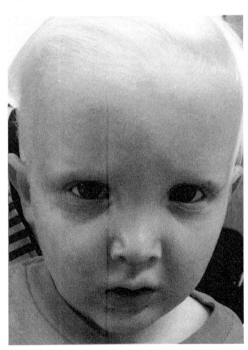

Hypohidrotic ectodermal dysplasia reprinted with permission from Gru AA, Wick MR, Mir A, et al. *Pediatric Dermatopathology and Dermatology.* Wolters Kluwer; 2018.

- Ectodermal dysplasias demonstrate **abnormalities in ≥2 of the major ectodermally derived structures: sweat glands, hair, nails, and teeth.** Abnormalities may also occur in sebaceous and mucous glands, as well as nonectodermally derived structures.
- Over 180 **ectodermal dysplasias** have been described; the most classic are summarized in Table 2.57.
  - Ectodermal dysplasias demonstrate variable hypoplasia of adnexal structures.
- **Hyperthermia** in hypohidrotic ectodermal dysplasia may be life threatening. Current management focuses on controlling ambient temperatures and external cooling; however, protein therapy (in utero or postnatal administration of recombinant ectodysplasin A (EDA) protein) is on the horizon.

Table 2.57. ECTODERMAL DYSPLASIAS

Diagnosis[a]	Inheritance Pattern	Gene(s)	Classic Description	Notes
Hypohidrotic ectodermal dysplasia (anhidrotic ectodermal dysplasia, Christ-Siemens-Touraine syndrome)	XLR AD, AR	*EDA* encoding EDA *EDAR* encoding EDAR, *EDARADD* encoding EDAR-associated death domain	Hypohidrosis/anhidrosis with heat intolerance, hypotrichosis, and tooth hypoplasia (eg, absent or peg shaped). Other features include collodion-like membrane, periorbital hyperpigmentation and wrinkling, and altered facial appearance (saddle nose, full everted lips, frontal bossing).	Normal nails. Hypohidrotic ectodermal dysplasia has a variable phenotype in females due to lyonization.
Hypohidrotic ectodermal dysplasia with immune deficiency	XLR	*NEMO* encoding NF-κB essential modulator	Mild hypohidrotic ectodermal dysplasia (hypodontia, conical teeth, reduced sweating) with a poor antibody response to polysaccharide antigens, elevated IgM/IgA but decreased IgG levels, and defective NK cell activity. Patients with the AD form also have a severe T-cell deficiency.	Female carriers may have mild IP.
	AD	*NFKBIA* encoding NF-κB inhibitor α-component		
Hidrotic ectodermal dysplasia (Clouston syndrome)	AD	*GJB6* encoding connexin 30	Hypotrichosis and nail hypoplasia. Other features include diffuse transgradient PPK with pseudoainhum and multiple syringofibroadenomas.	Normal sweat glands and teeth.
Schöpf-Schulz-Passarge syndrome	AR	*WNT10A* encoding WNT10A	Hypotrichosis, nail hypoplasia, and tooth hypoplasia. Other features include PPK and neoplasms (eg, BCCs, syringofibroadenomas, periocular/eyelid hidrocystomas).	Sweat gland involvement is variable.
Witkop tooth and nail syndrome (hypodontia with nail dysgenesis, tooth and nail syndrome, Witkop syndrome)	AD	*MSX1* encoding MSX1	Nail hypoplasia and tooth hypoplasia.	Normal sweat glands ± hair.
Ankyloblepharon–ectodermal defects–cleft lip/palate syndrome (Hay-Wells syndrome, Rapp-Hodgkin syndrome)	AD	*TP63* encoding P63	Hypohidrosis/anhidrosis with heat intolerance, hypotrichosis, nail hypoplasia, and tooth hypoplasia. The characteristic hair shaft abnormality with increased fragility is pili torti. The characteristic hair shaft abnormality without increased fragility is pili trianguli et canaliculi. Shared features include cleft lip/palate, conductive hearing loss, and genitourinary features. Erythroderma/chronic erosive scalp dermatitis and ankyloblepharon adnatum filiforme are distinguishing features. The eyelids are bound together, while the lip/palate cleft apart.	Mutation in the sterile α motif domain of *TP63*.
Ectodermal dysplasia–ectrodactyly–clefting syndrome (split hand–split foot–ectodermal dysplasia–clefting syndrome)			Hypotrichosis, nail hypoplasia, and tooth hypoplasia. Shared features include cleft lip/palate, conductive hearing loss, and genitourinary features. Ectrodactyly is a distinguishing feature. Ectrodactyly (split-hand/foot) resembles a "lobster claw."	Mutation in the DNA-binding domain of *TP63*. Normal sweat glands.

AD, atopic dermatitis or autosomal dominant; AR, autosomal recessive; BCCs, basal cell carcinomas; DNA, deoxyribonucleic acid; EDA, ectodysplasin A; EDAR, ectodysplasin A receptor; MSX1, muscle segment homeobox 1; PPK, palmoplantar keratoderma; WNT10A, Wnt family member 10A; XLR, X-linked recessive.
[a]Illustrative examples provided.

MILIARIA

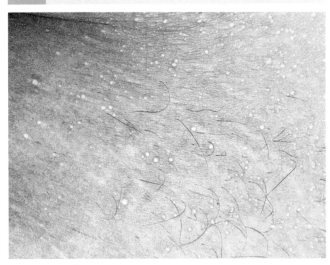

Miliaria crystallina.

- Miliaria refers to **obstruction of the eccrine duct.** It commonly affects individuals in **hot humid climates.**
  > **Miliaria** is frequent in **neonates** (whose eccrine ducts are not fully developed) and may rarely become infected, leading to multiple sweat gland abscesses.
- Miliaria classically favors **sites of occlusion and excessive sweating.** Lesion morphology depends on the depth of eccrine ductal occlusion:
  - **Miliaria crystallina** (miliaria sudamina), superficial: **clear vesicles.**
    - The vesicles of miliaria <u>crystal</u>lina are "<u>crystal</u> clear."
  - **Miliaria rubra (prickly heat),** intermediate: **erythematous papules and pustules.**
  - **Miliaria profunda** (miliaria mammillaria), deep: **white papules.**
    > In **infants,** miliaria is in the differential diagnosis for **diaper dermatitis.**
    - Miliaria is characterized by keratinous obstruction of the eccrine duct with sweat retention vesicle formation and periductal lymphocytic spongiosis. Eccrine duct obstructions occurs at the stratum corneum in miliaria crystallina, midepidermis in miliaria rubra, and DEJ in miliaria profunda.
- **Apocrine miliaria (Fox-Fordyce disease)** refers to **obstruction of the apocrine duct.** It commonly affects **young women** and is characterized by **intensely pruritic skin-colored follicular papules in the axillae, periareolar area, and anogenital area.**
- Miliaria self-resolves with relocation to a cooler environment. When relocation is not possible (eg, febrile hospitalized patient), techniques include frequent turning and cooling devices.

Disorders of the Hair and Nails

Basic Concepts

- **Hair disorders** arise from the hair follicle.
  - **Alopecia,** defined as **loss of hair follicles and/or hair shafts,** may be **nonscarring or scarring (cicatricial)** and **circumscribed, patterned, or diffuse.**
    - The histopathological evaluation of alopecia may involve horizontal and/or vertical sectioning (Figure 2.82).
  - **Hypertrichosis,** defined as **excessive hair growth,** may be **localized or generalized.**
- **Nail disorders** arise from the nail unit.

ALOPECIA AREATA
→ Diagnosis Group 1

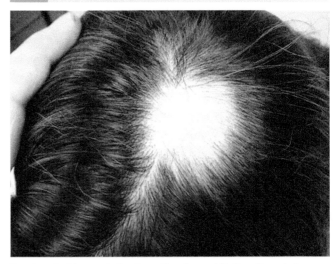

Reprinted with permission from Goodheart HP. *Goodheart's Same-Site Differential Diagnosis: A Rapid Method of Diagnosing and Treating Common Skin Disorders.* Wolters Kluwer Health/Lippincott Williams & Wilkins; 2011.

Epidemiology

- AA is an **autoimmune** nonscarring alopecia mediated by **CD8+ T cells** that engage in a primary attack against the hair follicle or a secondary attack following collapse of immune privilege.
- Associations include **atopy, vitiligo, IBD, and autoimmune thyroid disease. 20%** of patients have a **family history** of AA.
  > **AA** is a characteristic feature of **APECED/IPEX syndromes.**
- Drug associations include **ICIs.**

Clinicopathological Features

- AA classically presents with **nonscarring circumscribed hair loss**. **Madarosis** may occur.
- Nail unit involvement includes **small and geometrically distributed pits in the nail plate, red lunulae, and trachyonychia.**
- AA variants include **diffuse** AA, **patterned** AA such as the **ophiasis** (bandlike hair loss of the **posterolateral scalp**) and **sisaipho** (hair loss **sparing the posterolateral scalp**), **alopecia totalis** (hair loss of the **scalp**), and **alopecia universalis** (hair loss of the **scalp and body**). **Migratory poliosis** without hair loss may represent a *forme fruste* (incomplete manifestation) of AA.
  - Remember that the sisaipho pattern is the opposite of the ophiasis pattern because sisaipho is ophiasis spelled backward.
  - Figure 2.83.

Evaluation

- The differential diagnosis of AA varies based on the distribution of hair loss (circumscribed, patterned, or diffuse). The differential diagnosis of madarosis includes AD, AA, lepromatous leprosy, and **hypothyroidism**, which leads to preferential **madarosis of the lateral one third of the eyebrows.**
- **Trichoscopy** features include **exclamation point hairs, Pohl-Pinkus constrictions, and yellow dots.**
- Evaluation for associated diseases (eg, TSH) should be symptom driven.

Management

- AA may resolve spontaneously; however, **childhood onset, atopy, and diffuse distribution** are associated with a **poor prognosis.**

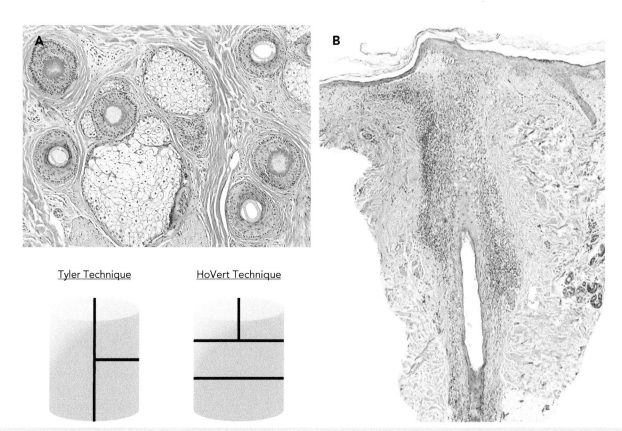

Figure 2.82. SIDE-BY-SIDE COMPARISON: HORIZONTAL AND VERTICAL SECTIONING. Benefits of horizontal sectioning include visualizing all hair follicles and deducing follicular counts, density, and ratio. Benefits of vertical sectioning include visualizing the full thickness of the hair follicle and assessing peribulbar inflammation and fibrosis. Horizontal sectioning is typically preferred for nonscarring alopecia, while vertical sectioning is typically preferred for scarring alopecia. The St. John's protocol calls for two specimens, while the Tyler and HoVert techniques combine horizontal and vertical sectioning in order to maximize the diagnostic yield of a single specimen. A, Horizontal sectioning: TE. B, Vertical sectioning: LPP. LPP, lichen planopilaris; TE, telogen effluvium.

(Histology images reprinted with permission from Elder DE, Elenitsas R, Rosenbach M, et al. *Lever's Histopathology of the Skin.* 11th ed. Wolters Kluwer; 2015.)

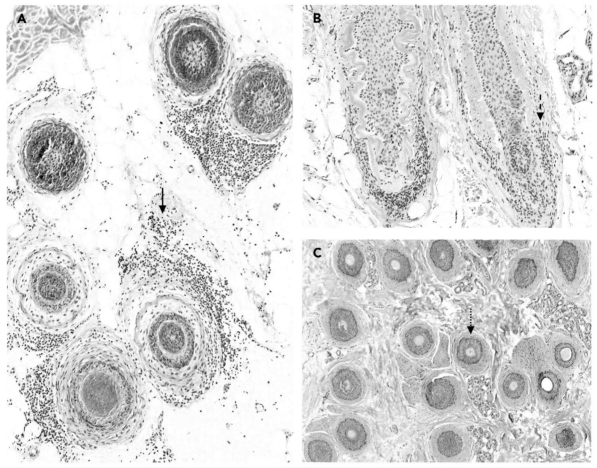

Figure 2.83. CLINICOPATHOLOGICAL CORRELATION: ALOPECIA AREATA. AA is characterized by a normal hair follicle count with a peribulbar lymphocytic ± eosinophilic infiltrate. Trichomalacia (pleated or twisted hair shafts within follicular infundibula) and marked hair shaft narrowing may also be observed. Overtime, there is a major (>50%) shift from anagen follicles to catagen and telogen follicles along with the appearance of numerous miniaturized, arrested, rapidly cycling nanogen follicles. A, High-power view (acute, horizontal). Solid arrow: lymphocytes surrounding an anagen follicle. B, High-power view (acute, horizontal). Dashed arrow: lymphocytes surrounding a catagen follicle with an eosinophilic glassy membrane. C, Low-power view (subacute, horizontal). Dotted arrow: telogen follicle with trichilemmal keratin. Bright-red trichilemmal keratin gives the club-shaped telogen hair a flamethrower-like appearance on vertical sections. AA, alopecia areata.

(Histology images reprinted with permission from Elder DE, Elenitsas R, Rosenbach M, et al. *Lever's Histopathology of the Skin.* 11th ed. Wolters Kluwer; 2015.)

Lymphocytes surrounding the follicle bulb resemble a "swarm of bees."

- Local therapies include **corticosteroids (topical, intralesional)**, immunotherapy (eg, squaric acid dibutyl ester [SADBE]), irritants (eg, anthralin), minoxidil, and PUVA/excimer laser.
- **Pulsed systemic corticosteroids** are often used in rapidly progressive AA. **JAK inhibitors** are an emerging treatment option. In a **young child** not bothered by AA, it is **reasonable not to treat** or to use **a low-potency topical corticosteroid.**

"Real World" Advice

- In AA and AE, hair "sheds" by breaking near the scalp. In TE, hair "comes out by the roots." In hair shaft abnormalities with increased fragility, hair "breaks" near the ends.
- It is important to recognize the **negative impact of AA on quality of life and psychosocial well-being.**

TRICHOTILLOMANIA

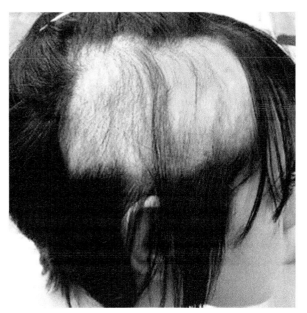

Reprinted with permission from Goodheart HP, Gonzalez ME. *Goodheart's Same-Site Differential Diagnosis: Dermatology for the Primary Health Care Provider.* 2nd ed. Wolters Kluwer; 2022.

- Trichotillomania is a nonscarring alopecia due to **hair pulling**, often in the setting of **impulse control disorder** (eg, body-focused repetitive behavior disorder). Trichotillomania commonly affects **preadolescent and adolescent children with a female preponderance.**

- Trichotillomania classically presents with **nonscarring circumscribed** hair loss with bizarre shapes and irregular borders. **Trichobezoar** is a potentially **life-threatening** complication.
  - ◈ Figure 2.84.

- Trichoscopy demonstrates **hair shafts of diverse lengths and black dots.** The diagnosis is supported by creating a **"hair growth window"** by repeatedly shaving a small area of involved scalp to demonstrate normal regrowth.

- Treatment options include **behavioral modification therapy**, hypnosis, insight-oriented psychotherapy, and pharmacologic therapy (eg, **clomipramine**).

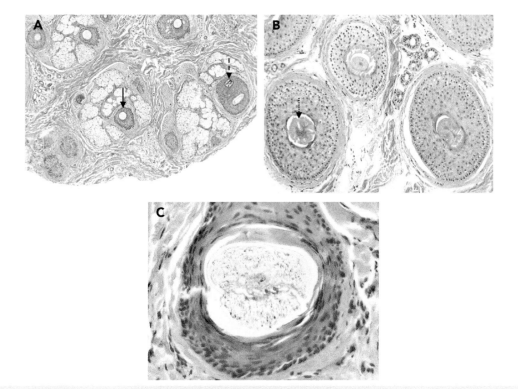

Figure 2.84. CLINICOPATHOLOGICAL CORRELATION: TRICHOTILLOMANIA. Trichotillomania is characterized by a normal hair follicle count with a major (>50%) shift from anagen follicles to catagen and telogen follicles. Empty anagen follicles may be observed. When the hair shaft is pulled, the IRS collapses and fills the void, forming a geometric configuration. Trichomalacia and pigment casts may be identified within follicular channels, with perifollicular hemorrhage. A, Low-power view (horizontal). Solid arrow: catagen follicle. Dashed arrow: pigment cast. B, High-power view (horizontal). Dotted arrow: collapsed IRS with a geometric configuration. C, High-power view ("hamburger sign," horizontal). IRS, inner root sheath.

(Histology images reprinted with permission from Elder DE, Elenitsas R, Rosenbach M, et al. *Lever's Histopathology of the Skin.* 11th ed. Wolters Kluwer; 2015.)

A rare but diagnostic finding in trichotillomania is longitudinal splitting of the hair shaft. When blood and proteinaceous debris are seen in the split, that is known as the "hamburger sign."

ANDROGENETIC ALOPECIA

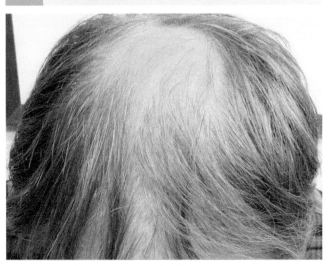

Male pattern alopecia courtesy of Kathie Huang, MD.

- AGA is a nonscarring alopecia due to **androgen-dependent follicular miniaturization** in genetically susceptible individuals. The primary mediator in men is **DHT.** Associations include **pregnancy (postpartum).**

- AGA classically presents in two patterns:
  - **Female pattern alopecia**: **nonscarring patterned** hair loss of the **vertex/midline scalp and widened part line > diffuse** hair loss graded by the **Ludwig system.**
    - The widened part line in female pattern alopecia resembles a "Christmas tree."
  - **Male pattern alopecia**: **nonscarring patterned** hair loss of the **frontotemporal and vertex scalp** graded by the **Hamilton-Norwood system.**

  In both male and female pattern alopecia, **eyebrows and eyelashes** are preserved because these hairs are not influenced by androgen signaling. In early AGA, the characteristic hair shaft abnormality without increased fragility is **acquired progressive kinking of the hair.**
    - Figure 2.85.
- **Trichoscopy** demonstrates **hair shafts with a diversity of diameters and brown halos.** In women, AGA may be a sign of hyperandrogenism and a male pattern may be a sign of virilization. Acquired progressive kinking of the hair is also associated with HIV infection.
- **Topical minoxidil** is first line. Alternative therapies are **5α-reductase inhibitors (eg, dutasteride, finasteride)** and hair restoration.

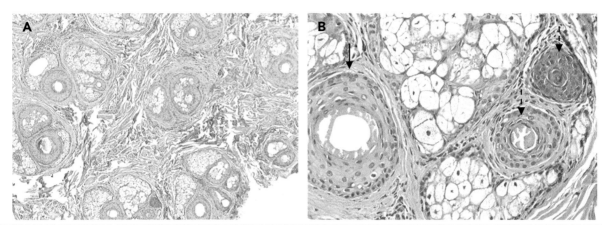

Figure 2.85. CLINICOPATHOLOGICAL CORRELATION: ANDROGENETIC ALOPECIA. AGA is characterized by a normal hair follicle count with follicular miniaturization. There is a diversity of diameters (anisotrichosis) ranging from terminal to intermediate to vellus follicles. Fibrous tract remnants have normal diameter and vascularity. A, Low-power view (horizontal). B, High-power view (horizontal). Solid arrow: terminal follicle. Dashed arrows: vellus follicles. AGA, androgenetic alopecia.

(Histology images reprinted with permission from Gru AA, Wick MR, Mir A, et al. *Pediatric Dermatopathology and Dermatology.* Wolters Kluwer; 2018.)

Fibrous tract remnants are sometimes called "fibrous streamers."

TRACTION ALOPECIA

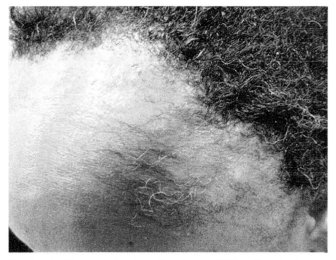

Reprinted with permission from Goodheart HP. *Goodheart's Same-Site Differential Diagnosis: A Rapid Method of Diagnosing and Treating Common Skin Disorders.* Wolters Kluwer Health/Lippincott Williams & Wilkins; 2011.

- Traction alopecia is a nonscarring alopecia due to **traction on the hair shaft.**
- Traction alopecia classically presents with **nonscarring patterned** hair loss of the **frontotemporal scalp and widened part line**; however, traction alopecia can **scar if chronic or severe (biphasic).**
  - Acute traction alopecia resembles trichotillomania on histopathology. Chronic traction alopecia resembles a noninflammatory scarring alopecia.
- **Avoid tight braids** and other forms of traumatic styling (eg, curlers).

ANAGEN EFFLUVIUM

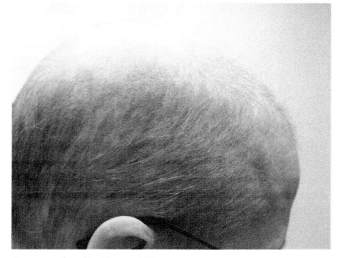

Courtesy of Kathie Huang, MD.

- AE is a nonscarring alopecia due to **shedding of anagen hairs after cessation of mitotic activity in rapidly dividing hair matrix cells.** Drug associations include **colchicine, alkylating agents, antimetabolites, and topoisomerase inhibitors.** Other triggers include **arsenic and thallium poisoning.**
  - AE of the hair is analogous to Beau lines of the nail.
  - Do NOT confuse AE due to cytotoxic chemotherapies with alopecia neoplastica, a secondary scarring alopecia due to solid organ metastases (eg, breast cancer).
- AE classically presents with **sudden-onset nonscarring diffuse** hair loss. While AE is typically reversible, it **may be irreversible** in some cases.
  - AE is differentiated from TE by the absence of a catagen/telogen shift.
- Trichoscopy demonstrates **Pohl-Pinkus constrictions.**
- Treatment options include **cooling (eg, cold caps)** before, during, and after chemotherapy infusion and topical minoxidil.

TELOGEN EFFLUVIUM

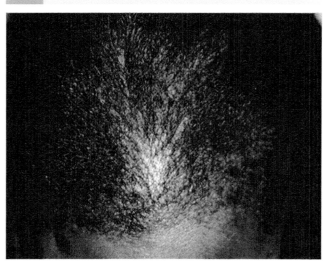

Reprinted with permission from Lugo-Somolinos A, McKinley-Grant L, Goldsmith LA, et al. *VisualDx: Essential Dermatology in Pigmented Skin.* Wolters Kluwer Health/Lippincott Williams & Wilkins; 2011.

- TE is a nonscarring alopecia due to **shedding of telogen hairs.** Associations include **chronic illness, marasmus, fever, severe infection, thyroid disorders, pregnancy (postpartum), surgery, and stress.** Drug associations include **systemic retinoids, SMO inhibitors, IFNs, minoxidil,** anticoagulants (eg, **heparin**), anticonvulsants, antithyroid drugs, **β-blockers,** and **discontinuation of OCPs.**

- Acute TE classically presents with **nonscarring diffuse** hair loss ~**3 months** after the trigger.
  - ◆ Figure 2.86.
- Trichoscopy demonstrates **hair shafts of equal diameter.** ≥**2 telogen hairs** on gentle hair pull test is suggestive of TE; >20% telogen hairs on unit area trichogram is diagnostic. Evaluation of chronic TE (>6 months) includes CMP, CBC, ESR, TFTs, and **ferritin** (should be ≥ **40 mg/dL).**
  - ◇ Telogen hairs are "club shaped."
- Patients should be reassured that **TE does not lead to baldness. Complete hair regrowth is expected**; however, **TE may unmask underlying patterned alopecia (eg, AGA).**

FRONTAL FIBROSING ALOPECIA/LICHEN PLANOPILARIS

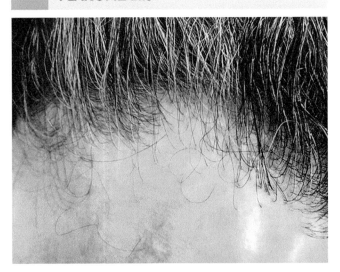

- Frontal fibrosing alopecia (FFA) and lichen planopilaris (LPP) are distinct presentations of a disorder of follicular keratinization that leads to scarring alopecia. The pathogenesis is unclear but may relate to **abnormal functioning of the peroxisome proliferator–activated receptor γ (PPAR-γ).** FFA and LPP commonly affect **Caucasian women.**
- **FFA** is characterized by **scarring circumscribed or patterned** hair loss of the **frontotemporal scalp ± eyebrows. LPP** is characterized by **scarring circumscribed > diffuse** hair loss. Pruritus and tenderness are often present. The terms "**Brocq alopecia**" **or "pseudopelade of Brocq**" refer to the end-stage of scarring alopecia with **polytrichia (tufting). Graham Little-Piccardi-Lassueur syndrome** is an **LPP variant** with **(1) patchy scarring alopecia of the scalp, (2) nonscarring alopecia of axillary and pubic areas, and (3) grouped spinous follicular papules** on the trunk and extremities.
  - ◇ "B̲rocq alopecia" is "b̲urnt out" scarring alopecia. Preserved areas of hair growth may resemble "footprints in the snow" and tufting may resemble "baby doll hair."
  - ◆ Figure 2.87.
- Trichoscopy of the periphery demonstrates **perifollicular erythema and hair casts**, while trichoscopy of the center demonstrates **white dots.** For scarring alopecia, it is preferable to biopsy the active border.
- First-line therapy combines **antimalarial with corticosteroid (topical, intralesional, or oral).** The PPAR-γ agonist pioglitazone is an emerging therapy.

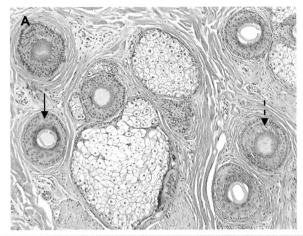
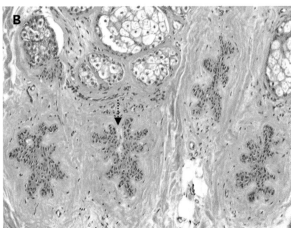

Figure 2.86. CLINICOPATHOLOGICAL CORRELATION: TELOGEN EFFLUVIUM. TE is characterized by a normal hair follicle count with a minor (20%-50%) shift from anagen follicles to catagen and telogen follicles. A, High-power view (horizontal). Solid arrow: anagen follicle. Dashed arrow: telogen follicle. B, High-power view (horizontal). Dotted arrow: telogen germinal unit. AA, alopecia areata; TE, telogen effluvium.

(Histology images reprinted with permission from Elder DE, Elenitsas R, Rosenbach M, et al. *Lever's Histopathology of the Skin.* 11th ed. Wolters Kluwer; 2015.)

The catagen/telogen shift in TE is less pronounced than in chronic AA and trichotillomania.

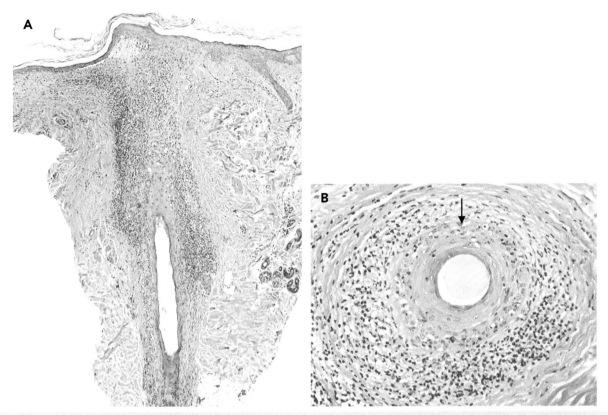

Figure 2.87. CLINICOPATHOLOGICAL CORRELATION: FRONTAL FIBROSING ALOPECIA/LICHEN PLANOPILARIS.
FFA/LPP is characterized by perifollicular ± epidermal lichenoid interface dermatitis concentrated at the lower infundibulum and isthmus. Fibrosis may lead to blurring of the junction between the follicular epithelium and the dermis. Fibrous tract remnants may be filled with colloid bodies. DIF is analogous to LP. A, LPP (vertical). B, LPP (horizontal). Solid arrow: perifollicular lichenoid inflammation at the lower infundibulum. DIF, direct immunofluorescence; DLE, discoid lupus erythematosus; FFA, frontal fibrosing alopecia; LP, lichen planus; LPP, lichen planopilaris

(Histology images reprinted with permission from Elder DE, Elenitsas R, Rosenbach M, et al. *Lever's Histopathology of the Skin.* 11th ed. Wolters Kluwer; 2015.)

Fibrosis at the lower infundibulum and isthmus may give rise to an "hourglass" configuration. The depth of interface dermatitis helps distinguish FFA/LPP (infundibulum > isthmus) from DLE (isthmus > infundibulum).

CENTRAL CENTRIFUGAL CICATRICIAL ALOPECIA

Synonyms: follicular degeneration syndrome, hot comb alopecia

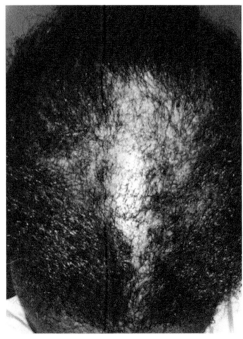

Reprinted with permission from Elder DE, Elenitsas R, Rubin AI, et al. *Atlas and Synopsis of Lever's Histopathology of the Skin.* 3rd ed. Wolters Kluwer Health/Lippincott Williams & Wilkins; 2012.

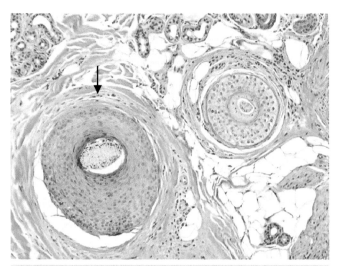

Figure 2.88. CLINICOPATHOLOGICAL CORRELATION: CENTRAL CENTRIFUGAL CICATRICIAL ALOPECIA. CCCA is characterized by premature desquamation of the IRS, eccentric atrophy of the ORS, and concentric lamellar fibroplasia of affected hair follicles. Variably dense perifollicular inflammation is concentrated at the lower infundibulum and isthmus. Folliculitis decalvans demonstrates intrafollicular and perifollicular infiltrates rich in neutrophils and lymphocytes. Solid arrow: lamellar fibroplasia. CCCA, central centrifugal cicatricial alopecia; IRS, inner root sheath; ORS, outer root sheath.

(Histology image reprinted with permission from Elder DE, Elenitsas R, Rosenbach M, et al. *Lever's Histopathology of the Skin.* 11th ed. Wolters Kluwer; 2015.)

- Central centrifugal cicatricial alopecia (CCCA) is a scarring alopecia. **Premature desquamation of the IRS is hypothesized to predispose to follicular injury related to caustic hair care products (eg, chemical hair relaxers), heat styling, and traction.** CCCA commonly affects **Black women of African heritage.**
- CCCA classically presents with **scarring circumscribed or patterned** hair loss of the **vertex/midline scalp.** It may co-occur with lipedematous alopecia of the scalp. At the end-stage, CCCA results in "Brocq alopecia" ± polytrichia. **Folliculitis decalvans** is a **highly inflammatory** CCCA variant characterized by **pustules** (may represent bacterial superinfection).
  - ◆ Figure 2.88.
- First-line therapy combines **tetracycline antibiotic with potent topical corticosteroid.** Clindamycin and rifampin are first line for folliculitis decalvans.

ACNE KELOIDALIS

Synonyms: folliculitis keloidalis

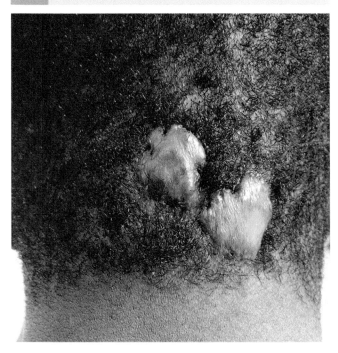

- Acne keloidalis is a deep folliculitis that leads to scarring alopecia. The pathogenesis is unclear but may be related to mechanical irritation from haircuts. Acne keloidalis commonly affects **Black men.**
- Acne keloidalis classically presents with **scarring circumscribed** hair loss that favors the **occipital scalp and posterior neck (acne keloidalis nuchae). Firm papules** coalesce to form **protuberant plaques.**
  - Figure 2.89.
- **Pseudofolliculitis barbae** is a closely related deep folliculitis in the **beard distribution.** The characteristic hair shaft abnormality without increased fragility is **pili recurvati.**
- **Avoid mechanical irritation of the posterior hairline.** First-line therapy combines **retinoid gel with high-potency corticosteroid gel** ± tetracycline antibiotic. If refractory, surgical excision can be beneficial.

DISSECTING CELLULITIS OF THE SCALP
Synonym: perifolliculitis capitis abscedens et suffodiens

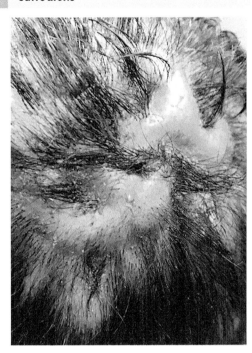

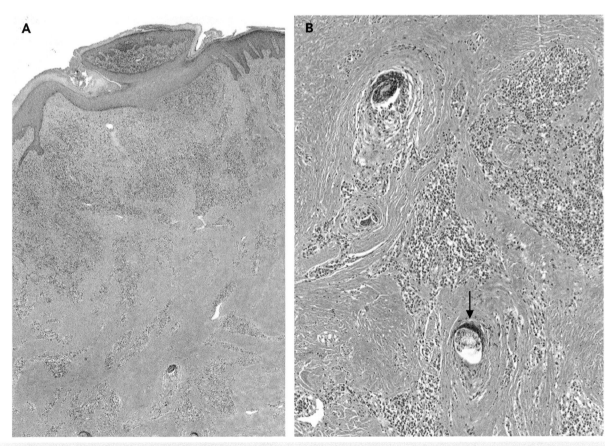

Figure 2.89. CLINICOPATHOLOGICAL CORRELATION: ACNE KELOIDALS. Acne keloidalis is characterized by a mixed perifollicular infiltrate concentrated at the lower infundibulum and isthmus. There is lamellar fibroplasia and free hair shafts may be present in the dermis. A, Low-power view. B, High-power view. Solid arrow: "naked hair shaft."

Free hair shafts in the dermis are commonly referred to as "naked hair shafts."

- Dissecting cellulitis of the scalp is an inflammatory disorder within the **follicular occlusion tetrad** that leads to scarring alopecia. Dissecting cellulitis of the scalp commonly affects **young adult Black men.**
- Dissecting cellulitis of the scalp classically presents with **scarring circumscribed** hair loss overlying **boggy, fluctuant, interconnected nodules with purulent drainage.**
  - ◆ Dissecting cellulitis of the scalp is characterized by perifollicular lymphocytic (early) to neutrophilic (late) inflammation extending from the dermis to the subcutaneous fat. Vascular proliferation, sinus tract formation, and fibrosis may occur.
- **Isotretinoin** is first line.

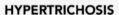

HYPERTRICHOSIS

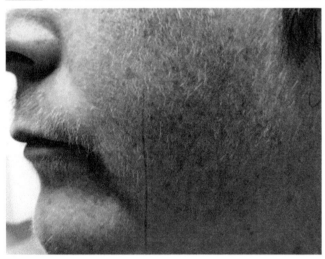

Acquired hypertrichosis lanuginosa.

- **Hypertrichosis** refers to **excessive hair growth. Hirsutism** refers to **excessive terminal hair growth in androgen-dependent sites of female individuals.** Similar to hormonal acne, hirsutism is caused by either increased end-organ sensitivity to androgens or hyperandrogenemia.
  - ◇ Hirsutism is NOT a synonym for hypertrichosis.
  - ◇ The distribution of hirsutism may provide a clue. Adrenal hirsutism favors the pubic triangle to upper abdomen and presternal area to neck/chin. Ovarian hirsutism favors the areolae and lateral face/neck. Idiopathic hirsutism favors the lateral face/back.
  - ◇ In PCOS, hirsutism (90%) is MORE common than acne (70%).
- **Acquired hypertrichosis** is summarized in Table 2.58. **Congenital hypertrichosis** is summarized in Table 2.59.
  - ◆ Hypertrichosis demonstrates an increased number of lanugo, vellus, or terminal hairs.
- The diagnosis of hirsutism is based on the modified **Ferriman and Gallwey scale,** which scores hair growth from 0 to 4 in nine locations: upper lip, chin, chest, upper back, lower back, upper abdomen, lower abdomen, upper arms, and thighs. A score of 9 to 14 indicates functional hirsutism, while a score >15 indicates organic hirsutism. Evaluation of hirsutism is similar to hormonal acne.
- Hypertrichosis treatments include bleaching, depilation, epilation, **eflornithine,** electrolysis, IPL therapy, and laser hair removal. Management of hirsutism is similar to hormonal acne.

Table 2.58. ACQUIRED HYPERTRICHOSIS

Diagnosis[a]	Classic Description	Notes
Localized		
Hirsutism	See above.	
Miscellaneous	Localized development of terminal hairs.	Associations include CRPS, porphyria (eg, PCT), and friction injury (eg, under plaster cast).
Generalized		
Acquired hypertrichosis lanuginosa	Generalized development of lanugo hairs.	Associations include nutritional deficiency (eg, marasmus) and malignancy (eg, breast, lung, colon).
Prepubertal hypertrichosis	Development of terminal hairs favoring peripheral face and back during early childhood.	Associations include Mediterranean or South Asian descent and hyperandrogenemia.
		Prepubertal hypertrichosis associated with Mediterranean or South Asian descent may create an "inverted fir tree" pattern on the back.
Miscellaneous	Generalized development of terminal hairs.	Associations include HIV infection and pregnancy. Drug associations include corticosteroids, cyclosporine, zidovudine, EGFR inhibitors, IFN, bimatoprost/latanoprost, minoxidil, phenytoin, and PUVA.

CRPS, complex regional pain syndrome; EGFR, epidermal growth factor receptor; HIV, human immunodeficiency virus; IFN, interferon; PCT, porphyria cutanea tarda; PUVA, psoralen ultraviolet A.
[a]Illustrative examples provided.

Table 2.59. CONGENITAL HYPERTRICHOSIS

Diagnosis[a]	Inheritance Pattern	Gene	Classic Description
Localized			
Nevoid hypertrichosis	Sporadic		Circumscribed hypertrichosis (primary) ± hemihypertrophy, lipodystrophy, scoliosis, and vascular abnormalities (secondary).
Hypertrichosis of specific anatomic sites	AD > AR		Hypertrichosis of the eyebrows, eyelashes (trichomegaly), nasal tip, auricle, neck (anterior cervical hypertrichosis or posterior cervical hypertrichosis), polythelia, elbows (hypertrichosis cubiti), or palms/soles ± other features.
Congenital melanocytic nevus	See Chapter 5: Melanocytic Neoplasms.		
Hair collar sign/faun tail nevus	See Chapter 5: Neural Malformations and Neoplasms.		
Plexiform neurofibroma	See Chapter 5: Neural Malformations and Neoplasms.		
Becker nevus	See Chapter 5: Other Malformations and Neoplasms.		
Cornelia de Lange syndrome	AD, XLD	*NIPBL*[b]	Dysmorphic syndrome with hypertrichosis of forehead, lateral face, shoulders, back; low anterior hairline, synophrys/trichomegaly.
Rubinstein-Taybi syndrome	AD	*CREBBP*	Dysmorphic syndrome with hypertrichosis of lateral face, shoulders, back; synophrys/trichomegaly; broad thumbs and great toes with brachyonychia (racquet nails) and macronychia.
Fetal alcohol syndrome/fetal hydantoin syndrome	N/A	N/A	Intrauterine exposure to alcohol/phenytoin with hypertrichosis of face, back, extremities.
Miscellaneous	Variable		Porphyria (eg, CEP, HEP).
Generalized[c]			
Congenital hypertrichosis lanuginosa	AD		Generalized lanugo hairs that may grow up to 10 cm in length and shed over the first year of life ± dental anomalies.
Universal hypertrichosis	AD		Generalized thick, long terminal hairs that persist.
Ambras syndrome	AD		Generalized fine, long hairs that persist with facial dysmorphism, dental anomalies, and polythelia.

AD, autosomal dominant; AR, autosomal recessive; CEP, congenital erythropoietic porphyria; HEP, hepatoerythropoietic porphyria; N/A, not applicable; XLD, X-linked dominant.
[a]Illustrative examples provided.
[b]Most common AD mutation.
[c]Increased hair is the major feature.

BEAU LINES
→ Diagnosis Group 2

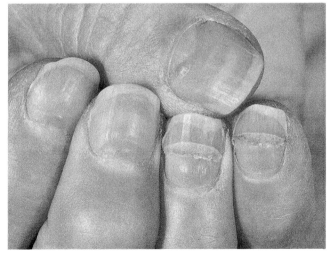

Courtesy of Adam Rubin, MD.

Epidemiology

- Beau lines result from **transient interruption of the mitotic activity of the proximal nail matrix.**
- Beau lines in a **single nail** often result from **disorders of the proximal nail fold (eg, AD, chronic paronychia) or mechanical injury. Friction injury** (eg, body-focused repetitive behavior disorder) may lead to multiple midline Beau lines in **habit-tic deformity,** a form of **median nail dystrophy.**
- Beau lines at the same level in **all nails** often result from a **systemic insult (eg, marasmus) or drugs (eg, cytotoxic chemotherapies).**
  - Beau lines of the nails are analogous to AE of the hair.

Clinicopathological Features

- Beau lines are **transverse depressions in the nail plate.**
  - Figure 2.90.
  - Beau lines demonstrate thinning of the nail plate.

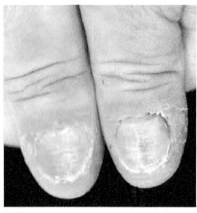
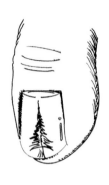

Figure 2.90. MEDIAN NAIL DYSTROPHY. Nail trauma may result in median nail dystrophy. Habit-tic deformity resembles a washboard: multiple midline Beau lines due to the nervous habit of rubbing and pushing back the midportion of the cuticle of the thumb with the index finger. Median canaliform dystrophy of Heller resembles an inverted fir tree: central longitudinal split due to friction.

(Median nail dystrophy image reprinted with permission from Schalock PC, Hsu JTS, Arndt KA. *Lippincott's Primary Care Dermatology.* Wolters Kluwer Health/Lippincott Williams & Wilkins; 2010. Illustration by Misha Rosenbach, MD.)

Evaluation

- Beyond Beau lines, the differential diagnosis of **transverse nail lines** includes:
  - **Mees lines: parallel bands of true leukonychia** of the nails. Associations include **cytotoxic chemotherapies, arsenic and thallium poisoning, and mechanical injury.**
  - **Muehrcke lines: parallel bands of apparent leukonychia** of the nails. Associations include **hypoalbuminemia, cirrhosis,** and **cytotoxic chemotherapies.**
  - **Lindsay nails: apparent leukonychia sparing the distal half** of the nails in the setting of **renal disease on hemodialysis.**
  - **Terry nails: apparent leukonychia sparing a distal 1 to 2 mm band** of the nails in **liver cirrhosis.**
    Figure 2.91.

Management

- Unless the matrix is reinjured, Beau lines grow out with the nail.

"Real World" Advice

- The **depth** of the Beau line indicates the **severity** of damage to the proximal nail matrix.
- The longitudinal **width** of the Beau line indicates the **duration** of damage to the proximal nail matrix.

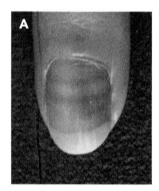
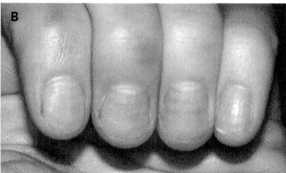
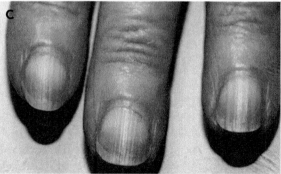
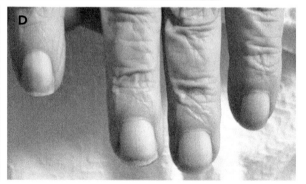

Figure 2.91. TRANSVERSE LEUKONYCHIA. To distinguish Mees lines from Muehrcke lines, compress the nail to determine whether the white discoloration remains (true leukonychia) or fades (apparent leukonychia). To distinguish Lindsay nails from Terry nails, determine whether apparent leukonychia spares the distal half of the nails ("half-and-half nails") or spares a distal 1-2 mm band of the nails. A, Mees lines. B, Muehrcke lines. C, Lindsay nails. D, Terry nails.

(A, Photo by Yannick Trotter, licensed under CC Attribution-Share Alike 3.0 Unported license. From Orient JM. *Sapira's Art & Science of Bedside Diagnosis.* 5th ed. Wolters Kluwer; 2019. B, Reprinted with permission from Orient JM. *Sapira's Art & Science of Bedside Diagnosis.* 5th ed. Wolters Kluwer; 2019. C, Image courtesy of Robert I. Rudolph, MD. From Goodheart HP, Gonzalez ME. *Goodheart's Same-Site Differential Diagnosis: Dermatology for the Primary Health Care Provider.* 2nd ed. Wolters Kluwer; 2022. D, Reprinted with permission from Mansoor AM. *Frameworks for Internal Medicine.* Wolters Kluwer; 2018.)

SPOTLIGHT ON PACHYONYCHIA CONGENITA

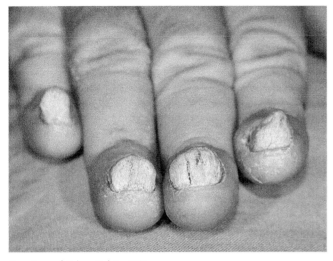

Courtesy of Adam Rubin, MD.

- Pachyonychia congenita (PC) is an AD hereditary disorder historically classified into two types:
  - **Type I (Jadassohn-Lewandowsky):** due to mutation of K6a and K16.
  - **Type II (Jackson-Lawlor):** due to mutation of K6b and K17.

  Today, PC is classified on the basis of the mutated gene: **PC-K6a, PC-K6b, PC-6c, PC-K16, PC-K17.**
- PC classically presents with **onychodystrophy (eg, pachyonychia, pincer deformity, subungual hyperkeratosis)** with frequent **paronychia.** Other manifestations include **follicular hyperkeratosis, focal PPK with pseudoainhum, steatocystomas/vellus hair cysts (PC-K17), and benign oral leukoplakia.**
  - ◈ PC is characterized by keratinocytes in the superficial epidermis and mucosal epithelium with pale cytoplasm and eosinophilic inclusions, which correlate at the ultrastructural level with perinuclear condensation of mutated keratin filaments.
- **Hereditary hair and nail disorders** not discussed elsewhere are summarized in Table 2.60.
  - Figure 2.92.
- Management of PC involves mechanical modalities (eg, filing) following soaking and application of emollients and keratolytics.

Table 2.60. HEREDITARY HAIR AND NAIL DISORDERS

Diagnosis[a]	Inheritance Pattern	Gene	Classic Description	Notes
Hair Disorders[b]				
Björnstad syndrome	AR	*BCS1L*	The characteristic hair shaft abnormality with increased fragility is pili torti. Systemic features include sensorineural hearing loss.	Crandall syndrome is Björnstad syndrome with hypogonadism.
Congenital atrichia with papules	AR	*Hairless, vitamin D receptor*	Loss of natal hair and development of follicular cysts and milia-like lesions. Systemic features include vitamin D–dependent rickets.	
Loose anagen hair syndrome			Loose anagen hair is a hair shaft abnormality without increased fragility. Alopecia results because hair can be easily and painlessly plucked.	The most common demographic is a young girl with blond hair.
Menkes kinky hair disease	XLR	*ATP7A,* encodes copper-transporting ATPase	Characteristic hair shaft abnormalities with increased fragility are pili torti and trichorrhexis nodosa. Other cutaneous features include a pudgy face with a "Cupid's bow" upper lip, doughy skin, and pigmentary dilution. Systemic features include tortuous arteries, musculoskeletal involvement (eg, metaphyseal widening of the long bone), and neurologic involvement (eg, seizures). Kinky hair resembles "steel wool." Remember pili <u>tort</u>i and <u>tort</u>uous arteries.	Check serum copper and ceruloplasmin to evaluate for copper deficiency.

(Continued)

Table 2.60. HEREDITARY HAIR AND NAIL DISORDERS (CONTINUED)

Diagnosis[a]	Inheritance Pattern	Gene	Classic Description	Notes
Monilethrix	AD > AR	*KRT81, KRT83, KRT86, DSG4,* encode K81, K83, K86, desmoglein 4	Monilethrix is a hair shaft abnormality with increased fragility. Other cutaneous features include KP and koilonychia. Systemic features include cataracts and abnormal teeth.	
Temporal triangular alopecia			Patterned nonscarring hair loss or vellus-like depigmented hairs of the temporal scalp.	Temporal triangular alopecia presents at birth or during the first decade of life.
Uncombable hair syndrome	AR > AD	*PADI3, TCHH, TMG3*	The characteristic hair shaft abnormality without increased fragility is pili trianguli et canaliculi.	
			Uncombable hair resembles "spun glass."	
Nail Disorders				
Coffin-Siris syndrome	AD	*ARID1A, ARID1B, SMARCA4, SMARCB1, SMARCE1*	Hypoplasia of the fifth nails. Other cutaneous features include sparse scalp hair and hypertrichosis. Systemic features include coarse facies, growth delay, and intellectual disability.	
COIF	Sporadic > AD		Hypoplasia of the second fingernails.	
Congenital malalignment of the great toes/congenital hypertrophy of the lateral fold of the hallux	Sporadic		Lateral deviation of the hallux nail plate/ hypertrophy of the lateral fold of the hallux.	Associated with onychocryptosis.
Nail-patella syndrome (HOOD)	AD	*LMX1B*	Triangular lunulae and nail hypoplasia. Systemic features include musculoskeletal involvement (eg, hypoplastic patella, iliac crest exostoses, radial head dysplasia), ocular involvement (eg, hyperpigmented pupillary margin known as Lester iris), and renal involvement (FSGS).	Obtain a UA.
			Figure 2.92.	
Pachydermoperiostosis (primary hypertrophic osteoarthropathy)	AR	*HPGD, SLCO2A1*	Pachydermia, clubbing, and periostosis.	Thyroid acropachy is a closely related acquired disorder characterized by acral soft-tissue swelling, clubbing, and periostosis.

AD, autosomal dominant; AR, autosomal recessive; COIF, congenital onychodysplasia of the index fingers; FSGS, focal segmental glomerulosclerosis; HOOD, hereditary osteo-onychodysplasia; K, keratin; KP, keratosis pilaris; US, urinalysis; XLR, X-linked recessive.
[a]Illustrative examples provided.
[b]Other hereditary hair shaft abnormalities without increased fragility include pili annulati, pili bifurcati, and pili multigemini (favors beard distribution).

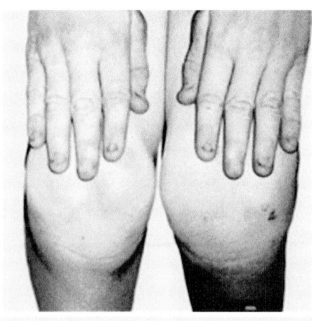

Figure 2.92. THE LUNULA. Examination of the lunula may provide a clue to the diagnosis of a systemic disorder. Absent lunulae is a characteristic feature of yellow nail syndrome. Triangular lunulae is pathognomonic for nail-patella syndrome. Blue lunulae may occur in the setting of Wilson disease or exogenous exposure to zidovudine, minocycline, or silver (argyria). Red lunulae may reflect an inflammatory or autoimmune disorder (eg, psoriasis, LP, SLE, DM, RA, AA) or exogenous CO poisoning. AA, alopecia areata; CO, carbon monoxide; DM, dermatomyositis; LP, lichen planus; RA, rheumatoid arthritis; SLE, systemic lupus erythematosus.

(Nail-patella syndrome image reprinted with permission from Staheli LT. *Fundamentals of Pediatric Orthopedics*. 5th ed. Wolters Kluwer; 2015.)

Neutrophilic and Eosinophilic Dermatoses

Basic Concepts

- **Neutrophilic dermatoses** are characterized by the presence of a **sterile, predominantly neutrophilic infiltrate** on histopathology.
- **Eosinophilic dermatoses** are characterized by the presence of an **eosinophilic infiltrate** on histopathology.

SWEET SYNDROME
→ **Diagnosis Group 2**
Synonym: acute febrile neutrophilic dermatosis

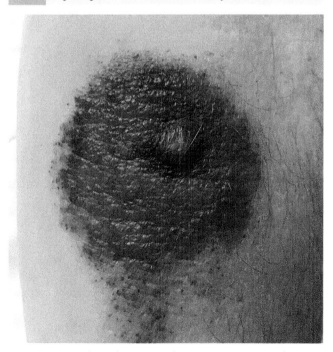

Note: Sweet syndrome has occurred at a venipuncture site due to pathergy.

Epidemiology

- Sweet syndrome is a neutrophilic dermatosis that typically presents in the fourth and fifth decades; **classic Sweet syndrome is female predominant.**
- Sweet syndrome may be divided into three subtypes:
  - **Classic:** URI (eg, *Streptococcus*) is the leading association, followed by **inflammatory disorders (eg, IBD, RA), pregnancy, and vaccinations (eg, BCG, influenza).**
  - **Malignancy-associated:** MDS and acute myeloid leukemia **(AML)** are the most common.
  - **Drug-induced: Filgrastim,** also known as **granulocyte colony-stimulating factor (G-CSF),** is the most commonly associated drug. Differentiation of malignant

clones into mature neutrophils is an established mechanism for Sweet syndrome induced by **all-trans retinoic acid (ATRA)** in acute promyelocytic leukemia (APL) and **FMS-like tyrosine kinase 3 (FLT3) inhibitors** in AML. Other drugs include **azathioprine, OCPs, sulfonamides (eg, TMP-SMX), tetracyclines, cytarabine, hypomethylators (eg, azacitidine), BRAF inhibitors, bortezomib, ICIs, and radiation therapy.**

Clinicopathological Features

- Sweet syndrome classically presents with **abrupt onset of painful edematous pseudovesicular erythematous plaques or nodules favoring the head and neck and upper extremities.** Sweet syndrome is characterized by **pathergy (new or worsening lesions secondary to trauma of the skin).**
  - Pseudovesicular lesions of Sweet syndrome are often called "juicy."
- Mucosal involvement (eg, conjunctivitis) may occur.
- Patients may exhibit **fever** and other constitutional symptoms. Systemic involvement including the **lungs** may result in death.
- **Diagnostic criteria** have been proposed (Table 2.61).
- Clinical Sweet syndrome variants include vesiculobullous and pustular, giant cellulitis-like, and necrotizing Sweet syndrome, as well as **neutrophilic dermatosis of the dorsal hands.**
  - Figure 2.93.

Evaluation

- The differential diagnosis for Sweet syndrome includes other inflammatory disorders (eg, Sweet syndrome–like neutrophilic dermatosis in SLE, RND, Wells syndrome), infections (eg, cellulitis), and malignancy (eg, leukemia cutis).

Table 2.61. DIAGNOSTIC CRITERIA FOR SWEET SYNDROME

Diagnostic criteria for Sweet Syndrome[a,b]

Major Criteria

1. Abrupt onset of typical cutaneous lesions
2. Histopathology consistent with Sweet syndrome

Minor Criteria

1. Preceded by one of the associated infections or vaccinations; accompanied by one of the associated malignancies or inflammatory disorders; associated with drug exposure or pregnancy
2. Presence of fever and constitutional signs and symptoms
3. Leukocytosis
4. Excellent response to systemic corticosteroids

[a]Both of the major and two minor criteria are required for diagnosis.
[b]Alternative diagnostic criteria have been proposed for drug-induced Sweet syndrome.

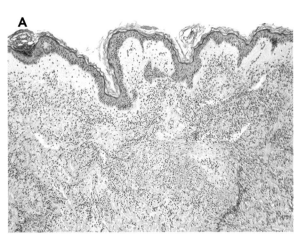 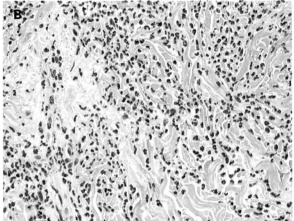

Figure 2.93. CLINICOPATHOLOGICAL CORRELATION: SWEET SYNDROME. Characteristic features are papillary dermal edema and a predominantly neutrophilic infiltrate in the dermis. Secondary vasculitis may be present. A, Low-power view. B, High power view. * Histiocytoid Sweet syndrome is controversial. Some contend that it is a variant of leukemia cutis. MPO, myeloperoxidase.

- **Histiocytoid variant:** predominantly mononuclear cell infiltrate in the dermis mimicking histiocytes but of myeloid lineage (MPO positive).*
- **Lymphocytic variant:** predominantly lymphocytic infiltrate in the dermis with immature granulocytes.
- **Subcutaneous variant:** predominantly neutrophilic infiltrate in the subcutis, often in a lobular pattern.

Marshall syndrome is a rare pediatric disorder with **Sweet syndrome–like cutaneous lesions and acquired cutis laxa.**

- There is no established guideline for the evaluation of Sweet syndrome. At a minimum, some experts recommend obtaining **sterile skin biopsy and tissue culture extending into the subcutis, CBC, and age-appropriate malignancy screening.**

Management

- Sweet syndrome may resolve spontaneously or with treatment of an associated disease or discontinuation of an associated medication; however, disease-targeted therapy is often required.
- **Systemic corticosteroids** are first line. Steroid-sparing therapies include **colchicine, dapsone, and SSKI.**
  - Excellent response to systemic corticosteroids is IN the diagnostic criteria.

"Real World" Advice

- **Age, vesiculobullous morphology,** cytopenias, elevated ESR, absence of arthralgia, and the **histiocytoid, lymphocytic, and subcutaneous variants** are reported in **association with malignancy.**
- Cutaneous lesions are often purpuric in patients with underlying malignancy due to thrombocytopenia.

NEUTROPHILIC ECCRINE HIDRADENITIS

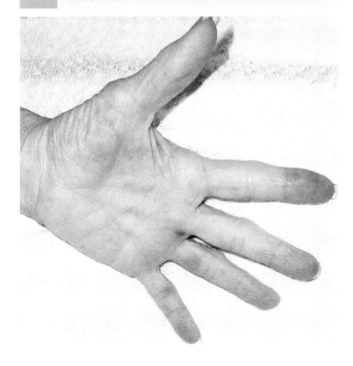

- Neutrophilic eccrine hidradenitis (NEH) classically presents 7 to 14 days after initiation of cytotoxic chemotherapies (eg, a patient with **AML** receiving **cytarabine**).
  - **Idiopathic palmoplantar hidradenitis is an NEH variant described in children.** It typically follows **vigorous physical activity** and is hypothesized to relate to eccrine gland rupture.
- NEH classically presents with **erythematous papules and plaques favoring the axillae, palms, and soles.**
  - Figure 2.94.
- NEH resolves spontaneously but may recur in subsequent chemotherapy cycles. Systemic corticosteroids and NSAIDs may reduce pain or fever; dapsone may prevent recurrences.

RECURRENT APHTHOUS STOMATITIS
Synonym: canker sores

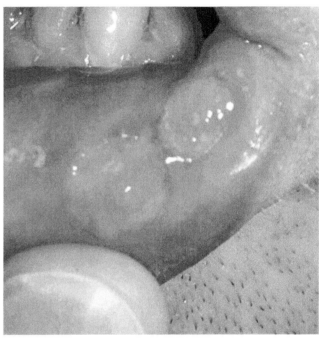

Reprinted with permission from Marder VJ, Aird WC, Bennett JS, et al. *Hemostasis and Thrombosis: Basic Principles and Clinical Practice.* 6th ed. Wolters Kluwer Health/Lippincott Williams & Wilkins; 2012.

- **Simple aphthosis** is common (20%-50% of the general population) and likely multifactorial. There are three forms: **minor, major (>1 cm),** and **herpetiform** (grouped). **Complex aphthosis** is defined by **nearly constant ≥ 3 oral aphthae or recurrent oral and genital aphthae** AND exclusion of Behçet disease. Other associated conditions include **IBD, folate and vitamin B$_{12}$ deficiencies, and HIV infection.**
  - Recurrent aphthous stomatitis occurs in hereditary disorders (eg, **cyclic neutropenia, mevalonate kinase deficiency [MKD]/hyper-IgD syndrome [HIDS]**).
- Aphthous ulcers are **painful creamy-white ulcerations surrounded by an erythematous halo favoring nonkeratinized mucosa.**
  - Figure 2.95.
  - Recurrent aphthous stomatitis is characterized by a central neutrophilic infiltrate with epithelial necrosis and a peripheral lymphocytic infiltrate.
- Local therapies include anesthetics, **corticosteroids,** and tacrolimus.

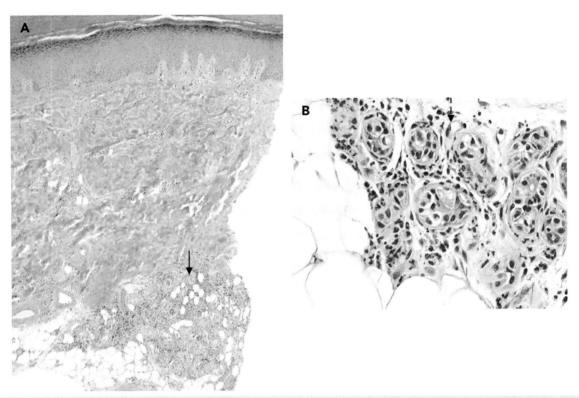

Figure 2.94. CLINICOPATHOLOGICAL CORRELATION: NEUTROPHILIC ECCRINE HIDRADENITIS. Characteristic features are degenerative vacuolar changes within secretory > ductal eccrine gland cells ± eccrine squamous syringometaplasia and a predominantly neutrophilic inflammatory infiltrate. A, Low-power view (palmoplantar skin). Solid arrow: inflammatory infiltrate surrounding eccrine glands within the subcutaneous fat. B, High-power view. Dashed arrow: eccrine necrosis with increased cytoplasmic eosinophilia and pyknotic nuclei and neutrophils and lymphocytes in the perieccrine adventitia and eccrine coil.

(Histology images reprinted with permission from Elder DE, Elenitsas R, Rosenbach M, et al. *Lever's Histopathology of the Skin.* 11th ed. Wolters Kluwer; 2015.)

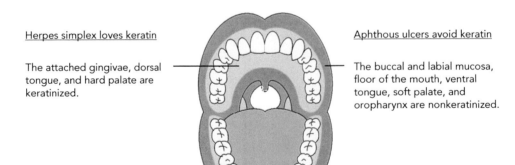

Herpes simplex loves keratin

The attached gingivae, dorsal tongue, and hard palate are keratinized.

Aphthous ulcers avoid keratin

The buccal and labial mucosa, floor of the mouth, ventral tongue, soft palate, and oropharynx are nonkeratinized.

Figure 2.95. MUCOSAL ULCERS.
(Illustration by Caroline A. Nelson, MD.)

BEHÇET DISEASE

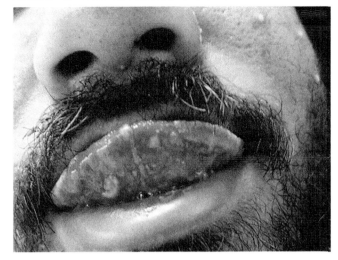

- Behçet disease is a neutrophilic dermatosis that primarily occurs along the **ancient Silk Route extending from Japan and the Korean peninsula to the Mediterranean Sea**, where **HLA-B51** is an important risk factor. **Turkey** has the highest prevalence.
- Mucocutaneous and ocular findings are summarized in the **diagnostic criteria for Behçet disease** (Table 2.62). **Aphthous stomatitis** is usually the first symptom; however, ocular involvement is the leading cause of morbidity. While **panuveitis** is most common, retinal vasculitis poses the greatest risk for blindness. Behçet disease may affect multiple other organ systems from the circulatory system (eg, **coronary arteritis, superior vena cava [SVC] thrombosis**) to the digestive system (eg, **bowel perforation**) to the joints (**asymmetric nonerosive mono- or polyarthritis**). Behçet disease may **overlap with relapsing polychondritis in MAGIC syndrome.**
  - ◈ Behçet disease exhibits vasculopathy that may affect arterial and venous vessels of all sizes in the dermis and subcutis. Early lesions are characterized by a neutrophilic vascular reaction or CSVV, while chronic lesions are characterized by a lymphocytic infiltrate.
- In 2018, the European League Against Rheumatism (EULAR) published updated treatment recommendations. For mucocutaneous involvement, strength A recommendations were:
  - ○ **Topical measures such as corticosteroids** should be used for the treatment of oral and genital ulcers. **Colchicine is first line for the prevention of recurrent mucocutaneous lesions** especially when the dominant lesion is erythema nodosum or genital ulcer.
    - ◈ Colchicine works like <u>MAGIC</u> in Behçet disease.
  - ○ Drugs such as azathioprine, thalidomide, IFN-α, TNFα inhibitors, or apremilast should be considered in selected cases.

Table 2.62. DIAGNOSTIC CRITERIA FOR BEHÇET DISEASE

The International Study Group for Behçet's Disease Criteria[a,b]

Major Criterion

Recurrent oral ulceration: minor aphthous, major aphthous, or herpetiform ulceration observed by physician or patient, which recurred at least three times in one 12-month period

Minor Criteria

1. Recurrent genital ulceration: aphthous ulceration or scarring, observed by physician or patient
2. Eye lesions: anterior uveitis, posterior uveitis, or cells in vitreous on slit lamp examination; or retinal vasculitis observed by ophthalmologist
3. Skin lesions: erythema nodosum observed by physician or patient, pseudofolliculitis, or papulopustular lesions; or acneiform nodules observed by physician in postadolescent patients not on corticosteroid treatment
4. A positive pathergy test[c]

[a]One major and two minor criteria are required for diagnosis applicable only in the absence of other clinical explanations.
[b]The International Criteria for Behçet's Disease are alternative diagnostic criteria.
[c]A papule >2 mm in size developing 24 to 48 h after oblique insertion of a 20- to 25-gauge needle 5 mm into the skin, generally performed on the forearm.

PYODERMA GANGRENOSUM
→ Diagnosis Group 1

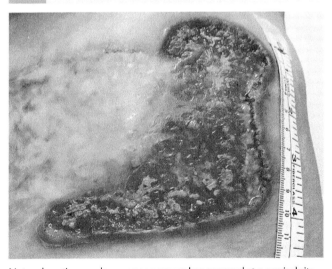

Note: ulcerative pyoderma gangrenosum has occurred at a surgical site due to pathergy.

Epidemiology

- PG is a neutrophilic dermatosis that most commonly affects middle-age women.
- Disease associations include **IBD**, inflammatory arthritis (eg, **RA**), hematologic disorders (eg, **IgA monoclonal gammopathy**), and malignancies (eg, **MDS, AML**).

Clinicopathological Features

- PG may be divided into **five subtypes:**
  - **Ulcerative: pustule that rapidly expands into an ulcer with violaceous, undermined borders, and an overhanging epidermal edge,** favoring the **pretibial** region. **Pediatric ulcerative PG** is more likely to involve the **head and anogenital region.**
  - **Bullous** (atypical): blue-gray bullae that develop rapidly and quickly erode leaving behind superficial ulcers. **Associated with hematologic malignancies.**
  - **Pustular**: multiple, tender pustules with an erythematous halo in a symmetric distribution.
  - **Vegetative** (superficial granulomatous): single superficial ulcer with verrucous growths.
  - **Peristomal**: ulcerative PG occurring around a stoma site. PG is characterized by **pathergy.** Ulcers heal with atrophic **cribriform** pigmented scars.
    - ◈ A <u>cri</u>briform scar has multiple holes, like the "slats of a <u>crib</u>."
- **Pyostomatitis vegetans** presents with **creamy-yellow tiny pustules arranged in a linear configuration** on a background of diffuse intense erythema. It favors the **labial, gingival, and buccal mucosa** and is associated with **IBD.**
  - ◈ The linear configuration of pyostomatitis vegetans may resemble a "snail track."
- Systemic involvement including the lungs is rare.
- Historically, the proposed **diagnostic criteria** classified PG as a diagnosis of exclusion (Table 2.63). More recently, this has become a subject of controversy with publication of alternative criteria (Delphi of International Experts and the PARACELSUS scoring system).
  - ◈ Figure 2.96.

Evaluation

- The differential diagnosis for ulcerative PG includes other inflammatory disorders (eg, cutaneous Crohn disease), vasculitis (eg, ANCA vasculitis, Takayasu arteritis), vascular disorders (eg, venous stasis ulcers), infections (eg, ecthyma gangrenosum), arthropod assault (eg, brown recluse spider bite), and malignancies (eg, SCC).
  - ◈ People love to blame spiders... but they are usually innocent! Brown <u>recluse</u> spiders are <u>reclusive</u>.
- There is no established guideline for the evaluation of PG; however, an **age-focused initial evaluation for PG** (Table 2.64) has been proposed. Tests should be tailored to the clinical setting.

Management

- Treatment of PG is typically divided into two stages: stopping the inflammation and healing the wound.

Table 2.63. DIAGNOSTIC CRITERIA FOR PYODERMA GANGRENOSUM

Diagnostic criteria for PG[a,b]

Major Criteria

1. Rapid progression of a painful, necrotic cutaneous ulcer with an irregular, violaceous, and undermined border[c]
2. Other causes of cutaneous ulceration have been excluded

Minor Criteria

1. History suggestive of pathergy or clinical finding of cribriform scarring
2. Systemic disease associated with PG
3. Histopathology consistent with PG
4. Treatment response[c]

PG, pyoderma gangrenosum.
[a]Both of the major and two minor criteria are required for diagnosis.
[b]The Delphi of International Experts and the PARACELSUS scoring system are alternative diagnostic criteria.
[c]Note that rapid response means decreased exudate, pain, edema, and erythema/inflammation, and not rapid wound healing; regardless of the response of the neutrophilic inflammation, wounds still take a long time to heal.

- **Systemic corticosteroids** were historically considered first line; however, the STOP-GAP clinical trial suggested equivalent efficacy for cyclosporine with fewer serious adverse events, especially infection. **Cyclosporine, TNFα inhibitors**, and the **IL-1β inhibitor canakinumab** are now also considered first line.

"Real World" Advice

- Beware of PG masquerading as "culture-negative necrotizing fasciitis."
- There is a small but clinically meaningful risk for postsurgical recurrence or exacerbation of PG, particularly with more invasive procedures and in chronic PG patients. Avoid surgical wound debridement, if possible, and exercise caution with compression wraps. If surgery is indicated, consider prophylactic immunosuppression on a case-by-case basis.
- For patients with PG and IBD, treatments with dual efficacy (eg, TNFα inhibitors) may be preferable to IBD treatments that lack efficacy for PG (eg, vedolizumab).
- For PCP prophylaxis, consider dapsone given its dual efficacy for PG.
- To evaluate treatment response in PG, look for decreasing signs of inflammation (*calor, dolor, rubor, tumor*) NOT rapid wound healing.

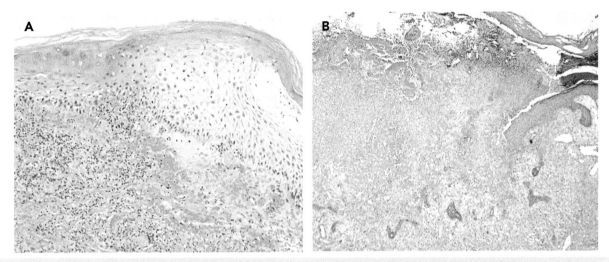

Figure 2.96. CLINICOPATHOLOGICAL CORRELATION: ULCERATIVE PYODERMA GANGRENOSUM. The border is characterized by an undermined epidermis with spongiosis or pustulation, while the center is characterized by an ulcerated epidermis with a predominantly neutrophilic infiltrate in early lesions versus a predominantly mononuclear infiltrate in chronic lesions. Secondary vasculitis may be present. A, Border. B, Center. This biopsy is from a patient with Crohn disease, as evidenced by the presence of multinucleated histiocytes within the infiltrate.

(Histology images reprinted with permission from Elder DE, Elenitsas R, Rosenbach M, et al. *Lever's Histopathology of the Skin.* 11th ed. Wolters Kluwer; 2015.)

Table 2.64. AGE-FOCUSED INITIAL EVALUATION FOR PG

Age Group	Recommended Work-Up
All patients	• A thorough history and physical examination focused on associated comorbidities and symptoms • Skin biopsy with tissue culture (bacterial, fungal, and mycobacterial) • CBC with differential • Age-appropriate malignancy screening
Targeted evaluation based on history and physical examination	• Inflammatory arthritis evaluation including anti-CCP and/or RF • Autoimmune and vasculitis evaluation including ANA and ANCA
Age < 65 y	• A thorough history and physical examination to evaluate for IBD • Low threshold for referral to gastroenterology for evaluation of IBD (including endoscopy and colonoscopy)
Age ≥ 65 y	• A thorough history and physical examination to evaluate for malignancies and hematologic disorders • Blood smear • Monoclonal gammopathy evaluation including SPEP, UPEP, and IFE • Low threshold for referral to hematology and oncology for consideration of bone marrow biopsy

ANA, antinuclear antibody; ANCA, antineutrophil cytoplasmic antibody; CBC, complete blood count; CCP, cyclic citrullinated peptide antibody; IBD, inflammatory bowel disease; IFE, immunofixation electrophoresis; PG, pyoderma gangrenosum; RF, rheumatoid factor; SPEP, serum protein electrophoresis; UPEP, urine protein electrophoresis; y, years.

SPOTLIGHT ON SYNDROMIC PYODERMA GANGRENOSUM

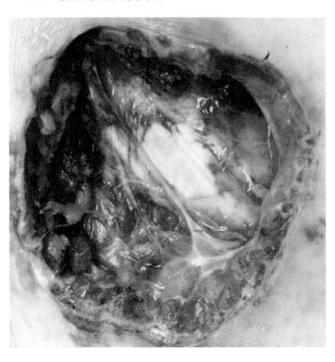

- Syndrome PG is a constellation of autoinflammatory syndromes due to mutations in proteins that form or regulate the **inflammasome** complex (eg, the *PSTPIP1* gene encoding CD2-binding protein in PAPA syndrome). The common pathway is overactivation of the innate immune system leading to increased production of **IL-1** and sterile neutrophil-rich cutaneous inflammation.
- Syndrome PG is divided into three primary disorders: **PAPA; PG, acne, and suppurative hidradenitis (PASH); and pyogenic arthritis, acne, PG, and suppurative hidradenitis (PAPASH).**
    - The histopathology of syndromic PG is similar to PG.
- Other hereditary disorders with PG-like lesions include synovitis, acne, pustulosis, hyperostosis, and osteitis (SAPHO) syndrome and primary immunodeficiencies such as leukocyte adhesion deficiency (LAD).
- Treatment of syndromic PG is similar to PG.

BOWEL-ASSOCIATED DERMATOSIS-ARTHRITIS SYNDROME
Synonym: bowel bypass syndrome

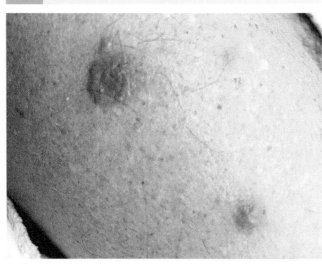

- Bowel-associated dermatosis-arthritis syndrome (BADAS) is a neutrophilic dermatosis that classically presents after **bowel bypass surgery** or in patients with **blind bowel loops.**
- BADAS **resembles serum sickness** (eg, fever, arthralgias, myalgias). The dermatosis is characterized by erythematous macules that evolve into papules and purpuric vesiculopustules and may **recur** at 4 to 6 week intervals. Patients may also develop **subcutaneous nodules.** The arthritis is typically asymmetric nonerosive polyarthritis. Diarrhea can provide a diagnostic clue.
    - The papules and vesiculopustules of BADAS overlap with Sweet syndrome, while the subcutaneous nodules may resemble erythema nodosum or exhibit lobular neutrophilic dermatosis.
- Treatment includes **antibiotics** (eg, tetracyclines), **bowel reanastamosis** (curative), and anti-inflammatories.
    - Bowel reanastamosis is <u>BADAS</u> because, by stopping bacterial overgrowth in the blind bowel loops, it stops immune complex deposition and cures <u>BADAS</u>.

GRANULOMA FACIALE

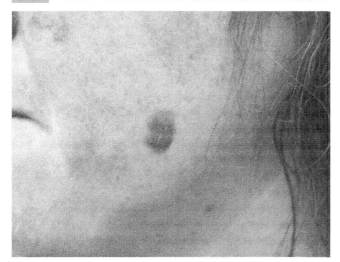

Reprinted with permission from Stedman TL. *Stedman's Medical Dictionary for the Health Professions and Nursing.* 6th ed. Wolters Kluwer Health/Lippincott Williams & Wilkins; 2007.

- Granuloma faciale most often presents as a localized cutaneous disease; however, it may be a cutaneous manifestation of immunoglobulin G4–related disease (IgG4-RD). It is classified as both a variant of CSVV and an eosinophilic dermatosis.
- Granuloma faciale classically presents with a **single asymptomatic red-brown plaque on the face**, but lesions may be multiple and extrafacial. **Follicular prominence**, a *peau d'orange* appearance, and telangiectasias have been described.
  - Figure 2.97.

- Treatment includes **corticosteroids, calcineurin inhibitors, and dapsone.** Destructive therapies (eg, cryosurgery) have been reported, but efficacy is limited and the risk of scarring is significant. **Vascular lasers** may be efficacious.

EOSINOPHILIC PUSTULAR FOLLICULITIS

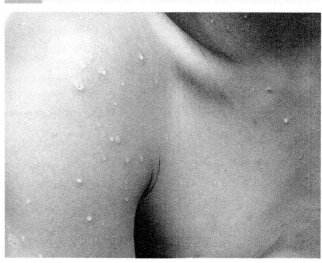

- Eosinophilic pustular folliculitis (EPF) is classified as both a superficial folliculitis and an eosinophilic dermatosis. Variants include:
  - **Ofuji disease**: primarily occurs in **Japan** with a **male:female ratio of ~5:1.**
    - Figure 2.98.

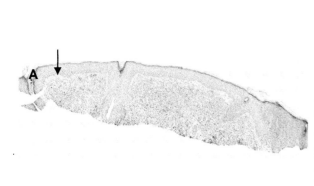
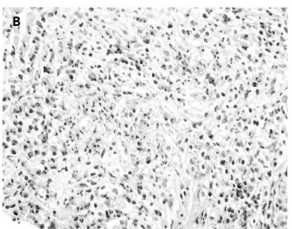

Figure 2.97. CLINICOPATHOLOGICAL CORRELATION: GRANULOMA FACIALE. A mixed dermal infiltrate with eosinophils, neutrophils, lymphocytes, and plasma cells spares the papillary dermis (Grenz zone). Early lesions often demonstrate CSVV, while chronic lesions often demonstrate concentric fibrosis. A, Low-power view. Solid arrow: Grenz zone. B, High-power view. CSVV, cutaneous small-vessel vasculitis; EED, erythema elevatum diutinum.

(Histology images reprinted with permission from Elder DE, Elenitsas R, Rosenbach M, et al. *Lever's Histopathology of the Skin.* 11th ed. Wolters Kluwer; 2015.)

Concentric fibrosis may be described as "onion skinning."
Granuloma faciale is a misnomer. Remember "Grenz faciale." Apart from the facial location, granuloma faciale can NOT be distinguished from EED on histopathology.

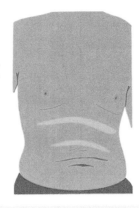

Do NOT confuse <u>Ofuji</u> disease with papuloerythroderma of <u>Ofuji</u>. Both are eosinophilic dermatoses that primarily occur in Japanese men, but the classic lesions of papuloerythroderma of Ofuji are red-brown papules that may coalesce into erythroderma sparing the skin folds.

If you see the "deck-chair sign," beware of associated infections (eg, HCV, HIV), malignancies (eg, T cell lymphoma, gastric carcinoma), and drugs (eg, NSAIDs).

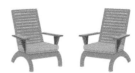

Figure 2.98. THE DECK-CHAIR SIGN. HCV, hepatitis C virus; HIV, human immunodeficiency virus; NSAIDs, nonsteroidal anti-inflammatory drugs.

(Illustration by Caroline A. Nelson, MD.)

○ **HIV-associated EPF:** primarily occurs with **CD4 count < 250 cells/mm³** or in immune reconstitution inflammatory syndrome (IRIS).

   EPF of infancy.

- EPF classically presents with **recurrent crops of intensely pruritic, grouped, follicular pustules and papulopustules in a seborrheic distribution.** EPF may be associated with **peripheral hypereosinophilia.**

   EPF of infancy favors the **scalp** and resolves spontaneously.
   ◆ Figure 2.99.

- **Papular pruritic eruption (PPE) of HIV** is characterized by **severe pruritus and skin-colored to erythematous, nonfollicular papules symmetrically distributed on the trunk and extremities.** It primary occurs with **CD4 count < 50 cells/mm³.** Some authors consider PPE of HIV to be on the same spectrum as HIV-associated EPF.

- **Indomethacin** is first line for Ofuji disease. **Antiretroviral therapy (ART)** improves HIV-associated EPF and should be continued, even in IRIS.

   EPF of infancy is self-limited.

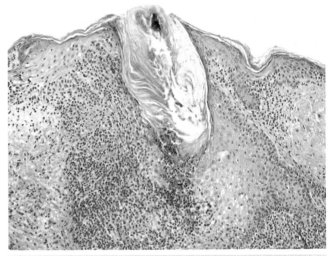

Figure 2.99. CLINICOPATHOLOGICAL CORRELATION: EOSINOPHILIC PUSTULAR FOLLICULITIS. Characteristic features are exocytosis of eosinophils and lymphocytes into the follicular epithelium and infundibular eosinophilic pustules.

(Histology image reprinted with permission from Elder DE, Elenitsas R, Rosenbach M, et al. *Lever's Histopathology of the Skin.* 11th ed. Wolters Kluwer; 2015.)

WELLS SYNDROME
Synonym: eosinophilic cellulitis

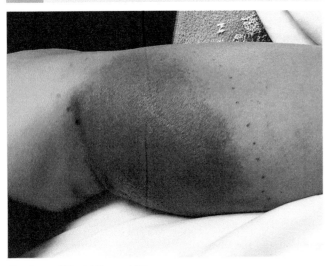

Courtesy of Daniel Yanes, MD.

- Wells syndrome is an eosinophilic dermatosis. Some experts consider Wells syndrome a manifestation of persistent bite reaction.

- **Prodromal pruritus** is typically followed by the eruption of **edematous erythematous plaques or nodules favoring the extremities.** Patients may exhibit constitutional symptoms, and Wells syndrome may be associated with **peripheral hypereosinophilia.**
   ◆ Figure 2.100.

- **Topical and/or systemic corticosteroids** are first line depending on disease severity.

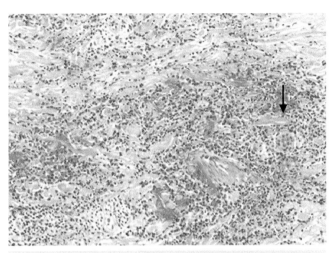

Figure 2.100. CLINICOPATHOLOGICAL CORRELATION: WELLS SYNDROME. Characteristic features are papillary dermal edema and a predominantly eosinophilic infiltrate in the dermis. Collagen fibers are coated with eosinophil granule proteins (eg, MBP). Solid arrow: "flame figure." MBP, major basic protein.

(Histology image reprinted with permission from Elder DE, Elenitsas R, Rubin AI, et al. *Atlas of Dermatopathology: Synopsis and Atlas of Lever's Histopathology of the Skin.* 4th ed. Wolters Kluwer; 2020.)

> Collagen fibers coated with eosinophil granule proteins are called "flame figures."

HYPEREOSINOPHILIC SYNDROME

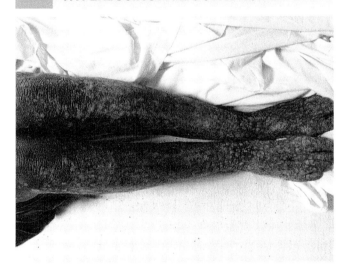

Lymphoid variant courtesy of Douglas Pugliese, MD, MPH.

- Hypereosinophilic syndrome (HES) was classified by the Working Conference on Eosinophil Disorders and Syndromes into three variants:
  - **Primary (neoplastic) HES$_N$:** underlying stem cell, myeloid, or eosinophilic neoplasm. Rearranged *PDGFRA*, *PDGFRB*, or *FGFR1* genes are classic, specifically *FIP1L1/ PDGFRA* + **chronic eosinophilic leukemia.**
  - **Secondary (reactive) HES$_R$:** underlying condition/disease in which eosinophils are considered nonclonal cells.

In **lymphoid variant HES**, cytokine production (eg, IL-4, IL-5, and IL-13) by clonal T cells leads to **peripheral hypereosinophilia and elevated IgE.** This variant is benign but carries an **increased risk of lymphoma.**
  - **Idiopathic HES:** no underlying cause.
- A diversity of cutaneous lesions has been observed, ranging from pruritic erythematous macules, papules, plaques, or nodules to urticaria to angioedema. **Mucosal ulcers are a poor prognostic sign.** Patients may exhibit constitutional symptoms. The proposed **diagnostic criteria** for HES are:
  - **Peripheral hypereosinophilia:** >1500/µL (on two examinations at a ≥1 month interval except when immediate therapy is required because of hypereosinophilia-related organ dysfunction) and/or tissue hypereosinophilia.
  - AND **organ damage and/or dysfunction** attributable to tissue hypereosinophilia.
  - AND exclusion of other disorders or conditions as major reason for organ damage.

Mucocutaneous involvement is included in the definition of eosinophil-related organ damage, along with **fibrosis (eg, endomyocardial fibrosis)**, thrombosis ± thromboembolism, neuropathy, and other less common organ manifestations. **CHF is the leading cause of death.**

  ◈ HES has nonspecific histopathology. Papules and plaques often resemble Wells syndrome, while wheels resemble urticaria.

- **Imatinib** (in combination with systemic corticosteroids to prevent cardiac exacerbation) is often effective in patients with HES$_N$ due to *PDGFR* fusion genes. **Systemic corticosteroids** are first line for HES$_R$.

  Analogous to imatinib for *BCR/ABL* + CML (the infamous "Philadelphia chromosome").

Noninfectious Granulomas, Histiocytoses, and Xanthomas

Basic Concepts

- **Noninfectious granulomas** are characterized by **sterile, histiocytic inflammation. Upregulation of CD4+ T helper cells of the Th1 subtype** is a key pathogenetic mechanism in granuloma formation.

  ◈ Granulomas may be classified as sarcoidal (epithelioid histiocytes with a paucity of surrounding infiltrate), tuberculoid (histiocytes with a peripheral lymphocytic infiltrate ± central caseous necrosis), palisading (histiocytes enclosing altered collagen, mucin, and/or foreign body), or suppurative (histiocytes with a central collection of neutrophils [stellate abscess]).

- **Histiocytoses** are characterized by **abnormal accumulation of histiocytes.** Histiocytes derive from a **common CD34+ progenitor cell in the bone marrow.** Class I refers to LCH, class II refers to non-LCHs, and class III refers to malignant histiocytoses (eg, Langerhans cell sarcoma).

◆ Histiocytoses are primarily distinguished by immunohistochemistry (IHC). While LCH is positive for CD1a, Langerin (CD207), and S100, non-LCHs are negative for CD1a, Langerin, and S100 and positive for CD68, CD163, and factor XIIIa (variable). Exceptions include indeterminate cell histiocytosis (CD1a and S100+) and Rosai-Dorfman disease (S100+).

- **Xanthomas** are characterized by **intracellular and dermal lipid deposition.**
  ◆ Xanthomas demonstrate lipid-laden macrophages (foam cells) in the dermis.

SARCOIDOSIS
→ Diagnosis Group 2

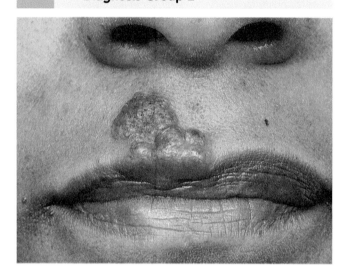

Epidemiology

- Sarcoidosis is a systemic granulomatous disorder that has not been definitively linked to a trigger such as a pathogen or foreign body.
- Sarcoidosis has a bimodal age distribution. In the United States, the incidence is highest in **African American women.**
- Drug associations with sarcoidal granulomatous eruptions include **TNFα inhibitors, BRAF inhibitors, IFNs, ICIs, and alemtuzumab.**

Clinicopathological Features

- Cutaneous sarcoidosis, in up to one third of patients, classically presents with **red-brown to violaceous papules and plaques favoring the face** (periorificial) **and sites of prior injury** (eg, scars, tattoos).
- Sarcoidosis may be associated with secondary **scarring alopecia.**
- EN is a nonspecific cutaneous manifestation and portends a **good prognosis. Ichthyosis vulgaris** may also occur.
- The **lung is the most common site** of systemic involvement (90%-95%), with end-stage **honeycombing** of the

parenchyma. Other sites include the heart (eg, **palpitations, sudden death, CHF**), endocrine system (eg, **hypercalcemia due to sarcoidal calcitriol synthesis**), lymph nodes (eg, **hilar and/or paratracheal lymphadenopathy**), liver and spleen, musculoskeletal system, nervous system, eyes (eg, **anterior > posterior uveitis**), kidneys (eg, **nephrolithiasis/hypercalciuria**), and upper respiratory tract.

- Sarcoidosis variants are summarized in Table 2.65.
- Tattoo reactions are summarized in Table 2.66.
  ◆ Table 2.67; Figure 2.101.

Evaluation

- Sarcoidosis is a diagnosis of exclusion. **Noncaseating granulomas**, an important clue, may be present in foreign body reactions and other granulomatous disorders, most notably **cutaneous Crohn disease and granulomatous cheilitis.** The former is characterized by erythematous plaques, lymphedema, and **cobblestoning/ulcers of the oral and anogenital mucosa**, while the latter is characterized by **persistent lip swelling. Melkersson-Rosenthal syndrome describes the triad of granulomatous cheilitis with a fissured tongue and facial nerve palsy.**
  ◆ Ulcers in cutaneous Crohn disease are often described as "knifelike."
  Umbilical granuloma is the most common neonatal umbilical abnormality, often treated with **silver nitrate cauterization or topical corticosteroids.**
- Upon **diascopy**, sarcoidosis lesions have the color of **apple jelly.**
- Historically, the **Kveim-Sitzbach test** was used to demonstrate sarcoidal granuloma formation in the skin following injection of a tissue suspension prepared from sarcoidal spleen. It is now rarely performed.
- An algorithm for the evaluation of cutaneous sarcoidosis patients has been proposed. Initial testing may include **punch biopsy with special stains ± tissue culture, CMP, CBC, TFTs, UA, PPD or IFN-γ release assay, vitamin D$_{25}$, vitamin D$_{1,25}$, CXR, PFTs with DLCO, ECG ± Holter monitor, TTE and cardiac PET/CT or MRI, and ophthalmology referral.**

Management

- The treatment of cutaneous sarcoidosis may be dictated by the severity of other organ system involvement. For example, pulmonary sarcoidosis is typically treated with **systemic corticosteroids.**
- A stepwise approach to the treatment of cutaneous sarcoidosis has been proposed. Mild disease may be controlled with local therapies (eg, **high-potency topical or intralesional corticosteroids**). Steroid-sparing agents progress from immunomodulatory agents (eg, **antimalarials, tetracycline antibiotics**) to immunosuppressive agents (eg, **methotrexate**) to biologic agents (eg, **TNFα inhibitors**). **JAK inhibitors** are an emerging treatment option.

Table 2.65. SARCOIDOSIS VARIANTS

Variant[a]	Classic Description	Notes
Darier-Roussy (sarcoidal panniculitis)	Painless firm subcutaneous nodules.	
Heerfordt syndrome (uveoparotid fever)	Fever, parotid gland enlargement, CN palsy (eg, facial), and uveitis.	
Löfgren syndrome	Triad of EN, bilateral hilar lymphadenopathy, and acute polyarthritis.	Most common in Scandinavian whites. Good prognosis.
Do NOT confuse Löfgren syndrome with Löffler syndrome.		
Lupus pernio	Violaceous papules and plaques on the nose and cheeks.	Associated with upper respiratory tract and lung involvement. Poor prognosis.
Do NOT confuse lupus pernio with lupus erythematosus, lupus miliaris disseminatus faciei, or lupus vulgaris.	Lupus pernio may have a "beaded" appearance along the nasal rim.	
Mikulicz syndrome	Bilateral enlargement of the parotid, sublingual, lacrimal, or submandibular glands ± sicca symptoms.	

CN, cranial nerve; EN, erythema nodosum.
[a]Illustrative examples provided.

Table 2.66. TATTOO REACTIONS

Tattoo[a]	Classic Description	Notes
Black	Carbon or iron oxide.	
Blue	Cobalt blue.	
Brown	Ferric oxide.	Amalgam and ferric subsulfate (Monsel solution) cause iatrogenic superficial brown tattoos due to accidental implantation during dental procedures or hemostasis, respectively.
Green	Chromic oxide.	Chromium leaching from cement or fresh concrete may cause ACD.
Purple	Manganese ammonium pyrophosphate.	
Red	Cinnabar/mercury sulfide or cadmium red.	Red tattoo pigment is the leading cause of eczematous, lichenoid, granulomatous, and pseudolymphomatous tattoo reactions.
White	Zinc oxide or titanium dioxide.	Laser-induced reduction of metallic compounds used in certain pigments (eg, titanium dioxide) may lead to tattoo darkening.
		Zinc oxide and titanium dioxide go ON white (physical sunscreens) and go IN white (tattoos).
Yellow	Cadmium yellow.	Yellow tattoo pigment is the leading cause of phototoxic tattoo reactions.
	Cadmium sulfide is yellow like the inside of a Cadbury cream egg.	Yellow is the color of the "sun."

ACD, allergic contact dermatitis.
[a]Illustrative examples provided.

Table 2.67. HISTOPATHOLOGICAL FEATURES OF SARCOIDOSIS AND FOREIGN BODY GRANULOMAS

Diagnosis[a]	Classic Description	Notes
Sarcoidosis		
Sarcoidosis	Epithelioid histiocytes with a paucity of surrounding infiltrate. Granulomas are typically noncaseating and may demonstrate asteroid bodies (eosinophilic "starburst" inclusions in giant cells) and/or Schaumann bodies (cytoplasmic, laminated calcifications).	The most common cause of sarcoidal granulomas is foreign body reaction.
	Due to the paucity of surrounding infiltrate, sarcoidal granulomas are often called "naked granulomas."	
Tissue Augmentation		
HA	Pale bluish material.	
Paraffin	Collection of vacuoles.	Sclerosing lipogranuloma refers to a predominantly lobular panniculitis typically due to self-injection of paraffin or silicone (eg, into penis).
	"Swiss cheese" appearance.	
Silicone	Collection of vacuoles.	
	"Swiss cheese" appearance.	
Crystals		
Silica	Colorless crystals. Birefringent.	Found in sand, soil, rocks, and glass. Associated with blast injuries.
Talc	Needle-shaped or round crystals. Birefringent.	Found in deodorant and dusting powders.
	"Maltese cross-like" appearance.	
Zinc	Rhomboidal crystals. Birefringent.	Iatrogenic (insulin-zinc injection sites).
Other Nonbiologic Foreign Bodies		
Aluminum	Basophilic granular material within the cytoplasm of histiocytes.	Iatrogenic (aluminum-containing vaccine injection sites and aluminum chloride hemostasis).
Beryllium		Found in fluorescent lamps (historical). Check BAL for lung involvement.
		Beryllium is berylliant.
Corticosteroid	Pale bluish material.	Found at sites of intralesional injection.
Gel foam	Blue-purple material.	Iatrogenic (hemostasis).
	"Arabesque net-like" pattern.	
Suture	Birefringent material.	Iatrogenic (surgery).
	Linear.	
Zirconium		Found in antiperspirants.
		Zirconium makes you smell zestfully clean.
Other Biologic Foreign Bodies		
Keratin	Birefringent material.	Found at sites of ruptured follicles, cysts, and ingrown hairs or nails.
Sea urchin spines	Calcite crystals. Birefringent.	Other animal foreign bodies include arthropod, jellyfish, and coral parts.
Starch	Ovoid basophilic granules. Birefringent. PAS positive.	Iatrogenic (surgery).
Wood splinter	Orderly arrangement of rectangular cells. Birefringent. PAS positive.	Obtain special stains to evaluate for infection. Other plant foreign bodies include cactus and prickly pear spines.

BAL, bronchoalveolar lavage; HA, hyaluronic acid; PAS, periodic acid-Schiff.
[a]Illustrative examples provided.

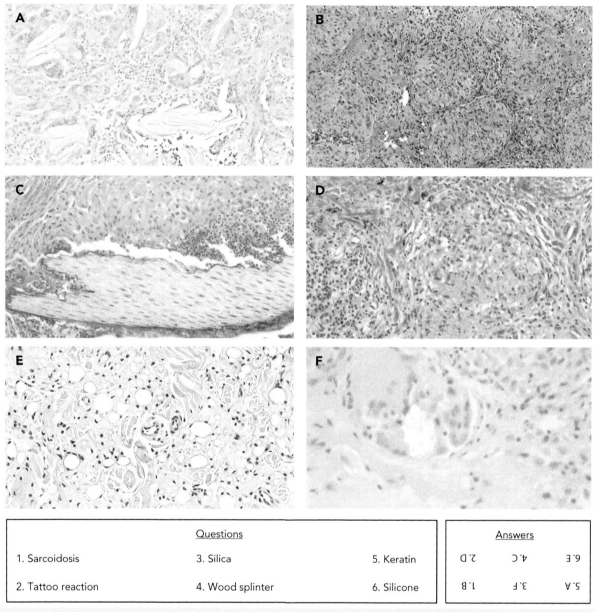

Questions			Answers		
1. Sarcoidosis	3. Silica	5. Keratin	6. E	4. C	2. D
2. Tattoo reaction	4. Wood splinter	6. Silicone	5. A	3. F	1. B

Figure 2.101. MATCHING EXERCISE: SARCOIDOSIS AND FOREIGN BODY GRANULOMAS. A, Keratin. Birefringent. Note the neutrophils and histiocytes surrounding cornified cells. B, Sarcoidosis. Note the epithelioid histiocytes with a paucity of surrounding infiltrate ("naked granulomas"). The granulomas of sarcoidosis are typically noncaseating and may demonstrate asteroid bodies (eosinophilic "starburst" inclusions in giant cells) and/or Schaumann bodies (cytoplasmic, laminated calcifications). C, Wood splinter. Note the orderly arrangement of rectangular cells, typical of plant material. Birefringent. PAS positive. D, Tattoo reaction. Note the granulomatous reaction to red tattoo pigment. E, Silicone. Note the Swiss cheese appearance. F, Silica. Birefringent. For the histopathology of aluminum chloride and Monsel solution, see Figure 8.21. For the histopathology of gel foam and suture, see Figure 8.22. PAS, periodic acid-Schiff.

(A, Histology image courtesy of Noel Turner, MD, MHS and Christine J. Ko, MD. C, Histology image reprinted with permission from Elder DE, Elenitsas R, Rosenbach M, et al. *Lever's Histopathology of the Skin*. 11th ed. Wolters Kluwer; 2015. D, Histology image reprinted with permission from Elder DE, Elenitsas R, Rosenbach M, et al. *Lever's Histopathology of the Skin*. 11th ed. Wolters Kluwer; 2015. F, Histology image reprinted with permission from Elder DE, Elenitsas R, Rosenbach M, et al. *Lever's Histopathology of the Skin*. 11th ed. Wolters Kluwer; 2015.)

"Real World" Advice

- The presence of a foreign body does not rule out sarcoidosis (eg, sarcoidosis often presents in tattoos).
- An elevated serum **angiotensin-converting enzyme (ACE)** level is present in ~**60%** of patients. While it may aid in the diagnosis (especially at 2-3 times the upper limit of normal), it is nonspecific and has a ~**10% false-positive rate.** As such, the ACE level has greater utility for monitoring disease progression.
- Granulomatous inflammation is slow to respond; therefore, patients should be advised to maintain a therapeutic regimen for at least 3 months before determining its efficacy.

SPOTLIGHT ON BLAU SYNDROME

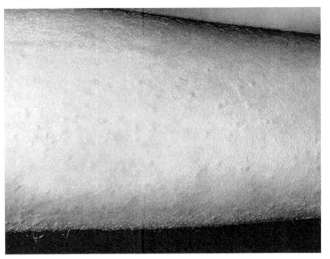

Courtesy of Lisa Arkin, MD. From Gru AA, Wick MR, Mir A, et al. *Pediatric Dermatopathology and Dermatology*. Wolters Kluwer; 2018.

- Blau syndrome (early-onset sarcoidosis) is an **NF-kβ–related autoinflammatory syndrome** due to **AD *NOD2/CARD15*** mutation.
- Blau syndrome classically presents in early childhood with a **triad of granulomatous dermatitis (widespread red-brown papules), arthritis, and uveitis.** The PIP joints may develop a contracture (**camptodactyly**). Extra-triad manifestations, such as fever, are also observed.
    - Blau syndrome demonstrates sarcoidal granulomas.
- Systemic corticosteroids are first line.

GRANULOMA ANNULARE
→ Diagnosis Group 1

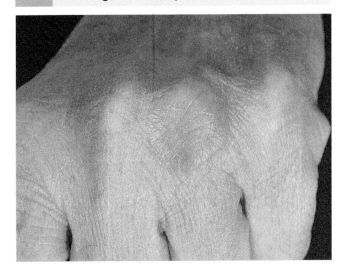

Epidemiology

- Granuloma annulare (GA) is a benign, typically self-limited granulomatous disorder.
- GA most often affects **children and young adults** with a **~2:1 female:male ratio.**

Clinicopathological Features

- The classic lesions of GA are **papules coalescing into arciform and annular plaques.** Macules, papules ± central perforation, and subcutaneous nodules have also been described.
- Lesion distribution varies based on the **clinical GA variant** (Table 2.68).
    - **Subcutaneous GA is the most common variant in children.**
    - Figure 2.102.

Table 2.68. CLINICAL GRANULOMA ANNULARE VARIANTS

Variant[a]	Distribution	Notes
Localized	Favors the dorsal hands and feet.	Most common. May develop within herpes zoster scars or at BCG vaccination sites.
Generalized	Favors the trunk and extremities.	Associated with diabetes mellitus, hyperlipidemia, thyroid disorders, and (rarely) infection (eg, HBV, HCV, HIV), vaccinations (eg, HBV), malignancy, or drugs (eg, TNFα inhibitors).
Subcutaneous	Favors the lower extremities.	

BCG, Bacillus Calmette-Guérin; HBV, hepatitis B virus; HCV, hepatitis C virus; HIV, human immunodeficiency virus.
[a]Illustrative examples provided.

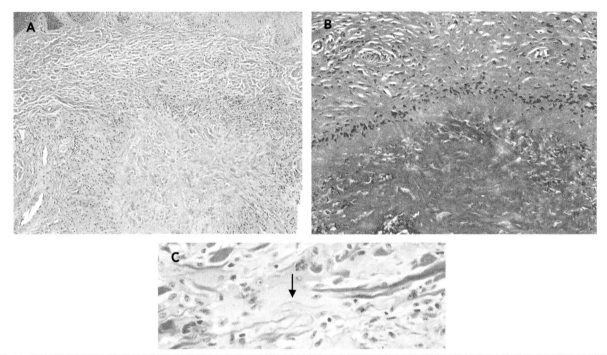

Figure 2.102. SIDE-BY-SIDE COMPARISON: GRANULOMA ANNULARE AND RHEUMATOID NODULE. Both GA and rheumatoid nodules display a nodular infiltrate of palisading granulomas. GA palisades around altered dermal collagen and mucin in the upper-to-mid reticular dermis. A rheumatoid nodule palisades around fibrin in the deep dermis and subcutis. Annular elastolytic giant cell granuloma, which some consider a GA variant, is characterized by solar elastosis, elastic fibers engulfed by palisading histiocytes, and central loss of elastic tissue. A, GA. B, Rheumatoid nodule. C. Annular elastolytic giant cell granuloma. Solid arrow: elastolysis. DF, dermatofibroma; GA, granuloma annulare.

(Histology images A and C reprinted with permission from Elder DE, Elenitsas R, Rosenbach M, et al. *Lever's Histopathology of the Skin.* 11th ed. Wolters Kluwer; 2015.)

GA:
- **Interstitial variant:** patchy interstitial histiocytes, lymphocytes, and mucin.
- **Deep variant:** histiocytes palisading around fibrin in the subcutis (pseudorheumatoid nodule).

GA is a blue granuloma. A rheumatoid nodule is a red granuloma.
The "busy dermis" of interstitial GA may also describe scleromyxedema, blue nevus, dermal Spitz nevus, DF, patch-stage Kaposi sarcoma, neurofibroma, and metastatic breast carcinoma.

Evaluation

- The differential diagnosis for classic GA includes annular sarcoidosis and **annular elastolytic giant cell granuloma**, which some consider a GA variant. Distribution is an important clue as this disorder occurs most often on **chronically sun-exposed sites (eg, the head and neck).**
- **Reactive granulomatous dermatitis** is an umbrella term used to describe two closely related disorders that, like GA, demonstrate palisading granulomas on histopathology:
  - **IGD with arthritis: annular plaques or linear cords** in patients with **RA or seronegative arthritis.**
    - Linear cords in IGD are termed the "rope sign."
    - IGD demonstrates rosettes of palisading histiocytes.

- **PNGD: symmetric umbilicated papules favoring the elbows and extensor digits** in patients with **SLE, RA, and GPA/EGPA.**
  - CSVV is present in early lesions of PNGD, while neutrophils and granulomatous inflammation are present in fully developed lesions.

Both of these disorders must be distinguished from **interstitial granulomatous drug eruption.** Drug associations include **CCBs > TNFα inhibitors and statins.**

Management

- **Spontaneous resolution (~50% of patients within 2 years)** is the norm for localized GA, but recurrence is common.

- Observation ± local therapies (eg, **high-potency topical or intralesional corticosteroids**) are first line. Steroid-sparing therapies for generalized GA include antimalarials, tetracyclines, dapsone, and phototherapy.

"Real World" Advice

- Patients are often concerned about cosmetic disfigurement; therefore, counseling that GA rarely spreads to the head and neck can provide reassurance.

NECROBIOSIS LIPOIDICA
→ **Diagnosis Group 2**
Synonym: necrobiosis lipoidica diabeticorum

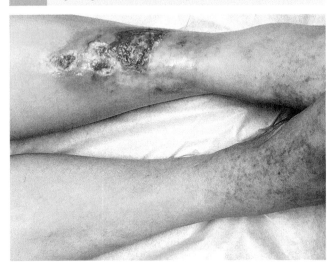

Epidemiology

- Necrobiosis lipoidica (NL) is a granulomatous disorder. The pathogenesis is unknown; however, a primary role for **immunologically mediated vascular disease leading to collagen degeneration and inflammation** has been hypothesized.
- NL is most common in **adult women.**
- **Diabetes mellitus is common in NL (~60%), but NL is rare in diabetes mellitus (~0.3%). There is no proven association between glycemic control and the likelihood of developing NL.** However, there is a higher reported rate of complications (eg, **limited joint mobility, peripheral neuropathy, retinopathy**). Other associations include hypertension, dyslipidemia, obesity, and thyroid disease.
  - The historical name for NL was necrobiosis lipoidica diabeticorum (NLD).

Clinicopathological Features

- NL classically presents with **yellow-orange, atrophic, telangiectatic plaques with a violaceous rim** that may ulcerate. Lesions are typically bilateral and favor the **pretibial** region. **Hypohidrosis** and secondary **scarring alopecia** can be observed, along with **decreased sensation to pinprick and fine touch.**

- Rarely, SCC may develop within NL lesions.
  - ◆ Figure 2.103.

Evaluation

- The differential diagnosis includes other granulomatous disorders (eg, GA), histiocytoses (eg, necrobiotic xanthogranuloma [NXG]), lipodermatosclerosis, and diabetic dermopathy.
- NL is a clinical diagnosis; however, a punch biopsy may be helpful in atypical cases.

Management

- Treatment should be directed toward the underlying disorder (eg, glycemic control).
- Local therapies (eg, **high-potency topical or intralesional corticosteroids**) are first line. Steroid-sparing therapies may be directed at the vascular disease component (eg, pentoxifylline) or the inflammation component (eg, antimalarials, tetracyclines).

"Real World" Advice

- Preventative measures (eg, elastic support stockings) are important to minimize trauma and ulceration.

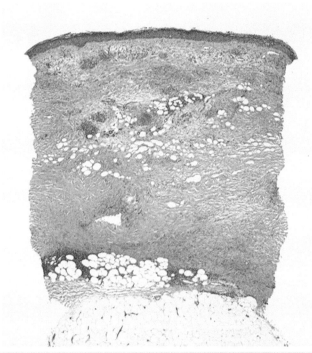

Figure 2.103. CLINICOPATHOLOGICAL CORRELATION: NECROBIOSIS LIPOIDICA. NL is characterized by horizontal layers of necrobiotic collagen and palisading granulomas. There is top-to-bottom, side-to-side involvement with sclerosis, resulting in a square punch. The inflammatory infiltrate is composed of histiocytes and lymphocytes with plasma cells located at the dermal subcutaneous junction. NL, necrobiosis lipoidica.

(Histology image reprinted with permission from Gru AA, Wick MR, Mir A, et al. *Pediatric Dermatopathology and Dermatology.* Wolters Kluwer; 2018.)

Horizontal layers of necrobiotic collagen and palisading granulomas may resemble "tiers of a layer cake."

LANGERHANS CELL HISTIOCYTOSIS
Synonyms: class I histiocytosis, histiocytosis X

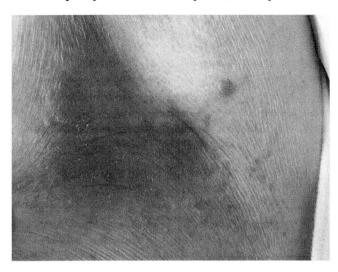

- LCH is a clonal proliferative disorder of Langerhans cells.
- LCH represents a disease spectrum **historically classified into four disorders** (Table 2.69). Today, LCH is generally considered one disease. Oral and anogenital mucosal involvement can occur. In **infants**, LCH is in the differential diagnosis for **diaper dermatitis.**
  ◈ Figure 2.104.
- At a minimum, all LCH patients should undergo **hematologic, pulmonary, hepatosplenic, renal, and skeletal evaluation.**
- **Prognosis depends on involvement of "risk organs"** (hematopoietic system, liver, lungs, and/or spleen). Local therapies (eg, high-potency topical corticosteroids) are first line. **BRAF inhibitors** are now included among the treatment options for refractory or multisystem LCH with *BRAF V600E* mutations.

Table 2.69. HISTORICAL CLASSIFICATION OF LANGERHANS CELL HISTIOCYTOSIS

Diagnosis	Classic Description	Notes
Letterer-Siwe disease	Onset between 0 and 2 years of age of skin-colored papules, pustules, and/or vesicles with frequent scale, crust, petechiae, and purpura. Lesions favor the scalp, flexural areas, and trunk with visceral and bone lesions.	Poor prognosis.
	Letterer-Siwe disease is littered in a seborrheic distribution.	
Hand-Schüller-Christian disease	Onset between 2 and 6 years of age with lesions similar to Letterer-Siwe disease. Systemic features include DI, bone lesions, and exophthalmos.	Treat DI with vasopressin.
	The three eponyms Hand, Schüller, and Christian describe a triad: DI, bone lesions, and exophthalmos.	
Eosinophilic granuloma	Onset between 7 and 12 years of age with rare skin involvement. Single osteolytic lesion of the cranium is characteristic.	Chronic otitis media may be the presenting sign.
Congenital self-healing reticulohistiocytosis (Hashimoto-Pritzker disease)	Congenital onset of widespread red-purple-brown papulonodules.	Typically self-limited.
	Congenital self-healing reticulohistiocytosis is in the differential diagnosis of "blueberry muffin" lesions.	

DI, diabetes insipidus.

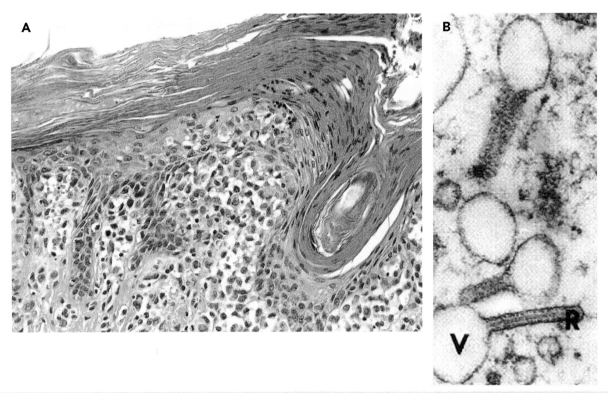

Figure 2.104. CLINICOPATHOLOGICAL CORRELATION: LANGERHANS CELL HISTIOCYTOSIS. Characteristic features are spongiosis and Langerhans cells accumulating at the DEJ. On electron microscopy, Birbeck or Langerhans granules consist of a vesicle and a rod. A, H&E. B, EM. V: vesicle. R: rod. DEJ, dermal-epidermal junction; H&E, hematoxylin and eosin.

(Histology and electron microscopy images reprinted with permission from Elder DE, Elenitsas R, Rosenbach M, et al. *Lever's Histopathology of the Skin.* 11th ed. Wolters Kluwer; 2015.)

Langerhans cells have "kidney bean–shaped" nuclei and "tennis racquet–shaped" granules on electron microscopy.

NECROBIOTIC XANTHOGRANULOMA

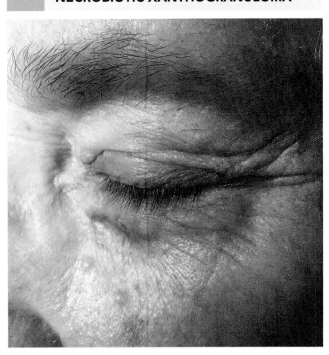

- NXG is a **non-LCH.** NXG typically presents in the sixth decade in association with **monoclonal gammopathy (most often IgG-κ), due to plasma cell dyscrasias or lymphoproliferative disorders.**
    - κ resembles the "X" in N<u>X</u>G.
  Non-LCHs in adults are summarized in Table 2.70.
    - Figure 2.105.
      Non-LCHs in children are summarized in Table 2.71.
- Cutaneous findings are summarized in the proposed **diagnostic criteria for NXG** (Table 2.72). NXG patients may exhibit a low high-density lipoprotein cholesterol (HDL-C) phenotype. Systemic involvement including the heart, gastrointestinal tract, liver, **eye**, and lung may result in death.
    - Figure 2.106.
- NXG exists on a spectrum with **normolipemic plane xanthoma.**
- Low-dose corticosteroids plus chlorambucil were historically considered to be the most effective treatment for NXG; however, **IVIG** is an emerging therapeutic option.

Table 2.70. NON-LANGERHANS CELL HISTIOCYTOSES IN ADULTS

Diagnosis[a]	Classic Description	Notes
Erdheim-Chester disease	Red-brown to yellow nodules and indurated plaques with visceral and bone lesions.	Poor prognosis. Associated with *BRAF* V600E mutations.
Generalized eruptive histiocytoma	Recurrent crops of numerous, small, red-brown papules.	Associated with leukemia. Self-limited.
HLH (secondary)	Protean cutaneous manifestation. 5/8 diagnostic criteria required: (1) fever for >7 days; (2) splenomegaly; (3) cytopenias; (4) hypertriglyceridemia or hypofibrinogenemia; (5) histologic evidence of hemophagocytosis (in the bone marrow, lymph nodes, or spleen); (6) low or absent NK cell activity; (7) hyperferritinemia; and (8) elevated soluble CD25, plus evidence of an associated disease. Ferritin and heme bind iron. Hyperferritinemia is an important clue to the diagnosis of hemophagocytic lymphohistiocytosis.	Associated with MAS in autoimmune CTD (eg, SLE), infection (eg, EBV), and malignancy (eg, lymphoma).
Indeterminate cell histiocytosis	Solitary or generalized red-brown papules with rare visceral involvement.	Associated with leukemia and lymphoma.
NXG	See above.	
Reticulohistiocytosis	Giant cell reticulohistiocytoma favors the head, while MRH favors the head, elbows, hands, and nail folds with variable mucous membrane and/or visceral involvement. Figure 2.105.	MRH is associated with destructive arthritis and solid organ malignancies.
Rosai-Dorfman disease	Massive, painless bilateral cervical lymphadenopathy with cutaneous lesions in ~10% cases. Patients may exhibit fever, neutrophilia, anemia, elevated ESR, and polyclonal hypergammaglobulinemia. A skin-limited variant is also recognized.	Linked to IgG4-RD. Typically self-limited.
Xanthoma disseminatum (Montgomery syndrome)	Classic triad of cutaneous xanthomas favoring flexural and intertriginous areas, mucous membrane xanthomas (eg, ocular leading to blindness), and diabetes insipidus. Montgomery syndrome involves mucous membranes.	Normolipemic.

CD, cluster of differentiation; CTD, connective tissue disease; EBV, Epstein-Barr virus; ESR, erythrocyte sedimentation rate; IgG4-RD, immunoglobulin G4–related disease; HLH, hemophagocytic lymphohistiocytosis; MAS, macrophage activation syndrome; MRH, multicentric reticulohistiocytosis; NK, natural killer; NXG, necrobiotic xanthogranuloma
[a]Illustrative examples provided.

Table 2.71. NON-LANGERHANS CELL HISTIOCYTOSES IN CHILDREN

Diagnosis[a]	Classic Description	Notes
Benign cephalic histiocytosis	Infants or young children, typically <1 year of age, with red-brown macules and papules favoring the face.	Rarely associated with DI. Self-limited. Benign cephalic histiocytosis demonstrates "comma-shaped" or "worm-shaped" bodies on ultrastructure.
HLH (primary)	Infants or young children, typically 0-2 years of age. See above.	Familial or associated with other hereditary disorders (eg, Chédiak–Higashi syndrome, Griscelli syndrome type 2).
JXG	Infants or young children, typically <1 year of age, with solitary or multiple yellow nodules favoring the head and neck and variable mucous membrane and/or visceral involvement (eg, ocular, pulmonary). Ocular complications (eg, glaucoma, hyphema) uniquely occur in patients with multiple cutaneous lesions and may lead to blindness. Early referral to an ophthalmologist is critical.	Association with JMML in patients with NF1 (20-fold increased risk). Self-limited.

DI, diabetes insipidus; HLH, hemophagocytic lymphohistiocytosis; JMML, juvenile myelomonocytic leukemia; JXG, juvenile xanthogranuloma; NF1, neurofibromatosis 1.
[a]Illustrative examples provided.

Table 2.72. DIAGNOSTIC CRITERIA FOR NECROBIOTIC XANTHOGRANULOMA

Diagnostic criteria for NXG[a]

Major Criteria

1. Cutaneous papules, plaques, and/or nodules, most often yellow or orange in color.
2. Histopathological features demonstrating palisading granulomas with lymphoplasmacytic infiltrate and zones of necrobiosis. Characteristic features that are variably present include cholesterol clefts and/or giant cells (Touton or foreign body).

Minor Criteria

1. Paraproteinemia, most often IgG-κ, plasma cell dyscrasia, and/or other associated lymphoproliferative disorder.
2. Periorbital distribution of cutaneous lesions.

Ig, immunoglobulin; NXG, necrobiotic xanthogranuloma
[a]Both of the major and one minor criterion are required for diagnosis, applicable only in the absence of foreign body, infection, or other identifiable cause.

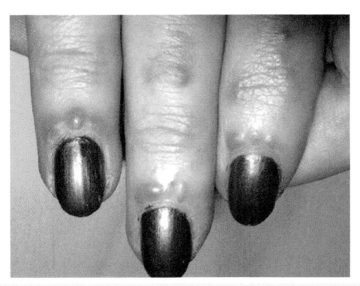 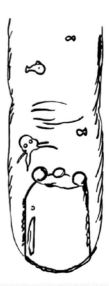

Figure 2.105. CORAL BEAD PAPULES. Periungual papules in MRH may resemble coral beads. MRH, multicentric reticulohistiocytosis.

(MRH image reprinted with permission from Requena L, Kutzner H. *Cutaneous Soft Tissue Tumors.* Wolters Kluwer Health; 2014. Illustration by Misha Rosenbach, MD.)

XANTHOMA

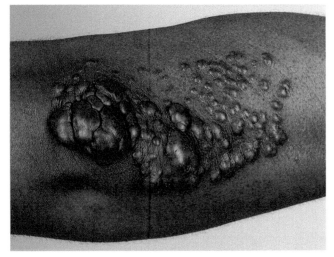

Tuberous xanthomas courtesy of Jennifer Nevas, CRNP.

- Xanthomas arise in the setting of disordered lipid metabolism.
- **Xanthoma variants** are summarized in Table 2.73.

  Xanthoma variants may be associated with **familial hyperlipoproteinemia** (Table 2.74) and other hereditary disorders. **Eruptive** xanthomas occur in **types I, IV, and V. Plane** xanthomas occur in **types II (eg, interdigital) and III (eg, xanthoma striatum palmare)** and **cholestasis** (eg, Alagille syndrome, biliary atresia). **Tendinous and tuberous/tuberoeruptive** xanthomas occur in **types II and III. Verruciform** xanthomas are associated with **congenital hemidysplasia with ichthyosiform erythroderma and limb defects (CHILD) syndrome.**
  - Figure 2.107.
  - Figure 2.108.
- In addition to **fasting lipid panel**, screening tests for secondary hyperlipidemia include **fasting glucose (diabetes mellitus), LFTs (cholestasis), albumin (nephrotic syndrome), and TSH (hypothyroidism).**
- Treatment should be directed at the underlying disorder. Lipid-lowering therapy includes **dietary measures**

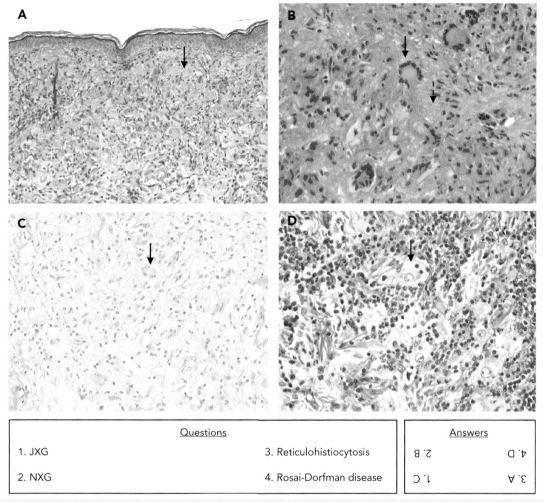

Questions	
1. JXG	3. Reticulohistiocytosis
2. NXG	4. Rosai-Dorfman disease

Answers	
2. B	4. D
1. C	3. A

Figure 2.106. MATCHING EXERCISE: NON-LANGERHANS CELL HISTIOCYTOSES. A, Reticulohistiocytosis. Solid arrow: histiocyte with characteristic "ground glass" appearance. B, NXG. Solid arrow: foreign body giant cell. Dashed arrow: necrobiosis. Note the typical pattern of palisading granulomas with lymphoplasmacytic infiltrate and zones of necrobiosis. Cholesterol clefts and/or giant cells (Touton or foreign body) may also be observed. C, JXG. Solid arrow: Touton giant cell with a "wreath" of nuclei around a central eosinophilic core and a xanthomatous periphery. D, Rosai-Dorfman disease. Note the typical pattern of pale sinusoidal macrophages admixed with darker-staining lymphocytes. Plasma cells stain positive for κ and λ light chains, and fibrosis is a common feature. Solid arrow: emperipolesis (histiocytes ingest lymphocytes and/or plasma cells). JXG, juvenile xanthogranuloma; NXG, necrobiotic xanthogranuloma

(C, Histology image courtesy of Noel Turner, MD, MHS and Christine J. Ko, MD.)

(eg, decreasing total caloric intake with fat restriction to <30% and majority monounsaturated fats, alcohol avoidance) **and medications (eg, statins).** Xanthelasma and other xanthomas may also be treated with **excision or destruction (eg, cryosurgery, chemical skin resurfacing, lasers).**

Depositional Disorders, Porphyrias, and Nutritional Deficiencies

Basic Concepts

- **Depositional disorders** are characterized by deposition of **primarily endogenous substances** within the dermis and/

or subcutis, such as mucinoses, amyloidosis, colloid milium, and gout.

- **Porphyrias** arise from dysfunction of specific enzymes in the **heme biosynthetic pathway.** They are classified into **acute** versus **nonacute** and **cutaneous** versus **noncutaneous.** Porphyrins absorb light energy most efficiently within the **Soret band (400-410 nm)**, enter into an excited molecular state, and generate ROS that induce cellular and tissue damage.

- **Nutritional deficiencies** often manifest in the skin, mucous membranes, hair, and nails. Nutrients are categorized as **macronutrients (carbohydrates, proteins, and fats)** or **micronutrients (vitamins and trace elements).** Protein-energy deficient nutrition leads to **protein-energy malnutrition. Primary** protein-energy malnutrition results from insufficient and/or inadequate food ingestion with risk factors

Table 2.73. XANTHOMA VARIANTS

Variant[a]	Classic Description	Notes
Eruptive xanthoma	Pink to yellow papules favoring the buttocks, extensor extremities, and hands.	Associated with hypertriglyceridemia (often >3000-4000 mg/dL) (eg, diabetes mellitus, hypothyroidism, obesity, alcohol abuse) and cholestasis (eg, PBC). Drug associations include systemic retinoids and OCPs.
		The serum in hypertriglyceridemia has a "creamy" top layer.
Plane xanthoma	Yellow to orange macules, papules, patches, and plaques. Normolipemic plane xanthomas favor the upper body. Xanthelasma are plane xanthomas of the eyelid.	Associations include hyperlipidemia (~50% of patients with xanthelasma), cholestasis (eg, PBC), and monoclonal gammopathy due to plasma cell dyscrasias or lymphoproliferative disorders.
Tendinous xanthoma	Nodules favoring elbow, knee, Achilles and extensor hand tendons.	Associated with hyperlipidemia (eg, hypothyroidism).
Tuberous/tuberoeruptive xanthoma	Pink to yellow papules favoring elbows and knees.	Associated with hyperlipidemia (eg, hypothyroidism).
Verruciform xanthoma	Solitary planar or verrucous plaque favoring periorificial, oral, or anogenital areas.	Associations include EBA and lymphedema.

EBA, epidermolysis bullosa acquisita; OCPs, oral contraceptive pills; PBC, primary biliary cholangitis.
[a]Illustrative examples provided.

Table 2.74. FAMILIAL HYPERLIPOPROTEINEMIA TYPES

Type[a]	Subtype	Inheritance Pattern	Pathogenesis	Classic Description	Notes
Type I	a	AR	Deficient or abnormal LPL	Eruptive xanthomas, recurrent pancreatitis. No increased risk of CAD.	Hypertriglyceridemia.
Type II (familial hypercholesterolemia)	a	AD	LDL receptor defect	Plane xanthomas (xanthelasma, intertriginous, interdigital), tendinous xanthomas, tuberous/ tuberoeruptive xanthomas, atherosclerosis.	Hypercholesterolemia.
	b	AD	Reduced affinity of LDL for LDL receptor due to apoB-100 (ligand) dysfunction		
Type III (familial dysbetalipoproteinemia)		AR > AD	Hepatic remnant clearance impaired due to apo E abnormality	Plane xanthomas (xanthoma striatum palmare), tendinous xanthomas, tuberous/ tuberoeruptive xanthomas, atherosclerosis.	Hypercholesterolemia. Hypertriglyceridemia.
Type IV			Elevated VLDL production associated with glucose intolerance and hyperinsulinemia	Eruptive xanthomas.	Hypertriglyceridemia. Associations include diabetes mellitus.
Type V			Elevated chylomicrons and VLDLs	Eruptive xanthomas.	Hypertriglyceridemia. Associations include diabetes mellitus.

AD, autosomal dominant; AR, autosomal recessive; CAD, coronary artery disease; LDL, low density lipoprotein; LPL, lipoprotein lipase; VLDL, very-low-density lipoprotein.
[a]Illustrative examples provided.

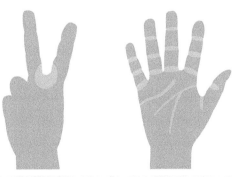

To remember the association between <u>interdigital</u> plane xanthomas and homozygous familial hyperlipoproteinemia type <u>II</u>, note that an <u>interdigital</u> webspace lies between <u>two</u> fingers.

To remember the association between xanthoma <u>striatum palmare</u> and familial hyperlipoproteinemia type <u>III</u>, note that <u>three palmar creases</u> are most common.

Figure 2.107. XANTHOMAS AND HYPERLIPOPROTEINEMIA. As a general rule, eruptive xanthomas are associated with hypertriglyceridemia (eg, familial hyperlipoproteinemia types I, IV, and V), while plane, tendinous, tuberoeruptive, and tuberous xanthomas are associated with hypercholesterolemia (eg, familial hyperlipoproteinemia types II and III). Atherosclerosis, a common complication of familial hypercholesterolemia, is also associated with diagonal earlobe crease (<u>Frank</u> sign). To remember this association, note that <u>Frank</u>furters are high in cholesterol.

(Illustration by Caroline A. Nelson, MD.)

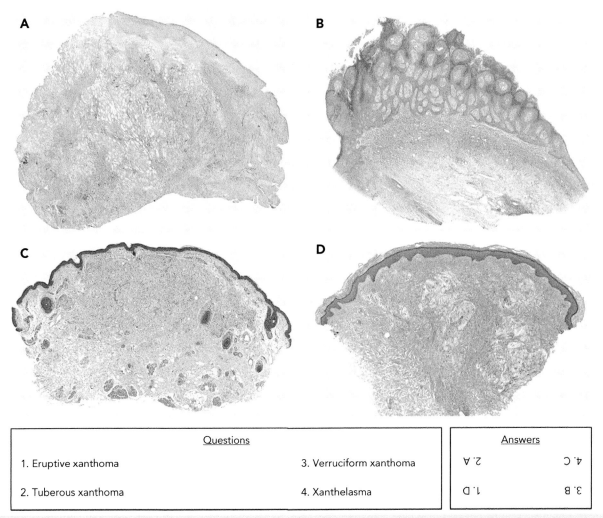

Questions		Answers	
1. Eruptive xanthoma	3. Verruciform xanthoma	4. C	2. A
2. Tuberous xanthoma	4. Xanthelasma	3. B	1. D

Figure 2.108. MATCHING EXERCISE: XANTHOMAS. Adipophilin IHC may be helpful to detect lipid accumulation in xanthomas. A, Eruptive xanthoma. Note the foam cells and extracellular lipid (the phagocytic capacity of histiocytes is overwhelmed by the pace of lipid deposition) in the reticular dermis. B, Verruciform xanthoma. Note the papillomatosis foam cells in the dermal papillae, and orange "V-shaped" columns of parakeratosis. C, Xanthelasma. Note the band of foam cells in the superficial dermis. Thin epidermis and muscle fibers at the base, when present, may be clues to an eyelid location. D, Tendinous xanthoma. Note the foam cells and cholesterol clefts in the dermis. Tendinous xanthomas are histologically similar to tuberous xanthomas except for location (fasciae, ligaments, and tendons). Adipophilin IHC may be helpful to detect lipid accumulation in xanthomas. IHC, immunohistochemistry.

(Histology images courtesy of Noel Turner, MD, MHS and Christine J. Ko, MD.)

including **restrictive diets, alcoholism, poverty, and psychiatric disorders (eg, anorexia nervosa, bulimia). Secondary** protein-energy malnutrition results from inadequate food absorption and/or metabolism or increased nutritional requirements with risk factors including **intestinal malabsorption and bariatric surgery, particularly the Roux-en-Y procedure.** Protein-energy excessive nutrition leads to **obesity (body mass index [BMI] ≥ 30 kg/m²). Primary** obesity results from excessive and/or high-calorie food ingestion. **Secondary** obesity results from metabolic alterations.

SCLEROMYXEDEMA
Synonyms: diffuse/generalized and scleroder-moid lichen myxedematosus, papular mucinosis

Courtesy of Victoria Werth, MD.

- Scleromyxedema is a **primary cutaneous mucinosis** (Table 2.75) associated with **monoclonal gammopathy (most often IgG-λ).**
  - λ resembles the "y" in scleromyxedema inverted.
    In **cutaneous mucinosis of infancy**, papules favor the neck, upper trunk, and extremities. **Self-healing cutaneous mucinosis and primary follicular mucinosis are more common in children** than adults.
- Scleromyxedema classically presents with **numerous, symmetric, 2 to 3 mm, firm, waxy, closely aligned papules favoring the head and neck, upper trunk, thighs, forearms, and hands.** Other cutaneous features include **deep longitudinal furrowing (eg, of the glabella), skin stiffening, sclerodactyly, and decreased motility of the mouth and joints.** Systemic involvement including cardiovascular, rheumatologic (arthropathies, carpel tunnel syndrome), muscular (dysphagia, myositis), neurologic (coma, peripheral neuropathy), renal, and pulmonary (restrictive or obstructive lung disease) may result in death.

Severe involvement of the face leads to "leonine facies." Deep furrowing on the trunk and extremities is called the "Shar-Pei sign." A central depression with an elevated rim overlying a proximal interphalangeal (PIP) joint is called the "doughnut sign."
  - Figure 2.109.
- Work-up includes **skin biopsy, TFTs, SPEP/IFE, and UPEP/IFE.**
- **IVIG** is first line.

SCLEREDEMA
Synonyms: scleredema adultorum of Buschke, scleredema diabeticorum

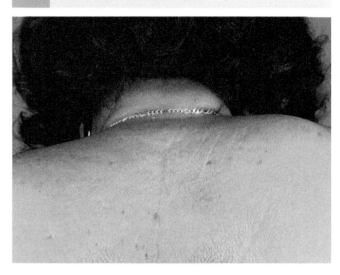

- Scleredema is a primary cutaneous mucinosis classically divided into three types:
  - **Type I:** associated with **infection (eg, streptococcal);**
  - **Type II:** associated with **monoclonal gammopathy (most often IgG-κ);**
    - κ resembles the "k" in Busch<u>k</u>e.
  - **Type III:** associated with **insulin-dependent diabetes mellitus.**
- Scleredema **types I and II** classically present with **hardening of the skin of the cervicofacial region** with extension to the trunk and proximal upper extremities. Hallmark features are an **expressionless face and difficulty opening the mouth and swallowing** due to tongue and pharynx involvement. Scleredema **type III** classically presents with **erythema and induration of the posterior neck and back with a *peau d'orange* appearance of the skin** ± cheiroarthropathy.
  - Figure 2.110.
- Scleredema **type I is typically self-limited**, while **types II and III are typically chronic. Phototherapy (UVA1, PUVA)** is first line.

Table 2.75. PRIMARY CUTANEOUS MUCINOSES

Diagnosis[a]	Classic Description	Notes
Degenerative Inflammatory Mucinoses: Dermal		
Scleromyxedema	See above.	
Lichen myxedematosus (localized variants)	Papules favoring the limbs and trunk (discrete papular lichen myxedematosus); papules favoring the distal extremities (acral persistent papular mucinosis); nodules favoring the trunk and extremities (nodular lichen myxedematosus).	
Self-healing cutaneous mucinosis	Acute eruption of papules coalescing into linear infiltrated plaques on the head and neck, abdomen, and thighs along with nodules on the face (periorbital swelling) and periarticular areas ± constitutional symptoms.	
Scleredema	See below.	
Mucinoses associated with altered thyroid function	Erythematous to skin-colored waxy indurated nodules or plaques with a *peau d'orange* appearance favoring the anterolateral lower legs or feet (localized [pretibial] myxedema); pale, cool, waxy, dry skin (generalized myxedema).	Localized (pretibial) myxedema is most often associated with hyperthyroidism (eg, Graves disease). Generalized myxedema is most often associated with hypothyroidism (eg, Hashimoto thyroiditis), along with macroglossia. Teprotumumab is a novel therapy.
Reticular erythematous mucinosis	Pink to red macules and papules in reticulated and annular patterns favoring the chest and mid back.	May overlap with LE tumidus and lymphocytic infiltrate of Jessner.
Papulonodular mucinosis associated with autoimmune CTDs	Skin-colored to erythematous papules and nodules favoring the "V" of the chest, back, and upper extremities.	Associations include SLE > DM, SSc.
Cutaneous focal mucinosis	Focal skin-colored papule or nodule.	Associations include trauma.
Digital mucous cyst	See Chapter 5: Cysts and Pseudocysts.	
Degenerative Inflammatory Mucinoses: Follicular		
Follicular mucinosis (Pinkus)	Pink plaques, often composed of grouped follicular papules, on the scalp or face associated with alopecia.	Associations with secondary follicular mucinosis include AD and CTCL.
Urticaria-like follicular mucinosis	Pruritic urticarial papules or plaques favoring seborrheic areas on the head and neck.	
Hamartomatous-Neoplastic Mucinoses		
Mucinous nevus	Plaque with a unilateral linear nevoid pattern.	Congenital or acquired.
Superficial (angio)myxoma	Nodule favoring the head and neck, trunk, and genital area.	Multiple superficial (angio)myxomas are associated with the Carney complex.

AD, atopic dermatitis; CTCL, cutaneous T-cell lymphoma; CTD, connective tissue disease; DM, dermatomyositis; HCV, hepatitis C virus; SLE, lupus erythematosus; SSc, systemic sclerosis.
[a]Illustrative examples provided.

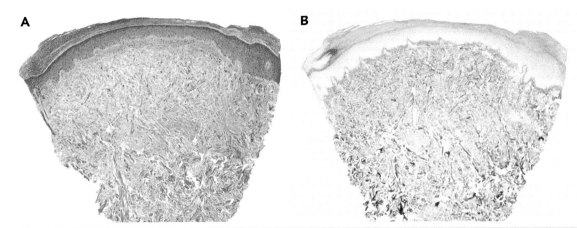

Figure 2.109. CLINICOPATHOLOGICAL CORRELATION: SCLEROMYXEDEMA. Characteristic features are a thickened upper and mid reticular dermis with increased space between collagen fibers containing mucin, CD34+ and procollagen 1–positive fibroblast-like cells, and increased factor XIIIa positive cells. Mucin may appear blue or may leave empty spaces on H&E. A, H&E. B, Colloidal iron stain. CD, cluster of differentiation; H&E, hematoxylin and eosin; NSF, nephrogenic systemic fibrosis.

For mucinoses, fixation in absolute alcohol is preferable to formalin. ABSOLUT MUCIN.
Scleromyxedema can NOT be distinguished from NSF on histopathology. Unlike scleromyxedema, however, NSF tends to involve the subcutis.

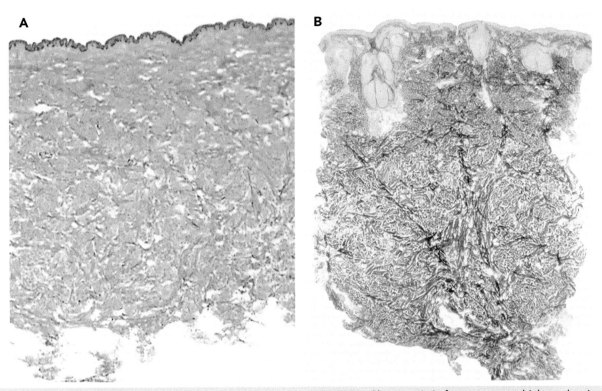

Figure 2.110. CLINICOPATHOLOGICAL CORRELATION: SCLEREDEMA. Characteristic features are a thickened reticular dermis with increased space between collagen fibers containing mucin. A, H&E. B, Colloidal iron stain. H&E, hematoxylin and eosin.

(Histology images reprinted with permission from Elder DE, Elenitsas R, Rosenbach M, et al. *Lever's Histopathology of the Skin*. 11th ed. Wolters Kluwer; 2015.)

AMYLOIDOSIS

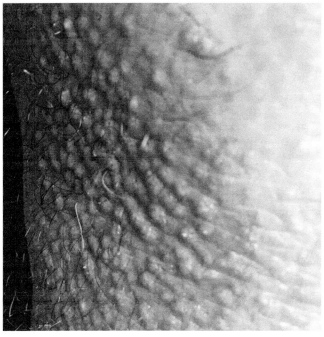

Lichen amyloidosis.

- Amyloidosis describes abnormal deposition of amyloid. Properties of amyloid include congophilia **and green birefringence under polarized light**, a distinctive fibrillar ultrastructure, and a **cross-β-pleated sheet configuration** by X-ray crystallography.
- **Amyloidosis** (Table 2.76) may be **cutaneous or systemic. Macular and lichen amyloidosis** may be observed in **multiple endocrine neoplasia (MEN) type 2A. Secondary systemic amyloidosis** is associated with autoinflammatory disorders such as **FMF, MWS, and TNF receptor–associated periodic syndrome (TRAPS). Amyloid transthyretin (ATTR)** amyloidosis due to *TTR* **mutations** occurs in **familial amyloid polyneuropathy and cardiomyopathy.**
  - Figure 2.111.
- Treatment of macular or lichen amyloidosis should be directed at breaking the itch-scratch cycle (eg, topical corticosteroids). Treatment of systemic amyloidosis should be directed at the underlying cause.

Table 2.76. AMYLOIDOSIS

Diagnosis[a]	Protein[b]	Classic Description	Notes
Cutaneous Amyloidosis			
Macular amyloidosis	Keratinocyte-derived (also seen as an incidental finding within skin tumors)	Confluent or rippled hyperpigmentation favoring the upper back (scapular) and extensor extremities.	Primary cutaneous amyloidosis is associated with prolonged friction. It commonly occurs in Southeast Asia, Central and South America (macular amyloidosis), and China (lichen amyloidosis). Macular amyloidosis overlaps with pigmented notalgia paresthetica.
Lichen amyloidosis		Hyperpigmented papules, often in a rippled pattern, favoring the shins and extensor extremities.	
Nodular amyloidosis	AL (most often λ) λ resembles the "y" in amyloidosis inverted.	Waxy nodules favoring the trunk and extremities.	~7% of patients progress to systemic involvement.
Systemic Amyloidosis			
Primary systemic amyloidosis	AL (most often λ) >> AH	Waxy papulonodules and plaques, ecchymoses > hemorrhagic bullae; macroglossia; alopecia; koilonychia. Systemic involvement may affect the heart (eg, restrictive cardiomyopathy), liver, joints (eg, carpel tunnel syndrome), nerves, and kidneys (eg, nephrotic syndrome).	Primary systemic amyloidosis is associated with plasma cell dyscrasia. If specific mucocutaneous lesions are not present for biopsy, aspirate the abdominal fat pad. Screen with SPEP/IFE, UPEP/IFE, and serum-free light chains.
		Periorbital purpura, known as "raccoon eyes," may result from increased intra-abdominal pressure. "Pinch purpura" may result from pinching the skin. The "shoulder pad sign" may result from amyloid deposition in periarticular soft tissue.	
Secondary systemic amyloidosis	AA	Skin involvement is rare. Systemic involvement may affect the heart, liver, spleen, adrenals, and kidneys.	Secondary systemic amyloidosis is associated with inflammatory disorders (eg, RA) and chronic infections. If specific mucocutaneous lesions are not present for biopsy, aspirate the abdominal fat pad.

Table 2.76. AMYLOIDOSIS

Diagnosis[a]	Protein[b]	Classic Description	Notes
HD-associated amyloidosis	Aβ2MG	Skin involvement is rare. Systemic involvement primarily affects the musculoskeletal system (eg, carpal tunnel syndrome).	Due to decreased excretion of Aβ2MG in patients on chronic HD.
ATTR amyloidosis (wild-type, senile systemic amyloidosis, senile cardiac amyloidosis)	ATTR	Skin involvement is rare. Systemic involvement primarily affects the heart.	

AA, amyloid A; Aβ2MG, amyloid β2-microglobulin; AH, amyloid heavy chain; AL, amyloid light chain; ATTR, amyloid transthyretin; HD, hemodialysis; IFE, immunofixation electrophoresis; RA, rheumatoid arthritis; SPEP, serum protein electrophoresis; UPEP, urine protein electrophoresis.
[a]Illustrative examples provided.
[b]Amyloid deposits consist of three components: protein-derived amyloid fibers, amyloid P, and ground substance.

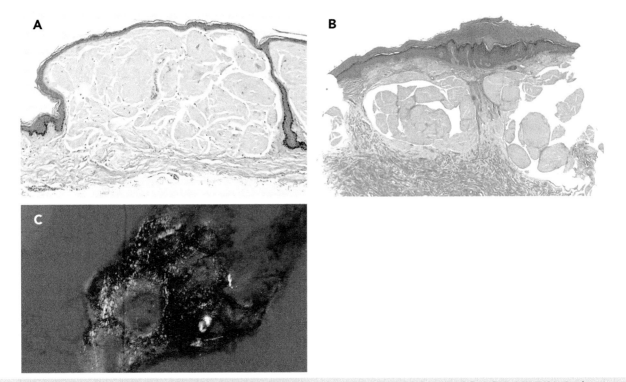

Figure 2.111. SIDE-BY-SIDE COMPARISON: PRIMARY SYSTEMIC AMYLOIDOSIS AND COLLOID MILIUM. Both primary systemic amyloidosis and colloid milium demonstrate amorphous pale-pink fissured deposits. Amyloid stains include Congo red, crystal violet, methyl violet, pagoda red, PAS (diastase-resistant), Sirius red, and thioflavin T. IHC may also be helpful (eg, amyloid P protein). Colloid milium may stain weakly with amyloid stains except for pagoda red (the most specific) and features prominent solar elastosis. A, Primary systemic amyloidosis. B, Colloid milium. C, Primary systemic amyloidosis Congo red with green birefringence under polarized light (abdominal fat pad aspirate). IHC, immunohistochemistry; PAS, periodic acid-Schiff.

(Histology images reprinted with permission from Elder DE, Elenitsas R, Rosenbach M, et al. *Lever's Histopathology of the Skin.* 11th ed. Wolters Kluwer; 2015.)

On Congo red stain, amyloid is "brick red" with "apple green" birefringence under polarized light.

Primary Cutaneous Amyloidosis:
- **Macular amyloidosis variant**: amyloid deposits in the papillary dermis ± melanophages and a sparse perivascular lymphohistiocytic infiltrate.
- **Lichen amyloidosis variant**: hyperkeratosis, acanthosis, amyloid deposits in the papillary dermis ± melanophages, and a sparse perivascular lymphohistiocytic infiltrate.
- **Nodular amyloidosis variant**: diffuse amyloid deposits in the reticular dermis, subcutis, and vessel walls with a perivascular plasma cell infiltrate that may be monoclonal.

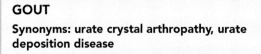

GOUT
Synonyms: urate crystal arthropathy, urate deposition disease

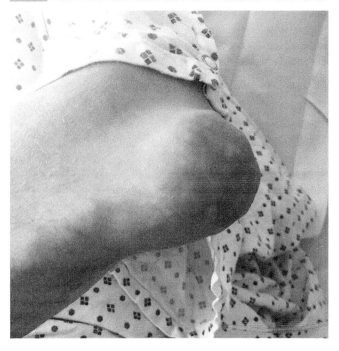

- Gout is an acquired depositional disorder due to **hyperuricemia. Monosodium urate (MSU) crystals deposit in the skin (tophi) and joints.** Uric acid overproduction may be idiopathic or result from excessive dietary purine intake and obesity, increased nucleotide turnover (eg, tumor lysis syndrome), and/or accelerated ATP degradation (eg, alcohol abuse). Decreased excretion of uric acid may be idiopathic or may result from renal insufficiency, enhanced tubular urate reabsorption (eg, diuretics), drug ingestion (eg, cyclosporine), toxins (eg, lead-induced nephropathy), and other causes. Gout is **male predominant.**

  Hereditary enzyme deficiencies and other depositional disorders are summarized in Table 2.77.

- Gout classically progresses through four clinical stages: (1) asymptomatic hyperuricemia, (2) acute gouty arthritis, (3) intercritical gout, and (4) chronic tophaceous gout. On the skin, **acute gouty arthritis** is characterized by **tenderness, erythema, warmth, and swelling overlying a painful joint,** most commonly the **first metatarsophalangeal (MTP) joint (podagra),** while **chronic tophaceous gout** is characterized by **firm variably ulcerated/draining dermal or subcutaneous papules and nodules or fusiform swelling overlying ear helices or joints. Uric acid nephrolithiasis** may cause acute renal failure.

  ◆ Figure 2.112.

- **Pseudogout** resembles gout but results from deposition of **calcium pyrophosphate dihydrate (CPPD) crystals** in large joints, most commonly the **knee joint.** Associations include **osteoarthritis.**

- Treatments for **acute gouty arthritis** include **NSAIDs (eg, indomethacin) and colchicine.** Treatments for **chronic tophaceous gout** include **xanthine oxidase inhibitors (eg, allopurinol, febuxostat) and uricosuric agents (eg, probenecid).**

Table 2.77. HEREDITARY ENZYME DEFICIENCIES AND OTHER DEPOSITIONAL DISORDERS

Diagnosis[a]	Inheritance Pattern	Gene Product	Classic Description	Notes
Alkaptonuria (endogenous ochronosis)	AR	Homogentisate 1,2-dioxygenase	Cutaneous features include blue-grey pigmentation of skin (eg, axillae), sclerae (Osler sign), and cartilage (eg, ear helices). Systemic features include valvular heart disease and arthritis.	Due to deposition of HGA. The urine darkens on standing. Exogenous ochronosis occurs secondary to hydroquinone application.
Argininosuccinic aciduria	AR	Argininosuccinate lyase	Characteristic hair shaft abnormalities with increased fragility are pili torti and trichorrhexis nodosa. Systemic features include liver dysfunction and neurocognitive deficits.	Due to hyperammonemia.
Biotinidase and holocarboxylase synthetase deficiencies (late- and early-onset multiple carboxylase deficiency)	AR	Biotinidase, holocarboxylase synthetase	Cutaneous features resemble zinc deficiency. Systemic features include metabolic acidosis and neurologic involvement (eg, optic atrophy in biotinidase deficiency).	Biotinidase deficiency presents in juveniles. Holocarboxylase synthetase deficiency presents in neonates. Both disorders are treated with vitamin B_7 (biotin).
Citrullinemia Type 1 (classic) Type 2 (adult-onset)	AR	Argininosuccinate synthase 1 (type 1), citrin (type 2)	Characteristic hair shaft abnormalities with increased fragility are pili torti and trichorrhexis nodosa. Systemic features include liver dysfunction and neurocognitive deficits.	Due to hyperammonemia.

(Continued)

Table 2.77. HEREDITARY ENZYME DEFICIENCIES AND OTHER DEPOSITIONAL DISORDERS (CONTINUED)

Diagnosis[a]	Inheritance Pattern	Gene Product	Classic Description	Notes
Fabry disease	XLR	α-galactosidase A	Cutaneous features include angiokeratoma corporis diffusum; hypohidrosis. Systemic features include acral pain and paresthesias, coronary and renal insufficiency, and whorled corneal opacities (cornea verticillata).	Due to deposition of neutral glycosphingolipids. Polarizing microscopy of the urine reveals birefringent lipid globules. Enzyme replacement therapy is available.
			Angiokeratomas favor the "bathing trunk" distribution.	Birefringent lipid globules are called "Maltese crosses."
Gaucher disease Type 1 (adult) Type 2 (infant) Type 3 (juvenile)	AR	Glucocerebrosidase	Cutaneous features include diffuse hyperpigmentation/easy tanning and petechiae/ecchymoses (type 1) and collodion baby or other ichthyosiform features (type 2). Systemic features include HSM, cytopenias and bone pain (type 1), and neurologic involvement (type 2, 3).	Due to deposition of glucocerebroside. Infiltration of the bone marrow with glycolipid-filled macrophages (Gaucher cells) results in the radiographic finding of metaphyseal flaring. Enzyme replacement therapy is available.
				Metaphyseal flaring is also known as the "Erlenmeyer flask" deformity.
Hartnup disease	AR	Neutral amino acid transporter in the kidneys and intestines encoded by SLC6A19	Cutaneous features resemble vitamin B₃ deficiency. Systemic features include neurologic involvement (eg, ataxia).	Due to decreased renal reabsorption and intestinal absorption of neutral amino acids including tryptophan, which is required to make niacin.
Lesch-Nyhan syndrome	XLR	HGPRT	Cutaneous features include gout and self-mutilation (eg, onychophagia, onychotillomania). Systemic features include dystonia and intellectual disability.	Due to hyperuricemia and deposition of MSU crystals. Uric acid in the urine leaves orange deposits in the diaper.
				Deposits in the diaper are often described as "orange sand."
Lipoid proteinosis	See below.			
Mitochondrial disorders	Maternal (mtDNA mutations) or Mendelian (nuclear DNA mutations)	Respiratory chain components and other mitochondrial proteins	Cutaneous features include pigmentary changes. Systemic features include cardiomyopathy, myopathy, and encephalopathy.	
MPS I (Hurler)	AR	α-L-iduronidase	Cutaneous features include coarse facies and dermal melanocytosis; macroglossia. Systemic features include cardiovascular, musculoskeletal, and respiratory involvement, HSM, intellectual disability, and corneal clouding.	Due to deposition of GAGs (eg, dermatan sulfate, heparan sulfate). Dermal melanocytosis is observed in other hereditary disorders (eg, GM1 gangliosidosis).
MPS II (Hunter)	XLR For the hunter, "X marks the spot" (XLR).	Iduronidase-2-sulfatase	Cutaneous features include coarse facies, dermal melanocytosis, and skin-colored to white papules over the scapulae; macroglossia. Systemic features include cardiovascular and musculoskeletal involvement, HSM, intellectual disability, and retinal degeneration.	
Niemann-Pick disease	AR	Acid sphingomyelinase	Cutaneous features include generalized ochre or brownish-yellow discoloration and papules favoring the face and upper extremities (type A). Systemic features include FTT, HSM, neurologic involvement, and cherry-red retinal spots.	Due to deposition of sphingomyelin and other phospholipids. Cherry-red retinal spots are observed in other hereditary disorders (eg, Tay-Sachs disease).

Table 2.77. HEREDITARY ENZYME DEFICIENCIES AND OTHER DEPOSITIONAL DISORDERS (CONTINUED)

Diagnosis[a]	Inheritance Pattern	Gene Product	Classic Description	Notes
Phenylketonuria	AR	Phenylalanine hydroxylase	Cutaneous features include atopic-like dermatitis, pigmentary dilution, and sclerodermatous skin changes. Systemic features include neurologic involvement (eg, intellectual disability).	Pigmentary dilution occurs because phenylalanine is a competitive inhibitor of tyrosinase. Sweat has a musty odor (eccrine bromhidrosis). Treat with a phenylalanine-restricted diet (eg, avoid aspartame). The musty odor is sometimes described as "mousy." Remember that mice prefer coke over diet coke.
Prolidase deficiency	AR	Prolidase	Cutaneous features include premature canities, recalcitrant leg ulcers, and telangiectasias.	
Wilson disease (hepatolenticular degeneration)	AR	Copper transporter in the liver encoded by *ATP7B*	Cutaneous features include pretibial hyperpigmentation; blue lunulae. Systemic features include hepatomegaly, cirrhosis, neurologic symptoms, and Kayser-Fleischer corneal rings (Descemet membrane).	Due to deposition of copper. Diagnose with low serum ceruloplasmin, increased urinary copper excretion, increased hepatic copper content, and/or genetic testing. Treatments include copper-chelating agents (eg, D-penicillamine, trientine), zinc acetate, and liver transplantation.

AR, autosomal recessive; ATP, adenosine triphosphate; DNA, deoxyribonucleic acid; FTT, failure to thrive; GAG, glycosaminoglycan; HGA, homogentisic acid; HGPRT, hypoxanthine-guanine phosphoribosyltransferase; HSM, hepatosplenomegaly; MPS, mucopolysaccharidosis; MSU, monosodium urate; mtDNA, mitochondrial DNA; XLR, X-linked recessive.
[a]Illustrative examples provided.

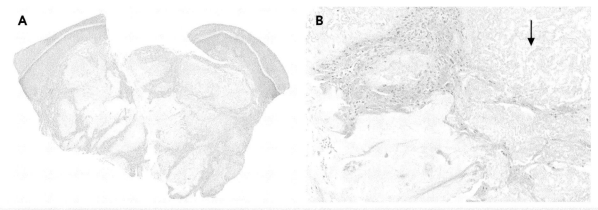

Figure 2.112. CLINICOPATHOLOGICAL CORRELATION: GOUT. Gout is characterized by giant cells surrounding MSU crystals deposited in a radial array in the dermis and subcutis. MSU crystals exhibit negative birefringence under polarized light in contrast to the rhomboid CPPD crystals of pseudogout, which exhibit weakly positive birefringence under polarized light. A, Low-power view. B, High-power view. Solid arrow: needlelike clefts. CPPD, calcium pyrophosphate dihydrate; MSU, monosodium urate.

(Histology images courtesy of Noel Turner, MD, MHS and Christine J. Ko, MD.)

MSU crystals, destroyed by formalin fixation, leave behind "needlelike" clefts. The best fixative to preserve MSU crystals is ethanol based (Carnoy's fluid).

SPOTLIGHT ON LIPOID PROTEINOSIS

Synonyms: hyalinosis cutis et mucosae, Urbach-Wiethe disease

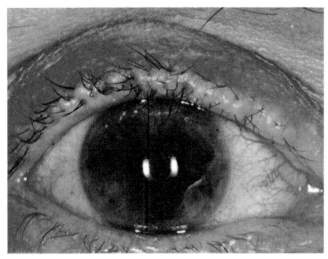

Reprinted with permission from Shields JA, Shields CL. *Eyelid, Conjunctival, and Orbital Tumors: An Atlas and Textbook.* 3rd ed. Wolters Kluwer; 2015.

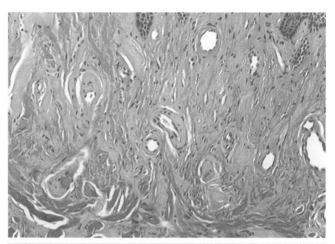

Figure 2.113. CLINICOPATHOLOGICAL CORRELATION: LIPOID PROTEINOSIS. Characteristic features are hyaline deposits and cuffs around vessels ± appendages in the dermis. Deposits are derived from the basement membrane (PAS positive, diastase resistant). Electron microscopy demonstrates reduplication of the basement membrane. PAS, periodic acid-Schiff.

(Histology image courtesy of Travis Vandergriff, MD. From Gru AA, Wick MR, Mir A, et al. *Pediatric Dermatopathology and Dermatology.* Wolters Kluwer; 2018.)

- Lipoid proteinosis is a hereditary depositional disorder of amorphous hyaline material due to **AR mutation in ECM-1.**
- Cutaneous features include **papules, nodules, and pitted scars favoring the face and diffuse waxy thickening of the skin favoring the elbows, knees, and hands. Macroglossia with restricted tongue motion** may occur. Systemic features include **neurologic involvement (eg, seizures) and laryngeal involvement (eg, weak cry, hoarseness).**
  - Eyelid papules are often described as a "string of pearls."
  - Scars are often described as "ice pick like."
  - Macroglossia with restricted tongue motion is often described as a "wooden tongue."
  - Figure 2.113.
- **Bilateral intracranial calcification within the amygdalae** is a pathognomonic radiographic finding.
  - Calcifications are often described as "bean shaped" or "sickle shaped."
- There is no known cure or effective treatment for lipoid proteinosis.

PORPHYRIA CUTANEA TARDA
→ Diagnosis Group 2

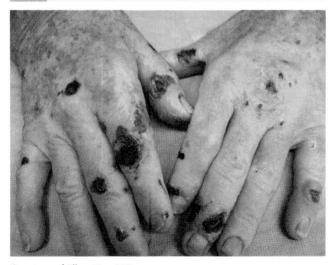

Courtesy of Ellen Kim, MD.

Epidemiology

- PCT, the **most common porphyria**, arises due to decreased activity of **uroporphyrinogen decarboxylase.**
- PCT is **more often acquired** (type I, liver only) than hereditary (type II, all tissues).
  - The **heme biosynthetic pathway** is illustrated in Figure 2.114.
  - **Hereditary porphyrias** are summarized in Table 2.78.
- PCT typically presents in the **third and fourth decades.**
  - Remember that PCT does not present until later in life because tarda is derived from the Latin word *tardus* meaning "late."
- Associations include **hemochromatosis (homozygosity for the *HFE* gene mutation C282Y associated with earlier onset), viral infections (eg, HCV, HIV), and malignancy (eg, hepatocellular carcinoma).**
- Drug associations include **antimalarials, OCPs, rifampin, sulfonamides, and tetracyclines.** Other triggers include

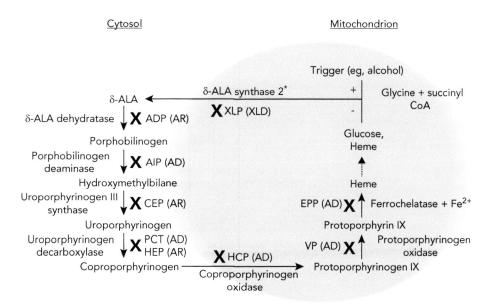

Figure 2.114. HEME BIOSYNTHETIC PATHWAY. * Rate-limiting step. Illustrative examples of activators and inhibitors provided. AD, autosomal dominant; ADP, ALA-D deficiency porphyria; AIP, acute intermittent porphyria; ALA, aminolevulinic acid; AR, autosomal recessive; CEP, congenital erythropoietic porphyria; CoA, coenzyme A; EPP, erythropoietic protoporphyria; HCP, hereditary coproporphyria; HEP, hepatoerythropoietic porphyria; OCTs, oral contraceptive pills; PCT, porphyria cutanea tarda; VP, variegate porphyria; XLD, X-linked dominant; XLP, X-linked dominant protoporphyria.

alcohol (most common), iron, dialysis, and polychlorinated hydrocarbons.

Clinicopathological Features

- PCT classically presents with **photosensitivity with skin fragility, blistering, erosions, crusts, milia, scarring, morpheaform and sclerodermoid changes, and hyperpigmentation in sun-exposed areas.** Adnexal involvement may manifest as **hypertrichosis and scarring alopecia.**
    - Figure 2.115.

Evaluation

- The differential diagnosis of PCT includes other porphyrias most notably hepatoerythropoietic porphyria (HEP) and variegate porphyria (VP), pseudoporphyria, and EBA. **Pseudoporphyria** resembles PCT but lacks detectable biochemical abnormalities in porphyrin metabolism. Associations include **stage 4 or 5 CKD including dialysis (hemodialysis > peritoneal dialysis) and tanning bed use.** Drug associations include **systemic retinoids, quinolones, tetracyclines, voriconazole, amiodarone, diuretics (eg, furosemide), and NSAIDs.**

- The **urine** of PCT patients turns red to brown after several hours of exposure to natural light and it has a **pink to red fluorescence** when exposed to a UVA light source (eg, **Wood's lamp**).
- **Screen for PCT with urinary uro- and copro-porphyrins, aminolevulinic acid (ALA), and porphobilinogen.** If normal, consider pseudoporphyria or EBA. If elevated, perform additional testing (eg, plasma, stool) to differentiate PCT from other porphyrias.

Management

- The cornerstones of prevention are **avoiding triggers (eg, alcohol) and photoprotection.**
- **Therapeutic phlebotomy** is first line for patients with iron overload.
- **Low-dose antimalarials** have demonstrated efficacy, except in patients homozygous for C2382Y.

"Real World" Advice

- **Physical sunscreens** (eg, titanium dioxide, zinc oxide) are more effective than chemical sunscreens at blocking visible light, which includes the Soret band (400-410 nm).
- Pay attention to antimalarial dose, as higher doses (eg, for cutaneous LE) can lead to hepatotoxicity.

Table 2.78. HEREDITARY PORPHYRIAS

Diagnosis	Inheritance Pattern	Gene Product	Classic Description	Notes
XLP	XLD	δ-ALA synthase 2	Resembles EPP.	
ADP	AR	δ-ALA dehydratase	Resembles AIP.	
AIP	AD	Porphobilinogen deaminase	Noncutaneous porphyria. Systemic features include tachycardia, colicky abdominal pain, nausea and vomiting, paresthesias, and motor and sensory peripheral neuropathy. AIP = Abdomen Is Painful	Treatments include avoiding triggers (eg, alcohol), heme arginate or hematin infusions, and glucose infusions (if heme preparations unavailable).
CEP (Günther disease)	AR	Uroporphyrinogen III synthase	Cutaneous features include vesicles and bullae, erosions, ulcerations, crusts, milia, scarring, hyperpigmentation, and mutilation; hypertrichosis in sun-exposed areas. Systemic features include hemolytic anemia, HSM, and porphyrin deposition in bones and teeth (erythrodontia).	Porphyrins present in the urine (uroporphyrinogen > coproporphyrinogen) stain the diaper pink, red, or violet. Photoprotection is critical. Treatments include vitamins C and E (antioxidants), splenectomy, and bone marrow or HSCT. CEP = Colorful Exotic Pee
HEP	AR	Uroporphyrinogen decarboxylase	Overlap between CEP and PCT.	
PCT	AD		See above.	
HCP	AD	Coproporphyrinogen oxidase	Overlap between AIP and PCT.	
VP	AD	Protoporphyrinogen oxidase		
EPP	AD	Ferrochelatase	Cutaneous features include erythema, edema, crusts, purpura, skin thickening, and waxy scars favoring the face and dorsal hands. Systemic features include liver disease and cholelithiasis. EPP = Empty Pee Pee	Most common porphyria in children. Associations include solar urticaria. Porphyrins are absent from the urine. Photoprotection is critical. Treatments include β-carotene, afamelanotide, and cholestyramine or charcoal.

AD, autosomal dominant; ADP, ALA-D deficiency porphyria; AIP, acute intermittent porphyria; ALA, aminolevulinic acid; AR, autosomal recessive; CEP, congenital erythropoietic porphyria; EPP, erythropoietic protoporphyria; HCP, hereditary coproporphyria; HEP, hepatoerythropoietic porphyria; HSCT, hematopoietic stem cell transplantation; HSM, hepatosplenomegaly; PCT, porphyria cutanea tarda; VP, variegate porphyria; XLD, X-linked dominant; XLP, X-linked dominant protoporphyria.

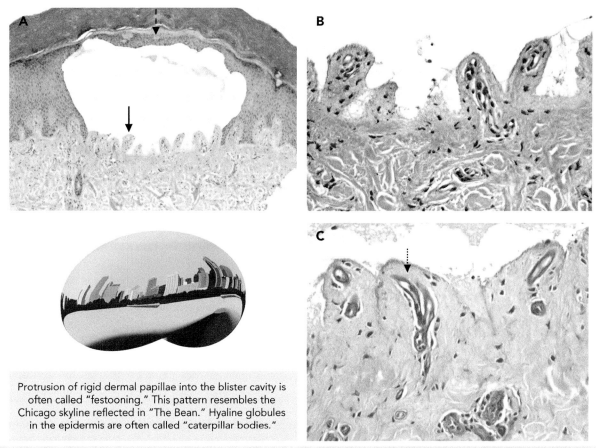

Protrusion of rigid dermal papillae into the blister cavity is often called "festooning." This pattern resembles the Chicago skyline reflected in "The Bean." Hyaline globules in the epidermis are often called "caterpillar bodies."

Figure 2.115. CLINICOPATHOLOGICAL CORRELATION: PORPHYRIA CUTANEA TARDA. Characteristic features are a subepidermal split with protrusion of rigid dermal papillae into the blister cavity and a pauci-inflammatory infiltrate. Hyaline globules in the epidermis and cuffs around vessels ± appendages in the dermis are derived from the basement membrane (PAS positive, diastase resistant). DIF classically demonstrates homogenous deposition of IgG, C3, IgA, and IgM along the DEJ and in vessels. A, H&E low-power view. Solid arrow: festooning. Dashed arrow: caterpillar body. B, H&E high-power view. C, PAS stain. Dotted arrow: PAS-positive, diastase-resistant hyaline cuff around a vessel in the dermis. C, complement; DEJ, dermal-epidermal junction; DIF, direct immunofluorescence; H&E, hematoxylin and eosin; Ig, immunoglobulin; PAS, periodic acid-Schiff; PCT, porphyria cutanea tarda.

(Histology images A and B reprinted with permission from Elder DE, Elenitsas R, Rosenbach M, et al. *Lever's Histopathology of the Skin.* 11th ed. Wolters Kluwer; 2015. Illustration by Caroline A. Nelson, MD.)

PCT can NOT be distinguished from pseudoporphyria.

ZINC DEFICIENCY

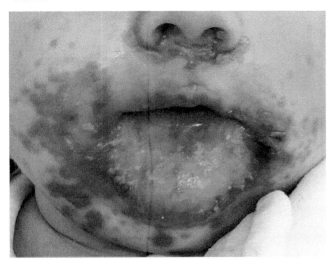

Acrodermatitis enteropathica courtesy of Sa Rang Kim, MD.

- Zinc deficiency occurs in the following four scenarios:
  - **AR hereditary disorder (acrodermatitis enteropathica):** presents **1 to 2 weeks after weaning from breast milk** (cow's milk has zinc-binding proteins) or at 4 to 8 weeks of age if bottle-fed due to mutations in *SLC39A4* (encodes a zinc transporter in the intestine and kidney).
  - **Premature infants after weaning from breast milk.**
  - **Babies breastfed with zinc-deficient breastmilk.**
  - **Inadequate zinc intake** due to primary or secondary malnutrition.
    - In **adults**, inadequate zinc intake may result from diets high in mineral-binding phytate (eg, **Middle Eastern diets**), **vegan diets**, chronic renal failure, HIV infec-

tion, pregnancy, and drugs (eg, D-penicillamine). Mucocutaneous and adnexal features of **acquired nutritional deficiencies** are summarized in Table 2.79.
  - Figure 2.116.
- Zinc deficiency classically presents with **erythema, scale crusts, and erosions ± vesicles**, bullae, and psoriasiform plaques **favoring the perioral, anogenital, and acral areas.** In **infants**, zinc deficiency is in the differential diagnosis for **diaper dermatitis.** Mucous membrane involvement (eg, **angular cheilitis**) is often observed. Adnexal involvement may manifest as **alopecia, paronychia**, and onychodystrophy. The **complete triad** of zinc deficiency—**dermatitis, diarrhea, and depression**—is only present in **20% of patients. Cutaneous superinfection (eg, *staphylococci, Candida* species)** is common.
  - Figure 2.117.
- The constellation of findings in zinc deficiency is shared by **CF and the hereditary enzyme deficiencies, biotinidase deficiency and holocarboxylase synthetase deficiency.** These disorders are often mistaken for more common pediatric dermatoses such as seborrheic dermatitis, resulting in diagnostic delay. **If zinc is normal, low serum alkaline phosphatase** (a zinc-dependent enzyme) may suggest the diagnosis. Other nutritional deficiencies in children include:
  - **Rickets (vitamin D deficiency).**
  - **Hemorrhagic disease of the newborn (vitamin K deficiency).**
  - **Copper deficiency** is observed in **Menkes kinky hair disease. Copper excess** is observed in **Wilson disease.**
  - **Iron deficiency** is observed in **hereditary hemorrhagic telangiectasia (HHT).**
- **Zinc supplementation** is first line.

Table 2.79. ACQUIRED NUTRITIONAL DEFICIENCIES

Deficiency[a]	Classic Description	Notes
Macronutrients		
Marasmus	Cutaneous features include dry, thin, pale, lax, wrinkled skin with loss of subcutaneous fat and muscle, pityriasis rotunda, aquagenic PPK, and ichthyosis vulgaris; TE and acquired hypertrichosis lanuginosa; Beau lines. In anorexia nervosa, the characteristic hair shaft abnormality with increased fragility is pili torti. In bulimia, calluses or scars on the knuckles or dorsal hands (Russel sign) are associated with salivary gland enlargement and tooth enamel erosion. Systemic features include bradycardia, hypotension, and hypothermia.	Marasmus is due to decreased energy intake. Slowly replace proteins and calories monitoring for cardiorespiratory failure and hypophosphatemia.
	The term "monkey facies" is used to describe an "aged" appearance due to loss of buccal fat pads.	
Kwashiorkor	Cutaneous features include dyschromia, pallor, and erosion of the skin, xerosis; cheilitis, vulvovaginitis and xerophthalmia/xerostomia; brittle hair; and hapalonychia. Systemic features include edema and acquired immunodeficiency.	Kwashiorkor is due to decreased protein intake (eg, stress and diets consisting primarily of rice or rice-based beverages).

Table 2.79. ACQUIRED NUTRITIONAL DEFICIENCIES (CONTINUED)

Deficiency[a]	Classic Description	Notes
	Erosion of the skin is often likened to "flaky paint." The "flag sign" refers to bands of light and dark hair coloration reflecting intermittent malnutrition. Edema may manifest as a "pot belly."	
Essential fatty acids (eg, linoleic, linolenic, arachidonic)	Cutaneous features include dry, scaly, leathery skin with underlying erythema and intertriginous erosions; alopecia. Systemic features include neurologic damage.	Essential fatty acid deficiency is due to decreased fat intake (eg, parenteral nutrition without lipid supplementation) or malabsorption, nephrotic syndrome, and inborn errors of metabolism.

Fat Soluble Vitamins—Easily Accumulate and Lead to Toxicity

Deficiency[a]	Classic Description	Notes
A (retinol)	Cutaneous features include ichthyosis vulgaris, phrynoderma, and xerosis; Bitot spots (gray-white conjunctival patches), xerophthalmia, xerostomia. Systemic features include night blindness and keratomalacia.	Vitamin A deficiency increases mortality related to measles, diarrheal, and respiratory illnesses. Vitamin A excess resembles the side effect profile of systemic retinoids. ß-carotene, a natural provitamin of vitamin A, causes yellow-orange discoloration due to carotenemia, leukopenia, or inability to convert to vitamin A (eg, hypothyroidism).
	Phrynoderma, a disorder of follicular keratinization, is derived from the Greek words *phrúnē* meaning "toad" and *derma* meaning "skin."	
D (D_2 ergocalciferol, D_3 cholecalciferol)	Systemic features include muscle weakness and osteomalacia.	For recommended dietary allowance of vitamin D, see Chapter 1: Photobiology. Features of vitamin D excess include nephrolithiasis and nephrocalcinosis. Vitamin D analogues are used to treat a variety of skin disorders including psoriasis.
E (derivative tocopherol)	Systemic features include muscle weakness and pigmentary retinopathy.	Features of vitamin E excess include hemorrhage due to reduced platelet aggregation and vitamin K function.
K (K_1 phytonadione, K_2 menaquinone)	Cutaneous features include ecchymoses and retiform purpura.	Vitamin K is required to activate factors II, VII, IX, X, and proteins C and S. Deficiency prolongs the PT > PTT. Risk factors include broad-spectrum antibiotics, which reduce vitamin K synthesis by gut bacteria. Vitamin K may be associated with sclerosis (injection sites), also known as Texier disease.

Water Soluble Vitamins—Less Likely to Accumulate and Lead to Toxicity

Deficiency[a]	Classic Description	Notes
B_1 (thiamin, thiamine)	Cutaneous features include skin breakdown due to edema; glossitis. Systemic features include cardiac failure (wet) and peripheral neuropathy (dry).	Vitamin B_1 deficiency is termed "beriberi." Risk factors include a polished rice diet.
B_2 (riboflavin, lactoflavin)	Cutaneous features include seborrheic dermatitis–like periorificial eruption; conjunctivitis, angular cheilitis, and glossitis. Systemic features include superficial keratitis and photophobia.	Vitamin B_2 deficiency may lead to oro-oculo-genital syndrome.
B_3 (niacin, nicotinic acid)	Cutaneous features include photodistributed erythema ± scale or crust and painful palmoplantar fissures. Systemic features include diarrhea, dementia, and peripheral neuropathy.	Vitamin B_3 deficiency is called pellagra. Other causes of pellagra include tryptophan deficiency, carcinoid syndrome, Hartnup disease, and drugs (eg, INH). UVR is a trigger. Flushing may occur with niacin supplementation.
	The three Ds of pellagra are dermatitis, diarrhea, and dementia. A well-demarcated band around the neck is called "Casal necklace" after Gasper Casal, who described pellagra in 1762.	
B_6 (pyridoxine, pyridoxamine, pyridoxal)	Cutaneous features resemble vitamin B_2 deficiency. Systemic features include sideroblastic anemia, peripheral neuropathy, and seizures.	Risk factors include cirrhosis and drugs (eg, INH). UVR is a trigger.
B_7 (biotin)	Resembles zinc deficiency.	Risk factors include ingestion of raw egg whites rich in avidin (binds B_7).
		Rocky, an avid drinker of raw eggs, is at risk of B_7 deficiency due to avidin.

(Continued)

Table 2.79. ACQUIRED NUTRITIONAL DEFICIENCIES (CONTINUED)

Deficiency[a]	Classic Description	Notes
B₉ (folic acid)	Cutaneous features include diffuse hyperpigmentation with photoaccentuation; recurrent aphthous stomatitis, glossitis. Systemic features include megaloblastic anemia.	Risk factors include drugs that interfere with folate metabolism (eg, methotrexate).
B₁₂ (cyanocobalamin)	Cutaneous features resemble vitamin B₉ deficiency. Systemic features include megaloblastic anemia, ataxia, and peripheral neuropathy.	Risk factors include strict vegetarianism/veganism, celiac disease, and pernicious anemia. Folate can reverse the megaloblastic anemia but not the neurologic damage of vitamin B₁₂ deficiency. Vitamin B₁₂ may be associated with acne and sclerosis (injection sites).
C (ascorbic acid)	Cutaneous features include petechiae and ecchymoses, follicular hyperkeratosis, and impaired wound healing; spongy gingivae with bleeding and erosions; corkscrew hairs with perifollicular erythema or hemorrhage. Systemic features include hemorrhage (eg, subperiosteal), hematologic abnormalities, and hypochondriasis.	Vitamin C deficiency is called scurvy. Features primarily relate to impaired collagen synthesis.
	The four <u>H</u> of scurvy are <u>h</u>yperkeratosis, <u>h</u>emorrhage, <u>h</u>ematologic abnormalities, and <u>h</u>ypochondriasis.	
Trace Elements		
Copper	Cutaneous features include pigmentary dilution of the skin and hair. Systemic features include cytopenias.	Copper-dependent enzymes include tyrosinase and lysyl oxidase.
Iron	Cutaneous features include pruritus; alopecia; platonychia; and koilonychia. Systemic features include microcytic anemia.	Risk factors include ancylostomiasis. Ferritin should be ≥ 40 ng/dL.
	Figure 2.116.	
Selenium	Cutaneous features include pigmentary dilution of the skin and hair. Systemic features include cardiomyopathy, hypothyroidism, and muscle degeneration.	Selenium sulfide is used to treat seborrheic dermatitis.
Zinc	See above.	

INH, isoniazid; PPK, palmoplantar keratoderma; PT, prothrombin time; PTT, partial thromboplastin time; TE, telogen effluvium; UVR, ultraviolet radiation.
[a]Illustrative examples provided.

Platonychia, like <u>plat</u>ypus, is derived from the Greek word <u>plat</u>us meaning flat.

Koilonychia is derived from the Greek word <u>koilos</u> meaning hollow.

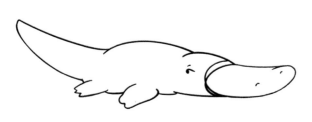

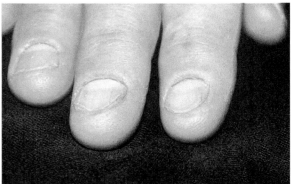

Figure 2.116. PLATONYCHIA AND KOILONYCHIA. In iron deficiency, nails first become flat (platonychia) and then hollow or "spoon shaped" (koilonychia). Koilonychia may also be observed in primary systemic amyloidosis and hyperthyroidism. (Koilonychia image reprinted with permission from Goodheart HP, Gonzalez ME. *Goodheart's Same-Site Differential Diagnosis: Dermatology for the Primary Health Care Provider.* 2nd ed. Wolters Kluwer; 2022. Illustration by Misha Rosenbach, MD.)

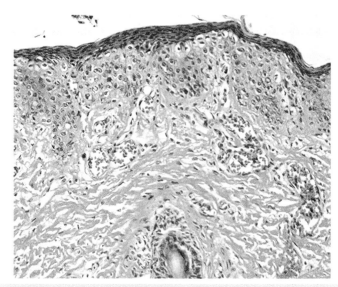

Figure 2.117. CLINICOPATHOLOGICAL CORRELATION: ZINC DEFICIENCY. Early zinc deficiency is characterized by pallor and ballooning of the upper half of the epidermis. Late zinc deficiency is characterized by parakeratosis, psoriasiform epidermal hyperplasia, and necrosis of the superficial one third of the epidermis.

(Histology image reprinted with permission from Elder DE, Elenitsas R, Rosenbach M, et al. *Lever's Histopathology of the Skin.* 11th ed. Wolters Kluwer; 2015.)

Zinc deficiency, pellagra, and necrolytic migratory erythema share the same histopathological pattern.

FURTHER READING

Abréu-Vélez AM, Reason IJd M, Howard MS, Roselino AM. Endemic pemphigus foliaceus over a century: Part I. *N Am J Med Sci.* 2010;2(2):51-59.

Ahluwalia J, Correa-Selm LM, Rao BK. Vitiligo: not simply a skin disease. *Skinmed.* 2017;15(2):125-127.

Ahmad M, Hassan I, Masood Q. Papillon-lefevre syndrome. *J Dermatol Case Rep.* 2009;3(4):53-55. doi:10.3315/jdcr.2009.1039

Aizawa T, Shiomi H, Kitano K, Kimura T. Frank's sign: diagonal earlobe crease. *Eur Heart J.* 2018;39(40):3653. doi:10.1093/eurheartj/ehy414

Alavi A, Sibbald RG, Phillips TJ, et al. What's new: management of venous leg ulcers – treating venous leg ulcers. *J Am Acad Dermatol.* 2016;74(4): 643-664. quiz 665-6. doi:10.1016/j.jaad.2015.03.059

Alavi A, Sibbald RG, Phillips TJ, et al. What's new: management of venous leg ulcers – approach to venous leg ulcers. *J Am Acad Dermatol.* 2016;74(4):627-640. quiz 641-2. doi:10.1016/j.jaad.2014.10.048

Al-Breiki SH, Al-Zoabi NM. Scurvy as the tip of the iceberg. *J Dermatol Dermatologic Surg.* 2014;18(1):46-48. doi:10.1016/j.jdds.2014.06.005

Aldana PC, Khachemoune A. Grover disease: review of subtypes with a focus on management options. *Int J Dermatol.* 2020;59(5):543-550. doi:10.1111/ijd.14700

Al-Khenaizan S. Lichen planus occurring after hepatitis B vaccination: a new case. *J Am Acad Dermatol.* 2001;45(4):614-615. doi:10.1067/mjd.2001.114590

Allanore Y, Wung P, Soubrane C, et al. A randomised, double-blind, placebo-controlled, 24-week, phase II, proof-of-concept study of romilkimab (SAR156597) in early diffuse cutaneous systemic sclerosis. *Ann Rheum Dis.* 2020;79(12):1600-1607. doi:10.1136/annrheumdis-2020-218447

Anhalt GJ, Kim SC, Stanley JR, et al. Paraneoplastic pemphigus. An autoimmune mucocutaneous disease associated with neoplasia. *N Engl J Med.* 1990;323(25):1729-1735. doi:10.1056/nejm199012203232503

Antia C, Baquerizo K, Korman A, Alikhan A, Bernstein JA. Urticaria: a comprehensive review – treatment of chronic urticaria, special populations, and disease outcomes. *J Am Acad Dermatol.* 2018;79(4):617-633. doi:10.1016/j.jaad.2018.01.023

Aringer M, Costenbader K, Daikh D, et al. 2019 European League against Rheumatism/American College of Rheumatology classification criteria for systemic lupus erythematosus. *Ann Rheum Dis.* 2019;78(9):1151-1159. doi:10.1136/annrheumdis-2018-214819

Arpita R, Monica A, Venkatesh N, Atul S, Varun M. Oral pemphigus vulgaris: case report. *Ethiop J Health Sci.* 2015;25(4):367-372.

Ashchyan HJ, Nelson CA, Stephen S, James WD, Micheletti RG, Rosenbach M. Neutrophilic dermatoses: pyoderma gangrenosum and other bowel- and arthritis-associated neutrophilic dermatoses. *J Am Acad Dermatol.* 2018;79(6):1009-1022. doi:10.1016/j.jaad.2017.11.063

Ashchyan HJ, Butler DC, Nelson CA, et al. The association of age with clinical presentation and comorbidities of pyoderma gangrenosum. *JAMA Dermatol.* 2018;154(4):409-413. doi:10.1001/jamadermatol.2017.5978

Azarchi S, Bienenfeld A, Lo Sicco K, Marchbein S, Shapiro J, Nagler AR. Androgens in women: hormone-modulating therapies for skin disease. *J Am Acad Dermatol.* 2019;80(6):1509-1521. doi:10.1016/j.jaad.2018.08.061

Bachmeyer C, Aractingi S. Neutrophilic eccrine hidradenitis. *Clin Dermatol.* 2000;18(3):319-330.

Bajaj S, Sharma PK, Sachdev IS, Bhardhwaj M. A novel presentation of cutaneous angiosarcoma: a case report and review. *Indian J Med Paediatr Oncol.* 2017;38(3):363-366. doi:10.4103/ijmpo.ijmpo_81_16

Barron SJ, Del Vecchio MT, Aronoff SC. Intravenous immunoglobulin in the treatment of Stevens-Johnson syndrome and toxic epidermal necrolysis: a meta-analysis with meta-regression of observational studies. *Int J Dermatol.* 2015;54(1):108-115. doi:10.1111/ijd.12423

Bassi A, Campolmi P, Cannarozzo G, et al. Tattoo-associated skin reaction: the importance of an early diagnosis and proper treatment. *BioMed Res Int.* 2014;2014:354608. doi:10.1155/2014/354608

Bastuji-Garin S, Fouchard N, Bertocchi M, Roujeau JC, Revuz J, Wolkenstein P. SCORTEN: a severity-of-illness score for toxic epidermal necrolysis. *J Invest Dermatol.* 2000;115(2):149-153. doi:10.1046/j.1523-1747.2000.00061.x

Bayers S, Shulman ST, Paller AS. Kawasaki disease: part II. Complications and treatment. *J Am Acad Dermatol.* 2013;69(4):513.e1-8. quiz 521-2. doi:10.1016/j.jaad.2013.06.040

Bayers S, Shulman ST, Paller AS. Kawasaki disease: part I. Diagnosis, clinical features, and pathogenesis. *J Am Acad Dermatol.* 2013;69(4):501.e1-11. quiz 511-2. doi:10.1016/j.jaad.2013.07.002

Bell S, Kolobova I, Crapper L, Ernst C. Lesch-nyhan syndrome: models, theories, and therapies. *Mol Syndromol.* 2016;7(6):302-311. doi:10.1159/000449296

Berger TG, Shive M, Harper GM. Pruritus in the older patient: a clinical review. *JAMA.* 2013;310(22):2443-2450. doi:10.1001/jama.2013.282023

Bernstein JA, Lang DM, Khan DA, et al. The diagnosis and management of acute and chronic urticaria: 2014 update. *J Allergy Clin Immunol.* 2014;133(5):1270-1277. doi:10.1016/j.jaci.2014.02.036

Beyer V, Wolverton SE. Recent trends in systemic psoriasis treatment costs. *Arch Dermatol.* 2010;146(1):46-54. doi:10.1001/archdermatol.2009.319

Bienenfeld A, Azarchi S, Lo Sicco K, Marchbein S, Shapiro J, Nagler AR. Androgens in women: androgen-mediated skin disease and patient evaluation. *J Am Acad Dermatol.* 2019;80(6):1497-1506. doi:10.1016/j.jaad.2018.08.062

Bohnett MC, Heath M, Mengden S, Morrison L. Arterial hand ulcer: a common disease in an uncommon location. *JAAD Case Rep.* 2019;5(2):147-149. doi:10.1016/j.jdcr.2018.12.001

Bolduc C, Sperling LC, Shapiro J. Primary cicatricial alopecia: other lymphocytic primary cicatricial alopecias and neutrophilic and mixed primary cicatricial alopecias. *J Am Acad Dermatol.* 2016;75(6):1101-1117. doi:10.1016/j.jaad.2015.01.056

Bolduc C, Sperling LC, Shapiro J. Primary cicatricial alopecia: lymphocytic primary cicatricial alopecias, including chronic cutaneous lupus erythematosus, lichen planopilaris, frontal fibrosing alopecia, and Graham-Little syndrome. *J Am Acad Dermatol.* 2016;75(6):1081-1099. doi:10.1016/j.jaad.2014.09.058

Bolognia JL, Schaffer JV, Cerroni L. *Dermatology.* 4th ed. Elsevier Saunders; 2018.

Bolotin D, Petronic-Rosic V. Dermatitis herpetiformis. Part II. Diagnosis, management, and prognosis. *J Am Acad Dermatol.* 2011;64(6):1027-1033. quiz 1033-4. doi:10.1016/j.jaad.2010.09.776

Bolotin D, Petronic-Rosic V. Dermatitis herpetiformis. Part I. Epidemiology, pathogenesis, and clinical presentation. *J Am Acad Dermatol.* 2011;64(6):1017-1024. quiz 1025-6. doi:10.1016/j.jaad.2010.09.777

Boulton AJM, Cutfield RG, Abouganem D, et al. Necrobiosis lipoidica diabeticorum: a clinicopathologic study. *J Am Acad Dermatol.* 1988;18(3):530-537. doi:10.1016/S0190-9622(88)70076-6

Brown F, Tanner LS. *Lofgren syndrome. StatPearls.* StatPearls Publishing; 2019. StatPearls Publishing LLC.

Buzi F, Badolato R, Mazza C, et al. Autoimmune polyendocrinopathy-candidiasis-ectodermal dystrophy syndrome: time to review diagnostic criteria? *J Clin Endocrinol Metab.* 2003;88(7):3146-3148. doi:10.1210/jc.2002-021495

Buzney E, Sheu J, Buzney C, Reynolds RV. Polycystic ovary syndrome: a review for dermatologists – Part II. Treatment. *J Am Acad Dermatol.* 2014;71(5):859.e1-859.e15. quiz 873-4. doi:10.1016/j.jaad.2014.05.009

Byrd JA, Davis MDP, Bruce AJ, Drage LA, Rogers RS,IIIrd. Response of oral lichen planus to topical tacrolimus in 37 patients. *Arch Dermatol.* 2004;140(12):1508-1512. doi:10.1001/archderm.140.12.1508

Cale CM, Morton L, Goldblatt D. Cutaneous and other lupus-like symptoms in carriers of X-linked chronic granulomatous disease: incidence and autoimmune serology. *Clin Exp Immunol.* 2007;148(1):79-84. doi:10.1111/j.1365-2249.2007.03321.x

Chan LS, Cooper KD. A novel immune-mediated subepidermal bullous dermatosis characterized by IgG autoantibodies to a lower lamina lucida component. *Arch Dermatol.* 1994;130(3):343-347.

Chang Y, Dabiri G, Damstetter E, Baiyee Ebot E, Powers JG, Phillips T. Coagulation disorders and their cutaneous presentations: pathophysiology. *J Am Acad Dermatol.* 2016;74(5):783-792. quiz 793-4. doi:10.1016/j.jaad.2015.08.072

Chaowattanapanit S, Silpa-Archa N, Kohli I, Lim HW, Hamzavi I. Postinflammatory hyperpigmentation: a comprehensive overview—treatment options and prevention. *J Am Acad Dermatol.* 2017;77(4):607-621. doi:10.1016/j.jaad.2017.01.036

Chen L, Tsai TF. HLA-Cw6 and psoriasis. *Br J Dermatol.* 2018;178(4):854-862. doi:10.1111/bjd.16083

Chitkara RK, Krishna G. Parasitic pulmonary eosinophilia. *Semin Respir Crit Care Med.* 2006;27(2):171-184. doi:10.1055/s-2006-939520

Cho YT, Lin JW, Chen YC, et al. Generalized bullous fixed drug eruption is distinct from Stevens-Johnson syndrome/toxic epidermal necrolysis by immunohistopathological features. *J Am Acad Dermatol.* 2014;70(3):539-548. doi:10.1016/j.jaad.2013.11.015

Chung SA, Langford CA, Maz M, et al. 2021 American College of rheumatology/vasculitis foundation guideline for the management of antineutrophil cytoplasmic antibody-associated vasculitis. *Arthritis Rheumatol.* 2021;73:1366-1383. doi:10.1002/art.41773

Chung SA, Gorelik M, Langford CA, et al. 2021 American College of rheumatology/vasculitis foundation guideline for the management of polyarteritis nodosa. *Arthritis Rheumatol.* 2021;73:1384-1393. doi:10.1002/art.41776

Chuquilin M, Alghalith Y, Fernandez KH. Neurocutaneous disease: cutaneous neuroanatomy and mechanisms of itch and pain. *J Am Acad Dermatol.* 2016;74(2):197-212. doi:10.1016/j.jaad.2015.04.060

Cohen PR, Grossman ME, Almeida L, Kurzrock R. Tripe palms and malignancy. *J Clin Oncol.* 1989;7(5):669-678. doi:10.1200/jco.1989.7.5.669

Colboc H, Moguelet P, Bazin D, et al. Localization, morphologic features, and chemical composition of calciphylaxis-related skin deposits in patients with calcific uremic arteriolopathy. *JAMA Dermatol.* 2019;155(7):789-796. doi:10.1001/jamadermatol.2019.0381

Anonymous, 1990 Criteria for diagnosis of Behcet's disease. International study group for Behcet's disease. *Lancet (London, England).* 1990;335(8697):1078-1080.

Coulombe PA. The molecular revolution in cutaneous biology: keratin genes and their associated disease—diversity, opportunities, and challenges. *J Invest Dermatol.* 2017;137(5):e67-e71. doi:10.1016/j.jid.2016.04.039

Cowper SE, Rabach M, Girardi M. Clinical and histological findings in nephrogenic systemic fibrosis. *Eur J Radiol.* 2008;66(2):191-199. doi:10.1016/j.ejrad.2008.01.016

Creadore A, Watchmaker J, Maymone MBC, Pappas L, Lam C, Vashi NA. Cosmetic treatment in patients with autoimmune connective tissue diseases: best practices for patients with morphea/systemic sclerosis. *J Am Acad Dermatol.* 2020;83(2):315-341. doi:10.1016/j.jaad.2019.12.081

Creadore A, Watchmaker J, Maymone MBC, Pappas L, Vashi NA, Lam C. Cosmetic treatment in patients with autoimmune connective tissue diseases: best practices for patients with lupus erythematosus. *J Am Acad Dermatol.* 2020;83(2):343-363. doi:10.1016/j.jaad.2020.03.123

Cugno M, Borghi A, Marzano AV. PAPA, PASH and PAPASH syndromes: pathophysiology, presentation and treatment. *Am J Clin Dermatol.* 2017;18(4):555-562. doi:10.1007/s40257-017-0265-1

Curtis C, Ogbogu P. Hypereosinophilic syndrome. *Clin Rev Allergy Immunol.* 2016;50(2):240-251. doi:10.1007/s12016-015-8506-7

Dabiri G, Damstetter E, Chang Y, Baiyee Ebot E, Powers JG, Phillips T. Coagulation disorders and their cutaneous presentations: diagnostic work-up and treatment. *J Am Acad Dermatol.* 2016;74(5):795-804. quiz 805-6. doi:10.1016/j.jaad.2015.08.071

Damsky W, Thakral D, Emeagwali N, Galan A, King B. Tofacitinib treatment and molecular analysis of cutaneous sarcoidosis. *N Engl J Med.* 2018;379(26):2540-2546. doi:10.1056/NEJMoa1805958

Dave S, Thappa DM, Dsouza M. Clinical predictors of outcome in vitiligo. *Indian J Dermatol Venereol Leprol.* 2002;68(6):323-325.

de Castro JL, Freitas JP, Brandão FM, Themido R. Sensitivity to thimerosal and photosensitivity to piroxicam. *Contact Dermatitis.* 1991;24(3):187-192. doi:10.1111/j.1600-0536.1991.tb01696.x

DeRossi SS, Ciarrocca KN. Lichen planus, lichenoid drug reactions, and lichenoid mucositis. *Dent Clin North Am.* 2005;49(1):77-89. viii. doi:10.1016/j.cden.2004.08.004

Dev T, Thami T, Longchar M, Sethuraman G. Lupus miliaris disseminatus faciei: a distinctive facial granulomatous eruption. *BMJ Case Rep.* 2017;2017:bcr2017221118. doi:10.1136/bcr-2017-221118

DeWane ME, Waldman R, Lu J. Dermatomyositis: clinical features and pathogenesis. *J Am Acad Dermatol.* 2020;82(2):267-281. doi:10.1016/j.jaad.2019.06.1309

Dicken CH. Trigeminal trophic syndrome. *Mayo Clin Proc.* 1997;72(6):543-545. doi:10.4065/72.6.543

Dimitriades VR, Brown AG, Gedalia A. Kawasaki disease: pathophysiology, clinical manifestations, and management. *Curr Rheumatol Rep.* 2014;16(6):423. doi:10.1007/s11926-014-0423-x

Duong TA, Valeyrie-Allanore L, Wolkenstein P, Chosidow O. Severe cutaneous adverse reactions to drugs. *Lancet.* 2017;390(10106):1996-2011. doi:10.1016/S0140-6736(16)30378-6

Eichenfield LF, Tom WL, Berger TG, et al. Guidelines of care for the management of atopic dermatitis: section 2. Management and treatment of atopic dermatitis with topical therapies. *J Am Acad Dermatol.* 2014;71(1):116-132. doi:10.1016/j.jaad.2014.03.023

Eichenfield LF, Tom WL, Chamlin SL, et al. Guidelines of care for the management of atopic dermatitis: section 1. Diagnosis and assessment of atopic dermatitis. *J Am Acad Dermatol.* 2014;70(2):338-351. doi:10.1016/j.jaad.2013.10.010

Elder DE. *Lever's Histopathology of the Skin.* 11th ed. Wolters Kluwer; 2015.

Ellebrecht CT, Bhoj VG, Nace A, et al. Reengineering chimeric antigen receptor T cells for targeted therapy of autoimmune disease. *Science (New York, NY).* 2016;353(6295):179-184. doi:10.1126/science.aaf6756

Elmets CA, Leonardi CL, Davis DMR, et al. Joint AAD-NPF guidelines of care for the management and treatment of psoriasis with awareness and attention to comorbidities. *J Am Acad Dermatol.* 2019;80(4):1073-1113. doi:10.1016/j.jaad.2018.11.058

mets CA, Lim HW, Stoff B, et al. Joint American Academy of Dermatology~National Psoriasis Foundation guidelines of care for the management and treatment of psoriasis with phototherapy. *J Am Acad Dermatol.* 2019;81(3):775-804. doi:10.1016/j.jaad.2019.04.042

Elmets CA, Korman NJ, Prater EF, et al. Joint AAD-NPF Guidelines of care for the management and treatment of psoriasis with topical therapy and alternative medicine modalities for psoriasis severity measures. *J Am Acad Dermatol.* 2021;84(2):432-470. doi:10.1016/j.jaad.2020.07.087

Elston DM, Ferringer T. *Dermatopathology.* 2nd ed. Elsevier Saunders; 2014.

Elston DM, Clayton AS, Meffert JJ, McCollough ML. Migratory poliosis: a forme fruste of alopecia areata? *J Am Acad Dermatol.* 2000;42(6):1076-1077. doi:10.1016/s0190-9622(00)90307-4

Estokova A, Palascakova L, Kanuchova M. Study on Cr(VI) leaching from cement and cement composites. *Int J Environ Res Public Health.* 2018;15(4):824. doi:10.3390/ijerph15040824

Feldman SR, Krueger GG. Psoriasis assessment tools in clinical trials. *Ann Rheum Dis.* 2005;64(suppl 2):ii65-ii68; discussion ii69-73. doi:doi:10.1136/ard.2004.031237.

Fett N, Werth VP. Update on morphea: part II. Outcome measures and treatment. *J Am Acad Dermatol.* 2011;64(2):231-242. quiz 243-4. doi:10.1016/j.jaad.2010.05.046

Fett N, Werth VP. Update on morphea: part I. Epidemiology, clinical presentation, and pathogenesis. *J Am Acad Dermatol.* 2011;64(2):217-228. quiz 229-30. doi:10.1016/j.jaad.2010.05.045

Filipovich AH, Weisdorf D, Pavletic S, et al. National Institutes of Health consensus development project on criteria for clinical trials in chronic graft-versus-host disease: I. Diagnosis and staging working group report. *Biol Blood Marrow Transplant.* 2005;11(12):945-956. doi:10.1016/j.bbmt.2005.09.004

Fine JD, Mellerio JE. Extracutaneous manifestations and complications of inherited epidermolysis bullosa: part II. Other organs. *J Am Acad Dermatol.* 2009;61(3):387-402. quiz 403-4. doi:10.1016/j.jaad.2009.03.053

Fine JD, Mellerio JE. Extracutaneous manifestations and complications of inherited epidermolysis bullosa: part I. Epithelial associated tissues. *J Am Acad Dermatol.* 2009;61(3):367-384. quiz 385-6. doi:10.1016/j.jaad.2009.03.052

Flåm ST, Gunnarsson R, Garen T; Norwegian MCTD Study Group, Lie BA, Molberg O. The HLA profiles of mixed connective tissue disease differ distinctly from the profiles of clinically related connective tissue diseases. *Rheumatology (Oxford, England).* 2015;54(3):528-535. doi:10.1093/rheumatology/keu310

Fonda-Pascual P, Vano-Galvan S, Garcia-Hernandez MJ, Camacho F. Alopecia areata sisaipho: clinical and therapeutic approach in 13 patients in Spain. *Int J Trichology.* 2016;8(2):99-100. doi:10.4103/0974-7753.188039

Forlino A, Marini JC. Osteogenesis imperfecta. *Lancet (London, England).* 2016;387(10028):1657-1671. doi:10.1016/S0140-6736(15)00728-X

Freites-Martinez A, Shapiro J, Goldfarb S, et al. Hair disorders in patients with cancer. *J Am Acad Dermatol.* 2019;80(5):1179-1196. doi:10.1016/j.jaad.2018.03.055

Freites-Martinez A, Shapiro J, van den Hurk C, et al. Hair disorders in cancer survivors. *J Am Acad Dermatol.* 2019;80(5):1199-1213. doi:10.1016/j.jaad.2018.03.056

Frew JW, Murrell DF. Current management strategies in paraneoplastic pemphigus (paraneoplastic autoimmune multiorgan syndrome). *Dermatol Clin.* 2011;29(4):607-612. doi:10.1016/j.det.2011.06.016

Fritsch C, Bolsen K, Ruzicka T, Goerz G. Congenital erythropoietic porphyria. *J Am Acad Dermatol.* 1997;36(4):594-610. doi:10.1016/s0190-9622(97)70249-4

Gantz M, Butler D, Goldberg M, Ryu J, McCalmont T, Shinkai K. Atypical features and systemic associations in extensive cases of Grover disease: a systematic review. *J Am Acad Dermatol.* 2017;77(5):952-957.e1. doi:10.1016/j.jaad.2017.06.041

Garcia MA, Ramonet M, Ciocca M, et al. Alagille syndrome: cutaneous manifestations in 38 children. *Pediatr Dermatol.* 2005;22(1):11-14. doi:10.1111/j.1525-1470.2005.22102.x

Gelfand JM, Neimann AL, Shin DB, Wang X, Margolis DJ, Troxel AB. Risk of myocardial infarction in patients with psoriasis. *JAMA.* 2006;296(14):1735-1741. doi:10.1001/jama.296.14.1735

Gerson D, Sriganeshan V, Alexis JB. Cutaneous drug eruptions: a 5-year experience. *J Am Acad Dermatol.* 2008;59(6):995-999. doi:10.1016/j.jaad.2008.09.015

Goldburg SR, Strober BE, Payette MJ. Hidradenitis suppurativa: epidemiology, clinical presentation, and pathogenesis. *J Am Acad Dermatol.* 2020;82(5):1045-1058. doi:10.1016/j.jaad.2019.08.090

Goldburg SR, Strober BE, Payette MJ. Hidradenitis suppurativa: current and emerging treatments. *J Am Acad Dermatol.* 2020;82(5):1061-1082. doi:10.1016/j.jaad.2019.08.089

Gorouhi F, Davari P, Fazel N. Cutaneous and mucosal lichen planus: a comprehensive review of clinical subtypes, risk factors, diagnosis, and prognosis. *Sci World J.* 2014;2014:742826. doi:10.1155/2014/742826

Gottenberg J-E, Busson M, Loiseau P, et al. In primary Sjögren's syndrome, HLA class II is associated exclusively with autoantibody production and spreading of the autoimmune response. *Arthritis Rheum.* 2003;48(8):2240-2245. doi:10.1002/art.11103

Grada AA, Phillips TJ. Lymphedema: pathophysiology and clinical manifestations. *J Am Acad Dermatol.* 2017;77(6):1009-1020. doi:10.1016/j.jaad.2017.03.022

Grada AA, Phillips TJ. Lymphedema: diagnostic workup and management. *J Am Acad Dermatol.* 2017;77(6):995-1006. doi:10.1016/j.jaad.2017.03.021

Haimovic A, Sanchez M, Judson MA, Prystowsky S. Sarcoidosis: a comprehensive review and update for the dermatologist – part II. Extracutaneous disease. *J Am Acad Dermatol.* 2012;66(5):719.e1-10. quiz 729-30. doi:10.1016/j.jaad.2012.02.003

Haimovic A, Sanchez M, Judson MA, Prystowsky S. Sarcoidosis: a comprehensive review and update for the dermatologist – part I. Cutaneous disease. *J Am Acad Dermatol.* 2012;66(5):699.e1-18. quiz 717-8. doi:10.1016/j.jaad.2011.11.965

Halevy S, Shai A. Lichenoid drug eruptions. *J Am Acad Dermatol.* 1993;29(2 pt 1):249-255. doi:10.1016/0190-9622(93)70176-t

Harita Y, Kitanaka S, Isojima T, Ashida A, Hattori M. Spectrum of LMX1B mutations: from nail-patella syndrome to isolated nephropathy. *Pediatr Nephrol.* 2017;32(10):1845-1850. doi:10.1007/s00467-016-3462-x

Hashemi DA, Brown-Joel ZO, Tkachenko E, et al. Clinical features and comorbidities of patients with necrobiosis lipoidica with or without diabetes. *JAMA Dermatol.* 2019;155(4):455-459. doi:10.1001/jamadermatol.2018.5635

Hatemi G, Christensen R, Bang D, et al. 2018 update of the EULAR recommendations for the management of Behçet's syndrome. *Ann Rheum Dis.* 2018;77(6):808-818. doi:10.1136/annrheumdis-2018-213225

Haynes D, Strunck JL, Topham CA, et al. Evaluation of ixekizumab treatment for patients with pityriasis rubra pilaris: a single-arm trial. *JAMA Dermatol.* 2020;156(6):668-675. doi:10.1001/jamadermatol.2020.0932

He Y, Sawalha AH. Drug-induced lupus erythematosus: an update on drugs and mechanisms. *Curr Opin Rheumatol.* 2018;30(5):490-497. doi:10.1097/BOR.0000000000000522

Hirschmann JV, Raugi GJ. Blue (or purple) toe syndrome. *J Am Acad Dermatol.* 2009;60(1):1-20. quiz 21-2. doi:10.1016/j.jaad.2008.09.038

Hoegler KM, John AM, Handler MZ, Schwartz RA. Generalized pustular psoriasis: a review and update on treatment. *J Eur Acad Dermatol Venereol.* 2018;32(10):1645-1651. doi:10.1111/jdv.14949

Hon KL, Leung AKC. Neonatal lupus erythematosus. *Autoimmune Dis.* 2012;2012:301274. doi:10.1155/2012/301274

Housman E, Reynolds RV. Polycystic ovary syndrome: a review for dermatologists – Part I. Diagnosis and manifestations. *J Am Acad Dermatol.* 2014;71(5):847.e1-847.e10. quiz 857-8. doi:10.1016/j.jaad.2014.05.007

Huang AH, Williams KA, Kwatra SG. Prurigo nodularis: epidemiology and clinical features. *J Am Acad Dermatol.* 2020;83(6):1559-1565. doi:10.1016/j.jaad.2020.04.183

Hunder GG, Arend WP, Bloch DA, et al. The American College of Rheumatology 1990 criteria for the classification of vasculitis. Introduction. *Arthritis Rheum.* 1990;33(8):1065-1067. doi:10.1002/art.1780330802

Hunter L, Burry AF. Necrobiotic xanthogranuloma: a systemic disease with paraproteinemia. *Pathology.* 1985;17(3):533-536.

Husain Z, Reddy BY, Schwartz RA. DRESS syndrome: part II. Management and therapeutics. *J Am Acad Dermatol.* 2013;68(5):709.e1-709.e9. quiz 718-20. doi:doi:10.1016/j.jaad.2013.01.032.

Husain Z, Reddy BY, Schwartz RA. DRESS syndrome: part I. Clinical perspectives. *J Am Acad Dermatol.* 2013;68(5):693.e1-14. quiz 706-8. doi:10.1016/j.jaad.2013.01.033

Husein-ElAhmed H, Steinhoff M. Efficacy of topical ivermectin and impact on quality of life in patients with papulopustular rosacea: a systematic review and meta-analysis. *Dermatol Ther.* 2020;33(1):e13203. doi:10.1111/dth.13203

Hymes SR, Alousi AM, Cowen EW. Graft-versus-host disease: part II. Management of cutaneous graft-versus-host disease. *J Am Acad Dermatol.* 2012;66(4):535.e1-16. quiz 551-2. doi:10.1016/j.jaad.2011.11.961

Hymes SR, Alousi AM, Cowen EW. Graft-versus-host disease: part I. Pathogenesis and clinical manifestations of graft-versus-host disease. *J Am Acad Dermatol.* 2012;66(4):515.e1-18. quiz 533-4. doi:10.1016/j.jaad.2011.11.960

Inamoto Y, Pidala J, Chai X, et al. Assessment of joint and fascia manifestations in chronic graft-versus-host disease. *Arthritis Rheumatol.* 2014;66(4):1044-1052. doi:10.1002/art.38293

International Team for the Revision of the International Criteria for Behcet's Disease ITR-ICBD. The International Criteria for Behcet's Disease (ICBD): a collaborative study of 27 countries on the sensitivity and specificity of the new criteria. *J Eur Acad Dermatol Venereol.* 2014;28(3):338-347. doi:10.1111/jdv.12107

Jachiet M, Flageul B, Deroux A, et al. The clinical spectrum and therapeutic management of hypocomplementemic urticarial vasculitis: data from a French nationwide study of fifty-seven patients. *Arthritis Rheumatol.* 2015;67(2):527-534. doi:10.1002/art.38956

Jagasia MH, Greinix HT, Arora M, et al. National Institutes of health consensus development project on criteria for clinical trials in chronic graft-versus-host disease: I. The 2014 diagnosis and staging working group report. *Biol Blood Marrow Transplant.* 2015;21(3):389-401.e1. doi:10.1016/j.bbmt.2014.12.001

James WD, Elston DM, Treat JR, Rosenbach MA, Neuhaus IM. *Andrews' Diseases of the Skin: Clinical Dermatology.* 13th ed. Elsevier; 2020.

Jedlowski PM, Fazel M, Foshee JP, Curiel-Lewandrowski C. A patient with concurrent prurigo nodularis and squamous cell carcinomas of keratoacanthoma type: the role of aprepitant in diagnostic clarity. *JAAD Case Rep.* 2020;6(1):3-5. doi:10.1016/j.jdcr.2019.10.014

Jennette JC, Falk RJ, Bacon PA, et al. 2012 revised International Chapel Hill consensus Conference Nomenclature of vasculitides. *Arthritis Rheum.* 2013;65(1):1-11. doi:10.1002/art.37715

Jockenhofer F, Wollina U, Salva KA, Benson S, Dissemond J. The PARACELSUS score: a novel diagnostic tool for pyoderma gangrenosum. *Br J Dermatol.* 2019;180(3):615-620. doi:10.1111/bjd.16401

Joly P, Courville P, Lok C, et al. Clinical criteria for the diagnosis of bullous pemphigoid: a reevaluation according to immunoblot analysis of patient sera. *Dermatology (Basel, Switzerland).* 2004;208(1):16-20. doi:10.1159/000075040

Jordan WP, Jr. Bourlas MC. Allergic contact dermatitis to underwear elastic: chemically transformed by laundry bleach. *Arch Dermatol.* 1975;111(5):593-595. doi:10.1001/archderm.1975.01630170051006

Juhl P, Bay-Jensen A-C, Hesselstrand R, Siebuhr AS, Wuttge DM. Type III, IV, and VI collagens turnover in systemic sclerosis: a longitudinal study. *Sci Rep.* 2020;10(1):7145. doi:10.1038/s41598-020-64233-8

Kardaun SH, Sekula P, Valeyrie-Allanore L, et al. Drug reaction with eosinophilia and systemic symptoms (DRESS): an original multisystem adverse drug reaction. Results from the prospective RegiSCAR study. *Br J Dermatol.* 2013;169(5):1071-1080. doi:10.1111/bjd.12501

Kasparis C, Loffeld A. Childhood acne in a boy with XYY syndrome. *BMJ Case Rep.* 2014;2014:bcr2013201587. doi:10.1136/bcr-2013-201587

Kasperkiewicz M, Ellebrecht CT, Takahashi H, et al. Pemphigus. *Nat Rev Dis Primers.* 2017;3:17026. doi:10.1038/nrdp.2017.26

Kaushik SB, Lebwohl MG. Psoriasis: which therapy for which patient – psoriasis comorbidities and preferred systemic agents. *J Am Acad Dermatol.* 2019;80(1):27-40. doi:10.1016/j.jaad.2018.06.057

Kaushik SB, Lebwohl MG. Psoriasis: which therapy for which patient – focus on special populations and chronic infections. *J Am Acad Dermatol.* 2019;80(1):43-53. doi:10.1016/j.jaad.2018.06.056

Kaye A, Gordon SC, Deverapalli SC, Her MJ, Rosmarin D. Dupilumab for the treatment of recalcitrant bullous pemphigoid. *JAMA Dermatol.* 2018;154(10):1225-1226. doi:10.1001/jamadermatol.2018.2526

Kern JS, Technau-Hafsi K, Schwacha H, et al. Esophageal involvement is frequent in lichen planus: study in 32 patients with suggestion of clinicopathologic diagnostic criteria and therapeutic implications. *Eur J Gastroenterol Hepatol.* 2016;28(12):1374-1382. doi:10.1097/meg.0000000000000732

Khalil S, Bardawil T, Kurban M, Abbas O. Tissue-resident memory T cells in the skin. *Inflamm Res.* 2020;69(3):245-254. doi:10.1007/s00011-020-01320-6

Kim J, Chavel S, Girardi M, McNiff JM. Pemphigoid vegetans: a case report and review of the literature. *J Cutan Pathol.* 2008;35(12):1144-1147. doi:10.1111/j.1600-0560.2008.01016.x

Kimura Y, Pawankar R, Aoki M, Niimi Y, Kawana S. Mast cells and T cells in Kimura's disease express increased levels of interleukin-4, interleukin-5, eotaxin and RANTES. *Clin Exp Allergy.* 2002;32(12):1787-1793.

Kirchhof MG, Miliszewski MA, Sikora S, Papp A, Dutz JP. Retrospective review of Stevens-Johnson syndrome/toxic epidermal necrolysis treatment comparing intravenous immunoglobulin with cyclosporine. *J Am Acad Dermatol.* 2014;71(5):941-947. doi:10.1016/j.jaad.2014.07.016

Knowles SR, Shapiro LE, Shear NH. Anticonvulsant hypersensitivity syndrome: incidence, prevention and management. *Drug Saf.* 1999;21(6):489-501. doi:10.2165/00002018-199921060-00005

Kossard S, Winkelmann RK. Necrobiotic xanthogranuloma. *Australas J Dermatol.* 1980;21(2):85-88.

Kremer N, Snast I, Cohen ES, et al. Rituximab and omalizumab for the treatment of bullous pemphigoid: a systematic review of the literature. *Am J Clin Dermatol.* 2019;20(2):209-216. doi:10.1007/s40257-018-0401-6

Kreuter A, Kryvosheyeva Y, Terras S, et al. Association of autoimmune diseases with lichen sclerosus in 532 male and female patients. *Acta Derm Venereol.* 2013;93(2):238-241. doi:10.2340/00015555-1512

Kridin K, Ahmed AR. Anti-p200 pemphigoid: a systematic review. *Front Immunol.* 2019;10:2466. doi:10.3389/fimmu.2019.02466

Kridin K, Patel PM, Jones VA, Cordova A, Amber KT. IgA pemphigus: a systematic review. *J Am Acad Dermatol.* 2020;82(6):1386-1392. doi:10.1016/j.jaad.2019.11.059

Kuhn H, Mennella C, Magid M, Stamu-O'Brien C, Kroumpouzos G. Psychocutaneous disease: clinical perspectives. *J Am Acad Dermatol.* 2017;76(5):779-791. doi:10.1016/j.jaad.2016.11.013

Kuhn H, Mennella C, Magid M, Stamu-O'Brien C, Kroumpouzos G. Psychocutaneous disease: pharmacotherapy and psychotherapy. *J Am Acad Dermatol.* 2017;76(5):795-808. doi:10.1016/j.jaad.2016.11.021

Kumar N, Davis MDP. Erythromelalgia: an underrecognized manifestation of small-fiber neuropathy. *Mayo Clin Proc.* 2006;81(8):1001. doi:10.4065/81.8.1001

Lacouture ME. *Dermatologic Principles and Practice in Oncology: Conditions of the Skin, Hair, and Nails in Cancer Patients.* John Wiley & Sons, Inc.; 2014.

Landers M, Law S, Storrs FJ. Contact urticaria, allergic contact dermatitis, and photoallergic contact dermatitis from oxybenzone. *Am J Contact Dermat.* 2003;14(1):33-34. doi:10.2310/6620.2003.38769

Landry M, Winkelmann RK. Multiple clear-cell acanthoma and ichthyosis. *Arch Dermatol*. 1972;105(3):371-383. doi:10.1001/archderm.1972.01620060013003

Langley RGB, Walsh N, Nevill T, Thomas L, Rowden G. Apoptosis is the mode of keratinocyte death in cutaneous graft-versus-host disease. *J Am Acad Dermatol*. 1996;35(2, part 1):187-190. doi:10.1016/S0190-9622(96)90320-5

Laurberg G, Geiger JM, Hjorth N, et al. Treatment of lichen planus with acitretin. A double-blind, placebo-controlled study in 65 patients. *J Am Acad Dermatol*. 1991;24(3):434-437. doi:10.1016/0190-9622(91)70067-c

Lazarov A. Sensitization to acrylates is a common adverse reaction to artificial fingernails. *J Eur Acad Dermatol Venereol*. 2007;21(2):169-174. doi:10.1111/j.1468-3083.2006.01883.x

Lebwohl M, Hecker D, Martinez J, Sapadin A, Patel B. Interactions between calcipotriene and ultraviolet light. *J Am Acad Dermatol*. 1997;37(1):93-95. doi:10.1016/s0190-9622(97)70217-2

Leccese P, Ozguler Y, Christensen R, et al. Management of skin, mucosa and joint involvement of Behcet's syndrome: a systematic review for update of the EULAR recommendations for the management of Behcet's syndrome. *Semin Arthritis Rheum*. 2019;48(4):752-762. doi:10.1016/j.semarthrit.2018.05.008

Lee A, Bradford J, Fischer G. Long-term management of adult vulvar lichen sclerosus: a prospective cohort study of 507 women. *JAMA Dermatol*. 2015;151(10):1061-1067. doi:10.1001/jamadermatol.2015.0643

Letsinger JA, McCarty MA, Jorizzo JL. Complex aphthosis: a large case series with evaluation algorithm and therapeutic ladder from topicals to thalidomide. *J Am Acad Dermatol*. 2005;52(3 pt 1):500-508. doi:10.1016/j.jaad.2004.10.863

Leung AKC, Leong KF, Lam JM. Erythema nodosum. *World J Pediatr*. 2018;14(6):548-554. doi:10.1007/s12519-018-0191-1

Levin C, Warshaw E. Protein contact dermatitis: allergens, pathogenesis, and management. *Dermatitis*. 2008;19(5):241-251.

Lindhaus C, Elsner P. Granuloma faciale treatment: a systematic review. *Acta Derm Venereol*. 2018;98(1):14-18. doi:10.2340/00015555-2784

Ling ML, Yosar J, Lee BW, et al. The diagnosis and management of temporal arteritis. *Clin Exp Optom*. 2020;103(5):572-582. doi:10.1111/cxo.12975

Lipner SR, Scher RK. Evaluation of nail lines: color and shape hold clues. *Cleve Clin J Med*. 2016;83(5):385-391. doi:10.3949/ccjm.83a.14187

Lipowicz S, Sekula P, Ingen-Housz-Oro S, et al. Prognosis of generalized bullous fixed drug eruption: comparison with Stevens-Johnson syndrome and toxic epidermal necrolysis. *Br J Dermatol*. 2013;168(4):726-732. doi:10.1111/bjd.12133

Lomaga MA, Polak S, Grushka M, Walsh S. Results of patch testing in patients diagnosed with oral lichen planus. *J Cutan Med Surg*. 2009;13(2):88-95. doi:10.2310/7750.2008.08017

Lombardi ML, Mercuro O, Ruocco V, et al. Common human leukocyte antigen alleles in pemphigus vulgaris and pemphigus foliaceus Italian patients. *J Invest Dermatol*. 1999;113(1):107-110. doi:10.1046/j.1523-1747.1999.00626.x

Long H, Zhang G, Wang L, Lu Q. Eosinophilic skin diseases: a comprehensive review. *Clin Rev Allergy Immunol*. 2016;50(2):189-213. doi:10.1007/s12016-015-8485-8

Lutz J, Huwiler KG, Fedczyna T, et al. Increased plasma thrombospondin-1 (TSP-1) levels are associated with the TNF alpha-308A allele in children with juvenile dermatomyositis. *Clin Immunol*. 2002;103(3 pt 1):260-263. doi:10.1006/clim.2001.5212

Maaloul I, Talmoudi J, Chabchoub I, et al. Chediak–Higashi syndrome presenting in accelerated phase: a case report and literature review. *Hematol Oncol Stem Cell Ther*. 2016;9(2):71-75. doi:10.1016/j.hemonc.2015.07.002

Maderal AD, Lee Salisbury P,IIIrd, Jorizzo JL. Desquamative gingivitis: clinical findings and diseases. *J Am Acad Dermatol*. 2018;78(5):839-848. doi:10.1016/j.jaad.2017.05.056

Maderal AD, Lee Salisbury P,IIIrd, Jorizzo JL. Desquamative gingivitis: diagnosis and treatment. *J Am Acad Dermatol*. 2018;78(5):851-861. doi:10.1016/j.jaad.2017.04.1140

Magin P, Pond D, Smith W. Isotretinoin, depression and suicide: a review of the evidence. *Br J Gen Pract*. 2005;55(511):134-138.

Maguire GA, Ginawi A, Lee J, et al. Clinical utility of ANA measured by ELISA compared with ANA measured by immunofluorescence. *Rheumatology*. 2009;48(8):1013-1014. doi:10.1093/rheumatology/kep137

Mankad AK, Shah KB. Transthyretin cardiac amyloidosis. *Curr Cardiol Rep*. 2017;19(10):97. doi:10.1007/s11886-017-0911-5

Marino A, Tirelli F, Giani T, Cimaz R. Periodic fever syndromes and the autoinflammatory diseases (AIDs). *J Transl Autoimmun*. 2020;3:100031. doi:10.1016/j.jtauto.2019.100031

Marvi U, Chung L, Fiorentino DF. Clinical presentation and evaluation of dermatomyositis. *Indian J Dermatol*. 2012;57(5):375-381. doi:10.4103/0019-5154.100486

Marzano AV, Damiani G, Genovese G, Gattorno M. A dermatologic perspective on autoinflammatory diseases. *Clin Exp Rheumatol*. 2018;36 suppl 110(1):32-38.

Mauskar MM, Marathe K, Venkatesan A, Schlosser BJ, Edwards L. Vulvar diseases: approach to the patient. *J Am Acad Dermatol*. 2020;82(6):1277-1284. doi:10.1016/j.jaad.2019.07.115

Mauskar MM, Marathe K, Venkatesan A, Schlosser BJ, Edwards L. Vulvar diseases: conditions in adults and children. *J Am Acad Dermatol*. 2020;82(6):1287-1298. doi:10.1016/j.jaad.2019.10.077

Maverakis E, Ma C, Shinkai K, et al. Diagnostic criteria of ulcerative pyoderma gangrenosum: a Delphi consensus of international experts. *JAMA Dermatol*. 2018;154(4):461-466. doi:10.1001/jamadermatol.2017.5980

May NC, Lester RS. Elastosis perforans serpiginosa associated with systemic sclerosis. *J Am Acad Dermatol*. 1982;6(5):945. doi:10.1016/s0190-9622(82)80131-x

Maz M, Chung SA, Abril A, et al. 2021 American College of rheumatology/vasculitis foundation guideline for the management of giant cell arteritis and Takayasu arteritis. *Arthritis Rheumatol*. 2021;73:1349-1365. doi:10.1002/art.41774

Mazariegos GV, Abu-Elmagd K, Jaffe R, et al. Graft versus host disease in intestinal transplantation. *Am J Transplant*. 2004;4(9):1459-1465. doi:10.1111/j.1600-6143.2004.00524.x

Mease PJ, Armstrong AW. Managing patients with psoriatic disease: the diagnosis and pharmacologic treatment of psoriatic arthritis in patients with psoriasis. *Drugs*. 2014;74(4):423-441. doi:10.1007/s40265-014-0191-y

Mellerio JE, Robertson SJ, Bernardis C, et al. Management of cutaneous squamous cell carcinoma in patients with epidermolysis bullosa: best clinical practice guidelines. *Br J Dermatol*. 2016;174(1):56-67. doi:10.1111/bjd.14104

Menter A, Strober BE, Kaplan DH, et al. Joint AAD-NPF guidelines of care for the management and treatment of psoriasis with biologics. *J Am Acad Dermatol*. 2019;80(4):1029-1072. doi:10.1016/j.jaad.2018.11.057

Menter A, Cordoro KM, Davis DMR, et al. Joint American Academy of Dermatology-National Psoriasis Foundation guidelines of care for the management and treatment of psoriasis in pediatric patients. *J Am Acad Dermatol*. 2020;82(1):161-201. doi:10.1016/j.jaad.2019.08.049

nter A, Gelfand JM, Connor C, et al. Joint American Academy of Dermatology-National Psoriasis Foundation guidelines of care for the management of psoriasis with systemic nonbiologic therapies. *J Am Acad Dermatol*. 2020;82(6):1445-1486. doi:10.1016/j.jaad.2020.02.044

Michaels JD, Hoss E, DiCaudo DJ, Price H. Prurigo pigmentosa after a strict ketogenic diet. *Pediatr Dermatol*. 2015;32(2):248-251. doi:10.1111/pde.12275

Micheletti RG, Chiesa-Fuxench Z, Noe MH, et al. Stevens-johnson syndrome/toxic epidermal necrolysis: a multicenter retrospective study of 377 adult patients from the United States. *J Invest Dermatol*. 2018;138(11):2315-2321. doi:10.1016/j.jid.2018.04.027

Mina R, Brunner HI. Pediatric lupus--are there differences in presentation, genetics, response to therapy, and damage accrual compared with adult lupus? *Rheum Dis Clin North Am*. 2010;36(1):53-80, vii-viii. doi:10.1016/j.rdc.2009.12.012

Mirmirani P, Karnik P. Lichen planopilaris treated with a peroxisome proliferator-activated receptor gamma agonist. *Arch Dermatol*. 2009;145(12):1363-1366. doi:10.1001/archdermatol.2009.283

Misidou C, Papagoras C. Complex regional pain syndrome: an update. *Mediterr J Rheumatol*. 2019;30(1):16-25. doi:10.31138/mjr.30.1.16

Montagnon CM, Lehman JS, Murrell DF, Camilleri MJ, Tolkachjov SN. Intraepithelial autoimmune bullous dermatoses disease activity assessment and therapy. *J Am Acad Dermatol*. 2021;84(6):1523-1537. doi:10.1016/j.jaad.2021.02.073

Montagnon CM, Tolkachjov SN, Murrell DF, Camilleri MJ, Lehman JS. Intraepithelial autoimmune blistering dermatoses: clinical features and diagnosis. *J Am Acad Dermatol.* 2021;84(6):1507-1519. doi:10.1016/j.jaad.2020.11.075

Montagnon CM, Lehman JS, Murrell DF, Camilleri MJ, Tolkachjov SN. Subepithelial autoimmune bullous dermatoses disease activity assessment and therapy. *J Am Acad Dermatol.* 2021;85(1):18-27. doi:10.1016/j.jaad.2020.05.161

Montagnon CM, Tolkachjov SN, Murrell DF, Camilleri MJ, Lehman JS. Subepithelial autoimmune blistering dermatoses: clinical features and diagnosis. *J Am Acad Dermatol.* 2021;85(1):1-14. doi:10.1016/j.jaad.2020.11.076

Morton LM, Phillips TJ. Wound healing and treating wounds: differential diagnosis and evaluation of chronic wounds. *J Am Acad Dermatol.* 2016;74(4):589-605. quiz 605-6. doi:10.1016/j.jaad.2015.08.068

Mowad CM, Anderson B, Scheinman P, Pootongkam S, Nedorost S, Brod B. Allergic contact dermatitis: patient management and education. *J Am Acad Dermatol.* 2016;74(6):1043-1054. doi:10.1016/j.jaad.2015.02.1144

Mowad CM, Anderson B, Scheinman P, Pootongkam S, Nedorost S, Brod B. Allergic contact dermatitis: patient diagnosis and evaluation. *J Am Acad Dermatol.* 2016;74(6):1029-1040. doi:10.1016/j.jaad.2015.02.1139

Mubki T, Rudnicka L, Olszewska M, Shapiro J. Evaluation and diagnosis of the hair loss patient: part II. Trichoscopic and laboratory evaluations. *J Am Acad Dermatol.* 2014;71(3):431.e1-431.e11. doi:10.1016/j.jaad.2014.05.008

Mubki T, Rudnicka L, Olszewska M, Shapiro J. Evaluation and diagnosis of the hair loss patient: part I. History and clinical examination. *J Am Acad Dermatol.* 2014;71(3):415.e1-415.e15. doi:10.1016/j.jaad.2014.04.070

Muller SA, Henderson ED. Melorheostosis with linear scleroderma. *Arch Dermatol.* 1963;88(2):142-145. doi:10.1001/archderm.1963.01590200030005

Navarini AA, Burden AD, Capon F, et al. European consensus statement on phenotypes of pustular psoriasis. *J Eur Acad Dermatol Venereol.* 2017;31(11):1792-1799. doi:10.1111/jdv.14386

Nawrocki S, Cha J. The etiology, diagnosis, and management of hyperhidrosis: a comprehensive review—etiology and clinical work-up. *J Am Acad Dermatol.* 2019;81(3):657-666. doi:10.1016/j.jaad.2018.12.071

Nawrocki S, Cha J. The etiology, diagnosis, and management of hyperhidrosis: a comprehensive review – therapeutic options. *J Am Acad Dermatol.* 2019;81(3):669-680. doi:10.1016/j.jaad.2018.11.066

Neale H, Garza-Mayers AC, Tam I, Yu J. Pediatric allergic contact dermatitis. Part I: clinical features and common contact allergens in children. *J Am Acad Dermatol.* 2021;84(2):235-244. doi:10.1016/j.jaad.2020.11.002

Neale H, Garza-Mayers AC, Tam I, Yu J. Pediatric allergic contact dermatitis. Part 2: patch testing series, procedure, and unique scenarios. *J Am Acad Dermatol.* 2021;84(2):247-255. doi:10.1016/j.jaad.2020.11.001

Nelson CA, Stephen S, Ashchyan HJ, James WD, Micheletti RG, Rosenbach M. Neutrophilic dermatoses: pathogenesis, Sweet syndrome, neutrophilic eccrine hidradenitis, and Behcet disease. *J Am Acad Dermatol.* 2018;79(6):987-1006. doi:10.1016/j.jaad.2017.11.064

Nelson CA, Noe MH, McMahon CM, et al. Sweet syndrome in patients with and without malignancy: a retrospective analysis of 83 patients from a tertiary academic referral center. *J Am Acad Dermatol.* 2018;78(2):303-309.e4. doi:10.1016/j.jaad.2017.09.013

Nelson CA, Zhong CS, Hashemi DA, et al. A multicenter cross-sectional study and systematic review of necrobiotic xanthogranuloma with proposed diagnostic criteria. *JAMA Dermatol.* 2020;156(3):270-279. doi:10.1001/jamadermatol.2019.4221

Nguyen E, Yanes D, Imadojemu S, Kroshinsky D. Evaluation of cyclosporine for the treatment of DRESS syndrome. *JAMA Dermatol.* 2020;156(6):704-706. doi:10.1001/jamadermatol.2020.0048

NIAID-Sponsored Expert Panel; Boyce JA, Assa'ad A, et al. Guidelines for the diagnosis and management of food allergy in the United States: report of the NIAID-sponsored expert panel. *J Allergy Clin Immunol.* 2010;126(6 suppl):S1-S58. doi:10.1016/j.jaci.2010.10.007

Nigwekar SU, Bloch DB, Nazarian RM, et al. Vitamin K-dependent carboxylation of matrix Gla protein influences the risk of calciphylaxis. *J Am Soc Nephrol.* 2017;28(6):1717-1722. doi:10.1681/asn.2016060651

Niu Z, Zhang P, Tong Y. Value of HLA-DR genotype in systemic lupus erythematosus and lupus nephritis: a meta-analysis. *Int J Rheum Dis.* 2015;18(1):17-28. doi:10.1111/1756-185x.12528

Noe MH, Rosenbach M, Hubbard RA, et al. Development and validation of a risk prediction model for in-hospital mortality among patients with Stevens-Johnson syndrome/toxic epidermal necrolysis-ABCD-10. *JAMA Dermatol.* 2019;155(4):448-454. doi:10.1001/jamadermatol.2018.5605

Nomura K, Umeki K, Sawamura D, Hashimoto I. Dominant dystrophic epidermolysis bullosa albopapuloidea Pasini: ultrastructural observations of albopapuloid lesions and a type VII collagen DNA polymorphism study of a family. *Acta Derm Venereol.* 1997;77(4):277-280. doi:10.2340/0001555577277280

NXG P.

Ogawa C, Sato Y, Suzuki C, et al. Treatment with silver nitrate versus topical steroid treatment for umbilical granuloma: a non-inferiority randomized control trial. *PLoS One.* 2018;13(2):e0192688. doi:10.1371/journal.pone.0192688

Ormerod AD, Thomas KS, Craig FE, et al. Comparison of the two most commonly used treatments for pyoderma gangrenosum: results of the STOP GAP randomised controlled trial. *BMJ (Clinical research ed).* 2015;350:h2958. doi:10.1136/bmj.h2958

Ovadja ZN, Schuit MM, van der Horst CMAM, Lapid O. Inter- and intrarater reliability of Hurley staging for hidradenitis suppurativa. *Br J Dermatol.* 2019;181(2):344-349. doi:10.1111/bjd.17588

Palo S, Biligi DS. Utility of horizontal and vertical sections of scalp biopsies in various forms of primary alopecias. *J Lab Physicians.* 2018;10(1):95-100. doi:10.4103/JLP.JLP_4_17

Paolino G, Didona D, Magliulo G, et al. Paraneoplastic pemphigus: insight into the autoimmune pathogenesis, clinical features and therapy. *Int J Mol Sci.* 2017;18(12):E2532. doi:10.3390/ijms18122532

Paradisi A, Abeni D, Bergamo F, Ricci F, Didona D, Didona B. Etanercept therapy for toxic epidermal necrolysis. *J Am Acad Dermatol.* 2014;71(2):278-283. doi:10.1016/j.jaad.2014.04.044

Partridge ACR, Bai JW, Rosen CF, Walsh SR, Gulliver WP, Fleming P. Effectiveness of systemic treatments for pyoderma gangrenosum: a systematic review of observational studies and clinical trials. *Br J Dermatol.* 2018;179(2):290-295. doi:10.1111/bjd.16485

Pascoe VL, Fenves AZ, Wofford J, Jackson JM, Menter A, Kimball AB. The spectrum of nephrocutaneous diseases and associations: inflammatory and medication-related nephrocutaneous associations. *J Am Acad Dermatol.* 2016;74(2):247-270. quiz 271-2. doi:10.1016/j.jaad.2015.05.042

Pastori D, Carnevale R, Cangemi R, et al. Vitamin E serum levels and bleeding risk in patients receiving oral anticoagulant therapy: a retrospective cohort study. *J Am Heart Assoc.* 2013;2(6):e000364. doi:10.1161/JAHA.113.000364

Patel N, Spencer LA, English JC,IIIrd, Zirwas MJ. Acquired ichthyosis. *J Am Acad Dermatol.* 2006;55(4):647-656. doi:10.1016/j.jaad.2006.04.047

Patel S, John AM, Handler MZ, Schwartz RA. Fixed drug eruptions: an update, emphasizing the potentially lethal generalized bullous fixed drug eruption. *Am J Clin Dermatol.* 2020;21(3):393-399. doi:10.1007/s40257-020-00505-3

Penneys NS, Ziboh V, Simon P, Lord J. Pathogenesis of Woronoff ring in psoriasis. *Arch Dermatol.* 1976;112(7):955-957.

Pesonen M, Suuronen K, Suomela S, Aalto-Korte K. Occupational allergic contact dermatitis caused by colophonium. *Contact Dermatitis.* 2019;80(1):9-17. doi:10.1111/cod.13114

Petri M, Orbai AM, Alarcón GS, et al. Derivation and validation of the systemic lupus international collaborating clinics classification criteria for systemic lupus erythematosus. *Arthritis Rheum.* 2012;64(8):2677-2686. doi:10.1002/art.34473

Piaggesi A, Viacava P, Rizzo L, et al. Semiquantitative analysis of the histopathological features of the neuropathic foot ulcer: effects of pressure relief. *Diabetes Care.* 2003;26(11):3123-3128. doi:10.2337/diacare.26.11.3123

Piette EW, Rosenbach M. Granuloma annulare: pathogenesis, disease associations and triggers, and therapeutic options. *J Am Acad Dermatol.* 2016;75(3):467-479. doi:10.1016/j.jaad.2015.03.055

Piette EW, Rosenbach M. Granuloma annulare: clinical and histologic variants, epidemiology, and genetics. *J Am Acad Dermatol.* 2016;75(3):457-465. doi:10.1016/j.jaad.2015.03.054

Powers JG, Higham C, Broussard K, Phillips TJ. Wound healing and treating wounds: chronic wound care and management. *J Am Acad Dermatol.* 2016;74(4):607-625. quiz 625-6. doi:10.1016/j.jaad.2015.08.070

Provost TT, Watson R. Anti-Ro(SS-A) HLA-DR3-positive women: the interrelationship between some ANA negative, SS, SCLE, and NLE mothers and SS/LE overlap female patients. *J Invest Dermatol.* 1993;100(1, supplement):S14-S20. doi:10.1038/jid.1993.18

Rapp SR, Feldman SR, Exum ML, Fleischer AB, Jr. Reboussin DM. Psoriasis causes as much disability as other major medical diseases. *J Am Acad Dermatol.* 1999;41(3 pt 1):401-407. doi:10.1016/s0190-9622(99)70112-x

Räßler F, Lukacs J, Elsner P. Treatment of eosinophilic cellulitis (Wells syndrome): a systematic review. *J Eur Acad Dermatol Venereol.* 2016;30(9):1465-1479. doi:10.1111/jdv.13706

Reiter N, El-Shabrawi L, Leinweber B, Berghold A, Aberer E. Calcinosis cutis: part II. Treatment options. *J Am Acad Dermatol.* 2011;65(1):15-22. quiz 23-4. doi:10.1016/j.jaad.2010.08.039

Reiter N, El-Shabrawi L, Leinweber B, Berghold A, Aberer E. Calcinosis cutis: part I. Diagnostic pathway. *J Am Acad Dermatol.* 2011;65(1):1-12. quiz 13-4. doi:10.1016/j.jaad.2010.08.038

Requena L, Requena C. Erythema nodosum. *Dermatol Online J.* 2002;8(1):4.

Reyes-Habito CM, Roh EK. Cutaneous reactions to chemotherapeutic drugs and targeted therapies for cancer: part I. Conventional chemotherapeutic drugs. *J Am Acad Dermatol.* 2014;71(2):203.e1-203.e12. quiz 215-216. doi:10.1016/j.jaad.2014.04.014

Reynolds TB. The "butterfly" sign in patients with chronic jaundice and pruritus. *Ann Intern Med.* 1973;78(4):545-546. doi:10.7326/0003-4819-78-4-545

Rodrigues M, Ezzedine K, Hamzavi I, Pandya AG, Harris JE; Vitiligo Working Group. New discoveries in the pathogenesis and classification of vitiligo. *J Am Acad Dermatol.* 2017;77(1):1-13. doi:10.1016/j.jaad.2016.10.048

Rodrigues M, Ezzedine K, Hamzavi I, Pandya AG, Harris JE; Vitiligo Working Group. Current and emerging treatments for vitiligo. *J Am Acad Dermatol.* 2017;77(1):17-29. doi:10.1016/j.jaad.2016.11.010

Rosenbach MW, Karolyn A, Micheletti RG, Taylor LA. *Inpatient Dermatology.* Springer; 2018.

Roujeau JC, Stern RS. Severe adverse cutaneous reactions to drugs. *N Engl J Med.* 1994;331(19):1272-1285. doi:10.1056/nejm199411103311906

Rozas-Muñoz E, Lepoittevin JP, Pujol RM, Giménez-Arnau A. Allergic contact dermatitis to plants: understanding the chemistry will help our diagnostic approach. *Actas Dermosifiliogr.* 2012;103(6):456-477. doi:10.1016/j.ad.2011.07.017

Rubin BY, Anderson SL. IKBKAP/ELP1 gene mutations: mechanisms of familial dysautonomia and gene-targeting therapies. *Appl Clin Genet.* 2017;10:95-103. doi:10.2147/TACG.S129638

Rubin CB, Brod B. Natural does not mean safe-the dirt on clean beauty products. *JAMA Dermatol.* 2019;155(12):1344-1345. doi:10.1001/jamadermatol.2019.2724

Rucker Wright D, Gathers R, Kapke A, Johnson D, Joseph CLM. Hair care practices and their association with scalp and hair disorders in African American girls. *J Am Acad Dermatol.* 2011;64(2):253-262. doi:10.1016/j.jaad.2010.05.037

Sadeghian A, Rouhana H, Oswald-Stumpf B, Boh E. Etiologies and management of cutaneous flushing: malignant causes. *J Am Acad Dermatol.* 2017;77(3):405-414. doi:10.1016/j.jaad.2016.12.032

Sadeghian A, Rouhana H, Oswald-Stumpf B, Boh E. Etiologies and management of cutaneous flushing: nonmalignant causes. *J Am Acad Dermatol.* 2017;77(3):391-402. doi:10.1016/j.jaad.2016.12.031

Sadler E, Lazarova Z, Sarasombath P, Yancey KB. A widening perspective regarding the relationship between anti-epiligrin cicatricial pemphigoid and cancer. *J Dermatol Sci.* 2007;47(1):1-7. doi:10.1016/j.jdermsci.2007.02.012

Saleem MD, Oussedik E, Picardo M, Schoch JJ. Acquired disorders with hypopigmentation: a clinical approach to diagnosis and treatment. *J Am Acad Dermatol.* 2019;80(5):1233-1250.e10. doi:10.1016/j.jaad.2018.07.070

Saleem MD, Oussedik E, Schoch JJ, Berger AC, Picardo M. Acquired disorders with depigmentation: a systematic approach to vitiliginoid conditions. *J Am Acad Dermatol.* 2019;80(5):1215-1231.e6. doi:10.1016/j.jaad.2018.03.063

Sardana K, Sarkar R, Sehgal VN. Pigmented purpuric dermatoses: an overview. *Int J Dermatol.* 2004;43(7):482-488. doi:10.1111/j.1365-4632.2004.02213.x

Sartor L, Forteza A. Strategies to prevent aortic complications in Marfan syndrome. *J Thorac Dis.* 2017;9(suppl 6):S434-S438. doi:10.21037/jtd.2017.04.69

Schmitt SK. Reactive arthritis. *Infect Dis Clin North Am* 2017;31(2):265-277. doi:10.1016/j.idc.2017.01.002

Schwartz RA, McDonough PH, Lee BW. Toxic epidermal necrolysis: part II. Prognosis, sequelae, diagnosis, differential diagnosis, prevention, and treatment. *J Am Acad Dermatol.* 2013;69(2):187.e1-16. quiz 203-4. doi:10.1016/j.jaad.2013.05.002

Schwartz RA, McDonough PH, Lee BW. Toxic epidermal necrolysis: part I. Introduction, history, classification, clinical features, systemic manifestations, etiology, and immunopathogenesis. *J Am Acad Dermatol.* 2013;69(2):173.e1-13. quiz 185-6. doi:10.1016/j.jaad.2013.05.003

Seminario-Vidal L, Kroshinsky D, Malachowski SJ, et al. Society of Dermatology Hospitalists supportive care guidelines for the management of Stevens-Johnson syndrome/toxic epidermal necrolysis in adults. *J Am Acad Dermatol.* 2020;82:1553-1567. doi:10.1016/j.jaad.2020.02.066

Shaffer MP, Belsito DV. Allergic contact dermatitis from glutaraldehyde in health-care workers. *Contact Dermatitis.* 2000;43(3):150-156. doi:10.1034/j.1600-0536.2000.043003150.x

Shanmugam VK, Tsagaris KC, Attinger CE. Leg ulcers associated with Klinefelter's syndrome: a case report and review of the literature. *Int Wound J.* 2012;9(1):104-107. doi:10.1111/j.1742-481X.2011.00846.x

Shao S, Tsoi LC, Sarkar MK, et al. IFN-γ enhances cell-mediated cytotoxicity against keratinocytes via JAK2/STAT1 in lichen planus. *Sci Transl Med.* 2019;11(511):eaav7561. doi:10.1126/scitranslmed.aav7561

Sharma A, Sharma K. Hepatotropic viral infection associated systemic vasculitides-hepatitis B virus associated polyarteritis nodosa and hepatitis C virus associated cryoglobulinemic vasculitis. *J Clin Exp Hepatol.* 2013;3(3):204-212. doi:10.1016/j.jceh.2013.06.001

Sheth VM, Pandya AG. Melasma: a comprehensive update – part II. *J Am Acad Dermatol.* 2011;65(4):699-714. doi:10.1016/j.jaad.2011.06.001

Sheth VM, Pandya AG. Melasma: a comprehensive update—part I. *J Am Acad Dermatol.* 2011;65(4):689-697. doi:10.1016/j.jaad.2010.12.046

Shiohara T, Iijima M, Ikezawa Z, Hashimoto K. The diagnosis of a DRESS syndrome has been sufficiently established on the basis of typical clinical features and viral reactivations. *Br J Dermatol.* 2007;156(5):1083-1084. doi:10.1111/j.1365-2133.2007.07807.x

Shumway NK, Cole E, Fernandez KH. Neurocutaneous disease: neurocutaneous dysesthesias. *J Am Acad Dermatol.* 2016;74(2):215-228. quiz 229-30. doi:10.1016/j.jaad.2015.04.059

Sidbury R, Davis DM, Cohen DE, et al. Guidelines of care for the management of atopic dermatitis: section 3. Management and treatment with phototherapy and systemic agents. *J Am Acad Dermatol.* 2014;71(2):327-349. doi:10.1016/j.jaad.2014.03.030

Sidbury R, Tom WL, Bergman JN, et al. Guidelines of care for the management of atopic dermatitis: section 4. Prevention of disease flares and use of adjunctive therapies and approaches. *J Am Acad Dermatol.* 2014;71(6):1218-1233. doi:10.1016/j.jaad.2014.08.038

Sidoroff A, Halevy S, Bavinck JN, Vaillant L, Roujeau JC. Acute generalized exanthematous pustulosis (AGEP): a clinical reaction pattern. *J Cutan Pathol.* 2001;28(3):113-119.

Silpa-Archa N, Kohli I, Chaowattanapanit S, Lim HW, Hamzavi I. Postinflammatory hyperpigmentation: a comprehensive overview – epidemiology, pathogenesis, clinical presentation, and noninvasive assessment technique. *J Am Acad Dermatol.* 2017;77(4):591-605. doi:10.1016/j.jaad.2017.01.035

Simpson EL, Chalmers JR, Hanifin JM, et al. Emollient enhancement of the skin barrier from birth offers effective atopic dermatitis prevention. *J Allergy Clin Immunol.* 2014;134(4):818-823. doi:10.1016/j.jaci.2014.08.005

Singal A, Arora R. Nail as a window of systemic diseases. *Indian Dermatol Online J.* 2015;6(2):67-74. doi:10.4103/2229-5178.153002

Stander S, Weisshaar E, Mettang T, et al. Clinical classification of itch: a position paper of the international forum for the study of itch. *Acta Derm Venereol.* 2007;87(4):291-294. doi:10.2340/00015555-0305

Stashower J, Bruch K, Mosby A, et al. Pregnancy complications associated with pityriasis rosea: a multicenter retrospective study. *J Am Acad Dermatol.* 2021;85(6):1648-1649. doi:10.1016/j.jaad.2020.12.063

Stawczyk-Macieja M, Szczerkowska-Dobosz A, Nowicki R, Majewska H, Dubowik M, Sokołowska-Wojdyło M. Malignant acanthosis nigricans, florid cutaneous papillomatosis and tripe palms syndrome associated with gastric adenocarcinoma. *Postepy Dermatol Alergol.* 2014;31(1):56-58. doi:10.5114/pdia.2014.40663

Stone JH, Zen Y, Deshpande V. IgG4-related disease. *N Engl J Med.* 2012;366(6):539-551. doi:10.1056/NEJMra1104650

Strazzulla LC, Wang EHC, Avila L, et al. Alopecia areata: an appraisal of new treatment approaches and overview of current therapies. *J Am Acad Dermatol.* 2018;78(1):15-24. doi:10.1016/j.jaad.2017.04.1142

Strazzulla LC, Wang EHC, Avila L, et al. Alopecia areata: disease characteristics, clinical evaluation, and new perspectives on pathogenesis. *J Am Acad Dermatol.* 2018;78(1):1-12. doi:10.1016/j.jaad.2017.04.1141

Su WP, Liu HN. Diagnostic criteria for Sweet's syndrome. *Cutis.* 1986;37(3):167-174.

Su WPD, Davis MDP, Weenig RH, Powell FC, Perry HO. Pyoderma gangrenosum: clinicopathologic correlation and proposed diagnostic criteria. *Int J Dermatol.* 2004;43(11):790-800. doi:10.1111/j.1365-4632.2004.02128.x

Sudy E, Urbina F, Gubelin W, Misad C, Espinoza A. Pseudoatrophoderma colli: distinct entity or just a variant of confluent and reticular papilomatosis of Gougerot-Carteaud. *Dermatol Online J.* 2020;26(10):13030/qt9q40r8v8.

Szalat R, Pirault J, Fermand JP, et al. Physiopathology of necrobiotic xanthogranuloma with monoclonal gammopathy. *J Intern Med.* 2014;276(3):269-284. doi:10.1111/joim.12195

Szczerkowska-Dobosz A, Placek W, Szczerkowska Z, Roszkiewicz J. Psoriasis vulgaris with the early and late onset: HLA phenotype correlations. *Arch Immunol Ther Exp.* 1996;44(4):265-269.

Takeshita J, Grewal S, Langan SM, et al. Psoriasis and comorbid diseases: epidemiology. *J Am Acad Dermatol.* 2017;76(3):377-390. doi:10.1016/j.jaad.2016.07.064

Takeshita J, Grewal S, Langan SM, et al. Psoriasis and comorbid diseases: implications for management. *J Am Acad Dermatol.* 2017;76(3):393-403. doi:10.1016/j.jaad.2016.07.065

Teo WL. Diagnostic and management considerations for "Maskne" in the Era of COVID-19. *J Am Acad Dermatol.* 2021;84(2):520-521. doi:10.1016/j.jaad.2020.09.063

Thiboutot DM, Dreno B, Abanmi A, et al. Practical management of acne for clinicians: an international consensus from the global alliance to improve outcomes in acne. *J Am Acad Dermatol.* 2018;78(2 suppl 1):S1-S23.e1. doi:10.1016/j.jaad.2017.09.078

Thomas MG, Betsy A. Linear lichen planus: continuum from skin to mucosa. *J Cutan Med Surg.* 2018;22(2):232-233. doi:10.1177/1203475417733463

Tracey EH, Elston C, Feasel P, Piliang M, Michael M, Vij A. Erythrodermic presentation of psoriasis in a patient treated with dupilumab. *JAAD Case Rep.* 2018;4(7):708-710. doi:10.1016/j.jdcr.2018.05.014

Tunçbilek E, Alanay Y. Congenital contractural arachnodactyly (Beals syndrome). *Orphanet J Rare Dis.* 2006;1:20. doi:10.1186/1750-1172-1-20

Two AM, Wu W, Gallo RL, Hata TR. Rosacea: part II. Topical and systemic therapies in the treatment of rosacea. *J Am Acad Dermatol.* 2015;72(5):761-770. quiz 771-2. doi:10.1016/j.jaad.2014.08.027

Two AM, Wu W, Gallo RL, Hata TR. Rosacea: part I. Introduction, categorization, histology, pathogenesis, and risk factors. *J Am Acad Dermatol.* 2015;72(5):749-758. quiz 759-760. doi:10.1016/j.jaad.2014.08.028

Tziotzios C, Lee JYW, Brier T, et al. Lichen planus and lichenoid dermatoses: clinical overview and molecular basis. *J Am Acad Dermatol.* 2018;79(5):789-804. doi:10.1016/j.jaad.2018.02.010

Tziotzios C, Brier T, Lee JYW, et al. Lichen planus and lichenoid dermatoses: Conventional and emerging therapeutic strategies. *J Am Acad Dermatol.* 2018;79(5):807-818. doi:10.1016/j.jaad.2018.02.013

Ugurlu S, Bartley GB, Gibson LE. Necrobiotic xanthogranuloma: long-term outcome of ocular and systemic involvement. *Am J Ophthalmol.* 2000;129(5):651-657.

Valent P, Klion AD, Horny HP, et al. Contemporary consensus proposal on criteria and classification of eosinophilic disorders and related syndromes. *J Allergy Clin Immunol.* 2012;130(3):607-612.e9. doi:10.1016/j.jaci.2012.02.019

van Zuuren EJ, Fedorowicz Z. Interventions for rosacea: abridged updated Cochrane systematic review including GRADE assessments. *Br J Dermatol.* 2015;173(3):651-662. doi:10.1111/bjd.13956

Vanoni F, Lava SAG, Fossali EF, et al. Neonatal systemic lupus erythematosus syndrome: a comprehensive review. *Clin Rev Allergy Immunol.* 2017;53(3):469-476. doi:10.1007/s12016-017-8653-0

Viljoen DL, Beatty S, Beighton P. The obstetric and gynaecological implications of pseudoxanthoma elasticum. *Br J Obstet Gynaecol.* 1987;94(9):884-888. doi:10.1111/j.1471-0528.1987.tb03760.x

Waldman R, DeWane ME, Lu J. Dermatomyositis: diagnosis and treatment. *J Am Acad Dermatol.* 2020;82(2):283-296. doi:10.1016/j.jaad.2019.05.105

Walker DC, Cohen PR. Trimethoprim-sulfamethoxazole-associated acute febrile neutrophilic dermatosis: case report and review of drug-induced Sweet's syndrome. *J Am Acad Dermatol.* 1996;34(5 pt 2):918-923.

Walsh SN, Santa Cruz DJ. Lipodermatosclerosis: a clinicopathological study of 25 cases. *J Am Acad Dermatol.* 2010;62(6):1005-1012. doi:10.1016/j.jaad.2009.08.006

Wanat KA, Rosenbach M. A practical approach to cutaneous sarcoidosis. *Am J Clin Dermatol.* 2014;15(4):283-297. doi:10.1007/s40257-014-0079-3

Wang CW, Yang LY, Chen CB, et al. Randomized, controlled trial of TNF-α antagonist in CTL-mediated severe cutaneous adverse reactions. *J Clin Invest.* 2018;128(3):985-996. doi:10.1172/jci93349

Watanabe T, Tsuchida T, Kanda N, Mori K, Hayashi Y, Tamaki K. Anti-α-Fodrin antibodies in Sjögren syndrome and lupus erythematosus. *Arch Dermatol.* 1999;135(5):535-539. doi:10.1001/archderm.135.5.535

Weaver J, Bergfeld WF. Grover disease (transient acantholytic dermatosis). *Arch Pathol Lab Med.* 2009;133(9):1490-1494. doi:10.1043/1543-2165-133.9.1490

Williams RC, McKenzie AW, Roger JH, Joysey VC. HL-A antigens in patients with guttate psoriasis. *Br J Dermatol.* 1976;95(2):163-167. doi:10.1111/j.1365-2133.1976.tb00820.x

Williams KA, Huang AH, Belzberg M, Kwatra SG. Prurigo nodularis: pathogenesis and management. *J Am Acad Dermatol.* 2020;83(6):1567-1575. doi:10.1016/j.jaad.2020.04.182

Winkelmann RK, Litzow MR, Umbert IJ, Lie JT. Giant cell granulomatous pulmonary and myocardial lesions in necrobiotic xanthogranuloma with paraproteinemia. *Mayo Clin Proc.* 1997;72(11):1028-1033. doi:10.1016/s0025-6196(11)63542-8

Wisuthsarewong W, Soongswang J, Chantorn R. Neonatal lupus erythematosus: clinical character, investigation, and outcome. *Pediatr Dermatol.* 2011;28(2):115-121. doi:10.1111/j.1525-1470.2011.01300.x

Wojnarowska F, Calnan CD. Contact and photocontact allergy to musk ambrette. *Br J Dermatol.* 1986;114(6):667-675. doi:10.1111/j.1365-2133.1986.tb04874.x

Wouters CH, Maes A, Foley KP, Bertin J, Rose CD. Blau syndrome, the prototypic auto-inflammatory granulomatous disease. *Pediatr Rheumatol Online J.* 2014;12:33. doi:10.1186/1546-0096-12-33

Wu H, Wang ZH, Yan A, et al. Protection against pemphigus foliaceus by desmoglein 3 in neonates. *N Engl J Med.* 2000;343(1):31-35. doi:10.1056/nejm200007063430105

Wu TP, Miller K, Cohen DE, Stein JA. Keratoacanthomas arising in association with prurigo nodules in pruritic, actinically damaged skin. *J Am Acad Dermatol.* 2013;69(3):426-430. doi:10.1016/j.jaad.2013.03.035

Xia FD, Liu K, Lockwood S, et al. Risk of developing pyoderma gangrenosum after procedures in patients with a known history of pyoderma gangrenosum-A retrospective analysis. *J Am Acad Dermatol*. 2018;78(2):310-314.e1. doi:10.1016/j.jaad.2017.09.040

Yeon HB, Lindor NM, Seidman JG, Seidman CE. Pyogenic arthritis, pyoderma gangrenosum, and acne syndrome maps to chromosome 15q. *Am J Hum Genet*. 2000;66(4):1443-1448. doi:10.1086/302866

Yorulmaz A, Akin F, Sert A, Agir MA, Yilmaz R, Arslan S. Demographic and clinical characteristics of patients with serum sickness-like reaction. *Clin Rheumatol*. 2018;37(5):1389-1394. doi:10.1007/s10067-017-3777-4

Zachariae H, Overgaard Petersen H, Kissmeyer Nielsen F, Lamm L. HL-A antigens in pustular psoriasis. *Dermatol*. 1977;154(2):73-77. doi:10.1159/000251035

Zaenglein AL, Pathy AL, Schlosser BJ, et al. Guidelines of care for the management of acne vulgaris. *J Am Acad Dermatol*. 2016;74(5):945-973.e33. doi:10.1016/j.jaad.2015.12.037

Zuberbier T, Aberer W, Asero R, et al. The EAACI/GA²LEN/EDF/WAO guideline for the definition, classification, diagnosis and management of urticaria. *Allergy*. 2018;73(7):1393-1414. doi:10.1111/all.13397

Infections, Infestations, and Other Animal Kingdom Encounters

Jeff Gehlhausen, MD, PhD

Viral Diseases

Basic Concepts

- **Viruses** utilize host subcellular machinery for replication. All viruses have a basic structure of a genome as well as a protein capsid. Broadly, they can be divided into DNA- or RNA-based genomes as well as enveloped or nonenveloped structures based on the presence or absence of a membrane surrounding the protein capsid. Enveloped viruses are less resistant to environmental changes and disinfectants.
- **Viral classification and associations** (for dermatology-relevant viruses) are summarized in Table 3.1.
- **The skin's strongest protection against infectious diseases is the mechanical barrier.** This is well demonstrated by the propensity for patients with AD, Hailey-Hailey disease, and Darier disease to develop secondary herpetic infections (Kaposi varicelliform eruption). Acquired immunodeficiency may result from viral infections (eg, HIV), other medical disorders (eg, Kwashiorkor, Cushing disease/Cushing syndrome, diabetes mellitus, nephrotic syndrome, cancer), aging (immunosenescence), pregnancy, and medications.
- **Mucocutaneous signs of HIV infection** are summarized in Table 3.2.

HIV may present as a **congenital infection**. **Hereditary immunodeficiency syndromes** are summarized in Table 3.3.

HERPES SIMPLEX
→ Diagnosis Group 1

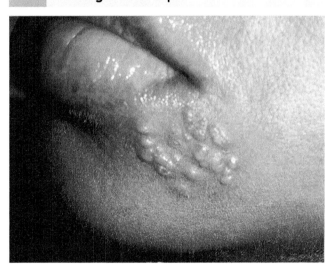

Table 3.1. VIRAL CLASSIFICATION AND ASSOCIATIONS

Type	Family	Virus	Diagnosis[a]	Association(s)[a]
dsDNA	Adenoviruses	Adenovirus	Adenovirus infection	Conjunctivitis
	Hepadnaviruses (e)	HBV	HBV infection, Gianotti-Crosti syndrome	Urticaria, CSVV, mixed cryoglobulinemia, PAN, generalized GA
	Herpesviruses (e)	HSV-1 (HHV-1)	Herpes simplex	EM
		HSV-2 (HHV-2)		
		VZV (HHV-3)	Varicella, herpes zoster	Pruritus, localized GA (in herpes zoster scars)
		EBV (HHV-4)	Infectious mononucleosis, Gianotti-Crosti syndrome, Lipschutz ulcer, oral hairy leukoplakia, papular purpuric gloves and socks syndrome	DRESS syndrome, HLH, HV, extranodal NK/T-cell lymphoma, nasal type (includes HV-like CTCL), PTLD, lymphomatoid granulomatosis, Hodgkin lymphoma, endemic Burkitt lymphoma, nasopharyngeal carcinoma
		CMV (HHV-5)	CMV infection	DRESS syndrome
		HHV-6	Roseola	PR, DRESS syndrome
		HHV-7		
		HHV-8	HHV-8 infection	KS, multicentric Castleman disease, primary effusion lymphoma
	Papovaviruses (papillomaviruses)	HPV	Wart	Verrucous carcinoma, SCC/cervical cancer/vulvar cancer/vaginal cancer/penile cancer/anal cancer
	Papovaviruses (polyomaviruses)	JC virus	PML	
		MCPyV	Merkel cell polyomavirus infection	MCC
		TSPyV	Trichodysplasia spinulosa	
	Poxviruses (e)	Molluscipox (MCV-1, MCV-2)	Molluscum contagiosum, Gianotti-Crosti syndrome–like reaction	AD, conjunctivitis
		Orthopoxvirus	Variola, vaccinia, monkeypox, cowpox	
		Parapoxvirus	Orf, paravaccinia	
ssDNA	Parvoviruses	Parvovirus B19	Erythema infectiosum, papular purpuric gloves and socks syndrome	
dsRNA	Reoviruses	Rotavirus	Rotavirus infection	
ssRNA	Coronaviruses (e)	SARS-CoV-2	COVID-19	
	Flaviviruses (e)	Dengue virus[b]	Dengue	
		HCV	HCV infection	LP, urticaria, necrolytic acral erythema, CSVV, mixed cryoglobulinemia, PAN, pruritus, generalized GA, PCT
		West Nile virus[b]	West Nile infection	
		Yellow fever virus[b]	Yellow fever	
		Zika virus[b]	Zika	
	Orthomyxoviruses (e)	Influenza virus	Influenza	
	Paramyxoviruses (e)	Morbillivirus	Rubeola	
		Paramyxovirus	Mumps	
		RSV	RSV infection	

Type	Family	Virus	Diagnosis[a]	Association(s)[a]
	Picornaviruses (enteroviruses)	Coxsackievirus	HFMD, herpangina	
		HAV	HAV infection	
		Poliovirus	Polio	
	Picornaviruses (rhinoviruses)	Rhinovirus	Common cold	
	Retroviruses (e)	HIV	HIV infection/AIDS	See Table 3.2
		HTLV-1/HTLV-2	ATLL	Ichthyosis vulgaris, HTLV-associated infective dermatitis
	Rhabdoviruses (e)	Rabies lyssavirus[c]	Rabies	
	Togaviruses (e)	Chikungunya virus[b]	Chikungunya	
		Rubella virus	Rubella	

[a]Illustrative examples provided.
[b]Arbovirus transmitted by mosquitoes, ticks, or other arthropods.
[c]Dermatologists may be consulted to perform a nuchal biopsy to assess for presence of rabies virus as it moves in a rostral direction through nerves toward brain.
(e), enveloped virus; AD, atopic dermatitis; AIDS, acquired immunodeficiency syndrome; ATLL, adult T-cell leukemia/lymphoma; CMV, cytomegalovirus; COVID-19, coronavirus disease 2019; CSVV, cutaneous small vessel vasculitis; CTCL, cutaneous T-cell lymphoma; EM, erythema multiforme; DNA, deoxyribonucleic acid; DRESS, drug reaction with eosinophilia and systemic symptoms; ds, double-stranded; EBV, Epstein-Barr virus; GA, granuloma annulare; HAV, hepatitis A virus; HBV, hepatitis B virus; HCV, hepatitis C virus; HFMD, hand-foot-and-mouth disease; HHV, human herpesvirus; HIV, human immunodeficiency virus; HLH, hemophagocytic lymphocytic histiocytosis; HPV, human papillomavirus; HSV, herpes simplex virus; HTLV, human T-lymphotropic virus; HV, hydroa vacciniforme; JC, John Cunningham; LP, lichen planus; MCC, Merkel cell carcinoma; MCPyV, Merkel cell polyomavirus; MCV, molluscum contagiosum virus; NK, natural killer; PAN, polyarteritis nodosa; PCT, porphyria cutanea tarda; PML, progressive multifocal leukoencephalopathy; PR, pityriasis rosea; PTLD, post-transplant lymphoproliferative disorder; RNA, ribonucleic acid; RSV, respiratory syncytial virus; ss, single-stranded; SARS-CoV-2, severe acute respiratory syndrome coronavirus 2; TSPyV, trichodysplasia spinulosa–associated polyomavirus; VZV, varicella zoster virus.

Table 3.2. MUCOCUTANEOUS SIGNS OF HUMAN IMMUNODEFICIENCY VIRUS INFECTION

Type	Association(s)[a]
Inflammatory	Psoriasis, reactive arthritis, PRP type VI, seborrheic dermatitis, ichthyosis vulgaris, HIV/ART-associated lipodystrophy syndrome, CSVV, EED, mixed cryoglobulinemia, pruritus, acquired progressive kinking of the hair, hypertrichosis, recurrent aphthous stomatitis, HIV-associated EPF, PPE of HIV, papuloerythroderma of Ofuji, generalized GA, PCT, zinc deficiency, angular cheilitis, linear gingival erythema, mucosal erosions/ulcers
Infectious	Viral: acute retroviral syndrome (infectious mononucleosis-like syndrome), longitudinal melanonychia, oral hairy leukoplakia, HSV (chronic ulcerative), VZV (herpes zoster), CMV (perianal ulcers), HPV (extensive warts, acquired EDV), molluscum contagiosum (MCV-2, extensive face and genital involvement, giant mollusca)
	Bacterial: bacillary angiomatosis, syphilis, TB, atypical mycobacteria
	Fungal: proximal subungual onychomycosis, white superficial onychomycosis due to *Tinea rubrum*, candidiasis (eg, oropharyngeal candidiasis due to *Candida dubliniensis*), disseminated dimorphic fungal infection, angioinvasive fungal infection
	Parasitic: atypical disseminated leishmaniasis
Neoplastic	Verrucous carcinoma, SCC, eruptive melanocytic nevi/melanoma, multiple DFs, KS, extra-nodal NHL (oral cavity)
Drug-associated	Cutaneous adverse reactions (eg, erythroderma, SJS/TEN)

[a]Illustrative examples provided.
ART, antiretroviral therapy; CMV, cytomegalovirus; CSVV, cutaneous small vessel vasculitis; DFs, dermatofibromas; EDV, epidermodysplasia verruciformis; EED, erythema elevatum diutinum; EPF, eosinophilic pustular folliculitis; GA, granuloma annulare; HIV, human immunodeficiency virus; KS, Kaposi sarcoma; HPV, human papillomavirus; HSV, herpes simplex virus; MCV, molluscum contagiosum virus; NHL, non-Hodgkin lymphoma; PCT, porphyria cutaneous tarda; PPE, pruritic papular eruption; PRP, pityriasis rubra pilaris; SCC, squamous cell carcinoma; SJS/TEN, Stevens-Johnson syndrome/toxic epidermal necrolysis; TB, tuberculosis; VZV, varicella zoster virus.

Table 3.3. HEREDITARY IMMUNODEFICIENCY SYNDROMES

Diagnosis[a]	Inheritance pattern	Gene(s)	Classic description	Notes
Autoinflammatory syndromes	See Chapter 2: Interface Dermatoses and Other Connective Tissue Disorders.			
A-T	See Chapter 4: Photodermatoses.			
Bloom syndrome	See Chapter 4: Photodermatoses.			
CGD	See Chapter 3: Bacterial Diseases.			
CMC	See Chapter 3: Fungal Diseases.			
CVID	Variable	Variable	Infections, autoimmune disorders.	
DKC	See Chapter 2: Pigmentary Disorders.			
Disorders of complement	See Chapter 1: Immunology and Inflammation.			
EDV	See below.			
HPS/CHS/GS	See Chapter 2: Pigmentary Disorders.			
Hypohidrotic ectodermal dysplasia with immune deficiency	See Chapter 2: Disorders of Sebaceous, Apocrine, and Eccrine Glands.			
Hyper-IgE syndromes	See Chapter 3: Parasitic Diseases and Other Animal Kingdom Encounters.			
Hyper-IgM syndrome	XLR >AR	*CD40LG* encoding CD40 ligand (XLR)[a]	Sinopulmonary and gastrointestinal infections, oral and anogenital ulcerations, warts.	
IgA deficiency	AD, AR	Variable	Bacterial sinopulmonary infections, autoimmune disorders.	Most common hereditary immunodeficiency syndrome. Higher risk of anaphylaxis to IVIG.
IgM deficiency	Unknown	Unknown	Bacterial infections, autoimmune disorders.	
LAD	AR	Variable	Delayed cord separation, poor wound healing.	
Netherton syndrome	See Chapter 2: Eczematous Dermatoses and Related Disorders.			
SCID	XLR > AR	*IL2RG* gene encoding IL-2Rγ (XLR); *ADA* encoding ADA, *IL-7R* encoding IL-7R, *JAK3* encoding JAK3 (AR)[a]	Seborrheic dermatitis–like or morbilliform eruptions (maternofetal GVHD), infections, chronic diarrhea, FTT.	Defective humoral and cell-mediated immunity. Absent tonsillar buds and palpable lymphoid tissue.
SCID (Omenn syndrome)	AR	*RAG1/RAG2* encoding RAG1/RAG2	SCID with erythroderma; diffuse alopecia.	IgM deficiency. Increased IgA, IgD, and IgE. Normal IgG.
WAS	XLR	*WASP* gene encoding WASP	Atopic predisposition and IgE-mediated sequelae with eczematous dermatitis, urticaria, food allergies, and asthma. Thrombocytopenia. Recurrent pyogenic bacterial infections (eg, otitis media).	Deficiency in surface glycoprotein sialophorin. Increased risk of NHL. Treat with bone marrow transplantation.
WHIM	AD	*CXCR4* encoding CXCR4	Warts, hypogammaglobulinemia, infections, and myelokathexis.	Myelokathexis refers to retention of neutrophils in bone marrow.

TABLE 3.3. HEREDITARY IMMUNODEFICIENCY SYNDROMES (CONTINUED)

Diagnosis[a]	Inheritance pattern	Gene(s)	Classic description	Notes
WILD	AD	*GATA2* encoding the GATA2 transcription factor	Warts, immunodeficiency, lymphedema, and anogenital dysplasia.	
X-linked agammaglobulinemia	XLR	*BTK* encoding BTK	Recurrent bacterial infections.	

[a]Illustrative examples provided.

AA, alopecia areata; AD, atopic dermatitis or autosomal dominant; ADA, adenosine deaminase; AR, autosomal recessive; A-T, ataxia-telangiectasia; BTK, Bruton tyrosine kinase; CD, cluster of differentiation; CGD, chronic granulomatous disease; CHS, Chédiak-Higashi syndrome; CMC, chronic mucocutaneous candidiasis; CVID, common variable immunodeficiency; CXCR4, C-X-C chemokine receptor type 4; DKC, dyskeratosis congenita; EDV, epidermodysplasia verruciformis; FTT, failure to thrive; GS, Griscelli syndrome; GVHD, graft-versus-host disease; JAK, Janus kinase; HPS, Hermansky-Pudlak syndrome; Ig, immunoglobulin; IL-2Rγ, interleukin-2 receptor γ, IL-7R, interleukin-7 receptor; IP, incontinentia pigmenti; IVIG, intravenous immune globulin; LAD, leukocyte adhesion deficiency; NF-κB, nuclear factor κ-light-chain-enhancer of activated B cells; NHL, non-Hodgkin lymphoma; NK, natural killer; PV, pemphigus vulgaris; SCID, severe combined immunodeficiency syndrome; Tregs, T regulatory cells; WAS, Wiskott-Aldrich syndrome; WASP, Wiskott-Aldrich syndrome protein; WHIM, warts, hypogammaglobulinemia, infections, and myelokathexis; WILD, warts, immunodeficiency, lymphedema, dysplasia; XLR, X-linked recessive.

Epidemiology

- Herpes simplex is an infection caused by **HSV-1 (HHV-1)** and **HSV-2 (HHV-2)**. ~50% and ~15% of the US population have been infected with HSV-1 and HSV-2, respectively, though the minority manifest clinical disease. **HSV-1 is the major cause of orolabial herpes, while HSV-2 is the major cause of genital herpes.** However, HSV-1 is a more common cause of genital herpes than HSV-2 in young adults.
- HSV can be transmitted by subclinical shedding at mucous membranes in addition to overt clinical lesions. Risk factors for genital herpes include increased number of sexual partners, homosexuality, and lower socioeconomic status and education. **Genital herpes increases risk of HIV infection (and vice versa).**
- Herpes simplex is the **leading association with EM (80% of cases).**

  HSV may present as a **congenital infection (15%)** due to transplacental transmission or a **neonatal infection (85%)** due to perinatal transmission. The **majority of women** with active HSV infection at the time of delivery are **asymptomatic.** The nature of maternal infection, **primary** vs **recurrent**, is the most important risk factor. Risk increases with **vaginal delivery (8%)** vs **C-section (1%).**

  Recall congenital infections with the TORCH acronym: Toxoplasmosis, Other, Rubella, CMV infection, Herpes simplex. The "other" category includes varicella, parvovirus B19 infection, mumps, zika, HIV infection, and syphilis.

  In children, HSV infection is primarily due to HSV-1.

Clinicopathological Features

- Primary HSV can be preceded by 3 to 7 days of fever, malaise, and lymphadenopathy, with eventual tingling, burning, and mucocutaneous lesion formation. Characteristic HSV lesions are **grouped vesicles on an erythematous base.** After primary infection, HSV establishes residency in sensory ganglia and reactivation leads to recurrent local infection. Recurrent HSV is frequently asymptomatic but can feature a sensory prodrome (~24 hours) prior to vesicle formation. Systemic symptoms are not generally observed and severity is typically less than primary infection.
- **Herpes simplex variants in adults** are summarized in Table 3.4.

  Congenital HSV infection lesions range from vesicles to scars. Systemic manifestations include **limb abnormalities, microcephaly, seizures, and chorioretinitis.**

  Neonatal HSV infection is divided into three types: (1) localized **skin, eye, and mouth (SEM)** disease; (2) CNS ± localized SEM disease; and (3) disseminated disease with multiorgan involvement.

  Primary herpetic gingivostomatitis is the most common herpes simplex variant in children.

  Figure 3.1.

Evaluation

- The differential diagnosis of orolabial herpes includes EM, SJS/TEN, recurrent aphthous stomatitis, Behçet disease, viral pharyngitis, and oropharyngeal candidiasis.

Table 3.4. HERPES SIMPLEX VARIANTS IN ADULTS

Variant[a]	Classic description	Notes
Primary		
Primary herpetic gingivostomatitis	Gingivitis, stomatitis.	
Primary genital herpes	Most common site is the glans and shaft of the penis in men and the vulva and vagina in women.	
Recurrent		
Recurrent herpes labialis (cold sore, fever blister)	Less severe than primary infection. Most common sites are the vermillion border, buccal mucosa, and gingiva.	Triggers include stress, immunosuppression, sun exposure or phototherapy (especially nbUVB), chemical peels, and laser.
Recurrent genital herpes	Less severe than primary infection.	Frequency of HSV shedding decreases in the first year after initial infection but persists at high rate.
Miscellaneous variants		
Chronic ulcerative HSV	Polycyclic well-defined ulcerations with friable tissue and a scalloped border. Most common sites are the perianal area and buttocks.	Seen in HIV-infected and other immunocompromised patients.
Eczema herpeticum	See below.	
Herpes encephalitis	Fever, confusion, focal neurologic deficits, and seizures.	Dormant HSV in trigeminal ganglion, travels retrograde to the brain, targets temporal region. Association with natalizumab.
Herpes folliculitis (herpes sycosis)	Erythematous papules and plaques ± vesicopustules.	VZV > HSV.
Herpes gladiatorum	Grouped vesicles and erosions on exposed sites (eg, face, neck, arms).	Wrestlers.
Herpetic whitlow	Acute paronychia.	Primarily HSV-1 in children and HSV-2 in adults.
Keratoconjunctivitis	Eyelid edema, chemosis, and photophobia.	Dendritic corneal ulcerations are visible with fluorescein staining.

[a]Illustrative examples provided.
AD, atopic dermatitis; HIV, human immunodeficiency virus; HSV, herpes simplex virus; nbUVB, narrowband ultraviolet B; VZV, varicella zoster virus.

- The differential diagnosis of genital herpes includes Behçet disease, chancroid, gonococcal urethritis/cervicitis, granuloma inguinale, lymphogranuloma venereum (LGV), and primary syphilis.
- Diagnostic tests for herpes simplex include:
  - **Tzanck smear**: reveals **multinucleated** keratinocytes with nuclear **molding** and **margination** of basophilic chromatin to the periphery.
    - Tzanck smear reveals the "3 Ms": multinucleation, molding, and margination ("eggshell" chromatin). It can NOT distinguish between HSV and varicella zoster virus (VZV).
  - **Skin biopsy**: helpful in unclear cases.
  - **Viral culture**: viral culture can help identify treatment resistance.
  - **Serologies**: IgG can identify previous infection; IgM not recommended as not type specific and can be positive in primary or recurrent infection.
  - **Direct fluorescent antibody (DFA)**: rapid but poor sensitivity compared to reverse transcriptase (RT) polymerase chain reaction (PCR) and not type specific.
  - **RT-PCR: most sensitive and specific; type-specific.**
- Ophthalmological evaluation is indicated if there is concern for eye involvement.
  Congenital and neonatal HSV infections mandate CNS workup with lumbar puncture, neurologic imaging, and ophthalmologic evaluation.

Management

- **Antiviral therapy decreases lesion duration, viral shedding, and pain.** Oral antivirals include **acyclovir, famciclovir, and valacyclovir.** Acyclovir and penciclovir are available in topical formulations. **IV acyclovir** is indicated in HIV-infected and other immunocompromised patients with severe disease.

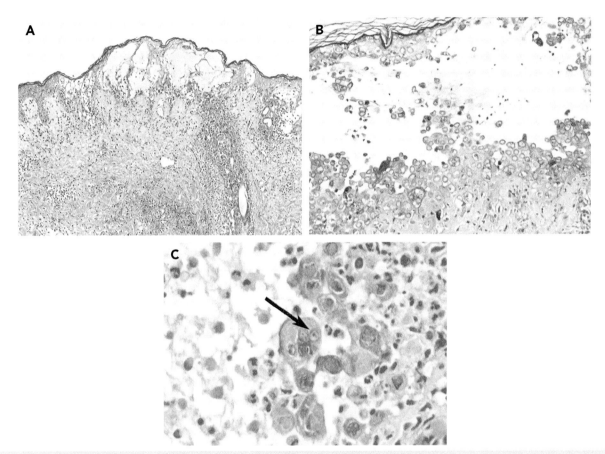

Figure 3.1. CLINICOPATHOLOGICAL CORRELATION: HERPES SIMPLEX. Herpes simplex is characterized by an intraepidermal vesicle with acantholysis and ballooning and reticular degeneration of keratinocytes. Mild CSVV may be present. IHC can detect HSV. Keratinocytes (balloon cells) are multinucleated with nuclear molding and margination of basophilic chromatin to the periphery. While most keratinocytes exhibit homogenous pale chromatin, some exhibit Cowdry A bodies: eosinophilic intranuclear inclusion bodies surrounded by a halo. A, Low-power view. B, Medium-power view. C, High-power view. Solid arrow: eosinophilic intranuclear inclusion body (Cowdry A body) surrounded by a halo within a "balloon cell." CMV, cytomegalovirus; CSVV, cutaneous small vessel vasculitis; HSV, herpes simplex virus; IHC, immunohistochemistry; VZV, varicella zoster virus.

(Histology images reprinted with permission from Elder DE, Elenitsas R, Rosenbach M, et al. *Lever's Histopathology of the Skin.* 11th ed. Wolters Kluwer; 2015.)

> Keratinocytes demonstrate "3 Ms": multinucleation, molding, and margination ("eggshell" chromatin). Do NOT confuse the Cowdry A bodies of HSV and VZV with the Cowdry B bodies of CMV and poliovirus.

- For episodic therapy, regimens of acyclovir, famciclovir, and valacyclovir appear equally efficacious. More than 10 outbreaks per year may require suppressive therapy.
- **Foscarnet** may be used in case of **acyclovir resistance.**
  Neonatal HSV has a >50% mortality rate if untreated. **C-section is indicated for active maternal genital herpes.** Acyclovir suppressive therapy after neonatal HSV with CNS involvement improves neurodevelopmental outcomes.

"Real World" Advice

- Skin biopsy with IHC, viral culture, and RT-PCR are tests that can differentiate between HSV and VZV.
- Valacyclovir 2 g twice daily or famciclovir 1 g single dose can be very effective at aborting orolabial HSV recurrence when administered in the prodrome period.
- HSV prophylaxis should be administered for moderate/deep chemical peels and laser resurfacing.

ECZEMA HERPETICUM

Synonym: Kaposi varicelliform eruption

→ **Diagnosis Group 1**

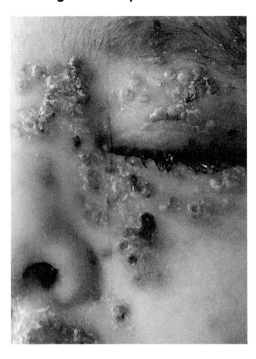

Epidemiology

- Eczema herpeticum refers to dissemination of HSV due to disrupted skin barrier in **AD.** Secondary herpetic infections can be seen in other disorders of skin barrier function. The most common cause is HSV-1.
- Eczema herpeticum is associated with filaggrin deficiency and younger age (<5 years).

Clinicopathological Features

- Eczema herpeticum most often presents on the head and neck but can progress to widespread involvement of **monomorphic umbilicated vesiculopustules and punched out erosions with crusting.** Fevers, malaise, and lymphadenopathy can be observed and can be life threatening.
- Staphylococcal and streptococcal superinfections are common.
  - Eczema herpeticum shares the histopathological features of herpes simplex.

Evaluation

- The differential diagnosis of eczema herpeticum includes AGEP, varicella, disseminated herpes zoster, eczema vaccinatum, eczema coxsackium, and GAS infection.
- Tzanck smear and RT-PCR are commonly employed to detect HSV, along with superficial wound culture to evaluate for bacterial superinfection.

Management

- **IV acyclovir** is first line in severe cases.
- Addition of a penicillinase-resistant antibiotic is reasonable given the propensity for staphylococcal superinfection (>70%).
- Ophthalmological evaluation is indicated if there is periocular involvement.

"Real World" Advice

- An acute, widespread flare in patients with severe AD should prompt consideration of eczema herpeticum, molluscum contagiosum, eczema coxsackium, and *Staphylococcus aureus.*
- GAS infection closely mimics eczema herpeticum due to erosions and crusting; however, the lesions are not as uniform in size.

VARICELLA

Synonym: chickenpox

→ **Diagnosis Group 1**

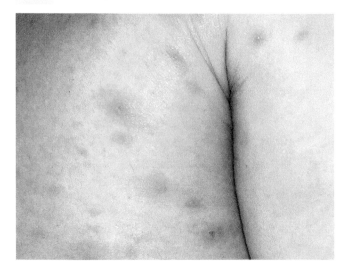

Epidemiology

- Varicella is an infection caused by **VZV (HHV-3).** Varicella refers to primary VZV infection, whereas herpes zoster refers to latent VZV reactivation.
- 98% of the worldwide population is seropositive for VZV. Varicella incidence has declined dramatically since introduction of the vaccine in 1995.
- **Airborne respiratory droplets** are the most common route of transmission. The incubation period after exposure is up to 3 weeks. Varicella is extremely contagious (>90% attack rate in susceptible hosts). Individuals are **infectious from 1 to 2 days before skin lesions occur until all are crusted over.**
- Varicella may present as a **congenital infection.** The highest risk of complications occurs with **primary infection in the first 20 weeks of pregnancy.**

- **Neonatal varicella is seen 5 days before to 2 days after delivery.** It is associated with **high mortality (30%)** due to lack of maternal antibody protection.

Clinicopathological Features

- A prodrome of fever and malaise can precede the varicella rash. **Pruritic macules and papules progress in a cephalocaudal distribution and rapidly evolve into vesicles and vesiculopustules followed by erosions** in ~12 hours. Lesions in **all stages of development** are seen simultaneously. Keratoconjunctivitis and mucosal ulcers may occur (the enanthem may precede the exanthem by 1-3 days).
    - Vesicles on a red base are classically described as "dew drops on a rose petal."
- Complications include **hepatitis, meningoencephalitis, and pneumonitis. Thrombocytopenia and idiopathic thrombocytopenic purpura (ITP)** can occur acutely and postinfection; anti-platelet antibodies have been observed.
    - Varicella is **more severe in adolescents and adults**, and adults have an increased risk of complications. **Elderly or immunocompromised** patients may manifest confusion, fatigue, headache, loss of appetite, and **seizures** due to **syndrome of inappropriate antidiuretic hormone secretion (SIADH).**
- **Congenital varicella** is characterized by **stellate cicatricial lesions at birth.** Complications include **limb abnormalities (hypoplasia, paresis), CNS involvement (hydrocephalus, intellectual disability), and ocular involvement (cataracts, chorioretinitis).**
- **Neonatal varicella** is characterized by **generalized varicella at birth.**
    - Varicella shares the histopathological features of herpes simplex (Cowdry A bodies) with occasional CSVV and more frequent follicular involvement. IHC can detect VZV.

Evaluation

- The differential diagnosis of varicella includes PLEVA, AGEP, disseminated herpes simplex, disseminated herpes zoster, hand-foot-mouth disease (HFMD), and scabies.
- Diagnostic evaluation includes the same battery of tests as for HSV.
- Ophthalmological evaluation is indicated if there is concern for eye involvement. In complicated disease, consider additional evaluation for hepatitis, meningoencephalitis, and pneumonitis.

Management

- Healthy children with uncomplicated varicella do not require therapy. **IV acyclovir** is indicated in HIV-infected and other immunocompromised patients with severe or complicated disease.
    - Even for uncomplicated varicella, adults should receive oral antivirals given the increased risk of complications.
- The **live attenuated varicella vaccine** confers protection to patients whose antibody levels are undetectable. **Postexposure vaccination is indicated within 3 to 5 days if > 12 months of age, not pregnant, and not immunocompromised** (these populations should receive **VZV-Ig**).

"Real World" Advice

- A common sequela of pediatric varicella is scarring as a result of scratching given the degree of pruritus associated with the exanthem. Soothing baths with colloidal oatmeal and antipruritic drugs (eg, antihistamines, camphor, menthol, pramoxine [>2 years of age]) can be helpful.

HERPES ZOSTER

Synonym: shingles
→ **Diagnosis Group 1**

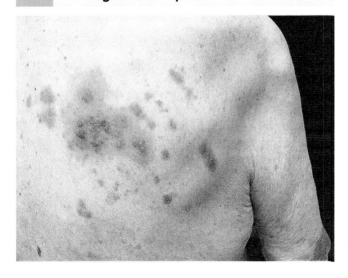

Epidemiology

- Herpes zoster refers to **latent VZV reactivation** in sensory ganglia.
- Varicella vaccination in childhood appears to confer less risk for development of herpes zoster than natural infection with varicella, although the risk is still present with the vaccine VZV strain.
- Associations include older age and immunosuppression. The risk of herpes zoster is **3%/y in HIV-infected patients** and **70% in the first year in leukemia or bone marrow transplant patients.**
    - There is no risk to the fetus in maternal herpes zoster.

Clinicopathological Features

- Herpes zoster classically follows a **sensory prodrome** of pruritus, tingling, and burning with the development of **grouped vesicles on an erythematous base in a dermatomal distribution.** Individual lesions evolve rapidly over 1 to 2 days. Classic herpes zoster can involve adjacent dermatomes and can rarely cross the midline. The most common location is the **trunk**; however, the single most common nerve is the **trigeminal nerve.** Keratoconjunctivitis and mucosal ulcers may occur.

- Neuropathic complications are dependent on location. For example, lumbar involvement can lead to motor neuropathy of the leg, while sacral involvement can lead to obstructive urinary symptoms.
  - **Hutchinson sign** (herpes zoster involving the **nasal tip**) may indicate **ocular involvement** since the external nasal branch of the anterior ethmoidal nerve and the ciliary nerve are both branches of the nasociliary nerve. **Uveitis** > keratitis can lead to **visual loss.**
    - ◈ Do NOT confuse <u>Hutchinson</u> sign of herpes zoster with <u>Hutchinson</u> sign of nail unit melanoma or <u>Hutchinson</u> teeth in <u>Hutchinson</u> triad of late congenital syphilis.
  - **Bell palsy** is due to herpes zoster of the facial nerve with **ipsilateral paralysis/paresis.**
  - **Ramsey-Hunt syndrome** is due to herpes zoster of the facial nerve affecting the **geniculate ganglion** with **ipsilateral paralysis/paresis, hearing loss/vestibular dysfunction,** and **loss of taste from the anterior two-thirds of the tongue.**
- **Disseminated herpes zoster (> 20 vesicles outside the dermatome)** is typically seen in HIV-infected and other immunocompromised patients with **hepatitis, meningoencephalitis, and pneumonitis.**
- The most common complication of herpes zoster is **postherpetic neuralgia (PHN).** This manifests in up to 20% of cases, with an increased incidence and severity with age.
- Pruritus and localized GA may occur in herpes zoster scars.
  - ◈ Herpes zoster shares the histopathological features of varicella.

Evaluation

- The differential diagnosis of herpes zoster includes contact dermatitis, herpes simplex, and bullous impetigo.
- Tzanck smear and RT-PCR are commonly employed to detect VZV. A fourfold increase in IgG serology titers over baseline is also diagnostic.
- Ophthalmological evaluation is indicated if there is concern for eye involvement. In disseminated disease, consider additional evaluation for hepatitis, meningoencephalitis, and pneumonitis.

Management

- For herpes zoster prevention, Zostavax (live attenuated vaccine, approved ≥50 years of age, 50% decrease in disease, 67% decrease in PHN) has been superseded by **Shingrix (recombinant vaccine, approved ≥50 years of age, >90% effective at prevention of zoster and PHN).** Shingrix is a subunit vaccine (HZ/su) containing recombinant VZV glycoprotein E and the AS01B adjuvant system.
- **Antiviral therapy decreases the severity and duration of skin lesions and pain, as well as the frequency and duration of PHN.** Oral antivirals include **acyclovir, famciclovir, and valacyclovir. IV acyclovir** is indicated in **disseminated herpes zoster.**
- **Gabapentin**, pregabalin, or TCAs are first line for **PHN.**

"Real World" Advice

- Antivirals are most effective if initiated within **48 to 72 hours.**
- **Concomitant systemic corticosteroids have no effect on the frequency or duration of PHN** but may decrease acute pain.

INFECTIOUS MONONUCLEOSIS
Synonym: glandular fever

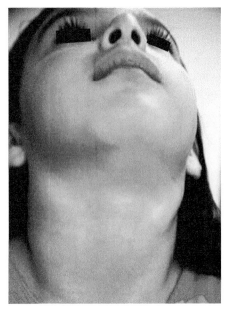

- Infectious mononucleosis is caused by **EBV (HHV-4).** By early adulthood, 95% of individuals have been infected with EBV. While the virus is most commonly transmitted through saliva, it can be transmitted through blood and other body fluids as well as organ transplants. The **incubation period is 3 to 7 weeks.** EBV infects mucosal epithelial cells and B-cells (mediated by **CD21 binding**). After acute infection, EBV can establish latent infection in B-cells (mediated by Epstein-Barr nuclear antigen 1 [EBNA1] and lateral membrane protein 2 [LMP2]). Immunocompetent hosts generally prevent cellular transformation from EBV; however, in susceptible hosts, latent infection in B-cells can lead to EBV-positive lymphoproliferative disorders (LPDs) and lymphomas.
- Though EBV infection is commonly asymptomatic in children, **~50% of adolescents and young adults develop infectious mononucleosis** (fever, fatigue, lymphadenopathy, pharyngitis). An exanthem (morbilliform, urticarial, or purpuric eruption 4-6 days after symptom onset) is seen in 70% of hospitalized patients and 10% of patients overall. An enanthem of **palatal petechiae (Forchheimer spots)** may occur. **Dermatologic signs of EBV infection** are summarized in Table 3.5.
  - ◈ EBV reactivation has been implicated in **DRESS syndrome, HLH, hydroa vacciniforme (HV), extranodal NK/T-cell lymphoma, nasal type (includes**

Table 3.5. DERMATOLOGIC SIGNS OF EPSTEIN-BARR VIRUS INFECTION

Diagnosis[a]	Classic description	Notes
Gianotti-Crosti syndrome (papular acrodermatitis of childhood)	Asymptomatic skin-colored or pink-red edematous papules favoring the cheeks, buttocks, and extensor extremities and monomorphic, flat-topped acral papules. Systemic features include diarrhea, low-grade fever, and lymphadenopathy.	Onset between 3 months and 15 years of age. Viral associations include HBV (most common in Europe), EBV (most common in the United States), CMV, and enterovirus. Vaccination associations include HBV. Self-limited over 2-3 weeks (do not treat with oral corticosteroids).
Infectious mononucleosis	See above.	
Lipschutz ulcer	Acute anogenital ulcer.	Nonvenereal.
Oral hairy leukoplakia	White patch favoring the lateral tongue. Oral hairy leukoplakia is often described as having a "corrugated" surface.	Viral associations include HIV infection and EBV infection.
Papular purpuric gloves and socks syndrome	Lacy eruption associated with burning, pruritus, edema of the hands and feet.	Viral associations include parvovirus B19 infection > EBV infection.

[a]Illustrative examples provided.

CMV, cytomegalovirus; EBV, Epstein-Barr virus; HBV, hepatitis B virus; HIV, human immunodeficiency virus; US, United States.

HV-like CTCL), posttransplant lymphoproliferative disorder (PTLD), lymphomatoid granulomatosis, Hodgkin lymphoma, endemic Burkitt lymphoma, and nasopharyngeal carcinoma.

- ⬥ Infectious mononucleosis has nonspecific histopathology.
- Infectious mononucleosis-like syndromes include acute retroviral syndrome and CMV infection. Transaminitis and lymphocytosis are common. Diagnostic tests include the heterophile antibody test (Monospot), EBV-specific serologies, and PCR.
- Treatment of infectious mononucleosis is supportive. **Morbilliform eruption may occur with amoxicillin/ampicillin administration.** Patients are recommended to avoid contact sports for 4 weeks given the risk of splenic rupture.

CYTOMEGALOVIRUS INFECTION

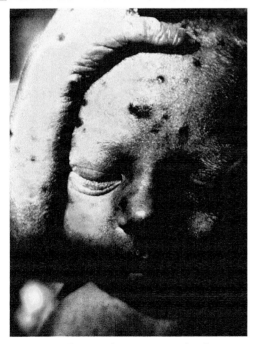

Congenital cytomegalovirus infection reprinted with permission from Sweet RL, Gibbs RS. *Atlas of Infectious Diseases of the Female Genital Tract.* Lippincott Williams & Wilkins; 2004.

- **CMV (HHV-5)** may be transmitted via body fluids, transplanted tissues, and fomites. The seroprevalence increases with age, averaging 60% in adults and over 90% in patients >80 years of age. Infection rate is **inversely proportional to socioeconomic status** (increased in low-income countries). The pathogenesis involves an incubation period of 4 to 8 weeks followed by viremia and multiorgan dissemination. Recurrent infection may occur due to **reactivation of latent CMV (eg, immunosuppression)** or reinfection with a different antigenic type.
  CMV is the leading cause of congenital infection. The highest risk of complications occurs with **primary infection in the first trimester.**
- **>90% of CMV infections are subclinical or asymptomatic.** In immunocompetent patients, CMV infection may present as an **infectious mononucleosis-like syndrome.** In immunosuppressed patients, CMV has protean manifestations including cutaneous vasculitis, morbilliform eruption, and **chronic perineal ulcers (eg, HIV-infected patients with CD4 < 50 cells/mm³).** Sequelae of multiorgan involvement include **esophagitis, colitis, chorioretinitis, and pneumonitis.** CMV reactivation has been implicated in **DRESS syndrome.**
  - ⬥ The perineal location of CMV ulcers is easy to recall based on proximity to colitis.

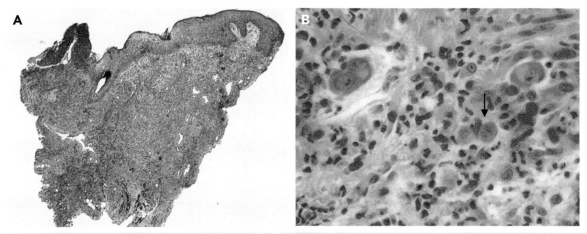

Figure 3.2. CLINICOPATHOLOGICAL CORRELATION: CYTOMEGALOVIRUS INFECTION. CMV infection is characterized by a superficial perivascular lymphocytic infiltrate in the dermis with prominent vessels. Endothelial cells are large and irregularly shaped with Cowdry B bodies: homogenous amphophilic glassy intranuclear inclusion bodies surrounded by a halo. IHC can detect CMV. A,Low-power view. B, High-power view. Solid arrow: crystalline intranuclear inclusion bodies surrounded by a clear halo ("owl's eyes"). CMV, cytomegalovirus; HSV, herpes simplex virus; IHC, immunohistochemistry; VZV, varicella zoster virus.

(Histology images courtesy of Anjela Galan, MD.)

In CMV, intranuclear inclusion bodies surrounded by a clear halo may resemble "owl's eyes." Do NOT confuse the Cowdry B bodies of CMV and poliovirus with the Cowdry A bodies of HSV and VZV.

Congenital CMV infection classically presents with **petechiae, purpura, and vesicles** along with **extramedullary hematopoiesis** (purpuric papules and nodules due to bone marrow dysfunction). It is the **leading infectious cause of deafness and intellectual disability** in the United States, which may be delayed.
- Congenital CMV is in the differential diagnosis of "blueberry muffin" lesions.
- Figure 3.2.
• Viral culture is the diagnostic gold standard, but more rapid tests include skin biopsy, CMV-specific serologies, assays to detect CMV antigens within leukocytes, and PCR. Diagnosis of cutaneous CMV should prompt **ophthalmologic evaluation for chorioretinitis.**

• Treatment of CMV mononucleosis-like syndrome is supportive. Organs and hematopoietic stem cells from seronegative donors are preferentially transplanted into seronegative recipients. For prophylaxis or treatment of CMV in immunosuppressed patients, **IV ganciclovir or oral valganciclovir** is first line. Alternatives include **cidofovir and foscarnet.**

RUBEOLA, RUBELLA, AND ROSEOLA

Rubeola synonyms: 1st disease, 14-day measles, measles

Rubella synonyms: 3rd disease, 3-day measles, German measles

Roseola synonyms: 6th disease, 3-day fever, baby measles, exanthem subitum, roseola infantum

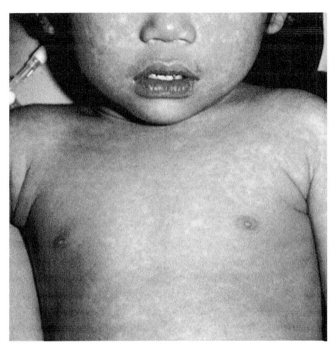

Rubeola reprinted with permission from Lugo-Somolinos A, McKinley-Grant L, Goldsmith LA, et al. *VisualDx: Essential Dermatology in Pigmented Skin*. Wolters Kluwer Health/Lippincott Williams & Wilkins; 2011.

- **Rubeola** is due to **morbillivirus; rubella** is due to **rubella virus;** and **roseola** is due to HHV-6 and HHV-7. **Rubella** may present as a **congenital infection**. The highest risk of complications occurs with **primary infection in the first trimester.**
- **Rubeola, rubella, and roseola** are summarized in Table 3.6. **Congenital rubella** classically presents with **petechiae, purpura, and vesicles** along with **extramedullary hematopoiesis.** Complications include cardiac defects, hepatosplenomegaly, cataracts, and deafness.
  - Congenital rubella is in the differential diagnosis of "blueberry muffin" lesions.
  - **Rubella** has been associated with **granulomatous eruptions** in immunocompromised patients. **HHV-6 and HHV-7** infection has been associated with **PR** and reactivation has been implicated in **DRESS syndrome.**
  - Rubeola, rubella, and roseola exanthems have nonspecific histopathology.
- Rubeola, rubella, and roseola can be diagnosed with serologies for IgM/IgG or PCR.
- **The measles, mumps, rubella (MMR) vaccine is the cornerstone of prevention.** Unfortunately, there has been a resurgence of outbreaks with increased vaccine hesitancy. Treatment is supportive, which may involve **vitamin A supplementation for acute rubeola.**

Table 3.6. RUBEOLA, RUBELLA, AND ROSEOLA

Diagnosis	Classic description
Rubeola	Exanthem: cephalocaudal spread of erythematous macules and papules coalescing into patches and plaques. Enanthem: gray papules on buccal mucosa (Koplik spots) precede the exanthem. Systemic features: myocarditis, fever, lymphopenia, encephalitis ± subacute sclerosing panencephalitis, conjunctivitis, coryza, cough. The "3 Cs" of rubeola are <u>c</u>onjunctivitis, <u>c</u>oryza, and <u>c</u>ough.
Rubella	Exanthem: morbilliform eruption. Enanthem: palatal petechiae (Forchheimer spots). Systemic features: mild prodrome. tender lymphadenopathy (occipital, postauricular, cervical).
Roseola	Exanthem: circular to elliptical red macules or papules ± white halo favoring the trunk > extremities. Enanthem: red papules on the soft palate and uvula (Nagayama spots). Systemic features: sudden-onset high fever ± seizures (exanthem begins as fever subsides). The exanthem of <u>rose</u>ola is "<u>rose</u> red."

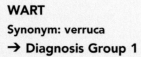

WART
Synonym: verruca
→ Diagnosis Group 1

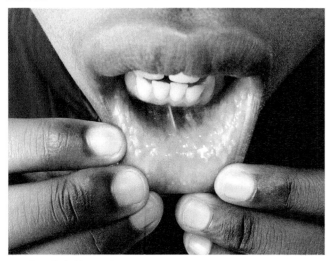

Focal epithelial hyperplasia.

Epidemiology

- A wart is an infection caused by **HPV.** Alpha HPV types are generally involved with clinically evident papillomas (less so with beta and gamma types).
- The HPV genome includes E (early) and L (late) genes, encoding respective gene products important for early (replication and growth) and late (capsid) parts of the HPV life cycle. **E6 binds to and promotes the degradation of P53, thereby abrogating its tumor suppressor function. E7**

binds to RB, leading to de-repression of E2F family transcription factors and cell division. The affinity of E7 for Rb may explain the increased oncogenic behavior in higher risk (16, 18) vs lower risk (6, 11) HPV types.
- Transmission of nongenital HPV types occurs via skin-skin contact and indirect contact with fomites. Sexual transmission of genital warts may occur.
    In infants, the most common mode of HPV transmission is vertical.
- As HPV is primarily controlled by cell-mediated immunity, extensive warts may be observed in HIV-infected and other immunocompromised patients. For example, anal HPV is present in >90% of HIV-infected men who have sex with men (MSM), and there is a 30- to 50-fold higher risk of anal cancer.
    Warts are associated with hereditary immunodeficiency syndromes including epidermodysplasia verruciformis (EDV); hyper-IgM syndrome; warts, hypogammaglobulinemia, infections, and myelokathexis (WHIM); and warts, immunodeficiency, lymphedema, dysplasia (WILD).

Clinicopathological Features

- **Wart variants** are summarized in Table 3.7.
    Focal epithelial hyperplasia is more common in children than in adults.
- Warts can **pseudo-koebnerize**, which describes local spread at sites of cutaneous trauma.
- There is a risk of malignant degeneration into **verrucous carcinoma and SCC/cervical cancer/vulvar cancer/vaginal cancer/penile cancer/anal cancer.** The risk is governed by HPV type (see Chapter 5: Epidermal Neoplasms) and depth of dysplasia.
    ◆ Figure 3.3.

Table 3.7. WART VARIANTS

Variant[a]	HPV types[a]	Classic description	Notes
Common wart (verruca vulgaris)	1, 2, 4	Verrucous papule favoring the hands and fingers, including periungual.	
Flat wart (verruca plana)	3, 10	Flat topped skin colored papules, often in linear array, favoring the face and dorsal hands.	Triggered by sun exposure.
Focal epithelial hyperplasia (Heck disease)	13, 32	Oral mucosal flat warts.	
Recurrent respiratory papillomatosis	6, 11	Hoarseness, stridor.	
Genital wart (condyloma acuminatum)	6, 11	Skin colored or white exophytic papillomas on anogenital skin; may be discrete or coalesce.	Most common STD.
Flat genital wart (condyloma plana)	2, 4	Subtle skin colored sessile papillomas on anogenital skin.	
Butcher wart	2, 7	Verrucous papules favoring the hands and fingers.	
Palmoplantar wart (verrucae palmares et plantares)	1, 2, 27, 57	Thick endophytic papules and plaques on the palms and soles.	

[a]Illustrative examples provided.
HPV, human papillomavirus; STD, sexually transmitted disease.

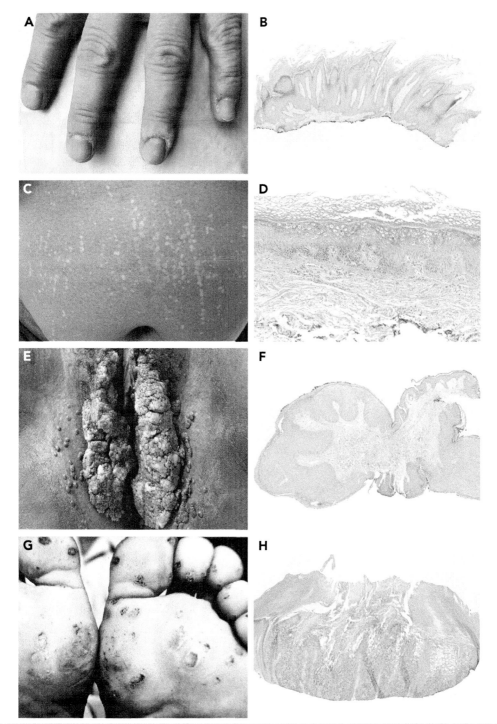

Figure 3.3. CLINICOPATHOLOGICAL CORRELATION: WART. A and B, Common wart. C and D, Flat wart. E and F, Genital wart. G and H, Palmoplantar wart.

(G, Histology image reprinted with permission from Elder DE, Elenitsas R, Rosenbach M, et al. *Lever's Histopathology of the Skin.* 11th ed. Wolters Kluwer; 2015. H, Histology images courtesy of Noel Turner, MD, MHS and Christine J. Ko, MD.)

- **Common wart:** compact hyperkeratosis, parakeratosis on peaks alternating with hypergranulosis in valleys, acanthosis, and papillomatosis (exophytic). Koilocytes (vacuolated cells with hyperchromatic nuclei) are pathognomonic for wart but variably present.
- **Flat wart:** hyperkeratosis, hypergranulosis, acanthosis, and vacuolated keratinocytes.
- **Focal epithelial hyperplasia:** hyperkeratosis, parakeratosis, and epithelial pallor.
- **Genital wart:** hyperkeratosis, parakeratosis, hypergranulosis, acanthosis, papillomatosis, and vacuolated keratinocytes (exophytic).
- **Palmoplantar wart:** compact hyperkeratosis, eosinophilic cytoplasmic inclusion bodies, and eosinophilic nuclear inclusion bodies (endophytic).

Flat wart differs from common wart due to the "basket weave" *stratum corneum* and absence of parakeratosis and papillomatosis. Palmoplantar wart is called "myrmecia" based on its resemblance to an "ant hill."

Evaluation

- The differential diagnosis of wart includes calluses and corns, molluscum contagiosum, seborrheic keratosis (SK), actinic keratosis (AK), SCCis, and SCC. Condyloma lata may mimic genital warts.
- Detection of subtle genital HPV infection can be performed with **5% acetic acid** treatment, which leads to whitening of lesions (though not specific).
- Skin biopsy may be helpful in unclear cases.

Management

- Destructive therapies are the most commonly utilized. Home-based therapies include salicylic acid (typically first line) along with podophyllotoxin, retinoids, and sinecatechins. Office-based therapies include **cryotherapy** (typically first line) along with cantharidin, podophyllin, intralesional 5-FU or bleomycin, electrosurgery, shave removal, high-concentration TCA, and PDL and CO_2 lasers. Immunotherapies include **imiquimod** (typically first line) and intralesional candida antigen.
  - **Spontaneous clearance of common warts** is seen in 70% to 75% of children within 2 years.
- Vaccines targeting L1 capsid protein are incredibly effective at preventing the neoplastic sequela of HPV infection. There are three FDA-approved vaccines: Cervarix vaccine (HPV 16, 18); Gardasil 4-valent vaccine (HPV 6, 11, 16, 18); and Gardasil 9-valent vaccine (HPV 6, 11, 16, 18, 31, 33, 45, 52, 68). The Gardasil 9-valent vaccine is approved for males and females ages 9 to 45 years. Vaccines can be administered regardless of history of abnormal Papanicolaou (PAP) smear.

"Real World" Advice

- Calluses emphasize dermatoglyphs, whereas warts and corns interrupt them. Paring of a wart will reveal thrombosed capillaries, whereas paring of a callus will reveal layers of yellow keratin and paring of a corn will reveal a yellow core.

SPOTLIGHT ON EPIDERMODYSPLASIA VERRUCIFORMIS

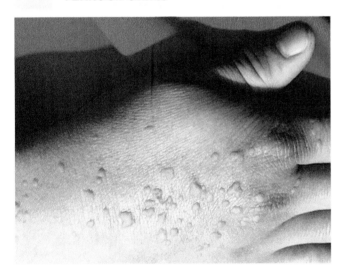

- EDV is an **AR** hereditary disorder due to *EVER1* and *EVER2* mutations. Evidence suggests that *EVER1*- and *EVER2*-encoded proteins function as keratinocyte-specific restriction factors antagonizing HPV replication. The predominant oncogenic HPV subtypes are **HPV 5 and 8.**
  - ◆ EDV can be acquired in the setting of HIV infection.
- EDV is characterized by **flat topped, scaly white or red/brown papules and plaques** with variable verrucous change. EDV warts typically favor sun-exposed areas but often generalize. **30% to 50% of patients develop skin cancers (typically SCC).**

◆ Figure 3.4.
- Skin biopsy may be helpful to establish the diagnosis.
- Patients should be counseled regarding sun protection. Treatment options for EDV warts are analogous to other warts; however, the widespread distribution presents a challenge.

MOLLUSCUM CONTAGIOSUM
→ **Diagnosis Group 1**

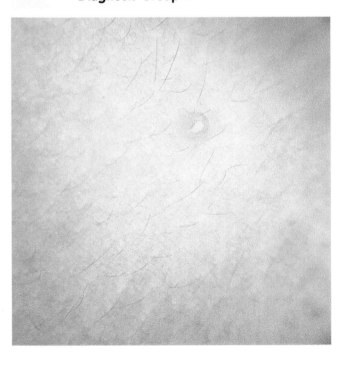

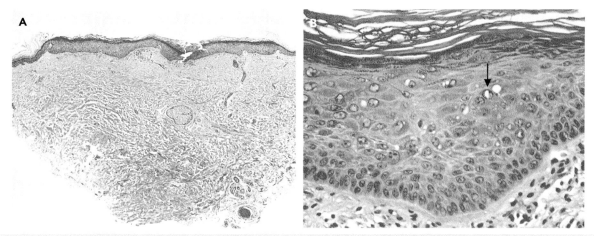

Figure 3.4. CLINICOPATHOLOGICAL CORRELATION: EPIDERMODYSPLASIA VERRUCIFORMIS. Flat warts in EDV are characterized by hyperkeratosis, hypergranulosis, acanthosis, and vacuolated keratinocytes with swollen abundant blue-gray cytoplasm. A, Low-power view. B, High-power view. EDV, epidermodysplasia verruciformis.

Epidemiology

- Molluscum contagiosum is a common self-limited infection due to **molluscipox.** Poxviruses use the **IL-18-binding protein to suppress the Th1 response.**
- Transmission of molluscum contagiosum primarily occurs via skin-skin contact and indirect contact with fomites. Sexual transmission may occur.
- Molluscum contagiosum is frequently observed in children with **AD** and other disorders of skin barrier function; however, it is also observed in HIV-infected and other immuno-compromised patients. While molluscum contagiosum virus 1 (MCV-1) is the most common subtype overall, **MCV-2 is the most common subtype in HIV-infected patients.**

Clinicopathological Features

- Molluscum contagiosum classically presents with **shiny skin-colored umbilicated papules.** Lesions may occur anywhere on body but have a predilection for skin folds. **Extensive facial/genital involvement and giant mollusca are observed in HIV-infected and other immunocompromised patients.** A Gianotti-Crosti syndrome–like reaction has been reported.
- Molluscum contagiosum can **pseudo-koebnerize.**
- **Molluscum dermatitis** refers to lesional attack by the host immune response, which causes papules to become inflamed and acquire a pustular component with surrounding dermatitis.
- Molluscum contagiosum has also been associated with conjunctivitis.

- **Poxvirus infections** are summarized in Table 3.8.
- Figure 3.5.

Evaluation

- The differential diagnosis of molluscum contagiosum includes JXG, wart, and pyogenic granuloma (PG). In immunocompromised patients, opportunistic fungal infections with **molluscum contagiosum–like lesions** include **coccidioidomycosis, cryptococcosis, histoplasmosis, and penicilliosis.**
- **Dermoscopy** reveals **central umbilication with polylobular white-yellow amorphous structures surrounded by arborizing vessels.**
- Diagnostic tests for molluscum contagiosum include:
  - **Tzanck smear or KOH:** reveals monomorphic, cuboidal, pathognomonic 30 to 35 μm virally transformed cells.
  - **Skin biopsy:** helpful in unclear cases.

Management

- Treatment of molluscum contagiosum is similar to wart. While curettage remains the most direct and effective treatment, compliance can be challenging in pediatric patients.

"Real World" Advice

- Reversal of skin barrier dysfunction can help prevent autoinoculation and spread of molluscum contagiosum through scratching.

Table 3.8. POXVIRUS INFECTIONS

Diagnosis[a]	Virus	Classic description	Notes
Molluscipox			
Molluscum contagiosum	See above.		
Orthopoxvirus			
Variola (smallpox)	Variola virus	Papules progress to vesiculopustules (same stage of development) and crust over leaving behind pitted scars. The distribution favors the face, trunk, and extremities including the palms and soles and the mucosa. Systemic features include fever, lymphadenopathy, arthritis, encephalitis, panophthalmitis, and pneumonitis.	Animal reservoir: humans. Individuals at high risk of exposure include military personnel and health care workers. Potential bioterrorism agent. Incubation period 7-17 days. Vaccinia vaccination is the cornerstone of prevention. Antivirals include tecovirimat.
Vaccinia	Vaccinia virus	Resembles variola at the vaccine injection site.	Animal reservoir: humans. For mucocutaneous adverse events of the vaccine, see Chapter 6: Immunosuppressants and Immunomodulators.
Monkeypox	Monkeypox virus	Resembles variola (multiple stages of development), often involving the face, chest, hands, feet, oral cavity, and anogenital area.	Animal reservoirs: humans, monkeys, rodents. JYNNEOS is a preventative vaccine. Tecovirimat is indicated for severe disease and high-risk patients
Cowpox	Cowpox virus	Resembles variola.	Animal reservoirs: humans, cats, cattle (rare), rodents.
Parapox			
Orf (contagious pustular dermatosis, ecthyma contagiosum, infectious pustular dermatosis)	Orf virus	Six clinical stages (maculopapular, targetoid, weeping nodule, regenerative dry stage with black dots, papillomatosis, regression with a dry crust, evolves into a crusted nodule prior to resolution). The distribution favors the hands. Systemic features include fever and lymphadenopathy/lymphangitis.	Animal reservoirs: humans, goat, reindeer, sheep (vaccine in livestock can lead to human transmission). Lives in soil for 6 months. Self-limited over 7-10 weeks.
Paravaccinia (milker's nodule, pseudocowpox)	Paravaccinia virus	Resembles an isolated orf lesion.	Animal reservoirs: cattle, humans.

[a]Illustrative examples provided.

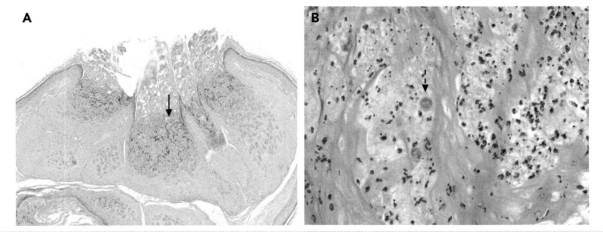

Figure 3.5. SIDE-BY-SIDE COMPARISON: MOLLUSCUM CONTAGIOSUM AND ORF. Both molluscum contagiosum and orf are characterized by inclusion bodies. Inclusion bodies in molluscum contagiosum (Henderson-Patterson bodies, molluscum bodies) are eosinophilic-to-basophilic and cytoplasmic. Inclusion bodies in orf are eosinophilic and either cytoplasmic or intranuclear. A, Molluscum contagiosum. Solid arrow: eosinophilic cytoplasmic inclusion body. B, Orf. Dashed arrow: eosinophilic cytoplasmic inclusion body.

(A, Histology image courtesy of Noel Turner, MD, MHS and Christine J. Ko, MD.)

Eosinophilic cytoplasmic inclusion bodies (Guarnieri bodies) ± eosinophilic intranuclear inclusion bodies are also present in variola and other poxvirus infections.

ERYTHEMA INFECTIOSUM
Synonyms: 5th disease

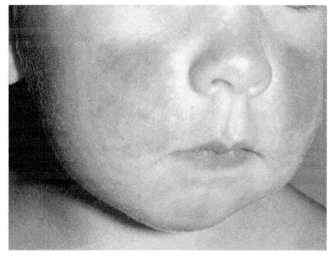

Reprinted with permission from Burkhart CN, Morrell DS, Goldsmith LA, et al. *VisualDx: Essential Pediatric Dermatology*. Wolters Kluwer Health/Lippincott Williams & Wilkins; 2009.

- Erythema infectiosum is due to **parvovirus B19. Transmission primarily occurs** via **respiratory droplets** but also via blood and other secretions. It **peaks in children during the winter and spring.** Through vertical transmission, parvovirus B19 may also present as a **congenital infection** (hydrops fetalis), with the highest risk of fetal death in the second trimester.
- Erythema infectiosum classically presents with **bright red macular erythema over the cheeks followed by a lacy eruption of the extremities (signals conversion of IgM to IgG and an end to the infectious state).** The enanthem is characterized by **erythema of the tonsils and pharynx.** There is a **risk for aplastic crisis**, especially in patients with **hereditary spherocytosis** and patients on **dapsone. Symmetrical polyarthritis** can be observed with or without rash. **Hydrops fetalis** results in abnormal fluid buildup in fetal compartments and is associated with **anemia and high-output CHF.**
    - The colloquial name for erythema infectiosum is "slapped cheek disease."
    - **Papular purpuric gloves and socks syndrome** (see above) is a distinct presentation of parvovirus B19 infection that primarily occurs in **adolescents and young adults.** Unlike the lacy eruption in erythema infectiosum, **patients are infectious.**
    - Erythema infectiosum has nonspecific histopathology.
- CBC typically reveals leukopenia and anemia with **decreased reticulocyte count** due to transient effects of parvovirus B19 on erythroid progenitors. **If a pregnant woman is exposed, check IgM and IgG levels.**
- Treatment of erythema infectiosum is supportive. **Aplastic crisis may require blood transfusion.**

CORONAVIRUS DISEASE 2019

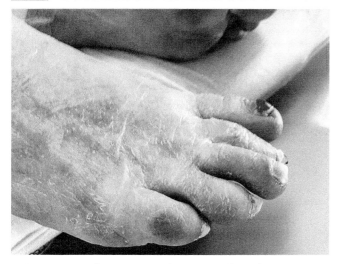

- Coronavirus disease 2019 (COVID-19) is due to **severe acute respiratory syndrome coronavirus 2 (SARS-CoV-2).** Since its emergence in 2019, the COVID-19 global pandemic has resulted in the deaths of over 6 million people and counting.
- One report found that 20% of hospitalized patients had a skin rash attributed to SARS-CoV-2. Analysis of 171 cases in the international registry from the AAD and International League of Dermatological Societies with laboratory-confirmed COVID-19 revealed the most common morphologies to be morbilliform (22%), pernio-like (18%), urticarial (16%), macular erythema (13%), vesicular (11%), papulosquamous (9.9%), and retiform purpura (6.4%). **Pernio-like lesions** affected patients with **mild disease**, whereas **retiform purpura** affected **ill, hospitalized patients.** The association between pernio-like lesions and COVID-19 remains controversial as only a minority of these patients have laboratory-confirmed COVID-19. Alternate hypotheses include changes in behavior during quarantine (eg, not wearing socks and shoes).
    - **Pernio-like skin lesions** may occur in **interferonopathies** such as familial chilblain lupus, Aicardi-Goutières syndrome, chronic atypical neutrophilic dermatosis with lipodystrophy and elevated temperature (CANDLE) syndrome, and SAVI. Because these lesions are attributed to systemic elevations in type I IFN signaling, COVID-19-associated pernio-like lesions have been hypothesized to result from a similar underlying pathophysiology.
    - Pernio-like lesions related to SARS-CoV-2 share the histopathological features of pernio. However, some studies have identified unique features including tight cuffing of lymphocytes around vessels and Spike glycoprotein detection by IHC.
- Lymphopenia is the most common laboratory finding. Diagnosis of COVID-19 requires detection of SARS-CoV-2 RNA or antigen in respiratory specimens.

- **Vaccination is the cornerstone of prevention.** Antivirals include nirmatrelvir with ritonavir, remdesivir, and molnupiravir. Antithrombotic therapy may be indicated in select patients. Clinical trials are ongoing.

DENGUE

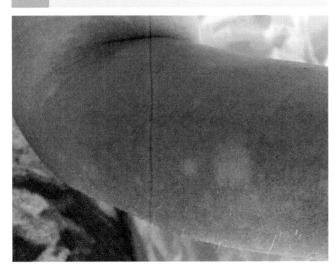

- Dengue is due to **dengue virus**, an **arbovirus** transmitted by *Aedes* mosquitoes. Dengue is most common in Asia and the Caribbean; however, geographic shifts are occurring due to climate change.
- 50% of dengue patients develop a **morbilliform eruption sparing discrete areas of skin.** Asymptomatic and mild cases manifest with a nonspecific viral syndrome. Classical dengue fever leads to **arthralgias, myalgias, headaches, and retro-orbital pain.** Prior infection from a different viral serotype can predispose patients to **dengue hemorrhagic fever** (shock, hemorrhage, confusion, respiratory distress) mediated by nonneutralizing antibodies against the prior viral serotype.
  - Skin lesions in dengue may be described as "white islands in a sea of red."
  - Dengue has nonspecific histopathology.
- Diagnostic tests include serologies or PCR. Other arboviruses that cause **morbilliform eruptions** include **West Nile virus** (transmitted by *Culex* mosquitoes, associated with **encephalitis**), **zika virus** (transmitted by *Aedes* mosquitoes and as a **sexually transmitted disease [STD]**), and **chikungunya virus** (transmitted by *Aedes* mosquitoes, associated with **arthritis**).
  - **Zika** may present as a **congenital infection** resulting in **microcephaly.**
- Skin application of **diethyltoluamide (Deet)** is widely used for protection from biting arthropods including mosquitoes. Treatment is supportive.

HAND-FOOT-MOUTH DISEASE
→ Diagnosis Group 2

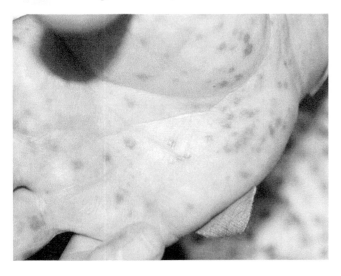

Epidemiology

- The most common enterovirus serotypes to cause hand-foot-mouth disease (HFMD) are **coxsackieviruses A16 and A10 and enterovirus 17.** The recent emergence of HFMD caused by **highly infective coxsackievirus A6** has led to several large outbreaks in the United States and worldwide.

- Initial infection occurs in the oropharynx or gut and subsequently spreads to other organs in a viremic phase of illness. Transmission may occur via the **fecal-oral route or respiratory droplets.** The incubation period is up to 6 days.
- HFMD is more likely to affect children and is primary observed in the summer and early fall. However, HFMD caused by coxsackievirus A6 has also been observed in the winter.
  - While HFMD caused by coxsackievirus A6 is overall more common in children, it may also affect adults.

Clinicopathological Features

- HFMD classically presents with **oral vesicles or erosions on a red base along with elliptical grayish vesicles or pustules favoring the buttocks, hands, and feet.** The rash follows the fever by 1 to 2 days.
  - The elliptical lesions of HFMD resemble American "footballs." "Hand-foot-mouth-butt" disease would be a more accurate descriptor.
- Complications include **eczema coxsackium** and **onychomadesis (nail shedding)** after 1 to 2 months.
  - Figure 3.6.
- **HFMD caused by coxsackievirus A6** is characterized by an **atypical, more widespread, eruption with vesicular and bullous lesions.**
  - HFMD histopathology demonstrates ballooning and reticular degeneration of keratinocytes.

Evaluation

- The differential diagnosis of HFMD includes **herpangina.** This infection, due to **group A and B coxsackieviruses and echovirus,** classically presents with **painful gray vesicles on the palatal, buccal, and tonsillar mucosa.** Other mimickers include autoimmune blistering disorders, EM, herpes simplex, varicella, disseminated herpes zoster, and Gianotti-Crosti syndrome.
- Diagnosis of HFMD may be accomplished through PCR of vesicle fluid, throat, and/or anus.
- Skin biopsy may be helpful in unclear cases.

Management

- HFMD **self-resolves in 1 to 2 weeks.** Treatment is supportive.

"Real World" Advice

- Eczema herpeticum and eczema coxsackium can have a similar clinical appearance. Generally, evaluation for both entities is recommended. Eczema coxsackium does not respond to antivirals that target HSV.

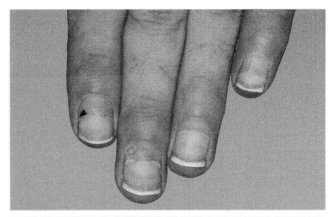

Figure 3.6. ONYCHOMADESIS. Onychomadesis (nail shedding) describes detachment of the nail plate from the proximal nail fold. It occurs most often due to mechanical or friction injury; however, involvement of multiple nails may indicate a systemic insult (eg, antecedent HFMD). HFMD, hand-foot-mouth disease.

Bacterial Diseases

- **Bacteria** are single-celled organisms that have evolved to inhabit nearly all environments on the planet. They can be broadly separated into groups on the basis of staining pattern under the microscope:
  - **Gram-positive (GP)** bacteria possess a thick peptidoglycan layered cell wall and lack an outer cell membrane layer. They stain **purple on Gram stain.**
  - **Gram-negative (GN)** bacteria only possess a very thin peptidoglycan layer in addition to an outer membrane. They stain **red on Gram stain.**
  - **Acid-fast bacilli (AFB)** require special stains given the lipid content of their cell wall. *Nocardia* are partially acid-fast GP bacteria not considered AFB.
- Though traditionally considered pathogenic, there is a growing appreciation for the essential homeostatic interplay between commensal bacteria of the skin and gut and how the microbiome impacts human health. The normal skin flora is colonized by aerobic cocci, aerobic and anaerobic corynebacteria, GN bacteria, and yeast in homeostatic conditions; however, dysbiosis develops in pathogenic states and has been implicated as a potential cause or cofactor in skin diseases (eg, *S. aureus* in AD; GAS species in guttate psoriasis and EN).
- **Bacterial classification** (for dermatology-relevant bacteria) is summarized in Table 3.9.

Table 3.9. BACTERIAL CLASSIFICATION

Type	Family	Bacterium	Diagnosis[a]
GPCs	*Staphylococcus* species	*Staphylococcus aureus*	Infectious eczematous dermatitis, impetigo (nonbullous, bullous), SSSS, staphylococcal TSS, cellulitis, abscess/furuncle/carbuncle, botryomycosis, folliculitis, acute paronychia, staphylococcal sepsis (septic vasculitis)
	Streptococcus species	GAS (*Streptococcus pyogenes*)	Impetigo (nonbullous), ecthyma, scarlet fever, streptococcal TSS, erysipelas, cellulitis, infection-induced panniculitis, necrotizing fasciitis, purpura fulminans
		GBS (*Streptococcus agalactiae*)	Impetigo (neonates)
		Streptococcus iniae	Hand cellulitis
	Kytococcus species	*Kytococcus sedentarius* (formerly *Micrococcus sedentarius*)	Pitted keratolysis

(Continued)

Table 3.9. BACTERIAL CLASSIFICATION (CONTINUED)

Type	Family	Bacterium	Diagnosis[a]
GPRs	*Cutibacterium* species	*Cutibacterium acnes* (formerly *Propionibacterium acnes*)	Acne
	Clostridium species	*Clostridium perfringens*	Necrotizing fasciitis
	Corynebacterium species	*Corynebacterium minutissimum*	Erythrasma
		Corynebacterium tenuis	Trichomycosis axillaris
		Corynebacterium diphtheriae	Diphtheria
	Bacillus species	*Bacillus anthracis*	Anthrax
GP filamentous bacteria	*Actinomyces* species	*Actinomyces israelii*	Actinomycetoma
	Nocardia species	*Nocardia asteroides, Nocardia brasiliensis*	Superficial cutaneous nocardiosis, lymphocutaneous nocardiosis, actinomycetoma
	Actinomadura species	*Actinomadura madurae, Actinomadura pelletieri*	Actinomycetoma
	Streptomyces species	*Streptomyces somaliensis*	Actinomycetoma
GNCs	*Neisseria* species	*Neisseria gonorrhoeae*	Gonococcal urethritis/cervicitis, gonococcemia (septic vasculitis)
		Neisseria meningitidis	Meningococcemia (septic vasculitis)
GNRs	*Bartonella* species	*Bartonella bacilliformis*	Oroya fever/verruga peruana
		Bartonella henselae	Bacillary angiomatosis, cat-scratch disease
		Bartonella quintana	Bacillary angiomatosis, trench fever
	Brucella species	Variable	Brucellosis
	Burkholderia species	*Burkholderia mallei*	Glanders
		Burkholderia pseudomallei	Melioidosis
	Capnocytophaga species	*Capnocytophaga canimorsus*	Dog bites
	Eikenella species	*Eikenella corrodens*	Human bites
	Escherichia species	*Escherichia coli*	Malakoplakia
	Hemophilus species	*Haemophilus influenzae*	Hemophilus infection
	Klebsiella species	*Klebsiella granulomatis*	Granuloma inguinale
		Klebsiella rhinoscleromatis	Rhinoscleroma
	Salmonella species	*Salmonella typhi*	Typhoid fever
	Pasteurella species	*Pasteurella canis*	Dog bites
		Pasteurella multocida	Cat bites, dog bites
	Proteus species	*Proteus mirabilis*	Black nail syndrome
	Pseudomonas species	*Pseudomonas aeruginosa*	Pseudomonal pyoderma, pseudomonal hot foot syndrome, ecthyma gangrenosum, pseudomonal folliculitis, green nail syndrome, otitis externa, pseudomonal sepsis (septic vasculitis)
	Streptobacillus species	*Streptobacillus moniliformis*	Rate-bite fever
	Vibrio species	*Vibrio vulnificus*	Vibriosis
	Yersinia species	*Yersinia pestis*	Plague

Table 3.9. BACTERIAL CLASSIFICATION (CONTINUED)

Type	Family	Bacterium	Diagnosis[a]
GN pleomorphic bacteria	*Anaplasma* species	*Anaplasma phagocytophilum*	Anaplasmosis (granulocytic)
	Chlamydia species	*Chlamydia trachomatis*	LGV
	Coxiella species	*Coxiella burnetii*	Q fever
	Ehrlichia species	*Ehrlichia chaffeensis*	Ehrlichiosis (monocytic)
		Ehrlichia phagocytophilum	Ehrlichiosis (granulocytic)
	Francisella species	*Francisella tularensis*	Tularemia
	Haemophilus species	*Haemophilus ducreyi*	Chancroid
	Helicobacter species	*Helicobacter pylori*	Urticaria
	Mycoplasma species	*Mycoplasma pneumoniae*	MIRM
	Orientia species	*Orientia tsutsugamushi*	Typhus (scrub)
	Rickettsia species	*Rickettsia akari*	Rickettsialpox
		Rickettsia conorii	Mediterranean spotted fever
		Rickettsia felis	Typhus (endemic)
		Rickettsia prowazekii	Typhus (epidemic)
		Rickettsia rickettsii	RMSF
		Rickettsia typhi	Typhus (endemic)
GN spirochetes	*Borrelia* species	*Borrelia afzelii*	Lyme disease
		Borrelia burgdorferi	Lyme disease
		Borrelia duttonii	Relapsing fever (tick-borne)
		Borrelia garinii	Lyme disease
		Borrelia hermsii	Relapsing fever (tick-borne)
		Borrelia lonestari	STARI
		Borrelia parkeri	Relapsing fever (tick-borne)
		Borrelia recurrentis	Relapsing fever (louse-borne)
	Leptospira species	*Leptospira interrogans*	Leptospirosis
	Treponema species	*Treponema carateum*	Pinta
		Treponema pallidum endemicum	Syphilis (endemic)
		Treponema pallidum pertenue	Yaws
		Treponema pallidum pallidum	Syphilis (venereal)
AFBs	*Mycobacterium* species	*Mycobacterium tuberculosis*	TB
		Atypical mycobacteria	Buruli ulcer, fish tank granuloma
		Mycobacterium leprae	Leprosy

[a]Illustrative examples provided.

AFBs, acid-fast bacilli; GAS, group A β-hemolytic *Streptococcus*; GBS, group B *Streptococcus*; GNCs, gram-negative cocci; GNRs, gram-negative rods; GP, gram-positive; GPCs, gram-positive cocci; GPRs, gram-positive rods; LGV, lymphogranuloma venereum; MIRM, *Mycoplasma pneumoniae*–induced rash and mucositis; RMSF, Rocky Mountain spotted fever; SSSS, staphylococcal scalded skin syndrome; STARI, southern tick associated rash illness; TB, tuberculosis; TSS, toxic shock syndrome.

IMPETIGO
→ Diagnosis Group 1

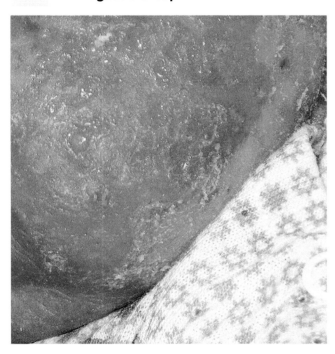

Epemiology

- Impetigo is the **most common skin infection in children.** It is primarily due to *Staphylococcus* > GAS species; however, **group B *Streptococcus* (GBS)** is an important cause of impetigo in **neonates.**
  - *Staphylococcus* species are **facultative aerobic catalase-positive gram-positive cocci (GPCs).** *S. aureus*, a common pathogen, is divided into **methicillin-sensitive *Staphylococcus aureus* (MSSA)** and **methicillin-resistant *Staphylococcus aureus* (MRSA).** Methicillin resistance primarily arises due to staphylococcal chromosome cassette (SCC) mec, specifically the ***mecA*** gene encoding the alternative **penicillin-binding protein (PBP) 2α.** Panton-Valentine leukocidin (PVL) is a MRSA virulence factor.
  - GAS species are **facultative aerobic GPCs. M proteins** are GAS virulence factors that can prevent phagocytosis, among other functions.
- Impetigo is contagious through both direct and indirect contact. While nasal carriage of *S. aureus* is the major risk factor, pharyngeal, axillary, and perineal carriage also increases risk. Other risk factors include AD, skin injury, contact sports, warm and humid climates, and poor hygiene.
- There are two major types of impetigo:
  - **Nonbullous impetigo:** 70% of cases.
  - **Bullous impetigo:** due to <u>*S. aureus*</u> **phage II types 55 or 71** that express **exfoliative toxin (ET)-A (chromosome)** and **ET-B (plasmid),** which **cleave desmoglein 1 in the granular layer causing acantholysis and a subcorneal split.**
- **Ecthyma** is a deep variant of nonbullous impetigo **due to GAS but rapidly colonized with** <u>*S. aureus*</u>.
  - Do NOT confuse <u>ecthyma</u> with <u>ecthyma</u> gangrenosum.

Clinicopathological Features

- The classic presentation of impetigo varies based on type:
  - **Nonbullous:** erythematous macules that evolve into eroded vesicles or pustules with golden crust.
    - The Latin word *aureus* means "golden." Golden crust in impetigo is alternatively called "honey-colored crust."
  - **Bullous:** small vesicles that evolve into superficial bullae, eventually giving rise to larger flaccid bullae that rupture leaving behind a collarette of scale.
  - **Ecthyma:** ulcer with a necrotic base and surrounding erythema favoring the lower extremities.
    - Ecthyma has a "punched out" appearance.
- Impetigo favors the face but may also affect the anogenital area. In **infants,** impetigo is in the differential diagnosis for **diaper dermatitis.**
- Complications of impetigo include **poststreptococcal glomerulonephritis (GAS);** risk is not altered with antibacterial therapy.
  - Figure 3.7.

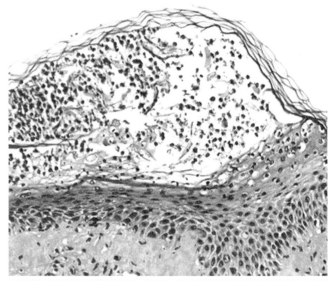

Figure 3.7. CLINICOPATHOLOGICAL CORRELATION: IMPETIGO. Impetigo is characterized by GPCs within small neutrophilic vesiculopustules in the epidermis and a superficial mixed infiltrate in the dermis. DIF, direct immunofluorescence; GPCs, gram-positive cocci; PF, pemphigus foliaceus; SSSS, staphylococcal scalded skin syndrome.

(Reprinted with permission from Husain AN, Stocker JT, Dehner LP. *Stocker and Dehner's Pediatric Pathology.* 4th ed. Wolters Kluwer; 2015.)

- Bullous impetigo: subcorneal split with acantholysis.
- Ecthyma: GPCs within neutrophilic crust overlying an ulcer and a neutrophilic infiltrate in the dermis

Bullous impetigo can NOT be distinguished from PF or SSSS on histopathology. GPCs may be evident in bullous impetigo. DIF is positive in PF and negative in bullous impetigo and SSSS.

Evaluation

- The differential diagnosis of nonbullous impetigo includes eczematous dermatitis, herpes simplex, varicella, tinea, candidiasis, and arthropod bites. The differential diagnosis of bullous impetigo further includes autoimmune bullous disorders (eg, PF) and SSSS.
- Diagnostics include **Gram stain and bacterial culture.**

Management

- Topical antibacterial therapy is first line (eg, **bacitracin, mupirocin, retapamulin**) for most cases.
    - Polymyxin B is NOT a treatment for impetigo.
- Oral antibacterial therapy can be employed for a 7-day course if infection is extensive (eg, **dicloxacillin, cephalexin**). For **MRSA**, **oral** options include **TMP-SMX, clindamycin, linezolid, and tetracyclines** and **IV** options include **daptomycin and vancomycin.**
- *S. aureus* **decolonization** is indicated for recurrent disease.

"Real World" Advice

- **Culture-positivity for *S. aureus* from the bullae** distinguishes bullous impetigo from SSSS.

STAPHYLOCOCCAL SCALDED SKIN SYNDROME
Synonym: 4th disease, Ritter disease

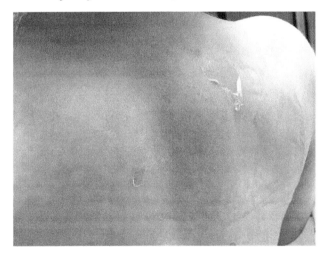

- SSSS is due to *S. aureus* **phage II types 55 or 71. ET-A and ET-B cleave desmoglein 1 in the granular layer causing acantholysis and a subcorneal split.** In SSSS, the clinical features are due to hematogenous spread of the toxins, whereas bullous impetigo is due to local toxin-mediated effects. **Infants** and **young children are at highest risk of SSSS due to lack of toxin-neutralizing antibodies and relatively decreased renal toxin clearance.**
    - At-risk adult populations for SSSS include those with renal disease and immunosuppression.
- SSSS classically presents with **skin tenderness** and a prodrome of constitutional symptoms including fever and either rhinorrhea or conjunctivitis. **Erythema first occurs on the head and intertriginous areas** before generalizing. Formation of **superficial flaccid bullae leads to a wrinkled appearance and a positive Nikolsky sign. Periorificial crusting** and **radial fissuring** is characteristic. There is no mucosal involvement. Re-epithelialization without scarring occurs in 1 to 2 weeks.
    - In SSSS, an unhappy child with superficial flaccid bullae leading to a wrinkled appearance is sometimes described as having "sad man facies." Periorificial crusting may resemble a child after dunking their face in a bowl of oatmeal.
    - SSSS can NOT be distinguished from PF or bullous impetigo on histopathology. GPCs may be evident in bullous impetigo. DIF is positive in PF and negative in bullous impetigo and SSSS.
- A helpful clue to distinguish SSSS from SJS/TEN is **absence of mucosal involvement.** "Jelly roll" preparation will show an intraepidermal split. Bacterial cultures should be obtained from the conjunctivae, nasopharynx, perianal area, and/or injured skin. Blood cultures are typically negative in children but can be positive in adults.
- The mortality rate for SSSS in children is low (<4%). **Age < 5 years is the most important prognostic factor.** SSSS is treated with a **penicillinase-resistant penicillin (eg, dicloxacillin) or cephalexin plus clindamycin (clindamycin is added to target toxin production).** In severe cases, IV fluids are used to correct insensible losses. *S. aureus* decolonization is indicated after acute treatment.
    - The mortality rate for SSSS in adults is up to 60%.

SCARLET FEVER
Synonym: 2nd disease, scarlatina

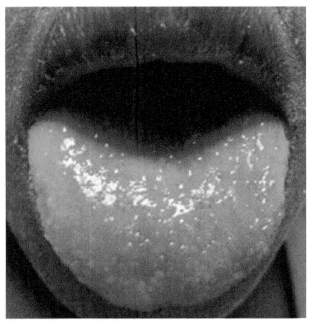

Reprinted with permission from Sherman SC, Cico SJ, Nordquist E, et al. *Atlas of Clinical Emergency Medicine*. Wolters Kluwer; 2016.

- Scarlet fever is due to **GAS** species, typically **pharyngitis or tonsillitis**, and is mediated by **streptococcal pyrogenic exotoxin (SPE)-A, SPE-B, and SPE-C**. It most commonly affects **children 1 to 10 years old** during the fall, winter, and spring months in temperate climates.

- Scarlet fever occurs in <u>children</u> learning their "<u>A</u>, <u>B</u>, <u>C</u>s" (SPE-<u>A</u>, SPE-<u>B</u>, SPE-<u>C</u>).
- Scarlet fever classically presents with sore throat, malaise, nausea, and fevers 1 to 2 days prior to the skin eruption. The skin eruption is characterized by **macular erythema of the neck, chest, and axillae, which generalizes to small papules**. Other clinical features include **circumoral pallor** and **Pastia lines (linear petechial streaks in body folds)**. Palmoplantar and fingertip desquamation may occur ≥1 week after the skin eruption. The enanthem includes **Forchheimer spots on the soft palate and a tongue that is initially white with red papilla followed by evolution into a bright red appearance**. Complications of scarlet fever include **rheumatic fever** and **poststreptococcal glomerulonephritis**. The **revised Jones criteria for acute rheumatic fever** are presented in Table 3.10.
  - Colloquial descriptions of scarlet fever include "sandpaper skin" and "strawberry tongue."
  - Scarlet fever is characterized by perifollicular dilated capillaries and lymphatics, dermal edema, perivascular neutrophilic infiltrates, and hemorrhagic foci. The desquamative stage is characterized by parakeratosis and spongiosis.
- CBC frequently shows leukocytosis with a left shift. **Nasal and/or throat bacterial cultures are the gold standard** for GAS diagnosis, but antigen and RT-PCR-based approaches are increasingly employed. **ASO and anti-DNase B or streptozyme titer** can be used for confirmation of recent GAS infection.
- **Penicillin or amoxicillin** for 10 to 14 days is the typical treatment.

Table 3.10. REVISED JONES CRITERIA FOR ACUTE RHEUMATIC FEVER[a]

Major Criteria

1. Carditis
2. Polyarthritis
3. Chorea
4. Subcutaneous nodules
5. Erythema marginatum

Minor Criteria

1. Fever
2. Arthralgia
3. Elevated ESR or CRP
4. Prolonged PR interval on ECG

[a]Evidence of streptococcal infection and two major or one major and two minor criteria are required for diagnosis.
CRP, C-reactive protein; ECG, electrocardiogram; ESR, erythrocyte sedimentation rate.

TOXIC SHOCK SYNDROME

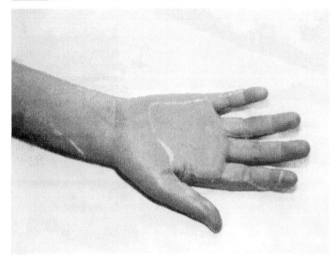

Reprinted with permission from Engleberg NC, DiRita V, Dermody TS. *Schaechter's Mechanisms of Microbial Disease.* 5th ed. Wolters Kluwer Health/Lippincott Williams & Wilkins; 2012.

- TSS is due to **superantigens** that **crosslink the Vβ region of TCR on T-cells and MHC II on APCs** resulting in nonspecific polyclonal activation of large T-cell populations in affected hosts and significant cytokine elaboration. TSS typically affects young healthy individuals. TSS can be divided into two groups:
  - **Staphylococcal TSS:** *S. aureus* elaborates **toxic shock syndrome toxin 1 (TSST-1)** (especially "menstrual TSS" caused by superabsorbent tampons) and **enterotoxins B and C** (especially "nonmenstrual TSS" caused by nasal packing or other implanted foreign bodies).
  - **Streptococcal TSS: GAS species (mainly M types 1 and 3)** elaborate **SPE-A and SPE-B**, often in the setting of **necrotizing fasciitis.**
- Four clinical features of TSS are **fever, hypotension (100%), scarlatiniform exanthem, and involvement of ≥ 3 organ systems (especially renal). Staphylococcal TSS is more likely to manifest with a scarlatiniform exanthem than streptococcal TSS.** Desquamation of the hands and feet 1 to 3 weeks after TSS is classically observed.
  - TSS is characterized by a neutrophilic and lymphocytic infiltrate in the superficial dermis ± exocytosis, epidermal spongiosis, and papillary dermal edema.
- **Staphylococcal TSS has a lower blood culture-positivity rate than streptococcal TSS.**
- **Staphylococcal TSS has a lower mortality rate (< 3%) than Streptococcal TSS (30%-60%).** Management includes intensive monitoring and supportive therapy. Any possible culprit **foreign bodies must be removed**, and for relevant cases, **consider surgical debridement.** Antibacterial therapy for staphylococcal TSS is similar to SSSS. Antibacterial therapy for streptococcal TSS is **IV penicillinase G plus clindamycin.** IVIG can be employed in severe cases for toxin neutralization.

CELLULITIS
→ Diagnosis Group 1

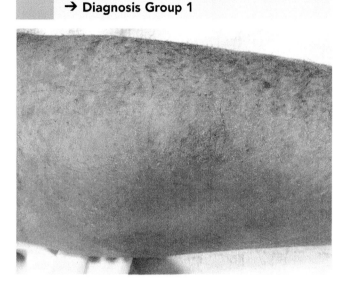

Epidemiology

- Cellulitis in adults is primarily due to **GAS species > S. aureus.**
  Cellulitis in children is primarily due to *S. aureus.*
- Rarer pathogens include *Streptococcus iniae* **(hand cellulitis from fresh fish)** and GNRs (see below).
- Risk factors include **lymphedema**, PAD, immunocompromise, diabetes mellitus, alcoholism, and intravenous drug use (IVDU).

Clinicopathological Features

- **Cellulitis** classically presents with **erythema with a poorly defined border ± lymphangitis.** Four hallmark features are **warmth (*calor*), pain (*dolor*), erythema (*rubor*), and swelling (*tumor*).** While cellulitis favors the **lower extremities,** cellulitis associated with IVDU favors the upper extremities. Cellulitis of the **volar tips of the fingers or toes** is called **blistering distal dactylitis.**
- Following periapical abscess and osteomyelitis, cellulitis may occur as a sequela of dental caries leading to an intraoral dental sinus tract (erosion to oral mucosa) or a cutaneous sinus of dental origin (erosion to facial skin). **Ludwig angina** (swelling of the submandibular, submental, and sublingual spaces) is a life-threatening complication that may result in **airway obstruction** due to rapid spread to the retropharyngeal space ± mediastinum. **Cavernous sinus thrombosis** (retrograde spread of infection from the nasal area to the brain) is a life-threatening complication that may result in meningitis or brain abscesses.
  In **children**, cellulitis most commonly involves the **head and neck** but also occurs in axillary and inguinal folds and the perianal area. The most common demographic is **preschool age boys (>4 years of age).**

In **infants**, **perianal streptococcal infection** is in the differential diagnosis for **diaper dermatitis.**

- Complications of cellulitis include **lymphedema**, infection-induced panniculitis (mixed septal and lobular neutrophilic panniculitis characterized by tender erythematous subcutaneous nodules ± ulceration), endocarditis, and poststreptococcal glomerulonephritis (GAS).
  - ◈ Cellulitis is characterized by diffuse edema, capillary and lymphatic dilation, and predominantly neutrophilic inflammation in the dermis and often the subcutis.

Evaluation

- The differential diagnosis of cellulitis includes stasis dermatitis, lipodermatosclerosis, erysipelas, and drug-related etiologies of cellulitis (eg, talimogene laherparepvec [T-VEC]), recall reactions (eg, methotrexate, pemetrexed, doxorubicin), and pseudocellulitis (eg, gemcitabine in patients with lower extremity edema).
- **Sterile tissue culture in immunocompetent hosts has poor sensitivity,** but may be considered to exclude rare pathogens, particularly in immunocompromised patients. **Blood cultures** may be positive. Alternatives for confirmation of recent GAS infection include **ASO and anti-DNase B or streptozyme titer.**
  - In cases of **perianal streptococcal infection**, both **throat and perianal bacterial cultures** should be obtained.

Management

- First-line therapy for cellulitis includes **dicloxacillin, cephalexin, or clindamycin**, which target both GAS species and MSSA (clindamycin also targets MRSA but resistance can be high in certain areas**).** Duration of therapy is at least 5 days and depends on the clinical response; complicated cases may require up to 14 days of therapy. Factors that indicate empiric MRSA coverage (see above) include history of MRSA infection, known MRSA risk factors (eg, hospitalization, recent surgery), proximity to an indwelling device, systemic findings (eg, fever), and poor response to non-MRSA coverage.
- **Diabetic or decubitus ulcers are often polymicrobial. Piperacillin-tazobactam** is first line given its broad coverage of GAS, MSSA, GN bacteria, and anaerobes.
- **Incision and drainage (I&D)** in combination with topical or oral antibacterial therapy is indicated for **blistering distal dactylitis.**
  - **Penicillin or cefuroxime** is first line for **perianal streptococcal infection.**

"Real World" Advice

- Presence of a pyogenic focus is a helpful clue to distinguish staphylococcal and streptococcal cellulitis.
- **Unilateral** distribution is a helpful clue to distinguish cellulitis from inflammatory mimickers (eg, stasis dermatitis, lipodermatosclerosis) with bilateral distribution.
- **Poorly defined border** is a helpful clue to distinguish cellulitis from erysipelas.

ERYSIPELAS
Synonym: Saint Anthony's fire

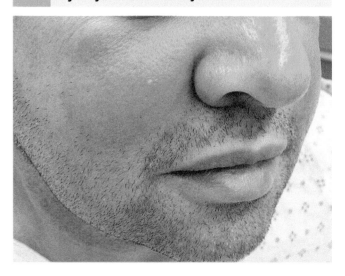

- Erysipelas is due to **GAS** > other streptococcal groups (eg, B, G). Most cases are seen in children and elderly individuals with comorbidities. Risk factors overlap with cellulitis.
  - ◈ Do NOT confuse <u>erysipel</u>as with <u>erysipel</u>oid.
- Erysipelas classically presents with **erythema with a sharply defined border ± lymphangitis.** Erysipelas **favors the lower extremities > face.**
  - ◈ Erysipelas is characterized by diffuse edema, capillary and lymphatic dilation, and predominantly neutrophilic inflammation in the dermis.
- Evaluation is similar to cellulitis.
- **Oral penicillin** is first line. Macrolides can be used in penicillin-allergic patients; however, resistance has been reported. Duration of therapy is at least 5 days and depends on the clinical response.
  - ◈ Penicillin is the treatment of choice for <u>erysipel</u>as and <u>erysipel</u>oid.

NECROTIZING FASCIITIS

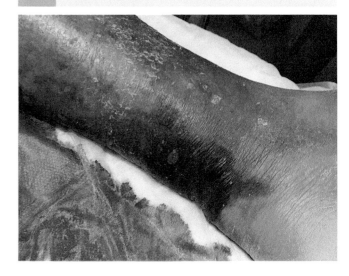

- Necrotizing fasciitis is divided into two major types:
  - **Type 1: polymicrobial** infection with ≥1 anaerobe (eg, *Bacteroides* species, *Clostridium* species) and ≥1 facultative anaerobe (eg, *Enterobacter* species, *Escherichia coli*). ***Clostridium perfringens* is a spore-forming gram-positive rod (GPR)** that produces **α-toxin** (phospholipase C) and **perfringolysin** (cholesterol-dependent cytolysin disrupting endothelial cell integrity and causing platelet aggregation). Type 1 necrotizing fasciitis tends to occur in elderly individuals with comorbidities.
  - **Type 2: GAS (M types 1 and 3) infection. GAS M protein** is a key virulence factor that promotes attachment to epithelial cells and antagonizes both phagocytosis and innate immune host responses. **SPE-A, SPE-B, and SPE-C** also play a pathogenic role with both superantigen and proteinase functions. Type 2 necrotizing fasciitis cases can occur in any age group.
    - In children, GAS infection is the most common cause of necrotizing fasciitis.
  Risk factors overlap with cellulitis.
- Necrotizing fasciitis classically presents with **rapidly evolving erythema with a poorly defined border that progresses to duskiness, tense edema, crepitus, and a foul-smelling brown exudate. Pain out of proportion to examination** is an alarming clinical feature. Necrotizing fasciitis may occur in the anogenital area (**Fournier gangrene**).
  - Necrotizing fasciitis is colloquially known as "flesh-eating bacteria syndrome." The exudate in necrotizing fasciitis has been compared to "dirty dishwater."
  - Early necrotizing fasciitis demonstrates fibrinoid necrosis of the media of fascial vessels with fibrin thrombi. Late necrotizing fasciitis demonstrates coagulative necrosis of overlying skin with infiltration of bacteria, neutrophils, and lymphocytes.
- **Soft-tissue gas on XR, CT scan (most sensitive), or MRI** is diagnostic. Sterile tissue culture and blood cultures may be positive.
- Mortality rates are up to 60%. Negative prognostic factors include **older age, female sex, increased extent, increased lactic acid, AKI, and increased time to surgical debridement. Rapid and extensive surgical debridement with broad-spectrum IV antibacterial therapy** is standard of care.

- **Abscesses** are walled-off purulent collections. **Furuncles** refer to abscesses centered on hair follicles. **Carbuncles** refer to coalescing adjacent furuncles. **Botryomycosis** refers to **abscesses ± sinus tracts with yellow grains.** Abscesses, furuncles, carbuncles, and botryomycosis are primarily due to *S. aureus* (especially MRSA)** in combination with skin injury. Rarer causes of botryomycosis include *Corynebacterium, Pseudomonas, Proteus,* and *Serratia* species. Risk factors overlap with cellulitis. Disseminated botryomycosis is associated with HIV infection and other immunocompromised states.
  - Botryomycosis is derived from the Greek word *botrys* meaning "bunch of grapes" and "mycosis" (a misnomer due to the presumed fungal etiology).
  - **Multiple abscesses** are associated with hereditary immunodeficiency syndrome (eg, **CGD, hyper-IgE syndromes**).
- Abscesses classically present as **fluctuant nodules. Sporotrichoid spread** is rare. **Pyomyositis** extends to skeletal muscle. **Hordeolum ("stye")** occurs on the eyelid in association with an obstructed sebaceous or apocrine gland. **Necrotizing ulcerative gingivitis** (due to oral bacteria) leads to hemorrhagic painful gingiva. Furuncles and carbuncles are located on hair-bearing sites; carbuncles favor areas of thicker skin (eg, the nape of the neck, back, and thighs).
  - Remember that <u>car</u>buncles are comprised of <u>fur</u>uncles and that both are located on hair-bearing sites with the phrase, "The <u>car</u> is full of <u>fur</u>."
  - Bacterial abscess is characterized by a dense neutrophilic infiltrate in the subcutis. Gram stain may reveal the pathogenic organism. Botryomycosis is characterized by an abscess containing bacterial grains, often with a Splendore–Hoeppli reaction.
- Diagnostics include **Gram stain and bacterial culture.**
- Simple abscesses and furuncles may resolve with warm compresses; however, **I&D** is often required. The decision to administer empiric MRSA coverage (see above) depends on additional clinical information including the extent of infection and systemic findings. Antibacterial therapy should be tailored based on bacterial culture and sensitivities. ***S. aureus* decolonization** is indicated for recurrent disease.

BACTERIAL ABSCESS

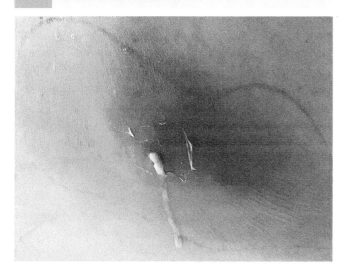

SPOTLIGHT ON CHRONIC GRANULOMA-TOUS DISEASE

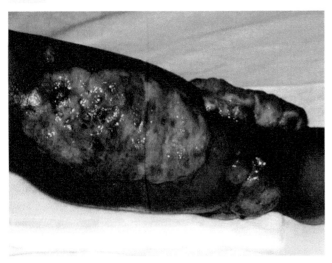

Reprinted with permission from Gru AA, Wick MR, Mir A, et al. *Pediatric Dermatopathology and Dermatology*. Wolters Kluwer; 2018.

- CGD is an umbrella term that describes hereditary immunodeficiency disorders caused by the inability of host phagocytes to destroy certain microbes. 90% of CGD patients are males and 75% of cases are **XLR**, primarily due to mutations in the **CYBB gene encoding the gp91 subunit of NADPH oxidase.** Macrophages and neutrophils use NADPH oxidase to generate ROS that destroy microbes. Catalase catalyzes the breakdown of hydrogen peroxide in phagosomes. Therefore, **decreased NADPH oxidase activity in CGD leads to increased risk of infection, particularly with catalase-positive microbes (eg, *S. aureus*** and *Nocardia*, *Burkholderia*, *Serratia*, *Candida*, and *Aspergillus* species). CGD patients have a high risk of **disseminated *Mycobacterium bovis* infection after BCG vaccination.**

- CGD classically presents with ***S. aureus* infections around the nose and ears. Suppurative granulomas and abscesses** are characteristic. Multiorgan involvement including the lymph nodes, liver, spleen, and lungs is common. A **lupus-like syndrome**, in particular DLE, has been observed in both **XLR CGD patients and female carriers.**
  - CGD histopathology demonstrates suppurative granulomas and abscesses. Lupus-like skin lesions in carriers of X-linked CGD resemble DLE on histopathology; however, vacuolar interface dermatitis is variable and lesional DIF is typically negative.

- Diagnosis is made with the **nitro blue tetrazolium test**, in which phagocytes are unable to reduce yellow dye to blue dye.

- Chronic antimicrobial prophylaxis with TMP-SMX and itraconazole reduces infectious complications. Patients can require immunomodulatory agents for inflammatory granulomatous disease. HSCT can provide a cure for CGD. Gene therapy approaches are under investigation and hold great promise.

BACTERIAL FOLLICULITIS

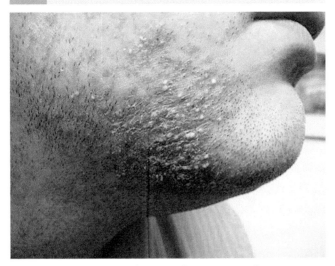

Reprinted with permission from Goodheart HP. *Goodheart's Same-Site Differential Diagnosis: A Rapid Method of Diagnosing and Treating Common Skin Disorders*. Wolters Kluwer Health/Lippincott Williams & Wilkins; 2011.

- Folliculitis refers to suppurative inflammation of the hair follicle. The most common bacterium is ***S. aureus.*** GN folliculitis (eg, *Pseudomonas aeruginosa*) develops in patients with acne on chronic topical or oral antibacterial therapy and in association with water exposure.

- Clinical features of folliculitis depend on depth:
  - **Superficial folliculitis (most common)**: papulopustules and background erythema.
  - **Deep folliculitis (sycosis)**: indurated nodules and plaques.
    - Bacterial folliculitis is characterized by follicular and perifollicular inflammation with neutrophils. Follicular rupture elicits a granulomatous response. The hair follicle may not be visible in every plane of section. Gram stain may reveal the pathogenic organism.

- Diagnostics include **Gram stain and bacterial culture.**

- Management includes prevention with antimicrobial wash (eg, **benzoyl peroxide, chlorhexidine**) and topical antibacterial therapy.

PARONYCHIA

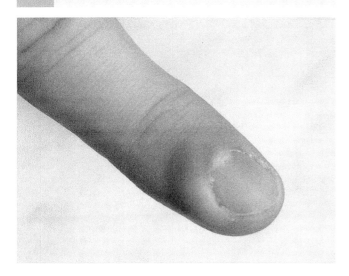

PITTED KERATOLYSIS
→ **Diagnosis Group 2**

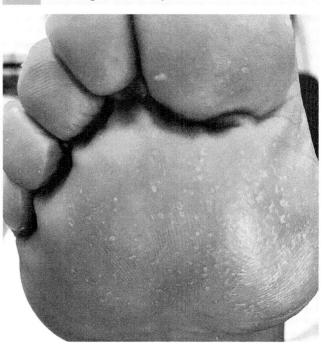

- **Acute paronychia** is most often due to *S. aureus* or GAS species. **Recurrent** acute paronychia may result from **herpetic whitlow. Chronic paronychia** is most often due to an inflammatory dermatosis (eg, contact dermatitis) with **secondary pseudomonal or candidal infection.** Associations include mechanical injury. Drug associations ± excessive periungual granulation tissue include NRTIs/NtRTIs (eg, lamivudine) and protease inhibitors (eg, indinavir). Drug associations ± pseudopyogenic granulomas include cytotoxic chemotherapies (eg, capecitabine) and targeted antineoplastic therapies (eg, EGFR inhibitors, MEK 1/2 inhibitors).
- Paronychia classically presents with a **red and swollen nail fold** associated with **pain (acute)** or **absent cuticle (chronic). There is a risk of spread to adjacent tissue/bone due to lack of subcutaneous tissue between nail dermis and bone.**
  - The histopathology of paronychia is nonspecific.
- Diagnostics for acute paronychia include **Gram stain and bacterial culture.** If recurrent, HSV testing is indicated. If chronic, KOH and fungal culture are indicated.
- Management includes I&D (in case of abscess) and topical antibacterial therapy.

Epidemiology

- Pitted keratolysis is a noninflammatory infectious dermatosis involving volar skin. It is primarily due to the GP bacteria *Kytococcus sedentarius* > *Corynebacterium*, *Actinomyces*, or *Streptomyces* species.
- Pathogenic bacteria produce **keratin-degrading proteases that form pits in the *stratum corneum.*** Hyperhidrosis and associated moisture of occluded skin is a critical cofactor for development.

Clinicopathological Features

- Pitted keratolysis is characterized by **small pits that coalesce into large crater-like areas on the soles > palms (typically in weight-bearing areas).** While generally there is an absence of inflammation and symptoms, there is associated **malodor.**
  - Figure 3.8.

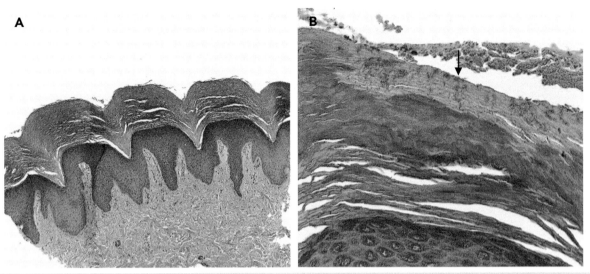

Figure 3.8. CLINICOPATHOLOGICAL CORRELATION: PITTED KERATOLYSIS. Pitted keratolysis is characterized by GPCs or GPRs within pits in the *stratum corneum*. A, Low-power view. B, High-power view. Solid arrow: GP cocci within a pit in the *stratum corneum*. GPCs, gram-positive cocci; GPRs, gram-positive rods.

In pitted keratolysis, acral skin is a helpful diagnostic clue.

Evaluation

- The differential diagnosis of pitted keratolysis includes punctate PPK, circumscribed palmar or plantar hyperkeratosis, warts, and tinea pedis.

Management

- Treatments include topical antibacterials (eg, **erythromycin, clindamycin**), antimicrobials (eg, **benzoyl peroxide**), and antifungals (eg, **triazoles**). Oral antibacterial therapy is rarely necessary.

"Real World" Advice

- In addition to managing the pitted keratolysis, it is equally important to manage the hyperhidrosis to prevent future outbreaks.

ERYTHRASMA

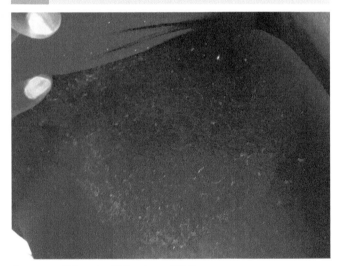

Courtesy of Veronica Richardson, CRNP

- Erythrasma is a superficial skin infection due to overgrowth of *Corynebacterium minutissimum*. Risk factors include warmth and humidity, poor hygiene, hyperhidrosis, immunocompromise, diabetes mellitus, and obesity. **Corynebacterial infections** are summarized in Table 3.11.
- Erythrasma is characterized by **pink-to-red patches with fine scale ± pruritus. Interdigital erythrasma (especially of the third and fourth toe web spaces)** is the most common location; other sites include the **axillae, inframammary folds, groin (sparing penis), and gluteal creases.**
    - Figure 3.9.

Table 3.11. CORYNEBACTERIAL INFECTIONS

Diagnosis[a]	Bacterium	Classic description	Notes
Diphtheria	*Corynebacterium diphtheriae*	Ulcer with a punched out appearance and adherent pseudomembrane at the base.	Skin injury usually precedes the infection.
		The pseudomembrane has a "leathery" appearance.	
Erythrasma	*Corynebacterium minutissimum*	See above.	
Trichomycosis axillaris	*Corynebacterium tenuis*	Concretions along hair shafts.	Shaving is the most effective treatment.
		Concretions give hair shafts a "frosted" appearance.	

[a]Illustrative examples provided. For pitted keratolysis, see above.

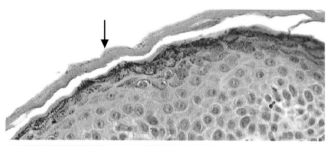

Figure 3.9. CLINICOPATHOLOGICAL CORRELATION: ERYTHRASMA. Erythrasma is characterized by GPRs forming vertical filaments in the *stratum corneum*. Solid arrow: GPRs. GPRs, gram-positive rods.

- **Coral red fluorescence due to coproporphyrin III on Wood's lamp** helps distinguish erythrasma from important mimickers (eg, granular parakeratosis).
- Topical treatment of erythrasma is similar to pitted keratolysis. For severe cases oral antibacterial therapy (eg, **erythromycin**) can be administered.

ANTHRAX
Synonym: woolsorter's disease

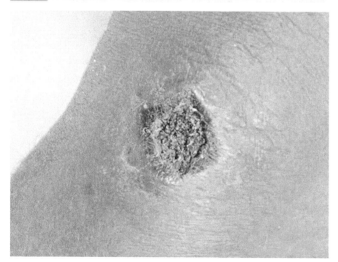

Courtesy of James H. Steele and the CDC. From Engelkirk PG, Duben-Engelkirk JL. *Burton's Microbiology for the Health Sciences.* 10th ed. Wolters Kluwer; 2014.

- **Anthrax** is due to *Bacillus anthracis,* **a spore-forming GPR.** *B. anthracis* spores are stable for decades. Virulence factors include a capsule and two exotoxins: **edema toxin increases cyclic adenosine monophosphate (cAMP) levels; lethal toxin increases TNFα and IL-1β levels.** Types of anthrax infection include **cutaneous** (**most common,** transmitted by contact with spores from **infected animals or animal products like wool**), **gastrointestinal** (transmitted by spore ingestion), and **pulmonary** (transmitted by spore inhalation). **Miscellaneous GPR infections** are summarized in Table 3.12.

Table 3.12. MISCELLANEOUS GRAM-POSITIVE ROD INFECTIONS

Diagnosis[a]	Bacterium	Classic description	Notes
Anthrax	*Bacillus anthracis*	See above.	
Erysipeloid (of Rosenbach) (fish handler's disease)	*Erysipelothrix rhusiopathiae*	Finger webs often involved, sparing terminal phalanges.	At-risk populations include butchers (pork) and fishermen (fish). Penicillin is first line.
Do NOT confuse erysipeloid with erysipelas.			Penicillin is the treatment of choice for erysipeloid and erysipelas.
Listeria	*Listeria monocytogenes*	Papules and pustules.	At-risk populations include infants. Ampicillin is first line.
Necrotizing fasciitis	*Clostridium perfringens*	See above.	

[a]Illustrative examples provided.

- **Cutaneous anthrax** classically presents with **nonpitting edema surrounding an eschar.** Gastrointestinal anthrax can cause a myriad of upper and lower gastrointestinal symptoms including bleeding and ulceration. Pulmonary anthrax can cause hilar fullness, widened mediastinum, and pleural effusions.
  - ◆ Anthrax is characterized by spongiosis and papillary dermal edema, hemorrhage, a predominantly neutrophilic superficial and deep infiltrate; GPRs can also be observed on Gram stain. Ulceration and coagulative necrosis may develop over time.
- The **ulceroglandular differential diagnosis** includes anthrax (*B. anthracis*), glanders (*Burkholderia mallei*), melioidosis (*Burkholderia pseudomallei*), plague (*Yersinia Pestis*), rat-bite fever (*Streptobacillus moniliformis*), tularemia (*Francisella tularensis*), and tuberculoid chancre (*Mycobacterium tuberculosis*).
- **Cutaneous anthrax** has the **lowest mortality risk (20% if untreated).** Treatments are **ciprofloxacin, levofloxacin, or doxycycline,** which can be used for **postexposure prophylaxis.** Anthrax is considered a **potential bioterrorism agent.** An attack in the United States via the mail service in 2001 killed five people.

ACTINOMYCOSIS
Cervicofacial actinomycosis synonym: lumpy jaw

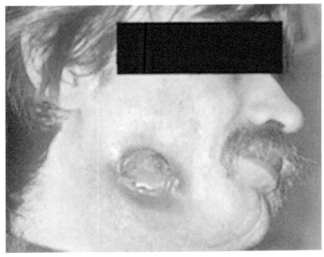

Cervicofacial actinomycosis reprinted with permission from Humphrey PA, Dehner LP, Pfeifer JD. *The Washington Manual of Surgical Pathology.* Wolters Kluwer Health/Lippincott Williams & Wilkins; 2008..

- Actinomycosis is due to ***Actinomyces israelii,*** a **filamentous GP anaerobe.** Types of actinomycosis include **cervicofacial, gastrointestinal, and pulmonary.** *A. israelii* is part of **normal oral flora** and **dental procedures** are a known risk factor for cervicofacial infection.
- **Cervicofacial actinomycosis** classically presents with a **firm nodule or bluish swelling at the angle of the jaw** that

progresses to form **multiple nodules and sinus tracts with yellow grains (actinomycetoma).**
  - ◇ Yellow grains of *A. israelii* are commonly termed "sulfur granules."
  - ◆ Figure 3.10.
- **Nocardiosis** is a closely related infection due to *Nocardia* **species,** which are **filamentous GP partially acid-fast aerobes.** Three types of cutaneous nocardiosis are **superficial cutaneous, lymphocutaneous, and actinomycetoma.** Traumatic implantation of *Nocardia* species (eg, gravel, soil) can lead to **sporotrichoid spread.** *Nocardia* species also infect immunocompromised patients resulting in a TB-like syndrome with CNS and pulmonary infection.
- While a sulfonamide (eg, TMP-SMX) is first line for nocardiosis, **penicillin** (or ampicillin) is first line for actinomycosis. Treatment typically requires weeks of IV therapy followed by months of oral therapy.
  - ◇ SNAP: Sulfonamide Nocardiosis, Actinomycosis Penicillin.

SEPTIC VASCULITIS AND INFECTIVE ENDOCARDITIS

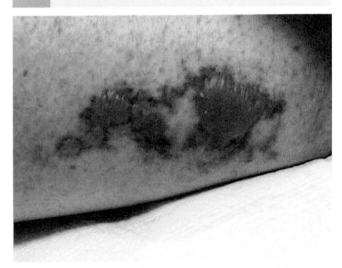

Staphylococcal septic vasculitis courtesy of Sotonye Imadojemu, MD, MBE.

- **Septic vasculitis** is a small and medium vessel vasculitis seen in septic patients with specific infections including *S. aureus, Neisseria gonorrhoeae, Neisseria meningitidis,* **and *P. aeruginosa.*** The mechanism of vessel damage in septic vasculitis may include direct damage by bacteria and immune-mediated destruction, principally by neutrophils. Risk factors include **immunocompromise and IVDU.** On the other hand, **infective endocarditis** with skin involvement is primarily due to *S. aureus.* Risk factors include **CHF, prosthetic valves, and IVDU. Miscellaneous GN cocci infections** are summarized in Table 3.13.
- The presentation depends on the diagnosis:
  - ○ **Septic vasculitis** is characterized by **palpable purpura, inflammatory retiform purpura, and proximal splinter**

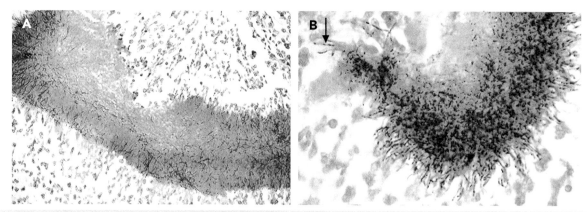

Figure 3.10. CLINICOPATHOLOGICAL CORRELATION: ACTINOMYCOSIS. Actinomycosis is characterized by an abscess with grains of branching filamentous GPRs, often with a Splendore–Hoeppli reaction. GMS, a stain primarily used to identify fungus, is also positive. The Splendore–Hoeppli reaction involves deposition of brightly eosinophilic Ig and fibrin at the periphery of bacterial or fungal grains. A, H&E. B, Gram stain. Solid arrow: grain edge demonstrating branching filamentous GPRs. H&E, hematoxylin & eosin; GMS, Grocott methenamine silver; GPRs, gram-positive rods; Ig, immunoglobulin.
(Histology images reprinted with permission from Elder DE, Elenitsas R, Rosenbach M, et al. *Lever's Histopathology of the Skin.* 11th ed. Wolters Kluwer; 2015.)

Table 3.13. MISCELLANEOUS GRAM-NEGATIVE COCCUS INFECTIONS

Diagnosis[a]	Bacterium	Classic description	Notes
Gonococcemia	*Neisseria gonorrhoeae*	Septic vasculitis with hallmark pustular purpuric skin lesions. Systemic symptoms include fever, arthralgias, and joint swelling.	Encapsulated diplococcus. Facultative intracellular bacteria. Associated with disorders in late complement components (C5-C9). Dual therapy (eg, IV ceftriaxone plus oral azithromycin) is preferred.
Meningococcemia	*Neisseria meningitidis*	Septic vasculitis. Systemic features include fever and CNS involvement. Rarely can have chronic disease.	Encapsulated diplococcus. Elaborates an endotoxin. Bacterial carriage via the nasopharynx. Male predominance. Associated with disorders in late complement components (C5-C9) and asplenia. 10%-15% mortality. IV penicillin is first line and used for contact prophylaxis.

[a]Illustrative examples provided.
C, complement; CNS, central nervous system; IV, intravenous.

hemorrhages, most commonly on pressure sites and extremities.

○ **Infective endocarditis** is characterized by **noninflammatory retiform purpura, Janeway lesions (painless purpuric macules on the palms and soles), Osler nodes (painful purpuric nodules on the distal fingers and toes), and proximal splinter hemorrhages.** Involvement of the mucous membranes with **conjunctival and palatal petechiae** may occur.

Janeway lesions are painless, while Osler nodes are painful ("ouch"). Figure 3.11.

- Septic vasculitis demonstrates CSVV. Organisms may be identified within microabscesses (eg, *S. aureus*) or endothelial cells (eg, *N. meningitidis*). Infective endocarditis demonstrates septic microemboli.
- Diagnostics for both septic vasculitis and infective endocarditis include skin biopsy, Gram stain and sterile tissue culture, and blood cultures.
- In both septic vasculitis and infective endocarditis, management is multidisciplinary and centered around treatment of the pathogenic cause with antibacterial therapy and supportive care.

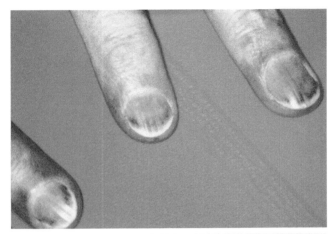

Figure 3.11. SPLINTER HEMORRHAGES. The differential diagnosis of splinter hemorrhages depends on their location within the nail. Proximal splinter hemorrhage associations include APLS, vasculitis, endocarditis, and trichinosis. Distal splinter hemorrhage associations include psoriasis, onychomycosis, and mechanical injury. Splinter hemorrhages in GPA. APLS, antiphospholipid antibody syndrome, GPA, granulomatosis with polyangiitis.

(Reprinted with permission from Koopman WJ, Moreland LW. *Arthritis and Allied Conditions: A Textbook of Rheumatology.* 15th ed. Lippincott Williams & Wilkins; 2004.)

ECTHYMA GANGRENOSUM

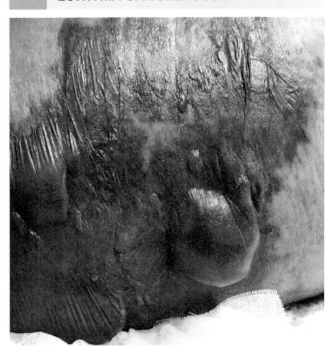

- Ecthyma gangrenosum is due to **GNR invasion of the vessels and perivascular space** leading to direct cellular damage and necrosis. Immunosuppression is a risk factor, especially **neutropenia**, is required. *P. aeruginosa*, the leading cause of ecthyma gangrenosum, is an encapsulated GNR that produces multiple pigments: fluorescein (yellow-green), pyocyanin (green-blue), and pyomelanin (brown-black). **Pseudomonal infections** are summarized in Table 3.14.

Table 3.14. PSEUDOMONAL INFECTIONS

Diagnosis[a]	Classic description	Notes
Pseudomonal pyoderma	Maceration, blue-green purulence, and eroded borders.	Commonly involved in mixed GN toe web infections.
Pseudomonal hot foot syndrome	Exquisitely tender plantar nodules.	Exposure to pool water contaminated by *Pseudomonas aeruginosa*. Self-limited in immunocompetent host.
Ecthyma gangrenosum	See above.	
Pseudomonal folliculitis (hot tub folliculitis)	Folliculitis in areas covered by bathing suit.	Exposure to pool water contaminated by *P. aeruginosa*. Self-limited in immunocompetent host.
Green nail syndrome	Green discoloration of the nail plate.	Chronic subungual pseudomonal infection. Frequent washing is a risk factor. Topical ciprofloxacin or gentamicin is first line. Treatment may lead to complete resolution.
Otitis externa	Severe pain on pinna manipulation.	Portal of entry may be injury or infectious perichondritis. "Malignant" otitis externa occurs in patients with immunocompromise or diabetes mellitus. Fluoroquinolone is first line. Surgery may be required.

[a]Illustrative examples provided.
GN, gram negative.

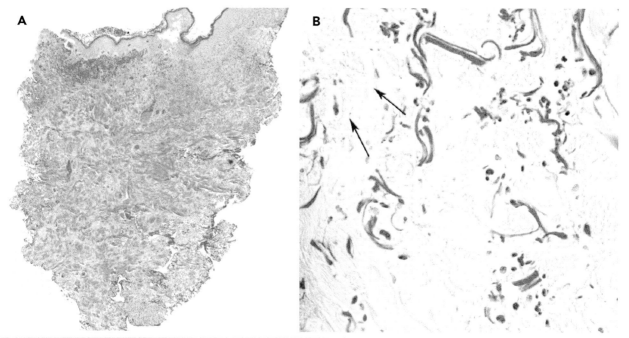

Figure 3.12. CLINICOPATHOLOGICAL CORRELATION: ECTHYMA GANGRENOSUM. Ecthyma gangrenosum is characterized by amphophilic bacilli surrounding necrotic deep dermal vessels with fibrin thrombi ± hemorrhage and coagulation necrosis of overlying skin. Gram stain highlights the pathogenic organism. A, H&E. B, Gram stain. Solid arrows: GNRs isolated as *Pseudomonas* species by culture. GNRs, gram-negative rods; H&E, hematoxylin & eosin.

(Histology images reprinted with permission from Elder DE, Elenitsas R, Rosenbach M, et al. *Lever's Histopathology of the Skin.* 11th ed. Wolters Kluwer; 2015.)

Amphophilic bacilli envelop necrotic deep dermal vessels in a "light blue haze."

Do NOT confuse <u>ecthyma</u> gangrenosum with <u>ecthyma</u>.

P. aeruginosa has a "grape-like" or "mousy" odor.

- Ecthyma gangrenosum classically presents with **erythematous nodules with dusky-gray centers favoring the anogenital area and extremities that evolve into eschars.**
  - Figure 3.12.
- Bedside diagnostics such as **touch preparation with Gram stain** may be helpful to speed the diagnosis. **Skin biopsy**, often with an additional **frozen section** for rapid evaluation, is helpful. **Sterile tissue culture** is also critical.
- **Poor prognostic factors include neutropenia, number of lesions, and diagnostic delay.** A common antibacterial approach is double coverage with **IV aminoglycoside and antipseudomonal penicillin/cephalosporin.** Antipseudomonal **fluoroquinolone prophylaxis** is frequently employed in immunocompromised hematology/oncology patients.

VIBRIOSIS

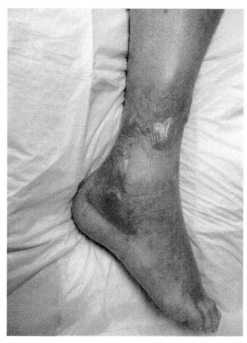

Reprinted with permission from McNichol LL, Ratliff C, Yates S. *Wound, Ostomy, and Continence Nurses Society Core Curriculum: Wound Management.* 2nd ed. Wolters Kluwer; 2021.

- Vibriosis is due to *Vibrio vulnificus*, a GNR transmitted through either cutaneous exposure to contaminated seawater/shellfish or consumption of contaminated raw/undercooked seafood (e.g. oysters). Infection typically occurs in men > 40 years of age. Risk factors include immunosuppression, chronic liver disease, and diabetes mellitus. **Miscellaneous GNR infections** are summarized in Table 3.15.
- Vibriosis classically presents with **hemorrhagic bullae with cellulitis**. It may cause necrotizing fasciitis and ecthyma gangrenosum

- ◆ Vibriosis is characterized by subepidermal bullae, necrosis of the superficial dermis, and numerous organisms clustering around vessels.
- ◆ Malakoplakia is characterized by foamy histiocytes containing GNRs, fine eosinophilic granules, and Michaelis-Gutmann bodies (basophilic inclusions that are round or ovoid and homogenous or targetoid due to concentric laminations). The staining pattern includes periodic acid-Schiff (PAS) positive, diastase resistant, and von Kossa positive.

Table 3.15. MISCELLANEOUS GRAM-NEGATIVE ROD INFECTIONS

Diagnosis[a]	Bacterium	Classic description	Notes
Animal bite	Cat: *Pasteurella multocida* Dog: *Capnocytophaga canimorsus*, *Pasteurella canis*, *Pasteurella multocida* Human: *Eikenella corrodens*	*Capnocytophaga canimorsus* and *Pasteurella* species may lead to sepsis in immunocompromised hosts, particularly those with disorders in late complement components (C5-C9).	Dog bites are most common. Augmentin is first line, along with tetanus prophylaxis.
Black nail syndrome	*Proteus mirabilis*	Black discoloration of the nail plate.	
Brucellosis (Malta fever, undulant fever)	*Brucella species*	Rare skin involvement (20%).	Transmitted by goats and sheep. Doxycycline and rifampin are first line.
Glanders	*Burkholderia mallei*	(1) Localized, (2) pulmonary, (3) bloodstream, (4) chronic.	Transmitted by horses. Surgical excision and streptomycin plus tetracycline is first line.
		Swollen lymph nodes in glanders are called "Farcy buds."	
Haemophilus infection	*Haemophilus influenzae*	Blue-red indurated plaque favoring the periorbital area or cheek. May lead to sepsis.	*Haemophilus influenzae* type B vaccination is preventative.
Malakoplakia	*Escherichia coli* > other bacteria	Perianal plaque or polypoid mass.	Surgical excision is first line.
Melioidosis (Whitmore disease)	*Burkholderia pseudomallei*	Nodule, ulcer, or abscess.	Transmitted by soil and water.
Plague (bubonic plague, black death)	*Yersinia pestis*	Lymphadenopathy.	The transmission vector is *Xenopsylla cheopis* (oriental rat flea). Streptomycin is first line.
		Swollen lymph nodes in plague are called "buboes."	
Rat-bite fever (Haverhill fever)	*Streptobacillus moniliformis*	Acral morbilliform eruption (palms/soles). Systemic features include fever and arthritis.	Transmitted by cats, dogs, rodents, and contaminated food, most often in urban settings. 15% mortality. Penicillin is first line.
Rhinoscleroma Do NOT confuse rhinoscleroma with rhinosporidiosis. Rhino is derived from the Greek word *rhino* meaning "nose," and both infections favor this site.	*Klebsiella rhinoscleromatis*	Catarrhal phase: rhinitis and edema. Granulomatous infiltrative phase: destruction of nasal cartilage with possible associated dysphonia/anesthesia of the soft palate. Sclerotic phase: fibrous tissue and scarring.	Tropical climates in Africa, Asia, and Central and South America. The required culture medium is MacConkey agar. Tetracycline is first line.
Typhoid fever	*Salmonella typhi*	Pink blanching papules favoring the anterior trunk.	Transmitted by reptiles (eg, iguanas). Fluoroquinolone is first line.
		Pink blanching papules in typhoid fever are called "rose spots."	
Vibriosis	*Vibrio vulnificus*	See above.	

[a]Illustrative examples provided.
C, complement; PAS, periodic acid-Schiff.

"Foamy histiocytes are present in malakoplakia, rhinoscleroma, and lepromatous leprosy.

◆ Rhinoscleroma is characterized by foamy histiocytes (Mikulicz cells) containing GNRs along with plasma cells containing brightly eosinophilic Ig (Russell bodies). Warthin-Starry stain reveals the presence of *Klebsiella rhinoscleromatis.*

Russell bodies are sometimes called "pregnant plasma cells".

- Skin biopsy and sterile tissue culture can confirm the diagnosis.
- **Doxycycline with a third generation cephalosporin** is first line ± surgical debridement

CAT SCRATCH DISEASE

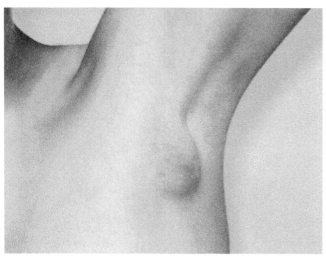

Reprinted with permission from Scheld WM, Whitley RJ, Marra CM. *Infections of the Central Nervous System.* 4th ed. Wolters Kluwer Health; 2014.

- Cat scratch disease is due to *Bartonella henselae*, a small, pleomorphic, **facultative intracellular GNR that activates endothelial cells.** The transmission vector is *Ctenocephalides felis* **(cat flea).** Transmission occurs most commonly via **cat scratch** with inoculation of flea feces. The incubation period is 2 to 4 weeks. *Bartonella* **infections** are summarized in Table 3.16.
- Cat scratch disease is characterized by **unilateral tender lymphadenopathy. Parinaud oculoglandular syndrome** refers to **unilateral conjunctivitis** with associated ipsilateral tender lymphadenopathy. Cat scratch disease may be complicated by **chronic infective endocarditis** and **peliosis hepatis** (proliferation of the sinusoidal hepatic capillaries resulting in cystic blood-filled cavities). Immunosuppressed patients may have more severe disease.
  ◆ The cat scratch disease inoculation site demonstrates palisading granulomas with central necrosis and peripheral lymphocytic infiltrate. The Warthin-Starry silver stain reveals *B. henselae.*
- **Serologies and PCRs** are the most common diagnostics; culture is performed on **chocolate agar.**
- Cat scratch disease frequently **self-resolves** without the need for active treatment, though antibacterial therapy may

decrease duration of symptoms and risk of complications. Azithromycin is first line.

Azithro-<u>meow</u>-cin is first line for <u>cat</u>-scratch disease.

ROCKY MOUNTAIN SPOTTED FEVER

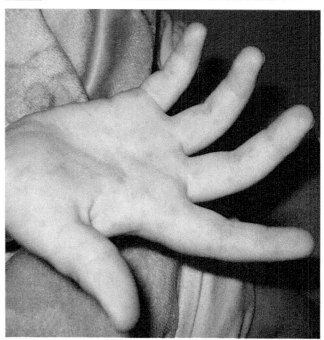

- Rocky Mountain spotted fever (RMSF) is due to *Rickettsia rickettsii*, which is an **obligate intracellular GN bacterium that infects endothelial cells.** Transmission vectors include *Amblyomma americanum* **lone star tick** (southeastern United States), *Dermacentor andersoni* **Rocky Mountain wood tick** (western United States), *Dermacentor variabilis* **dog tick** (eastern United States, most common), and *Rhipicephalus sanguineus* **brown dog tick** (worldwide). **Rickettsial and related infections** are summarized in Table 3.17.
- RMSF classically presents with fever, malaise, nausea/vomiting, and headaches followed after 3 to 5 days by **purpuric macules and papules favoring the wrists/ankles with centripetal spread to the trunk (80%-90% of patients) ± noninflammatory retiform purpura.** Other systemic features include **thrombocytopenia, meningoencephalitis, and pulmonary edema/pneumonitis.**
  RSMF is <u>spotless</u> in 10% to 20% of patients.
  ◆ RMSF demonstrates vascular damage with minimal inflammation. PCR is one of a variety of methods to reveal the presence of *R. rickettsii.*
- Historically, the **Weil-Felix test** was used for diagnosis by detecting rickettsial antibodies in the serum through agglutination. Current diagnostics include skin biopsy and testing of the blood via serology or PCR; however, **empiric treatment in cases with reasonable suspicion is the standard of care.**
- RMSF carries a **15% to 25% mortality if untreated. Doxycycline** is first line in all patients; however, some sources still suggest **chloramphenicol** as first line in **pregnant women.**
  Doxycycline is first line, even in **children < 8 years of age with RMSF.**

Table 3.16. *BARTONELLA* INFECTIONS

Diagnosis[a]	Bacterium	Vector(s)	Classic description	Notes
Bacillary angiomatosis	*Bartonella henselae*, *Bartonella quintana*	*Ctenocephalides felis* cat flea, *Pediculus humanus var corporis* body louse	Erythematous tender papules and nodules with collarettes of scale resembling PGs. Similar to cat scratch disease, bacillary angiomatosis due to *Bartonella henselae* may be complicated by chronic infective endocarditis and peliosis hepatis.	HIV/AIDS (CD4 < 250 cells/mm³). Azithromycin or rifampin is first line.
Cat scratch disease	*Bartonella henselae*	*Ctenocephalides felis* cat flea	See above.	
Oroya fever/ verruga peruana (Carrión disease)	*Bartonella bacilliformis*	*Lutzomyia verrucarum* phlebotomine sandfly	Acute stage (Oroya fever): fever and hemolytic anemia. Chronic stage (verruga peruana): erythematous papules and nodules that may self-resolve or persist for years.	Acute stage: chloramphenicol is first line (covers salmonella coinfection, the most frequent cause of death). Chronic stage: penicillin or tetracycline is first line.
			Daniel Carrión was a Peruvian medical student who fatally inoculated himself to prove Oroya fever and verruga peruana represented two stages of the same infection.	
Trench fever (shinbone fever)	*Bartonella quintana*	*Pediculus humanus var corporis* body louse	Truncal-predominant red macules. Systemic features include fevers, myalgias, shin pain, and headaches.	Erythromycin or doxycycline is first line.

[a]Illustrative examples provided.
AIDS, acquired immunodeficiency syndrome; CD, cluster of differentiation; HIV, human immunodeficiency virus; PGs, pyogenic granulomas.

LYME DISEASE

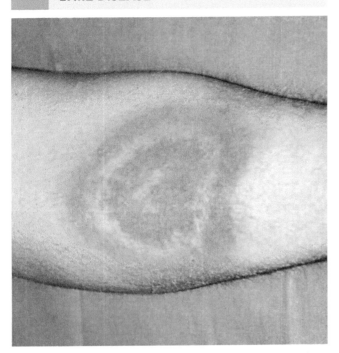

Reprinted with permission from Scheld WM, Whitley RJ, Marra CM. *Infections of the Central Nervous System.* 4th ed. Wolters Kluwer Health; 2014.

- Lyme disease is due to **Borrelia afzelli (Europe)**, *Borrelia burgdorferi* **(United States), and *Borrelia garinii* (Europe).** Transmission vectors include **A. americanum lone star tick** (southeastern United States), **Ixodes scapularis deer tick** (Eastern United States), **Ixodes pacificus western black-legged tick** (western United States), and **Ixodes ricinus castor bean tick** (Europe). Animal reservoirs include the **white-footed mouse and white-tailed deer.** Transmission primarily occurs in **late spring and early summer**, requiring >1 day of tick attachment, with increased risk after 48 hours. Spirochete infections are summarized in Table 3.18.
  - ◊ Spirochetes are spiral-shaped resembling a "corkscrew."
- Lyme disease can be divided into **three stages**:
  - **Early localized (90%)**: single erythema migrans lesion develops 1 to 2 weeks after tick bite.
  - **Early disseminated (25%)**: multiple erythema migrans lesions. Systemic features include **atrioventricular block, arthralgias, and Bell palsy.**
  - **Chronic**: prevalence and symptomatology are controversial. More objective findings in chronic Lyme disease include **arthritis, encephalopathy, and neuropathy.**
  In Europe, Lyme disease is characterized by **larger erythema migrans lesions, borrelial lymphocytoma, and acrodermatitis chronica atrophicans.** The risk of arthritis is lower; however, the risk of encephalopathy and neuropathy is higher.
  - ◈ Erythema migrans is characterized by a superficial and deep perivascular predominantly lymphocytic infiltrate. Warthin-Starry stain or PCR reveals the presence of *B. burgdorferi*.
- Skin biopsy may be helpful for diagnosis. The required culture medium is **Barbour-Stoenner-Kelly agar.** The primary mode of diagnosis is **ELISA with western blot validation.** The **peak IgM is seen after 3 to 6 weeks**; therefore, **serology is unreliable for early Lyme disease.**

Table 3.17. RICKETTSIAL AND RELATED INFECTIONS

Diagnosis[a]	Bacterium	Vector(s)	Classic description	Notes
Rickettsial Infections				
Mediterranean spotted fever (Boutonneuse fever)	*Rickettsia conorii*	*Rhipicephalus sanguineus* brown dog tick (worldwide)	Necrotic ulcer at the tick bite site and purpuric macules and papules favoring the lower extremities "Tache noir" refers to the necrotic ulcer at the tick bite site.	Doxycycline is first line.
Rickettsialpox	*Rickettsia akari*	*Liponyssoides sanguineus* mouse mite	Necrotic ulcer at the tick bite site and a generalized papulovesicular eruption. "Tache noir" refers to the necrotic ulcer at the tick bite site.	Self-resolves. Doxycycline is first line.
RMSF	*Rickettsia rickettsii*	*Amblyomma americanum* lone star tick (southeastern US), *Dermacentor andersoni* wood tick (western US), *Dermacentor variabilis* American dog tick (eastern US), *Rhipicephalus sanguineus* brown dog tick (worldwide)	See above.	
Typhus (endemic, flea-borne)	*Rickettsia felis* *Rickettsia typhi*	*Ctenocephalides felis* cat flea *Xenopsylla cheopis* Oriental rat flea	Erythematous papules.	1% mortality if untreated. Doxycycline is first line.
Typhus (epidemic, louse-borne)	*Rickettsia prowazekii*	*Pediculus humanus var corporis* body louse Reservoir: flying squirrel Epidemic typhus is due to *Rickettsia prowazekii* transmitted by *Pediculus humanus var corporis*.	Erythematous papules.	15% mortality if untreated. Doxycycline is first line. May relapse years later (Brill-Zinsser disease).
Related Infections				
Anaplasmosis (granulocytic)	*Anaplasma phagocytophilum*	*Dermacentor andersoni* wood tick (western US), *Dermacentor variabilis* American dog tick (eastern US), *Ixodes scapularis* deer tick (eastern US), *Ixodes pacificus* western black-legged tick (western US).	Highly variable exanthem.	Obligate intracellular bacteria. Infects neutrophils. Doxycycline is first line.
Ehrlichiosis (granulocytic)	*Ehrlichia phagocytophilum*	*Dermacentor andersoni* wood tick (western US), *Dermacentor variabilis* American dog tick (eastern US), *Ixodes scapularis* deer tick (eastern US), *Ixodes pacificus* western black-legged tick (western US). Reservoir: white-tailed deer	Highly variable exanthem.	Obligate intracellular bacteria. Infects neutrophils. Doxycycline is first line.

(Continued)

Table 3.17. RICKETTSIAL AND RELATED INFECTIONS (CONTINUED)

Diagnosis[a]	Bacterium	Vector(s)	Classic description	Notes
Ehrlichiosis (monocytic)	*Ehrlichia chaffeensis*	*Amblyomma americanum* lone star tick (southeastern US)	Highly variable exanthem.	Obligate intracellular bacteria. Infects monocytes. Doxycycline is first line.
Q fever	*Coxiella burnetii*	*Amblyomma americanum* lone star tick (southeastern US), *Dermacentor andersoni* Rocky Mountain wood tick (western US) Reservoir: cattle and sheep	Rare exanthem.	Obligate intracellular bacteria. Infects monocytes. Doxycycline is first line.
Tularemia	*Francisella tularensis*	*Chrysops* species deer flies, *Aedes* and *Culex* species mosquitoes, *Amblyomma americanum* lone star tick (southeastern US), *Dermacentor andersoni* wood tick (western US), *Dermacentor variabilis* American dog tick (eastern US) plus direct skin contact with infected animal (eg, rabbit).	Ulceroglandular (most common). Systemic symptoms include fever and lymphadenopathy.	Facultative intracellular bacteria. Infects monocytes. At-risk populations include hunters. Culture with buffered charcoal and yeast extract. Live-attenuated vaccine is preventative. Streptomycin is first line. Potential bioterrorism agent.
Typhus (scrub)	*Orientia tsutsugamushi*	*Trombiculid* species chigger mites	Eschars favoring the axillae and ankles.	Obligate intracellular bacteria. Infects monocytes. At-risk populations include outdoor workers in Asia. Doxycycline is first line.

[a]Illustrative examples provided.
RMSF, Rocky Mountain spotted fever; US, United States.

Table 3.18. SPIROCHETE INFECTIONS

Diagnosis[a]	Bacterium	Vector(s)	Classic description	Notes
Borrelia Species				
Acrodermatitis chronica atrophicans	*Borrelia afzelii* (Europe), *Borrelia garinii* (Europe)	*Ixodes ricinus* castor bean tick (Europe)	Inflammatory stage: unilateral violet discoloration favoring the extensor extremities. Atrophic stage: skin atrophy with vessel dilatation. Acrodermatitis chronica atrophicans has a "cigarette paper" appearance.	Manifestation of chronic Lyme disease in up to 10% of patients (Europe).
Borrelial lymphocytoma	*Borrelia afzelii* (Europe), *Borrelia garinii* (Europe)	*Ixodes ricinus* castor bean tick (Europe)	Small, bluish-red nodule or plaque favoring the earlobe, nipple, or scrotum.	Rare manifestation of early localized Lyme disease (Europe).
Lyme disease	*Borrelia afzelii* (Europe), *Borrelia burgdorferi* (US), *Borrelia garinii* (Europe)	*Amblyomma americanum* lone star tick (southeastern US), *Ixodes scapularis* deer tick (eastern US), *Ixodes pacificus* western black-legged tick (western US), *Ixodes ricinus* castor bean tick (Europe) Reservoirs: white-footed mouse, white-tailed deer	See above.	

Table 3.18. SPIROCHETE INFECTIONS (CONTINUED)

Diagnosis[a]	Bacterium	Vector(s)	Classic description	Notes
Relapsing fever (louse-borne)	*Borrelia recurrentis*	*Pediculus humanus var corporis* body louse	Petechial eruption. Systemic features include fevers, fatigue, myalgias, and headache.	Louse-borne relapsing fever is more severe than tick-borne relapsing fever. Doxycycline is first line.
Relapsing fever (tick-borne)	*Borrelia duttonii, Borrelia hermsii, Borrelia parkeri*	*Ornithodoros* species soft ticks	Variable exanthem.	
STARI	*Borrelia lonestari*	*Amblyomma americanum* lone star tick (southeastern US)	Erythema migrans–like lesions.	Doxycycline is first line; however, it is unknown whether treatment speeds recovery.
Leptospira Species				
Leptospirosis (Fort Bragg fever, pretibial fever, Weil disease)	*Leptospira interrogans*	N/A (direct skin contact with water contaminated by urine of infected animal)	Painful pretibial plaques.	Doxycycline or penicillin is first line.
Treponema Species				
Pinta (Carate)	*Treponema carateum*	N/A (direct skin contact)	Primary: inoculation site papule favoring the lower extremity. Secondary: red, blue, brown, gray, black psoriasiform papules and plaques (pintids). Tertiary: vitiligo-like lesions. Pinta is derived from the Spanish word *pinta* meaning "painted."	IM benzathine penicillin G 2.4 million units is first line.
Syphilis (endemic, Bejel)	*Treponema pallidum endemicum*	N/A (direct skin contact)	Similar to venereal syphilis except the inoculation site is usually the mouth and there is no congenital infection or cardiovascular/neurologic involvement.	IM benzathine penicillin G 2.4 million units is first line.
Syphilis (venereal, Lues)	*Treponema pallidum pallidum*	N/A (direct skin contact)	See below.	
Yaws (Frambesia)	*Treponema pallidum pertenue*	N/A (direct skin contact)	Primary: inoculation site papule (mother yaw) favoring the lower extremity that evolves into an ulcer and heals with scarring. Secondary: symmetric smaller papules (daughter yaws). Tertiary: nodules and abscesses.	IM benzathine penicillin G 2.4 million units is first line.

[a]Illustrative examples provided.

IM, intramuscular; N/A, not applicable; STARI, southern tick associated rash illness; US, United States.

- A single 200 mg dose of doxycycline is used as prophylaxis if administered within 72 hours of exposure to a nymphal or adult *I. scapularis* tick that was attached for at least 36 hours in endemic areas. **Erythema migrans typically resolves in 4 weeks without treatment.** Doxycycline is first line. **Amoxicillin** is first line in **pregnant women.**

  Amoxicillin is first line in **children < 8 years of age with Lyme disease**, although there are some data supporting the use of doxycycline in this age group.

SYPHILIS

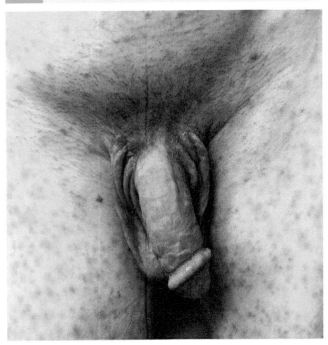

Secondary syphilis courtesy of Jake Wang, MD.

- Syphilis is divided into endemic and venereal syphilis. Risk factors for venereal syphilis include **male gender and MSM. Syphilis increases the risk of HIV infection** due to decreased epithelial barrier and increased macrophages and T cells with receptors for HIV. **HIV infection also increases** the risk of ulcer formation in secondary syphilis and the risk of neurosyphilis. **Venereal bacterial infections** are summarized in Table 3.19.

  Syphilis may present as a **congenital infection**.
- Syphilis can be divided into three stages:
  - **Primary**: inoculation site papule favoring the anogenital area that evolves into a **painless indurated ulcer (chancre) ± lymphadenopathy** in 10 days to 3 months and **self-resolves over an average of 3 weeks.**
  - **Secondary**: presents **3 to 10 weeks** after primary syphilis. Patients experience prodromal symptoms (eg, fever) and develop **copper-, ham-, or salmon-colored papulosquamous lesions** extending onto the **palms and soles with collarettes of scale. Split papules** occur at the oral commissures. **Mucous patches** are moist white plaques in the oropharynx, while **condyloma lata** are moist white plaques, often with a verrucous appearance, in the anogenital area. **Nonscarring circumscribed** hair loss may occur.
    - The appearance of alopecia in secondary syphilis is often called "moth-eaten."
  - **Tertiary**: presents **2 to 20 years** after secondary syphilis. Locally destructive **gumma** (plural: gummata) formation occurs in the skin, mucous membranes, bones, and other organs. **Cardiovascular syphilis** may lead to aortitis. **Neurosyphilis** may lead to the **Argyll Robertson pupil,** dementia, meningitis, and **tabes dorsalis.**

Latent syphilis refers to **positive serology without symptoms** and may be **early <1 year** or **late ≥1 year.**

Congenital syphilis can be divided into **early (birth to 2 years of age) and late (≥2 years of age)** stages. Early

Table 3.19. VENEREAL BACTERIAL INFECTIONS

Diagnosis[a]	Bacterium	Classic description	Notes
Chancroid (soft chancre)	*Haemophilus ducreyi*	Anogenital papule evolves into painful nonindurated ulcer (soft chancre) with ragged undermined borders ± regional lymphadenopathy with suppuration.	Facultative intracellular bacteria. Four CDC-approved regimens: azithromycin, ceftriaxone, ciprofloxacin, or erythromycin.
Gonococcal urethritis/cervicitis	*Neisseria gonorrhoeae*	Urethritis/cervicitis with dysuria/purulent discharge. Ascending acute salpingitis and PID (Fitz-Hugh-Curtis syndrome).	Facultative intracellular bacteria. The required culture medium is chocolate agar or Thayer-Martin. Azithromycin and ceftriaxone are first line (*Chlamydia trachomatis* co-infection is common).
Granuloma inguinale (Donovanosis)	*Klebsiella granulomatis*	Anogenital papule evolves into painful ulcer with red granulation tissue.	Obligate intracellular bacteria. Azithromycin is first line.
LGV (tropical bubo)	*Chlamydia trachomatis*	Stage I: anogenital painless papule that evolves into an ulcer. Stage II: unilateral inguinal lymphadenopathy. Stage III: proctocolitis. The "groove sign" refers to lymphadenopathy above and below Poupart ligament.	Obligate intracellular bacteria. L1-L3 serotypes. Men > women. Doxycycline is first line (*Neisseria gonorrhoeae* co-infection is common).
Syphilis	*Treponema pallidum*	See above.	

[a]Illustrative examples provided.

CDC, Centers for Disease Control and Prevention; CO₂, carbon dioxide; LGV, lymphogranuloma venereum; PID, pelvic inflammatory disease; TMP-SMX, trimethoprim-sulfamethoxazole.

congenital syphilis is characterized by **papulosquamous lesions, rhagades** (perioral furrows), **mucous patches, and condyloma lata.** Systemic features include hepatomegaly, lymphadenopathy, **pseudoparalysis of Parrot** (osteochondritis with limited ROM), **Wimberger sign** (sawtooth appearance of proximal tibia), and **snuffles** (bloody or purulent nasal discharge). Late congenital syphilis is characterized by **Parrot lines** (from rhagades) and **palatal gummata.** Systemic features include **saddle nose, Hutchinson teeth** (widely spaced peg-shaped upper incisors), **mulberry molars** (multiple rounded rudimentary enamel cusps on the permanent first molars), **Higoumenakis sign** (thickening of the medial aspect of the clavicle)**, Clutton joints** (joint effusions and synovitis, especially of the knees), **saber shins** (pronounced anterior bowing of the tibial bones), **CN VIII deafness,** and **interstitial keratitis.** In infants, congenital syphilis is in the differential diagnosis for **diaper dermatitis.** Congenital syphilis is the only form with **bullous lesions (pemphigus syphiliticus).**

In late congenital syphilis, Hutchinson teeth with interstitial keratitis and CN VIII sensorineural hearing loss is called "Hutchinson triad." Do NOT confuse Hutchinson teeth in Hutchinson triad of late congenital syphilis with Hutchinson sign of herpes zoster or Hutchinson sign of nail unit melanoma.

- Figure 3.13.
- Chancroid is characterized by organisms clumping in long parallel strands.
- In chancroid, organisms clumping in long parallel strands resemble a "school of fish."
- Granuloma inguinale is characterized by pseudoepitheliomatous hyperplasia (PEH) and histiocytes containing Donovan bodies (bipolar intracellular inclusions) on Giemsa and Warthin-Starry stains.
- In granuloma inguinale, Donovan bodies are "safety pin"-shaped.
- LGV is characterized by endothelial cells containing Gamma-Favre bodies (large intracytoplasmic basophilic inclusion bodies).

- Skin biopsy may be helpful. The **diagnosis of syphilis** primarily relies on the nontreponemal and treponemal tests summarized in Table 3.20. Increasingly, a **"reverse algorithm"** of testing is employed with the fluorescent treponemal antibody absorption (FTA-ABS) treponemal test as an initial screen and a nontreponemal test, either rapid plasma reagin (RPR) or venereal disease research laboratory (VDRL) as a confirmatory test. **Both nontreponemal and treponemal tests lack reactivity in early primary syphilis; therefore, dark field microscopy is the most sensitive and specific diagnostic test. Every patient with syphilis should be tested for HIV infection.**
- Syphilis treatment:
  - A single dose of **IM benzathine penicillin G 2.4 million units** is first line for primary, secondary, and early latent syphilis. **Neurosyphilis in HIV-infected patients** is treated with **11 to 24 million units aqueous crystalline penicillin G for 10 to 14 days.**

  - In penicillin-allergic patients, alternatives are azithromycin, doxycycline, or tetracycline. **Penicillin desensitization** is required in certain forms of syphilis (**pregnant woman, gummata, neurosyphilis**).

    Congenital syphilis is treated with **aqueous crystalline penicillin G 10,000 to 15,000 units/kg/d for 10 days.** In penicillin-allergic patients, **penicillin desensitization** is required.
  - The **Jarisch-Herxheimer reaction** is due to increased proinflammatory cytokines (eg, **TNFα**) after initiation of antibacterial therapy. It can also be seen in other spirochete infections.

TUBERCULOSIS

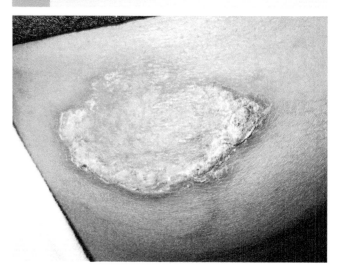

- Cutaneous TB is due to **M. tuberculosis** and rarely **M. bovis**, which are aerobic **AFBs.** TB can result from exogenous inoculation or endogenous lymphatic or hematogenous spread. **M. tuberculosis** infection risk is increased in immigrants from areas with high rates of TB, close quarters living (eg, homelessness, incarceration), HIV-infected and other immunocompromised patients, and IVDU. Iatrogenic **M. bovis** infection may occur after **BCG vaccination or intravesical installation of BCG for bladder cancer.** Individuals with impaired Th1 immunity are at particularly high risk of systemic disease. **Tuberculids** describe a set of disorders characterized by a robust cell-mediated immune response to TB antigen, presumably related to a previous systemic infection and dissemination to the skin. TB is also associated with **pityriasis rotunda.**
- The protean clinical features of **cutaneous TB variants and tuberculids** are presented in Table 3.21. Primary cutaneous TB may be associated with secondary **scarring alopecia.**
  - Figure 3.14.
- While the **PPD** skin test is commonly used to screen for TB exposure, **IFN-γ release assays** such as QuantiFERON Gold and T-SPOT have similar sensitivity and improved specificity and do not cause false positive results in BCG-vaccinated individuals. Skin biopsy and sterile tissue culture can con-

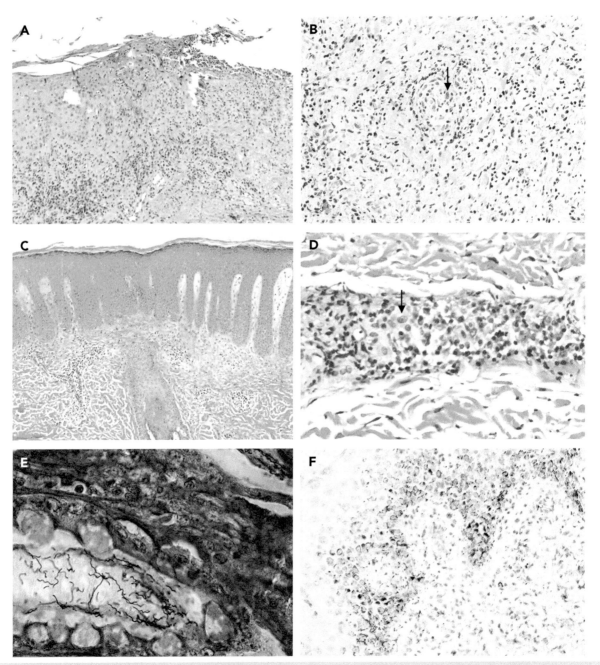

Figure 3.13. CLINICOPATHOLOGICAL CORRELATION: SYPHILIS. A, Primary syphilis. B, Primary syphilis (endarteritis obliterans). C, Secondary syphilis. D, Secondary syphilis (endarteritis obliterans). Solid arrows: plasma cells. E, Silver stain. F, *Treponema pallidum* IHC. IHC, immunohistochemistry.

(A-F, Histology images reprinted with permission from Elder DE, Elenitsas R, Rosenbach M, et al. *Lever's Histopathology of the Skin.* 11th ed. Wolters Kluwer; 2015. E, Illustration courtesy of Dr. David Elder. From Elder DE, Elenitsas R, Rosenbach M, et al. *Lever's Histopathology of the Skin.* 11th ed. Wolters Kluwer; 2015.)

- **Primary syphilis:** ulcer with granulation tissue, plasma cell–rich infiltrate, and endarteritis obliterans.
- **Secondary syphilis:** slender psoriasiform acanthosis, neutrophils in the *stratum corneum*, vacuolar interface dermatitis, perivascular lymphohistiocytic infiltrate ± plasma cells, and endarteritis obliterans.
- **Tertiary syphilis:** granulomas ("gummas") and endarteritis obliterans.

Warthin-Starry stain or IHC reveal the presence of *Treponema pallidum.*

The appearance of slender psoriasiform acanthosis has been compared to "icicles" or "icepicks." Plasma cells help distinguish syphilis from psoriasis.

Table 3.20. DIAGNOSIS OF SYPHILIS

Test	Notes
Nontreponemal tests	**Key utility in detection of recurrence and response to treatment**
RPR, VDRL	Detects IgM/IgG antibodies against cardiolipins from an ox heart extract; both tests detect the same antigen and report a titer. 4× increase in titer indicates recurrence, 4x decrease indicates cure. Both RPR and VDRL may not be reactive in early primary syphilis (4-5 weeks) and may become nonreactive in late stage and treated syphilis. False positives occur in SLE, lepromatous leprosy, malaria, increasing age, and pregnancy. False negatives occur with the prozone phenomenon when high antibody titers prevent flocculation and visualization of a positive result in the assay. This requires serum dilution.
Treponemal tests	**More sensitive and specific than nontreponemal tests. Do not differentiate between past and prior infection (positive for life) unless IgM antibody isotypes are tested.**
FTA-ABS	Most sensitive serology in all stages of disease; ideal initial screening test (after 3 weeks).
MHA-TP	Detects antibodies directed against surface proteins of *Treponema pallidum* attached to rabbit erythrocytes.
Treponemal IgM ELISA	First test to become reactive and therefore useful for congenital and primary syphilis. Can also aid in diagnosis of recurrent infection and neurosyphilis (positive, low titer).

ELISA, enzyme-linked immunosorbent assay; FTA-ABS, fluorescent treponemal antibody absorption test; Ig, immunoglobulin; MHA-TP, microhemagglutination assay for *Treponema pallidum* antibodies; RPR, rapid plasma reagin; SLE, systemic lupus erythematosus; VDRL, venereal disease research laboratory.

Table 3.21. CUTANTEOUS TUBERCULOSIS VARIANTS AND TUBERCULIDS

Diagnosis	Classic description	Notes
Variant[a]		
Lupus vulgaris Do NOT confuse lupus vulgaris with lupus erythematosus, lupus miliaris disseminatus faciei, or lupus pernio.	Gelatinous red-brown nodules involving the face or neck.	Immunity: sensitized with moderate-to-high immunity. Route: contiguous from hematogenous or lymphatic spread. Upon diascopy, lupus vulgaris lesions have the color of apple jelly.
Miliary TB	Small blue-red papules.	Immunity: nonsensitized, low immunity. Route: hematogenous.
Scrofuloderma	Suppurative nodule evolves into draining ulcer over cervical lymph node.	Immunity: sensitized with low immunity. Route: continuous (underlying lymphadenitis, bone, or lung).
TB gumma	Necrotic plaque with abscess formation.	Immunity: low. Route: hematogenous.
TB chancre	Painless papulonodule 2-4 weeks after inoculation that erodes and ulcerates.	Immunity: nonsensitized. Route: exogenous (direct inoculation at site of trauma).
TB cutis orificialis	Edematous papule on mucosal site that ulcerates.	Immunity: sensitized with low immunity. Route: autoinoculation.
TB verrucosa cutis	Indurated wart-like papule or plaque. "Prosector's wart" refers to TB verrucosa cutis due to inoculation in lab or medical personnel in contact with autopsy or tissue from a TB patient.	Immunity: sensitized with moderate-to-high immunity. Route: exogenous (direct inoculation at site of trauma).
Tuberculid[a]		
Lichen scrofulosorum	Clustered perifollicular pink to yellow brown papules.	Immunity: sensitized. Route: hypersensitivity reaction to distant focus of TB.
Nodular vasculitis/EI of Bazin	See Chapter 2: Panniculitis and Lipodystrophy.	
Papulonecrotic tuberculid	Widely distributed red papules and pustules.	Immunity: sensitized. Route: hypersensitivity reaction to distant focus of TB.

[a]Illustrative examples provided.
EI, erythema induratum; TB, tuberculosis.

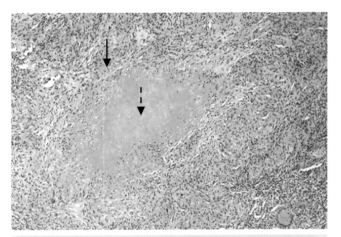

Figure 3.14. CLINICOPATHOLOGICAL CORRELATION: TUBERCULOSIS. Primary cutaneous TB is characterized by neutrophilic inflammation with numerous organisms followed by the development of tuberculoid granulomas (histiocytes with a peripheral lymphocytic infiltrate ± central caseous necrosis) with reduction in organisms. AFB stains include Ziehl-Neelsen, Fite-Faraco, and Truant (auramine-rhodamine), which is fluorescent and the most sensitive. PCR can also identify *Mycobacterium tuberculosis*. Primary cutaneous TB. Solid arrow: histiocytes with a peripheral lymphocytic infiltrate. Dashed arrow: central caseous necrosis. AFB, acid-fast bacillus; PCR, polymerase chain reaction; TB, tuberculosis.

(Histology image reprinted with permission from Elder DE, Elenitsas R, Rosenbach M, et al. *Lever's Histopathology of the Skin.* 11th ed. Wolters Kluwer; 2015.)

firm the diagnosis. **Fine needle aspiration (FNA)** may reveal AFB. The selective culture medium for mycobacteria is **Lowenstein-Jensen. Atypical mycobacterial infections** are summarized in Table 3.22.

- First-line TB antibacterials include **ethambutol, isoniazid (INH), pyrazinamide, rifabutin, rifapentine, and rifampin.** Regimens for prevention of active TB in patients with latent disease typically use INH, rifapentine, or rifampin for up to 9 months; newer, shorter courses are increasingly employed. Regimens for treatment of active TB typically involve a shorter intensive phase with multiple agents followed by a longer continuation phase with fewer agents. **Directly observed therapy is critical.**
  - The RIPE acronym is often used for the most classic regimen: rifampin, INH, pyrazinamide, and ethambutol combination therapy.

Table 3.22. ATYPICAL MYCOBACTERIAL INFECTION

Diagnosis[a]	Bacterium	Classic description	Notes
Slow-Growing			
Buruli ulcer	*Mycobacterium ulcerans*	Ulcer > 15 cm favoring the extremities, especially the legs.	Transmitted by spiky tropical vegetation in Africa. Excision is first line.
Fish tank granuloma (swimming pool granuloma)	*Mycobacterium marinum*	Plaque, nodule, or ulcer with sporotrichoid spread.	Photochromagen.[b] Ideal growth temperature 30 °C. Transmitted by contaminated fish tanks and swimming pools. Minocycline is first line. Clarithromycin is second line.
MAI complex infection	*Mycobacterium avium* and *Mycobacterium intracellulare* symbiosis	Myriad presentations.	Transmitted via ingestion or inhalation. Risk increased in HIV-infected and other immunocompromised patients.
Rapid-Growing			
Mycobacterium fortuitum complex infection	*Mycobacterium abscessus, Mycobacterium chelonae, Mycobacterium fortuitum*	Plaque, nodule, or ulcer with sporotrichoid spread.	Transmitted by contaminated tap water (surgical wounds). Excision is first line.
Mycobacterium kansasii infection	*Mycobacterium kansasii*	Plaque, nodule, or ulcer with sporotrichoid spread.	Photochromagen.[b] Transmitted by blackberries. Rifampin is first line.

[a]Illustrative examples provided.
[b]Pigmentation upon exposure to light.
HIV, human immunodeficiency virus; I&D, incision and drainage; MAI, *mycobacterium avium-intracellulare* complex.

LEPROSY

Synonym: Hansen disease

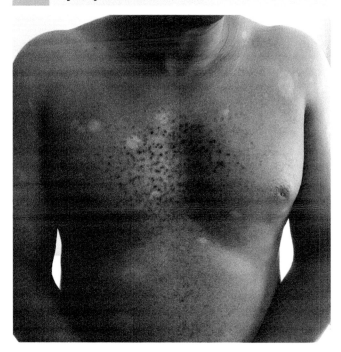

Courtesy of Victoria Williams, MD

- Leprosy is due to *Mycobacterium leprae*, an obligate intracellular **AFB**. The major cell targets are macrophages and Schwann cells in the skin, mucous membranes, and peripheral nerves; however, visceral organ involvement may occur. Cooler regions of the body are preferred including the nose, ears, testicles, and extremities. The subtype of leprosy skin disease is dictated by the degree of cell-mediated immunity: a **Th1** response is seen in **tuberculoid leprosy**, whereas a **Th2** response is seen in **lepromatous leprosy**. Transmission of leprosy primarily occurs via **respiratory droplets** and infrequently via cutaneous inoculation. The **nine-banded** armadillo is the major animal vector in the southern United States. There is a **prolonged incubation period of at least 4 to 10 years.**
- The leprosy spectrum (based on the **Ridley and Jopling classification**) includes:
  - **Indeterminate leprosy (I): earliest stage** characterized by solitary or few **hypopigmented macules**, typically **lacks enlargement of peripheral nerves.**
  - **Tuberculoid leprosy (TT):** solitary or few **well-demarcated, infiltrative erythematous slow-growing anesthetic plaques.** Tuberculoid leprosy may be associated with **anhidrosis** and secondary **scarring alopecia.**
  - **Mid-borderline leprosy (BB):** asymmetrically distributed plaques and dome-shaped lesions with diminished sensation. There are two additional types of borderline disease that have more polarized Th1 response **borderline tuberculoid (BT)** or Th2 response **borderline lepromatous (BL).**
  - **Lepromatous leprosy (LL): diffuse poorly demarcated sensate plaques. Madarosis** may occur. Complications include **claw hand, neuropathic ulcers, stocking-glove anesthesia, ocular damage (eg, corneal anesthesia, lagophthalmos), and orchitis.**
    - Severe involvement of the face in lepromatous leprosy leads to "leonine facies."

  Anesthesia is associated with tuberculoid leprosy; however, all forms can be associated with peripheral nerve enlargement. **Leprosy reactions** (Table 3.23) are acute-onset eruptions of the skin that occur in 50% of patients after starting therapy. Upgrading reactions refer to increased cell-mediated immunity and a shift toward tuberculoid leprosy, whereas downgrading reactions refer to decreased cell-mediated immunity and a shift toward lepromatous leprosy. **Borderline forms are unstable; polar forms are stable.**
    - Figure 3.15.
- **Slit-skin** smear or skin biopsy can confirm the diagnosis. There is no culture medium for leprosy, which can only be grown in a **mouse foot pad or nine-banded armadillo.**

Table 3.23. LEPROSY REACTIONS

Diagnosis[a]	Classic description	Notes
Type 1 (reversal) reaction	Increased inflammation of established lesions with pain and neuritis.	Upgrading Th1 cell–mediated response from preexisting BL or LL state. BL leprosy is the highest risk state. Systemic corticosteroids are first line.
Type 2 reaction (ENL) Do NOT confuse erythema nodosum leprosum with erythema nodosum.	Nodular, infiltrative skin lesions with fevers, myalgias, and joint pain.	Immune complex-mediated reaction in LL and BL patients. LL is the highest risk state, particularly in patients with a high bacterial load when initiating treatment. Thalidomide is first line.
Type 3 (Lucio) reaction	Noninflammatory retiform purpura.	Immune complex-dependent (type III) reaction. Western Mexico is the most common location. Systemic corticosteroids are first line.

[a]Illustrative examples provided.
BL, borderline lepromatous; ENL, erythema nodosum leprosum; LL, lepromatous leprosy; Th1, T helper type 1.

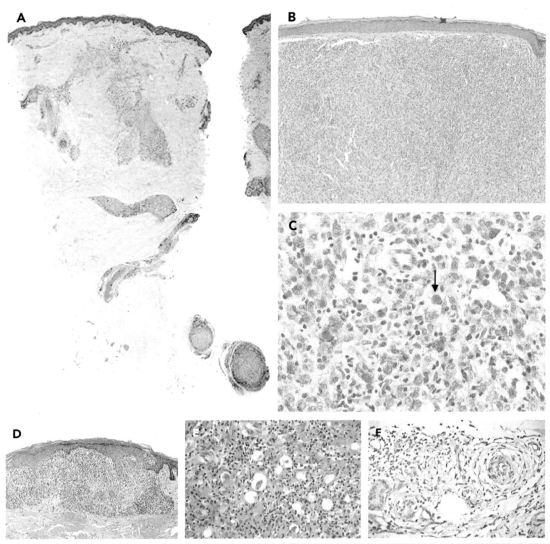

Figure 3.15. SIDE-BY-SIDE COMPARISON: TUBERCULOID AND LEPROMATOUS LEPROSY. Both tuberculoid and lepromatous leprosy demonstrate histiocytic inflammation. Epithelioid histiocytes in tuberculoid leprosy follow deep neurovascular bundles. Foamy histiocytes (Virchow cells) containing clumped organisms (globi) in lepromatous leprosy spare the papillary dermis (Grenz zone). Fite-Faraco is preferred over Ziehl-Neelsen. PCR can also identify *Mycobacterium leprae* in lepromatous > tuberculoid leprosy. A, Tuberculoid leprosy H&E. B, Lepromatous leprosy H&E. C, Lepromatous leprosy Fite-Faraco stain. Solid arrow: AFB. D, Type 1 (reversal) reaction. E, Type 2 reaction (ENL). F, Type 3 (Lucio) reaction. AFB, acid-fast bacillus; CSVV, cutaneous small vessel vasculitis; ENL, erythema nodosum leprosum; H&E, hematoxylin & eosin; PCR, polymerase chain reaction.

(A, Histology image reprinted with permission from Elder DE, Elenitsas R, Rosenbach M, et al. *Lever's Histopathology of the Skin.* 11th ed. Wolters Kluwer; 2015. B, Histology image courtesy of Noel Turner, MD, MHS and Christine J. Ko, MD. C, Histology image courtesy of Noel Turner, MD, MHS and Christine J. Ko, MD. D, Histology image reprinted with permission from Elder DE, Elenitsas R, Rosenbach M, et al. *Lever's Histopathology of the Skin.* 11th ed. Wolters Kluwer; 2015. E, Histology image reprinted with permission from Elder DE, Elenitsas R, Rosenbach M, et al. *Lever's Histopathology of the Skin.* 11th ed. Wolters Kluwer; 2015. F, Histology image reprinted with permission from Elder DE, Elenitsas R, Rosenbach M, et al. *Lever's Histopathology of the Skin.* 11th ed. Wolters Kluwer; 2015.)

> "Sausage-shaped" granulomas in tuberculoid leprosy are oriented "east-to-west."
> Foamy histiocytes are present in malakoplakia, rhinoscleroma, and lepromatous leprosy.

- **Indeterminate leprosy:** mild lymphohistiocytic inflammation.
- **Borderline leprosy:** intermediate between tuberculoid and lepromatous leprosy.
- **Histoid leprosy:** well circumscribed spindle cell proliferation and globi.
- **Leprosy reactions:**
  - **Type 1 (reversal) reaction:** preexisting leprosy with prominent lymphohistiocytic inflammation.
  - **Type 2 reaction (ENL):** preexisting leprosy with CSVV.
  - **Type 3 (Lucio) reaction:** preexisting leprosy with necrotizing CSVV.

Tuberculoid leprosy demonstrates a positive **lepromin test**, in which intradermal injection of heat-killed *M. leprae* leads to a nodular reaction 3 to 4 weeks later.

- The terms **"paucibacillary (PB)"** and **"multibacillary (MB)"** leprosy are primarily used in the context of treatment. PB patients are slit-skin negative and lack organisms on skin biopsy (eg, I, TT, BT stages). MB patients are slit-skin positive and demonstrate organisms on skin biopsy (eg, LL, BL, BB stages). The World Health Organization (WHO) regimens with multidrug therapy are as follows:
  - ○ **PB leprosy**: rifampin 600 mg monthly + dapsone 100 mg daily; duration is 6 months.
  - ○ **MB leprosy**: rifampin 600 mg monthly + dapsone 100 mg daily + clofazimine 300 mg once per month/50 mg daily; duration is 12 months.

Resistance develops rapidly with rifampin monotherapy; therefore, multidrug therapy is essential. If a leprosy reaction develops, it is critical to continue treatment while managing the reaction to prevent long-term disability. Leprosy treatment is effective and curative (patients are considered noninfectious 72 hours after starting appropriate multidrug therapy); however, it is important to recognize the negative impact of complications and social stigmatization on quality of life and psychosocial well-being.

Fungal Diseases

Basic Concepts

- **Fungi** are ubiquitous eukaryotic organisms that exist in two basic forms: yeast and mold.
  - ○ **Yeast**: **unicellular**, reproduces via **budding or binary fission forming moist colonies**, may demonstrate **pseudohyphae** (long chains of yeast cells with **constrictions**).
  - ○ **Mold**: **multicellular, filamentous**, reproduces via **spore** development and dispersal, may demonstrate **hyphae** (transverse walls).
  - ○ **Hyalohyphomycosis**: *Acremonium* species, *Aspergillus* species (*flavus*), *Fusarium* species, *Penicillium* species, and *Scopulariopsis* species.
  - ○ **Phaeohyphomycosis (dematiaceous, pigmented)**: *Alternaria* species, *Bipolaris* species, *Curvularia* species, and *Exophiala* species.
- Along with bacteria, fungi are important contributors to the microbiome, and dysbiosis has been implicated as a potential cause or cofactor in skin diseases (eg, *Malassezia* species in CARP, seborrheic dermatitis, and neonatal acne; *Coccidioides immitis* in EN; *Histoplasma capsulatum* in EM, particularly in patients with concomitant EN).
- **Fungal classification** (for dermatology-relevant fungi) is summarized in Table 3.24.

Superficial Mycoses

TINEA VERSICOLOR
→ **Diagnosis Group 1**

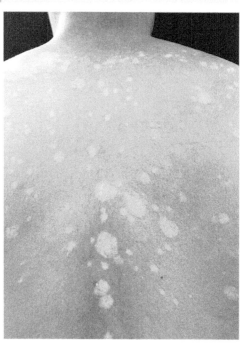

Epidemiology

- TV is a noninflammatory superficial mycosis due to *Malassezia* species such as *Malassezia furfur* and *Malassezia globosa*. These fungi produce **azelaic acid**, a **dicarboxylic acid** that **competitively inhibits tyrosinase** causing hypopigmentation.
  - Topical azelaic acid is FDA-approved for acne and rosacea.
- TV is more common during **pregnancy and postpartum**.

Clinicopathological Features

- TV classically presents with **hypo- and hyperpigmented macules and patches with fine scale in sebum-rich areas**, giving it a seborrheic distribution that favors the **trunk**.
  - The **face** is a common location for TV in **children**.
- *Malassezia* **folliculitis** may occur with or without concomitant TV. It is characterized by **monotonous folliculocentric papules favoring the chest, shoulders, and back**.
  - Figure 3.16.

Evaluation

- The differential diagnosis of TV includes CARP, seborrheic dermatitis, disorders of hypopigmentation/depigmentation and hyperpigmentation, tinea corporis, and CTCL.

Table 3.24. FUNGAL CLASSIFICATION

Type	Type	Fungus	Diagnosis[a]
Superficial mycoses	Noninflammatory	*Malassezia furfur* (formerly *Pityrosporum ovale*), *Malassezia globosa*	TV, *Malassezia* folliculitis
		Hortaea werneckii	Tinea nigra (dematiaceous)
		Piedraia hortae	Black piedra (dematiaceous)
		Trichosporon species	White piedra
	Inflammatory	*Epidermophyton*, *Microsporum*, and *Trichophyton* species	Tinea, tinea capitis, onychomycosis
		Trichophyton mentagrophytes > *Acremonium*, *Aspergillus*, *Fusarium*, and *Scopulariopsis* species	Superficial white onychomycosis
		Scytalidium dimidiatum	Dematiaceous onychomycosis
		Candida species	Primary total dystrophic onychomycosis
Superficial and deep mycoses	Inflammatory, yeast	*Candida* species	Candidiasis
Deep mycoses	Dimorphic fungi	*Blastomyces dermatitidis*	Blastomycosis
		Cladosporium carrionii, *Fonsecaea pedrosoi*, *Fonsecaea compacta*, *Phialophora verrucosa*, *Rhinocladiella aquaspersa*	Chromoblastomycosis (dematiaceous)
		Paracoccidioides brasiliensis	Paracoccidioidomycosis
		Coccidioides immitis	Coccidioidomycosis
		Histoplasma capsulatum	Histoplasmosis
		Penicillium marneffei	Penicilliosis
		Cryptococcus neoformans	Cryptococcosis
		Lacazia loboi	Lobomycosis
		Sporothrix schenckii	Sporotrichosis
	Miscellaneous fungi	*Aspergillus* species	Aspergillosis (angioinvasive)
		Fusarium species	Fusariosis (angioinvasive)
		Mucor and *Rhizopus* species	Zygomycosis (angioinvasive)
		Pseudallescheria boydii > *Acremonium*, *Aspergillus*, and *Fusarium* species	Eumycotic mycetoma
		Curvularia species, *Exophiala jeanselmei*, *Madurella* species, *Leptosphaeria* species, *Pyrenochaeta romeroi*	Eumycotic mycetoma (dematiaceous)
	Algae[b]	*Prototheca wickerhamii*	Protothecosis

[a]Illustrative examples provided.
[b]Protothecosis is not a fungus.
TV, tinea versicolor.

In children, the differential diagnosis of TV includes pityriasis alba and neonatal acne.

- TV has an **orange fluorescence** when exposed to a UVA light source (eg, **Wood's lamp**).
- KOH demonstrates **short hyphae with round spores.**
  - Short hyphae resemble "ziti" and round spores resemble "meatballs."
- Skin biopsy is rarely performed but may be helpful.

- Fungal culture may confirm the diagnosis but requires an **olive oil overlay** for lipid enrichment.

Management

- Initial therapy includes **antifungal shampoo** several times per week (eg, ketoconazole, selenium sulfide, zinc pyrithione) with the addition of a **topical azole cream** (eg, ketoconazole) for 2 weeks.

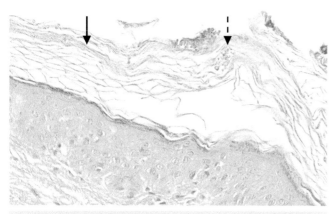

Figure 3.16. CLINICOPATHOLOGICAL CORRELATION: TINEA VERSICOLOR. TV is characterized by hyperkeratosis with short hyphae and round spores in the *stratum corneum*. GMS and PAS highlight the pathogenic organism. Solid arrow: hypha ("ziti"). Dashed arrow: spore ("meatball"). GMS, Grocott-Gomori methenamine silver; PAS, periodic acid-Schiff; TV, tinea versicolor.

(Histology image courtesy of Noel Turner, MD, MHS and Christine J. Ko, MD.)

Short hyphae resemble "ziti" and round spores resemble "meatballs."

- Widespread or recalcitrant eruptions may indicate oral fluconazole or itraconazole.
- For individuals predisposed to chronic tinea infections, weekly pulsed fluconazole can be considered.

"Real World" Advice

- TV often comes to patients' attention when **involved skin fails to tan in the summer.**

TINEA NIGRA

Synonym: superficial phaeohyphomycosis

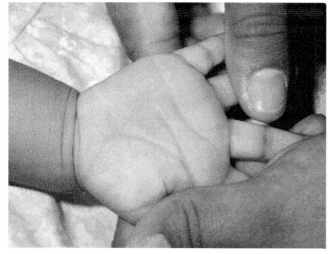

Reprinted with permission from Lugo-Somolinos A, McKinley-Grant L, Goldsmith LA, et al. *VisualDx: Essential Dermatology in Pigmented Skin.* Wolters Kluwer Health/Lippincott Williams & Wilkins; 2011.

- Tinea nigra is a noninflammatory superficial mycosis due to *Hortaea werneckii*, a **dematiaceous** fungus found in soil, sewage, and other humid environments.
- Tinea nigra classically presents with a **well-demarcated brown to gray macule or patch with mild scaling** favoring the extremities, particularly the **palms.**
  - Figure 3.17.

- **KOH** demonstrates **brown-to-yellow hyphae and spores.** Skin biopsy is rarely performed but may be helpful. Fungal culture can confirm the diagnosis.
- Topical azole cream for 2 to 4 weeks typically leads to resolution.

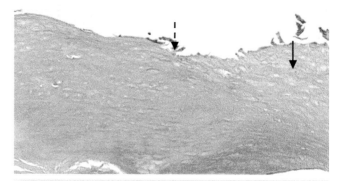

Figure 3.17. CLINICOPATHOLOGICAL CORRELATION: TINEA NIGRA. Tinea nigra is characterized by brown-to-yellow hyphae and spores in the *stratum corneum*. GMS, PAS, and Fontana-Mason highlight the pathogenic dematiaceous organism. Solid arrow: hypha. Dashed arrow: spore. GMS, Grocott-Gomori methenamine silver; PAS, periodic acid-Schiff.

(Histology image courtesy of Noel Turner, MD, MHS and Christine J. Ko, MD.)

Acral skin is a helpful diagnostic clue.

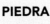

PIEDRA
Synonym: trichomycosis nodularis

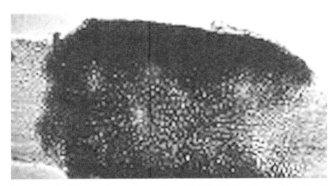

Reprinted with permission from Gru AA, Wick MR, Mir A, et al. *Pediatric Dermatopathology and Dermatology*. Wolters Kluwer; 2018.

- Piedra is a noninflammatory superficial mycosis that forms adherent nodules on the hair shaft and is most commonly found in tropical climates.
  - **Black piedra** is due to *Piedraia hortae*, a **dematiaceous** fungus.
  - **White piedra** is due to *Trichosporon* **species**, most often *Trichosporon asahii.*
    - Do NOT confuse Trichosporon species (white piedra) with Trichophyton species (tinea).
- Black and white piedra have distinct clinical features:
  - **Black piedra: black velvety colonies forming concretions that are fixed to the hair shaft**, especially on the **scalp and face.**
  - **White piedra: white velvety colonies that move freely along the hair shaft**, especially on the **face, axillae, and pubic hair.** Immunocompromised patients are susceptible to *Trichophyton cutaneum* **fungemia.**
    - Piedra is not evaluated via skin biopsy.
- KOH **"crush preparation" of cut hair shafts** or fungal culture can be used to diagnose piedra.
- Treatment involves **cutting affected hair along with antifungal shampoo**, most commonly ketoconazole. Widespread or recalcitrant cases may indicate oral fluconazole or itraconazole.

TINEA
Synonym: ringworm
→ Diagnosis Group 1

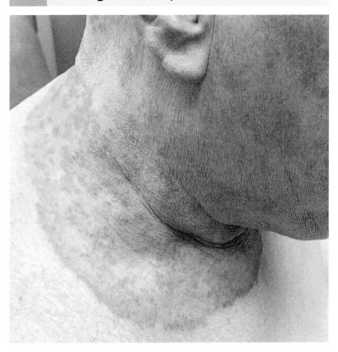

Epidemiology

- Tinea is an inflammatory superficial mycosis due to *Epidermophyton, Microsporum,* and *Trichophyton* species, which invade and proliferate in the skin, hair, and nail unit. *Trichophyton rubrum* is the leading cause overall.
  - Do NOT confuse Trichophyton species (tinea) with Trichosporon species (white piedra).
- Transmission depends on the fungus:
  - **Anthropophilic (human-to-human transmission):** for example, *T. rubrum.*
  - **Geophilic (soil-to-human transmission):** for example, *Microsporum gypseum.*
  - **Zoophilic (animal-to-human transmission):** for example, *Microsporum canis.*
  Anthropophilic fungi tend to be the least inflammatory; zoophilic fungi tend to be the most inflammatory.
- Tinea is associated with **EAC.**

Clinicopathological Features

- **Tinea corporis (ringworm)** classically presents with an **annular centrifugally spreading plaque with "leading scale" along the border.**
- **Tinea variants** are summarized in Table 3.25.
    - **Tinea faciei** is seen more often in **children** than adults.
    - Figure 3.18.

Table 3.25. TINEA VARIANTS

Diagnosis[a]	Classic description	Notes
Location-Specific Tinea Variants		
Tinea faciei	Resembles tinea corporis with pustules on the face.	Most commonly due to *Microsporum canis*.
Tinea barbae (barber's itch, tinea sycosis)	Resembles tinea corporis on the face with pustules in the beard distribution.	
Tinea cruris (gym itch, jock itch)	Resembles tinea corporis in the groin with scrotal sparing.	
Tinea manus	Variable, most commonly erythema and scale accentuating palmar lines (moccasin).	Tinea may involve one hand and two feet.
Tinea pedis (athlete's foot)	Variable, three variants are tense vesicles on the instep and forefoot (bullous), white and macerated web spaces (interdigital), and erythema and scale accentuating plantar lines (moccasin). Disseminated eczema may occur.	Bullous tinea pedis is most commonly due to *Trichophyton mentagrophytes*. For refractory tinea pedis, consider *Scytalidium dimidiatum*.
Other Tinea Variants		
Majocchi granuloma	Resembles tinea corporis with perifollicular papules, nodules, and pustules.	Granulomatous folliculitis.
Tinea corporis gladiatorum	Resembles tinea corporis.	Tinea in wrestlers. Most commonly due to *Trichophyton tonsurans*.
Tinea imbricata	Scale in concentric rings with hypopigmentation.	Due to *Trichophyton concentricum*.
Tinea incognita	Resembles tinea corporis but less raised and scaly and more pustular, extensive, and irritated.	Tinea following topical corticosteroid use.
Tinea profunda	Resembles tinea corporis but more inflamed.	Analogous to kerion on the scalp.

[a]Illustrative examples provided. For tinea capitis and onychomycosis, see below.

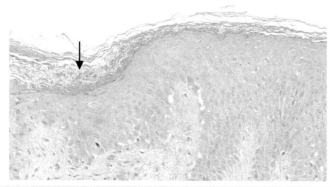

Figure 3.18. CLINICOPATHOLOGICAL CORRELATION: TINEA. Tinea is characterized by orthokeratosis, parakeratosis, and hyphae and spores in the *stratum corneum*. GMS and PAS highlight the pathogenic organism. solid arrow: hypha. GMS, Grocott-Gomori methenamine silver; PAS, periodic acid-Schiff.

(Histology image courtesy of Noel Turner, MD, MHS and Christine J. Ko, MD.)

The "sandwich sign" refers to hyphae sandwiched between loose orthokeratosis above and compact orthokeratosis/parakeratosis below. Hyphae in tinea tend to orient horizontally, while pseudohyphae in candidiasis tend to orient vertically.

- **Bullous tinea pedis**: resembles tinea with papillary dermal edema.
- **Majocchi granuloma**: resembles tinea capitis.

Evaluation

- The differential diagnosis of tinea corporis includes other inflammatory mycoses (eg, candidiasis), papulosquamous disorders (eg, psoriasis), eczematous disorders (eg, nummular eczema), autoimmune CTDs (eg, SCLE), erythemas (eg, EAC), and CTCL.
- **KOH** demonstrates **hyphae and spores. Dermatophyte test medium (DTM)** is another bedside diagnostic for tinea.
- Skin biopsy is rarely performed but may be helpful.
- Fungal cultures are less sensitive but can confirm the diagnosis and offer speciation. Tests to distinguish dermatophytes include **colony morphology, fluorescence, growth temperature, and nutritional requirements.**

The details of these tests are beyond the scope of this chapter.

Management

- Uncomplicated localized tinea can be treated with **topical terbinafine or azole cream** for 2 to 4 weeks.
- **Widespread tinea, tinea involving hair follicles, and Majocchi granuloma** are indications for oral **terbinafine.** Alternatives include oral fluconazole or itraconazole.

"Real World" Advice

- **Scrotal sparing** is a clinical clue to differentiate tinea cruris from candidiasis.

TINEA CAPITIS
Synonym: ringworm of the scalp / hair

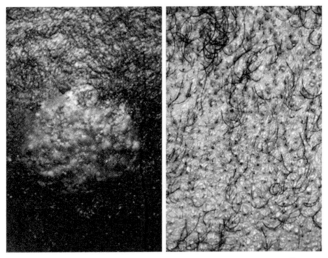

Ectothrix tinea capitis (kerion) (left) reprinted with permission from Lugo-Somolinos A, McKinley-Grant L, Goldsmith LA, et al. *VisualDx: Essential Dermatology in Pigmented Skin.* Wolters Kluwer Health/ Lippincott Williams & Wilkins; 2011.

Endothrix tinea capitis (right) courtesy of Anne W. Lucky, MD. From Marino BS, Fine KS. *Blueprints Pediatrics.* 7th ed. Wolters Kluwer; 2019.

- Tinea capitis refers to dermatophyte infection of scalp hair. It more often affects **children** with **curly hair.**
  - **Ectothrix** tinea capitis is characterized by **arthroconidia outside the hair shaft** with **variable fluorescence. *M. canis*** is the leading cause of tinea capitis worldwide, often transmitted from **cats and dogs.**
  - **Endothrix** tinea capitis is characterized by **arthroconidia inside the hair shaft. *Trichophyton tonsurans*** is the leading cause of tinea capitis in the United States.
    - Endothrix tinea capitis may be recalled with the mnemonic "<u>R</u>ingo gave <u>Y</u>oko <u>t</u>wo <u>s</u>queaky <u>v</u>iolins": *Trichophyton <u>r</u>ubrum* (variable), *<u>g</u>ourvilli, <u>y</u>aoundei, <u>t</u>onsurans, <u>s</u>oudanense,* and *<u>v</u>iolaceum.*
  - **Favus** is a special form of endothrix tinea capitis with **yellow crusted masses (scutula)** comprised of hyphae and

keratin debris instead of arthroconidia that is **fluorescent.** *Trichophyton schoenleinii* is the leading cause of favus.
  - In favus, *Trichophyton <u>schoenleinii</u> <u>shines light</u>.*
- Tinea capitis classically presents with **nonscarring circumscribed** hair loss; however, it can **scar if chronic or severe (biphasic). Kerion** is a severe pustular reaction to tinea capitis leading to **boggy plaques and abscesses** (more often with ***M. canis*** infection than *T. tonsurans* infection). **Lymphadenopathy** is common and can help distinguish tinea capitis from other causes of circumscribed hair loss.
  - Figure 3.19.

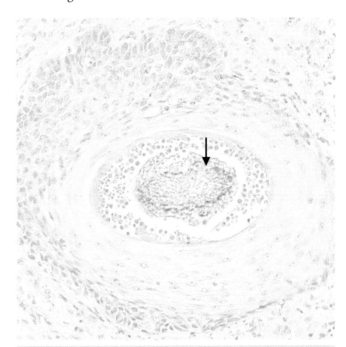

Figure 3.19. CLINICOPATHOLOGICAL CORRELATION: TINEA CAPITIS. Tinea capitis is characterized by hyphae and spores outside the hair shaft (ectothrix) or inside the hair shaft (endothrix). GMS and PAS highlight the pathogenic organism. Endothrix tinea capitis. Solid arrow: spore. GMS, Grocott-Gomori methenamine silver; PAS, periodic acid-Schiff.

(Histology image courtesy of Noel Turner, MD, MHS and Christine J. Ko, MD.)

- In tinea capitis, trichoscopy features include **black dots** (endothrix) and **comma hairs** (ectothrix and endothrix). **KOH** (often obtained with a toothbrush), skin biopsy, or fungal culture can be used to diagnose tinea capitis. **Fluorescence** when exposed to a UVA light source (eg, **Wood's lamp**) depends on whether the fungus produces **pteridine** (selected ectothrix tinea capitis, favus).

    Endothrix tinea capitis is also known as "black dot ringworm."

Fluorescent tinea capitis may be recalled with the mnemonic "c̲ats a̲nd d̲ogs f̲ight and g̲rowl s̲ometimes": *Microsporum c̲anis, a̲udouinii, d̲istortum, f̲errugineum,* and *g̲ypseum* (variable); *Trichophyton s̲choenleinii.*

- **Oral griseofulvin (>2 years of age)** is first line for **ectothrix** tinea capitis, whereas **oral terbinafine (>4 years of age)** is first line for **endothrix** tinea capitis. Disseminated eczema can occur after initiation of oral griseofulvin and may be confused with cutaneous adverse reactions given the timing.

ONYCHOMYCOSIS
Synonyms: ringworm of the nail, tinea unguium
→ **Diagnosis Group 1**

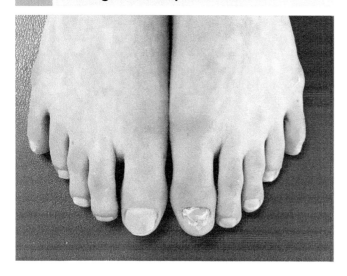

Epidemiology

- Onychomycosis refers to dermatophyte infection of the nail unit. *T. rubrum* is the leading cause overall. Notable exceptions include:
  - **White superficial onychomycosis:** due to *Trichophyton mentagrophytes* > *Acremonium, Aspergillus, Fusarium,* and *Scopulariopsis* species.
    - In white superficial onychomycosis, *Trichophyton rubrum* is a <u>red</u> flag for HIV infection.
  - **Dematiaceous onychomycosis:** due to *Scytalidium dimidiatum.*
  - **Primary total dystrophic onychomycosis:** due to **Candida species.**

Clinicopathological Features

- Onychomycosis is associated with **onycholysis, distal splinter hemorrhages, and subungual hyperkeratosis.** Other clinical features vary based on anatomic location:
  - **Proximal subungual onychomycosis:** involvement of the proximal nail bed, underside of the proximal nail plate, and proximal nail fold leads to **proximal beige nail plate opacity.**

    Proximal subungual onychomycosis, most commonly due to *Trichophyton* <u>rubrum</u>, is a <u>red</u> flag for HIV infection.
  - **Distal subungual onychomycosis (most common):** involvement of the distal nail bed, underside of the distal nail plate, and hyponychium leads to **distal beige nail plate opacity.**
  - **White superficial onychomycosis:** involvement of the superficial nail plate leads to **pseudoleukonychia.**
  - **Dematiaceous onychomycosis:** involvement by dematiaceous fungus leads to **longitudinal melanonychia.**
  - **Primary total dystrophic onychomycosis:** simultaneous involvement of the entire nail unit leads to **paronychia and proximal and distal beige nail plate opacity.**
    - Figure 3.20.

Evaluation

- The differential diagnosis of distal subungual onychomycosis includes inflammatory disorders (eg, psoriasis), injury (eg, mechanical), and drug-induced onycholysis.

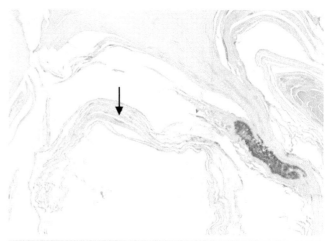

Figure 3.20. CLINICOPATHOLOGICAL CORRELATION: ONYCHOMYCOSIS. Onychomycosis is characterized by hyphae and spores in the nail plate and subungual debris. GMS and PAS highlight the pathogenic organism. Solid arrow: hypha. GMS, Grocott-Gomori methenamine silver; PAS, periodic acid-Schiff.

(Histology image courtesy of Noel Turner, MD, MHS and Christine J. Ko, MD.)

- **KOH, nail plate biopsy (clipping), and fungal culture** can be used to diagnose onychomycosis. Nail plate biopsy (clipping) with PAS stain is the most sensitive.
- **PCR** is an emerging diagnostic with high sensitivity. While PCR offers speciation (similar to fungal culture), it cannot indicate fungal viability.

Management

- **Oral terbinafine** is the most effective treatment for onychomycosis. The standard regimen is **250 mg daily for 6 weeks (fingernails) or 12 weeks (toenails).** Alternatives include pulsed dosing of oral terbinafine or fluconazole or itraconazole.
- Topical options include allylamines (eg, terbinafine), azoles (eg, efinaconazole), or ciclopirox. These options require long duration of therapy and offer low cure rates.
- *S. dimidiatum* is refractory to most antifungals.

"Real World" Advice

- Some data suggest that laboratory monitoring of terbinafine and griseofulvin may not be required.

Superficial and Deep Mycoses

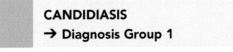

CANDIDIASIS
→ **Diagnosis Group 1**

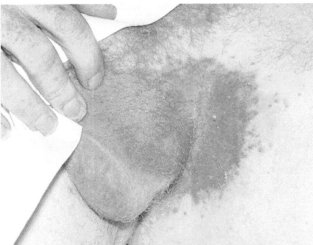

Reprinted with permission from Goodheart HP. *Goodheart's Photoguide of Common Skin Disorders: Diagnosis and Management.* 2nd ed. Lippincott Williams & Wilkins; 2003.

Epidemiology

- Candidiasis is typically an inflammatory superficial mycosis; however, it can become a deep mycosis in HIV-infected and other immunocompromised patients (opportunistic infection).
- Beyond **immunocompromise**, associations include **diabetes mellitus**, obesity, moisture, and occlusion. Xerostomia is associated with oropharyngeal candidiasis.

  Candidiasis may present as a **congenital or neonatal infection** and is associated with **CMC.**
- Drug associations include systemic immunosuppressants, particularly **IL-17 inhibitors.**

Clinicopathological Features

- Candidiasis classically presents with **erythematous papules and plaques, often studded with pustules. Mucocutaneous candidiasis variants** and **candida species** are summarized in Tables 3.26 and 3.27.

  Congenital candidiasis classically presents with **small monomorphous papules and pustules. Neonatal candidiasis** can present with **either classic mucocutaneous candidiasis (eg, intertrigo) or candidemia.** In **infants,** candidiasis is in the differential diagnosis for **diaper dermatitis.**
  - Figure 3.21.

Evaluation

- The differential diagnosis of candidiasis includes other inflammatory mycoses (eg, tinea), papulosquamous disorders (eg, psoriasis), eczematous disorders (eg, ICD), impetigo, erythrasma, and CTCL.
- **KOH** demonstrates **pseudohyphae and budding yeast.**
- Skin biopsy is rarely performed but may be helpful.
- Fungal cultures are less sensitive but can confirm the diagnosis and offer speciation.

Management

- Treatment for the most common mucocutaneous candidiasis variants:
  - **Oropharyngeal candidiasis:** clotrimazole troche, nystatin suspension, oral fluconazole.
  - **Candidal intertrigo:** azole cream, nystatin powder, oral fluconazole.
  - **Candidal balanitis/vulvovaginitis:** azole cream, nystatin suppository, oral fluconazole.
- Fluconazole-resistant candidiasis may be treated with an alternative azole (eg, itraconazole, voriconazole, posaconazole, isavuconazole) or an echinocandin (eg, **anidulafungin, caspofungin, micafungin**).

"Real World" Advice

- **Scrotal involvement** is a clinical clue to differentiate candidiasis from tinea cruris.

Table 3.26. MUCOCUTANEOUS CANDIDIASIS VARIANTS

Diagnosis[a]	Classic description	Notes
Oropharyngeal candidiasis (thrush)	Loosely adherent leukoplakia (scrapes off with a tongue blade) and friable mucosa.	May extend to involve the esophagus in HIV-infected and other immunocompromised patients.
Median rhomboid glossitis	Smooth, red, atrophic plaque on the dorsal tongue.	Most commonly due to *Candida albicans*.
Angular cheilitis (perlèche)	Erythematous fissured skin at the oral commissures.	May occur in the setting of ill-fitting dentures due to saliva accumulation.
Erosio interdigitalis blastomycetica	Maceration between finger web spaces (especially the third web space) and/or toe web spaces (especially the fourth toe web space).	
Candidal intertrigo	Macerated erythematous plaques with satellite papules and pustules.	Strongly associated with diabetes mellitus and obesity.
Candidal balanitis/vulvovaginitis	Erythematous papules, plaques, and pustules often in occluded areas on the glans penis and vulva/vagina.	Strongly associated with diabetes mellitus and obesity.
Candidal folliculitis	Folliculocentric papules.	Immunocompromised host.
Primary total dystrophic onychomycosis	See above.	Immunocompromised host.
Candidemia	Disseminated erythematous papules, plaques, pustules, and nodules.	Immunocompromised host.

[a]Illustrative examples provided.
HIV, human immunodeficiency virus.

Table 3.27. CANDIDA SPECIES

Species[a]	Notes
Candida albicans	Most common species. Increasing incidence of fluconazole resistance.
Candida auris	Emerging drug-resistant species that can colonize skin and spread in healthcare settings. Lethal in the setting of systemic infection.
Candida dubliniensis	Oropharyngeal candidiasis in HIV-infected and other immunocompromised patients.
Candida glabrata	Fungemia in immunocompromised patients. Fluconazole resistance.
Candida krusei	Endocarditis in the setting of IVDU. Fluconazole resistance.
Candida parapsilosis	Chronic paronychia. Endocarditis in the setting of IVDU.
Candida tropicalis	Most likely to cause disseminated candidiasis, including skin lesions.
	Candida <u>tropic</u>alis disseminates far and wide like tourists visiting the <u>tropics</u>.

[a]Illustrative examples provided.
HIV, human immunodeficiency virus; IVDU, intravenous drug use.

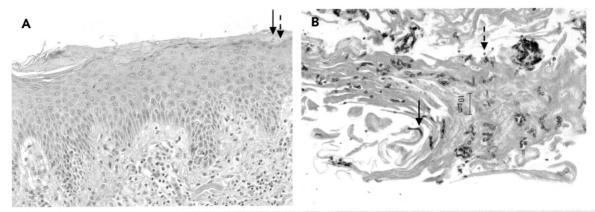

Figure 3.21. CLINICOPATHOLOGICAL CORRELATION: CANDIDIASIS. Candidiasis is characterized by hyperkeratosis, neutrophils, and pseudohyphae and budding yeast in the *stratum corneum*. GMS and PAS highlight the pathogenic organism. A, H&E. B, GMS. Solid arrows: pseudohyphae. Dashed arrows: yeast. GMS, Grocott-Gomori methenamine silver; H&E, hematoxylin & eosin; PAS, periodic acid-Schiff.

(A, Histology image courtesy of Noel Turner, MD, MHS and Christine J. Ko, MD. B, Histology image reprinted with permission from Elder DE, Elenitsas R, Rosenbach M, et al. *Lever's Histopathology of the Skin.* 11th ed. Wolters Kluwer; 2015.)

Pseudohyphae in candidiasis tend to orient vertically, while hyphae in tinea tend to orient horizontally.

SPOTLIGHT ON CHRONIC MUCOCUTANEOUS CANDIDIASIS

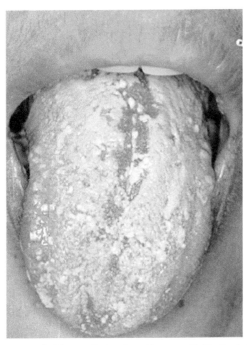

Thrush reprinted with permission from Harpavat S, Nissim S. *Lippincott's Microcards.* 3rd ed. Wolters Kluwer Health/Lippincott Williams & Wilkins; 2011.

- CMC describes a heterogeneous set of hereditary immunodeficiency disorders. Underlying gene mutations often involve the **IL-17 signaling pathway** or the **STAT1 signaling pathway**. **AD gain-of-function mutation in** *STAT1* is the leading cause overall. **APECED syndrome** is due to **AR** mutation in *AIRE* **encoding Autoimmune Regulator.** IPEX syndrome is due to **AR** mutation in *FOXP3* **encoding a transcription factor controlling Tregs.** Both syndromes are associated with CMC.
- CMC is characterized by **recurrent candidiasis.** The oral mucosa and nail unit are common sites. Patients with **APECED/IPEX syndromes** must satisfy **2/3 diagnostic criteria: CMC, chronic hypoparathyroidism, and Addison disease.** Other autoimmune associations include **vitiligo, AA, and pernicious anemia.**
    - CMC demonstrates candidiasis with a high burden of pseudohyphae and budding yeast.
- 70% of CMC patients have direct evidence of immunodeficiency including impaired cytokine and T-cell responses to *Candida* species.
- CMC is challenging to treat. Most patients require long-term therapy with fluconazole or itraconazole and eventual management with alternative antifungals for resistant *Candida* species.

Deep Mycoses

Dimorphic Fungi

- Dimorphic fungi are yeast at 37 °C (tissue) and molds at 25 °C (ambient environment).
- Dimorphic fungi are important causes of **opportunistic infection in HIV-infected and other immunocompromised patients.**
- The **distribution of selected dimorphic fungi in the United States** is illustrated in Figure 3.22.
- **KOH preparation of a "touch prep"** from a biopsy can facilitate rapid bedside diagnosis and initiation of treatment. The exception is sporotrichosis, which typically has a negative KOH. **Tzanck smear** may identify **cryptococcosis.**
- **Skin biopsy and sterile tissue culture** can confirm the diagnosis. The exception is lobomycosis, which has never been cultured in vivo.

BLASTOMYCOSIS, CHROMOBLASTOMYCOSIS, AND PARACOCCIDIOIDOMYCOSIS

Blastomycosis synonym: North American blastomycosis

Chromoblastomycosis synonym: chromomycosis

Paracoccidioidomycosis synonym: South American blastomycosis

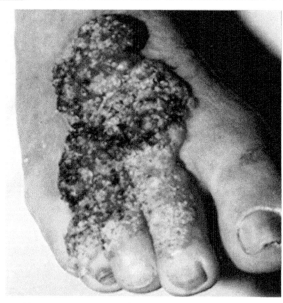

Chromoblastomycosis reprinted with permission from Engleberg NC, DiRita V, Dermody TS. *Schaechter's Mechanisms of Microbial Disease.* 5th ed. Wolters Kluwer Health/Lippincott Williams & Wilkins; 2012.

- Blastomycosis, chromoblastomycosis, and paracoccidioidomycosis are deep mycoses:
  - **Blastomycosis** is due to the dimorphic fungus *Blastomyces dermatitidis*, which is endemic to the **Great Lakes, Ohio River Basin, and Mississippi River** and transmitted primarily by inhalation. **Dogs** are a known animal

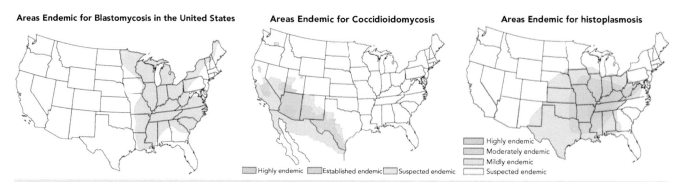

Figure 3.22. DISTRIBUTION OF SELECTED DIMORPHIC FUNGI IN THE UNITED STATES.
(Images reprinted with permission from LoCicero J III, Feins RH, Colson YL, et al. *Shields' General Thoracic Surgery.* 8th ed. Wolters Kluwer; 2018.)

reservoir. **Secondary cutaneous blastomycosis after dissemination from a primary pulmonary infection** is more common than primary cutaneous blastomycosis.

◆ Blastomycosis <u>blasts</u> off from the lungs to the skin.

○ **Chromoblastomycosis** is due to **five dimorphic dematiaceous fungi**: *Cladosporium carrionii, Fonsecaea pedrosoi* **(most common)**, *Fonsecaea compacta, Phialophora verrucosa,* **and** *Rhinocladiella aquaspersa* transmitted primarily by traumatic inoculation.

○ **Paracoccidioidomycosis** is due to the dimorphic fungus *Paracoccidioides brasiliensis*, which is endemic to **Central and South America** and transmitted primarily by inhalation. **Male agricultural workers** are an at-risk population.

● The characteristic presentation depends on the mycosis:

○ **Blastomycosis** classically presents with **well-demarcated plaques with a verrucous border with crusting and pustules ± central ulceration.**

◆ The verrucous border correlates with PEH and is often referred to as "stadium seating."

○ **Chromoblastomycosis** classically presents with a **granulomatous or verrucous plaque**, typically on an extremity.

○ **Paracoccidioidomycosis** classically presents with **ulcerative or verrucous plaques in the nasal or oral mucosa. Cervical lymphadenopathy** may result from lymphangitic spread.

◆ Figure 3.23.

● **Itraconazole** is first line. **Amphotericin B** is required for more severe systemic disease.

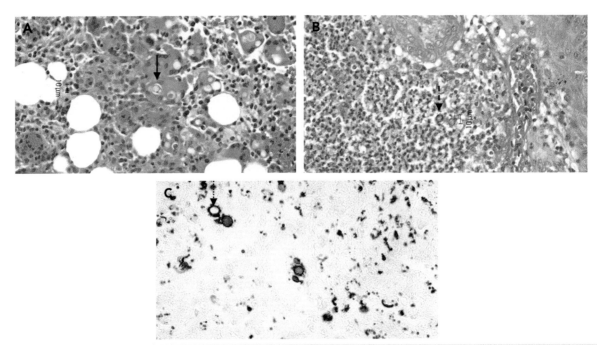

Figure 3.23. SIDE-BY-SIDE COMPARISON: BLASTOMYCOSIS, CHROMOBLASTOMYCOSIS, AND PARACOCCIDIOIDOMYCOSIS. Blastomycosis, chromoblastomycosis, and paracoccidioidomycosis all demonstrate PEH and intraepidermal pustules and multinucleated giant cells. Blastomycosis is characterized by broad-based budding yeast. Chromoblastomycosis is characterized by Medlar bodies: pigmented clumps of dematiaceous organisms highlighted by Fontana-Mason stain. Paracoccidioidomycosis is characterized by narrow-based budding yeast. A, Blastomycosis. Solid arrow: broad-based budding yeast. B, In chromoblastomycosis. Dashed arrow: Medlar body resembling a "copper penny." C, paracoccidioidomycosis (GMS). Dotted arrow: narrow-based budding yeast with multiple buds radiating outward resembling a "mariner's wheel." GMS, Grocott-Gomori methenamine silver; PAS, periodic acid-Schiff; PEH, pseudoepitheliomatous hyperplasia.

(Histology images reprinted with permission from Elder DE, Elenitsas R, Rosenbach M, et al. *Lever's Histopathology of the Skin.* 11th ed. Wolters Kluwer; 2015.)

Medlar bodies in chromoblastomycosis resemble "copper pennies."
Narrow-based budding yeast with multiple buds radiating outward in paracoccidioidomycosis resemble a "mariner's wheel."
Beyond deep mycoses, the differential diagnosis of PEH includes pemphigus vegetans, halogenoderma, granuloma inguinale, and leishmaniasis.

COCCIDIOIDOMYCOSIS
Synonym: San Joaquin valley fever

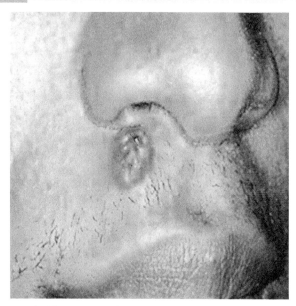

Reprinted with permission from Gru AA, Wick MR, Mir A, et al. *Pediatric Dermatopathology and Dermatology.* Wolters Kluwer; 2018.

- Coccidioidomycosis is a deep mycosis due the dimorphic fungus *Coccidioides immitis*, which is endemic to the **southwestern United States and parts of Mexico and Central and South America** and transmitted primarily by inhalation. **Individuals of African American or Southeast Asian descent and pregnant women** are at-risk populations. Coccidioidomycosis is associated with **EN.**
- Coccidioidomycosis classically presents with **papules, plaques, and pustules. Molluscum-type central umbilicated papules** may occur. Beyond **cutaneous coccidioidomycosis**, coccidioidomycosis may be restricted to the lungs (**pulmonary coccidioidomycosis**) or may involve multiple organ systems (**disseminated coccidioidomycosis**) including the skin, skeletal system, and CNS.
    - Figure 3.24.
- **EN is a positive prognostic factor** suggesting a robust host immune response. **Itraconazole** is first line. **Amphotericin B** is required for more severe systemic disease or **pregnant women.**

HISTOPLASMOSIS AND TALAROMYCOSIS
Histoplasmosis synonym: Ohio valley disease

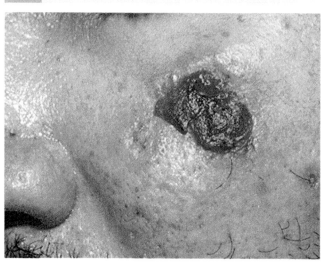

Histoplasmosis reprinted with permission from Lugo-Somolinos A, McKinley-Grant L, Goldsmith LA, et al. *VisualDx: Essential Dermatology in Pigmented Skin.* Wolters Kluwer Health/Lippincott Williams & Wilkins; 2011.

- Histoplasmosis and penicilliosis are deep mycoses:
    - **Histoplasmosis** is due to the dimorphic fungus *H. capsulatum*, which is endemic to the **central and southeastern United States** and transmitted primarily by inhalation. **Birds, fowl, and bats** are known animal reservoirs. African histoplasmosis is due to *H. capsulatum* var. *duboisii*. Histoplasmosis is associated with **EM**, particularly in patients with concomitant **EN.**
    - Talaromycosis (formerly penicilliosis) is due to *Talaromyces marneffei* (formerly *Penicillium marneffei*), which is endemic to **Southeast Asia** and transmitted primarily by inhalation. **Healthy bamboo rats** are a known animal reservoir.
- The characteristic presentation depends on the mycosis:
    - Histoplasmosis classically presents with **molluscum-type central umbilicated papules.** Involvement of the **nasal and oral mucosa** is common.
    - **Talaromycosis** classically presents with **molluscum-type central umbilicated papules.**
        - Figure 3.25.
        - Talaromycosis is challenging to differentiate from histoplasmosis. Yeast do not bud, but rather divide by fission.
- **Itraconazole** is first line. **Amphotericin B** is required for opportunistic infections.

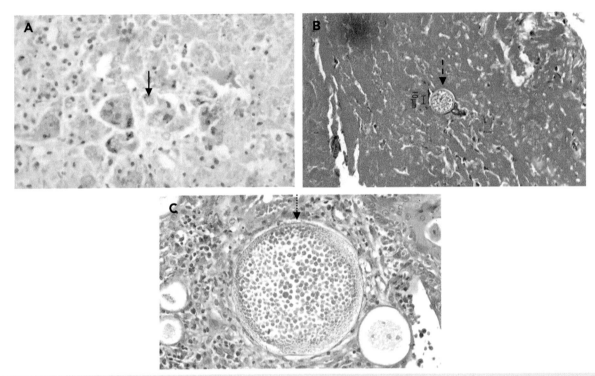

Figure 3.24. SIDE-BY-SIDE COMPARISON: PROTOTHECOSIS, COCCIDIOIDOMYCOSIS, AND RHINOSPORIDIOSIS.
Protothecosis, coccidioidomycosis, and rhinosporidiosis all demonstrate multinucleated giant cells. Protothecosis is characterized by 8-20 μm morula-like clusters of organisms. Coccidioidomycosis is characterized by PEH with intraeptihelial pustules and 10-80 μm double-walled refractile spherules containing endospores. Rhinosporidioisis is characterized by 250-325 μm sporangia containing endospores. GMS and PAS highlight the pathogenic organisms. A, Protothecosis. Solid arrow: morula-like cluster of organisms resembling a "soccer ball." B, Coccidioidomycosis. Dashed arrow: spherule containing endospores. C, Rhinosporidiosis. Dotted arrow: sporangium containing endospores. GMS, Grocott-Gomori methenamine silver; PAS, periodic acid-Schiff; PEH, pseudoepitheliomatous hyperplasia.

(Histology images reprinted with permission from Elder DE, Elenitsas R, Rosenbach M, et al. *Lever's Histopathology of the Skin.* 11th ed. Wolters Kluwer; 2015.)

Protothecosis is an algae NOT a fungus. Morula-like clusters of organisms resemble "soccer balls."
Rhinosporidiosis is a protozoan NOT a fungus.

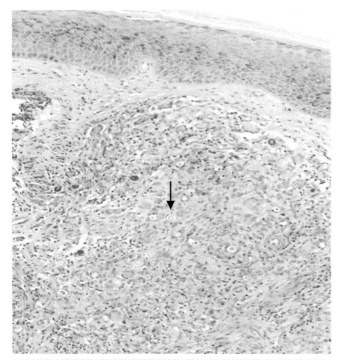

Figure 3.25. CLINICOPATHOLOGICAL CORRELATION: HISTOPLASMOSIS. Histoplasmosis is characterized by PEH with intraepidermal pustules and intracellular yeast. Yeast are evenly spaced within histiocytes and surrounded by pseudocapsules. Giemsa, GMS, PAS highlight the pathogenic organism. Solid arrow: intracellular yeast surrounded by a pseudocapsule. GMS, Grocott-Gomori methenamine silver; PAS, periodic acid-Schiff; PEH, pseudoepitheliomatous hyperplasia.

(Histology image reprinted with permission from Edward S, Yung A. *Essential Dermatopathology*. Wolters Kluwer Health/Lippincott Williams & Wilkins; 2011.)

• **African histoplasmosis:** multinucleated giant cells, large intracellular yeast.

The differential diagnosis of "parasitized histiocytes" includes rhinoscleroma, granuloma inguinale, histoplasmosis, penicilliosis, and leishmaniasis. Helpful histopathological features to differentiate histoplasmosis from leishmaniasis include spacing within histiocytes, presence of a pseudocapsule, and absence of a kinetoplast. Note that *Histoplasma capsulatum* is a misnomer as the pseudocapsule is due to shrinkage artifact.

CRYPTOCOCCOSIS

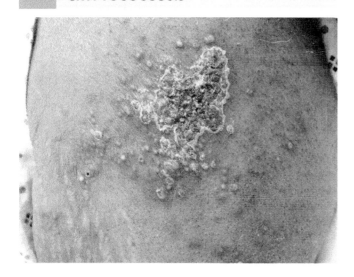

• Cryptococcosis is a deep mycosis due to the dimorphic fungus *Cryptococcus neoformans.* The organism, found in **pigeon droppings** and psittacine birds like the **cockatoo**, is transmitted primarily by inhalation.

• Cryptococcus has protean manifestations ranging from **molluscum-type central umbilicated papules** to **nodules** to **cellulitis-like, granulomatous, herpetiform, and ulcerative plaques.** Involvement of the **nasal and oral mucosa** is common. Beyond **cutaneous cryptococcosis**, cryptococcosis may be restricted to the lungs (**pulmonary cryptococcosis**) or may involve multiple organ systems (**disseminated cryptococcosis**) including the skin, skeletal system, and CNS.

◈ Figure 3.26.

• Disseminated cryptococcosis to the skin portends a poor prognosis with an 80% mortality rate if untreated. An oral azole (eg, **fluconazole, itraconazole, voriconazole, posaconazole, isavuconazole**) is first line. **Amphotericin B** is required for more severe systemic disease and is combined with **flucytosine** in cases with **CNS involvement.**

LOBOMYCOSIS
Synonym: keloidal blastomycosis

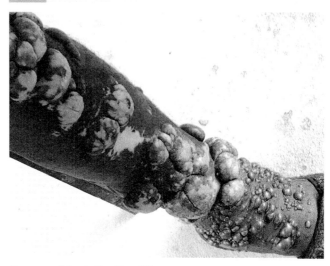

Courtesy of Justin Bandino, MD

• Lobomycosis is a deep mycosis due to the dimorphic fungus *Lacazia loboi*, which is endemic to the **Amazon basin** and transmitted primarily by traumatic inoculation. **Dolphins** are a known animal reservoir.

• Lobomycosis classically presents with **keloid-like firm nodules** that are frequently asymptomatic and favor the face, ears, and distal extremities. Beyond **lymphadenopathy**, there is **no systemic involvement.**

◈ Figure 3.27.

• Antifungals are typically ineffective. **Surgical excision** is the treatment of choice.

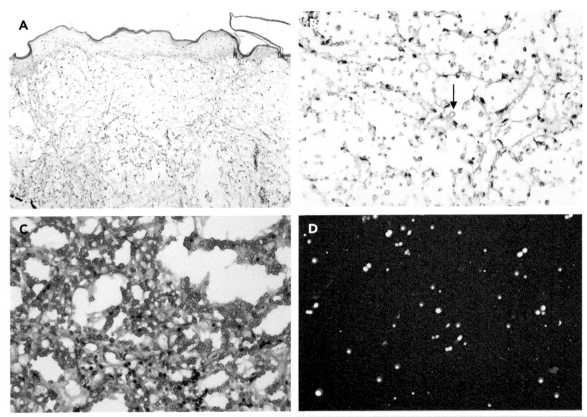

Figure 3.26. CLINICOPATHOLOGICAL CORRELATION: CRYPTOCOCCOSIS. Cryptococcosis is characterized by pleomorphic encapsulated yeast. GMS and PAS highlight the central yeast. India ink preparation colors the central yeast purple and the dark background reveals the presence of a clear capsule. The capsule contains sialomucin (mucicarmine positive; PAS-positive, diastase resistant). A, Gelatinous cryptococcosis, low-power H&E. B, Gelatinous cryptococcosis, high-power H&E. Solid arrow: encapsulated yeast. C, Mucicarmine. D, India Ink preparation. GMS, Grocott-Gomori methenamine silver; H&E, hematoxylin-eosin; PAS, periodic acid-Schiff.

(A, Histology image reprinted with permission from Elder DE, Elenitsas R, Rosenbach M, et al. *Lever's Histopathology of the Skin.* 11th ed. Wolters Kluwer; 2015. B, Histology image reprinted with permission from Elder DE, Elenitsas R, Rosenbach M, et al. *Lever's Histopathology of the Skin.* 11th ed. Wolters Kluwer; 2015. C, Histology image reprinted with permission from Vigorita VJ. *Orthopaedic Pathology.* 3rd ed. Wolters Kluwer; 2015. D, Histology image reprinted with permission from Vigorita VJ. *Orthopaedic Pathology.* 3rd ed. Wolters Kluwer; 2015.)

- Gelatinous cryptococcosis: relatively more organisms and less inflammation.
- Granulomatous cryptococcosis: relatively fewer organisms and more inflammation ± necrosis.

Cryptococcus neoformans lives together in a "gelatinous condominium."

SPOROTRICHOSIS
→ Diagnosis Group 2

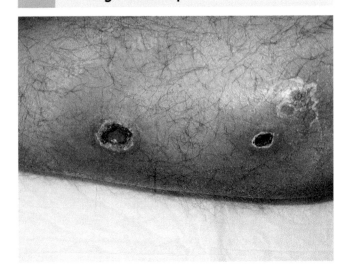

Epidemiology

- Sporotrichosis is a deep mycosis due to the dimorphic fungus ***Sporothrix schenckii.***
- The organism, found in **grasses, sphagnum moss, thorns, and wood splinters**, is transmitted primarily by traumatic inoculation.
- **Alcoholics, florists, and gardeners** are at-risk populations.

Clinicopathological Features

- There are three main types of cutaneous sporotrichosis:
  ○ **Lymphocutaneous**: subcutaneous nodules following along path of lymphatic drainage (**sporotrichoid spread**).
  ○ **Fixed cutaneous (seen with prior exposure and host immune response)**: granulomatous plaque with ulceration.
  ○ **Disseminated**: widespread subcutaneous nodules.
    ◆ Figure 3.28.

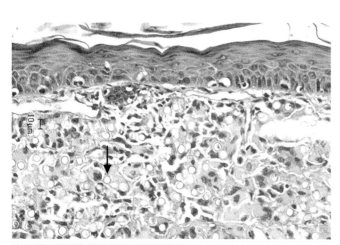

Figure 3.27. CLINICOPATHOLOGICAL CORRELATION: LOBOMYCOSIS. Lobomycosis is characterized by thick collagen fibers and multinucleated giant cells containing yeast with tubular connections between cells. GMS and PAS highlight the pathogenic organism. solid arrow: yeast with tubular connections between cells resembling a child's "pop-beads." GMS, Grocott-Gomori methenamine silver; PAS, periodic acid-Schiff.

(Histology image reprinted with permission from Elder DE, Elenitsas R, Rosenbach M, et al. *Lever's Histopathology of the Skin.* 11th ed. Wolters Kluwer; 2015.)

> Yeast with tubular connections between cells resemble a child's "pop-beads."

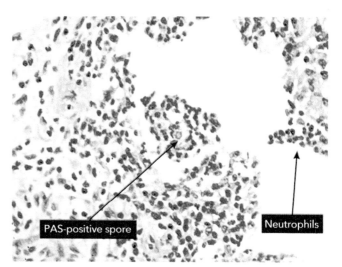

Figure 3.28. CLINICOPATHOLOGICAL CORRELATION: SPOROTRICHOSIS. Sporotrichosis is characterized by PEH with intraepithelial pustules and suppurative granulomas containing rare pleomorphic yeast ± a Splendore–Hoeppli reaction (asteroid body). GMS and PAS highlight the pathogenic organism. GMS, Grocott-Gomori methenamine silver; PAS, periodic acid-Schiff; PEH, pseudoepitheliomatous hyperplasia.

(Histology image reprinted with permission from Elder DE, Elenitsas R, Rubin AI, et al. *Atlas of Dermatopathology: Synopsis and Atlas of Lever's Histopathology of the Skin.* 4th ed. Wolters Kluwer; 2020.)

> Yeast may be round or "cigar-shaped."

Evaluation

- The differential diagnosis of sporotrichosis depends on the type.
    - To remember the differential diagnosis of sporotrichoid spread, use the <u>SLANT</u> mnemonic: <u>S</u>porotrichosis, <u>L</u>eishmaniasis, <u>A</u>typical Mycobacterial infections, <u>N</u>ocardiosis, <u>T</u>ularemia.

Management

- **SSKI** can be effective; however, multicenter trial data better support the use of **itraconazole** for lymphocutaneous or fixed cutaneous sporotrichosis.

"Real World" Advice

- Despite the moniker "sporotrichoid spread," it is important not to assume that sporotrichosis is the cause, as nocardiosis and atypical mycobacterial infections are other common causes in the United States.

Miscellaneous Fungi

ANGIOINVASIVE FUNGAL INFECTION

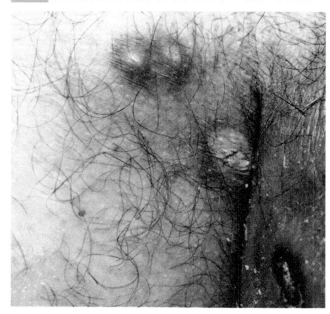

Aspergillosis courtesy of Sotonye Imadojemu, MD, MBE

- Angioinvasive fungal infection is primarily divided into:
  - **Aspergillosis**: *Aspergillus flavus* and *Aspergillus fumigatus* are the most common pathogens.
  - **Fusariosis**: *Fusarium* **species** may infect **burn wounds**.
  - **Zygomycosis**: *Mucor* **species** and *Rhizopus* **species** may cause **rhinocerebral infection** in patients with **diabetes mellitus**.

  HIV-infected and other immunocompromised patients, particularly those with **prolonged neutropenia**, are at high risk for all pathogens.
- Angioinvasive fungal infection classically presents with **noninflammatory retiform purpura** as well as **necrotic plaques and papulonodules**.
  - ◆ Figure 3.29.
- Bedside diagnostics such as **touch preparation with KOH** may be helpful to speed the diagnosis. **Skin biopsy**, often with an additional **frozen section** for rapid evaluation, is helpful. **Sterile tissue culture** is also critical. *Fusarium* **species** is one of the few mold species that can yield **positive blood cultures**.
- Angioinvasive fungal infection is highly lethal; **fusariosis has a nearly 100% mortality rate in the setting of prolonged neutropenia**. Susceptible patients should receive fungal prophylaxis. While **voriconazole** continues to be a common choice, it **lacks activity against mucormycosis**. Posaconazole has broad activity and isavuconazole lacks activity against fusariosis. **Amphotericin B** has broad activity and is historically considered the treatment of choice (though other agents may be more effective against specific pathogens such as voriconazole for aspergillosis). Echinocandins (eg, anidulafungin, caspofungin, micafungin) lack activity against fusariosis and mucormycosis.

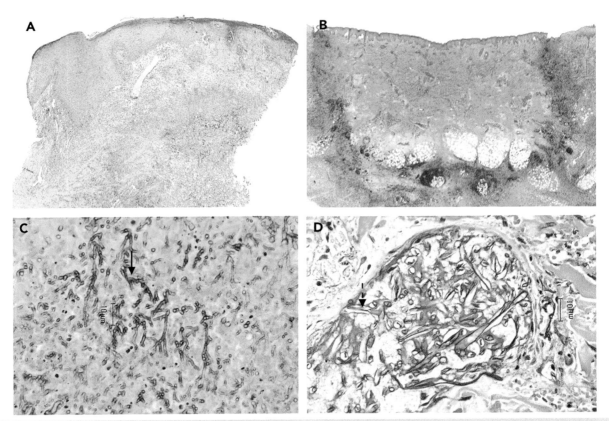

Figure 3.29. SIDE-BY-SIDE COMPARISON: ASPERGILLOSIS AND ZYGOMYCOSIS. Both aspergillosis and zygomycosis demonstrate hyphae invading blood vessels leading to tissue necrosis. Hyphae in aspergillosis are septate and typically branch at 45° angles. Hyphae in zygomycosis are nonseptate and typically branch at 90° angles. GMS and PAS highlight the pathogenic organisms. A and C, Aspergillosis. Solid arrow: septate hypha with blue "bubbly" cytoplasm and 45° branching. B and D, Zygomycosis. Dashed arrow: nonseptate "hollow," "ribbon-like" hypha with 90° branching. GMS, Grocott-Gomori methenamine silver; PAS, periodic acid-Schiff.

(Histology images reprinted with permission from Elder DE, Elenitsas R, Rosenbach M, et al. *Lever's Histopathology of the Skin.* 11th ed. Wolters Kluwer; 2015.)

In aspergillosis, septate hyphae retain blue "bubbly" cytoplasm.
In zygomycosis, nonseptate hyphae appear "hollow" and "ribbon-like."

MYCETOMA

Synonym: Madura foot

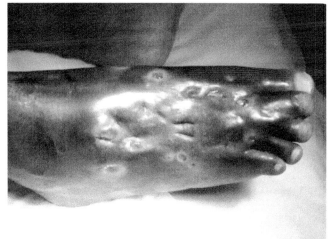

Courtesy of Leslie-Castelo-Soccio, MD, PhD.

- Mycetoma is divided into two types: **actinomycetoma (bacterial)** and **eumycetoma (fungal)** (Table 3.28). Transmission often occurs via traumatic implantation (eg, gravel, soil). While actinomycetoma has a worldwide distribution, eumycetoma is more prevalent in tropical climates such as in Africa, India, and Central and South America.
- Mycetoma is characterized by **tumefaction and sinus tracts with discharge of grains**. The **foot** is the most common location. **Extension to fascia, muscle, bone** may occur.
  - Mycetoma is characterized by an abscess containing grains often with a Splendore–Hoeppli reaction.
- Skin biopsy and sterile tissue culture can confirm the diagnosis.

- Mycetoma is not self-limited. Actinomycetoma requires antibacterial therapy; eumycetoma requires antifungal therapy ± surgical debridement. To avoid deep extension, early treatment is paramount.

PROTOTHECOSIS

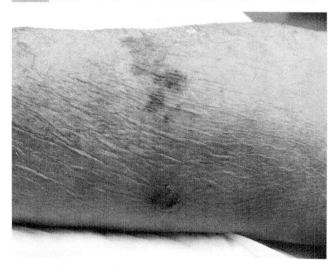

- Protothecosis is due to *Prototheca wickerhamii*, an **algae found in stagnant water.** It is endemic to **Southeast Asia** and infections are due to traumatic inoculation in contaminated water.
- Protothecosis classically presents with **plaques and ulcers.** It may be complicated by **olecranon bursitis.**
  - For the histopathology of protothecosis, see Figure 3.24.
- Skin biopsy and sterile tissue culture can confirm the diagnosis.
- Immunocompromised hosts can develop widespread disease. Management is challenging and often requires a multimodal medical and surgical approach.

Table 3.28. MYCETOMA

Grain Color	Actinomycetoma organisms[a]	Eumycetoma organisms[a]
Red	*Actinomadura pelletieri*	
Pink-to-cream	*Actinomadura madurae*	
Yellow-to-brown	*Actinomyces israelii, Streptomyces somaliensis*	
Yellow-to-white		*Pseudallescheria boydii* (leading cause in the US, *Scedosporium apiospermum* is the asexual mold form)
White	*Nocardia asteroides, Nocardia brasiliensis* (leading cause in the US)	*Acremonium* species, *Aspergillus* species, *Fusarium* species
Black		*Curvularia* species, *Exophiala jeanselmei, Madurella* species, *Leptosphaeria* species, *Pyrenochaeta romeroi*

[a]Illustrative examples provided.
US, United States.

Parasitic Diseases and Other Animal Kingdom Encounters

Basic Concepts

- **Parasites** are organisms that live on or within a host and at the expense of the host.
- Some organisms exist in a commensal relationship with humans without a clear pathogenic role. *Demodex* **mites** are commonly found in hair follicles on the face in association with sebaceous glands and have been implicated in the pathogenesis of rosacea. Some degree of controversy exists over their designation as a commensal organism versus a parasite.
- **Parasite classification** (for dermatology-relevant parasites) is summarized in Table 3.29.
- **Vectors in dermatology** are summarized in Table 3.30.
  - Figure 3.30.

LEISHMANIASIS

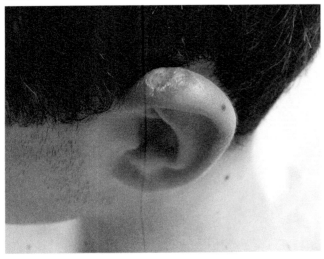

- **Leishmaniasis** is due to the *Leishmania* species of protozoa, an **obligate intracellular parasite.** Infections are divided into **old world leishmaniasis transmitted by the** *Phlebotomus* **species of sandfly** (Africa, Asia, the Mediterranean, the Middle East) and **new world leishmaniasis transmitted by the** *Lutzomyia* **species of sandfly** (Central and South America, southern United States). **Protozoan infections** are summarized in Table 3.31.
  - **Congenital toxoplasmosis infection** classically presents with **petechiae, purpura, and vesicles** along with **extramedullary hematopoiesis.** Complications include **hydrocephalus, intracranial calcifications, and chorioretinitis.**
  - Congenital toxoplasmosis is in the differential diagnosis of "blueberry muffin" lesions.

- There are three major clinical types of leishmaniasis:
  - **Cutaneous leishmaniasis**: classically presents as a **verrucous or ulcerated plaque on an exposed site**, frequently with isolated lesions though also an important cause of **sporotrichoid spread.** Most acute infections resolve spontaneously with scarring. New world leishmaniasis has a wider clinical spectrum including disseminated cutaneous and mucocutaneous disease (especially *Leishmania brasiliensis* infection).
    - Localized cutaneous leishmaniasis involving the ear (primarily due to *Leishmania mexicana*) is sometimes called "Chiclero ulcer" in reference to its occurrence in workers who gathered chicle latex for gum (*chicleros*).
  - **Mucocutaneous leishmaniasis (espundia)**: classically presents with mild edema that progresses to **infiltrative and ulcerative plaques of the nasal or oral mucosa.** Local tissue destruction may lead to **perforation of the nasal septum.**
    - The nasal appearance in mucocutaneous leishmaniasis is sometimes called "tapir face."
  - **Visceral leishmaniasis (kala-azar)**: classically presents with **nonspecific skin lesions (eg, hyperpigmented patches, purpura)** with spread to the bone marrow, liver, and spleen. Systemic symptoms include fever, lymphadenopathy, hepatosplenomegaly, diarrhea, and cough.
    - The combination of hyperpigmented patches and fever in visceral leishmaniasis is sometimes called "black fever."

  Leishmaniasis recidivans refers to a chronic, recurrent destructive granulomatous response that develops at the edge of a previously healed ulcer.
    - Figure 3.31. For the histopathology of rhinosporidiosis, see Figure 3.24.

- Skin biopsy and sterile tissue culture can confirm the diagnosis. The required culture medium is **Novy-McNeal-Nicolle**, but culture is unreliable (positive in <50% of cases). Bedside diagnostics such as the **"thick drop method" (modified Tzanck smear) or touch preparation followed by Tzanck smear** may be helpful to speed the diagnosis. The **Montenegro-Leishman test** can identify host responses to *Leishmania* species antigens but has limited utility in endemic areas. **PCR** is most sensitive and can render the diagnosis from formalin-fixed skin biopsy specimens. Upon **diascopy**, leishmaniasis recidivans lesions have the color of **apple jelly.**
- Cutaneous leishmaniasis is treated with **antimony compounds (meglumine antimonate, sodium stibogluconate),** miltefosine, or pentamidine. Mucocutaneous leishmaniasis can be more challenging to treat with better responses to amphotericin B than antimony compounds. **Visceral leishmaniasis leads to death within 2 years if untreated.** Amphotericin B is first line.

Table 3.29. PARASITE CLASSIFICATION

Type	Family	Parasite	Diagnosis[a]
Protozoa	Ciliophora	*Trypanosoma brucei gambiense* (west), *Trypanosoma brucei rhodesiense* (east)	African trypanosomiasis (sleeping sickness)
		Trypanosoma cruzi	American trypanosomiasis (Chagas disease)
	Flagellates	*Leishmania aethiopica*[b], *Leishmania donovani*,[c] *Leishmania infantum*,[c] *Leishmania major*, *Leishmania tropica*.	Leishmaniasis (old world)
		Leishmania amazonensis, *Leishmania brasiliensis*,[b] *Leishmania chagasi*,[c] *Leishmania mexicana*, *Leishmania peruviana*.[b]	Leishmaniasis (new world)
	Sarcodina	*Acanthamoeba* genus	Amebiasis
		Balamuthia mandrillaris	
		Entamoeba histolytica	
		Naegleria fowleri	
	Sporozoans	*Babesia* species	Babesiosis
		Plasmodium falciparum, *Plasmodium malariae*, *Plasmodium ovale*, *Plasmodium vivax*	Malaria
		Rhinosporidium seeberi[d]	Rhinosporidiosis
		Toxoplasma gondii	Toxoplasmosis
Helminths	Roundworms (nematodes)	*Ancylostoma braziliense*, *Ancylostoma carinum*	Cutaneous larva migrans (creeping eruption)
		Dracunculus medinensis	Dracunculiasis (Guinea worm disease)
		Wuchereria bancrofti	Filariasis
		Gnathostoma dolorosi, *Gnathostoma spinigerum*	Gnathostomiasis
		Ancylostoma duodenale, *Necator americanus*	Ground itch
		Loa loa	Loiasis (Calabar swelling)
		Onchocerca volvulus	Onchocerciasis (river blindness)
		Enterobius vermicularis	Pinworm infection
		Strongyloides stercoralis	Strongyloidiasis (larva currens, racing larva)
		Trichinella spiralis	Trichinosis (trichinellosis)
	Flukes (trematodes)	*Trichobilharzia* species (avian schistosomes)	Cercarial dermatitis (clam digger's itch, duck itch, swimmer's itch)
		Schistosoma haematobium, *Schistosoma japonicum*, *Schistosoma mansoni*	Schistosomiasis (snail fever)
	Tapeworms (cestodes)	*Taenia solium*	Cysticercosis

(Continued)

Table 3.29. PARASITE CLASSIFICATION (CONTINUED)

Type	Family	Parasite	Diagnosis[a]
Ectoparasites	Fleas	*Pulex irritans* (human flea)	Pulicosis
		Tunga penetrans	Tungiasis
	Flies	*Dermatobia hominis* (botfly larva)	Myiasis
	True bugs	*Cimex lectularius* (bed bug)	Bed bug infestation
	Mites	*Acarus siro* (grain mite)	Baker's itch
		Cheyletiella species	Cheyletiellosis
		Trombiculid species (chigger mites)	Chigger bites
		Demodex folliculorum (skin mites)	Demodicosis
		Tyrophagus casei (cheese mite)	Grocer's itch
		Sarcoptes scabiei var hominis (itch mite)	Scabies
	Lice	*Pediculus humanus var capitis* (head louse)	Pediculosis capitis (cooties)
		Pediculus humanus var corporis (body louse)	Pediculosis corporis
		Pthirus pubis (crab louse, pubic louse)	Pediculosis pubis (crabs)
	Ticks	*Amblyomma americanum* (lone star tick), *Dermacentor andersoni* (Rocky Mountain wood tick), *Dermacentor variabilis* (American dog tick), *Ixodes pacificus* (western black-legged tick), *Ixodes ricinus* (castor bean tick), *Ixodes scapularis* (deer tick), *Ornithodoros* species (soft ticks), *Rhipicephalus sanguineus* (brown dog tick)	Tick bites

[a]Illustrative examples provided.
[b]Mucocutaneous leishmaniasis.
[c]Visceral leishmaniasis.
[d]The classification of *Rhinosporidium seeberi* is controversial as it is alternatively classified as a fungus.

CUTANEOUS LARVA MIGRANS
→ Diagnosis Group 2
Synonym: creeping eruption

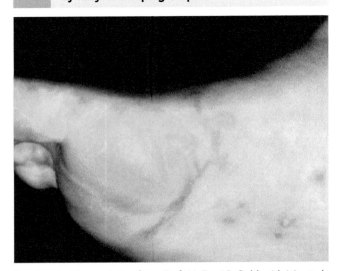

Reprinted with permission from Craft N, Fox LP, Goldsmith LA, et al. *VisualDx: Essential Adult Dermatology.* Wolters Kluwer Health/Lippincott Williams & Wilkins; 2010.

Epidemiology

- Cutaneous larval migrans is due to the **helminths *Ancylostoma braziliense* and *Ancylostoma caninum***, which are roundworms (nematodes) that function as animal hookworms. Cutaneous larva migrans is most commonly seen in Africa, Central and South America, the southeastern United States, and other tropical climates.
- Infection occurs when **walking barefoot or lying down** in an area contaminated by animal feces containing the eggs, which hatch into larvae in the soil.
- **Helminth infections** are summarized in Table 3.32.

Clinicopathological Features

- Cutaneous larva migrans moves slowly (**2-10 mm/h**), creating **pink-red plaques appearing as serpiginous tracts.**
- Cutaneous larva migrans cannot leave the epidermis because it lacks collagenase; therefore, there is **no systemic involvement.** However, it is rarely associated with **Löffler syndrome**, which refers to **pulmonary eosinophilia due to larval migration through**

Table 3.30. VECTORS IN DERMATOLOGY

Type	Vector(s)[a]	Diagnosis[a]
Fleas	*Ctenocephalides felis* (cat flea)	Bacillary angiomatosis, cat scratch disease, typhus (endemic, flea-borne)
	Xenopsylla cheopis (oriental rat flea)	Plague, typhus (endemic, flea-borne)
Flies	*Chrysops* species (deer fly, mango fly)	Tularemia, loiasis
	Glossina species (tsetse fly)	African trypanosomiasis (sleeping sickness)
	Lutzomyia species (sandfly)	Oroya fever/verruga peruana (Carrión disease), leishmaniasis (new world)
	Phlebotomus species (sandfly)	Oroya fever/verruga peruana (Carrión disease), leishmaniasis (old world)
	Simulium species (black fly)	Fogo selvagem, onchocerciasis
Mosquitoes	*Aedes* species	Dengue, zika, chikungunya, tularemia, filariasis
	Anopheles species	Malaria, filariasis
	Culex species	West Nile infection, tularemia, filariasis
	Mansonia species	Filariasis
True bugs	*Triatoma* species (assassin bug, kissing bug, reduviid bug)	American trypanosomiasis (Chagas disease)
Mites	*Liponyssoides sanguineus* (mouse mite)	Rickettsialpox
	Trombiculid species (chigger mites)	Typhus (scrub)
Lice	*Pediculus humanus var corporis* (body louse)	Bacillary angiomatosis, trench fever (shinbone fever), typhus (epidemic, louse-borne), relapsing fever (louse-borne)
Ticks	*Amblyomma americanum* (lone star tick)	RMSF, ehrlichiosis (monocytic), Q fever, tularemia, Lyme disease, STARI
	Dermacentor andersoni (Rocky Mountain wood tick)	RMSF, anaplasmosis (granulocytic), ehrlichiosis (granulocytic), Q fever, tularemia
	Dermacentor variabilis (American dog tick)	RMSF, anaplasmosis (granulocytic), ehrlichiosis (granulocytic), tularemia
	Ixodes pacificus (western black-legged tick)	Babesiosis, anaplasmosis (granulocytic), ehrlichiosis (granulocytic), Lyme disease
	Ixodes ricinus (castor bean tick)	Borrelial lymphocytoma, Lyme disease
	Ixodes scapularis (deer tick)	Babesiosis, anaplasmosis (granulocytic), ehrlichiosis (granulocytic), Lyme disease
	Ornithodoros species (soft ticks)	Relapsing fever (tick-borne)
	Rhipicephalus sanguineus (brown dog tick)	Mediterranean spotted fever (Boutonneuse fever), RMSF
Crustaceans	*Cyclops* species	Dracunculiasis (Guinea worm disease)

[a]Illustrative examples provided.
RMSF, Rocky Mountain spotted fever; STARI, southern tick associated rash illness.

the lungs (seen with Ancylostomiasis, Ascariasis, and Strongyloidiasis).
- Do NOT confuse Löffler syndrome with Löfgren syndrome.
- Figure 3.32.

Evaluation

- The differential diagnosis of cutaneous larva migrans includes other helminth infections (eg, strongyloidiasis), myiasis, and arthropod bites.

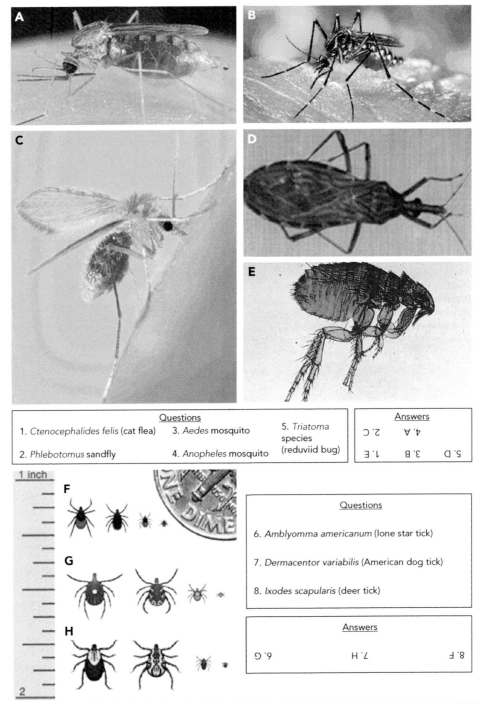

Questions

1. *Ctenocephalides felis* (cat flea)   3. *Aedes* mosquito   5. *Triatoma* species (reduviid bug)

2. *Phlebotomus* sandfly   4. *Anopheles* mosquito

Answers

2. C   4. A

3. B   1. E   5. D

Questions

6. *Amblyomma americanum* (lone star tick)

7. *Dermacentor variabilis* (American dog tick)

8. *Ixodes scapularis* (deer tick)

Answers

6. G   7. H   8. F

Figure 3.30. MATCHING EXERCISE: VECTORS IN DERMATOLOGY. A, The *Anopheles* mosquito is yellow and feeds with hind end pointing up. B, The *Aedes* mosquito has black with white patches and feeds with hind end pointing down. C, The *Phlebotomus* sandfly is hairy and yellow with black eyes. D, The *Triatoma* species (reduviid bug) has a long, thin head. E, *Xenopsylla cheopis* (oriental rat flea) has long, muscular legs and a "hunched" appearance F, *Ixodes scapularis* (deer tick). Adult female: red with dark brown scutum. Adult male: dark brown. G, *Amblyomma americanum* (lone star tick). Adult female: brown with dorsal white spot. Adult male: brown with white markings at the perimeter. H, *Dermacentor variabilis* (American dog tick). Adult female: red-brown with white scutum. Adult male: red brown with dorsal white markings. For each, from left, adult female and male, nymph and larva.

(A, Reprinted with permission from McDonagh DO, Micheli LJ, Frontera WR, et al. *FIMS Sports Medicine Manual: Event Planning and Emergency Care.* Wolters Kluwer Health/Lippincott Williams & Wilkins; 2011. B, Courtesy of James Gathany. From McDonagh DO, Micheli LJ, Frontera WR, et al. *FIMS Sports Medicine Manual: Event Planning and Emergency Care.* Wolters Kluwer Health/Lippincott Williams & Wilkins; 2011. C, Courtesy of James Gathany. From McDonagh DO, Micheli LJ, Frontera WR, et al. *FIMS Sports Medicine Manual: Event Planning and Emergency Care.* Wolters Kluwer Health/Lippincott Williams & Wilkins; 2011. D, Reprinted with permission from Louis ED, Mayer SA, Noble JM. *Merritt's Neurology.* 14th ed. Wolters Kluwer; 2021. E, Reprinted with permission from Procop GW, Church DL, Hall GS, et al. *Koneman's Color Atlas and Textbook of Diagnostic Microbiology.* 7th ed. Wolters Kluwer; 2016. H, Courtesy of the Centers for Disease Control and Prevention. From Scheld WM, Whitley RJ, Marra CM. *Infections of the Central Nervous System.* 4th ed. Wolters Kluwer Health; 2014.)

Table 3.31. PROTOZOAN INFECTIONS

Diagnosis[a]	Parasite	Vector	Classic description	Notes
Ciliophora				
African trypanosomiasis (sleeping sickness)	*Trypanosoma brucei gambiense* (west), *Trypanosoma brucei rhodesiense* (east)	*Glossina* species (tsetse fly)	First stage: chancre at the site of inoculation heals spontaneously with subsequent periodic fever and annular erythema. Winterbottom sign (West African trypanosomiasis): posterior cervical lymphadenopathy. Second stage: daytime somnolence (Kerandel deep delayed hyperesthesia). Winterbottom sign occurs in West African trypanosomiasis at the bottom of the scalp.	Pentamidine is first line.
American trypanosomiasis (Chagas disease)	*Trypanosoma cruzi*	*Triatoma* species (reduviid bug) Common names for the reduviid bug are the "assassin bug" and the "kissing bug."	First stage: erythema and edema at the site of inoculation (chagoma) and lymphadenopathy. Romaña sign: unilateral eyelid edema and conjunctivitis. Second stage: heart block, megaesophagus, megacolon.	Benznidazole is first line.
Flagellates				
Leishmaniasis (old world)	*Leishmania aethiopica,*[b] *Leishmania donovani,*[c] *Leishmania infantum,*[c] *Leishmania major,* *Leishmania tropica.*	*Phlebotomus* species (sandfly)	See above.	
Leishmaniasis (new world)	*Leishmania amazonensis,* *Leishmania brasiliensis,*[b] *Leishmania chagasi,*[c] *Leishmania mexicana,* *Leishmania peruviana.*[b]	*Lutzomyia* species (sandfly)	See above.	
Sarcodina				
Amebiasis	*Acanthamoeba* genus	N/A	Chronic ulcers.	
	Balamuthia mandrillaris	N/A	Painless plaque on the central face. CNS involvement.	
	Entamoeba histolytica	N/A	Perianal cysts, nodules, or ulcers. Colitis.	Can be transmitted as an STD. Metronidazole is first line.
	Naegleria fowleri	N/A	CNS involvement.	Almost invariably fatal.

(Continued)

Table 3.31. PROTOZOAN INFECTIONS (CONTINUED)

Diagnosis[a]	Parasite	Vector	Classic description	Notes
Sporozoans				
Babesiosis	*Babesia* species	*Ixodes scapularis* (deer tick) (Eastern US), *Ixodes pacificus* (western black-legged tick) (western US)	Rarely can develop an exanthem. Petechia can be seen if thrombocytopenic.	Obligate intracellular parasite. Endemic in the northeastern and upper mid-western US (eg, Martha's vineyard).
Malaria	*Plasmodium falciparum, Plasmodium malariae, Plasmodium ovale, Plasmodium vivax*	*Anopheles* species (mosquitoes)	Retiform purpura (rare).	Obligate intracellular parasite. Endemic in large areas of Africa, Asia, Central and South America, and Oceania.
Rhinosporidiosis[d]	*Rhinosporidium seeberi*	N/A	Papillomas favoring the nasal mucosa.	Aquatic fish parasite. Endemic in Africa, Asia (especially India and Sri Lanka), and South America.
Do NOT confuse <u>rhino</u>sporidiosis with <u>rhino</u>scleroma.			Papillomas in rhinosporidiosis are "raspberry-like."	
Toxoplasmosis	*Toxoplasma gondii*	N/A	Immunocompromised: CNS involvement.	Obligate intracellular parasite. Transmitted by cat feces.

[a]Illustrative examples provided.
[b]Mucocutaneous leishmaniasis.
[c]Visceral leishmaniasis.
[d]The classification of *Rhinosporidium seeberi* is controversial as it is alternatively classified as a fungus.
CNS, central nervous system; N/A, not applicable; STD, sexually transmitted disease; US, United States.

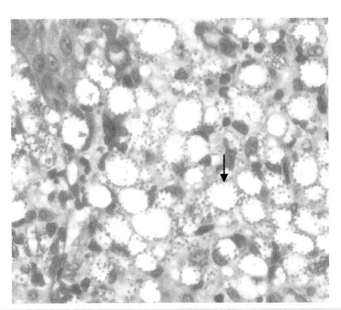

Figure 3.31. CLINICOPATHOLOGICAL CORRELATION: LEISHMANIASIS. Leishmaniasis is characterized by PEH with intraepidermal pustules and intracellular protozoa. Protozoa are randomly spaced within histiocytes or line the periphery of intracellular histiocyte vacuoles (Leishman-Donovan bodies). A kinetoplast is present. Giemsa, CD1a, and PCR highlight the pathogenic organism. Giemsa. Solid arrow: protozoa lining the periphery of intracellular histiocyte vacuoles ("marquee sign").

(Histology image reprinted with permission from Elder DE, Elenitsas R, Rosenbach M, et al. *Lever's Histopathology of the Skin*. 11th ed. Wolters Kluwer; 2015.)

Helpful histopathological features to differentiate leishmaniasis from histoplasmosis include spacing within histiocytes, absence of a pseudocapsule, and presence of a kinetoplast. Protozoa lining the periphery of intracellular histiocyte vacuoles resemble the cache of light bulbs surrounding a marquee ("marquee sign").

Table 3.32. HELMINTH INFECTIONS

Diagnosis[a]	Helminth	Vector	Classic description	Notes
Roundworms (Nematodes)				
Cutaneous larva migrans (creeping eruption)	*Ancylostoma braziliense, Ancylostoma carinum*	N/A	See below.	
Dracunculiasis (Guinea worm disease)	*Dracunculus medinensis*	*Cyclops* species (crustaceans)	Urticaria and pruritus precedes bulla formation, which erupts after ~1 year releasing the worm. The most common location is the lower extremity.	The worm migrates from the gastrointestinal tract to the skin. Use of straws to filter water is a public health measure.
Filariasis	*Wuchereria bancrofti*	*Aedes* species, *Anopheles* species, *Culex* species, *Mansonia* species (mosquitoes)	Acute: recurrent fever and lymphangitis. Chronic: lymphedema.	Diethylcarbamazine is first line.
Gnathostomiasis	*Gnathostoma dolorosi, Gnathostoma spinigerum*	N/A	Gnathostomiasis moves 1 cm/d, creating recurrent migratory erythematous urticarial plaques every 2-6 weeks.	Food-borne zoonosis from freshwater fish.
Ground itch	*Ancylostoma duodenale, Necator americanus*	N/A	Similar to cutaneous larva migrans with pulmonary involvement.	Human hookworms. Albendazole or mebendazole is first line.
Loiasis (Calabar swelling)	*Loa loa*	*Chrysops* species (deer flies, mango flies)	Subcutaneous edema primarily surrounding joints (Calabar swelling) ± conjunctivitis.	The patient may observe the adult worm migrating across the conjunctiva. Diethylcarbamazine is first line.
Onchocerciasis (river blindness)	*Onchocerca volvulus*	*Simulium* species (black fly)	Subcutaneous nodules (onchocercomas), dermatitis, and depigmentation on the lower extremities. Sclerosis keratitis may result in vision loss. ⬚ Depigmentation on the lower extremities is sometimes called "leopard skin."	Near fast-flowing rivers in Sub-Saharan Africa. Skin snip is the preferred bedside diagnostic. Ivermectin or diethylcarbamazine is first line; however, diethylcarbamazine treatment may be complicated by the Mazzotti reaction.
Pinworm infection	*Enterobius vermicularis*	N/A	Perianal pruritus.	The "scotch tape" test is the preferred bedside diagnostic. Albendazole or mebendazole is first line.
Strongyloidiasis (larva currens, racing larva)	*Strongyloides stercoralis*	N/A	Strongyloidiasis moves rapidly (5-10 cm/h), creating urticaria and periumbilical purpura. Diarrhea is common. ⬚ Periumbilical purpura in strongyloidiasis is called "thumbprint purpura."	The life cycle is complex and involves migration of larvae to the lungs, where they are coughed up, swallowed, and ultimately result in fecal transmission. Ivermectin is first line.
Trichinosis (trichinellosis)	*Trichinella spiralis*	N/A	Periorbital edema and proximal splinter hemorrhages.	Food-borne zoonosis from undercooked meat (eg, pork). Perform muscle biopsy.

(Continued)

Table 3.32. HELMINTH INFECTIONS (CONTINUED)

Diagnosis[a]	Helminth	Vector	Classic description	Notes
Flukes (trematodes)				
Cercarial dermatitis (clam digger's itch, duck itch, Swimmer's itch)	*Trichobilharzia* species (avian schistosome)	N/A	Pruritic erythematous macules and papules in exposed areas.	Transmission via contaminated water. Larvae die immediately but cause a short-term immune reaction.
Schistosomiasis (snail fever)	*Schistosoma haematobium*, *Schistosoma japonicum*, *Schistosoma mansoni*	N/A	Acute (Katayama fever). Chronic gastrointestinal and urogenital involvement.	Transmission via contaminated water.
Tapeworms (Cestodes)				
Cysticercosis	*Taenia solium*	N/A	Subcutaneous nodules.	

[a]Illustrative examples provided.
GI, gastrointestinal; N/A, not applicable.

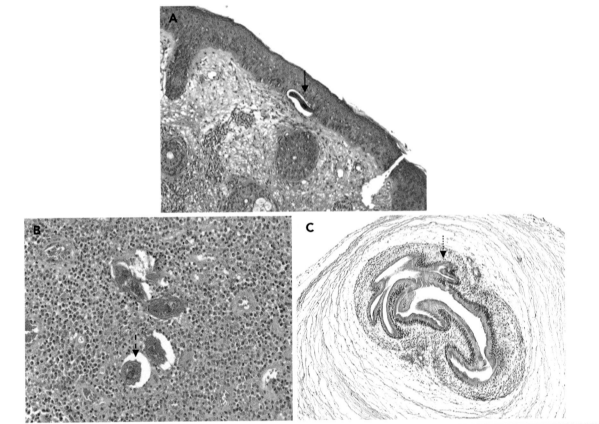

Figure 3.32. CLINICOPATHOLOGICAL CORRELATION: CUTANEOUS LARVA MIGRANS AND SELECTED OTHER HELMINTHS. A, Cutaneous larva migrans. Solid arrow: larva. B, Avian schistosomiasis. Dashed arrow: ovum. C, Cysticercosis. Dotted arrow: larva.

(A, Reprinted with permission from Mercado R, González-Chávez J, Sánchez JL, et al. Erythematous plaque in the cheek of an HIV patient. *Am J Dermatopathol.* 2016;38(7):531-532. Figure 3. B, Reprinted with permission from Edward S, Yung A. *Essential Dermatopathology.* Wolters Kluwer Health/Lippincott Williams & Wilkins; 2011. C, Histology image courtesy of Dieter Krahl, MD, Institut für DermatoHistoPathologie. From Elder DE, Elenitsas R, Rosenbach M, et al. *Lever's Histopathology of the Skin.* 11th ed. Wolters Kluwer; 2015.)

Selected roundworm (nematode)
• **Cutaneous larva migrans**: epidermis containing larvae (curvilinear and eosinophilic).
Selected fluke (trematode)
• **Schistosomiasis**: granuloma containing ova (chitinous wall ± apical or lateral spine and central stippling).
Selected tapeworm (cestode)
• **Cysticercosis**: cystic cavity containing larvae (scolex with hooklets and two pairs of suckers, double-layered eosinophilic membrane with duct-like invaginations, and body wall with myxoid matrix and calcareous bodies).

- Cutaneous larva migrans is primarily a clinical diagnosis; however, skin biopsy can be helpful.

Management

- Cutaneous larval migrans is usually self-limited.
- **Albendazole and ivermectin** are first line.

SPOTLIGHT ON HYPER-IMMUNOGLOBULIN E SYNDROMES

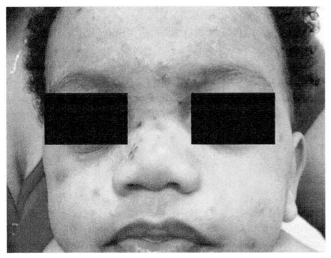

Autosomal dominant hyper immunoglobulin E syndrome courtesy of Barrett Zlotoff, MD. From Gru AA, Wick MR, Mir A, et al. *Pediatric Dermatopathology and Dermatology*. Wolters Kluwer; 2018.

"Real World" Advice

- A localized hypersensitivity reaction often leads to intense pruritus requiring anti-pruritic therapy (eg, topical corticosteroids, antihistamines).

- **Hyper-IgE syndromes** are a collection of genetically distinct disorders characterized by eczematous dermatitis, recurrent skin and sinopulmonary infections, and elevated IgE.
  - **AD hyper-IgE syndrome** is due to **loss-of-function *STAT3* mutations (Job syndrome).**
  - **AR hyper-IgE syndrome** is due to *DOCK8, PGM3,* and *TYK2* **mutations.**
- Clinical features of hyper-IgE syndromes include **eczematous dermatitis, papulopustular eruptions, viral infections, recurrent pyogenic infections (cold abscesses), and mucocutaneous candidiasis. Coarse facies and retained primary teeth** are characteristic of **AD** but not AR hyper-IgE syndrome.
  - Spongiotic dermatitis is a histopathological feature of hyper-IgE syndromes.
- **Increased polyclonal IgE (10-fold over normal level)** is characteristic. Patients also frequently have evidence of impaired cell-mediated immunity.
- Management is predicated on the control of infectious complications (eg, I&D and antibacterial therapy for cold abscesses). Recombinant IFN-γ and IVIG may improve some cutaneous and infectious complications.

SCABIES AND LICE
→ **Diagnosis Group 1**

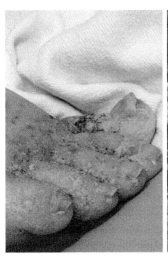 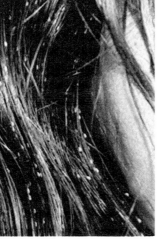

Scabies (left)
Lice (right) reprinted with permission from Lugo-Somolinos A, McKinley-Grant L, Goldsmith LA, et al. *VisualDx: Essential Dermatology in Pigmented Skin*. Wolters Kluwer Health/Lippincott Williams & Wilkins; 2011.

Epidemiology

- **Scabies** is due to the ectoparasite *Sarcoptes scabiei var hominis* **(itch mite).** Crusted scabies (Norwegian scabies) can be seen in elderly and immunosuppressed patients with significantly higher numbers of mites.
- **Lice infestation** is due to the ectoparasites *Pediculus humanus var corporis* **(body louse),** *Pediculus humanus var capitis* **(head louse), and** *Pthirus pubis* **(crab louse).**

Clinicopathological Features

- The characteristic presentation of **ectoparasite infestations** is summarized in Table 3.33.
  - In **infants, scabies** may involve the **scalp and face** is in the differential diagnosis for **diaper dermatitis.**
  - Figure 3.33.
  - Figure 3.34. For the histopathology of *Demodex folliculorum*, see Figure 2.80.

Evaluation

- The differential diagnosis of scabies includes ACD, BP, prurigo nodularis, and arthropod bites.

Table 3.33. ECTOPARASITE INFESTATIONS

Diagnosis[a]	Ectoparasite	Classic description	Notes
Fleas			
Pulicosis	*Pulex irritans* (human flea)	Red macules with central puncta.	Primarily in dogs and humans.
Tungiasis	*Tunga penetrans*	Nodules with central black dots (posterior end of the flea sticking out) favoring the soles, toe webs, and toenail folds.	Endemic in the Caribbean.
Flies			
Myiasis	*Dermatobia hominis* (botfly larva)	Small red papule evolves into a nodule with a central pore ± visible larva.	
True Bugs			
Bed bug infestation	*Cimex lectularius* (bed bug)	Grouped pruritic macules and papules on exposed skin.	
Mites[b]			
Baker's itch	*Acarus siro* (grain mite)	Pruritic papulovesicles favoring the upper extremities.	
Cheyletiellosis	*Cheyletiella* species	Walking dandruff.	Primarily in cats, dogs, and rabbits.
Chigger bites	*Trombiculid* species (chigger mites)	Pruritic papulovesicles favoring the belt line or lower extremities.	Etiology of summer penile syndrome in males.
Demodicosis	*Demodex folliculorum* (skin mites)	Rosacea, pityriasis folliculorum, and steroid-induced rosacea.	
Grocer's itch	*Tyrophagus casei* (cheese mite)	Pruritic papulovesicles favoring the upper extremities.	
Scabies	*Sarcoptes scabiei var hominis* (itch mite)	Pruritic papulovesicles and burrows sparing the scalp and face (except in infants and crusted scabies) and concentrated in folds, umbilicus, and groin.	Pruritus develops over 3-4 weeks (reflecting the 30-day life cycle).
		Scabies lesions resemble "grains of sand."	
Lice			
Pediculosis capitis (cooties)	*Pediculus humanus var capitis* (head louse)	Pruritic or asymptomatic. White lice eggs glued to the hair shaft (close to the scalp, posterior auricular, and nape of neck).	Insects can survive 36 h away from the host, enabling transmission through linen.
Pediculosis corporis	*Pediculus humanus var corporis* (body louse)	Pruritic papulovesicles.	
Pediculosis pubis (crabs)	*Pthirus pubis* (crab louse, pubic louse)	Blue macules (*maculae ceruleae*).	
Ticks			
Tick bites	*Amblyomma americanum* (lone star tick), *Dermacentor andersoni* (Rocky Mountain wood tick), *Dermacentor variabilis* (American dog tick), *Ixodes pacificus* (western black-legged tick), *Ixodes ricinus* (castor bean tick), *Ixodes scapularis* (deer tick), *Ornithodoros* species (soft ticks), *Rhipicephalus sanguineus* (brown dog tick)	Purpura at tick bite site.	

[a]Illustrative examples provided.
[b]*Dermatophagoides farinae* (dust mites) are an environmental trigger of AD.
AD, atopic dermatitis.

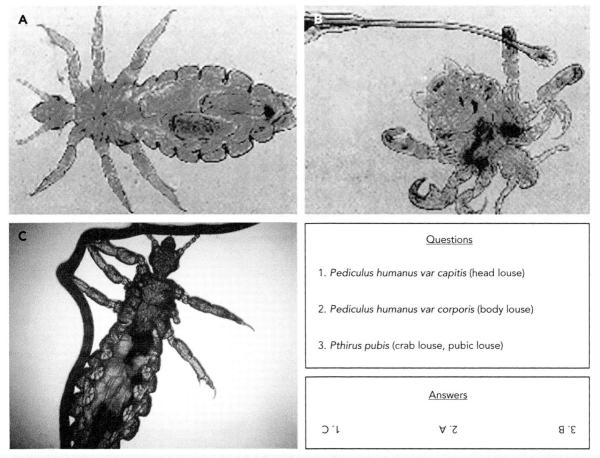

Figure 3.33. MATCHING EXERCISE: LICE. A, *Pediculus humanus var corporis* (body louse). B, *Pthirus pubis* (crab louse, pubic louse). C, *Pediculus humanus var capitis* (head louse).

(A, Reprinted with permission from Procop GW, Church DL, Hall GS, et al. *Koneman's Color Atlas and Textbook of Diagnostic Microbiology.* 7th ed. Wolters Kluwer; 2016. B, Reprinted with permission from Procop GW, Church DL, Hall GS, et al. *Koneman's Color Atlas and Textbook of Diagnostic Microbiology.* 7th ed. Wolters Kluwer; 2016. C, Reprinted with permission from Craft N, Fox LP, Goldsmith LA, et al. *VisualDx: Essential Adult Dermatology.* Wolters Kluwer Health/Lippincott Williams & Wilkins; 2010.)

In **infants**, the differential diagnosis of **scabies** includes **acropustulosis of infancy.** This disorder typically occurs between 6 months to 2 years of age and **resolves by 3 years of age. Recurrent crops of pruritic pustules on the distal extremities, especially the palms and soles that recur every 2 to 4 weeks with interval resolution,** is characteristic.

- Acropustulosis of infancy is an intraepidermal blister (split below the *stratum granulosum*).
- The differential diagnosis of lice includes hair casts, trichorrhexis nodosa, and white piedra.
- In **scabies, dermoscopy** reveals a **small dark brown triangular structure (corresponding to the anterior part of the mite) located at the end of a white line (corresponding to the burrow).**
  - The small dark brown triangular structure located at the end of a white line is called the "delta wing jet with contrail" sign.
- **Mineral oil preparation** is the preferred bedside diagnostic for scabies.

Management

- Scabies management includes **head to toe application of permethrin cream or oral ivermectin.** Treatment of crusted scabies involves a combination of both.
- Machine wash (>50 °C) and dry all bedding/clothes with suspected contamination 3 days before treatment initiation (as mites can only live off human hosts for 2-3 days).
- Topical permethrin is the preferred agent for use during pregnancy.
  - Permethrin is FDA-approved for scabies >2 months. Precipitated sulfur can be used for younger infants; however, it must be compounded and used 3 days in a row. It can also be irritating to the skin and malodorous.
- Treatments for head lice include malathion, lindane, permethrin, pyrethrins, and topical/oral ivermectin.

"Real World" Advice

- **Head lice nits are cemented to the hair shaft, while hair casts slide freely along the hair shaft.**

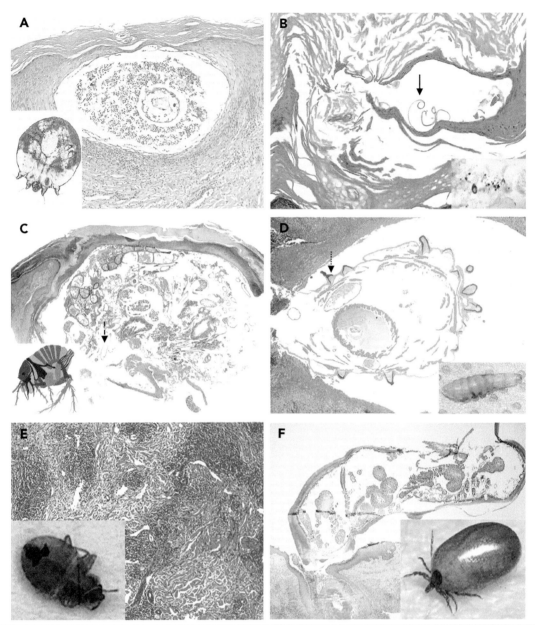

Figure 3.34. CLINICOPATHOLOGICAL CORRELATION: SCABIES AND SELECTED OTHER ECTOPARASITES. In scabies, the *Sarcoptes scabiei var hominis* itch mite, ova, and scybala are in the *stratum corneum*. In tungiasis, the gravid female *Tunga penetrans* flea is superficial within acral skin with red hollow tubules, striated muscle, and a blood-filled gut. In myiasis, the *Dermatobia hominis* botfly larva has a thick corrugated chitinous wall, pigmented setae, striated muscle, and a gut. In a bed bug bite, *Cimex lenticularis* induces an arthropod bite reaction, which is characterized by a wedge-shaped perivascular lymphoid infiltrate with eosinophils ± subepidermal bulla. In a tick bite, the tick induces a wedge-shaped area of neutrophilic inflammation and necrosis. The tick has a thick chitinous wall, striated muscle, pigmented mouthparts, and a blood-filled gut. A and B, Scabies. Solid arrow: "pigtails." C, Tungiasis. Dashed arrow: red hollow tubules. D, Myiasis. Dotted arrow: pigmented setae. E, Bed bug bite. F, Tick bite.

(A, Inset reprinted with permission from Elder DE, Elenitsas R, Rosenbach M, et al. *Lever's Histopathology of the Skin*. 11th ed. Wolters Kluwer; 2015; histology image courtesy of Noel Turner, MD, MHS and Christine J. Ko, MD. B, Inset reprinted with permission from Craft N, Fox LP, Goldsmith LA, et al. *VisualDx: Essential Adult Dermatology*. Wolters Kluwer Health/Lippincott Williams & Wilkins; 2010; histopathology image reprinted with permission from Elder DE, Elenitsas R, Rosenbach M, et al. *Lever's Histopathology of the Skin*. 11th ed. Wolters Kluwer; 2015. C, Inset illustration by Caroline A. Nelson, MD; histopathology image reprinted with permission from Elder DE, Elenitsas R, Rosenbach M, et al. *Lever's Histopathology of the Skin*, 11th ed. Wolters Kluwer; 2015. D, Inset reprinted with permission from Fleisher GR, Ludwig S, Baskin MN. *Atlas of Pediatric Emergency Medicine*. Lippincott Williams & Wilkins; 2004; histopathology image courtesy of Dieter Krahl, MD, Institut für DermatoHistoPathologie. From Elder DE, Elenitsas R, Rosenbach M, et al. *Lever's Histopathology of the Skin*. 11th ed. Wolters Kluwer; 2015. E, Histopathology image reprinted with permission from Elder DE, Elenitsas R, Rubin AI, et al. *Atlas of Dermatopathology: Synopsis and Atlas of Lever's Histopathology of the Skin*. 4th ed. Wolters Kluwer; 2020. F, Inset reprinted with permission from Onofrey BE, Skorin L Jr, Holdeman NR. *Ocular Therapeutics Handbook: A Clinical Manual*. 3rd ed. Wolters Kluwer Health/Lippincott Williams & Wilkins; 2012; histopathology image reprinted with permission from Elder DE, Elenitsas R, Rosenbach M, et al. *Lever's Histopathology of the Skin*. 11th ed. Wolters Kluwer; 2015.)

"Chitin scrolls" and "pigtails" (likely eggshell remnants) may provide a helpful clue to the diagnosis of scabies.

- So called "no nit" policies are impractical and lead to unnecessary absences from school for children. Children should return to the classroom after appropriate treatment for lice has begun.
- Resistance to permethrin and pyrethrins for head lice treatment is increasing worldwide.

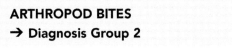

ARTHROPOD BITES
→ **Diagnosis Group 2**

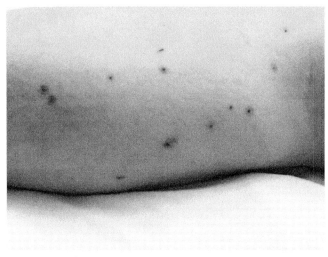

Epidemiology

- **Arthropod bites and stings** are a common occurrence worldwide, though they are more prevalent in warmer climates and a seasonal concern in temperate zones.
- **Bullous arthropod bites** are associated with hematologic disorders, particularly **CLL.**

Clinicopathological Features

- Arthropod bites classically present with **grouped, localized or disseminated, pink to red dermal papules** with associated **pruritus.**

Papular urticaria refers to a reaction pattern seen in **children** with a more widespread urticarial eruption to localized bites. It is presumed to be due to a lack of desensitization to arthropod antigens that occurs by adulthood.

- Less common clinical features include purpuric papules and nodules, vesicles, bullae, and targetoid lesions.
- The characteristic presentation of specific **animal bites and stings** is summarized in Table 3.34.
  - Figure 3.35.
  - For the histopathology of arthropod bites, see Figure 3.34.

Evaluation

- The differential diagnosis of arthropod bites includes ACD, impetigo, and furunculosis.
- History and physical examination are generally sufficient to make the diagnosis of arthropod bites; however, skin biopsy can be helpful.

Management

- N,N-diethyl-3-methylbenzamide (DEET) is the cornerstone of prevention for a wide range of arthropod bites and stings. As limited data support the use of DEET for tick bite prevention, 0.5% permethrin treatment of clothing and gear is often recommended.
- Antipruritic therapy typically entails the use of topical corticosteroids and antihistamines.

"Real World" Advice

- Lesion configuration is often a critical clue to the diagnosis of arthropod bites.
  - The common grouping of three bed bug bites in a linear configuration is called "breakfast, lunch, and dinner."

Table 3.34. ANIMAL BITES AND STINGS

Diagnosis[a]	Animal	Classic description	Notes
Arachnids			
Mites	See Table 3.33.		
Spiders	*Cheiracanthium* species (yellow sack spiders)	Painful bite.	Distinctive features: beige or pale yellow. Toxin: lipase. Treatment: supportive.
	Eratigena agrestis (hobo spider)	Painless bite ± necrosis and CNS involvement.	Distinctive features: brown and hairy with a herringbone pattern. Treatment: supportive.
	Latrodectus mactans (black widow spider)	Painful edematous bite with systemic symptoms mimicking acute abdomen and paralysis/spasms.	Distinctive features: black with a red hourglass-shaped marking. Toxin: α-latrotoxin (depolarizes neurons). Treatment: antivenin, benzodiazepine, IV calcium gluconate.
	Loxosceles reclusa (brown recluse spider)	Painful bite with necrosis ± DIC and shock.	Distinctive features: brown with a dark violin-shaped marking. Toxin: sphingomyelinase D. Treatment: ice, elevation, ± dapsone.
		A brown recluse spider bite is "red, white, and blue."	
	Lycosidae family (wolf spiders)	Painful bite ± eschar and lymphangitis.	Distinctive features: brown-gray with three rows of eyes (bottom row has four eyes) and a peach-colored stripe. Toxin: histamine. Treatment: supportive.
			Wolves howl, bark, and hiss (histamine).
	Peucetia viridans (green lynx spider)	Painful edematous bite.	Distinctive features: bright green with red spots and black spines. Treatment: supportive.
	Phidippus species (jumping spiders)	Painful bite.	Distinctive features: brown and hairy with two large eyes in the middle front row. Toxin: hyaluronidase. Treatment: supportive.
	Theraphosidae species (tarantulas)	Pruritic wheel or ophthalmia nodosa with risk of vision loss.	Distinctive features: large, brown, and hairy. Toxin: urticating hairs. Treatment: supportive.
Scorpions	*Centruroides* species	Painful sting with paresthesias ± cardiopulmonary/neurologic involvement.	Distinctive features: two poison glands open into two stingers. Treatment: remove stinger, cold compresses, elevation, analgesics, topical corticosteroids, antihistamines.
Ticks	See Table 3.33.		
Insects			
Ants	*Solenopsis* species (fire ants)	Painful sterile pustule with erythematous halo, pruritic wheel ± anaphylaxis and neurologic involvement (if multiple).	Distinctive features: red. Toxin: hemolytic factor, solenopsins (piperidine alkaloids that release histamine). Treatment: supportive.
Bees, wasps, hornets	*Hymenoptera* class	Anaphylaxis.	Distinctive features: yellow stripes. Toxin: phospholipase. Treatment: remove stinger; cold compresses, analgesics, topical corticosteroids, antihistamines.

Table 3.34. ANIMAL BITES AND STINGS (CONTINUED)

Diagnosis[a]	Animal	Classic description	Notes
Beetles	*Lytta vesicatoria* (blister beetle)	Vesicle or bulla.	Distinctive features: slender, soft-bodied beetle with metallic golden-green color. Toxin: cantharidin. Treatment: rinse off cantharidin; cold compresses, analgesics, topical corticosteroids.
	Anthrenus species, *Attagenus* species (carpet beetles)	Allergic papulovesicular dermatitis.	Distinctive features: oval shape beetle with white, yellow, and black scales. Treatment: topical corticosteroids, fumigation of infestation.
Caterpillars, butterflies, and moths	*Lonomia obliqua* (giant silkworm moth)	Sting with internal hemorrhage, hemolysis, and renal failure.	Distinctive features: stout, hairy body with feathery antennae and often bright colors. Treatment: supportive.
	Megalopyge opercularis (asp caterpillar, pus caterpillar, wholly slug)	Hemorrhagic burning painful linear track marks.	Distinctive features: woolly appearance, parallel rows of stiff hollow spines on dorsum. Treatment: adhesive tape to remove spines; cold compresses, analgesics.
Flies/fleas	See Table 3.33.		

Myriapods

Centipedes	*Chilopoda* class	Two hemorrhagic puncture wounds ± pain, edema, paresthesias. The two hemorrhagic puncture wounds make the "Chevron" shape.	Distinctive features: nocturnal carnivores with jaws. Toxin: neurotoxic venom. Treatment: symptomatic.
Millipedes	*Diplopoda* class	ICD with burning, blistering, or pigmentation ± conjunctivitis.	Distinctive features: harmless vegetarians. Treatment: topical corticosteroids.

Other Animals

Hedgehogs	*Erinaceidae* family	Urticaria.	Distinctive features: spines. Treatment: supportive.
Jellyfish	*Cyaneidae* family	Painful sting, flagellate erythema ± shock.	Distinctive features: tendrils coated with nematocysts that sting. Treatment: 5% acetic acid.
Sea cucumbers	*Holothuroidea* family	Conjunctivitis.	Distinctive features: tubules that are discharged when the sea cucumber is threatened. Toxin: holothurin. Treatment: supportive.
Sea lice	*Edwardsiella lineata* (sea anemone) *Linuche unguiculata* (thimble jellyfish larvae)	Seabather's eruption: pruritic papules on covered areas.	Distinctive features: sea lice trapped underneath the bathing suit. Treatment: 5% acetic acid can neutralize residual toxin; topical corticosteroids.
Sea urchins	*Echinoidea* class	ICD, synovitis and arthritis (near joints).	Distinctive features: spines. Treatment: 5% acetic acid.
Snakes	*Crotalidae* (pit vipers) family: copperhead, cottonmouth moccasin, rattlesnake.	*Crotalinae* bites typically cause local tissue and muscle damage as well as hematologic/cardiovascular complications.	Distinctive features: temperature-sensitive pit organ located on each side of the head. Treatment: tourniquet use/pressure immobilization may increase local tissue damage (controversial); antivenin.
	Elapidae family: coral snake.	Coral snake bites can cause neuromuscular weakness and resulting respiratory failure.	Distinctive features: black, yellow, and red stripes. Treatment: tourniquet use/pressure immobilization may prevent systemic spread of venom; antivenin.
			Venomous coral snake: "red touch yellow, kills a fellow." Nonvenomous king snake: "red touch black, safe for Jack."

[a]Illustrative examples provided.
CNS, central nervous system; DIC, disseminated intravascular coagulation; ICD, irritant contact dermatitis; IV, intravenous.

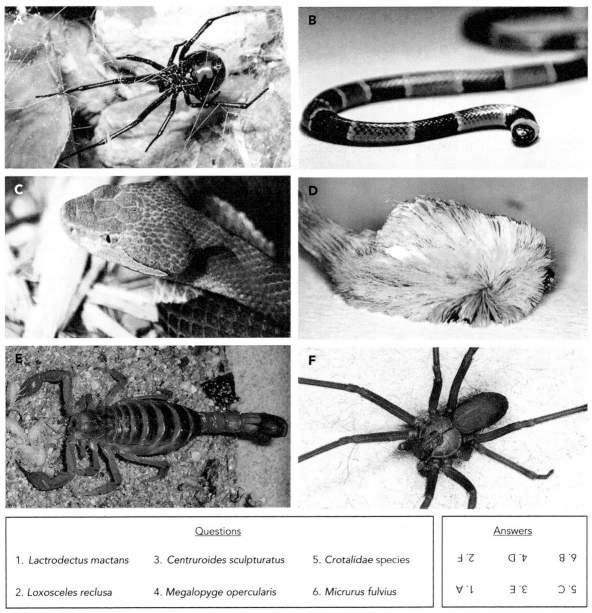

Questions

1. *Lactrodectus mactans*   3. *Centruroides sculpturatus*   5. *Crotalidae* species

2. *Loxosceles reclusa*   4. *Megalopyge opercularis*   6. *Micrurus fulvius*

Answers

6. B   4. D   2. F

5. C   3. E   1. A

Figure 3.35. MATCHING EXERCISE: ANIMALS. A, *Latrodectus mactans* (black widow spider). Note the red hourglass-shaped marking. B, *Micrurus fulvius* (Eastern coral snake). Note the characteristic pattern "red touch yellow, kills a fellow." C, *Crotalidae* (pit viper) species (copperhead snake). Note the temperature-sensitive pit organ located on each side of the head. D, *Megalopyge opercularis* (asp caterpillar, puss caterpillar, woolly slug). Note the woolly appearance. E, *Centruroides sculpturatus* (Arizona bark scorpion). Note the two stingers. F, *Loxosceles reclusa* (brown recluse spider). Note the dark violin-shaped marking.

(A, Reprinted with permission from Dimick JB, Upchurch GR Jr, Alam HB, et al. *Mulholland and Greenfield's Surgery: Scientific Principles and Practice.* 7th ed. Wolters Kluwer; 2021. B, Courtesy of Lt. Scott Mullin from Venom One. From Hawkins SC. *Wilderness EMS.* Wolters Kluwer; 2018. C, Courtesy of Ronald M. Stewart, MD. From Mulholland MW, Lillemoe KD, Doherty GM, et al. *Greenfield's Surgery: Scientific Principles and Practice.* 6th ed. Wolters Kluwer; 2016. D, Reprinted with permission from Dimick JB, Upchurch GR Jr, Alam HB, et al. *Mulholland and Greenfield's Surgery: Scientific Principles and Practice.* 7th ed. Wolters Kluwer; 2021. E, Reprinted with permission from Dimick JB, Upchurch GR Jr, Alam HB, et al. *Mulholland and Greenfield's Surgery: Scientific Principles and Practice.* 7th ed. Wolters Kluwer; 2021. F, Reprinted with permission from Mulholland MW, Lillemoe KD, Doherty GM, et al. *Greenfield's Surgery: Scientific Principles and Practice.* 6th ed. Wolters Kluwer; 2016.)

FURTHER READING

Awad MM, Ellemor DM, Boyd RL, Emmins JJ, Rood JI. Synergistic effects of alpha-toxin and perfringolysin O in Clostridium perfringens-mediated gas gangrene. *Infect Immun.* 2001;69(12):7904-7910. doi:10.1128/iai.69.12.7904-7910.2001

Baum MK, Lai S, Sales S, Page JB, Campa A. Randomized, controlled clinical trial of zinc supplementation to prevent immunological failure in HIV-infected adults. *Clin Infect Dis.* 2010;50(12):1653-1660. doi:10.1086/652864

Berger AP, Ford BA, Brown-Joel Z, Shields BE, Rosenbach M, Wanat KA. Angioinvasive fungal infections impacting the skin: diagnosis, management, and complications. *J Am Acad Dermatol.* 2019;80(4):883-898.e2. doi:10.1016/j.jaad.2018.04.058

Bhate C, Schwartz RA. Lyme disease: Part II. Management and prevention. *J Am Acad Dermatol.* 2011;64(4):639-653; quiz 654, 653. doi:10.1016/j.jaad.2010.03.047

Bhate C, Schwartz RA. Lyme disease: Part I. Advances and perspectives. *J Am Acad Dermatol.* 2011;64(4):619-636; quiz 637-638. doi:10.1016/j.jaad.2010.03.046

Böer A, Herder N, Winter K, Falk T. Herpes folliculitis: clinical, histopathological, and molecular pathologic observations. *Br J Dermatol.* 2006;154(4):743-746. doi:10.1111/j.1365-2133.2005.07118.x

Bolognia JL, Schaffer JV, Cerroni L. *Dermatology.* 4 ed. Elsevier Saunders; 2018.

Bradley H, Markowitz LE, Gibson T, McQuillan GM. Seroprevalence of herpes simplex virus types 1 and 2–United States, 1999-2010. *J Infect Dis.* 2014;209(3):325-333. doi:10.1093/infdis/jit458

Buzi F, Badolato R, Mazza C, et al. Autoimmune polyendocrinopathy-candidiasis-ectodermal dystrophy syndrome: time to review diagnostic criteria?. *J Clin Endocrinol Metab.* 2003;88(7):3146-3148. doi:10.1210/jc.2002-021495

Cale CM, Morton L, Goldblatt D. Cutaneous and other lupus-like symptoms in carriers of X-linked chronic granulomatous disease: incidence and autoimmune serology. *Clin Exp Immunol.* 2007;148(1):79-84. doi:10.1111/j.1365-2249.2007.03321.x

Carlson JA, Chen KR. Cutaneous vasculitis update: small vessel neutrophilic vasculitis syndromes. *Am J Dermatopathol.* 2006;28(6):486-506. doi:10.1097/01.dad.0000246646.45651.a2

Carlson A, Norwitz ER, Stiller RJ. Cytomegalovirus infection in pregnancy: should all women be screened? *Rev Obstet Gynecol.* 2010;3(4):172-179.

Caulfield AJ, Wengenack NL. Diagnosis of active tuberculosis disease: from microscopy to molecular techniques. *J Clin Tuberc Other Mycobact Dis.* 2016;4:33-43. doi:10.1016/j.jctube.2016.05.005

CDC. Accessed May 8, 2021. https://www.cdc.gov/vaccines/vpd/varicella/hcp/recommendations.html

Coates SJ, Thomas C, Chosidow O, Engelman D, Chang AY. Ectoparasites: Pediculosis and tungiasis. *J Am Acad Dermatol.* 2020;82(3):551-569. https://www.jaad.org/article/S0190-9622(19)32386-2/fulltext

Colmenero I, Santonja C, Alonso-Riaño M, et al. SARS-CoV-2 endothelial infection causes COVID-19 chilblains: histopathological, immunohistochemical and ultrastructural study of seven paediatric cases. *Br J Dermatol.* 2020;183(4):729-737. doi:10.1111/bjd.19327

Corey L, Bodsworth N, Mindel A, Patel R, Schacker T, Stanberry L. An update on short-course episodic and prevention therapies for herpes genitalis. *Herpes.* 2007;14(suppl 1):5a-11a.

Culora GA, Ramsay AD, Theaker JM. Aluminium and injection site reactions. *J Clin Pathol.* 1996;49(10):844-847. doi:10.1136/jcp.49.10.844

de Jong SJ, Créquer A, Matos I, et al. The human CIB1-EVER1-EVER2 complex governs keratinocyte-intrinsic immunity to β-papillomaviruses. *J Exp Med.* 2018;215(9):2289-2310. doi:10.1084/jem.20170308

de Oliveira WRP, Festa Neto C, Rady PL, Tyring SK. Clinical aspects of epidermodysplasia verruciformis. *J Eur Acad Dermatol Venereol.* 2003;17(4):394-398. doi:10.1046/j.1468-3083.2003.00703.x

Doorbar J, Egawa N, Griffin H, Kranjec C, Murakami I. Human papillomavirus molecular biology and disease association. *Rev Med Virol.* 2015;25(suppl 1):2-23. doi:10.1002/rmv.1822

Dorn JM, Patnaik MS, Van Hee M, et al. WILD syndrome is GATA2 deficiency: a novel deletion in the GATA2 gene. *J Allergy Clin Immunol Pract.* 2017;5(4):1149-1152.e1. doi:10.1016/j.jaip.2017.02.010

Elder DE. *Lever's Histopathology of the Skin.* 11 ed. Wolters Kluwer; 2015.

Elston DM, Ferringer T. *Dermatopathology.* 2 ed. Elsevier Saunders; 2014.

Eminger LA, Hall LD, Hesterman KS, Heymann WR. Epstein-Barr virus – dermatologic associations and implications—part II. Associated lymphoproliferative disorders and solid tumors. *J Am Acad Dermatol.* 2015;72(1):21-34; quiz 35-36. doi:10.1016/j.jaad.2014.07.035

Fitz-Gibbon S, Tomida S, Chiu BH, et al. Propionibacterium acnes strain populations in the human skin microbiome associated with acne. *J Invest Dermatol.* 2013;133(9):2152-2160. doi:10.1038/jid.2013.21

Forrestel AK, Kovarik CL, Katz KA. Sexually acquired syphilis: historical aspects, microbiology, epidemiology, and clinical manifestations. *J Am Acad Dermatol.* 2020;82(1):1-14. doi:10.1016/j.jaad.2019.02.073

Forrestel AK, Kovarik CL, Katz KA. Sexually acquired syphilis: laboratory diagnosis, management, and prevention. *J Am Acad Dermatol.* 2020;82(1):17-28. doi:10.1016/j.jaad.2019.02.074

Freeman EE, McMahon DE, Lipoff JB, et al. The spectrum of COVID-19-associated dermatologic manifestations: an international registry of 716 patients from 31 countries. *J Am Acad Dermatol.* 2020;83(4):1118-1129. doi:10.1016/j.jaad.2020.06.1016

Galván Casas C, Català A, Carretero Hernández G, et al. Classification of the cutaneous manifestations of COVID-19: a rapid prospective nationwide consensus study in Spain with 375 cases. *Br J Dermatol.* 2020;183(1):71-77. doi:10.1111/bjd.19163

Gormley RH, Kovarik CL. Human papillomavirus-related genital disease in the immunocompromised host: Part II. *J Am Acad Dermatol.* 2012;66(6):883.e1-17. quiz 899-900. doi:10.1016/j.jaad.2010.12.049

Gormley RH, Kovarik CL. Human papillomavirus-related genital disease in the immunocompromised host: Part I. *J Am Acad Dermatol.* 2012;66(6):867.e1-867.e14. quiz 881-882. doi:10.1016/j.jaad.2010.12.050

Haddad V Jr. Lupi O, Lonza JP, Tyring SK. Tropical dermatology: marine and aquatic dermatology. *J Am Acad Dermatol.* 2009;61(5):733-750; quiz 751-752. doi:10.1016/j.jaad.2009.01.046

Haddad V Jr. Cardoso JL, Lupi O, Tyring SK. Tropical dermatology—venomous arthropods and human skin—Part II. Diplopoda, Chilopoda, and Arachnida. *J Am Acad Dermatol.* 2012;67(3):347.e1-347.e7 quiz 355. doi:10.1016/j.jaad.2012.05.028.

Haddad V Jr. Cardoso JLC, Lupi O, Tyring SK. Tropical dermatology—venomous arthropods and human skin—Part I. Insecta. *J Am Acad Dermatol.* 2012;67(3):331.e1-331.e14; quiz 345. https://www.jaad.org/article/S0190-9622(12)00623-8/fulltext

Haley CT, Mui UN, Vangipuram R, Rady PL, Tyring SK. Human oncoviruses—mucocutaneous manifestations, pathogenesis, therapeutics, and prevention: papillomaviruses and Merkel cell polyomavirus. *J Am Acad Dermatol.* 2019;81(1):1-21. doi:10.1016/j.jaad.2018.09.062

Hall LD, Eminger LA, Hesterman KS, Heymann WR. Epstein-Barr virus—dermatologic associations and implications: part I. Mucocutaneous manifestations of Epstein-Barr virus and nonmalignant disorders. *J Am Acad Dermatol.* 2015;72(1):1-19; quiz 19-20. doi:10.1016/j.jaad.2014.07.034

Handler MZ, Handler NS, Majewski S, Schwartz RA. Human papillomavirus vaccine trials and tribulations: clinical perspectives. *J Am Acad Dermatol.* 2015;73(5):743-756; quiz 757-758. doi:10.1016/j.jaad.2015.05.040

Handler MZ, Patel PA, Kapila R, Al-Qubati Y, Schwartz RA. Cutaneous and mucocutaneous leishmaniasis: differential diagnosis, diagnosis, histopathology, and management. *J Am Acad Dermatol.* 2015;73(6):911-926; 927-928. 927-8. doi:10.1016/j.jaad.2014.09.014

Handler MZ, Patel PA, Kapila R, Al-Qubati Y, Schwartz RA. Cutaneous and mucocutaneous leishmaniasis: clinical perspectives. *J Am Acad Dermatol.* 2015;73(6):897-908; quiz 909-910. doi:10.1016/j.jaad.2014.08.051

Handler NS, Handler MZ, Majewski S, Schwartz RA. Human papillomavirus vaccine trials and tribulations: vaccine efficacy. *J Am Acad Dermatol.* 2015;73(5):759-767; quiz 767-768. doi:10.1016/j.jaad.2015.05.041

Herman A, Peeters C, Verroken A, et al. Evaluation of chilblains as a manifestation of the COVID-19 pandemic. *JAMA Dermatol.* 2020;156(9):998-1003. doi:10.1001/jamadermatol.2020.2368

Hirschmann JV, Raugi GJ. Lower limb cellulitis and its mimics: part II. Conditions that simulate lower limb cellulitis. *J Am Acad Dermatol.* 2012;67(2):177.e1-177.e9. quiz 185-186. doi:10.1016/j.jaad.2012.03.023

Hirschmann JV, Raugi GJ. Lower limb cellulitis and its mimics: part I. Lower limb cellulitis. *J Am Acad Dermatol.* 2012;67(2):163.e1-163.e2. quiz 175-176. doi:10.1016/j.jaad.2012.03.024

Hsu DY, Shinkai K, Silverberg JI. Epidemiology of eczema herpeticum in hospitalized U.S. Children: analysis of a nationwide cohort. *J Invest Dermatol.* 2018;138(2):265-272. doi:10.1016/j.jid.2017.08.039

James WD, Elston DM, Treat JR, Rosenbach MA, Neuhaus IM. *Andrews' Diseases of the Skin: Clinical Dermatology.* 13 ed. Elsevier; 2020.

Kalb RE, Grossman ME. Chronic perianal herpes simplex in immunocompromised hosts. *Am J Med.* 1986;80(3):486-490. doi:10.1016/0002-9343(86)90725-4

Kanitakis J, Carbonnel E, Delmonte S, Livrozet JM, Faure M, Claudy A. Multiple eruptive dermatofibromas in a patient with HIV infection: case report and literature review. *J Cutan Pathol.* 2000;27(1):54-56. doi:10.1034/j.1600-0560.2000.027001054.x

Kaplan MH, Sadick NS, McNutt NS, Talmor M, Coronesi M, Hall WW. Acquired ichthyosis in concomitant HIV-1 and HTLV-II infection: a new association with intravenous drug abuse. *J Am Acad Dermatol.* 1993;29(5 Pt 1):701-708. doi:10.1016/0190-9622(93)70234-k

Kimberlin DW, Whitley RJ, Wan W, et al. Oral acyclovir suppression and neurodevelopment after neonatal herpes. *N Engl J Med.* 2011;365(14):1284-1292. doi:10.1056/NEJMoa1003509

Kimberlin DW. Neonatal herpes simplex infection. *Clin Microbiol Rev.* 2004;17(1):1-13. doi:10.1128/cmr.17.1.1-13.2004

Ko CJ, Iftner T, Barr RJ, Binder SW. Changes of epidermodysplasia verruciformis in benign skin lesions: the EV acanthoma. *J Cutan Pathol.* 2007;34(1):44-48. doi:10.1111/j.1600-0560.2006.00579.x

Ko CJ, Harigopal M, Damsky W, et al. Perniosis during the COVID-19 pandemic: negative anti-SARS-CoV-2 immunohistochemistry in six patients and comparison to perniosis before the emergence of SARS-CoV-2. *J Cutan Pathol.* 2020;47(11):997-1002. doi:10.1111/cup.13830

Kollipara R, Peranteau AJ, Nawas ZY, et al. Emerging infectious diseases with cutaneous manifestations: fungal, helminthic, protozoan and ectoparasitic infections. *J Am Acad Dermatol.* 2016;75(1):19-30. doi:10.1016/j.jaad.2016.04.032

Krumm B, Meng X, Li Y, Xiang Y, Deng J. Structural basis for antagonism of human interleukin 18 by poxvirus interleukin 18-binding protein. *Proc Natl Acad Sci U S A.* 2008;105(52):20711-20715. doi:10.1073/pnas.0809086106

Lipner SR, Scher RK. Onychomycosis: clinical overview and diagnosis. *J Am Acad Dermatol.* 2019;80(4):835-851. doi:10.1016/j.jaad.2018.03.062

Lipner SR, Scher RK. Onychomycosis: treatment and prevention of recurrence. *J Am Acad Dermatol.* 2019;80(4):853-867. doi:10.1016/j.jaad.2018.05.1260

Lupi O, Downing C, Lee M, et al. Mucocutaneous manifestations of helminth infections: trematodes and cestodes. *J Am Acad Dermatol.* 2015;73(6):947-957; quiz 957-958. doi:10.1016/j.jaad.2014.11.035

Lupi O, Downing C, Lee M, et al. Mucocutaneous manifestations of helminth infections: Nematodes. *J Am Acad Dermatol.* 2015;73(6):929-944; quiz 945-946. doi:10.1016/j.jaad.2014.11.034

Magro CM, Mulvey JJ, Laurence J, et al. The differing pathophysiologies that underlie COVID-19-associated perniosis and thrombotic retiform purpura: a case series. *Br J Dermatol.* 2021;184(1):141-150. doi:10.1111/bjd.19415

Mayer JL, Beardsley DS. Varicella-associated thrombocytopenia: autoantibodies against platelet surface glycoprotein V. *Pediatr Res.* 1996;40(4):615-619. doi:10.1203/00006450-199610000-00017

McCredie MRE, Sharples KJ, Paul C, et al. Natural history of cervical neoplasia and risk of invasive cancer in women with cervical intraepithelial neoplasia 3: a retrospective cohort study. *Lancet Oncol.* 2008;9(5):425-434. doi:10.1016/s1470-2045(08)70103-7

McMillan DJ, Drèze PA, Vu T, et al. Updated model of group A *Streptococcus M* proteins based on a comprehensive worldwide study. *Clin Microbiol Infect.* 2013;19(5):E222-E229. doi:10.1111/1469-0691.12134

Mitteldorf C, Tronnier M. Histologic features of granulomatous skin diseases. *J Dtsch Dermatol Ges.* 2016;14(4):378-388. doi:10.1111/ddg.12955

Mui UN, Haley CT, Vangipuram R, Tyring SK. Human oncoviruses – mucocutaneous manifestations, pathogenesis, therapeutics, and prevention: hepatitis viruses, human T-cell leukemia viruses, herpesviruses, and Epstein-Barr virus. *J Am Acad Dermatol.* 2019;81(1):23-41. doi:10.1016/j.jaad.2018.10.072

Nawas ZY, Tong Y, Kollipara R, et al. Emerging infectious diseases with cutaneous manifestations: viral and bacterial infections. *J Am Acad Dermatol.* 2016;75(1):1-16. doi:10.1016/j.jaad.2016.04.033

Novelli VM, Atterton DJ. Eczema herpeticum (EH): clinical and epidemiologic features. *Pediatr Res.* 1987;21(4):260-260. doi:10.1203/00006450-198704010-00560

O'Loughlin RE, Roberson A, Cieslak PR, et al. The epidemiology of invasive group A streptococcal infection and potential vaccine implications: United States, 2000-2004. *Clin Infect Dis.* 2007;45(7):853-862. doi:10.1086/521264

Ornoy A, Ergaz Z. Parvovirus B19 infection during pregnancy and risks to the fetus. *Birth Defects Res.* 2017;109(5):311-323. doi:10.1002/bdra.23588

Patel M, Charlton R. First to seventh diseases: discarded diagnoses? *Br Med J (Clin Res Ed).* 2015;351:h3525. doi:10.1136/bmj.h3525

Phipps W, Saracino M, Magaret A, et al. Persistent genital herpes simplex virus-2 shedding years following the first clinical episode. *J Infect Dis.* 2011;203(2):180-187. doi:10.1093/infdis/jiq035

Pichard DC, Freeman AF, Cowen EW. Primary immunodeficiency update: Part II. Syndromes associated with mucocutaneous candidiasis and noninfectious cutaneous manifestations. *J Am Acad Dermatol.* 2015;73(3):367-381; quiz 381-382. doi:10.1016/j.jaad.2015.01.055

Pichard DC, Freeman AF, Cowen EW. Primary immunodeficiency update: Part I. Syndromes associated with eczematous dermatitis. *J Am Acad Dermatol.* 2015;73(3):355-364; quiz 365-366. doi:10.1016/j.jaad.2015.01.054

Recalcati S. Cutaneous manifestations in COVID-19: a first perspective. *J Eur Acad Dermatol Venereol.* 2020;34(5):e212-e213. doi:10.1111/jdv.16387

Servy A, Valeyrie-Allanore L, Alla F, et al. Prognostic value of skin manifestations of infective endocarditis. *JAMA Dermatol.* 2014;150(5):494-500. doi:10.1001/jamadermatol.2013.8727

Shields BE, Rosenbach M, Brown-Joel Z, Berger AP, Ford BA, Wanat KA. Angioinvasive fungal infections impacting the skin: background, epidemiology, and clinical presentation. *J Am Acad Dermatol.* 2019;80(4):869-880.e5. doi:10.1016/j.jaad.2018.04.059

Staras SAS, Dollard SC, Radford KW, Flanders WD, Pass RF, Cannon MJ. Seroprevalence of cytomegalovirus infection in the United States, 1988-1994. *Clin Infect Dis.* 2006;43(9):1143-1151. doi:10.1086/508173

Stevens DL, Bisno AL, Chambers HF, et al. Practice guidelines for the diagnosis and management of skin and soft tissue infections: 2014 update by the infectious diseases society of America. *Clin Infect Dis.* 2014;59(2):147-159. doi:10.1093/cid/ciu296

Stolmeier DA, Stratman HB, McIntee TJ, Stratman EJ. Utility of laboratory test result monitoring in patients taking oral terbinafine or griseofulvin for dermatophyte infections. *JAMA Dermatol.* 2018;154(12):1409-1416. doi:10.1001/jamadermatol.2018.3578

Thomas C, Coates SJ, Engelman D, Chosidow O, Chang AY. Ectoparasites: scabies. *J Am Acad Dermatol.* 2020;82(3):533-548. doi:10.1016/j.jaad.2019.05.109

Toro JR, Chu P, Yen TS, LeBoit PE. Granuloma annulare and human immunodeficiency virus infection. *Arch Dermatol.* 1999;135(11):1341-1346. doi:10.1001/archderm.135.11.1341

Wanat KA, Dominguez AR, Carter Z, Legua P, Bustamante B, Micheletti RG. Bedside diagnostics in dermatology: viral, bacterial, and fungal infections. *J Am Acad Dermatol.* 2017;77(2):197-218. doi:10.1016/j.jaad.2016.06.034

Williams MR, Gallo RL. The role of the skin microbiome in atopic dermatitis. *Curr Allergy Asthma Rep.* 2015;15(11):65. doi:10.1007/s11882-015-0567-4

Woellner C, Gertz EM, Schäffer AA, et al. Mutations in STAT3 and diagnostic guidelines for hyper-IgE syndrome. *J Allergy Clin Immunol.* 2010;125(2):424-432.e8. doi:10.1016/j.jaci.2009.10.059

Yim EK, Park JS. The role of HPV E6 and E7 oncoproteins in HPV-associated cervical carcinogenesis. *Cancer Res Treat.* 2005;37(6):319-324. doi:10.4143/crt.2005.37.6.319

Zuehlke RL, Taylor WB. Black nails with *Proteus mirabilis. Arch Dermatol.* 1970;102(2):154-155. Archives of Dermatology. doi:10.1001/archderm.1970.04000080026005 %J

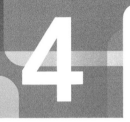

Disorders Due to Physical Agents

Caroline A. Nelson, MD

Photodermatoses

Basic Concepts

- **Abnormal cutaneous effects of UVR exposure** may be classified as idiopathic photodermatoses, defective DNA repair and chromosomal instability disorders, photoaggravated dermatoses, and chemical- and drug-induced photosensitivity (endogenous or exogenous).
- **Normal cutaneous effects of UVR exposure** may be acute/subacute or chronic.
- Evaluation of photodermatoses often includes:
  - **Phototesting**: use of a solar simulator (eg, an optically filtered xenon arc lamp) to calculate MEDs to UVB, UVA, and visible light.
  - **Photoprovocation testing**: exposure of one forearm to UVB light and one forearm to UVA light daily for 3 days.
  - **Photopatch testing**: placement of duplicate sets of photoallergens on the back followed by exposure of one set to UVA light.

POLYMORPHOUS LIGHT ERUPTION
→ **Diagnosis Group 2**

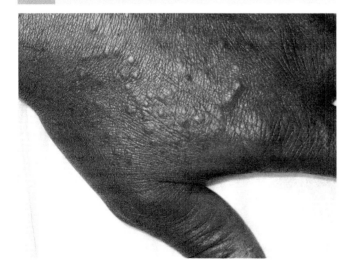

Epidemiology

- Polymorphous light eruption (PMLE) is the **most common idiopathic photodermatosis.** The hypothesized

pathogenesis is a **delayed-type, cell-mediated (type IV) reaction to endogenous cutaneous photoinduced antigens.**
- **Prevalence is inversely related to latitude** (highest in Scandinavia). Incidence peaks in the **second and third decades** and there is a **female predominance.** PMLE is most severe during the **spring and summer.**
  - The term "hardening" refers to UVR-induced immunologic tolerance, which is likely responsible for the low prevalence of PMLE at the Equator.
- **UVB > UVA > visible light** are triggers.
  - **Juvenile spring eruption** is a PMLE variant in children, especially **boys.**
  - **Actinic prurigo** is a PMLE variant primarily in **Native Americans.** Incidence peaks in the **first decade** and there is a **female predominance.** Actinic prurigo is most severe during the spring and summer but may persist year-round. It is often **familial**, with HLA associations including **-DR4 (DRB1*0401) and subtype DRB1*0407.**

Clinicopathological Features

- PMLE classically presents with **pruritic erythematous papules, papulovesicles, vesicles, or plaques in sun-exposed areas** within **hours** after light exposure. The face and other sites exposed year-round may be spared. Lesions **heal without scarring.**
  - **Juvenile spring eruption** is characterized by **vesicles favoring the ear helices.**
  - **Actinic prurigo** is characterized by **pruritic erythematous papules or nodules ± hemorrhagic crusts in both sun-exposed and covered areas.** Lesions **heal with scarring. Cheilitis ± conjunctivitis** is common.
  - Figure 4.1.

Evaluation

- The differential diagnosis of PMLE includes other photodermatoses and LE.
- **Skin biopsy** may be helpful to diagnose PMLE.
- Laboratory evaluation may include **ANA, anti-ro/la, plasma porphyrins, and HLA-DRB1*0407.**
- Phototesting typically demonstrates **normal MEDs** to UVB, UVA, and visible light. Photoprovocation testing to UVB and/or UVA is typically positive.

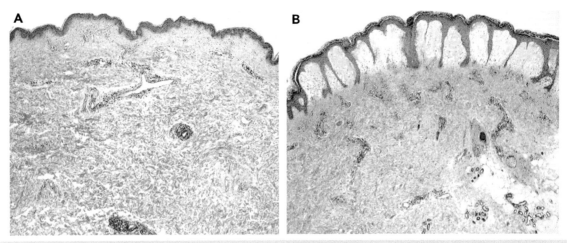

Figure 4.1. CLINICOPATHOLOGICAL CORRELATION: POLYMORPHOUS LIGHT ERUPTION. Characteristic features are papillary dermal edema ± epidermal spongiosis and a predominantly lymphocytic superficial and deep perivascular and periadnexal dermal infiltrate. A. Early PMLE. B. Late PMLE with marked papillary dermal edema. PMLE, polymorphous light eruption.
(Histology images reprinted with permission from Elder DE, Elenitsas R, Rosenbach M, et al. *Lever's Histopathology of the Skin.* 11th ed. Wolters Kluwer; 2015.)

Management

- **Photoprotection** is first line. In patients with severe PMLE, **prophylactic nbUVB phototherapy in the spring** may induce immunologic tolerance.
- Topical and/or systemic corticosteroids may be helpful for acute flares. Consider **hydroxychloroquine.**
    - **Actinic prurigo** often resolves by adolescence, but may persist. Consider **thalidomide.**

"Real World" Advice

- Clinical clues to differentiate PMLE from LE include pruritus and shorter duration (days to weeks as compared to weeks to months).
- PMLE is commonly mistaken for a "sunscreen allergy."
- When discussing photoprotection, remind patients that **light may trigger PMLE through window glass.**

HYDROA VACCINIFORME

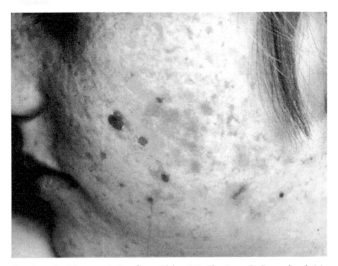

Reprinted with permission from Elder DE, Elenitsas R, Rosenbach M, et al. *Lever's Histopathology of the Skin.* 11th ed. Wolters Kluwer; 2015.

- HV is a rare idiopathic photodermatosis. It typically occurs in **light skin toned children** with an **increased incidence and severity in boys.** HV is most severe during the **spring and summer.** UVA light is the primary trigger. Associations include **EBV infection.**
- HV classically presents with **photodistributed macules** within **hours** after light exposure. Lesions evolve into **papules and plaques** that develop **umbilicated vesicles,** condense into **hemorrhagic crusts,** and ultimately **heal with varioliform scarring.**
    - HV progresses from epidermal spongiosis to vesiculation to necrosis to scarring. A predominantly lymphocytic perivascular dermal infiltrate demonstrates positive fluorescence *in situ* hybridization (FISH) for EBV RNA.
- Phototesting typically demonstrates lowered MEDs to UVB and UVA light. Photoprovocation testing to UVA light is typically positive. HV-like CTCL, a type of extranodal NK/T--cell lymphoma, nasal type, is an important consideration.
- **Photoprotection** is first line. While HV is **refractory to treatment,** it often **resolves** during adolescence or early adulthood.

CHRONIC ACTINIC DERMATITIS

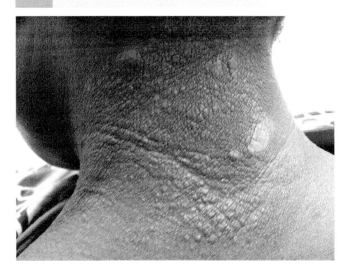

- CAD is a rare idiopathic photodermatosis. The hypothesized pathogenesis is a **delayed-type, cell-mediated (type IV) reaction to endogenous cutaneous photoinduced antigens.** CAD is most common in **men over 50 years of age. UVB and UVA > visible light** are triggers.
- CAD classically presents with a **photodistributed chronic eczematous eruption.** Generalization of CAD may lead to **erythroderma. Lymphadenopathy** is variably present. **Actinic reticuloid** is a severe CAD variant with **pseudolymphomatous papules and plaques.**
  - CAD can NOT be distinguished from MF on histopathology. However, psoriasiform acanthosis may be a helpful clue. There is a predominance of CD8+ T-cells in CAD versus CD4+ T-cells in MF. TCR gene rearrangement is often negative.
- Phototesting typically demonstrates **lowered MEDs to UVB and UVA > visible light.** CAD may coexist with airborne ACD (eg, **sesquiterpene lactones**) and photoallergic eruption/photoallergic contact dermatitis (eg, **benzophenones, musk ambrette**), yielding **positive photopatch testing.** Photoaggravated dermatoses (eg, AD) and CTCL are diagnostic considerations.
- CAD self-resolves in 10% of patients over 5 years and 20% of patients over 10 years. **Photoprotection** is first line. Topical and/or systemic corticosteroids and other immunosuppressive agents may be required.

SOLAR URTICARIA

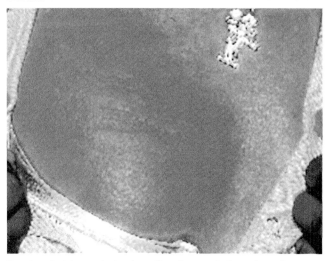

Reprinted with permission from Goodheart HP, Gonzalez ME. *Goodheart's Same-Site Differential Diagnosis: Dermatology for the Primary Health Care Provider.* 2nd ed. Wolters Kluwer; 2022.

- Solar urticaria is a rare idiopathic photodermatosis. The hypothesized pathogenesis is an **IgE-dependent (type I) reaction to endogenous cutaneous photoinduced antigens.** Solar urticaria is most common in women in the third decade. **Visible > UVA > UVB light** are triggers. Associations include **SLE and EPP.**
- Solar urticaria classically presents with **photodistributed urticaria ± anaphylaxis** within **minutes** after light exposure that resolves within hours.
  - Solar urticaria can NOT be distinguished from other urticarias on histopathology.
- Laboratory evaluation may include **ANA, anti-ro/la, and plasma porphyrins.** Phototesting typically demonstrates **wheals within minutes to visible > UVA > UVB light.**
- Solar urticaria self-resolves in 15% of patients over 5 years and 25% of patients over 10 years. While **photoprotection** is important, sunscreens often do not provide sufficient protection against visible and UVA light. **Oral nonsedating antihistamines** are first line.

SPOTLIGHT ON XERODERMA PIGMENTOSUM

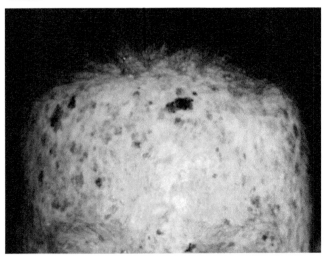

Reprinted with permission from Krakowski AC. *Procedural Pediatric Dermatology.* Wolters Kluwer; 2020.

- XP is classified under defective DNA repair and chromosomal instability disorders. It is due to hereditary defects in the **nucleotide excision repair (NER) pathway**, which repairs UVR damage to cellular DNA (eg, posaconazole-pyrimidine dimers).
- **XP and related disorders** are summarized in Table 4.1.
  - XP demonstrates UVR-associated histopathological changes (eg, solar lentigines).
- **Photoprotection** is first line.

Table 4.1. XERODERMA PIGMENTOSUM AND RELATED DISORDERS

Diagnosis[a]	Inheritance Pattern	Gene(s)	Classic Description	Notes
XP	AR	*XPA-XPG*	Photosensitivity/poikiloderma. Systemic features include neurologic degeneration (especially DeSanctis-Cacchione syndrome with dwarfism and hypogonadism) and ocular involvement (eg, conjunctivitis).	Impaired NER. Increased risk of BCC, SCC, and melanoma.
XP variant	AR	*pol*-η	Similar to XP without neurologic degeneration.	Impaired translational DNA synthesis. Increased risk of BCC, SCC, and melanoma.
Trichothiodystrophy with ichthyosis (IBIDS/PIBIDS, Tay syndrome)	AR	*ERCC2* encoding XPD > *ERCC3* encoding XPB[a] (DNA helicases)	Photosensitivity/poikiloderma (~50%). Ichthyosis (CIE-like) and brittle hair/nails. Characteristic hair shaft abnormalities with increased fragility are trichoschisis and trichothiodystrophy. Systemic features include short stature, intellectual disability, and hypogonadism.	Impaired transcription-coupled NER. Sulfur-deficient hair specifically due to deficiency of the sulfur-containing amino acids cysteine and methionine. Hypogammaglobulinemia. No increased risk of skin cancer.
			IBIDS is described by the name: ichthyosis, brittle hair, intellectual disability, decreased fertility, and short stature. PIBIDS adds photosensitivity.	
Cockayne syndrome	AR	*ERCC8* encoding CS-A, *ERCC6* encoding CS-B (proteins in the TCR complex that respond to DNA damage-stalled RNA polymerase II)	Periorbital atrophy, prominent ears, and photosensitivity/poikiloderma. Systemic features include cachectic dwarfism, neurologic degeneration, pigmentary retinal degeneration, and deafness.	Impaired transcription-coupled NER. Basal ganglia calcification. No increased risk of skin cancer.

(Continued)

Table 4.1. XERODERMA PIGMENTOSUM AND RELATED DISORDERS (CONTINUED)

Diagnosis[a]	Inheritance Pattern	Gene(s)	Classic Description	Notes
Progeria (Hutchinson-Gilford syndrome)	AD	*LMNA* encoding lamin A and lamin C (nuclear envelope proteins)	Premature aging (disproportionately large cranium with prominent scalp veins, beaked nose, micrognathia, sclerodermoid skin; alopecia). Systemic features include generalized atherosclerosis, poor growth, and high-pitched and piping voice.	Onset in the first year of life (median lifespan 14 years). Increased urine HA. Patients with progeria are "wasting" a soft-tissue dermal filler used to make people look young.
Adult progeria (Werner syndrome) Do NOT confuse adult progeria (Wer<u>ne</u>r syndrome) with MEN1 (Wer<u>me</u>r syndrome)	AR	*RECQL2* (*WRN*) encoding RECQ2 (DNA helicase)	Premature aging.	Onset in the second decade of life. Increased risk of malignancy (eg, melanoma, meningioma, sarcoma, thyroid cancer).
Bloom syndrome (congenital telangiectatic erythema)	AR	*RECQL3* (*BLM*) encoding RECQL3 (DNA helicase)	CALMs, malar erythema/telangiectasias, and photosensitivity/poikiloderma. Systemic features include short stature, prominent nose, and hypogonadism.	Increased sister chromatid exchanges. Immunodeficiency leading to recurrent otic and pulmonary infections (decreased IgA and IgM ± IgG). Increased risk of SCC, leukemia, lymphoma, and gastrointestinal cancer.
Rothmund-Thomson syndrome (poikiloderma congenitale)	AR	*RECQL4* encoding RECQL4 (DNA helicase)	EPS, photosensitivity/poikiloderma; scalp/eyebrow/eyelash alopecia. Systemic features include short stature, radial ray defects (eg, thumb aplasia), and hypogonadism.	Increased risk of SCC and osteosarcoma.
FA	AR > XLR	Variable	CALMs, diffuse hyperpigmentation. Systemic features include pancytopenia, short stature, radial ray defects (eg, thumb aplasia), and hypogonadism.	Enhanced chromosomal breakage and rearrangement. Increased risk of SCC and AML.
DKC (Zinsser-Engman-Cole syndrome)	XLR > AD, AR	*DKC1* encoding dyskerin[a]	Reticulated hyperpigmentation; premalignant leukoplakia; nail hypoplasia. Systemic features include liver cirrhosis, pancytopenia, epiphora (continuous lacrimation), and pulmonary fibrosis ± posterior fossa malformations (Hoyeraal-Hreidarsson syndrome).	Impaired ribosome activity and telomere maintenance. Bone marrow failure is the leading cause of death. Increased risk of SCC and AML.
A-T (Louis-Bar syndrome)	AR	*ATM* encoding ATM (kinase)	Cerebellar ataxia presents in infancy. Telangiectasias present between 3 and 6 years of age on the bulbar conjunctivae and spread to head/neck and acral sites. Other cutaneous features include CALMs, non-infectious granulomas, photosensitivity/poikiloderma, and premature aging; premature canities. Remember that ataxia precedes telangiectasia by the name: <u>ataxia-telangiectasia</u>.	Impaired DNA repair, particularly double strand breaks. Sensitivity to ionizing radiation. Defects in humoral and cell-mediated immunity (increased IgM, decreased IgA, IgG, IgE) leading to recurrent sinopulmonary infections. Bronchiectasis with respiratory failure is the leading cause of death. Decreased Purkinje cells in the cerebellum. Increased risk of leukemia and lymphoma. Carriers have an increased risk of breast cancer.

AD, autosomal dominant; AML, acute myelogenous leukemia; AR, autosomal recessive; A-T, ataxia telangiectasia; ATM, ataxia-telangiectasia mutated; BCC, basal cell carcinoma; CALMs, café-au-lait macules; CIE, congenital ichthyosiform erythroderma; CS-A, Cockayne syndrome A; CS-B, Cockayne syndrome B; DKC, dyskeratosis congenita; DNA, deoxyribonucleic acid; EPS, elastosis perforans serpiginosa; FA, Fanconi anemia; HA, hyaluronic acid; IBIDS, ichthyosis, brittle hair, intellectual impairment, decreased fertility, short stature; Ig, immunoglobulin; MEN, multiple endocrine neoplasia; NER, nucleotide excision repair; OCA, oculocutaneous albinism; PIBIDS, photosensitivity, ichthyosis, brittle hair, intellectual impairment, decreased fertility, short stature; RNA, ribonucleic acid; SCC, squamous cell carcinoma; XLR, X-linked recessive; XP, xeroderma pigmentosum.
[a]Illustrative examples provided. Hereditary disorders with photosensitivity/poikiloderma discussed elsewhere include OCA, Hailey-Hailey disease/Darier disease, Kindler syndrome, cutaneous porphyrias, and Hartnup disease.

PHOTOALLERGIC/PHOTOTOXIC ERUPTION
→ Diagnosis Group 2

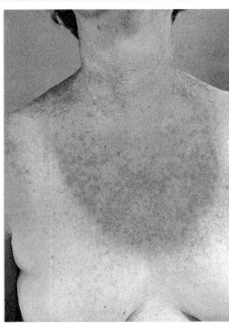

Reprinted with permission from Bobonich MA, Nolen ME, Honaker J, et al. *Dermatology for Advanced Practice Clinicians: A Comprehensive Guide to Diagnosis and Treatment.* 2nd ed. Wolters Kluwer; 2021.

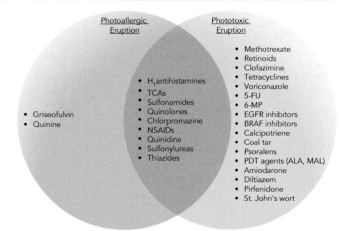

Figure 4.2. DRUG ASSOCIATIONS WITH PHOTOALLERGIC AND PHOTOTOXIC ERUPTIONS. Illustrative examples provided. 5-FU, 5-fluorouracil; 6-MP, 6-mercaptopurine; ALA, aminolevulinic acid; EGFR, epidermal growth factor receptor; H, histamine; MAL, methyl aminolevulinate; NSAIDs, non-steroidal anti-inflammatory drugs; PDT, photodynamic therapy; TCAs, tricyclic antidepressants.

Sulfur is yellow like sunlight. Drugs with sulfur moieties cause both photoallergic and phototoxic eruptions.

Drug associations with photoonycholysis include quinolones, tetracyclines, 6-MP, and psoralens.

Epidemiology

- Photoallergic and phototoxic eruptions are classified under exogenous chemical- and drug-induced photosensitivity.
  - **Photoallergic eruption** is a **delayed-type, cell-mediated (type IV) reaction** analogous to ACD.
  - **Phototoxic eruption** is a **dose-dependent** reaction analogous to ICD.
- **Phototoxic eruption is more common** than photoallergic eruption.
- **UVA light** is the primary trigger.
- **Drug associations with photoallergic and phototoxic eruptions** are illustrated in Figure 4.2.

Clinicopathological Features

- Photoallergic eruption classically presents with a **photodistributed eczematous or lichenoid eruption** within **hours to days** after light exposure.
- Phototoxic eruption classically presents with **photodistributed erythema ± vesiculation** within **minutes to hours** after light exposure. Lesions often heal with **hyperpigmentation. Pseudoporphyria and photoonycholysis** may occur. Patients may exhibit **fever** and other constitutional symptoms.
  - Photoallergic/phototoxic eruption exhibits spongiotic dermatitis. Photoallergic eruption is characterized by

a mixed dermal infiltrate with variable eosinophils. Phototoxic eruption is characterized by apoptotic keratinocytes.
- Apoptotic keratinocytes in phototoxic eruption are called "sunburn cells."

Evaluation

- The differential diagnosis of photoallergic eruption includes photoaggravated dermatoses (eg, AD).
- The differential diagnosis of phototoxic eruption includes LE and sunburn. Consider endogenous chemical-induced photosensitivity (eg, cutaneous porphyrias).

Management

- **Discontinuation of the suspected drug** along with all nonessential drugs is the first step. This step is particularly important in **photoallergic eruption** given the **risk of chronicity.** For a phototoxic drug with a short half-life, evening dosing may eliminate the eruption. **Photopatch testing** can detect photoallergy.
- **Photoprotection** is first line.
- Topical and/or systemic corticosteroids may be helpful for acute flares.

"Real World" Advice

- For phototoxic eruption to voriconazole, consider posaconazole substitution.

POIKILODERMA OF CIVATTE
→ **Diagnosis Group 2**

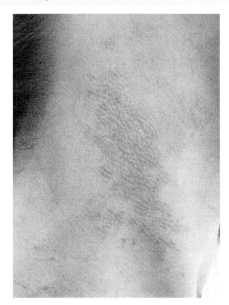

Epidemiology

- Poikiloderma of Civatte is classified under normal cutaneous effects of chronic UVR exposure. It is a **cutaneous sign of photoaging** (Table 4.2).

Clinicopathological Features

- Poikiloderma of Civatte classically presents with **reticulated pink-to-brown patches symmetrically distributed on the lateral face, neck, and upper chest.** It is characterized by **superficial atrophy, mottled hyperpigmentation, and telangiectasias sparing perifollicular skin.**
  - Poikiloderma of Civatte is characterized by epidermal atrophy/solar elastosis, melanophages, and telangiectasias. For the histopathology of colloid milium, see Figure 2.114.

Evaluation

- The differential diagnosis of poikiloderma of Civatte includes other poikiloderma, erythromelanosis follicularis faciei et colli, ACD (eg, Berloque dermatitis), pigmented ACD (Riehl melanosis), melasma, CTDs, chronic radiation dermatitis, and CTCL.

Management

- Treatment options include PDL, ablative fractional laser resurfacing, and **IPL.**

Table 4.2. CUTANEOUS SIGNS OF PHOTOAGING

Cutaneous Sign[a]	Classic Description
Acquired elastotic hemangioma	Erythematous plaque.
Acrokeratoelastoidosis	Bands of waxy or translucent papules and plaques favoring the ulnar side of the thumb and radial side of the forefinger.
Colloid milium	Numerous closely spaced translucent yellow papules.
Elastoma of Dubreuilh	Sharply marginated, thickened, yellow plaque.
Ephelides/solar lentigines	See Chapter 5: Melanocytic Neoplasms.
Erosive pustular dermatosis	Sterile pustules, crusts, erosions, and erythema favoring the bald scalp.
Favre-Racouchot syndrome[b]	Open comedones on a background of solar elastosis favoring the lateral and inferior periorbital skin.
Skin fragility	Skin tears.
IGH	See Chapter 2: Pigmentary Disorders.
Poikiloderma of Civatte	See below.
Pseudoscars	Irregularly shaped white scar-like patches.
Solar elastosis (includes cutis rhomboidalis nuchae, solar elastotic bands of the forearm, elastotic nodules of the ear)	Thickened yellow skin.
Solar purpura	See Chapter 2: Livedo Reticularis, Purpura, and Other Vascular Disorders.
Weathering nodules	Skin-colored or white papules favoring the ear helices.

IGH, idiopathic guttate hypomelanosis.
[a]Illustrative examples provided. For photocarcinogenesis, see Chapter 5: Epidermal Neoplasms and Melanocytic Neoplasms. Cutaneous signs of photoaging are attenuated in skin phototypes IV-VI.
[b]Cigarette smoking may be a cofactor.

"Real World" Advice

- An advantage of IPL is the ability to target multiple chromophores simultaneously, thereby addressing both mottled hyperpigmentation and telangiectasias in poikiloderma of Civatte.

Other Physical Agents

Basic Concepts

- The skin is the body's primary interface with the environment. Beyond photodermatoses, a variety of physical agents may lead to skin injury.
- **Heat injury**:
  - **Burn**: A burn may be thermal (contact, flame, scald), electrical, radiation, or chemical. Burn severity is based on **depth of injury** (Table 4.3) and BSA involvement. Initial burn evaluation should focus on respiratory and circulatory status. Superficial burns (first and superficial second degree) should be rinsed with cold running water for 20 minutes. All burns should be cleansed and treated with a topical agent (eg, silver sulfadiazine) under a sterile dressing. Deep burns (deep second, third, and fourth degree) may benefit from serial excision and autografting. Burn complications include **subepidermal delayed post-burn/post-graft blister** due to enhanced fragility of the newly synthesized DEJ, postthermal burn pruritus, and increased risk of skin cancer (**Marjolin ulcer**), particularly **SCC**. Arrhythmia is a known complication of electrical burns, which are often more extensive than the cutaneous burn wounds suggest.
    - Delayed bleeding from the labial artery is a known complication of oral commissure burns sustained by toddlers after biting into electrical cords.
    - Lichtenberg figures refer to a transient "fern-like" pattern of skin markings pathognomonic of lightning strikes.
  - *Skin disorder(s) discussed elsewhere*: EAI (see below), heat urticaria.
  - *Mucosal disorders*: Contact stomatitis, **nicotinic stomatitis** (gray-white mucosa with umbilicated papules).
  - *Gland disorders*: Tropical acne, miliaria.
  - *Hair disorders*: **Deep burns** may be associated with secondary **scarring alopecia**. After **heat styling**, the characteristic hair shaft abnormality **with increased fragility** is **bubble hair**.

- CCCA is also known as "hot comb alopecia"; however, premature desquamation of the IRS predisposing to follicular injury is now hypothesized to be central to its pathogenesis.
- **Cold injury**:
  - **Frostbite**: Frostbite occurs when skin temperature drops below approximately −2 °C (28 °F). Analogous to burn, frostbite severity is classified into 4° based on depth of injury. **First-degree frostbite (frost-nip)** is characterized by **erythema, edema, cutaneous anesthesia, and transient pain**, most commonly of the **nose and ears.** With progression, blistering and ulceration may occur. Rapid rewarming in a **warm water bath** is first line.
  - *Skin disorder(s) discussed elsewhere*: Hypopigmentation/ depigmentation and hyperpigmentation due to cryotherapy, chilblain lupus, Raynaud phenomenon, CAPS, cold panniculitis, sclerema neonatorum, subcutaneous fat necrosis of the newborn, cold urticaria, livedo reticularis/ acrocyanosis, cold-induced vascular occlusion, factitial dermatitis (salt and ice challenge), "COVID toes" (controversial), and pernio (see below).
- **Mechanical injury**:
  - **Hematoma**: Hematoma describes a collection of blood outside vessels. The cause is often traumatic (eg, **auricular hematoma in wrestlers**). For black heel and palm, see below.
    - Recurrent auricular hematoma produces the multinodular "cauliflower ear" deformity.
    - In neonates, extracranial injuries include **caput succedaneum** (serum accumulation above periosteum, crosses suture lines), **cephalohematoma** (blood accumulation beneath periosteum, respects suture lines), **subgaleal hemorrhage** (life-threatening blood accumulation under galea aponeurotica, crosses suture lines), and skull fractures.
  - *Skin disorders discussed elsewhere*: Mechanical ICD, panniculitis due to blunt trauma, ecchymoses, dystrophic calcification, cutaneous focal mucinosis, nodular fasciitis, solitary angiokeratoma, venous lake, epithelioid heman-

Table 4.3. BURN CLASSIFICATION BY DEPTH OF INJURY

Type	Depth of Injury	Classic Description	Prognosis
First degree	Epidermis	Dry, red, blanching, pain to touch.	Heals without scarring.
Superficial second degree	Epidermis and partial-thickness dermis (preserved adnexal structures)	Moist with serosanguinous bullae, red, blanching, severe pain to touch.	Heals with mild but variable scarring.
Deep second degree	Epidermis and partial-thickness dermis (destroyed adnexal structures)	Dry or moist with serosanguinous bullae, white or red, reduced blanching, decreased pain to touch (pain to deep pressure).	Heals with scarring and contraction.
Third degree	Epidermis and full-thickness dermis	Dry, white, nonblanching, absent pain to touch (pain to deep pressure).	Heals with scarring and contraction.
Fourth degree	Epidermis, full-thickness dermis, and fascia ± muscle ± bone	Exposed fascia ± muscle ± bone, absent pain to touch (pain to deep pressure).	Heals with scarring and contraction.

gioma, PG, schwannoma, traumatic neuroma, auricular pseudocyst, cutaneous lymphoid hyperplasia (CLH).
- *Mucosal disorders*: Bite fibroma/*morsicatio buccarum* (eg, body-focused repetitive behavior disorder), **eosinophilic ulcer of the oral mucosa**, necrotizing sialometaplasia (ischemic necrosis, often of the palate).

   Riga-fede disease is the childhood variant of eosinophilic ulcer of the oral mucosa that characteristically occurs on the **ventral tongue of nursing infants and toddlers with erupted mandibular incisor teeth** and in children with congenital insensitivity to pain.
- *Gland disorders*: Acne mechanica, Frey syndrome.
- *Hair disorders*: Trichotillomania (eg, body-focused repetitive behavior disorder), traction alopecia, acne keloidalis. After mechanical injury, the characteristic hair shaft abnormalities **with increased fragility** are **trichorrhexis nodosa** and **trichoschisis**, while the characteristic hair shaft abnormality without increased fragility is **trichoptilosis**. Trichonodosis may develop in curly hair after excessive combing or rustling.
- *Nail disorders*: Beau lines, leukonychia (true, punctate or transverse), onychocryptosis, onycholysis, onychomadesis, onychophagia/onychotillomania (eg, body-focused repetitive behavior disorder), paronychia, PG, splinter hemorrhages (distal), subungual exostosis, subungual hematoma.

- **Pressure injury**:
   Amniotic band syndrome occurs when amniotic bands exert pressure on the fetus, leading to congenital scarring and amputation (eg, **digit amputation**).
- **Coma bulla**: Coma bulla is a tense blister that favors pressure dependent areas.
   - Coma bulla is an intraepidermal or subepidermal blister with sweat gland necrosis.
- **Pressure ulcer (decubitus ulcer)**: Pressure ulcer occurs when soft tissue is compressed between a bony prominence and an external surface. Analogous to burn, pressure ulcer severity is classified into four degrees based on depth of injury. A **first-degree pressure ulcer** is characterized by **nonblanchable erythema**, most commonly of the **sacrum, ischial tuberosities, greater trochanters, lateral malleoli, and heels.** Ulceration occurs with progression. Intermittent pressure relief (eg, frequent position changes) is preventative.
   - The Latin word *decubitus* means "lying down."
- **Senile gluteal dermatosis**: Senile gluteal dermatosis typically occurs in elderly men of low body mass after prolonged sitting. Poorly defined, ridged brown plaques appear in a triangular distribution on the bilateral buttocks.
- *Skin disorders discussed elsewhere*: Acquired localized lipodystrophy, delayed pressure urticaria, Rumpel-Leede sign of a blood pressure cuff, chondrodermatitis nodularis helicis (CNH) (see below), piezogenic pedal papules.
- *Hair disorders*: **Pressure (postoperative) alopecia** classically presents with **nonscarring circumscribed or patterned** hair loss of the **occipital scalp.**

In neonates, the term "**halo scalp ring**" refers to a **band of alopecia** bordering a caput succedaneum due to **pressure necrosis during labor** that is usually **self-limited.**
- *Nail disorders*: Onychauxis, onychocryptosis, PG, pincer nails.

- **Friction injury**:
- **Acanthoma fissuratum**: Acanthoma fissuratum describes friction injury due to **ill-fitting eyeglass frames.** It is characterized by firm skin-colored to erythematous plaques or nodules on the upper lateral nose or upper postauricular sulci with central vertical fissure or groove.
- **Corn/callus**: Friction injury leads to hyperkeratosis, with high-risk demographics including athletes and musicians. **Hard corns** are firm, small, dome-shaped papules with translucent central cores favoring the **dorsal toes. Soft corns** are painful keratoses ± maceration favoring the **interdigital web spaces. Calluses** are broad keratotic plaques, most often **underlying the metatarsal heads.** For Russel sign, see Chapter 2: Depositional Disorders, Porphyrias, and Nutritional Deficiencies.
- **Friction bulla**: Friction bulla is a fragile blister that favors the soles > palms.
   - Friction bulla is an intraepidermal blister (split below the *stratum granulosum*).
   In infants, **suction blister** is a tense blister that favors the lips.
   - Suction blister is a subepidermal blister (split in the *lamina lucida*).
- **Nonvenereal sclerosing lymphangitis**: Nonvenereal sclerosing lymphangitis most often occurs after vigorous sexual activity. It is characterized by a minimally tender, indurated cord involving the coronal sulcus and is self-limited.
- **Zoon balanitis/vulvitis**: The pathogenesis of Zoon balanitis is unknown; however, friction injury and poor penile hygiene are hypothesized to play a role. Zoon balanitis/vulvitis classically presents with **discrete, erythematous, moist, speckled plaques on the glans penis or vulva** with frequent involvement of adjacent surfaces. Zoon balanitis is variably associated with pain, pruritus, dysuria, and/or dyspareunia. Skin biopsy demonstrating **plasma cell–rich lichenoid interface dermatitis** is helpful to confirm the diagnosis. For Zoon balanitis, **circumcision** is curative. The existence of Zoon vulvitis as an independent entity is controversial.
   - The speckled appearance of Zoon balanitis has been likened to "cayenne pepper." Involvement of adjacent surfaces is called "kissing" lesions.
- *Skin disorders discussed elsewhere*: Frictional lichenoid eruption, juvenile plantar dermatosis, dermatographism, macular/lichen amyloidosis.
- *Hair disorders*: Frictional alopecia/hypertrichosis. Friction may induce **rolled hairs.**
- *Nail disorders*: Longitudinal melanonychia (fourth/fifth digits), habit tic deformity (eg, body-focused repetitive

behavior disorder), median canaliform dystrophy of Heller, PG, onycholysis, onychomadesis, onychorrhexis, onychoschizia, subungual exostosis.
- **Vibration injury**:
  - *Skin disorders discussed elsewhere*: Secondary Raynaud phenomenon, vibratory angioedema.
- **Water exposure injury**:
  - **Immersion foot**: Continuous water exposure (eg, trench warfare) overhydrates the *stratum corneum*, inducing maceration. The **warm water variant** is characterized by **thickening, softening, and exaggerated wrinkling of the soles** with **painful ambulation**. The **tropical variant** extends to the dorsal feet with marked inflammation. The **cold water variant** is further complicated by cold-induced vasospasm injuring subcutaneous fat, muscle, bone, vessels, and nerves with the potential for **permanent peripheral neuropathy**. While thorough drying is first line, prevention (eg, "jungle boots") is ideal.
    - Immersion foot has multiple contextual descriptors, ranging from <u>foxhole</u> foot to <u>jungle</u> rot/<u>tropical jungle</u> foot to <u>paddy-field</u> foot to <u>shelter</u> foot to <u>swamp</u> foot to <u>trench</u> foot.
    - Painful ambulation in immersion foot has been likened to "walking on a rope."
  - *Skin disorders discussed elsewhere*: Aquagenic PPK, ICD due to water, aquagenic urticaria, aquagenic pruritus.
  - *Nail disorders* (repeated wet dry cycles): Onycholysis, onychorrhexis, onychoschizia.
- **Chemical exposure injury**:
  - *Skin disorders discussed elsewhere*: ICD due to acids, alcohols/glycols, alkalis, detergents and cleansers, disinfectants, and solvents; hyperpigmentation or discoloration due to heavy metals; hypopigmentation/depigmentation due to phenols/catechols and sulfhydryls; sclerodermoid reaction due to epoxy resins, organic solvents, pesticides, vinyl chloride; scombroid poisoning.
  - *Gland disorders*: Chromhidrosis.
  - *Hair disorders*: Chlorotrichosis (green hair, eg, due to copper or selenium exposure) and other chemical hair discoloration.
  - *Nail disorders*: Onycholysis (acrylic nails), onychorrhexis/onychoschizia (nail varnish solvents).
- The term "abuse" refers to either misuse (eg, drugs) or mistreatment (eg, child or elder abuse).
  - Local complications of drug injection include ecchymosis, scarring, and ulceration (eg, from accidental extravasation). Skin signs of drug abuse discussed elsewhere include APLS/anti-MPO ANCA vasculitis secondary to levamisole-adulterated cocaine, pruritus, formication, and infections (eg, HCV, HIV, abscess, necrotizing fasciitis, septic vasculitis).
    - IV drug injection leads to linear "skin tracks," while dermal or subcutaneous drug injection leads to circular or irregular "skin popping" scars. Chronic non-healing ulcers are called "shooter's patches." **Skin signs of child abuse** are summarized in Table 4.4. Beyond skin and mucosal examination, initial evaluation includes fundoscopic examination, otoscopic examination, and skeletal survey. When child abuse is suspected, an immediate referral should be made to child protective services.
  - Skin signs of elder abuse are variable. **Elder self-neglect** may lead to **dermatitis neglecta** (brown patches and plaques of retained skin due to poor skin hygiene) and **onychogryphosis** (hard, thick, and yellow-brown nail plate due to failure to cut nails).
    - Onychogryphosis has a "ram's horn" shape due to asymmetric growth.

Table 4.4. SKIN SIGNS OF CHILD ABUSE AND NEGLECT

Skin Sign[a]	Classic Description	Notes
Thermal burn	Characteristic patterns include round burns (cigarette), geometric burns (branding), and "donut-type sparing" on the buttocks or "stocking and glove distribution" on the extremities (dunking scald injuries).	Delay between the burn and seeking medical care should raise suspicion for child abuse.
Ecchymosis ± hematoma	Suspicious locations (not prone to accidental injury) include the head and neck > trunk, arms, and buttocks. Characteristic patterns include binding injuries, buckle imprints, hand imprints, human bite marks, loop marks, pinch marks, and traumatic alopecia.	Complementary and alternative medicine practices (eg, cupping, coining) may be mistaken for abuse. In cupping, vacuum devices produce circular areas of erythema or ecchymosis. In coining, rubbing heated oil on the skin followed by a coin produces symmetric linear erythema or ecchymosis.
Neglect	Poor health/nutrition/hygiene, infestations.	Neglect may be physical or emotional.
Sexual abuse	Attenuation of the hymen with loss of tissue, fresh tears or scars of the hymen, or anal margin extension onto perianal skin (diagnostic).	When anogenital LS occurs in children, subepidermal hemorrhagic bullae may be mistaken for sexual abuse.

LS, lichen sclerosis.
[a]Illustrative examples provided.

ERYTHEMA AB IGNE

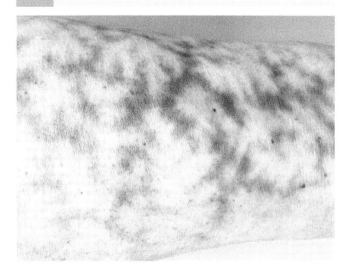

- EAI results from **chronic heat exposure** below the threshold for thermal burn.
- EAI classically presents with **reticulated erythema and hyperpigmentation.** Distribution depends on the heat source (eg, **lumbosacral from heating pads, abdomen/anterior thighs from laptop computers, shins from stoves/heaters**). Chronic EAI is associated with an increased risk of skin cancer (eg, **SCC**).
    - Early EAI exhibits epidermal atrophy, dermal pigmentation (both melanin and hemosiderin), and vasodilation. Interface dermatitis is variably present. Focal hyperkeratosis, dyskeratosis, and squamous atypia may develop over time.
- Removal of the offending heat source is first line.

PERNIO
Synonym: chilblains, perniosis

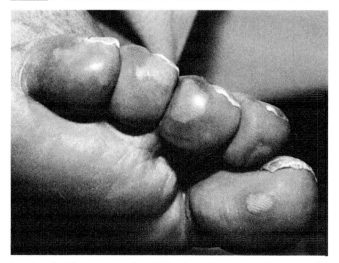

Reprinted with permission from Elder DE, Elenitsas R, Rubin AI, et al. *Atlas of Dermatopathology: Synopsis and Atlas of Lever's Histopathology of the Skin.* 4th ed. Wolters Kluwer; 2020.

- Pernio is an autoinflammatory disorder induced by **cold wet exposure** above the threshold for frostbite.
- Pernio classically presents with **erythematous to blue-violet macules, papules, or nodules** accompanied by **burning, pain, or pruritus.** Distribution favors the **distal fingers and toes** > nose, ears, and heels. Pernio may be complicated by angiokeratoma of Mibelli.
    - Figure 4.3.
- Laboratory evaluation to exclude important mimickers of pernio (chilblain lupus, acrocyanosis, cold-induced vascular occlusion) includes CBC, ANA, **cryoglobulins ± cryofibrinogen ± cold agglutinins**, and SPEP/IFE. The term "COVID toes" refers to the controversial association between COVID-19 and pernio.
    - **Pernio-like skin lesions** may occur in **interferonopathies** such as chronic atypical neutrophilic dermatosis with lipodystrophy and elevated temperature (CANDLE) syndrome and SAVI.
- Pernio typically self-resolves within 1 to 3 weeks but may recur. Avoidance of cold wet exposure is key. **Nifedipine** is an evidence-based treatment for moderate-to-severe pernio.

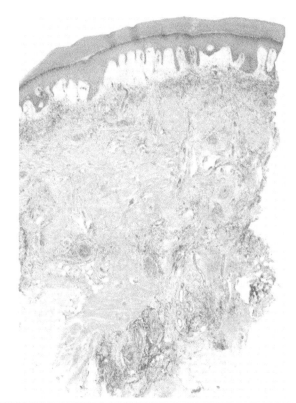

Figure 4.3. CLINICOPATHOLOGICAL CORRELATION: PERNIO. Characteristic features are papillary dermal edema and a predominantly lymphoplasmacytic perivascular and perieccrine infiltrate. Endothelial cells are often edematous and infiltrated by lymphocytes. Necrotic keratinocytes and vessel wall damage are variably present.

(Histology image reprinted with permission from Elder DE, Elenitsas R, Rosenbach M, et al. *Lever's Histopathology of the Skin.* 11th ed. Wolters Kluwer; 2015.)

Acral skin is a helpful diagnostic clue.

Cold panniculitis is a predominantly lobular panniculitis ± overlying histopathological features of pernio.

SPOTLIGHT ON SICKLE CELL DISEASE
Synonym: sickle cell anemia

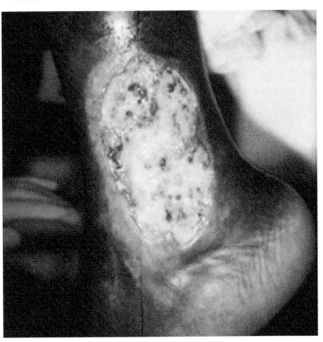

From Ballas SK. Sickle cell pain. In: *Progress in Pain Research and Management.* Vol 11. IASP Press; 1998. This figure has been reproduced with permission of the International Association for the Study of Pain® (IASP).

- Sickle cell disease is due to **homozygosity for the gene encoding sickle hemoglobin (HbS).** The prevalence is highest in **sub-Saharan Africa, the Mediterranean basin, the Middle East, and India** as sickle cell trait protects against severe malaria. When deoxygenated, HbS polymerization leads to hemolytic anemia and **vaso-occlusive crisis.** Triggers include **cold exposure,** dehydration, hypoxia, infections, and stress.
- Sickle cell disease is a multisystem disorder complicated by large vessel vasculopathy and progressive ischemic organ damage. Skin findings include **inflammatory retiform purpura and leg ulceration.**
  - Sickle cell disease has nonspecific histopathology.
- Early diagnosis, penicillin prophylaxis, blood transfusion, transcranial Doppler imaging, **hydroxyurea,** and HSCT can dramatically improve survival and quality of life for patients with sickle cell disease.

BLACK HEEL AND PALM
Black heel synonym: talon noir
Black palm synonym: paume noir

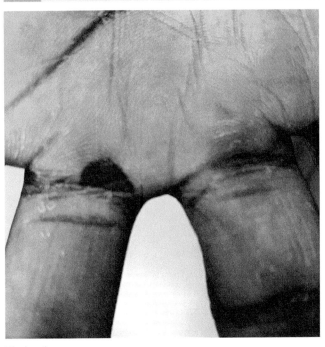

Black palm.

- Black heel and palm describes **intracorneal hematoma** most often in athletes due to mechanical injury.
- Black heel and palm classically presents with **black macules on the heel** > other palmoplantar location.
  - Black heel is commonly referred to by its French name "*talon noir,*" but do not forget the existence of "*paume noir.*"
  - Figure 4.4.
- Black heel and palm is self-limited. Gentle paring to remove the blood can be helpful to exclude a melanocytic lesion, most notably acral lentiginous melanoma.

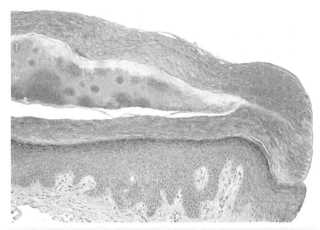

Figure 4.4. CLINICOPATHOLOGICAL CORRELATION: BLACK HEEL AND PALM. Characteristic features include hyperkeratosis, parakeratosis, and erythrocytes within the *stratum corneum*. Formation of a friction blister may occur. Hemoglobin stains are positive; however, iron stains are negative due to the absence of phagocytic or proteolytic activity within the *stratum corneum*.

(Histology image reprinted with permission from Elder DE, Elenitsas R, Rosenbach M, et al. *Lever's Histopathology of the Skin.* 11th ed. Wolters Kluwer; 2015.)

Acral skin is a helpful diagnostic clue.

CHONDRODERMATITIS NODULARIS HELICIS

→ **Diagnosis Group 2**

Synonyms: chondrodermatitis nodularis chronic helicis et antihelicis, ear corn

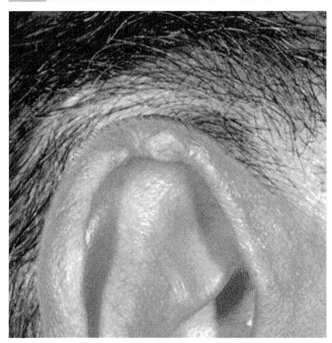

Reprinted with permission from Craft N, Fox LP, Goldsmith LA, et al. *VisualDx: Essential Adult Dermatology.* Wolters Kluwer Health/ Lippincott Williams & Wilkins; 2010.

Epidemiology

- CNH is an inflammatory disorder involving **collagen degeneration** due to physical agents, most notably **pressure injury.**
- CNH typically occurs in **older adults.**

Clinicopathological Features

- CNH classically presents with **painful or tender skin-colored to erythematous papules with central scale or crust.** The distribution favors the **helix in men** and the **antihelix in women.**
  - ◈ Figure 4.5.

Evaluation

- The differential diagnosis of CNH includes gouty tophus, BCC, AK, keratoacanthoma (KA), and SCC.
- Skin biopsy may be performed to confirm the diagnosis and exclude malignancy.

Management

- Pressure relief is first line. While donut pillows are often recommended, foam bandage and self-adhering foam are cheap, less bulky, and move with the patient while sleeping.
- Other treatment options include topical nitroglycerin, photodynamic therapy (PDT), and excision. Newer techniques (triangular window, retroauricular) are superior to wedge excision.

"Real World" Advice

- CNH is not life-threatening; however, it does impair quality of life by interfering with sleep.

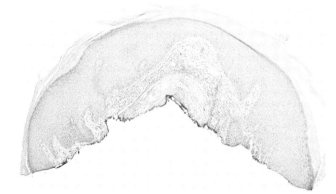

Figure 4.5. CLINICOPATHOLOGICAL CORRELATION: CHONDRODERMATITIS NODULARIS HELICIS. CNH is characterized by a central crater overlying fibrinoid degeneration of collagen. The surrounding epidermis demonstrates parakeratosis, hypergranulosis, and acanthosis. The surrounding dermis demonstrates granulation tissue, stellate fibroblasts, and a variable lymphohistiocytic infiltrate extending into thickened perichondrium.CNH, chondrodermatitis nodularis helicis.

(Histology image courtesy of Noel Turner, MD, MHS and Christine J. Ko, MD.)

Cartilage may be present but is NOT required for the diagnosis of CNH.

SUGGESTED READING

Austin E, Geisler AN, Nguyen J, et al. Visible light. Part I: properties and cutaneous effects of visible light. *J Am Acad Dermatol.* 2021;84(5):1219-1231. doi:10.1016/j.jaad.2021.02.048

Bittner EA, Shank E, Woodson L, Martyn JA. Acute and perioperative care of the burn-injured patient. *Anesthesiology.* 2015;122(2):448-464. doi:10.1097/aln.0000000000000559

Bolognia JL, Schaffer JV, Cerroni L. *Dermatology.* 4th ed. Elsevier Saunders; 2018.

Brooks BP, Thompson AH, Bishop RJ, et al. Ocular manifestations of xeroderma pigmentosum: long-term follow-up highlights the role of DNA repair in protection from sun damage. *Ophthalmology.* 2013;120(7):1324-1336. doi:10.1016/j.ophtha.2012.12.044

Campolmi P, Bonan P, Cannarozzo G, et al. Intense pulsed light in the treatment of non-aesthetic facial and neck vascular lesions: report of 85 cases. *J Eur Acad Dermatol Venereol.* 2011;25(1):68-73. doi:10.1111/j.1468-3083.2010.03700.x

Chantorn et al., 2012Chantorn R, Lim HW, Shwayder TA. Photosensitivity disorders in children: part I. *J Am Acad Dermatol.* 2012;67(6):1093.e1-18. quiz 1111-2. doi:10.1016/j.jaad.2012.07.033

Chantorn R, Lim HW, Shwayder TA. Photosensitivity disorders in children: part II. *J Am Acad Dermatol.* 2012;67(6):1113.e1-15. quiz 1128, 1127. doi:10.1016/j.jaad.2012.07.032

Diffey BL. Sources and measurement of ultraviolet radiation. *Methods.* 2002;28(1):4-13. doi:10.1016/s1046-2023(02)00204-9

Elder DE. *Lever's Histopathology of the Skin.* 11th ed. Wolters Kluwer; 2015.

Elston DM, Ferringer T. *Dermatopathology.* 2nd ed. Elsevier Saunders; 2014.

Evans TR, Kaye SB. Retinoids: present role and future potential. *Br J Cancer.* 1999;80(1-2):1-8. doi:10.1038/sj.bjc.6690312

Geisler AN, Austin E, Nguyen J, Hamzavi I, Jagdeo J, Lim HW. Visible light. Part II: photoprotection against visible and ultraviolet light. *J Am Acad Dermatol.* 2021;84(5):1233-1244. doi:10.1016/j.jaad.2020.11.074

James WD, Elston DM, Treat JR, Rosenbach MA, Neuhaus IM. *Andrews' Diseases of the Skin: Clinical Dermatology.* 13th ed. Elsevier; 2020.

Jones H, Blinder M, Anadkat M. Cutaneous manifestations of sickle cell disease. *Open J Blood Dis.* 2013;3(3):36934, 6. doi:10.4236/ojbd.2013.33019

Katoulis AC, Stavrianeas NG, Panayiotides JG, et al. Poikiloderma of Civatte: a histopathological and ultrastructural study. *Dermatology.* 2007;214(2):177-182. doi:10.1159/000098580

Martín JM, Jordá E, Alonso V, Villalón G, Montesinos E. Halo scalp ring in a premature newborn and review of the literature. *Pediatr Dermatol.* 2009;26(6):706-708. doi:10.1111/j.1525-1470.2009.01017.x

Mervis JS, Phillips TJ. Pressure ulcers: prevention and management. *J Am Acad Dermatol.* 2019;81(4):893-902. doi:10.1016/j.jaad.2018.12.068

Mervis JS, Phillips TJ. Pressure ulcers: pathophysiology, epidemiology, risk factors, and presentation. *J Am Acad Dermatol.* 2019;81(4):881-890. doi:10.1016/j.jaad.2018.12.069

Parker LA. Part 1: early recognition and treatment of birth trauma—injuries to the head and face. *Adv Neonatal Care.* 2005;5(6):288-297. quiz 298-300. doi:10.1016/j.adnc.2005.09.001

Piel FB, Steinberg MH, Rees DC. Sickle cell disease. *N Engl J Med.* 2017;376(16):1561-1573. doi:10.1056/NEJMra1510865

Rosen T, Hwong H. Sclerosing lymphangitis of the penis. *J Am Acad Dermatol.* 2003;49(5):916-918. doi:10.1016/s0190-9622(03)00464-x.

Shah S, Fiala KH. Chondrodermatitis nodularis helicis: a review of current therapies. *Dermatol Ther.* 2017;30(1):e12434. doi:10.1111/dth.12434

Udkoff J, Cohen PR. A report of 10 individuals with weathering nodules and review of the literature. *Indian J Dermatol.* 2016;61(4):433-436. doi:10.4103/0019-5154.185715

Wojnarowska F, Calnan CD. Contact and photocontact allergy to musk ambrette. *Br J Dermatol.* 1986;114(6):667-675. doi:10.1111/j.1365-2133.1986.tb04874.x

Vashi NA, Patzelt N, Wirya S, Maymone MBC, Kundu RV. Dermatoses caused by cultural practices: cosmetic cultural practices. *J Am Acad Dermatol.* 2018;79(1):19-30. doi:10.1016/j.jaad.2017.06.160

Vashi NA, Patzelt N, Wirya S, Maymone MBC, Zancanaro P, Kundu RV. Dermatoses caused by cultural practices: therapeutic cultural practices. *J Am Acad Dermatol.* 2018;79(1):1-16. doi:10.1016/j.jaad.2017.06.159

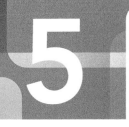

5 Neoplasms and Cysts

Hovik J. Ashchyan, MD and Daniel M. Klufas, MD

Epidermal Neoplasms

Basic Concepts

- Epidermal neoplasms encompass a group of benign and malignant tumors of the cornified stratified squamous epithelium. The majority are derived from keratinocytes, which are the most abundant cell type.

SEBORRHEIC KERATOSIS
→ **Diagnosis Group 1**

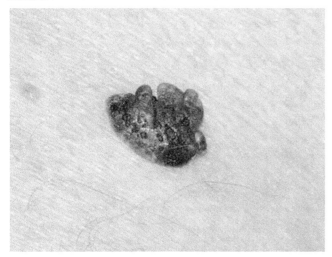

Reprinted with permission from Goodheart HP. *Goodheart's Same-Site Differential Diagnosis: A Rapid Method of Diagnosing and Treating Common Skin Disorders.* Wolters Kluwer Health/Lippincott Williams & Wilkins; 2011.

Epidemiology

- SK is a common benign epidermal neoplasm that can arise de *novo* or from a preexisting solar lentigo. While the exact pathogenesis is unknown, sun exposure and friction may play a role. Additionally, ~1/3 of cases harbor a **gain-of-function mutation in *FGFR3* or *PIK3CA*.**
- Though controversial, the **abrupt onset of numerous SKs** may be a cutaneous marker of an internal malignancy known as the **sign of Leser-Trélat.** It is most commonly associated with **colon or gastric adenocarcinoma, breast adenocarcinoma, and lymphoma.**

- Drug associations include **BRAF inhibitors.** Additionally, SKs may become **inflamed** with systemic antineoplastics (eg, **5-FU, cytarabine, ingenol mebutate**).

Clinicopathological Features

- SKs classically present as **oval-to-round, waxy or warty, papules or plaques that range in color from tan to black.** They can occur anywhere on the body but have a predilection for the **chest and back.**
    - SK has a "stuck-on" appearance.
    - On the back, the sign of Leser-Trélat creates a "Christmas tree" pattern.
- **Dermatosis papulosa nigra (DPN)** refers to **pigmented SKs favoring the central face,** primarily in **African American and Asian populations.**
- **Cutaneous melanoacanthoma** is a type of **heavily pigmented SK.** Oral melanoacanthoma is an unrelated reactive proliferation.
- **Stucco keratosis** is a type of **white or gray SK** favoring the ankles and feet. HPV (eg, **HPV23b**) has been implicated in the pathogenesis.
- SKs may become **inflamed. LK** represents an inflamed SK, solar lentigo, or AK that appears as a **pink-to-red brown scaly papule on a sun-exposed site.**
    - The histopathological features of SK variants are summarized in Table 5.1. Keratinocytes within pigmented SK contain melanin except in cutaneous melanoacanthoma, which is composed of both keratinocytes and pigmented dendritic melanocytes. Signs of irritation include areas of compact eosinophilic parakeratotic keratin, spindled keratinocytes, and squamous eddies (keratin pearls). Signs of inflammation include areas of compact eosinophilic parakeratotic keratin, crust, spongiosis, and lymphocytes ± lichenoid interface dermatitis. LK can NOT be distinguished from LP on histopathology.
    - Figure 5.1.

Evaluation

- The differential diagnosis of SK includes solar lentigo, nevocellular nevus, and melanoma. LK may clinically mimic psoriasis, eczematous dermatitis, superficial BCC, or SCCis.
- **Dermoscopy** features include **multiple (3+) milia-like cysts, comedo-like openings, and gyri and sulci (fissures and ridges).** Early SKs may demonstrate the **fingerprint-like structures and moth-eaten borders** characteristic of **solar lentigines.**

Management

- SKs do not require treatment. If inflamed or irritated, they are commonly treated with **cryotherapy.**

"Real World" Advice

- Care should be taken when using cryotherapy for SKs on hair-bearing areas (eg, the scalp) as this may result in alopecia. Consider performing gentle curettage instead.

Table 5.1. HISTOPATHOLOGICAL FEATURES OF SEBORRHEIC KERATOSIS VARIANTS AND RELATED DISORDERS

Diagnosis[a]	Histopathological Features
Acanthotic SK	Loose lamellar keratin, broad sheets of small keratinocytes of uniform depth, horn cysts (closed to the surface), and pseudohorn cysts (open to the surface).
	Loose lamellar keratin resembles "onion skin." The "string sign" refers to the ability to draw a horizontal line parallel to the epidermal surface underlying the lesion.
Clonal SK	Islands of small keratinocytes (often pigmented) within the epidermis.
	Absence of ducts helps distinguish clonal SK from hidroacanthoma simplex.
Hyperkeratotic SK (verrucous SK)	Resembles acanthotic SK with hyperkeratosis and variable papillomatosis.
	The combination of hyperkeratosis, papillomatosis, and acanthosis creates the appearance of "church spires."
Reticulated SK (adenoid SK)	Thin interlacing strands of keratinocytes (often pigmented) and horn cysts.
	Thin interlacing strands of epidermis are "lace-like."

SK, seborrheic keratosis.
[a]Illustrative examples provided.

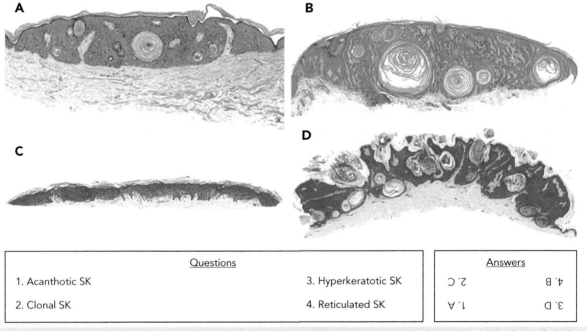

Questions		Answers	
1. Acanthotic SK	3. Hyperkeratotic SK	2. C	4. B
2. Clonal SK	4. Reticulated SK	1. A	3. D

Figure 5.1. MATCHING EXERCISE: SEBORRHEIC KERATOSIS VARIANTS. A, Acanthotic SK. Note the loose lamellar keratin, broad sheets of small keratinocytes of uniform depth (the "string sign"), horn cysts (closed to the surface), and pseudohorn cysts (open to the surface). B, Reticulated SK. Note the thin interlacing strands of keratinocytes and horn cysts. C, Clonal SK. Note the islands of small keratinocytes within the epidermis. D, Hyperkeratotic SK. Note the hyperkeratosis and papillomatosis. SK, seborrheic keratosis.

(Histology images reprinted with permission from Elder DE, Elenitsas R, Rubin AI, et al. Atlas of Dermatopathology: Synopsis and *Atlas of Lever's Histopathology of the Skin.* 4th ed. Wolters Kluwer; 2020.)

Without context, SK can NOT be distinguished from common epidermal nevus on histopathology.

EPIDERMAL NEVUS

Synonyms: keratinocytic nevus, verrucous nevus

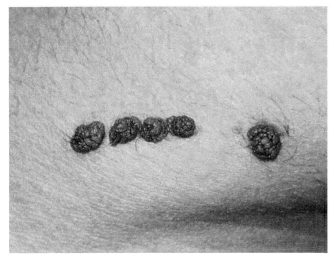

Reprinted with permission from Edward S, Yung A. *Essential Dermatopathology*. Wolters Kluwer Health/Lippincott Williams & Wilkins; 2011.

- Keratinocytic epidermal nevi are benign hamartomas caused by **postzygotic mutations in *HRAS* > *NRAS* > *KRAS* and *PIK3CA*** in the MAPK and PI3K signaling pathways, respectively. Occasionally, *FGFR3* mutations lead to epidermal nevi that can cause hypophosphatemic rickets. While most lesions are present at birth, some lesions may become more prominent or appear with age.

- Common epidermal nevus classically presents as a **linear or whorled, verrucous or hyperkeratotic, pink or brown plaque following lines of Blaschko.** Epidermal nevus variants include the following:
  - **Epidermolytic epidermal nevus** is caused by **postzygotic mutation in *K1* or *K10*** during embryogenesis. **If the mutation involves gonadal cells**, it can be transmitted to the patient's offspring, resulting in **generalized EI.**
  - **Epidermal nevus syndrome** is a **sporadic** association of epidermal nevus with systemic involvement, most commonly the skeletal, nervous, and ocular systems. CLOVES syndrome and Proteus syndrome are classified under the umbrella of epidermal nevus syndrome.
  - **ILVEN** classically presents as **chronic, pruritic, erythematous, scaly papules coalescing into a linear plaque.**
  - **Palisaded epidermal nevus with "skyline" basal cell layer (PENS)** is a newly described epidermal nevus with prominent basal cells.
    - Figure 5.2.
- **Skin biopsy is appropriate to exclude the epidermolytic epidermal nevus. White sponge nevus** is a closely related disorder to epidermal nevus caused by **AD mutations in *K4* and *K13*.** It is characterized by a **soft white plaque on the buccal mucosa.**
- Rarely, neoplasms such as BCC, SCC, and KA may arise within an epidermal nevus. Epidermal nevi are difficult to treat with a high rate of recurrence following cryotherapy, dermabrasion, electrodesiccation, or laser ablation. Surgical excision is advised only for smaller, localized lesions.

A

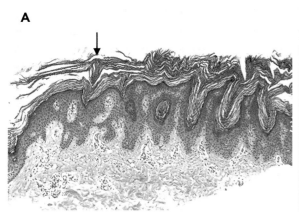

B

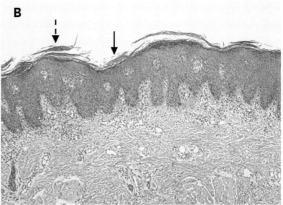

Figure 5.2. SIDE-BY-SIDE COMPARISON: COMMON EPIDERMAL NEVUS AND INFLAMMATORY LINEAR VERRUCOUS EPIDERMAL NEVUS. Both common epidermal nevus and ILVEN are characterized by a well-demarcated zone of hyperkeratosis, acanthosis, and papillomatosis. Common epidermal nevus demonstrates orthokeratosis. ILVEN demonstrates alternating orthokeratosis (granular layer present) and parakeratosis (granular layer absent). A, Common epidermal nevus. B, ILVEN. Solid arrows: orthokeratosis (granular layer present). Dashed arrow: parakeratosis (granular layer absent). ILVEN, inflammatory linear verrucous epidermal nevus; SK, seborrheic keratosis.

(Histology images reprinted with permission from Gru AA, Wick MR, Mir A, et al. *Pediatric Dermatopathology and Dermatology*. Wolters Kluwer; 2018.)

Without context, common epidermal nevus can NOT be distinguished from SK on histopathology.

- Epidermolytic epidermal nevus: demonstrates EHK (see Figure 2.8).

CLEAR CELL ACANTHOMA
Synonym: Degos acanthoma

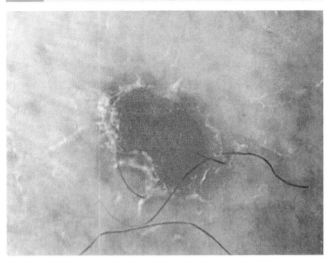

Reprinted with permission from Elder DE, Elenitsas R, Rubin AI, et al. *Atlas of Dermatopathology: Synopsis and Atlas of Lever's Histopathology of the Skin.* 4th ed. Wolters Kluwer; 2020

- Clear cell acanthoma is a rare benign epidermal neoplasm comprised of **clear glycogen-containing epithelial cells.** The most common demographic is middle-aged adults.
  - **Multiple or eruptive clear cell acanthomas** are associated with hereditary **ichthyosis vulgaris.**
- Clear cell acanthoma classically presents as a **well-circumscribed, pink-to-red brown, moist, shiny papule or nodule.** The lesion may be pigmented and have a collarette of scale. Typical locations include the thigh, shin, and calf. There is a small risk of malignant degeneration to SCC.
  - ◆ Figure 5.3.
  - ◆ Other benign epidermal neoplasms not discussed elsewhere are summarized in Table 5.2.

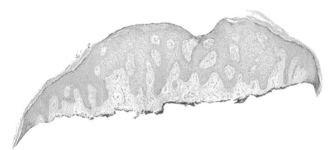

Figure 5.3. CLINICOPATHOLOGICAL CORRELATION: CLEAR CELL ACANTHOMA. Clear cell acanthoma is characterized by a well-demarcated zone of neutrophils and parakeratosis in the *stratum corneum* and acanthosis. Clear cells contain glycogen (PAS positive, diastase sensitive). PAS, periodic acid-Schiff.

(Histology image courtesy of Noel Turner, MD, MHS and Christine J. Ko, MD.)

> On high power, clear cell acanthoma can NOT be distinguished from psoriasis on histopathology.

- **Dermoscopy** features include **white superficial scales and dotted vessels in a uniform distribution against a light red background ± red globular rings.**
- While treatment is not necessary, options include cryotherapy, surgical excision, and CO_2 laser.

BASAL CELL CARCINOMA
→ Diagnosis Group 1

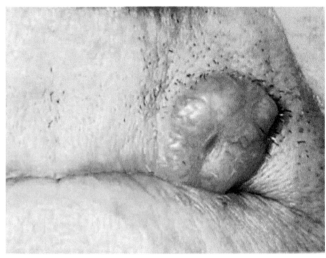

Nodulo-ulcerative basal cell carcinoma reprinted with permission from Elder DE, Elenitsas R, Rubin AI, et al. *Atlas of Dermatopathology: Synopsis and Atlas of Lever's Histopathology of the Skin.* 4th ed. Wolters Kluwer; 2020

Epidemiology

- BCC is the **most common nonmelanoma skin cancer (NMSC).** Technically, it is classified as a **malignant adnexal neoplasm with follicular matrical differentiation.**

Table 5.2. HISTOPATHOLOGICAL FEATURES OF OTHER BENIGN EPIDERMAL NEOPLASMS

Diagnosis[a]	Histopathological Features
Acantholytic acanthoma	Discrete acanthoma demonstrating acantholysis (resembles Hailey-Hailey disease).
Epidermolytic acanthoma	Discrete acanthoma demonstrating EHK (see Figure 2.8).
Large cell acanthoma	Discrete acanthoma demonstrating cells with large nuclei.
Warty dyskeratoma	Discrete endophytic growth of keratinocytes demonstrating acantholytic dyskeratosis (resembles Darier disease).

EHK, epidermolytic hyperkeratosis.
[a]Illustrative examples provided.

Table 5.3. HEREDITARY DISORDERS ASSOCIATED WITH BASAL CELL CARINOMA

Diagnosis[a]	Inheritance Pattern	Gene(s)	Classic Description
BCNS	See below.		
Bazex-Christol-Dupré syndrome	XLD	Gene mapped to Xq24-q27	Follicular atrophoderma, local hypohidrosis (above the neck), hypotrichosis, multiple BCCs, and milia. The characteristic hair shaft abnormality with increased fragility is pili torti.
Brooke-Spiegler syndrome	AD	*CYLD* (increased NFκB signaling)	Multiple BCCs, cylindromas, spiradenomas, and trichoepitheliomas.
MTS (BCCs with sebaceous differentiation)	See Chapter 5: Neoplasms of Sebaceous, Apocrine, and Eccrine Glands.		
OCA	See Chapter 2: Pigmentary Disorders.		
Rombo syndrome	AD		Atrophoderma vermiculatum, acrocyanosis, hypotrichosis (with loss of eyelashes), multiple BCCs, trichoepitheliomas, and milia.
Schöpf-Schulz-Passarge syndrome	See Chapter 2: Disorders of Sebaceous, Apocrine, and Eccrine Glands.		
XP and XP variant	See Chapter 4: Photodermatoses.		

AD, autosomal dominant; BCCs, basal cell carcinoma; BCNS, basal cell nevus syndrome; NFκB, nuclear factor κ-light-chain-enhancer of activated B cells; OCA, oculocutaneous albinism; XLD, X-linked dominant; XP, xeroderma pigmentosum.
[a]Illustrative examples provided.

- While **sun exposure, tanning bed use, and radiation therapy** are strongly associated with BCC, ~30% of sporadic BCCs are due to **somatic mutations in *PTCH1* encoding patched**, a member of the **SHH signaling pathway**.

  Hereditary disorders associated with BCC are summarized in Table 5.3.

Clinicopathological Features

- The most common location for BCC is the head and neck, particularly the **lower eyelid** and the **base of the nose**. However, BCC may occur anywhere on the body. Clinical presentation varies based on subtype:
  - **Nodular BCC (most common)**: pearly papule with arborizing blood vessels ± central ulceration.
  - **Pigmented BCC**: similar to nodular BCC with brown or black pigment.
  - **Superficial (multifocal) BCC**: scaly erythematous papule or plaque.
  - **Morpheaform (sclerosing) BCC**: white sclerotic plaque.
- Other BCC subtypes (eg, micronodular, infiltrative, adenoid, infundibulocystic) are distinguished histologically, not clinically.
- **Fibroepithelioma of Pinkus** is a **skin-colored, sessile lesion favoring the lumbosacral area.** While some classify this entity as a rare BCC subtype, others classify it as a **premalignant fibroepithelial tumor.**
- BCC metastasis is extremely rare. Tumors usually require **>15 years to develop metastases**, which typically spread to the **head and neck lymph node basin.**

Figure 5.4. For the histopathological differential diagnosis of morpheaform BCC, see Table 5.34.

Evaluation

- The differential diagnosis of nodular BCC includes SK, SCC, and sebaceous gland hyperplasia (SGH). Pigmented BCC may clinically mimic melanoma. Superficial BCC may clinically mimic psoriasis, eczematous dermatitis, LK, or SCCis. Morpheaform BCC may clinically mimic a scar.
- **Dermoscopy** features include **arborizing blood vessels, spoke wheel-like structures, leaf-like areas, large blue-gray ovoid nests, multiple nonaggregated blue-gray globules, ulceration, and shiny white blotches and strands.**
- If there is suspicion for extensive disease (deep structural involvement such as deep soft tissue, bone, or perineural disease), imaging studies are recommended. For suspected perineural disease, MRI is the preferred imaging modality.

Management

- High-risk BCCs have an increased risk for recurrence and metastasis. Factors include size (any size in a high-risk location [eg, the H area], ≥10 mm in moderate-risk locations, ≥20 mm in low-risk locations), ill-defined clinical borders, immunosuppression, sites of prior radiation, perineural disease, and aggressive growth patterns histologically (infiltrative, micronodular, morpheaform, sclerosing).
- **Surgical treatment is first line for localized BCC. For low-risk tumors**, surgical excision with **4 mm clinical margins**

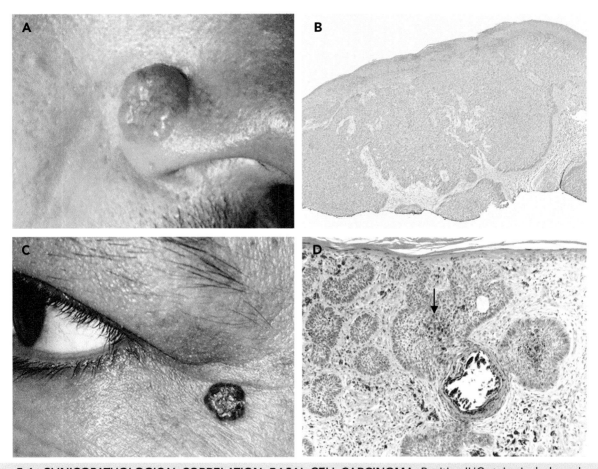

Figure 5.4. CLINICOPATHOLOGICAL CORRELATION: BASAL CELL CARCINOMA. Positive IHC stains include androgen receptor, BCL2 (diffuse), BerEP4, and toluidine blue (stroma). A and B, Nodular BCC. C and D, Pigmented BCC. Solid arrow: basophilic cells containing melanin. E and F, Superficial BCC. Dashed arrow: buds of basophilic cells. G and H, Morpheaform BCC. Dashed arrow: thin strands and small nests of basophilic cells "tadpole-shaped" with a "paisley-tie pattern." I, Fibroepithelioma of Pinkus. BCC, basal cell carcinoma; BCL2, B-cell lymphoma 2; IHC, immunohistochemistry.

(A, Reprinted with permission from Lugo-Somolinos A, McKinley-Grant L, Goldsmith LA, et al. *VisualDx: Essential Dermatology in Pigmented Skin.* Wolters Kluwer Health/Lippincott Williams & Wilkins; 2011. B, Histology image courtesy of Noel Turner, MD, MHS and Christine J. Ko, MD. C, Reprinted with permission from Lugo-Somolinos A, McKinley-Grant L, Goldsmith LA, et al. *VisualDx: Essential Dermatology in Pigmented Skin.* Wolters Kluwer Health/Lippincott Williams & Wilkins; 2011. D, Histology image reprinted with permission from Elder DE, Elenitsas R, Rosenbach M, et al. *Lever's Histopathology of the Skin.* 11th ed. Wolters Kluwer; 2015. E, Reprinted with permission from *Goodheart HP. Goodheart's Same-Site Differential Diagnosis: A Rapid Method of Diagnosing and Treating Common Skin Disorders.* Wolters Kluwer Health/Lippincott Williams & Wilkins; 2011. F, Histology image reprinted with permission from Elder DE, Elenitsas R, Rosenbach M, et al. *Lever's Histopathology of the Skin.* 11th ed. Wolters Kluwer; 2015. G, Reprinted with permission from Khan FM, Gerbi BJ. *Treatment Planning in Radiation Oncology.* 3rd ed. Wolters Kluwer Health/Lippincott Williams & Wilkins; 2011. H, Histology image reprinted with permission from Crowson N, Magro CM, Mihm MC Jr. *Biopsy Interpretation of the Skin: Primary Non-Lymphoid Cutaneous Neoplasia.* Wolters Kluwer Health/Lippincott Williams & Wilkins; 2010. I, Histology image courtesy of Noel Turner, MD, MHS and Christine J. Ko, MD.)

- **Nodular BCC:** nests of basophilic cells with peripheral palisading and clefting between basophilic cells and stroma. The stroma is fibromyxoid.
- **Micronodular BCC:** similar to nodular BCC with smaller nests of basophilic cells separated by thick dermal collagen bundles and an aggressive growth pattern.
- **Pigmented BCC:** similar to nodular BCC but basophilic cells contain melanin.
- **Superficial BCC:** multifocal buds of basophilic cells.
- **Morpheaform BCC:** thin strands and small nests of basophilic cells with limited peripheral palisading and minimal retractions around epithelial cells. The stroma is sclerotic. Perineural invasion is common.
- **Infiltrative BCC:** angulated nests of basophilic cells, often with focal squamous differentiation. The stroma is rich in fibroblasts with minimal mucin. Perineural invasion is common.
- **Adenoid BCC:** nest of basophilic cells with clear spaces.
- **Infundibulocystic BCC:** pink epithelial strands with buds of basophilic cells and horn cysts.
- **Fibroepithelioma of Pinkus:** anastomosing pink epithelial strands, often containing eccrine ducts, with buds of basophilic cells. Ample stroma is fibromyxoid.

Presence of clefting between basophilic cells and stroma helps distinguish BCC from trichoepithelioma.

Thin strands and small nests of basophilic cells in morpheaform BCC have been described as "tadpole-shaped" with a "paisley-tie pattern."

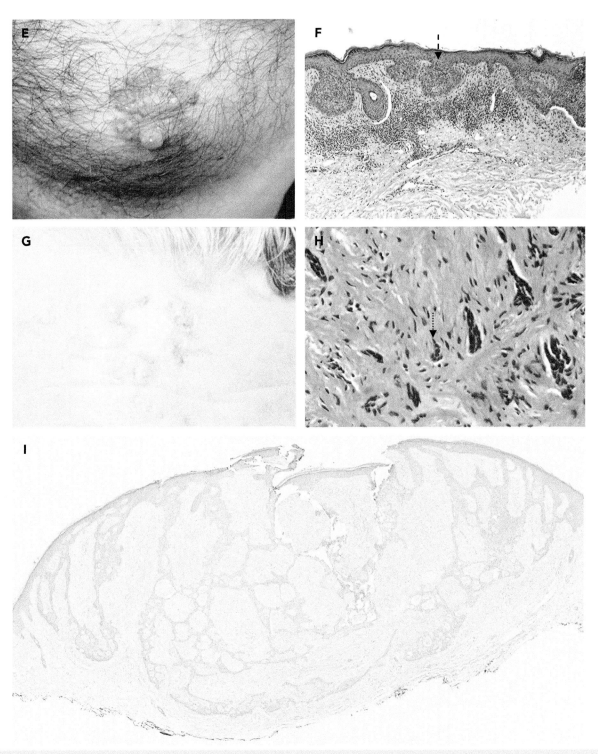

(**Figure 5.4.** Continued)

is recommended. While standard surgical excision may be considered for **high-risk tumors**, National Comprehensive Cancer Network (NCCN) guidelines recommend **Mohs micrographic surgery (MMS).** In 2012, a combined task force developed the **MMS appropriate use criteria (AUC),** which is a tool to determine whether MMS is the appropriate treatment for BCC. **Toluidine blue** may be used to stain serial frozen sections, thereby revealing the stromal change associated with BCC to visualize the margins.

- **Electrodesiccation and curettage (ED&C)** may be considered for **low-risk BCCs in nonterminal hair-bearing locations.**
- When a surgical approach is contraindicated or impractical, alternative therapies include **topical 5-FU or imiquimod, PDT, radiation therapy, or cryotherapy,** though the cure rate is lower.
- **SMO inhibitors (eg, vismodegib)** can be used in locally advanced or metastatic BCC.

"Real World" Advice

- Given the low risk of metastasis, goals of care discussion should be considered during the shared decision-making management plan of BCC in elderly patients with significant comorbidities. For example, **observation or radiation therapy may be appropriate for an elderly patient with Alzheimer dementia and a massive infiltrative BCC.**
- If a patient has a "scar" without history of trauma, consider biopsy to rule out morpheaform BCC.

SPOTLIGHT ON BASAL CELL NEVUS SYNDROME

Synonyms: Gorlin syndrome, nevoid basal cell carcinoma syndrome

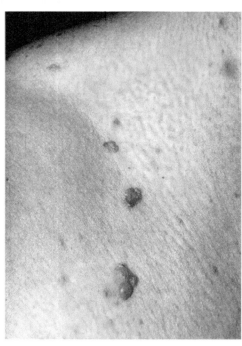

Reprinted with permission from Schaaf CP, et al. *Human Genetics.*

- Basal cell nevus syndrome (BCNS) is an **AD** syndrome due to mutations in *PTCH* encoding patched (loss-of-function) or *SMO* encoding smoothened (gain-of-function), which lead to constitutive activation of the **SHH signaling pathway.**
- The classic findings of BCNS are summarized in the **diagnostic criteria** (Table 5.4). BCCs in BCNS resemble acrochordons (skin tags); however, children rarely get acrochordons prior to puberty.
  - The histopathology of BCNS demonstrates BCCs, particularly nevoid BCCs.
- **Genetic testing** to confirm the diagnosis should be considered in specific situations: prenatal testing when there is a known family mutation, first-degree relatives of patients with the known mutation, and confirmation in a patient with an unclear diagnosis.
- After birth, patients with a known diagnosis of BCNS should have a yearly brain MRIs until age 8 to detect medulloblastoma. Other management options include echocardiogram to assess for cardiac fibromas, dental screening, head circumference and developmental monitoring, ophthalmological examinations, and vision and hearing screenings. In addition to age-appropriate malignancy screening, adult patients require yearly total body skin examinations (TBSEs). A more frequent interval can be considered after diagnosis of the first BCC. Treatment may require a multidisciplinary team. Genetic counseling is recommended for first-degree relatives. **SMO inhibitors (eg, vismodegib)** can be used in patients with numerous BCCs, locally invasive BCCs, or metastatic disease.

Table 5.4. DIAGNOSTIC CRITERIA FOR BASAL CELL NEVUS SYNDROME

Diagnostic criteria for BCNS[a]

Major criteria	Minor criteria
1. Calcification of the falx cerebri	1. Macrocephaly and frontal bossing (also agenesis of the corpus callosum)
2. Odontogenic keratocysts of jaw	2. Various ocular anomalies (eg, colobomas, hypertelorism)
3. ≥3 palmar or plantar pits	3. Vertebral/rib anomalies (eg, bifid ribs)
4. Multiple BCCs or a BCC before age 20, particularly nevoid BCCs.	4. Cleft palate/lip
5. First-degree relative with BCNS	5. Polydactyly
	6. Lymphomesenteric or pleural cysts
	7. Ovarian or cardiac fibromas
	8. Medulloblastoma

BCC, basal cell carcinoma; BCNS, basal cell nevus syndrome.

[a]2 major criteria OR 1 major criterion before 20 years of age OR 1 major and 2 minor criteria are required for diagnosis.

POROKERATOSIS
→ **Diagnosis Group 2**

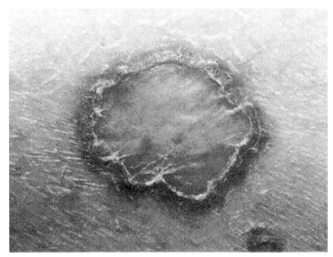

Disseminated superficial actinic porokeratosis reprinted with permission from Elder DE, Elenitsas R, Rubin AI, et al. *Atlas of Dermatopathology: Synopsis and Atlas of Lever's Histopathology of the Skin.* 4th ed. Wolters Kluwer; 2020.

Epidemiology

- Porokeratosis is thought to be a **premalignant disorder of cornification** caused by an abnormal clonal expansion of keratinocytes. Though the exact pathogenesis is unclear, heterozygous germline and sporadic mutations involving the **mevalonate pathway** (responsible for cholesterol synthesis) have been implicated.
- Eruptive disseminated porokeratosis is associated with gastrointestinal cancer (eg, hepatocellular carcinoma).

Clinicopathological Features

- Porokeratosis classically presents as an **annular papule or plaque with a furrowed keratotic rim** (correlates with the cornoid lamellae on histopathology).
- **Porokeratosis variants** are summarized in Table 5.5. **Risk of malignant degeneration into SCC** varies based on the variant. All forms of porokeratosis may be seen in pediatric patients though disseminated superficial actinic porokeratosis (DSAP) is rare.
  - Figure 5.5.

Evaluation

- The differential diagnosis of porokeratosis includes other annular lesions (eg, ring wart, tinea corporis) and AK. When linear, the differential diagnosis includes linear inflammatory disorders (eg, lichen striatus) and epidermal neoplasms (eg, epidermal nevus).

Management

- Photoprotection is recommended for patients with DSAP or linear porokeratosis.
- For symptomatic lesions, **cryotherapy, topical 5-FU,** topical retinoids, **imiquimod,** or PDT can be considered. Given the role of mutation in the **mevalonate pathway** in the pathogenesis of porokeratosis, **2% cholesterol/2% lovastatin** ointment or lotion has emerged as a novel therapy.

"Real World" Advice

- Porokeratosis tends to follow a chronic course and is often treatment refractory.

Table 5.5. POROKERATOSIS VARIANTS

Variant[a]	Classic Description	Notes
DSAP (most common)	Small skin-colored to pink-red hyperkeratotic papules. Favors sun-exposed skin (eg, extensor forearms, shins). Variably pruritic.	Associated with AD *SAR* mutation and UVR exposure. Rare malignant transformation.
Linear porokeratosis	Similar to porokeratosis of Mibelli though arranged in a Blaschko-linear array. Favors the extremities.	May be segmental or generalized, reflecting genetic mosaicism. Highest risk of malignant transformation.
Porokeratosis of Mibelli (classic)	Large annular plaque with a furrowed keratotic rim. Favors the extremities. Asymptomatic.	Associated with immunosuppression. Rare malignant transformation.
Porokeratosis ptychotropica	Red-brown hyperkeratotic papules and plaques. Favors the gluteal cleft and buttocks. Pruritic.	Associated with mechanical injury due to scratching. No reported risk of malignant transformation.
PPPD	Similar to porokeratosis of Mibelli though smaller and with a less keratotic rim. Favors the palms and soles.	PAON (encompasses both PEODDN and PPPD) is a rare adnexal hamartoma caused by mosaic mutation of *GJB2* encoding connexin 26. PPPD is also associated with UVR exposure. Rare malignant transformation.
Punctate porokeratosis	Depressed or spiculated keratotic papules. Favors the palms and soles.	No reported risk of malignant transformation.
	Punctate porokeratosis lesions are "seed-like."	

AD, autosomal dominant; DSAP, disseminated superficial actinic porokeratosis; PAON, porokeratotic adnexal ostial nevus; PEODDN, porokeratotic eccrine ostial and dermal duct nevus; PPPD, porokeratosis palmaris et plantaris et disseminata; UVR, ultraviolet radiation.
[a]Illustrative examples provided.

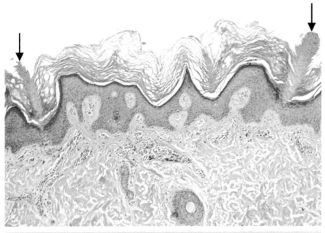

Figure 5.5. CLINICOPATHOLOGICAL CORRELATION: POROKERATOSIS. Porokeratosis is characterized by cornoid lamellae (columns of parakeratosis oriented at 45° angles toward the lesion center with underlying dyskeratosis). Intervening skin may appear psoriasiform or lichenoid. Disseminated superficial actinic porokeratosis. Solid arrows: cornoid lamellae.

ACTINIC KERATOSIS
→ Diagnosis Group 1

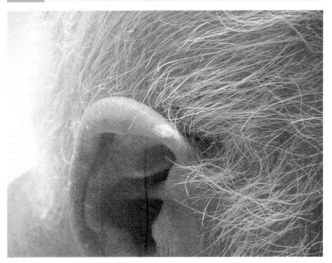

Reprinted with permission from Goodheart HP, Gonzalez ME. *Goodheart's Same-Site Differential Diagnosis: Dermatology for the Primary Health Care Provider.* 2nd ed. Wolters Kluwer; 2022.

Epidemiology

- AK is a **premalignant,** in situ dysplasia comprised of atypical keratinocytes.
- AKs develop due to **UVB-induced inactivating mutations in** *TP53* **encoding p53, an important regulator of the G1 (not S) phase of the cell cycle.** P53, when active, enhances the NER of UV-induced damage to cellular DNA (eg, **cyclobutene-pyrimidine dimers**), delays cell proliferation, and stimulates apoptosis. When inactivated, p53 cannot perform the critical role of inhibition of photocarcinogenesis.

- AKs predominate in lighter skin phototypes, particularly those with heavy cumulative **sun exposure, tanning bed use, and radiation therapy.**
- AKs are also associated with **arsenic poisoning,** which can result from contaminated drinking water, occupational exposures (eg, farming, glass manufacturing, recycling electronic waste), or foul-play.
- AKs may become **inflamed** with systemic antineoplastics (eg, **5-FU, cytarabine, ingenol mebutate**).

Clinicopathological Features

- AKs classically present as **erythematous papules or plaques with adherent scale in chronically sun-exposed areas** such as the scalp, face, ears, forearms, and dorsal hands.
    - AKs have a characteristic "gritty" scale that forms a "jagged" pattern after cryotherapy.
- **Arsenical keratoses** favor the **palms and soles,** usually with a latency of ~**20 years** following exposure.
- The presence of chronic actinic damage to the lower vermilion lip is termed **actinic cheilitis. Glandular cheilitis** refers to **inflammatory hyperplasia of the lower labial salivary glands** due to chronic irritation or in association with actinic cheilitis.
    - Figure 5.6.

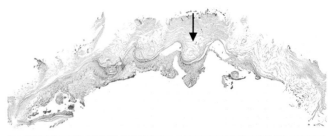

Figure 5.6. CLINICOPATHOLOGICAL CORRELATION: ACTINIC KERATOSIS. AK is characterized by loss of normal epidermal maturation with partial-thickness cytologic atypia (arising from the basal layer). Malignant keratinocytes can keratinize and integrate into the *stratum corneum,* forming malignant horn with parakeratosis. Solar elastosis is common. Solid arrow: "flag sign" indicating loose lamellar "onion skin" keratin arising from an adnexal structure. AK, actinic keratosis.

(Histology image courtesy of Noel Turner, MD, MHS and Christine J. Ko, MD.)

- Acantholytic AK: acantholysis.
- Bowenoid AK: SCCis without pagetoid scatter or full-thickness follicular involvement.
- Hypertrophic AK: prominent malignant horn and acanthosis.
- Lichenoid AK: lichenoid interface dermatitis.

The "flag sign" refers to malignant horn alternating with loose lamellar "onion skin" keratin arising from adnexal structures. Arsenical keratoses can NOT be distinguished from AK on histopathology.

Evaluation

- The differential diagnosis of AK includes PF, SK, SCC, and erosive pustular dermatosis.
- On the face, **dermoscopy** reveals **"strawberry" pattern vessels.**
- If an AK is presenting as a cutaneous horn (hypertrophic AK), biopsy to rule out underlying SCC.
- If arsenical keratoses are suspected, analysis of drinking water or blood, urine, hair, and nails is recommended.

Management

- For patients with AKs, the first step in management is sun protection.
- For isolated lesions, **cryotherapy** is recommended in conjunction with topical 5-FU or imiquimod over cryotherapy alone. It is not recommended to use cryotherapy in conjunction with diclofenac or adapalene.
- For diffuse, broad areas of involvement, field therapy with **topical 5-FU or imiquimod** is preferred. Diclofenac and PDT carry conditional recommendations based on recommendations from the 2021 AAD Working Group and may also be considered. Tirbanibulin is a new topical therapy. Of note, as of 2021, ingenol mebutate is no longer manufactured or marketed in the United States.

"Real World" Advice

- AKs are **easier to identify with palpation** than visual inspection.

SQUAMOUS CELL CARCINOMA
→ Diagnosis Group 1
Squamous cell carcinoma in situ synonym: Bowen disease

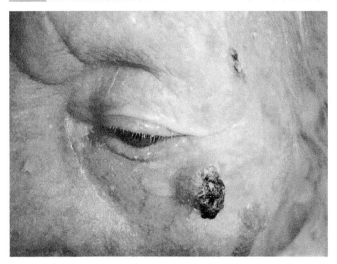

Reprinted with permission from Elder DE, Elenitsas R, Rosenbach M, et al. *Lever's Histopathology of the Skin.* 11th ed. Wolters Kluwer; 2015.

Epidemiology

- **SCC is the second most common NMSC.** It is classified as a malignant epidermal neoplasm derived from keratinocytes. The term "SCC in situ" is reserved for SCC without dermal invasion. The pathogenesis of SCC is similar to AK.
- SCC is the most common NMSC in **Asian Indian and Black populations.** Higher rates of SCC are also seen in the **Lesbian, gay, bisexual, and transgender (LGBT) population**, highlighting an important healthcare disparity. In **transplant patients**, the risk of **SCC is 65-fold higher** than the general population. By comparison, the risk of merkel cell carcinoma **MCC, BCC, and melanoma** is **23.8-, 10-, and 3- to 4-fold higher**, respectively, than the general population.
- In addition to **cumulative UVR exposure and arsenic poisoning**, associations with SCC include **increasing age, immunosuppression (CD4, not CD8, lymphopenia), scar or chronic ulcer (eg, Marjolin ulcer in a burn site), hypertrophic LP, hypertrophic LE, LS, HS, EAI, and HIV or HPV infection.** Occupational exposures that increase SCC risk include outdoor workers and those exposed to arsenic, polycyclic hydrocarbons, and radioactive materials.
  > SCC is further associated with OCA (see Chapter 2: Pigmentary Disorders); dystrophic EB (see Chapter 2: Vesiculobullous Disorders); EDV (see Chapter 3: Viral Diseases); and XP, XP variant, Bloom syndrome, Rothmund-Thomson syndrome, FA, and DKC (see Chapter 4: Photodermatoses).
- Drug associations include **azathioprine, cyclosporine, pimecrolimus/tacrolimus (controversial), rituximab, voriconazole, topical mechlorethamine, and BRAF inhibitors.** Other risk factors include PUVA and radiation therapy (often with a latency period > 20 years).
- **Oral SCC** is associated with **alcohol, tobacco, and betel nut** exposure.

Clinicopathological Features

- Invasive SCC classically presents as an **erythematous papule or nodule arising from an indurated, elevated base often on sun-exposed sites, particularly favoring the lower extremities in women,** and sites of preexisting AKs.
- SCC may occur on the oral mucosa.
- Periungual SCC may resemble a wart with erythema and scaling.
- **Premalignant SCC and verrucous carcinoma** are summarized in Table 5.6.
  - ⬦ Figure 5.7.

Evaluation

- The differential diagnosis of SCC includes hypertrophic AK, KA, and pseudoepitheliomatous hyperplasia (PEH), a reactive phenomenon. SCCis may clinically mimic

Table 5.6. PREMALIGNANT SQUAMOUS CELL CARCINOMA AND VERRUCOUS CARCINOMA.

Variant[a]	HPV Types[a]	Classic Description	Notes
Premalignant SCC			
SIL/CIN/VIN/VaIN/PIN/AIN	16, 18 Digital/nail: 16 EDV: 5, 8	Bowenoid papulosis: multiple red-brown smooth and warty papules on the external genitalia. Erythroplasia of Queyrat: red smooth plaque on glabrous vulvar, penile, or perianal skin.	Risk of malignant degeneration into SCC/ cervical cancer/vulvar cancer/vaginal cancer/penile cancer/anal cancer.
Leukoplakia	16, 18	White plaque favoring the floor of the mouth, lateral and ventral tongue, and soft palate.	Male predominant. Risk of malignant degeneration into SCC.
Erythroplakia	16, 18	Red patch or thin plaque favoring the floor of the mouth, lateral and ventral tongue, and soft palate.	Male predominant. Risk of malignant degeneration into SCC (less common but higher risk than leukoplakia).
Verrucous Carcinoma			
Papillomatosis cutis carcinoides (Gottron tumor)	6, 11	Vegetative, verrucous-like lesion on the trunk or extremities.	
Florid oral papillomatosis (Ackerman tumor)	6, 11	Verrucous lesions in the oral cavity.	
Giant condylomata acuminata (Buschke–Löwenstein tumor)	6, 11	Large exophytic condyloma-like plaques and tumors of the anogenital area.	Slow-growing mass that can invade the bone beneath the tumor.
Epithelioma cuniculatum	6, 11	Vegetative plaques on the plantar surface of the foot.	
Miscellaneous			
PVL	N/A	Multiple red and white patches on the oral mucosa with variable verrucous change.	Female predominant. Risk of malignant degeneration into SCC or verrucous carcinoma.
Pseudoepitheliomatous keratotic micaceous balanitis	N/A	Thick keratotic plaques on the glans penis.	Elderly circumscribed men. Risk of malignant degeneration into SCC or verrucous carcinoma.

[a]Illustrative examples provided.

AIN, anal intraepithelial neoplasia; CIN, cervical intraepithelial neoplasia; EDV, epidermodysplasia verruciformis; HPV, human papillomavirus; N/A, not applicable; PIN, penile intraepithelial neoplasia; PVL, proliferative verrucous leukoplakia; SCC, squamous cell carcinoma; SIL, squamous intraepithelial lesion; VaIN, vaginal intraepithelial neoplasia; VIN, vulvar intraepithelial neoplasia.

psoriasis, eczematous dermatitis, LK, or superficial BCC. The differential diagnosis of oral SCC includes salivary gland tumor, most commonly benign pleomorphic adenoma or malignant mucoepidermoid carcinoma. Location can be a helpful clue as salivary gland tumors favor the posterior hard palate/anterior soft palate.

- **Dermoscopy** features include **focal glomerular vessels, rosettes, keratin pearls (white circles), yellow scale, and brown dots aligned radially at the periphery.**
- A universally accepted staging system for risk stratification for cutaneous SCC does not exist. Stratification of localized SCC using the NCCN guidelines is recommended for clinical practice; however, the **Brigham and Women's Hospital tumor staging system for cutaneous SCC** is generally regarded as the best **prognostication** tool (Table 5.7). While there is an overall low risk of nodal and distant metastasis, imaging (CT, PET/CT, US) may be warranted for high-risk tumors (eg, Brigham and Women's Hospital ≥ T2b) and when there is concern for deep structural involvement.

Management

- Though SCC most commonly carries the risk of local, destructive infiltration, the risk of metastasis is approximately 4%. The **two highest risk factors for metastasis** are **depth of invasion > 4 mm and size ≥ 2 cm.** Additional poor prognostic factors include **comorbidities (eg, chronic**

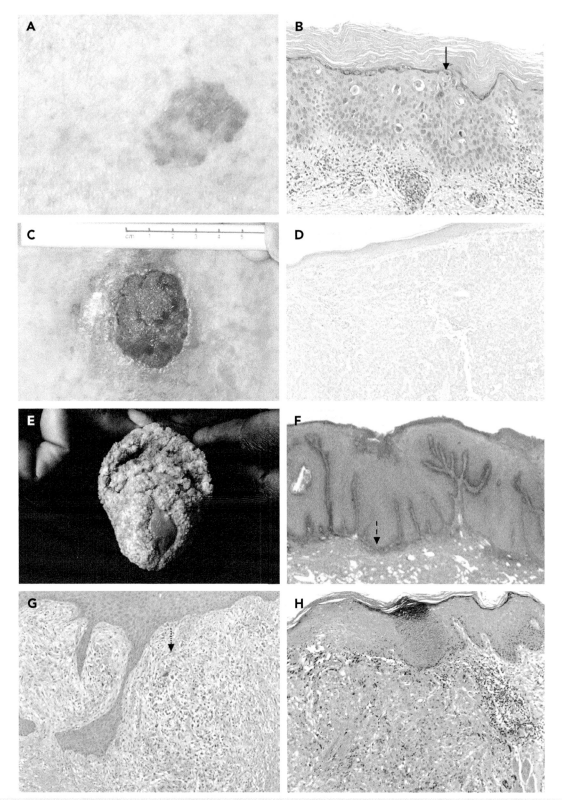

Figure 5.7. CLINICOPATHOLOGICAL CORRELATION: SQUAMOUS CELL CARCINOMA. A and B, SCCis. Solid arrow: loss of normal epidermal maturation ("wind-blown" appearance). C and D, SCC. E and F, Verrucous carcinoma. Dashed arrow: round "pushing" border "bulldozing" the underlying dermis. G, Spindle cell SCC. Dotted arrow: atypical spindle cells. H, Metastatic SCC. AK, actinic keratosis; CK, cytokeratin; EMA, epithelial membrane antigen; IHC, immunohistochemistry; PAS, periodic acid-Schiff; PEH, pseudoepitheliomatous hyperplasia; SCC, squamous cell carcinoma; SCCis, squamous cell carcinoma in situ.

(A, Reprinted with permission from Craft N, Fox LP, Goldsmith LA, et al. *VisualDx: Essential Adult Dermatology*. Wolters Kluwer Health/Lippincott

(Figure 5.7. Continued)

Williams & Wilkins; 2010. B, Histology image courtesy of Noel Turner, MD, MHS and Christine J. Ko, MD. C, Reprinted with permission from Elder DE, Elenitsas R, Rosenbach M, et al. *Lever's Histopathology of the Skin.* 11th ed. Wolters Kluwer; 2015. D, Histology image courtesy of Noel Turner, MD, MHS and Christine J. Ko, MD. F, Histology image reprinted with permission from Crowson N, Magro CM, Mihm MC Jr. *Biopsy Interpretation of the Skin: Primary Non-Lymphoid Cutaneous Neoplasia.* Wolters Kluwer Health/Lippincott Williams & Wilkins; 2010. G, Histology image reprinted with permission from Crowson N, Magro CM, Mihm MC Jr. *Biopsy Interpretation of the Skin: Primary Non-Lymphoid Cutaneous Neoplasia.* Wolters Kluwer Health/Lippincott Williams & Wilkins; 2010. H, Histology image reprinted with permission from Elder DE, Elenitsas R, Rosenbach M, et al. *Lever's Histopathology of the Skin.* 11th ed. Wolters Kluwer; 2015.)

- **SCCis:** loss of normal epidermal maturation with full-thickness cytologic atypia (the basement membrane remains intact). Malignant keratinocytes can keratinize and integrate into the *stratum corneum* forming malignant horn. Pagetoid spread is variably present. Follicular involvement is common.
- **SCC:** invasive. Malignant keratinocytes can keratinize and integrate into the *stratum corneum* forming malignant horn (well- or moderately differentiated). Hypergranulosis / PEH may occur at the periphery. Acantholysis and desmoplasia are variably present. Perineural invasion and plasma cells are common.
- **Verrucous carcinoma:** well-differentiated glassy eosinophilic keratinocytes with a round border.
- **Spindle cell SCC:** poorly differentiated SCC with atypical spindle cells abutting the epidermis.
- **Metastatic SCC:** lacks overlying in situ component, often deeper with a high degree of cytologic atypia.

Clear cells containing glycogen (PAS positive, diastase sensitive) are variably present. IHC is often required to diagnose poorly differentiated SCCs (eg., spindle cell). Positive stains include pan-CK and EMA.

Loss of normal epidermal maturation gives SCCis a "wind-blown" appearance.
The round "pushing" border of verrucous carcinoma "bulldozes" the dermis.

Table 5.7. BRIGHAM AND WOMEN'S HOSPITAL TUMOR STAGING SYSTEM FOR CUTANEOUS SQUAMOUS CELL CARCINOMA

TUMOR Classification System

Category	Definition	Risk Factors
T0	SCCis	Tumor diameter ≥ 2 cm
T1	0 risk factors.	Poorly differentiated histology Perineural invasion
T2a	1 risk factor.	Tumor invasion beyond subcutaneous fat (excluding bone which upgrades to T3)
T2b	2-3 risk factors.	
T3	4 risk factors or bone invasion.	

SCCis, squamous cell carcinoma in situ.

lymphocytic leukemia [CLL]); **location on the lip or ear; SCC arising within a scar or chronic ulcer, hypertrophic LP, hypertrophic LE, or LS; arsenical SCC; and poor histological differentiation or perineural invasion.**

- Per AAD guidelines, **surgical excision with 4 to 6 mm margins** to the depth of adipose tissue is recommended for low-risk SCC. ED&C may be considered for **low-risk SCCs on nonterminal hair-bearing sites.** Standard surgical excision can be considered for some high-risk SCC, though generally **MMS is preferred.** The MMS AUC is an excellent a tool to determine whether MMS is the appropriate treatment for SCC.
- When a surgical approach is contraindicated or impractical, **radiation therapy** may be considered, though the cure rate is lower.
- **PDT, cryotherapy, and ED&C** can be considered for the treatment of **SCCis.**
- Per AAD guidelines, there is insufficient evidence to recommend use of oral nicotinamide or celecoxib for chemoprevention in patients with a history of SCC. However, a phase III RCT did show that **niacinamide 500 mg twice daily reduced the incidence of keratinocytic skin cancer by ~25%** in a high-risk skin cancer population.
- For solid organ transplant recipients, **oral retinoids may be beneficial for chemoprevention.**

"Real World" Advice

- For solid organ transplant recipients, consider switching tacrolimus to sirolimus.

KERATOACANTHOMA

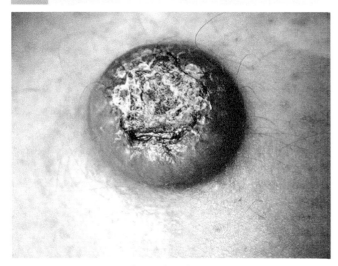

Reprinted with permission from Edward S, Yung A. *Essential Dermatopathology.* Wolters Kluwer Health/Lippincott Williams & Wilkins; 2011

- KA is generally regarded as a **low-grade form of SCC capable of regression** via **terminal differentiation.** Some KAs arise in the setting of trauma, suggesting a Koebner phenomenon. Drug associations with KAs include **BRAF inhibitors and ICIs.**

  KAs are associated with **Muir-Torre syndrome (MTS).**
- KA classically presents as a **rapidly growing papule, eventually forming a keratotic-filled crater.** The **Ferguson-Smith variant** due to AD mutation in *TGFBR1* is characterized by **multiple spontaneously regressing KAs** typically in younger, adolescent patients, while the **Grzybowski variant** is characterized by **thousands of widespread KA papules resembling milia** in older individuals.
  - Figure 5.8.
- Rapid growth, especially after a biopsy, is a helpful clinical clue to the diagnosis of KA.
- While some KAs will spontaneously regress, for those with persistent clinical disease, surgical excision is recommended. In cases where surgery may lead to poor cosmetic or functional outcome, intralesional 5-FU may be considered.

MAMMARY PAGET DISEASE AND EXTRAMAMMARY PAGET DISEASE

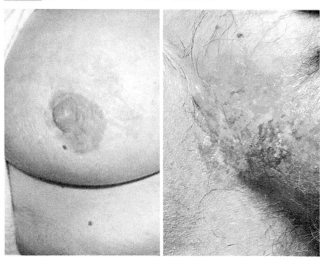

Mammary Paget disease (left) reprinted with permission from *Goodheart HP. Goodheart's Same-Site Differential Diagnosis: A Rapid Method of Diagnosing and Treating Common Skin Disorders.* Wolters Kluwer Health/Lippincott Williams & Wilkins; 2011. Extramammary Paget disease (right).

A

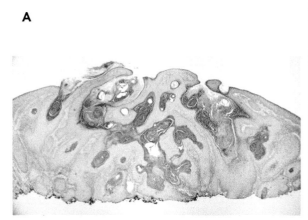

B

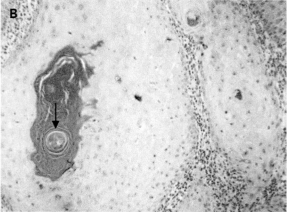

Figure 5.8. CLINICOPATHOLOGICAL CORRELATION: KERATOACANTHOMA. KA is characterized by a keratin-filled crater composed of glassy eosinophilic keratinocytes with mild cytologic atypia. Hypergranulosis / PEH may occur at the center; elastic trapping may occur at the periphery. Perineural invasion is common, along with lymphocytes ± lichenoid interface dermatitis with admixed neutrophilic microabscesses and eosinophils. A, Low-power view. B, High-power view. Solid arrow: squamous eddy (keratin pearl). KA, keratoacanthoma; PEH, pseudoepitheliomatous hyperplasia.

The classic teaching is that a KA should not demonstrate acantholysis.

• **Regressing KA:** keratin-filled crater, now involuted to a thin wall, and peripheral scar.

- **Mammary Paget disease (MPD)** is an intraepithelial condition of the **nipple and peri-areolar skin** associated with **underlying breast cancer.** In some cases, MPD may arise in the absence of underlying breast cancer from Toker cells. **Extramammary Paget disease (EMPD)** is an intraepithelial condition of the **apocrine gland** often located on **anogenital skin.** While patients most often present with **primary EMPD,** ~25% present with **secondary EMPD due to pagetoid spread of an adjacent or continuous malignancy (most commonly breast, colon, or bladder adenocarcinoma).**
- MPD and EMPD are each characterized by a **well-demarcated, erythematous expanding plaque** in the above distribution. Pruritus is common; erosion, bleeding, and pain are signs of late-stage disease.
  - The combination of <u>pink</u> erythema and <u>white</u> scale is sometimes called a "strawberries and cream" appearance.
  - Figure 5.9.
  - IHC for the differential diagnosis of pagetoid spread is summarized in Table 5.8.
- Skin biopsy is required to establish the diagnosis of MPD and EMPD, which are often mistaken for inflammatory eruptions (eg, eczematous dermatoses) or infections (eg, tinea).

- MPD prognosis is largely tied to the stage of the underlying breast adenocarcinoma; some studies suggest that MPD is a negative prognostic factor. Management is usually surgical excision or radiation therapy. EMPD can be invasive leading to metastasis and a poor prognosis; however, EMPD generally has a good prognosis with 5-year overall survival ranging from 75% to 95%. **MMS is superior to wide local excision (WLE)** with regard to higher recurrence-free survival, which is further enhanced by the use of **CK7 IHC. Topical cytotoxic chemotherapies (eg, 5-FU), imiquimod, and radiation therapy (eg, brachytherapy)** may be used for patients in whom surgery is not practical or contraindicated, and as adjunctive therapy.

Melanocytic Neoplasms

Basic Concepts

- Pigmented lesions can result from an increase in melanin production (for example, ephelis, café-au-lait macule [CALM]), or an increase in melanocytes (eg, lentigo simplex).
- Melanocytic lesions span a wide range of diagnoses ranging from benign etiologies (eg, lentigo simplex) to malignant etiologies (eg, melanoma).
- On dermoscopy, the four primary global features of melanocytic lesions are **reticular pattern, globular pattern, homogenous pattern, and starburst pattern.** For local and site-related features, see Appendix 4.

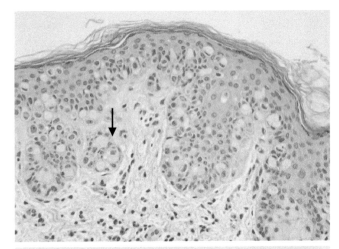

Figure 5.9. CLINICOPATHOLOGICAL CORRELATION: MAMMARY PAGET DISEASE AND EXTRAMAMMARY PAGET DISEASE. Both MPD and EMPD are characterized by large cells with abundant cytoplasm that scatter or form nests within the epidermis. Paget cells compress the basal layer and may spit out into the *stratum corneum.* Differentiation relies on staining pattern. Paget cells contain sialomucin (mucicarmine positive; PAS positive, diastase resistant). Solid arrow: Paget cell. EMPD, extramammary Paget disease; MPD, mammary Paget disease; PAS, periodic acid-Schiff; SCCis, squamous cell carcinoma in situ.

(Histology image courtesy of Kristin Smith, MD.)

Beyond MPD/EMPD, the differential diagnosis for pagetoid spread includes SCCis, Spitz nevus, melanoma, sebaceous carcinoma, and intraepithelial porocarcinoma.

LENTIGO SIMPLEX
→ **Diagnosis Group 1**
Synonyms: simple lentigo, lentiginosis (multiple)

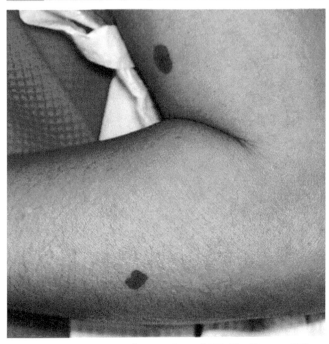

Table 5.8. IMMUNOHISTOCHEMISTRY FOR THE DIFFERENTIAL DIAGNOSIS OF PAGETOID SPREAD

Diagnosis	CK7	CK20	CAM 5.2	GCDFP-15	S100	Melan-A (MART-1)	EMA/CEA	Adipophilin/Androgen Receptor	HER-2/Neu
MPD	+		+				±		+
Primary EMPD	+		+	+			+		+
Secondary EMPD	+	+ (usually)	+				+		+
SCCis	±								
Spitz nevus					+	+			
Melanoma					+	+			
Sebaceous Carcinoma	+						+	+	
Intraepithelial porocarcinoma			±		±		+		

CEA, carcinoembryonic antigen; CK, cytokeratin; EMA, epithelial membrane antigen; EMPD, extramammary Paget disease; GCDFP-15, gross cystic disease fluid protein 15; MART-1, melanoma antigen recognized by T cells 1; MPD, mammary Paget disease; SCCis, squamous cell carcinoma in situ.

Epidemiology

- Lentigo simplex is a benign pigmented lesion that results from an **increase in melanocytes.**
    - **Hereditary syndromes associated with lentigines** are summarized in Table 5.9.

Clinicopathological Features

- Lentigo simplex classically presents as a **brown to black, well-circumscribed, oval macule**, either singly or in multiplicity.
- Lentigo variants include **ink-jet lentigo (very dark pigmentation), solar lentigo (sun-exposed sites), mucosal melanotic macule (oral, anogenital), nail unit lentigo (longitudinal melanonychia).**
- Lentigo simplex overlaps with junctional nevocellular nevus in lentiginous nevus.
    - Figure 5.10.

Evaluation

- The differential diagnosis of lentigo simplex includes ephelis, CALM, junctional melanocytic nevus, and lentigo maligna. In contradistinction to lentigo simplex, **ephelides and CALMs** are benign pigmented lesions that result from an **increase in melanin production.**
- The diagnosis of lentigo simplex can usually be made by clinical and dermatoscopic examination alone; however, skin biopsy may be helpful to confirm the diagnosis.

Management

- Treatment is not needed as lentigo simplex is benign. Cosmetic treatment options include cryotherapy, chemical peels, Q-switched lasers (ie, ruby, alexandrite, Nd:YAG), and IPL.

"Real World" Advice

- Lentigo simplex on a mucosal surface can have ill-defined borders and nonhomogenous pigment, which can mimic melanoma.

Table 5.9. HEREDITARY SYNDROMES ASSOCIATED WITH LENTIGINES

Diagnosis	Inheritance Pattern	Genes	Classic Description
Localized			
Peutz-Jeghers syndrome	AD	*STK11*	Lentigines favoring perioral skin, oral mucosa, and hands. Systemic features include hamartomatous gastrointestinal polyps, intussusception, and gastrointestinal hemorrhage. Increased risk for gastrointestinal, pancreatic, breast, and lung cancer.
Cowden syndrome/BRR syndrome	See Chapter 5: Adipose Neoplasms.		
Cronkite-Canada syndrome	Sporadic	Unknown	Lentigines on face, oral mucosa (often buccal), and acral skin, hypermelanosis, alopecia, onychoatrophy. Systemic features include weight loss, chronic diarrhea, and intestinal polyposis.
Laugier-Hunziker syndrome	Sporadic	Unknown	Lentigines in similar distribution as Peutz-Jeghers syndrome, genital melanosis, longitudinal melanonychia.
Generalized			
Noonan syndrome with lentigines (formerly LEOPARD)	AD	*PTPN11*	Lentigines present in early infancy, CALMs, low-set ears, KP atrophicans faciei. The characteristic hair shaft abnormality without increased fragility is woolly hair. Systemic features include growth retardation, ECG abnormalities (heart block), ocular hypertelorism, deafness, abnormal genitalia, and pulmonary stenosis. Increased risk for GCT.
		Remember that the gene implicated in <u>L</u>EOPARD is *PTPN11* with the phrase, "<u>L</u>EOPARD print <u>pants</u>."	<u>L</u>EOPARD is characterized by <u>l</u>entigines, <u>E</u>CG abnormalities, <u>o</u>cular hypertelorism, <u>p</u>ulmonary stenosis, <u>a</u>bnormal genitalia, growth <u>r</u>etardation, and <u>d</u>eafness.
Carney complex	AD	*PRKAR1A*	Superficial (angio)myxomas, lentigines, blue nevi, and psammomatous melanotic schwannomas. Systemic features include atria myxomas, pigmented nodular adrenocortical disease, myxoid mammary fibroadenomas, and testicular tumors.
		Remember that <u>PRKAR1A</u> is the gene implicated in <u>Car</u>ney complex with the phrase, "<u>park</u> your <u>car</u>."	

AD, autosomal dominant; BRR, Bannayan-Riley-Ruvalcaba; CALMs, café-au-lait macules; ECG, electrocardiogram; GCT, granular cell tumor; KP, keratosis pilaris.

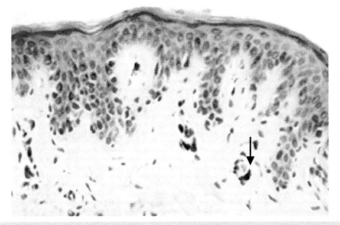

Figure 5.10. CLINICOPATHOLOGICAL CORRELATION: LENTIGO SIMPLEX. Lentigo simplex is characterized by epidermal acanthosis and a slight increase in melanocytes in the basal layer of the epidermis with hyperpigmentation. Melanophages may be observed in the upper dermis. Solid arrow: melanophage.

(Histology image reprinted with permission from Elder DE, Elenitsas R, Rosenbach M, et al. *Lever's Histopathology of the Skin*. 11th ed. Wolters Kluwer; 2015.)

- Ink-spot lentigo: marked hyperpigmentation.
- Solar lentigo: bulb-like elongation of rete ridges in a reticular pattern and solar elastosis in the dermis.
- Mucosal melanotic macule: mucosal location with less prominent epidermal acanthosis.
- Nail unit lentigo: nail matrix location.

DERMAL MELANOCYTOSIS

Synonyms: congenital dermal melanocytosis, Mongolian spot

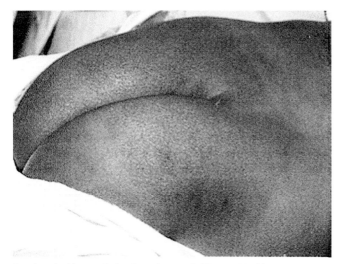

Reprinted with permission from Jensen S. *Nursing Health Assessment: A Best Practice Approach*. 3rd ed. Wolters Kluwer; 2018.

- Dermal melanocytosis is a benign melanocytic proliferation that is **usually present at birth.** It most commonly affects **Asian, Black, and Latino** patients. It is rarely associated with **GM1 gangliosidosis type 1, Hurler syndrome, and phakomatosis pigmentovascularis (*GNAQ* > *GNA11* mutations).**
- Dermal melanocytosis classically presents as **blue-gray macules or patches favoring the lumbosacral skin and buttocks** that fade over time. **Dermal melanocytosis variants** are summarized in Table 5.10.
    ◆ Figure 5.11.
- Dermal melanocytosis does not require treatment as it fades over time; however, nevus of Ota and Ito often persist. **Q-switched lasers (ruby, alexandrite, Nd:YAG)** can help minimize the pigmentation.

Table 5.10. DERMAL MELANOCYTOSIS VARIANTS

Diagnosis[a]	Classic Description	Notes
Nevus of Ota	Blue-gray patch in the V1 and V2 distribution on the face (often including the sclera of the eye). Can enlarge during puberty under the influence of hormones.	Patients with nevus of Ota are at risk for glaucoma (10%). They also have a slightly increased risk of uveal melanoma.
Nevus of Ito	Unilateral blue-gray patch on the scapular, supraclavicular, or shoulder region.	
Hori nevus (acquired nevus of Ota-like macules)	Bilateral blue-gray macules favoring the zygomatic skin.	

[a]Illustrative examples provided.

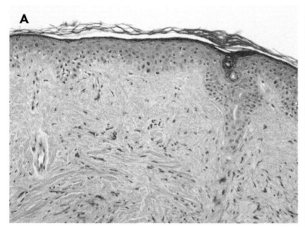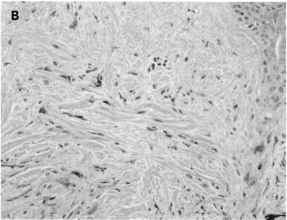

Figure 5.11. CLINICOPATHOLOGICAL CORRELATION: DERMAL MELANOCYTOSIS. Dermal melanocytosis is characterized by slender dendritic melanocytes in the dermis primarily oriented parallel to the epidermis ± melanophages. The stroma is nonsclerotic. A, Nevus of Ito low-power view. B, Nevus of Ito high-power view.

(Histology images reprinted with permission from Crowson AN, Magro CM, Mihm MC Jr. *Biopsy Interpretation of the Skin: Primary Non-Lymphoid Cutaneous Neoplasia*. 2nd ed. Wolters Kluwer; 2018.)

BLUE NEVUS
→ Diagnosis Group 2
Synonym: dermal melanocytoma

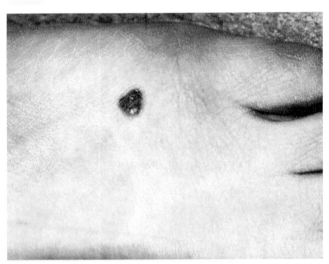

Reprinted with permission from Elder DE, Elenitsas R, Rubin AI, et al. *Atlas of Dermatopathology: Synopsis and Atlas of Lever's Histopathology of the Skin.* 4th ed. Wolters Kluwer; 2020.

Epidemiology

- Blue nevi are benign tumors of dermal melanocytes.
- **Most blue nevi present in childhood/adolescence**, but up to 25% develop in adulthood.
- The genetics of blue nevus most commonly include *GNAQ* **mutations** (also seen in nevus of Ota and uveal melanoma) in >50% of cases and *GNA11* **mutations** in ~10% of cases.
- Blue nevi, especially epithelioid blue nevi, are associated with the **Carney complex.**

Clinicopathological Features

- Blue nevi classically present as **solitary blue to blue-black papulonodules.**
- **Common blue nevi favor the distal extensor extremities (~50%) followed by the scalp.**
- Blue nevus variants include:
  - **Cellular blue nevus**: commonly occurs on the **buttocks.** There is a small risk of malignant degeneration to **malignant cellular blue nevus with *BAP-1* loss.**
  - **Epithelioid blue nevus**: favors the trunk and extremities. It is associated with **Carney complex.**
    - Figure 5.12.

Evaluation

- The differential diagnosis of blue nevus includes blue tattoo, dermal melanocytic nevus, vascular neoplasms (eg, angiokeratoma, venous lake), pigmented BCC, and melanoma.
- The diagnosis of blue nevus is often made by the clinical exam. If the diagnosis is uncertain, a blue nevus is changing, or there is concern for melanoma, a biopsy is indicated.

Management

- Common blue nevi do not require excision. However, complete surgical excision of cellular blue nevi is recommended because of the small risk of malignant transformation.

"Real World" Advice

- The **Tyndall effect** refers to optical scatter of different wavelengths of light encountering a clear substance. This effect, responsible for the **blue color of both dermal melanocytosis and blue nevus**, may also result in **bluish discoloration when an HA filler is injected too superficially into the dermis.**

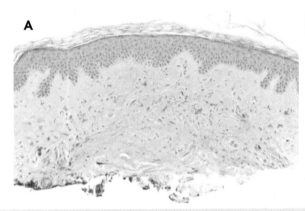
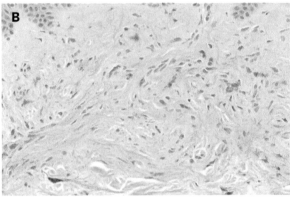

Figure 5.12. CLINICOPATHOLOGICAL CORRELATION: BLUE NEVUS. Common blue nevus is characterized by slender dendritic melanocytes in the dermis primarily oriented parallel to the epidermis ± melanophages. The stroma is sclerotic. A, Blue nevus low-power view. B, Blue nevus high-power view.

(Histology images reprinted with permission from Elder DE, Elenitsas R, Rosenbach M, et al. *Lever's Histopathology of the Skin.* 11th ed. Wolters Kluwer; 2015.)

- Cellular blue nevus: admixed large spindle-shaped or epithelioid cells.
- Malignant cellular blue nevus: cytologic atypia, mitotic activity, and necrosis.
- Epithelioid blue nevus: large epithelioid cells; nonsclerotic stroma.

In cellular blue nevus, a nodule may extend into the subcutis in a "dumbbell" pattern.

NEVOCELLULAR NEVUS AND ATYPICAL NEVUS

→ Diagnosis Group 1

Nevocellular nevus synonyms: common acquired melanocytic nevus, mole

Atypical nevus synonym: Clark nevus, dysplastic nevus

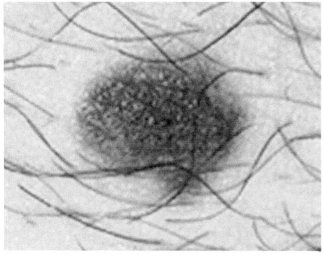

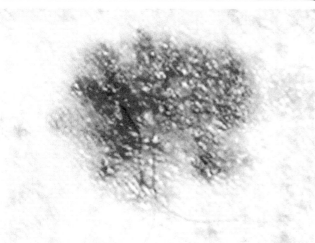

Nevocellular nevus (top) reprinted with permission from Gru AA, Wick MR, Mir A, et al. *Pediatric Dermatopathology and Dermatology.* Wolters Kluwer; 2018. Atypical nevus (bottom) reprinted with permission from Elder DE, Elenitsas R, Rosenbach M, et al. *Lever's Histopathology of the Skin.* 11th ed. Wolters Kluwer; 2015.

Epidemiology

- **Nevocellular nevi** are benign melanocytic neoplasms that come in three main varieties: **junctional, compound, and intradermal.**
- The genetics of common acquired nevocellular nevus most commonly include *BRAF* mutations in ~80% of cases and *NRAS* mutations in a minority of cases. **Gene mutations associated with melanocytic nevi** are summarized in Table 5.11.

    Cardiofaciocutaneous syndrome (AD mutation in *BRAF*, most commonly) is associated with **multiple**

Table 5.11. GENE MUTATIONS ASSOCIATED WITH MELANOCYTIC NEVI

Diagnosis[a]	Gene Associations[a]
Dermal melanocytosis	*GNAQ > GNA11*
Blue nevus	*GNAQ > GNA11*
Epithelioid blue nevus	*PRKAR1A*
Common acquired nevocellular nevus	*BRAF > NRAS*
Deep penetrating nevus	*CTNNB1* (β-catenin)
Atypical nevus	*CDKN2A* (p16)
Congenital melanocytic nevus	*NRAS*
Nevus spilus	*HRAS*
Spitz nevus	*HRAS*
Atypical epithelioid Spitz nevus	*BAP1, BRAF*

[a]Illustrative examples provided.

dark melanocytic nevi. Cardiofaciocutaneous syndrome is also associated with distinctive facial features (high forehead, short nose, hypertelorism, ptosis, and small chin), cardiac defects, and other cutaneous findings (ichthyosis, KP, and absent eyebrows/eyelashes).

- Nevi are more common in white patients. However, **nevi on acral surfaces, nails, and conjunctiva are more prevalent in black and Asian patients.**
- **Sun exposure (both intermittent intense and chronic moderate) and tanning bed use may trigger eruptive atypical melanocytic nevi.** Other triggers of eruptive melanocytic nevi include blistering conditions (ie, SJS/TEN), scarring conditions (ie, genital LS), and systemic immunosuppression (eg, HIV infection). Melanocytic nevi may darken under the influence of hormones (eg, pregnancy).
- Drug triggers include systemic immunosuppressants (eg, azathioprine, cyclosporine) and **BRAF inhibitors** (hypothesized role for paradoxical MAPK activation).

Clinicopathological Features

- **Junctional nevi are usually small (<5 mm), well-circumscribed, brown macules. Compound nevi show variable elevation but are usually thin papules that are lighter brown compared to junctional nevi. Finally, intradermal nevi are usually skin-colored to light brown papules.**
- **Atypical nevi** are often larger (>6 mm) and can have **irregular brown pigment and irregular borders.**
- There are several variants of nevocellular nevi which are summarized in Table 5.11 including **recurrent nevus** (often mistaken for melanoma given the atypia seen on histopathology), **longitudinal melanonychia, balloon cell nevus, and halo nevus.**

    Figure 5.13.

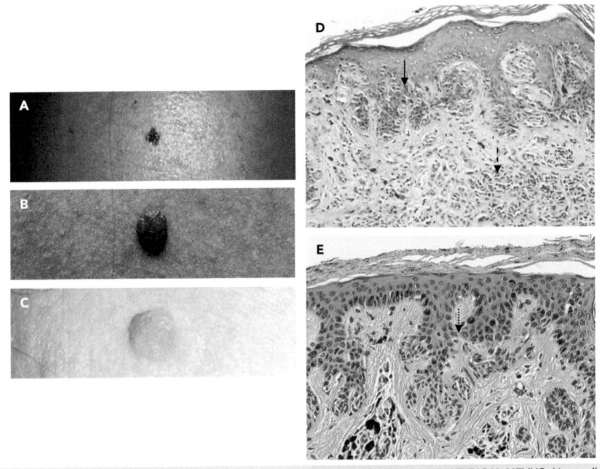

Figure 5.13. CLINICOPATHOLOGICAL CORRELATION: NEVOCELLULAR NEVUS AND ATYPICAL NEVUS. Nevocellular nevus is well-nested at the DEJ and demonstrates sharp lateral circumscription, left-right symmetry, maturation, and dispersion. Deep mitoses and deep pigment in nests are absent. Atypical nevus is well-nested at the DEJ and demonstrates maturation and dispersion. Deep mitoses and deep pigment in nests are absent. However, the junctional component extends ≥ 3 rete beyond the intradermal component (shoulder region), and there is left-right asymmetry. Irregular nests of junctional melanocytes ± cytologic atypia bridge adjacent rete. There is concentric papillary dermal fibrosis. Some dermatopathologists grade atypia as mild, moderate, or severe. A, Junctional nevus. B, Compound nevus. C, Dermal nevus. D, Compound nevus. Solid arrow: junctional component. Dashed arrow: intradermal component. E, Atypical compound nevus. Dotted arrow: bridging of adjacent retia.

(A, Reprinted with permission from Goodheart HP. *Goodheart's Same-Site Differential Diagnosis: A Rapid Method of Diagnosing and Treating Common Skin Disorders.* Wolters Kluwer Health/Lippincott Williams & Wilkins; 2011. B, Reprinted with permission from Gru AA, Wick MR, Mir A, et al. *Pediatric Dermatopathology and Dermatology.* Wolters Kluwer; 2018. C, Reprinted with permission from Edwards L, Lynch P. *Genital Dermatology Atlas and Manual.* 3rd ed. Wolters Kluwer; 2017. D, Histology image reprinted with permission from Crowson AN, Magro CM, Mihm MC Jr. *Biopsy Interpretation of the Skin: Primary Non-Lymphoid Cutaneous Neoplasia.* 2nd ed. Wolters Kluwer; 2018. E, Histology image reprinted with permission from Gru AA, Wick MR, Mir A, et al. *Pediatric Dermatopathology and Dermatology.* Wolters Kluwer; 2018.)

- **Junctional nevus:** melanocytic nests within the epidermis.
- **Compound nevus:** melanocytic nests within the epidermis and dermis.
- **Intradermal nevus:** melanocytic nests within the dermis.
- **Acral nevus:** elongated nests following dermatoglyphs.
- **Ancient nevus:** melanocytes with large hyperchromatic nuclei.
- **Balloon cell nevus:** melanocytes with swelling of cellular organelles (balloon cells).
- **Combined nevus:** contains ≥2 cell populations, most often nevocellular nevus and blue nevus.
- **Deep penetrating nevus:** heavily pigmented melanocytes penetrating toward or into the subcutis.
- **Neural nevus:** spindle melanocytes; nevic corpuscles resemble Meissner corpuscles.
- **Recurrent nevus:** confluent poorly and/or irregularly nested junctional melanocytic proliferation overlying a scar ± underlying residual nevocellular nevus.
- **Special site nevus (scalp, ear, breast, axilla, umbilicus, anogenital):** may appear atypical or demonstrate large junctional nests with poorly cohesive melanocytes.
- **Congenital melanocytic nevus / nevus spilus / halo nevus:** see below.

A "discount" is applied when grading the atypia of special site nevi.

Evaluation

- The differential diagnosis of junctional melanocytic nevus and atypical nevus includes lentigo simplex and melanoma. The differential diagnosis of compound nevus and intradermal nevus includes SK, Spitz nevus, dermatofibroma (DF), and neurofibroma.
- Biopsy is recommended to rule out melanoma if there are atypical features or if a lesion is changing.

Management

- Nevocellular nevi generally do not require treatment unless a biopsy reveals atypical features.

CONGENITAL MELANOCYTIC NEVUS

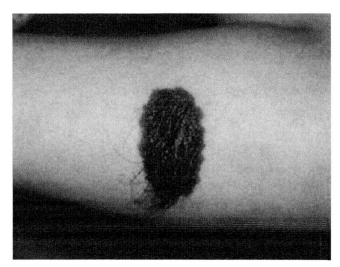

Reprinted with permission from Salimpour RR, Salimpour P, Salimpour P. *Photographic Atlas of Pediatric Disorders and Diagnosis.* Wolters Kluwer Health/Lippincott Williams & Wilkins; 2013.

- Congenital melanocytic nevi are melanocytic nevi that are **present at birth**. They are traditionally divided into four categories based on the adult size: **small (<1.5 cm), medium (1.5-20 cm), large (>20 cm), and giant (>40 cm).** The majority (~80%) are caused by *NRAS* mutations.
- Congenital melanocytic nevi classically present as **brown thin plaques ± hypertrichosis.** There may be **perifollicular hypo- or hyperpigmentation.** Lesions can become more elevated and pebbly (develop proliferative papules and nodules) with age. **Neurocutaneous melanosis (NCM)** is characterized by meningeal melanosis in the setting of a large/giant congenital melanocytic nevus or multiple (>3) medium congenital melanocytic nevi. Even in the absence of a large/giant congenital melanocytic nevus, having multiple satellite lesions confers the highest risk. NCM is associated with a **high mortality** in symptomatic patients. **Large and giant congenital melanocytic nevi have an increased risk for developing melanoma (~3%).** The majority of melanomas develop in the **first decade of life.**

- Surgical re-excision with narrow margins is generally recommended for severely atypical nevi.

"Real World" Advice

- Surgical re-excision of moderately atypical melanocytic nevi is an area of controversy. Recent data suggest that close observation of such nevi that have been excisionally biopsied with no residual clinical pigmentation but with histologically positive margins may be reasonable.

Figure 5.14.
- **Patients with medium or large congenital melanocytic nevi with ≥20 satellite lesions or giant congenital melanocytic nevi should get MRI of the brain and spine** to rule out NCM (though some argue for a lower satellite lesion threshold).
- Surgical excision of medium and large congenital nevi can be considered. However, **surgery has not been shown to decrease the risk of melanoma.** Surgery is usually done after 6 months of age to avoid the highest risk period for general anesthesia. Surgery is often staged and utilizes tissue expanders. An acceptable alternative to surgery is yearly TBSEs with photography. Any changing areas within the lesion should be biopsied to rule out melanoma.

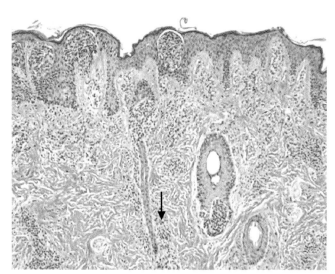

Figure 5.14. CLINICOPATHOLOGICAL CORRELATION: CONGENITAL MELANOCYTIC NEVUS. Congenital melanocytic nevus differs from acquired nevocellular nevus due to greater breadth and depth. Perivascular, periadnexal, and interstitial melanocytes extend into deeper tissues. Solid arrow: Periadnexal melanocytes.

(Histology image reprinted with permission from Husain AN. *Biopsy Interpretation of Pediatric Lesions.* Wolters Kluwer; 2014.)

NEVUS SPILUS
→ Diagnosis Group 2
Synonym: speckled lentiginous nevus

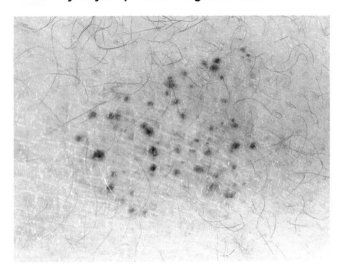

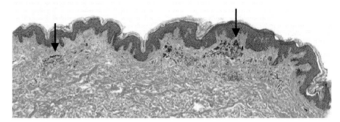

Figure 5.15. CLINICOPATHOLOGICAL CORRELATION: NEVUS SPILUS. Nevus spilus resembles a lentigo simplex with multifocal lentiginous nevi. Solid arrows: multifocal lentiginous nevi.

(Histology image reprinted with permission from Elder DE, Elenitsas R, Rubin AI, et al. *Atlas and Synopsis of Lever's Histopathology of the Skin.* 3rd ed. Wolters Kluwer Health/Lippincott Williams & Wilkins; 2012.)

- The diagnosis of nevus spilus is made clinically since it has very distinctive features.

Management

- Given the low risk of melanoma, patients should get periodic skin examinations for clinical monitoring. Macules or papules that are changing should be biopsied to rule out melanoma.

"Real World" Advice

- Photodocumentation with regular skin examination is helpful for monitoring nevus spilus.

Epidemiology

- Nevus spilus is increasingly being considered a type of congenital melanocytic nevus. It is associated with *HRAS* **mutations.**
- Nevus spilus is associated with **phakomatosis pigmentovascularis types III and IV** (see Chapter 5: Vascular Malformations and Neoplasms) and **phakomatosis pigmentokeratotica (rare neurocutaneous disorder due to *HRAS* mutation** characterized by the combination of **nevus spilus, nevus sebaceous,** and **hypophosphatemic vitamin-D-resistant rickets).**
  - Do NOT confuse <u>phakomatosis pigmento</u>vascularis with <u>phakomatosis pigmento</u>keratotica.

HALO NEVUS
Synonym: Sutton nevus

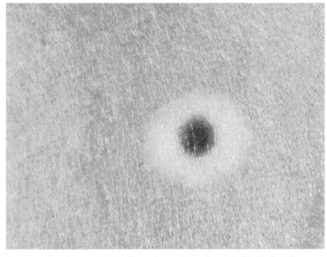

Reprinted with permission from *Lugo-Somolinos A, McKinley-Grant L, Goldsmith LA, et al. VisualDx: Essential Dermatology in Pigmented Skin.* Wolters Kluwer Health/Lippincott Williams & Wilkins; 2011.

Clinicopathological Features

- Nevus spilus classically presents as a **CALM-like light tan ovoid patch that is speckled with darker brown macules or papules.** There is often an increased degree of speckling over time.
  - The appearance of nevus spilus resembles a "chocolate chip cookie."
- While there are reports of melanoma arising within a nevus spilus, the overall risk is thought to be very low. Similar to congenital melanocytic nevus, the risk may be associated with lesion size.
  - Figure 5.15.

Evaluation

- The differential diagnosis of nevus spilus includes CALM and agminated nevus.

- Halo nevus is a **benign** variant of melanocytic nevus with surrounding hypopigmentation. The most common demographic is <**20 years of age.** Halo nevus is thought to be due to a cell-mediated response to altered melanocytes. Twenty percent of patients with halo nevi may develop **vitiligo.**

- Halo nevus classically presents as a **brown macule or papule surrounded by a well-marginated depigmented ring** favoring the trunk, especially the **upper back.** Halo nevi can demonstrate the **Koebner phenomenon.**
    - ◈ Figure 5.16.
- Halo nevi with atypical features should be biopsied to rule out melanoma.
    - ◈ **Adults with new onset multiple halo nevi should be evaluated for cutaneous and uveal melanoma.**

SPITZ NEVUS

→ Diagnosis Group 2

Synonyms: benign juvenile melanoma, Spitz juvenile melanoma

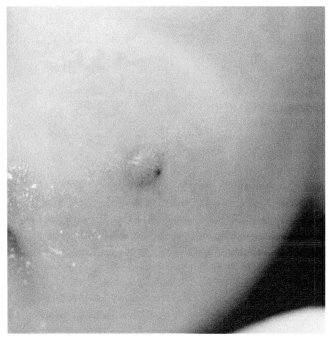

Reprinted with permission from Gru AA, Wick MR, Mir A, et al. *Pediatric Dermatopathology and Dermatology.* Wolters Kluwer; 2018.

Epidemiology

- **Spitz nevus** is a melanocytic neoplasm that typically occurs in **children.**

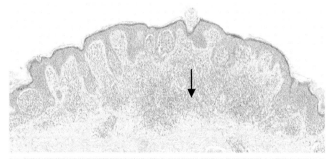

Figure 5.16. CLINICOPATHOLOGICAL CORRELATION: HALO NEVUS. Halo nevus is characterized by a dense lymphocytic infiltrate admixed with junctional and intradermal melanocytes. In the halo region, melanin and melanocytes are reduced or absent. Solid arrow: dense lymphocytic infiltrate.

(Histology image courtesy of Noel Turner, MD, MHS and Christine J. Ko, MD.)

- The genetics of Spitz nevus most commonly include *HRAS* **mutations,** *ALK1* **fusions, and gain of chromosome 11p.** Unlike common acquired nevocellular nevi, Spitz nevi do not harbor *BRAF* mutations. The one exception is the more recently described **atypical epithelioid Spitz nevus (BAPoma),** which often concurrently harbors **loss of** *BAP1* **and** *BRAF* **mutations.** *BAP1* mutation predisposes to a variety of malignancies including RCC (**clear cell variant**), **uveal melanoma, and mesothelioma.** Finally, Spitz nevi may harbor *CDKN2A* **mutations** leading to **focal loss of p16.** However, widespread loss of p16 should raise suspicion for Spitz melanoma.
    - ◈ **Pigmented spindle cell nevus of Reed** is a spindle cell variant of Spitz nevus that most commonly occurs in **young adult women.**

Clinicopathological Features

- **Common Spitz nevus** classically presents as a **pink or brown dome-shaped papule favoring the head and neck.**
    - ◈ **Pigmented spindle cell nevus of Reed** classically presents as a **dark brown dome-shaped papule favoring the thigh.**
- **Agminated Spitz nevus** is characterized by a variable number of grouped Spitz nevi in a localized or segmental distribution.
- **Atypical Spitz nevus** has ≥1 atypical feature that deviates from common Spitz nevus. These features include large size (>5 mm), asymmetry, involvement of deep dermis or

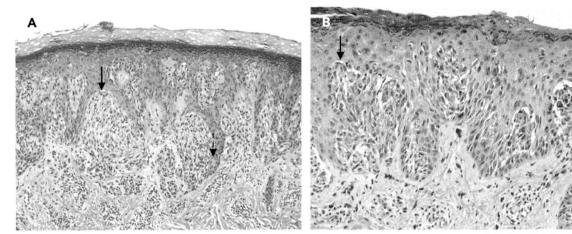

Figure 5.17. SIDE-BY-SIDE COMPARISON: SPITZ NEVUS AND PIGMENTED SPINDLE CELL NEVUS OF REED. Both classical Spitz nevus and the pigmented spindle cell nevus of Reed variant are well-nested at the DEJ and demonstrate sharp lateral circumscription, left-right symmetry, maturation, and dispersion. Deep mitoses and deep pigment in nests are absent. There is overlying hyperkeratosis, hypergranulosis, and PEH. Pagetoid spread, clefts around nests, pink Kamino bodies derived from the basement membrane (PAS positive, diastase resistant), and melanophages are variably present. In Spitz nevus, vertically oriented nests are comprised of epithelioid and spindled melanocytes and Kamino bodies are enriched. In pigmented spindle cell nevus of Reed, nests are comprised primarily of spindled melanocytes and melanophages are enriched.

A, Spitz nevus. B, Pigmented spindle cell nevus. Solid arrows: clefts around nests. Dashed arrow: Kamino body. DEJ, dermo-epidermal junction; PAS, periodic acid-Schiff; PEH, pseudoepitheliomatous hyperplasia.

(A, Histology image reprinted with permission from Husain AN. Biopsy Interpretation of Pediatric Lesions. Wolters Kluwer; 2014. B, Histology image reprinted with permission from Elder DE, Elenitsas R, Rosenbach M, et al. *Lever's Histopathology of the Skin.* 11th ed. Wolters Kluwer; 2015.)

Vertically oriented nests may be described as a "raining down pattern" or "bananas on the tree."

subcutis, ulceration, lack of maturation, pagetoid spread, or high mitotic rate (>2 mitoses/mm²).

- Atypical Spitz nevus has a risk of metastasis. **Features associated with risk of metastasis include ulceration, Breslow thickness, atypical mitotic figures, and loss of p16 (CDKN2A).**
  - ◆ Figure 5.17.

Evaluation

- The differential diagnosis of Spitz nevus includes intradermal nevus, melanoma, DF, and mastocytoma.
- There can often be a high clinical suspicion for a Spitz nevus from clinical and dermatoscopic examinations. However, given the difficulty in classifying Spitz nevus along with the variability in clinical presentation, a biopsy may be indicated to rule out atypical Spitz nevus or melanoma.
- While controversial, some recommend a sentinel lymph node biopsy (SLNB) for atypical Spitz nevus.

Management

- Treatment remains controversial. Historically, the recommendation was to excise all Spitz nevi. However, many pediatric dermatologists now favor monitoring lesions that do not display any clinical or histopathological atypia.
- There is mounting evidence that metastatic atypical Spitz nevi do not behave like metastatic melanoma and instead have a more benign course. Death is very rare. Patients with metastatic atypical Spitz nevi are often referred to oncology for co-management. Those with a positive SLNB are typically treated as having stage III melanoma with cytotoxic chemotherapy and immunotherapy.

"Real World" Advice

- Terminology can be confusing. "Spitz melanomas" have hallmark mutations of Spitz nevi, whereas "Spitzoid melanomas" have histopathologic morphology resembling Spitz nevi.

MELANOMA
→ Diagnosis Group 1

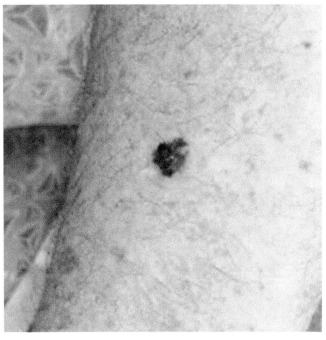

Superficial spreading melanoma

Epidemiology

- Melanoma is a malignant neoplasm that arises from melanocytes. Although it is **most commonly cutaneous in origin**, it can also arise on **mucosal surfaces and the uvea**.
- Initiating oncogenic mutations usually involve the **MAPK and PI3K signaling pathways. Genetic mutations associated with melanoma** are summarized in Table 5.12. Overall, *BRAF* **(V600E) is the most common mutation.**

Table 5.12. GENE MUTATIONS ASSOCIATED WITH MELANOMA

Diagnosis[a]	Gene Associations[a]
Superficial spreading melanoma	Non-CSD: *BRAF > NRAS* CSD: *c-KIT > BRAF, NRAS*
Lentigo maligna/lentigo maligna melanoma	*c-KIT > BRAF, NRAS*
Acral lentiginous melanoma	*c-KIT > BRAF > NRAS*
Nodular melanoma	*NRAS*
Uveal melanoma	*GNAQ, GNA11, BAP1*
Mucosal melanoma	*c-KIT > NRAS*

CSD, chronic sun-damaged.
[a]Illustrative examples provided.

- **Sun exposure (both intermittent intense and chronic moderate) and tanning bed use** may trigger the development of melanoma. Other triggers are similar to melanocytic nevi.

  Dysfunction of the MC1R can lead to **red hair**, inability to tan following UVR exposure, and increased risk of melanoma and NMSC. Melanoma is further associated with OCA (see Chapter 2: Pigmentary Disorders); XP, XP variant, and adult progeria (see Chapter 4: Photodermatoses); **Li Fraumeni syndrome (AD mutation in *TP53* encoding p53); and FAMMM syndrome** (see below).

Clinicopathological Features

- Melanoma can have a variety of clinical presentations based on subtype:
  - **Superficial spreading melanomas** initially present as **dark brown to black macules with color variation, asymmetry, and irregular borders.** A horizontal growth phase can develop into a more rapid vertical growth phase, which is clinically seen as papules forming within the macule. This subtype is most often seen on the **trunk of men and legs of women.**
  - **Lentigo maligna melanomas** are invasive melanomas that arise within **lentigo maligna**, a form of melanoma in situ (MIS). They present as **asymmetric brown to black macules with irregular, often ill-defined, borders.** This subtype is most often seen on **chronic sun-damaged (CSD) skin**, especially the **nose and cheeks.** Of note, lentigo maligna and lentigo maligna melanoma are controversial entities.
  - **Acral lentiginous melanomas** present as **asymmetric brown to black macules.** This subtype is the most common subtype seen in **skin of color.** A disproportionate number are **diagnosed at an advanced stage.**
  - **Nodular melanomas** present as **blue-black nodules.** They have minimal-to-no horizontal growth phase, but instead can have a **rapid vertical growth phase leading to ulceration.** This subtype is most often seen on the **head and neck and trunk.**
- Other melanoma variants include **amelanotic melanoma (pink), desmoplastic/neurotropic melanoma (head and neck), mucosal melanoma (oral, anogenital), and nail unit melanoma (longitudinal melanonychia).**

  The "ABCDE"s of melanoma are asymmetry, irregular borders, color variation, diameter > 6 mm, and evolution.

  The "ABCDEF"s of nail unit melanoma are age (50-70 years), band of black-brown color, change in size/growth, digits (thumb > big toe > index finger), extension of color onto cuticle, and family history of melanoma.

  Figure 5.18. Do NOT confuse Hutchinson sign of nail unit melanoma with Hutchinson sign of herpes zoster or Hutchinson teeth in Hutchinson triad of late congenital syphilis.

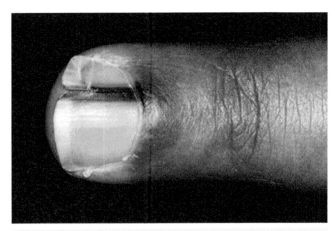

Figure 5.18. HUTCHINSON SIGN. Longitudinal mela-nonychia results from melanin production by nail unit melanocytes. Multiple bands, common in individuals with skin phototypes IV-VI, are typically due to melanocyte activation. A single band may be a sign of melanocyte hyperplasia (eg., lentigo, nevus, or melanoma). Hutchinson sign, periungual extension of pigmentation from longitudinal melanonychia onto the proximal and lateral nail folds, is an important indicator of nail unit melanoma.

(Hutchinson sign image reprinted with permission from Lugo-So-molinos A, McKinley-Grant L, Goldsmith LA, et al. *VisualDx: Essential Dermatology in Pigmented Skin.* Wolters Kluwer Health/Lippincott Williams & Wilkins; 2011.)

- **Clear cell sarcoma** ("melanoma of soft parts") is an aggressive soft tissue malignancy that is thought to be a melanoma variant. It usually presents as a **nodule on the distal extremities.** Unlike cutaneous melanoma, clear cell sarcoma is characterized by the **chromosomal transloca-tion t(12;22).**
- **Regression,** which is clinically seen as a **hypopigmented focus** within a melanoma, is observed in ~2/3 of superficial spreading melanomas.
- **Metastatic melanoma** to the skin usually presents as a **blue-black nodule.** The most common location is the **lower extremities.**
  - ◆ Figure 5.19.
  - ◆ IHC and FISH for melanocytic neoplasms are sum-marized in Table 5.13.

Evaluation

- The differential diagnosis of melanoma includes solar len-tigo, nevocellular nevus, atypical nevus, and Spitz nevus. On acral surfaces, hemorrhage within the skin (ie, black heel and palm) can be hard to differentiate from a melanoma without a dermatoscopic examination. The differential diagnosis of amelanotic melanoma includes wart, BCC, and SCC.
- Patients with suspected melanoma should get an **excisional biopsy (with 1-2 mm margins)** to evaluate the entire lesion. Sampling lesions with punch or shave biopsies can miss the diagnosis and is not advised. If an excisional biopsy is not possible, **saucerization biopsies are preferable over thin shave biopsies,** as thin shave biopsies may transect the mel-anoma and obscure the depth of invasion.

- **Nail matrix biopsy** is the gold standard to diagnose nail unit melanoma.
- Once the diagnosis of melanoma is made, evaluation depends on the clinical stage of the melanoma and symp-toms. The **American Joint Committee on Cancer (AJCC, 8th edition) TNM classification and staging for malig-nant melanoma** is summarized in Tables 5.14 and 5.15.
- Localized cutaneous melanoma (stage I and II) does not require laboratory or imaging evaluation in asymptomatic patients.
- Patients with **melanoma stage IB or higher** should undergo **SLNB.**
- Evaluation of stage III and IV melanomas usually includes imaging such as CT of the chest, abdomen, and pelvis or full body PET scan. Brain MRI is helpful in the assessment for intracranial metastases. Symptom-specific evaluation may also be helpful, such as colonoscopy for patients with gas-trointestinal symptoms/bleeding and bone scan for patients with bone pain.

Management

- The most important prognostic factor is **Breslow thickness,** which is measured from the **top of the *stratum granulosum* to the deepest invasive cell.** Historically, Clark's levels (five levels based on depth of invasion) were used for melanoma staging. However, Clark's level is no longer used in the AJCC TNM classification and staging for malignant melanoma as it is less prognostic and more subjective than Breslow thickness.
- **Other negative prognostic factors include male gender, increasing age, ulceration, head/neck/trunk location, pal-pable nodes, and increased tumor mitotic rate.**
- **Melanoma leukoderma is a positive prognostic factor.**
- **Treatment of melanoma is surgical for localized disease (stage I and II).** WLE is the most common surgical treatment for melanoma. The **recommended surgical margins** are:
  - ○ 0.5 to 1 cm for melanoma in situ.
  - ○ 1 cm for Breslow thickness of ≤1 mm.
  - ○ 1 to 2 cm for Breslow thickness of 1.01 to 2 mm.
  - ○ 2 cm for Breslow thickness >2 mm.
- **Adjuvant chemotherapy** (in particular, INFα and ipilim-umab) has been shown to improve survival in stage II and III melanoma after surgical resection.
- Advanced melanoma (stage III and IV) is typically treated with systemic immunotherapy. Historically, IFNα, IFNβ, and IL-2 were used. However, the discovery and success of ICIs such as **CTLA4 inhibitors (eg, ipilimumab) and PD1 inhibitors (eg, nivolumab, pembrolizumab)** has transformed the landscape of melanoma, such that ICIs have become the standard of care. **PD1 inhibitors are more effective than CTLA4 inhibitors.**
- In patients with *BRAF* mutations, targeted antineoplastics include **BRAF (V600E) inhibitors (eg, dabrafenib, vemu-rafenib) and MEK 1/2 inhibitors (eg, trametinib). Con-current BRAF and MEK inhibition prolongs the develop-ment of resistance.** In patients with known *BRAF* V600E mutations and a high tumor burden, BRAF and MEK inhib-itors are often used as first-line therapies.

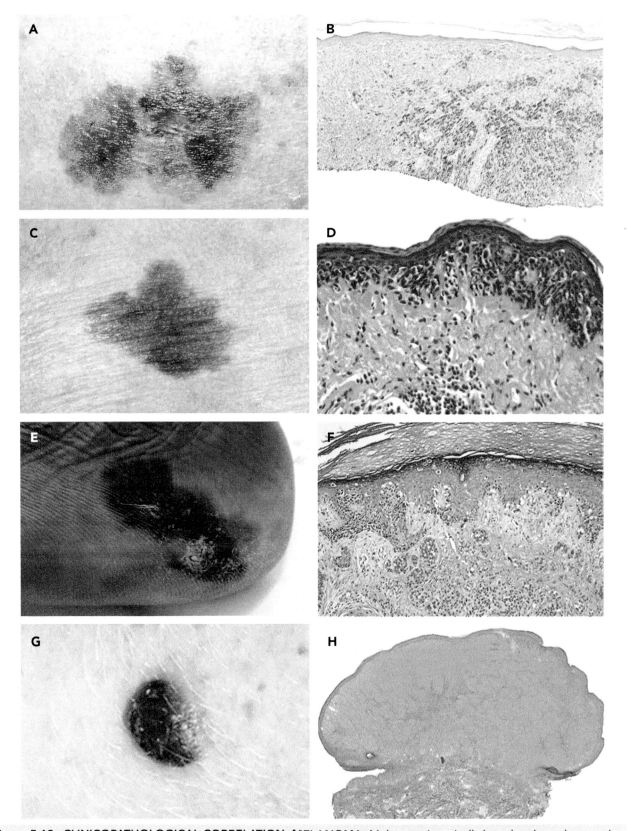

Figure 5.19. CLINICOPATHOLOGICAL CORRELATION: MELANOMA. Melanoma is typically broad and poorly nested at the DEJ. Irregular nests of junctional melanocytes extend from the tips and sides of rete to the tops of dermal papillae and display variable cytologic atypia. Lateral circumscription is variable, and there is left-right asymmetry, failure of maturation, and failure of dispersion. Deep mitoses and deep pigment in nests are variably present, along with pagetoid spread, melanophages, and a dense lymphocytic infiltrate at the base. Melanoma may enter both horizontal and vertical growth phases. A and B, Superficial spreading melanoma. C and D, Lentigo maligna E and F, Acral lentiginous melanoma. G and H, Nodular melanoma. DEJ, dermo-epidermal junction; MIS, melanoma in situ.

(Figure 5.19. Continued)

(A, Reprinted with permission from Elder DE, Elenitsas R, Rosenbach M, et al. *Lever's Histopathology of the Skin.* 11th ed. Wolters Kluwer; 2015. B, Histology image courtesy of Noel Turner, MD, MHS and Christine J. Ko, MD. C, Reprinted with permission from Craft N, Fox LP, Goldsmith LA, et al. *VisualDx: Essential Adult Dermatology.* Wolters Kluwer Health/Lippincott Williams & Wilkins; 2010. D, Histology image reprinted with permission from Crowson AN, Magro CM, Mihm MC Jr. *Biopsy Interpretation of the Skin: Primary Non-Lymphoid Cutaneous Neoplasia.* 2nd ed. Wolters Kluwer; 2018. F, Histology image reprinted with permission from Crowson AN, Magro CM, Mihm MC Jr. *Biopsy Interpretation of the Skin: Primary Non-Lymphoid Cutaneous Neoplasia.* 2nd ed. Wolters Kluwer; 2018. G, Reprinted with permission from Edwards L, Lynch P. *Genital Dermatology Atlas and Manual.* 3rd ed. Wolters Kluwer; 2017. H, Histology image reprinted with permission from Elder DE, Elenitsas R, Rosenbach M, et al. *Lever's Histopathology of the Skin.* 11th ed. Wolters Kluwer; 2015.)

- **Superficial spreading melanoma:** horizontal growth phase, pagetoid spread.
- **Lentigo maligna:** junctional MIS with adnexal extension, solar elastosis (controversial).
- **Lentigo maligna melanoma:** lentigo maligna with vertical growth phase (controversial).
- **Acral lentiginous melanoma:** junctional, acral location.
- **Nodular melanoma:** vertical growth phase, necrosis.
- **Amelanotic melanoma:** absence of melanin.
- **Desmoplastic melanoma:** spindle cells, desmoplastic stroma, nodular lymphoid aggregates.
- **Neurotropic melanoma:** desmoplastic melanoma with endoneurial invasion.
- **Mucosal melanoma:** mucosal location.
- **Nail unit melanoma:** nail matrix location.
- **Regressing melanoma:** zones of fibrosis and melanophages.
- **Metastatic melanoma:** radial symmetry or epidermotropic/nevoid, invasion of lymphatic vessels.

- Intralesional therapies include **IL-2** and the **oncolytic virus talimogene laherparepvec (T-VEC).**
- Some dermatologists treat lentigo maligna and lentigo maligna melanoma with MMS given that these melanomas are often located on the face and have ill-defined margins (controversial). **Melan-A (melanoma antigen recognized by T-cells 1 [MART-1])** is often utilized to stain serial frozen sections during in MMS for melanoma in order to better define the margins.

"Real World" Advice

- Amelanotic melanomas do not differ in prognosis than other melanomas of the same stage. However, the atypical appearance often results in a significant diagnostic delay.
- Terminology can be confusing. Cutaneous melanomas that are very difficult to diagnose are sometimes called "melanocytic tumor of unknown malignant potential (MELTUMP)."

Table 5.13. IMMUNOHISTOCHEMISTRY AND FLUORESCENCE IN SITU HYBRIDIZATION FOR MELANOCYTIC NEOPLASMS

Diagnosis	IHC[a]				FISH[a]	
	Melan-A (MART-1), MITF, S100, SOX-10	HMB-45	PRAME	p16 (CDKN2A)	ALK1 Fusions	Gain of Chromosome 11p
Nevocellular nevus	+	+ (top heavy)	-	+	-	-
Atypical nevus	+	+	-	+	-	-
Spitz nevus	+	+	-	± (negative or diminished in atypical Spitz nevus)	+	+
Melanoma[b]	+	+ (strong staining throughout)	+	-	-	-

ALK, anaplastic lymphoma kinase; CDKN2A, cyclin-dependent kinase inhibitor 2A; FISH, fluorescence in situ hybridization; HMB, human melanoma black; IHC, immunohistochemistry; MART-1, melanoma antigen recognized by T cells 1; MITF, microphthalmia-associated transcription factor; PRAME, preferentially expressed antigen of melanoma; SOX, Sry-related HMg-Box.
[a]Illustrative examples provided.
[b]Reliable IHC stains for desmoplastic melanoma include S100 and SOX-10.

Table 5.14. AMERICAN JOINT COMMITTEE ON CANCER TNM CLASSIFICATION FOR MALIGNANT MELANOMA

T Category	Thickness	Ulceration Status
Tis	N/A	N/A
T1	≤1.0 mm	Unknown or unspecified
T1a	<0.8 mm	Without ulceration
T1b	<0.8 mm	With ulceration
	0.8-1.0 mm	With or without ulceration
T2	>1-2 mm	Unknown or unspecified
T2a	>1-2 mm	Without ulceration
T2b	>1-2 mm	With ulceration
T3	>2-4 mm	Unknown or unspecified
T3a	>2-4 mm	Without ulceration
T3b	>2-4 mm	With ulceration
T4	>4 mm	Unknown or unspecified
T4a	>4 mm	Without ulceration
T4b	>4 mm	With ulceration

N Category	Number of Metastatic Nodes	Metastasis Status
N0	N/A	N/A
N1	0-1	a: clinically occult, no MSI
		b: clinically detected, no MSI
		c: 0 nodes, MSI present
N2	1-3	a: 2-3 clinically occult, no MSI
		b: 2-3 clinically detected, no MSI
		c: 1 node, clinical or occult, MSI present
N3	>1	a: >3 nodes, all clinically occult, no MSI
		b: >3 nodes, ≥1 clinically detected or matted, no MSI
		c: >1 node, clinical or occult, MSI present

M Category	Anatomic Site	LDH Level
M0	N/A	N/A
M1	Evidence of distant metastasis	
M1a	Distant metastasis to skin, soft tissue including muscles, and/or nonregional lymph node	
M1a (0)		0 = not elevated
M1a (1)		1 = elevated
M1b	Distant metastasis to lung with or without M1a sites of disease	
M1b (0)		0 = not elevated
M1b (1)		1 = elevated
M1c	Distant metastasis to non-CNS visceral sites with or without M1a or M1b sites of disease	
M1c (0)		0 = not elevated
M1c (1)		1 = elevated
M1d	Distant metastasis to CNS with or without M1a, M1b, or M1c sites of disease	
M1d (0)		0 = not elevated
M1d (1)		1 = elevated

CNS, central nervous system; LDH, lactate dehydrogenase; M, metastasis; MSI, microsatellite instability; N, node; N/A, not applicable; T, tumor.

Table 5.15. AMERICAN JOINT COMMITTEE ON CANCER STAGING FOR MALIGNANT MELANOMA

Clinical Staging				Pathologic Staging			
Stage 0	Tis	N0	M0	0	Tis	N0	M0
Stage IA	T1a	N0	M0	IA	T1a	N0	M0
Stage IB	T1b T2a	--	--	IB	T1b T2a	--	--
Stage IIA	T2b T3a	N0	M0	IIA	T2b T3a	N0	M0
Stage IIB	T3b T4a	--	--	IIB	T3b T4a	--	--
Stage IIC	T4b	--	--	IIC	T4b	--	--
Stage III	Any T	≥ N1	M0	IIIA	T1-2a T1-2a	N1a N2a	M0
				IIIB	T0 T1-2a T1-2a T2b-3a	N1b-c N1b-c N2b N1a-2b	--
				IIIC	T0 T0 T1-3a T3b-4a T4b	N2b-c N3b-c N2c-3c Any N N1a-2c	--
				IIID	T4b	N3a-c	M0
Stage IV	Any T	Any N	M1	IV	Any T	Any N	M1

SPOTLIGHT ON FAMILIAL ATYPIVAL MULTIPLE MOLE MELANOMA SYNDROME

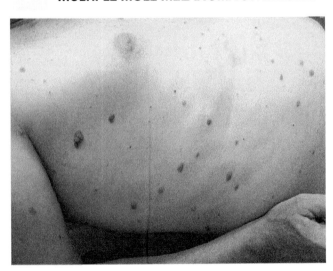

- **FAMMM syndrome** is an **AD** disorder due to mutations in *CDKN2A*, **which encodes p16** (tumor suppressor gene that inhibits CDK4). It is estimated that ~5% to 12% of melanomas are hereditary and about 40% of those are caused by *CDKN2A* mutations.
- FAMMM syndrome is associated with **multiple melanocytic nevi, atypical nevi, and a family history of melanoma.** The most common internal malignancies are **pancreatic cancer and astrocytoma.**
  - ◆ The histopathology of FAMMM syndrome demonstrates melanocytic nevi, atypical nevi, and melanoma.
- The NIH diagnostic criteria for FAMMM syndrome are **(1) ≥50 clinically atypical nevi, (2) malignant melanoma in ≥1st- or 2nd-degree relative, and (3) nevi with histologic features of atypia.** Patients with suspected FAMMM syndrome can get referred for **genetic testing.** However, this remains controversial as some clinicians believe testing positively will not change screening recommendations.
- In addition to age-appropriate malignancy screening, patients need TBSEs every 6 to 12 months. Screening for melanoma in FAMMM kindreds should begin at 10 years of age. There are no specific screening recommendations for pancreatic cancer. However, many physicians will offer screening with CT, MRI, or endoscopic US starting at 50 years of age or 10 years younger than the earliest family member with pancreatic cancer.

Fibrous Neoplasms

Basic Concepts

- Fibrous neoplasms comprise a diverse group of diagnoses that are generally characterized by an increased production of collagen in the skin.
- Fibrous neoplasms range from benign entities (eg, DF) to malignant entities (for example, dermatofibrosarcoma protuberans [DFSP]). The term "undifferentiated pleomorphic sarcoma" refers to a heterogeneous group of soft-tissue sarcomas.

KELOID
→ **Diagnosis Group 1**

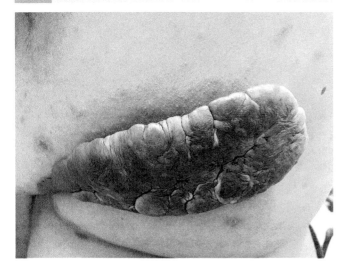

Epidemiology

- Keloids represent an abnormal wound healing response to skin injury. **TGFβ** plays a key role, stimulating fibroblasts to produce excessive collagen during the proliferative phase of wound healing. **Collagen III** is overrepresented in keloids.
- Keloids most commonly occur in patients <30 years of age. There is a higher prevalence in **Asian, black, and Latino populations.**

    Multiple keloids are associated with Rubinstein-Taybi syndrome.

Clinicopathological Features

- **Keloid** is characterized by a **smooth firm papule or plaque that extends beyond the boundaries of the original wound.** The color can range from pink to skin-colored to brown. Keloids favor areas of high tension such as the **shoulders, chest, and upper back.**
- In contrast, **hypertrophic scar** is characterized by a **smooth firm papule or plaque that is confined to the boundaries of the original wound.**
    - Figure 5.20.

Evaluation

- Beyond hypertrophic scar, the differential diagnosis of keloid includes xanthoma disseminatum and lobomycosis. **Hypertrophies and atrophies** are summarized in Table 5.16.

    Hypertrophies: for Beare-Stevenson cutis gyrata syndrome, see Chapter 2: Papulosquamous Disorders and

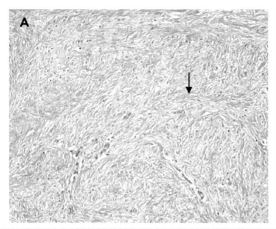
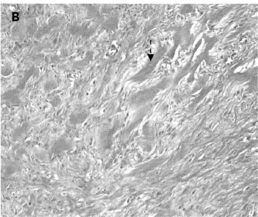

Figure 5.20. SIDE-BY-SIDE COMPARISON: HYPERTROPHIC SCAR AND KELOID. Scar is characterized by epidermal atrophy and proliferation of perpendicularly orientated fibroblasts (horizontal) and blood vessels (vertical) in the dermis with loss of elastic fibers and adnexal structures. Both hypertrophic scar and keloid demonstrate nodules and whorls of thick collagen fibers. Hypertrophic scar has thick collagen fibers. Keloid has thick hyalinized collagen fibers. IHC may be helpful. COX-1 expression increases with progression from scar to hypertrophic scar to keloid. CD34 and factor XIIIa are negative. A, Hypertrophic scar. Solid arrow: thick ("ropy") collagen fibers. B, Keloid. Dashed arrow: thick ("ropey") and hyalinized (pink "bubble gum") collagen fibers. CD, cluster of differentiation; COX-1, cyclooxygenase 1; IHC, immunohistochemistry.

(Histology images reprinted with permission from Fisher C, Montgomery EA, Thway K. *Biopsy Interpretation of Soft Tissue Tumors.* 2nd ed. Wolters Kluwer; 2015.)

Collagen fibers in hypertrophic scar are "ropy."
Collagen fibers in keloid are "ropy" and pink, Collagen fibers in hypertrophic scar are "ropy." resembling "bubble gum."

Table 5.16. HYPERTROPHIES AND ATROPHIES

Diagnosis[a]	Classic Description	Notes
Hypertrophies		
Cutis gyrata	Cerebriform folding of the skin on the scalp.	Primary or secondary. Associations include acromegaly, myxedema, Graves disease, and paraneoplastic syndrome due to metastatic carcinoma.
Fibromatosis	See below.	
Keloid/hypertrophic scar	See above.	
Atrophies		
Anetoderma	Well-circumscribed areas of flaccid skin that may be papular, macular, or depressed.	Primary or secondary. Associations include inflammation, infection, or skin tumor.
Atrophia maculosa varioliformis cutis	Varioliform or linear depressions resembling scars.	No history of trauma to the skin.
Atrophoderma of Pasini and Pierini	Depressed brown patches.	Most common in women. May be associated with *Borrelia burgdorferi* infection, but this remains controversial.
	The edge of atrophoderma resembles a "cliff drop."	
Diabetic dermopathy	Red to brown slightly depressed patches usually on the shins.	Associated with diabetes mellitus.
Mid-dermal elastolysis	Well-circumscribed symmetric areas of fine wrinkling.	Most common in Caucasian women 30-50 years of age.
Piezogenic pedal papules	Skin-colored papulonodules usually near the heels.	Induced by weight bearing. Disappear when leg is raised.
Striae	Well-circumscribed linear, atrophic plaques that range in color from purple to white.	Most common in women. Associations include puberty and pregnancy.
Elastic Tissue Disorders[b]		
Elastoma	Firm skin-colored to yellow papules favoring the trunk.	Type of connective tissue nevus.
Elastofibroma dorsi	Deep tumor/nodule on the mid-upper back.	Favors older women.
Late-onset focal dermal elastosis	Small skin-colored to yellow coalescing papules that favor the neck and intertriginous surfaces.	
Linear focal elastosis	Multiple, palpable linear plaques (striae-like) on the trunk.	

[a]Illustrative examples provided.
[b]Not discussed elsewhere.

Palmoplantar Keratodermas; for hyaline fibromatosis syndrome, see Chapter 5: Other Malformations and Neoplasms. Atrophies: for atrophoderma vermiculatum and follicular atrophoderma, see Chapter 2: Eczematous Dermatoses and Related Disorders.

- A skin biopsy is usually not required for keloid but can be helpful to confirm the diagnosis.

Management

- **ILK** is first line. It both flattens keloids and alleviates symptoms such as pruritus. In needle-averse patients, a potent topical corticosteroid under silicone dressing occlusion may have some benefit.

- Surgical excision should be undertaken with caution due to the high rate of recurrence. Postsurgical ILK may help reduce recurrence.
- **Cryotherapy** (needle > spray) done monthly for several months has some efficacy.
- Other therapies that have been shown to have some efficacy in treating keloid include topical 5-FU, PDL, silicone sheeting, and pressure therapy.
- **Radiation therapy** is reserved for treatment-resistant keloids.
- Newer therapies with promising results include **intralesional avotermin (recombinant TGFβ3), intralesional IL-10 (anti-inflammatory), and intralesional insulin (inhibits myofibroblasts).**

"Real World" Advice

- The management of keloids remains challenging, and a multimodal approach is often beneficial:
  - Cryotherapy causes tissue edema and may improve the penetration of ILK.
  - ILK or radiation therapy decreases the rate of recurrence after surgical excision.

ANGIOFIBROMA
→ **Diagnosis Group 2**
Synonyms: fibrous papule

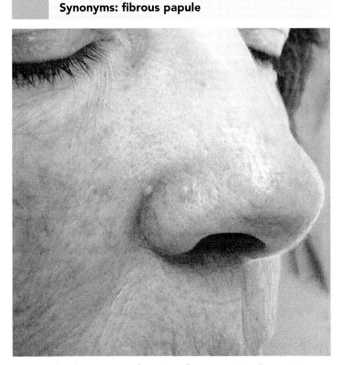

Reprinted with permission from Goodheart HP. *Goodheart's Same-Site Differential Diagnosis: A Rapid Method of Diagnosing and Treating Common Skin Disorders*. Wolters Kluwer Health/Lippincott Williams & Wilkins; 2011

Epidemiology

- Angiofibroma is a descriptive term to characterize a variety of fibrous neoplasms with overlapping histopathological features. **Multiple facial angiofibromas** are associated with **TSC and MEN1.**

Clinicopathological Features

- Angiofibroma classically presents as a **skin-colored to red dome-shaped papule.**
- Location-specific variants of angiofibroma include **facial angiofibromas, pearly penile papules (around the corona of the glans penis)**, and **periungual fibromas.**
  - Figure 5.21.

Evaluation

- The differential diagnosis of angiofibroma varies based on the variant. For example, a solitary facial angiofibroma may be mistaken for BCC, intradermal nevus, or an adnexal neoplasm, whereas pearly penile papules may be mistaken for condyloma acuminata.
- Patients with ≥3 facial angiofibromas and ≥2 ungual fibromas should be evaluated for TSC.

Management

- Treatment options for angiofibroma include PDL, fractional ablative laser, and electrosurgery.
- **Topical mTOR inhibitors (eg, sirolimus)** have also been successfully employed to treat angiofibromas.

"Real World" Advice

- Understanding the genetic basis of genodermatoses such as TSC has led to the discovery of targeted therapies. Examples of this include topical mTOR inhibitors (eg, sirolimus) for angiofibromas.

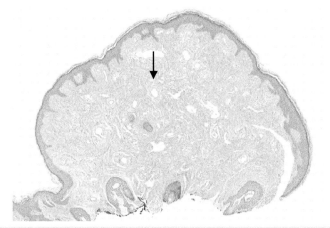

Figure 5.21. CLINICOPATHOLOGICAL CORRELATION: ANGIOFIBROMA. Angiofibroma is characterized by a dome-shaped dermal proliferation of dilated blood vessels with concentric perivascular fibrosis. Stellate stromal cells are factor XIIIa and stromolysin 3 positive. Solid arrow: dilated blood vessel with concentric perivascular fibrosis.
(Histology image courtesy of Noel Turner, MD, MHS and Christine J. Ko, MD.)

SPOTLIGHT ON TUBEROUS SCLEROSIS COMPLEX

Synonyms: Bourneville disease, Bourneville-Pringle disease

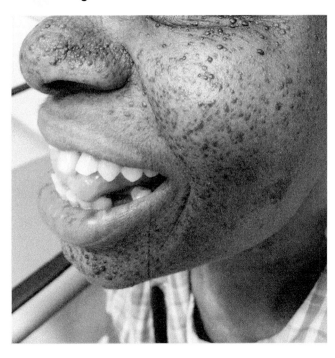

- TSC is an **AD** hereditary disorder due to mutations in *TSC1* **(hamartin)** and *TSC2* **(tuberin)**, which lead to activation of the **PI3K signaling pathway.**
- **Clinical features of TSC** are summarized in Table 5.17.
  - The histopathology of TSC demonstrates hypomelanotic macules, angiofibromas, CALMs, and collagenomas.
- **Diagnostic criteria for TSC** are summarized in Table 5.18. **MEN syndromes** (Table 5.19) have overlapping features with TSC.
- Given the multiple organ systems involved, evaluation of TSC patients requires a multidisciplinary approach. In addition to age-appropriate malignancy screening, patients need yearly TBSEs. Screening for systemic involvement in newly diagnosed patients includes chest CT (all women > 18 years old), brain MRI, abdominal MRI, ECG, echocardiogram, and dental and ophthalmological examinations. Depending on the screening results, patients will need to repeat these screening tests at regular intervals to assess for progression. **Topical mTOR inhibitors (eg, sirolimus)** have demonstrated efficacy in TSC patients with angiofibromas. Oral mTOR inhibitors (eg, everolimus) have also shown efficacy in the treatment of TSC-related tumors such as subependymal giant cell astrocytomas.

Table 5.17. CLINICAL FEATURES OF TUBEROUS SCLEROSIS COMPLEX

Cutaneous Features

Infancy:
- Hypomelanotic macules ("ash-leaf" macules) and "confetti" macules
- CALMs

Prepubertal:
- Facial angiofibromas
- Fibrous cephalic plaque (connective tissue nevus)
- Shagreen patch (connective tissue nevus)

Adolescence:
- Periungual fibromas (Koenen tumors)

Adulthood:
- Gingival/intraoral fibromas

Systemic Features

- Cardiac: myocardial rhabdomyomas
- Endocrine: precocious puberty
- Dental: enamel pits
- Nervous: cortical tubers, seizures (leading cause of mortality), subependymal giant cell astrocytomas, subependymal nodules
- Ocular: retinal hamartomas
- Renal: cysts, bilateral angiomyolipomas
- Respiratory lymphangioleiomyomatosis

CALMs, café-au-lait macules.

Table 5.18. DIAGNOSTIC CRITERIA FOR TUBEROUS SCLEROSIS COMPLEX

Clinical Diagnosis

- 2 major features OR 1 major feature and 2 minor features

Genetic Diagnosis

- Positive test for mutations in *TSC1* or *TSC2* from blood or normal tissue

Major Features

Cutaneous features:
- Hypomelanotic macules (≥3)
- Facial angiofibromas (≥3)
- Fibrous cephalic plaque (connective tissue nevus)
- Shagreen patch (connective tissue nevus)
- Periungual fibromas (Koenen tumors) (≥2)

Systemic features:
- Myocardial rhabdomyomas
- Cortical tubers
- Subependymal nodules
- Retinal hamartomas
- Angiomyolipomas
- Lymphangioleiomyomatosis

Minor Features

Cutaneous features:
- "Confetti" macules
- Gingival/intraoral fibromas

Systemic:
- Dental enamel pits
- Multiple renal cysts

TSC, tuberous sclerosis complex.

Table 5.19. MULTIPLE ENDOCRINE NEOPLASIA SYNDROMES

Diagnosis	Inheritance Pattern	Gene	Classic Description
MEN1 (Werner syndrome)	AD	*MEN1* encoding menin	Cutaneous: CALMs, collagenomas, angiofibromas, gingival/intraoral fibromas. Systemic: pituitary, parathyroid (hyperplasia or adenoma), and pancreatic tumors.
Do NOT confuse MEN1 (Wermer syndrome) with adult progeria (Werner syndrome).			The "3 Ps" of MEN1 are pituitary, parathyroid, and pancreatic tumors.
MEN2A (Sipple syndrome)	AD	*RET* encoding the RET protein	Cutaneous: macular and lichen amyloidosis Systemic: medullary thyroid carcinoma, parathyroid (hyperplasia or adenoma), pheochromocytoma.
MEN2B (multiple mucosal neuroma syndrome)	AD	*RET* encoding the RET protein	Cutaneous: marfanoid habitus, CALMs, circumoral hyperpigmentation/lentigines, mucosal neuromas on the tongue and lips, thickened lips. Systemic: medullary thyroid carcinoma, pheochromocytoma.

AD, autosomal dominant, CALMs, café au lait macules, MEN, multiple endocrine neoplasia; RET, rearranged during transfection.

DERMATOFIBROMA
→ Diagnosis Group 1
Synonyms: fibrous histiocytoma

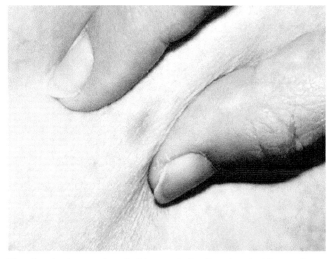

The dimple sign reprinted with permission Reprinted with permission from Goodheart HP. Goodheart's Photoguide of Common Skin Disorders: Diagnosis and Management. 2nd ed. Lippincott Williams & Wilkins; 2003.

Epidemiology

- DF is a common benign fibrous proliferation. The etiology of DFs is an area of controversy; it remains unclear whether they represent a reactive or truly neoplastic process.
- DFs are more common in **females.**
- Multiple DFs are associated with **SLE** and **HIV infection.**

Clinicopathological Features

- DFs are **firm, dome-shaped papules that favor the lower extremities.** They are often hyperpigmented.
  - Pinching a DF causes dimpling of the overlying skin due to downward displacement of the papule. This is referred to as the "dimple sign."
- Of the numerous DF histopathological variants, **cellular DF** is notable for **increased risk of local recurrence and rare metastasis.**
- DF may overlap with myofibroma (dermatomyofibroma).
  - Figure 5.22.
  - Other benign and borderline fibrous neoplasms not discussed elsewhere are summarized in Table 5.20.

Evaluation

- The differential diagnosis of DF incudes melanocytic lesions, hypertrophic scar, keloid, and DFSP.
- **Dermoscopy** reveals **central crystalline structure with a typical pseudonetwork at the periphery.**
- Skin biopsy is generally not required for diagnosis.

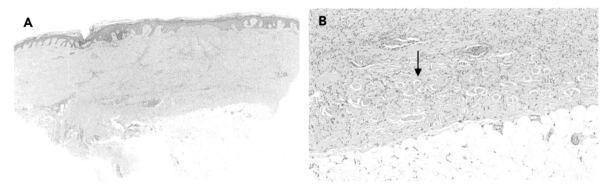

Figure 5.22. CLINICOPATHOLOGICAL CORRELATION: DERMATOFIBROMA. DF is characterized by epidermal acanthosis and a dermal spindle cell proliferation with collagen trapping and extension into the superficial subcutis. Folliculosebaceous induction is common. Ringed lipidized siderophages are pathognomonic. Factor XIIIa and stromolysin 3 are positive. CD34 is negative. A, Low-power view. B, High-power view. Solid arrow: collagen trapping. CD, cluster of differentiation; DF, dermatofibroma; SMA, smooth muscle actin; VVG, Verhoeff-van Gieson.

(Histology images courtesy of Noel Turner, MD, MHS and Christine J. Ko, MD.)

- **Cellular DF:** cell-rich DF.
- **Atypical DF:** DF with atypical (monster) cells.
- **Myofibroma:** myofibroblasts (SMA positive).
- **Dermatomyofibroma:** dermal spindle cell proliferation in a horizontal orientation respecting adnexal structures with myofibroblasts (SMA positive) and thick elastic fibers on VVG stain.

DF has a "curlicue" pattern and extends into the superficial subcutis in a "lacy" pattern.

Table 5.20. OTHER BENIGN AND BORDERLINE FIBROUS NEOPLASMS

Diagnosis[a]	Clinical Features	Histopathological Features	Notes
Benign			
Calcifying aponeurotic fibroma	Solitary, fixed subcutaneous nodule favoring the hands and feet.	Areas of calcification surrounded by palisading fibroblasts with a surrounding collagenous stroma.	Benign, but have a high recurrence rate after surgical excision (~50%).
Connective tissue nevus	Skin-colored papule or plaque, often with a pebbly surface.	Poorly demarcated dermal proliferation of collagen without an increase in fibroblasts.	Associated with Buschke-Ollendorff syndrome (dermatofibrosis lenticularis disseminata), TSC (fibrous cephalic plaque, Shagreen patch), and Proteus syndrome (palmoplantar cerebriform connective tissue nevus).
Superficial fascial fibromatosis	Dupuytren contracture: fascial nodule on the palm that extends into a thick cord, ultimately contracting the digits. Peyronie disease: scarred nodule on dorsal penis leading to abnormal curvature. Ledderhose plantar fibromatosis: skin-colored nodules, most commonly on the soles.	Nodular dermal proliferation of fibroblasts and myofibroblasts. Later stages are characterized by thicker collagen and fewer fibroblasts/myofibroblasts.	Deep variants are associated with increased morbidity and mortality. Treat with surgical excision and fasciotomy.
Fibromatosis colli	Proliferation of fibrous tissue at the lower 1/3 of the SCM muscle at birth.	Proliferation of fibroblasts, myofibroblasts, and bundles of collagen in muscle.	Hypothesized to relate to birth trauma leading to hemorrhage and fibromatosis.
Fibrous hamartoma of infancy	Painless, flesh-colored subcutaneous nodule or plaque favoring the upper extremity.	Composed of three elements: mature adipocytes, spindled myofibroblasts in fascicles, and aggregates of round mesenchymal cells in a myxoid stroma.	Most common <2 years of age and in males.
Giant cell tumor of the tendon sheath	Slow growing, firm papulonodule on the finger.	Sheets of epithelioid histiocytes with admixed multinucleated osteoclast-like giant cells. Tumors are often attached to the tendon.	Giant cell tumor of the tendon sheath without giant cells is called fibroma of the tendon sheath.

Table 5.20. OTHER BENIGN AND BORDERLINE FIBROUS NEOPLASMS (CONTINUED)

Diagnosis[a]	Clinical Features	Histopathological Features	Notes
Hyaline fibromatosis syndrome	Juvenile hyaline fibromatosis: small nodules on scalp, perinasal and perianal skin; gingival hyperplasia. Systemic features include joint contractures and osteopenia. Infantile systemic hyalinosis: Same as above, but with diffuse skin thickening and visceral involvement.	Nodules composed of dense, hyaline collagen (PAS positive, diastase resistant). Calcium deposits can also be seen (Von Kossa).	Associated with *CMG2* (*ANTXR2*) mutations. Infantile systemic hyalinosis is associated with a poor prognosis.
Infantile digital fibroma (inclusion body fibroma)	Dome-shaped papule favoring the dorsolateral finger or toe and sparing the thumb or great toe.	Proliferation of spindled myofibroblasts with pathognomonic actin bodies (round intracytoplasmic inclusion bodies that stain red with H&E and Masson-Trichrome; stain purple with PTAH; positive for SMA). Acral skin is a helpful diagnostic clue.	Most common in males. High recurrence rate after surgical excision.
Infantile myofibromatosis (infantile hemangiopericytoma)	Infantile myofibromatosis: flesh-colored to purple-red, firm or rubbery papules favoring the head. Congenital generalized myofibromatosis: scattered cutaneous and subcutaneous tumors with lytic bone lesions.	Nodular biphasic proliferation: myofibroblasts with abundant cytoplasm in fascicles in some areas and other areas with more cellular, smaller, round myofibroblasts associated with branching blood vessels. SMA is positive.	Most common in females. AD variant due to defective *PDGFRβ* encoding PDGFRβ. While cutaneous disease has an excellent prognosis, systemic disease may be fatal.
Nodular fasciitis	Rapidly growing subcutaneous nodule favoring the upper extremities in adults (proliferative variant) and the head and neck in children (cranial variant).	Well circumscribed subcutaneous proliferation of spindled fibroblasts and myofibroblasts in a myxoid and edematous stroma. Mitoses are common, as are erythrocyte extravasation and inflammatory cells. Fibroblasts have a "tissue culture" appearance.	Most common in young adults ± history of mechanical injury.
Pleomorphic fibroma	Solitary, skin-colored papule or plaque favoring the extremities.	Thin bundles of collagen with a proliferation of large mononucleated or multinucleated atypical fibroblasts. Stroma has abundant mucin.	
Sclerotic fibroma	Pearly papulonodules that can occur on the skin or mucous membranes.	Thick, sclerotic collagen bundles with intervening thin spaces containing sparse fibroblasts ± mucin. Sclerotic fibroma resembles "plywood" or Vincent Van Gogh's painting, *The Starry Night*.	Associated with Cowden syndrome and other PTEN hamartoma syndromes.
Borderline			
Desmoid tumor	Large nodules or tumors. Extra-abdominal variants can present in surgical scars or the abdominal wall.	Dermal and subcutaneous proliferation of bland-appearing fibroblasts in long fascicles. Often infiltrate surrounding fascia and muscle. β-catenin is positive.	Associated with Gardner syndrome. Trisomy of chromosome 8 and 14 may play a role in the pathogenesis.
Plexiform fibrohistiocytic tumor	Slow growing, painless nodule favoring the wrist or hand.	Multinodular dermal proliferation of histiocytes and fascicles of spindled cells intersecting in a plexiform pattern ± multinucleated giant cells.	Most common in children and young adults.

[a]Illustrative examples provided. For AFK, see Chapter 5: Other Malformations and Neoplasms.
AD, autosomal dominant; AFK, acral fibrokeratoma; CMG2, capillary morphogenesis protein 2; H&E, hematoxylin & eosin; PDGFRβ, platelet derived growth factor receptor-β; PTAH, phosphotungstic acid hematoxylin; PTEN, phosphatase and tensin homolog; SCM, sternocleidomastoid; SMA, smooth muscle actin; TSC, tuberous sclerosis complex.

Management

- Complete surgical excision is curative. However, given that DFs are benign, treatment is not necessary.

"Real World" Advice

- Avoid superficial shave biopsies of suspected DFs as folliculosebaceous induction may be mistaken for superficial BCC.

DERMATOFIBROSARCOMA PROTUBERANS

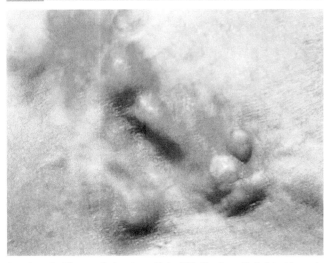

Reprinted with permission from Elder DE, Elenitsas R, Rubin AI, et al. *Atlas of Dermatopathology: Synopsis and Atlas of Lever's Histopathology of the Skin.* 4th ed. Wolters Kluwer; 2020

- DFSP is a locally aggressive sarcoma associated with **reciprocal translocation t(17;22)(q22;q13) leading to *COL1A1-PDGFB* fusion and supernumerary ring chromosomes containing sequences of chromosomes 17 and 22.**

   Giant cell fibroblastoma is the juvenile DFSP variant with *COL1A1-PDGFB* fusion. It most commonly occurs in **males.** Multiple DFSPs are associated with SCID.

- DFSPs usually begin as **small skin-colored papulonodules that expand into red to brown keloidal plaques and nodules.** They favor the trunk, especially the **shoulder.** In rare cases, DFSPs have been known to **metastasize to the lungs. Bednar tumor is a pigmented DFSP variant.** With *p53* **mutation,** there is a risk of progression to **fibrosarcoma,** which has a **higher rate of recurrence and metastasis.**

   ◆ Figure 5.23.

- **MMS is the treatment of choice for DFSP,** given the high recurrence rate and infiltrative growth pattern. If WLE is performed, surgical margins of 3 cm are recommended. **Imatinib (PDGFR inhibitor)** is used for unresectable or metastatic DFSP.

ATYPICAL FIBROXANTHOMA

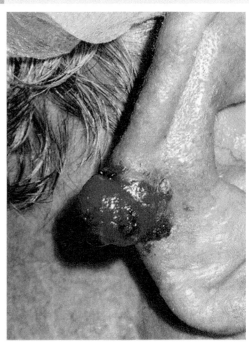

Reprinted with permission from Requena L, Kutzner H. *Cutaneous Soft Tissue Tumors.* Wolters Kluwer Health; 2014.

- Atypical fibroxanthoma (AFX) was historically classified as a sarcoma; however, the new WHO classification characterizes AFX as a benign growth of uncertain lineage. AFX typically occurs on **CSD skin in older patients.**
- AFX classically presents as a **rapidly growing, dome-shaped, red papule** with secondary erosion and **ulceration.** The most common location is the **head and neck. Pleomorphic dermal sarcoma** is a deep AFX variant.

   ◆ Figure 5.24.

- Complete surgical excision is curative. **Rates of local recurrence and metastasis are low, except in pleomorphic dermal sarcoma.**

EPITHELIOID SARCOMA

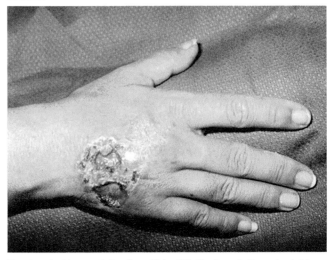

Reprinted with permission from Elder DE, Elenitsas R, Rosenbach M, et al. *Lever's Histopathology of the Skin.* 11th ed. Wolters Kluwer; 2015.

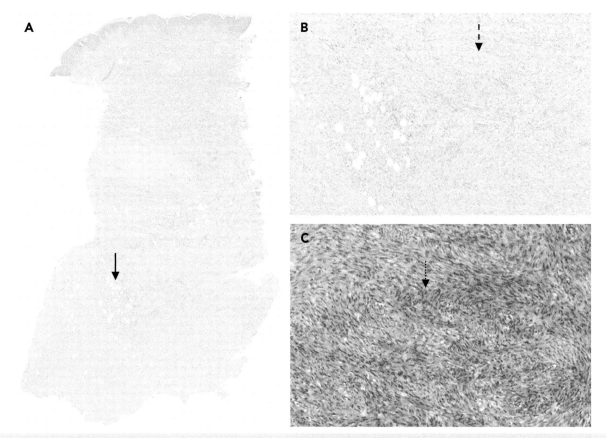

Figure 5.23. CLINICOPATHOLOGICAL CORRELATION: DERMATOFIBROSARCOMA PROTUBERANS. DFSP is characterized by epidermal effacement and a densely hypercellular dermal spindle cell proliferation with infiltration of the subcutis and formation of fibrous layers parallel to the epidermis. CD34, procollagen-1, vimentin are positive. Factor XIIIa and stromolysin 3 are negative. FISH can detect *COL1A1-PDGFB* fusion and supernumerary ring chromosomes containing sequences of chromosomes 17 and 22. A, DFSP low-power view. Solid arrow: infiltration of the subcutis in a "honeycomb" pattern. B, DFSP high-power view. Dashed arrow: spindle cell proliferation with a storiform "cartwheel" pattern. C, Fibrosarcoma. Dotted arrow: spindle cell proliferation with a "herringbone" pattern. CD, cluster of differentiation; DFSP, dermatofibrosarcoma protuberans; FISH, fluorescence in situ hybridization.

(A, Histology image courtesy of Noel Turner, MD, MHS and Christine J. Ko, MD. B, Histology image courtesy of Noel Turner, MD, MHS and Christine J. Ko, MD. C, Histology image reprinted with permission from Montgomery EA, James A. *Differential Diagnoses in Surgical Pathology: Soft Tissue and Bone.* Wolters Kluwer; 2020.)

- **Giant cell fibroblastoma:** multinucleated giant cells lining vascular-like spaces
- **Bednar tumor:** melanin pigment.
- **Fibrosarcoma:** cell-rich spindle cell proliferation with cytologic atypia and variable mitotic activity.

DFSP has a storiform "cartwheel" pattern and infiltrates the subcutis in a "honeycomb" pattern. Fibrosarcoma has a "herringbone" pattern.

- Epithelioid sarcoma is a rare soft-tissue sarcoma divided into two types: classic and proximal. Epithelioid sarcoma is associated with **mutations/deletions in *SMARCB1/INI1*** (tumor suppressor gene). The majority of affected patients are **young adults (20-40 years of age).**
- Epithelioid sarcoma is characterized by **skin-colored to brown, slow-growing, firm, multifocal nodules** on the **hands/fingers** (classic type) or the trunk (proximal type) ± secondary ulceration.
  - Figure 5.25.
- Historically, classic epithelioid sarcoma was treated aggressively with amputation. A more conservative approach is now recom-

mended with surgery and adjuvant radiation therapy. Proximal epithelioid sarcoma tends to be more aggressive; it has a higher rate of recurrence and a higher risk for metastasis (~50%).

Adipose Neoplasms

Basic Concepts

- Adipose neoplasms range from neoplasms of immature adipose tissue (eg, hibernoma) to neoplasms of mature adipose tissue (eg, lipoma).

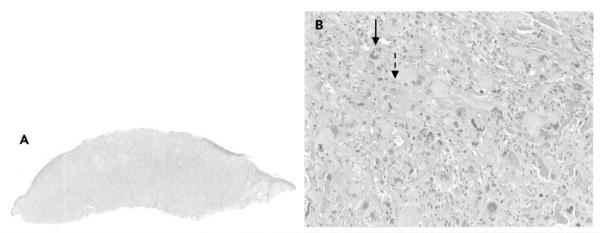

Figure 5.24. CLINICOPATHOLOGICAL CORRELATION: ATYPICAL FIBROXANTHOMA. AFX is characterized by a dome-shaped dermal proliferation of pleomorphic cells (bizarre multinucleated giant cells, histiocyte-like cells, spindle cells, xanthomatous cells) with cytologic atypia, mitotic activity, and necrosis. Nonspecific IHC stains include CD10, CD68, procollagen-1, and vimentin. A, Low-power view. B, High-power view. Solid arrow: bizarre multinucleated giant cell. Dashed arrow: spindle cell. AFX, atypical fibroxanthoma; CD, cluster of differentiation; EMA, epithelial membrane antigen; IHC, immunohistochemistry; SCC, squamous cell carcinoma; SMA, smooth muscle actin.

(Histology images courtesy of Noel Turner, MD, MHS and Christine J. Ko, MD.)

IHC is imperative to differentiate AFX from other neoplasms that "SLAM up" against the epidermis: spindle cell SCC (pan-CK and EMA positive), Leiomyosarcoma (desmin, SMA, and vimentin positive), AFX, and desmoplastic melanoma (S100 and SOX-10 positive).

• **Pleomorphic dermal sarcoma:** infiltration into the subcutis and lymphovascular/perineural invasion.

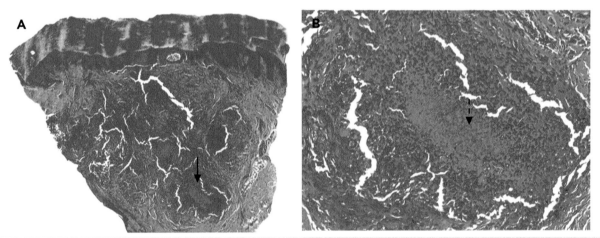

Figure 5.25. CLINICOPATHOLOGICAL CORRELATION: EPITHELIOID SARCOMA. Epithelioid sarcoma is characterized by a nodular proliferation of epithelioid cells and spindle cells with cytologic atypia, mitotic activity, and necrosis. CD34, pan-CK, and vimentin are positive; INI1 is negative. A, Low-power view. Solid arrow: nodular proliferation of epithelioid cells and spindle cells resembling a palisading granuloma. B, High-power view. Dashed arrow: necrosis. CD, cluster of differentiation; CK, cytokeratin; INI1, integrase interactor 1.

(Histology images reprinted with permission from Requena L, Kutzner H. *Cutaneous Soft Tissue Tumors*. Wolters Kluwer Health; 2014.)

On low power, epithelioid sarcoma mimics a palisading granuloma.

HIBERNOMA

Synonyms: lipoma of embryonic fat, lipoma of immature adipose tissue

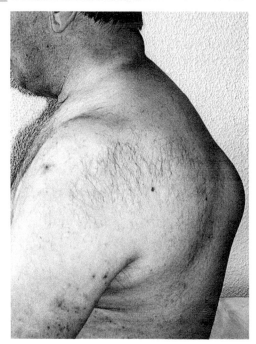

Reprinted with permission from Requena L, Kutzner H. *Cutaneous Soft Tissue Tumors*. Wolters Kluwer Health; 2014.

- Hibernoma is a rare benign neoplasm of **immature adipose cells (brown fat)** that may be associated with chromosomal rearrangements of 11q13 to 21. It usually develops during adulthood.
    - <u>Brown fat</u> produces heat in <u>hibern</u>ating animals.

- Hibernomas classically present as **slow growing subcutaneous nodules.** They have a predilection for the **neck, chest, interscapular area, and thighs.** They are usually larger than lipomas.
    - Figure 5.26.
- Complete surgical excision is curative.

LIPOMA

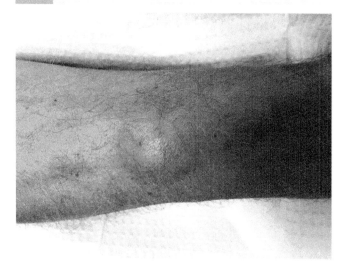

- Lipoma is a common benign neoplasm of **mature adipose cells (white fat)** that may be associated with cytogenetics deletions on chromosomes 13q and translocations on 12q 13 to 15. The incidence is slightly higher in men than women.
    - Multiple lipomas are associated with **adiposis dolorosa (Dercum disease)**, benign symmetric lipomato-

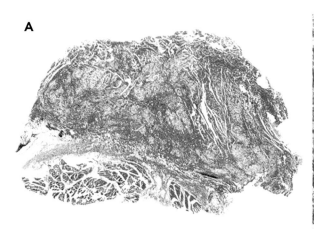

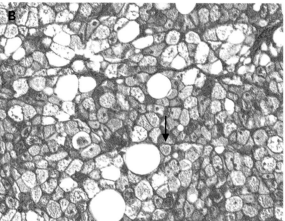

Figure 5.26. CLINICOPATHOLOGICAL CORRELATION: HIBERNOMA. Hibernoma is characterized by a well-circumscribed encapsulated proliferation of immature adipose cells (multivacuolated to granular eosinophilic cytoplasm, small central nucleus). A, Low-power view. B, High-power view. Solid arrow: multivacuolated "mulberry cell."

(Histology images reprinted with permission from Requena L, Kutzner H. *Cutaneous Soft Tissue Tumors*. Wolters Kluwer Health; 2014.)

Multivacuolated cells are often called "<u>mulberry</u> cells" and contain <u>mito</u>chondria.

sis (Madelung disease), diffuse congenital lipomatosis, familial multiple lipomatosis, **Cowden syndrome**, BRR syndrome, CLOVES syndrome, Proteus syndrome, neurofibromatosis (NF), and Gardner syndrome. A lipoma may signal a neural tube defect.

- Lipomas classically present as **mobile rubbery subcutaneous nodules.** They have a predilection for the **neck, buttocks, and upper extremities. Angiolipoma** is a **painful** lipoma variant that favors the forearms of women or patients on **protease inhibitors. Spindle cell lipoma and pleomorphic lipoma** are lipoma variants that favor the **neck, shoulder, or upper back of men. Liposarcoma** is thought to arise *de novo* rather than from a preexisting lipoma, most commonly in the retroperitoneum.

  - For painful neoplasms, remember ENGLAND: eccrine spiradenoma, traumatic neuroma, glomus tumor, leiomyoma, angiolipoma, neurilemmoma, and DF.
    Adiposis dolorosa classically presents in **postmenopausal women** with **multiple painful lipomas in periarticular regions** and is associated with **depression.**
    - Figure 5.27.
- Complete surgical excision is curative; however, lipomas often do not require treatment.

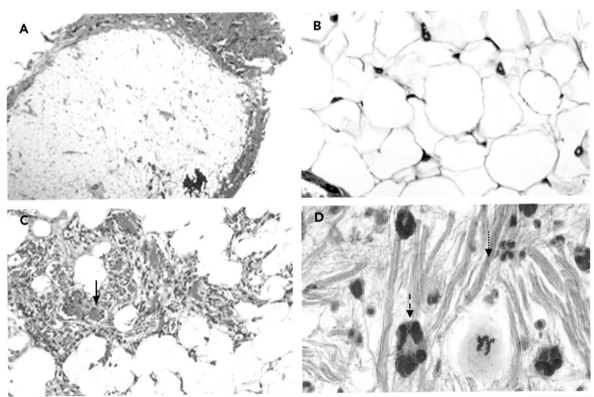

Figure 5.27. CLINICOPATHOLOGICAL CORRELATION: LIPOMA. Lipoma is characterized by a well-circumscribed encapsulated proliferation of mature adipose cells (univacuolated, eccentric nucleus). A, Low-power view. B, High-power view. C, Angiolipoma. Solid arrow: blood vessel filled with fibrin microthrombus. D, Pleomorphic lipoma. Dashed arrow: "floret-like" multinucleated cell. Dotted arrow: eosinophilic collagen bundles. CD, cluster of differentiation; CDK, cyclin-dependent kinase; MDM2, mouse double minute 2.

(Histology images reprinted with permission from Elder DE, Elenitsas R, Rosenbach M, et al. *Lever's Histopathology of the Skin.* 11th ed. Wolters Kluwer; 2015.)

- Angiolipoma: capillary-sized blood vessels filled with erythrocytes and fibrin microthrombi.
- Spindle cell lipoma: spindle cells (CD34+), eosinophilic collagen bundles, and myxoid stroma.
- Pleomorphic lipoma: multinucleated cells (CD34+) ± eosinophilic collagen bundles and myxoid stroma.
- Well-differentiated liposarcoma / atypical lipomatous tumor: lipoblasts (multivacuolated or univacuolated, indented or scalloped nucleus), cytologic atypia, and variable mitotic activity. *MDM2* and *CDK4* amplification may be observed.

In pleomorphic lipoma, overlapping nuclei at the periphery of multinucleated cells are "floret-like."

SPOTLIGHT ON COWDEN SYNDROME

Synonyms: Multiple hamartoma syndrome, *PTEN* hamartoma syndrome spectrum

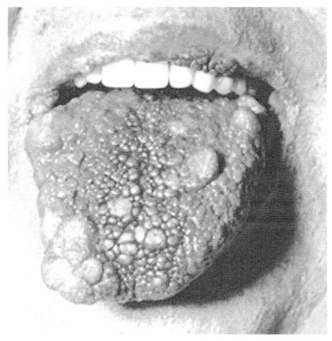

Reprinted with permission from Kazakov DV, Michal M, Kacerovska D, et al. *Cutaneous Adnexal Tumors.* Wolters Kluwer Health/Lippincott Williams & Wilkins; 2012

- Cowden syndrome is an **AD** hereditary disorder due to *PTEN* mutation. **Hypermethylation of the *KLLN* gene** may account for a small portion of Cowden syndrome. Cowden syndrome is characterized by the development of multiple hamartomatous tumors of the skin and internal organs. There is overlap with adult-onset **Lhermitte-Duclos disease** and other *PTEN* **hamartoma tumor syndromes.**
- **Clinical features of Cowden syndrome** are summarized in Table 5.21. Mucocutaneous features appear in >80% of patients and are often an early sign (typically the second decade). > 80% of patients with Cowden syndrome develop a malignancy, most commonly of the **breast or endometrium.** Adult-onset **Lhermitte-Duclos disease** is characterized by **dysplastic gangliocytoma of the cerebellum,** which causes stabbing pain in the back of the neck. **BRR syndrome** has overlapping features with Cowden syndrome including **penile lentigines, lipomas, tricholemmoma, and macrocephaly.**
  - Cowden syndrome is associated with trichilem<u>MOO</u>mas.
  - Penile lentigines in <u>Bannayan</u>-Riley-Ruvalcaba syndrome resemble a "spotted <u>banana</u>."

Table 5.21. CLINICAL FEATURES OF COWDEN SYNDROME

Mucocutaneous Features

- Acral keratoses
- Lipomas
- Mucosal cobblestoning
- Mucocutaneous neuromas
- Oral papillomas
- Penile lentigines
- Sclerotic fibromas
- Tricholemmomas

Systemic Features

- Digestive: multiple gastrointestinal polyps, colon adenocarcinoma (~10% lifetime risk)
- Endocrine: goiter, thyroid follicular carcinoma (~30% lifetime risk)
- Nervous: macrocephaly, intellectual disability
- Renal: RCC (~30% lifetime risk)
- Reproductive: breast fibroadenomas, breast carcinoma (>85% lifetime risk for females), and endometrial carcinoma (~30% lifetime risk for females)

RCC, renal cell carcinoma.

- The histopathology of Cowden syndrome demonstrates acral keratoses, lipomas, mucosal cobblestoning, mucocutaneous neuromas, oral papillomas, penile lentigines, sclerotic fibromas, and tricholemmomas.
- The diagnostic criteria for Cowden syndrome involve a combination of **pathognomonic criteria** (acral keratoses, mucosal neuromas/oral papillomas, papillomatous papules, and tricholemmomas), **major criteria** (breast adenocarcinoma, follicular thyroid carcinoma, adult-onset Lhermitte-Duclos disease, and macrocephaly), and **minor criteria** (fibromas, lipomas, gastrointestinal hamartomas, fibrocystic breast changes, intellectual disability, renal cell carcinoma (RCC)/genitourinary malignancies). Clinical diagnosis is made from cutaneous skin findings alone (≥3 tricholemmomas or ≥6 acral keratoses or oral papillomatosis), or 2 major criteria (must include macrocephaly and adult-onset Lhermitte-Duclos disease), or 1 major and 3 minor criteria, or 1 major and 3 minor criteria, or 4 minor criteria. **Genetic testing** can help confirm the diagnosis in uncertain cases.
- Management of patients with Cowden syndrome involves a multidisciplinary approach with dermatology, endocrinology, oncology, and surgery. In addition to age-appropriate malignancy screening, patients need **annual mammograms starting at age 30 to 35, annual thyroid US, baseline colonoscopy at age 35 years, and a referral to gynecologic oncology for discussion of endometrial cancer screening.**

Vascular Malformations and Neoplasms

ANGIOKERATOMA
→ Diagnosis Group 2

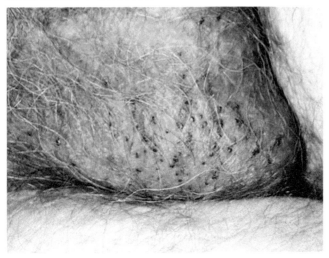

Reprinted with permission from Elder DE, Elenitsas R, Rubin AI, et al. *Atlas of Dermatopathology: Synopsis and Atlas of Lever's Histopathology of the Skin.* 4th ed. Wolters Kluwer; 2020.

Epidemiology

- Angiokeratoma is a benign vascular neoplasm of unclear etiology best categorized as a type of **telangiectasia (dilated capillary-type blood vessels)**.
- Associations with angiokeratoma depend on the variant.

Clinicopathological Features

- The clinical presentation of angiokeratoma depends on the variant:
  - **Solitary angiokeratoma: hyperkeratotic, dark blue or black papule favoring the lower extremities.** Associations include mechanical injury and chronic irritation.
  - **Angiokeratoma of the scrotum or vulva (Fordyce): numerous, small, bluish-purple papules along superficial vessels of the genitalia.**

    Angiokeratoma of Mibelli: single or multiple angiokeratomas on the **dorsal hands and feet in childhood/adolescence.** Associations include acrocyanosis and pernio.

    Angiokeratoma of Mibelli may form "grape-like clusters."

    Angiokeratoma circumscriptum: plaques of multiple discrete angiokeratomas in infancy/childhood.

    Angiokeratoma corpus diffusum: multiple, small angiokeratomas of the lower trunk and thighs in childhood/adolescence. Associations include **Fabry disease, fucosidosis, GM1 gangliosidosis, and sialidosis.**
    Figure 5.28.

Evaluation

- The differential diagnosis of angiokeratoma includes other telangiectasias. **Disorders associated with telangiectasia in adults** are summarized in Table 5.22.

Figure 5.28. CLINICOPATHOLOGICAL CORRELATION: ANGIOKERATOMA. Angiokeratoma is characterized by hyperkeratosis, acanthosis, and ectatic thin-walled blood vessels in the papillary dermis.
(Histology image courtesy of Noel Turner, MD, MHS and Christine J. Ko, MD.)

Table 5.22. DISORDERS ASSOCIATED WITH TELANGIECTASIA IN ADULTS

Diagnosis[a]	Classic Description	Notes
GET	Symmetrical generalized telangiectasia.	
Cutaneous collagenous vasculopathy	Similar to GET but involves the trunk and proximal extremities.	
Angioma serpiginosum	Rare vascular disorder with multiple, macular red-purple puncta in a clustered, serpiginous array favoring the extremities.	Female predominant. Vessels lack alkaline phosphatase activity.
Spider nevus	Erythematous, slightly raised papule with radiating telangiectasia.	Associated with cirrhosis, pregnancy, and OCPs. Cryotherapy is a treatment option.
Costal fringe	Band-like venous telangiectasias on the anterolateral thorax under the costal margins.	
Venous lake	Blue-purple papule favoring the lip.	Older adults. Associated with sun exposure and mechanical injury. Diascopy (performed by applying direct pressure against the lesion) will cause a venous lake to blanch, helping to differentiate it from neoplastic mimics (eg, melanoma).
TMEP	See Chapter 5: Hematolymphoid Neoplasms and Solid Organ Metastases.	

GET, generalized essential telangiectasia; OCPs, oral contraceptive pills; TMEP, telangiectasia macularis eruptive perstans.
[a]Illustrative examples provided.

Table 5.23. DISORDERS ASSOCIATED WITH TELANGIECTASIA IN CHILDREN

Diagnosis[a]	Inheritance Pattern	Gene(s)[a]	Classic Description	Notes
A-T	See Chapter 4: Photodermatoses.			
CMTC	See Chapter 2: Livedo Reticularis, Purpura, and Other Vascular Disorders.			
HHT (Osler-Weber-Rendu disease)	AD	HHT1: *endoglin* HHT2: *ALK1/ACVRL1* HHT5: *GDF2*	Mucocutaneous and gastrointestinal telangiectasias, epistaxis, pulmonary AVMs (type 1) and hepatic AVMs (type 2)	A rare variant of HHT caused by *SMAD4* gene mutation can present as HHT with juvenile gastrointestinal polyposis.
Hereditary benign telangiectasia	AD	Possibly *CMC1*	Similar to HHT without epistaxis or gastrointestinal involvement.	
Unilateral nevoid telangiectasia	Sporadic	Unknown	Telangiectasia in an upper cervical, trigeminal, or Blaschko-linear distribution.	Congenital or acquired, especially in females during puberty or pregnancy.

AD, autosomal dominant; A-T, ataxia-telangiectasia; CMTC, cutis marmorata telangiectasia congenita; HHT, hereditary hemorrhagic telangiectasia.
[a]Illustrative examples provided.

Disorders associated with telangiectasia in children are summarized in Table 5.23.

- **Dermoscopy** features include **red, blue, and black lacunae.**
- In general, no further evaluation is necessary for angiokeratoma.
  - If **angiokeratoma corporis diffusum** is suspected, then further evaluation for Fabry disease (eg, polarizing microscopy of the urine to look for birefringent lipid globules) and other associated disorders is recommended.

Management

- No treatment is necessary for angiokeratoma.
- If desired for cosmetic reasons, shave biopsy, PDL, or diathermy/electrosurgery may be considered.

"Real World" Advice

- If a thrombosis occurs in an angiokeratoma, it can mimic a melanoma. Dermoscopy may be helpful to distinguish these entities.

CAPILLARY MALFORMATION
→ Diagnosis Group 2

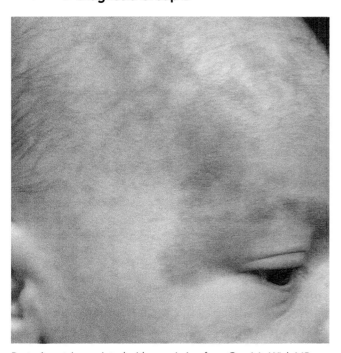

Port wine stain reprinted with permission from Gru AA, Wick MR, Mir A, et al. *Pediatric Dermatopathology and Dermatology.* Wolters Kluwer; 2018

Epidemiology

- A capillary malformation (CM) is a **slow-flow vascular malformation** consisting of **malformed capillaries.** CM is classified into multiple types:
  - **Salmon patch (nevus simplex):** very common finding in 30% to 80% of neonates felt to be a remnant of fetal circulation.
  - **Port-wine stain (PWS) (nevus flammeus):** broad, often segmental vascular malformation in 0.3% of neonates caused by somatic *GNAQ* mutation.
  - **Geometric purple CM:** associated with *PiK3CA* mutation and **Klippel-Trenaunay syndrome.**
  - **Reticulated CM:** associated with **PIK3CA-related segmental overgrowth spectrum.**
- CM can occur as an isolated cutaneous finding (salmon patch > PWS) or as a part of a broader syndrome (PWS > salmon patch). **Hereditary disorders associated with CM** are summarized in Table 5.24.

Clinicopathological Features

- **Salmon patch** classically presents as **red macules or patches at birth** that tend to **involve.**
  - The colloquial name for salmon patch is "stork bite," in reference to its presence at birth and characteristic location on the posterior neck.

Table 5.24. HEREDITARY DISORDERS ASSOCIATED WITH CAPILLARY MALFORMATION

Diagnosis[a]	Inheritance Pattern	Gene(s)	Classic Description	Notes
Beckwith-Wiedemann syndrome	Genomic imprinting	*CDKN1C, H19, IGF2, KCNQ1OT1*	Facial CM, ear abnormalities (circular depression over helical rims, linear earlobe creases). Systemic features include asymmetric overgrowth, macrosomia/gigantism, macroglossia. Visceromegaly, omphalocele, exomphalos, and Wilms tumor.	
Bonnet-Dechaume-Blanc syndrome	Unknown	Unknown	Facial vascular malformation. Systemic features include ipsilateral intracranial and retinal AVMs.	
CLOVES syndrome	Somatic, mosaic	*PIK3CA*	Epidermal nevi, lipomas, CMs. Systemic features include overgrowth of hands/feet, macrodactyly, sandal toe gap, scoliosis or spinal anomalies, and thoracic lipomatous hyperplasia.	
CM-AVM syndrome	AD (inactivating mutation)	*RASA1* or *EPHB4*	CMs and AVMs in a haphazard array. Systemic features include skeletal and soft-tissue hypertrophy and lytic bone lesions.	Recommend MRI/MRA of both spine and brain and duplex US.
Cobb syndrome	Unknown	*RASA1*	CM on posterior trunk. Systemic features include spinal AVM (neurologic deficits).	Recommend MRI/MRA of the corresponding region of the spinal cord.
Familial cerebral cavernous malformation (hyperkeratotic CVMs)	AD	*CCM1, CCM2, CCM3*	Characterized by vascular malformation of vertebrae, skin, or retina.	
Klippel-Trenaunay syndrome	Sporadic, mosaic	*PIK3CA*	Geographic CM of a limb. Systemic features include progressive soft-tissue swelling ± bony overgrowth of the affected extremity with lymphatic and deep venous insufficiency ± varicosities and gigantism.	Vascular malformations can be complicated by DVT, PE, superficial thrombophlebitis, and lymphedema with long-standing disease resulting in high-output CHF. Treatment involves sirolimus, compression stockings, and wound care.
Macrocephaly-CM syndrome	Somatic	*PIK3CA*	Nevus simplex of the mid-face, widespread reticulated CM. Systemic features include hemihypertrophy, syndactyly, and progressive neurologic dysfunction.	
Parkes Weber syndrome	Sporadic	*RASA1*	CM, fast-flow vascular malformations, LM. Systemic features include limb overgrowth with excess fat.	
Phakomatosis pigmentovascularis	Somatic, mosaic	*GNAQ or GNA11*	Five subtypes: I. PWS + epidermal nevus II. PWS + dermal melanocytosis ± nevus anemicus III. PWS + nevus spilus ± nevus anemicus IV. PWS + dermal melanocytosis + nevus spilus ± nevus anemicus V. CMTC + dermal melanocytosis	
Proteus syndrome	Sporadic	*AKT1* (part of mTOR pathway)	Palmoplantar cerebriform connective tissue nevi, lipomas, CM, VM. Systemic features include organomegaly, partial gigantism of the hands, hyperostosis (especially of external auditory canal), and various tumors (parotid adenomas, meningiomas, bilateral ovarian cystadenomas).	Life-threatening thromboembolic events may occur.

Do NOT confuse phakomatosis pigmentovascularis with phakomatosis pigmentokeratotica.

Proteus syndrome is named after the Greek god Proteus, who could change shape at will, in recognition of its protean manifestations.

Table 5.24. HEREDITARY DISORDERS ASSOCIATED WITH CAPILLARY MALFORMATION (CONTINUED)

Diagnosis[a]	Inheritance Pattern	Gene(s)	Classic Description	Notes
Rubinstein-Taybi syndrome	*De novo*	*CREBBP* or *EP300*	Brachyonychia, keloids, pilomatricomas. Systemic features include congenital heart defects, broad thumbs, and intellectual disability.	
Sturge-Weber Syndrome	Sporadic	*GNAQ*	PWS stain in V1 > V3, V2. Systemic features include TIAs, growth hormone deficiency, hyperthyroidism, skeletal hypertrophy, ADHD, seizures, and ipsilateral ocular involvement (anisometric amblyopia, choroid angioma, glaucoma).	The radiographic finding is parallel calcification of the cortex. Parallel calcification of the cortex is called "tram track" calcification.
Von Hippel-Lindau syndrome	AD	*VHL*	PWS (rarely of face). Systemic features include bilateral cerebellar/retinal hemangioblastomas, and various tumors (pancreatic, renal, pheochromocytoma).	

AD, autosomal dominant; ADHD, attention deficit hyperactivity disorder; AVM, arteriovenous malformation; CHF, congestive heart failure; CM, capillary malformation; CLOVES, Congenital *L*ipomatous asymmetric *O*vergrowth with lymphatic, capillary, venous, or combined-type *V*ascular malformation, *E*pidermal nevi, and *S*keletal anomalies/scoliosis; CMTC, cutis marmorata telangiectasia congenita; CVMs, capillary-venous malformations; DVT, deep venous thrombosis; LM, lymphatic malformation; MRA, magnetic resonance angiography; MRI, magnetic resonance imaging; PE, pulmonary embolus; PWS, port-wine stain; TIAs, transient ischemic attacks; VM, venous malformation.
[a]Illustrative example provided.

- **PWS** classically presents as a **unilateral, flat, irregular pink patch** that grows in proportion to body growth and **does not involute.** Over time, the skin changes from pink to deep purple and thickens with increased nodularity.
- Rarer CM variants include geographic CM and reticulated CM. Some characterize **nevus anemicus** as a CM variant. It presents as a congenital pale patch usually on the upper chest or back. It is believed to reflect a **localized hypersensitivity to catecholamines causing permanent vasoconstriction.**
    ◆ Figure 5.29.

Evaluation

- The differential diagnosis of CM includes infantile hemangioma (IH) but CM will not rapidly enlarge.
- No further evaluation is required for solitary CM.

Management

- No treatment is necessary for CM.
- If desired for cosmetic reasons, **PDL** can be used to treat discoloration.

"Real World" Advice

- CM can impact a child's cognitive and social development. Parents should be counseled that treatment can be considered early to minimize the developmental impact on the child and to reduce the amount of thickening and darkening over time.

VENOUS MALFORMATION

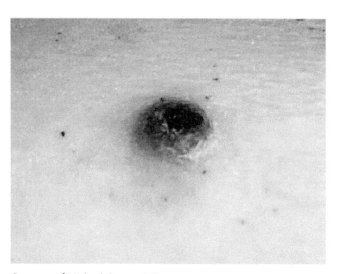

Courtesy of Michael Gowen, MD.

- Venous malformation (VM) is a **slow-flow vascular malformation** consisting of veins. Somatic mutations in *TEK (TIE2)* or *PIK3CA* are believed to cause 25% to 50% of sporadic VMs. While most VMs occur in isolation, associations include **blue-rubber-bleb nevus syndrome (Bean syndrome)** due to somatic activating mutations in *TEK* and **Maffucci syndrome** due to somatic mutations in *IDH-1* and *IDH-2.*

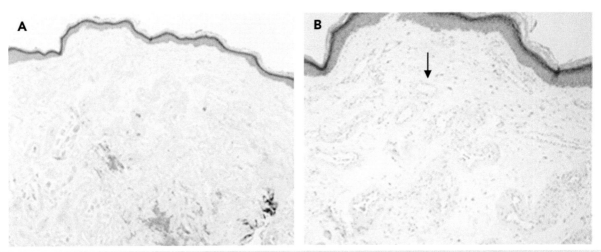

Figure 5.29. CLINICOPATHOLOGICAL CORRELATION: CAPILLARY MALFORMATION. CM is characterized by ectatic capillaries. A, Low-power view. B, High-power view. Solid arrow: ectatic capillary. CM, capillary malformation; PWS, port-wine stain.

(Histology image reprinted with permission from Gru AA, Wick MR, Mir A, et al. *Pediatric Dermatopathology and Dermatology.* Wolters Kluwer; 2018.)

- **Salmon patch:** ectatic capillaries in the papillary dermis.
- **PWS:** ectatic capillaries in the papillary dermis that gradually increase, sometimes extending into the reticular dermis/subcutis and filling with erythrocytes.

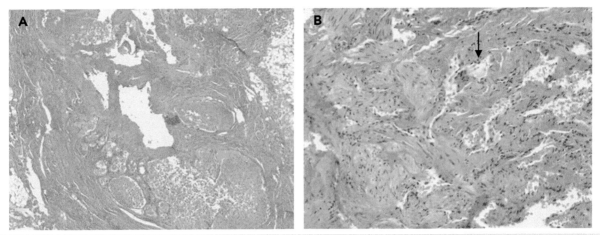

Figure 5.30. CLINICOPATHOLOGICAL CORRELATION: VENOUS MALFORMATION. VM is characterized by ectatic veins haphazardly arranged within the reticular dermis and subcutis. A, Low-power view. B, High-power view. Solid arrow: ectatic vein. VM, venous malformation.

(Histology images reprinted with permission from Gru AA, Wick MR, Mir A, et al. *Pediatric Dermatopathology and Dermatology.* Wolters Kluwer; 2018.)

VM was previously classified as "cavernous angioma" and "cavernous hemangioma." Verrucous venucapillary malformation (VCM) was previously classified as "verrucous hemangioma."

- VM classically presents as a **bluish-purple, nonpulsatile nodule**, sometimes with calcified phleboliths. While generally asymptomatic, VM may cause pain due to pressure on surrounding structures. Complications include **localized intravascular coagulation.**
  - **Blue-rubber-bleb nevus syndrome (Bean syndrome)** is characterized by **VMs favoring the trunk and upper extremities** that may exhibit **increased lesional hyper-** hidrosis and nocturnal pain. Gastrointestinal VMs, which appear after skin VMs, may cause gastrointestinal bleeding and intussusception.
  - **Maffucci syndrome is characterized by superficial VMs of the hands and feet, enchondromas, chondrosarcomas (central radiolucency on radiograph), short stature, and fractures.**
    - Figure 5.30.
- Treatment for VM is difficult. Conservative treatment may involve compression stocking. **Sclerotherapy** or surgical debulking may be considered.

LYMPHATIC MALFORMATION

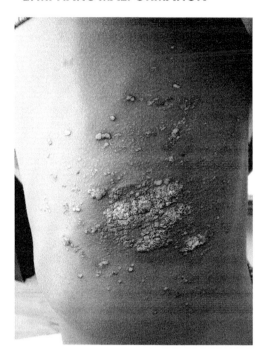

Verrucous lymphangioma circumscriptum

Lymphatic malformation (LM) is a **slow-flow vascular malformation** resulting from hyperplasia of a lymphatic network. LM variants are primarily divided into **macrocystic and microcystic** variants. **Hereditary disorders associated** with **macrocystic LMs** are summarized in Table 5.25. Somatic mutations in *PIK3CA* are associated with microcystic LMs.

- LM is characterized by **translucent nodules or papules** and may be complicated by **lymphedema and cellulitis.** The classic presentation of LM depends on the variant:
  - **Cystic hygroma (cavernous hemangioma)** is a **macrocystic LM** that presents as a large, translucent subcutaneous nodule favoring the **neck, axillae, and groin.**
  - **Lymphangioma circumscriptum** is a **microcystic LM** that presents as **aggregated translucent papules affecting a single anatomic region.** The surface may be verrucous.
    - Lymphangioma circumscriptum resembles "frog spawn."
    - **Acquired progressive lymphangioma (benign lymphangioendothelioma)** is a **microcystic LM** that presents as a **solitary well-circumscribed erythematous macule or plaque.**
    - **Targetoid hemosiderotic LM** is an acquired **microcystic LM** that presents as red-brown papule sometimes surrounded by a pale ring and ecchymotic halo **favoring the lower extremities,** often in a site of **mechanical injury.**
    - Targetoid hemosiderotic LM was previously classified as "targetoid hemosiderotic hemangioma" or "hobnail hemangioma." The clinical appearance is "target-like."
    - Figure 5.31.
- Treatment for both macrocystic and microcystic LM is surgical excision. Sclerotherapy may also be used to treat macrocystic LM. Sirolimus or PIK3CA inhibitors may be used to treat microcystic LM.

Table 5.25. HEREDITARY DISORDERS ASSOCIATED WITH MACROCYSTIC LYMPHATIC MALFORMATIONS

Diagnosis[a]	Inheritance Pattern	Gene(s)[a]	Classic Description	Notes
Noonan syndrome	AD	*PTPN11*	KP atrophicans faciei, macrocystic LM, GCT. Systemic features include congenital heart defects, facial dysmorphism, and short stature.	
Turner syndrome	Genomic imprinting	Missing X chromosome (45,X) or abnormal X chromosome	Macrocystic LM, pilomatricoma. Systemic features include aortic coarctation, webbed neck, short stature, shortened fourth and fifth metacarpal, and horseshoe kidney.	
Patau syndrome (trisomy 13)	Sporadic	Trisomy of chromosome 13	Macrocystic LM. Systemic features include congenital heart defects, cleft lip/palate, polydactyly, and intellectual disability.	Many infants die within the first day-to-weeks of life.
Edwards syndrome (trisomy 18)	Sporadic	Trisomy of chromosome 18	Macrocystic LM. Systemic features include congenital heart defects, cleft lip/palate, spina bifida, and intellectual disability.	Only 5%-10% of children live past the first year of life.
Down syndrome (trisomy 21)	Sporadic	Trisomy of chromosome 21	KP, EPS, primary systemic amyloidosis, macrocystic LM, syringomas, flat nipples, and single palmar crease. Systemic features include congenital heart defects, macroglossia, and intellectual disability.	Patients may have predilection for cutaneous infections and leukemia (ALL, AML).

AD, autosomal dominant; ALL, acute lymphocytic leukemia; AML, acute myelogenous leukemia; EPS, elastosis perforans serpiginosum; GCT, granular cell tumor; KP, keratosis pilaris; LM, lymphatic malformation.
[a]Illustrative examples provided.

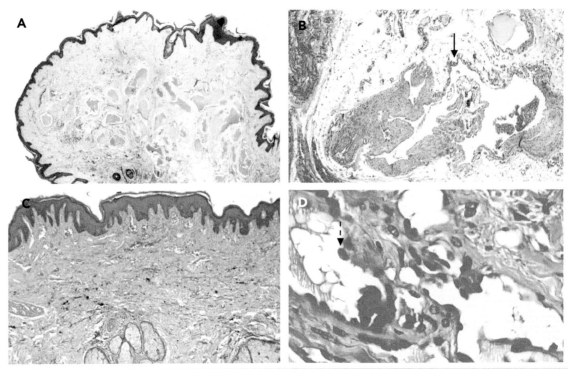

Figure 5.31. CLINICOPATHOLOGICAL CORRELATION: LYMPHATIC MALFORMATION. LM is characterized by ectatic lymphatics and is positive for podoplanin (D2-40). A, Lymphangioma circumscriptum low-power view. B, Lymphangioma circumscriptum high-power view. Solid arrow: ectatic lymphatic. C, Targetoid hemosiderotic LM low-power view. D, Targetoid hemosiderotic LM high-power view. Dashed arrow: superficial ectatic lymphatic with rounded "hobnail" nucleus that protrudes into the lumen. LM, lymphatic malformation.

(Histology images reprinted with permission from Elder DE, Elenitsas R, Rosenbach M, et al. *Lever's Histopathology of the Skin.* 11th ed. Wolters Kluwer; 2015.)

- **Cavernous lymphangioma/cystic hygroma:** large ectatic lymphatics in the dermis/subcutis.
- **Lymphangioma circumscriptum:** ectatic lymphatics in the papillary dermis.
- **Acquired progressive lymphangioma:** ectatic lymphatics in the papillary dermis that gradually increase, sometimes extending into the reticular dermis/subcutis.
- **Targetoid hemosiderotic LM:** superficial ectatic lymphatics with rounded nuclei that protrude into the lumina disappear in the deep dermis. There is erythrocyte extravasation and hemosiderin deposition.

In targetoid hemosiderotic LM, rounded nuclei resemble "hobnails" (short heavy-headed nails used to reinforce the soles of boots). "Hobnail nuclei" is a shared feature with epithelioid hemangioma.

ARTERIOVENOUS MALFORMATION

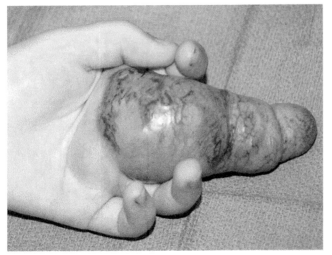

Reprinted with permission from Kransdorf MJ, Murphey MD. *Imaging of Soft Tissue Tumors.* 3rd ed. Wolters Kluwer Health/Lippincott Williams & Wilkins; 2013.

- Arteriovenous malformation (AVM) is a **fast-flow vascular malformation** consisting of both arterial and venous components, which leads to **arteriovenous shunting.** Other associations include **HHT, Bonnet-Dechaume-Blanc syndrome, CM-AVM syndrome, Cobb syndrome, and Parkes Weber syndrome.**
   - AVM is not the only vascular malformation with ≥2 blood vessel types. The alphabet soup of combined vascular malformations includes CVM, CLM, CLVM, LVM, C-AVM, and CL-AVM.
- AVM can have diverse clinical features ranging from macular erythema to a **large, pulsatile mass,** often favoring **cephalic** areas. A bruit may be heard on auscultation. **AVM grows in proportion to body growth and does not regress.** Complications due to arteriovenous shunting include **tachycardia and high-output CHF,** both of which may worsen during **pregnancy.**
   - Figure 5.32.
- **Arteriography** is the best imaging technique, though **MRI** and **US with color Doppler** may also be used.
- Treatment is difficult and requires **embolization or surgical excision.**

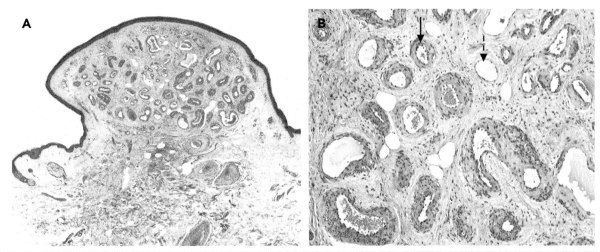

Figure 5.32. CLINICOPATHOLOGICAL CORRELATION: ARTERIOVENOUS MALFORMATION. AVM is characterized by a well-circumscribed proliferation of thick-walled blood vessels (arteries) and thin-walled blood vessels (veins) in the dermis. A, Low-power view. B, High-power view. Solid arrow: thick-walled vessel (artery). Dashed arrow: thin-walled vessel. AVM, arteriovenous malformation.

(Histology images reprinted with permission from Elder DE, Elenitsas R, Rosenbach M, et al. *Lever's Histopathology of the Skin.* 11th ed. Wolters Kluwer; 2015.)

HEMANGIOMA
→ Diagnosis Group 1

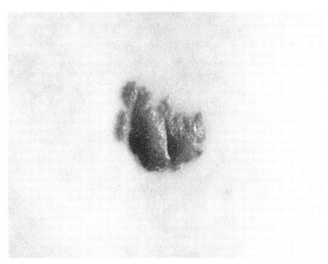

Infantile hemangioma reprinted with permission from Gru AA, Wick MR, Mir A, et al. *Pediatric Dermatopathology and Dermatology.* Wolters Kluwer; 2018

Epidemiology

- IH, comprised of blood vessels, is the most common benign soft-tissue neoplasm of childhood. When fully developed at birth, it is termed "congenital hemangioma (CH)." When minimally present at birth, it is termed "IH." The exact pathogenesis is not understood but **glucose transporter-1 (GLUT-1) is positive.**
- Risk factors include **female sex, Caucasian race, low-birth-weight/premature infants, advanced maternal age, multiple gestation, placental abnormalities, and chorionic villus sampling.**

- IH associations include **PHACE(S) and LUMBAR syn-dromes** (see below) and **diffuse neonatal hemangiomatosis (diffuse cutaneous hemangiomas with liver hemangiomas leading to high-output CHF and obstructive jaundice).**

Clinicopathological Features

- IH classically presents with a **pink or ecchymotic macule or patch with surrounding area of pallor ± telangiectasias** during the first few weeks of life that **evolves into a bright red, lobulated plaque or nodule** during the first months of life.

  The initial lesion of IH is sometimes called the "promontory mark."
- **Rapid growth occurs in the first 1 to 3 months,** followed by slow growth (complete by 5 months), then a period of no growth, and finally **involution (beginning as early as 1 year of age and continuing for several years).**
- IH may be **superficial (bright red plaque without a dermal component), deep (ill-defined, purple or blue mass without overlying surface change), or combined (bright red plaque with underlying mass). Color change from deep red to gray purple is often the first sign of involution.**

  Superficial IH is sometimes called "strawberry hemangioma" based on its bright red color resembling the fruit.
- Cutaneous hemangiomas may **ulcerate (especially over pressure points).** Regionally specific complications include **cosmetic disfigurement (nasal tip/lip/external ear/breast)** and **functional impairment such as obstruction of vision (periocular) and laryngeal hemangiomatosis with airway obstruction (beard area).**

Table 5.26. HEMANGIOMA VARIANTS

Diagnosis[a]	Classic Description	Notes
RICH	Presents fully formed at birth due to intrauterine proliferation. Rapid involution during first year.	Equal prevalence in the sexes. GLUT-1 negative.
PICH	Presents with regression like RICH but fails to completely involute.	
NICH	Presents fully formed at birth due to intrauterine proliferation, then grows in proportion to body growth and does not involute.	
IH	See above.	
IH-MAG	IH with a proliferative component <25% of total surface area. Most commonly presents with fine or coarse telangiectatic patches favoring the lower body.	GLUT-1 positive.
Epithelioid hemangioma (ALHE)	Tan/brown, red papules or nodules on the head and neck (especially the ear).	Associated with mechanical injury, AVMs, and fistulas. Rare reports of *TEK* mutations. Epithelioid hemangioma has overlapping histopathology with Kimura disease, which presents with unilateral, painless cervical lymphadenopathy, peripheral hypereosinophilia, and elevated IgE.
Glomeruloid hemangioma	Multiple, red-purple, firm papule or nodules favoring the trunk and extremities.	Favored to be reactive rather than neoplastic due to increased levels of VEGF in POEMS syndrome. Rarely associated with Castleman disease.
Microvenular hemangioma	Solitary, slow growing reddish nodules favoring the forearms.	May be a reactive condition.
Sinusoidal hemangioma	Solitary, slow-growing subcutaneous nodule.	Favored to be a sinusoidal growth of intravascular endothelial hyperplasia occurring within a low-flow VM.
Spindle cell hemangioma	Firm blue nodules favoring the extremities.	Spindle cell hemangioma was previously classified as "spindle cell hemangioendothelioma."

ALHE, angiolymphoid hyperplasia with eosinophilia; AVMs, arterio-venous malformations; GLUT-1, glucose transporter-1; IH, infantile hemangioma; IH-MAG, infantile hemangioma with minimal or arrested growth; Ig, immunoglobulin; NICH, noninvoluting congenital hemangioma; PICH, partially-involuting congenital hemangioma; POEMS, polyneuropathy, organomegaly, endocrinopathy, monoclonal gammopathy, and skin lesions; RICH, rapidly-involuting congenital hemangioma; VM, venous malformation.
[a]Illustrative examples provided.

- **Hemangioma variants** (IHs and distinct vascular neoplasms bearing the term "hemangioma") are summarized in Table 5.26. For PG and cherry angioma, see below.
  - ◆ **POEMS (Polyneuropathy, Organomegaly, Endocrinopathy, Monoclonal gammopathy, and Skin changes) syndrome** is a paraneoplastic syndrome characterized by **elevated VEGF level.** Skin changes include **hyperpigmentation, sclerodermoid skin, hypertrichosis, digital clubbing, cherry angiomas, and glomeruloid hemangiomas.** The monoclonal gammopathy is typically **IgA or IgG (λ > κ).** Glomeruloid hemangiomas may also occur in **Castleman disease.**
  - ◆ Figure 5.33.

Evaluation

- The differential diagnosis for IH includes telangiectasia, vascular malformation, and tufted angioma. The initial presentation may resemble nevus anemicus.
- **Dermoscopy** features include **red, blue, and black lacunae.**
- If ≥ 5 cutaneous IHs are present, abdominal US should be used to screen for hepatic IH (95% sensitivity). Abdominal US avoids the need for sedation and possible ionizing radiation of other imaging modalities.

Management

- 90% of IH involution is complete by 4 years of age; however, this does not imply that the skin will completely normalize. Parents should be advised that, even after involution, residual changes, such as telangiectasias, redundant skin, or a scar, may be left. In **diffuse neonatal hemangiomatosis, high-output CHF is the leading cause of death.**
- While IH without risk factors do not require therapy, there is a window of opportunity to treat problematic or high-risk IH, so early consultation (by 1 month of age) is recommended.
- **Topical timolol** can be used for small thin superficial IH.
- **Systemic propranolol (2-3 mg/kg/d for at least 6 months until ≥12 months of age)** can be considered for high-risk IH based on the following five risk factors:
  - (1) Life-threatening: "beard-area," ≥5 cutaneous hemangiomas.

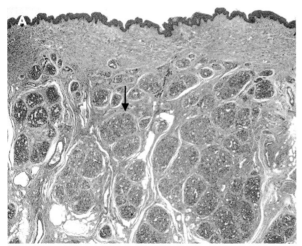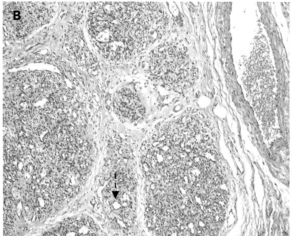

Figure 5.33. CLINICOPATHOLOGICAL CORRELATION: HEMANGIOMA. A, Early IH. Solid arrow: lobules of endothelial cells. B, Mature IH. Dashed arrow: lobules of dilated capillary-sized blood vessels. ALHE, angiolymphoid hyperplasia with eosinophilia; Fc, fragment crystallizable; GLUT-1, glucose transporter-1; IH, infantile hemangioma; IPEH, intravascular papillary endothelial hyperplasia; LM, lymphatic malformation; NICH, noninvoluting congenital hemangioma; PAS, periodic acid-Schiff; PICH, partially involuting congenital hemangioma; RICH, rapidly involuting congenital hemangioma.

(Histology images reprinted with permission from Elder DE, Elenitsas R, Rosenbach M, et al. *Lever's Histopathology of the Skin*. 11th ed. Wolters Kluwer; 2015.)

- **RICH / PICH / NICH:** lobules of capillary-sized blood vessels with intervening fibrotic bands in the subcutis. Larger blood vessels may be present in NICH > PICH > RICH. GLUT-1 staining is negative.
- **IH:** lobules of endothelial cells (early) produce dilated capillary-sized blood vessels (mature) that are gradually replaced by fibrosis (involution). IH may be located in the papillary dermis (superficial), reticular dermis and / or subcutis (deep), or both (combined). GLUT-1 staining is positive, along with other placenta-associated vascular proteins FcγRII, merosin, and Lewis Y antigen.
- **Epithelioid hemangioma:** lobules of capillary-sized blood vessels surrounding larger blood vessels with rounded nuclei that protrude into the lumina in the dermis and subcutis. There is a perivascular lymphocyte- and eosinophil-rich inflammatory infiltrate ± nodular lymphoid aggregates with eosinophils.
- **Glomeruloid hemangioma:** dilated blood vessels filled by capillary loops in the dermis with paraprotein-derived eosinophilic globules (PAS positive, diastase resistant).
- **Microvenular hemangioma:** branching capillaries and venules filling the reticular dermis.
- **Sinusoidal hemangioma:** lobules of dilated veins forming interconnected sieve-like spaces.
- **Spindle cell hemangioma:** hemorrhagic nodules containing both cavernous vascular spaces with organizing thrombi and spindle cell fascicles with intervening slit-like vascular spaces.

"Hobnail nuclei" is a shared feature between epithelioid hemangioma and targetoid hemosiderotic LM. Remember the presence of eosinophils in epithelioid hemangioma by its alternative name "ALHE." Capillary loops in glomeruloid hemangioma resemble the kidney glomeruli.

- ○ (2) Functional impairment: periocular >1 cm or involving lip or oral cavity.
- ○ (3) Increased risk of ulceration.
- ○ (4) Association with structural abnormalities.
- ○ (5) High-risk for permanent disfigurement: segmental on scalp or face, location on nasal tip or lip (any size) or ≥2 cm anywhere on face or scalp, >2 cm on neck, trunk, or extremities, anywhere on breast in female.

Though generally safe, propranolol can lead to **hypoglycemia, bronchospasm, hypothermia, hypotension, and bradycardia.** Due to the risk of hypoglycemia and hypoglycemia-related seizure, hold propranolol if a baby is having restricted oral intake. Pretreatment ECG is controversial. Of note, PHACE is technically a contraindication to the use of propranolol given risk of stroke; however, this is controversial as many authors have used it safely.

- For residual surface vascularity following involution or timolol/propranolol therapy, consider **PDL.**

"Real World" Advice

- Topical timolol gel is easier for parents to use than solution (spreads/runs over larger area).

SPOTLIGHT ON PHACE(S) SYNDROME AND LUMBAR SYNDROME

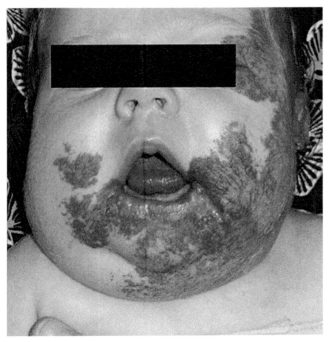

Facial segmental infantile hemangioma reprinted with permission from Johnson JT, Rosen CA. *Bailey's Head and Neck Surgery: Otolaryngology.* 5th ed. Wolters Kluwer Health/Lippincott Williams & Wilkins; 2013.

- PHACE(S) and LUMBAR syndromes are characterized by **facial and lower body segmental IH**, respectively, in association with systemic abnormalities. PHACE(S) has a **9:1 female:male ratio.**
- **PHACE(S)** syndrome presents with Posterior fossa malformations, Hemangioma, Arterial anomalies, Cardiac anomalies and aortic coarctation, Eye abnormalities, Sternal clefting and Supraumbilical abdominal raphe. The **highest risk segmental distributions are S1 (frontotemporal) and S2 (maxillary).** LUMBAR syndrome presents with Lower body hemangioma, Urogenital abnormalities, Myelopathy, Bony deformities, Anorectal malformations/arterial anomalies, and Renal anomalies.
  - ◆ The histopathology of PHACE(S) and LUMBAR syndromes demonstrates IH.
- **Diagnostic criteria for PHACE(S) syndrome** are detailed in Table 5.27. There are currently no consensus diagnostic criteria for LUMBAR syndrome. Evaluation for PHACE(S) syndrome includes MRI and/or MRA of the head and neck and echocardiogram. Screening for LUMBAR syndrome includes spinal US and Doppler US of the abdomen and pelvis; MRI will provide greater definition.
- Treatment for PHACE(S) and LUMBAR syndromes requires a multidisciplinary team. Depending on imaging studies and approval from cardiology and neurology, **propranolol** may be used to treat the segmental IH.

Table 5.27. DIAGNOSTIC CRITERIA FOR PHACE(S) SYNDROME

PHACE(S) Syndrome

- Hemangioma > 5 cm in diameter of the head including scalp PLUS 1 major criterion or 2 minor criteria
- Hemangioma of the neck, upper trunk, or trunk and proximal upper extremity PLUS 2 major criteria

Major Criteria

Arterial anomalies
- Anomaly of major cerebral and cervical arteries
- Dysplasia of large cerebral arteries
- Arterial stenosis or occlusion
- Persistent carotid-vertebrobasilar anastomosis

Structural brain
- Posterior fossa brain anomalies (Dandy-Walker complex most common)
- Other hypoplasia/displace of mid and/or hind brain

Cardiovascular
- Aortic arch anomalies
- Coarctation of the aorta
- Aberrant origin of subclavian ± vascular ring

Ocular
- Posterior segment anomalies—persistent hyperplastic primary vitreous/persistent fetal vasculature, retinal vascular anomalies, optic nerve hypoplasia, morning glory disc anomaly

Ventral or midline
- Sternal defect/pit/cleft
- Supraumbilical raphe

Minor Criteria

Arterial anomalies
- Aneurysm of any of the cerebral arteries

Structural brain
- Midline brain anomalies
- Malformation of cortical development

Cardiovascular
- Ventricular septal defect
- Right aortic arch/double aortic arch
- Systematic venous anomalies

Ocular
- Anterior segment anomalies (sclerocornea, cataract, coloboma, microphthalmia)

Ventral or midline
- Hypopituitarism
- Ectopic thyroid
- Midline sternal papule/hamartoma

PYOGENIC GRANULOMA
→ Diagnosis Group 2
Synonym: lobular capillary hemangioma

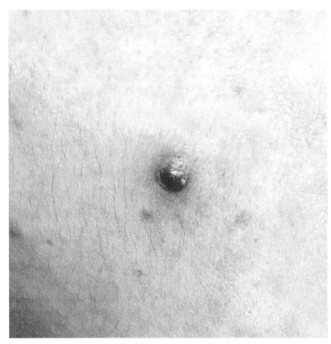

Courtesy of Cory Simpson, MD, PhD.

Epidemiology

- PG is a **benign, acquired vascular neoplasm.** The etiology is unclear though PG may be a form of reactive neovascu-larization. PG can occur at any age though is most common in children.
- Associations include **mechanical injury, pressure injury (onychocryptosis), friction injury, and pregnancy.**
- Drug associations include **systemic retinoids.**

Clinicopathological Features

- PG evolves with rapid growth into a **bleeding, friable, soft red papulonodule with an epidermal collarette.**
- PG may be mucosal or **periungual/subungual.**
  - ◆ Figure 5.34.

Evaluation

- The differential diagnosis of PG includes bacillary angiomatosis, amelanotic melanoma, KS, glomus tumor, and RCC metastasis.
- Given the potential for malignancies, especially amelanotic melanoma and RCC metastasis, to masquerade as PG, skin biopsy is required to confirm the diagnosis.

Management

- Shave excision with electrodesiccation of the base is the preferred treatment (though recurrence is common). PDL may be used for smaller lesions.

"Real World" Advice

- Remember that **NRTIs/NtRTIs (eg, lamivudine) and protease inhibitors (eg, indinavir)** cause **excessive periungual granulation tissue,** and **capecitabine, EGFR inhibitors, and MEK 1/2 inhibitors** cause **pseudopyogenic granulomas.**

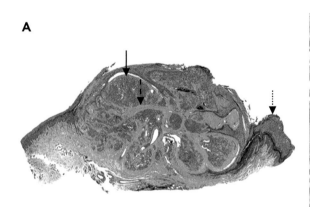

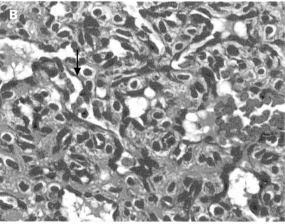

Figure 5.34. CLINICOPATHOLOGICAL CORRELATION: PYOGENIC GRANULOMA. In PG, lobules of endothelial cells (early) produce dilated capillary-sized blood vessels (mature) with intervening fibrotic bands in the dermis. Prominent epithelial collarettes may be observed at the periphery. A, PG low-power view. Solid arrow: dilated capillary-sized blood vessels. Dashed arrow: fibrotic band. Dotted arrow: epithelial collarette. B, PG high-power view. Solid arrow: dilated capillary-sized blood vessels. PG, pyogenic granuloma.

(Histology images reprinted with permission from Requena L, Kutzner H. *Cutaneous Soft Tissue Tumors.* Wolters Kluwer Health; 2014.)

Pyogenic granuloma is a misnomer. Granuloma refers to the resemblance of an early lesion, altered by ulceration and secondary inflammatory changes, to granulation tissue.

CHERRY ANGIOMA
Synonym: cherry hemangioma

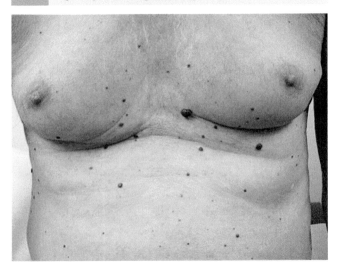

Reprinted with permission from Goodheart HP. *Goodheart's Same-Site Differential Diagnosis: A Rapid Method of Diagnosing and Treating Common Skin Disorders.* Wolters Kluwer Health/Lippincott Williams & Wilkins; 2011.

- Cherry angioma is the most common vascular proliferation in the skin. Cherry angiomas may appear as early as adolescence but commonly arise during the third decade of life and increase in number with age. Associations include POEMS syndrome and pregnancy.

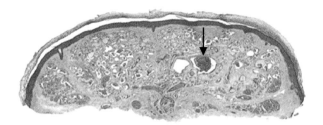

Figure 5.35. CLINICOPATHOLOGICAL CORRELATION: CHERRY ANGIOMA. Cherry angioma is characterized by a dome-shaped proliferation of capillary-sized blood vessels in the papillary dermis. Blood vessels have pink hyalinized walls and are filled with erythrocytes. Solid arrow: capillary-sized blood vessel.

(Histology image reprinted with permission from Elder DE, Elenitsas R, Rubin AI, et al. *Atlas of Dermatopathology: Synopsis and Atlas of Lever's Histopathology of the Skin.* 4th ed. Wolters Kluwer; 2020.)

- Cherry angiomas present as **round, sometimes elevated red papules, often on the trunk.**
    - Figure 5.35.
- Cherry angiomas are benign and do not require treatment. For cosmesis, shave excision, electrodesiccation, or PDL can be performed.

TUFTED ANGIOMA AND KAPOSIFORM HEMANGIOENDOTHELIOMA

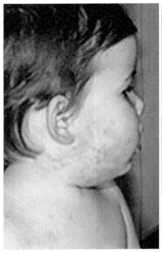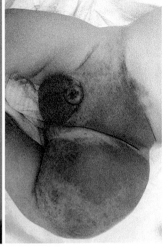

Tufted angioma (left) reprinted with permission from Thorne CH, Chung KC, Gosain AK, et al. *Grabb and Smith's Plastic Surgery.* 7th ed. Wolters Kluwer Health/Lippincott Williams & Wilkins; 2013. Kaposiform hemangioendothelioma (right) reprinted with permission from Husain AN, Stocker JT, Dehner LP. *Stocker and Dehner's Pediatric Pathology.* 4th ed. Wolters Kluwer; 2015.

- **Tufted angioma is a benign vascular neoplasm** comprised of capillaries. **Kaposiform hemangioendothelioma (KHE) is a borderline and low-grade malignant vascular neoplasm.** Tufted angioma is likely a superficial form of KHE. While the majority of both entities are acquired before 5 years of age, rare congenital cases occur.
- **Tufted angioma** classically presents as a **pink patch or ill-defined purple mass** favoring the neck and upper trunk, especially the **shoulders.** Tufted angioma may involve deeper structures like the soft tissue, bone, and retroperitoneum. Lesions are only locally aggressive. **KHE** classically presents as a **vascular patch or plaque or deep-seated purple nodule/mass.** Both tufted angioma and KHE (especially when congenital) may be complicated by **Kasabach-Merritt syndrome (localized intravascular coagulation** that may lead to **high-output CHF) and gastrointestinal bleeding.**
    - Figure 5.36.
- IH may clinically mimic tufted angioma; KS may clinically mimic KHE. Clinical evaluation should include skin biopsy, CBC, coagulation studies, and MRI.
- Tufted angioma usually remains stable in size but does not spontaneously regress. Surgical excision is the recommended treatment. KHE is a locally aggressive tumor that may infiltrate along lymphatics (though it does not truly metastasize).

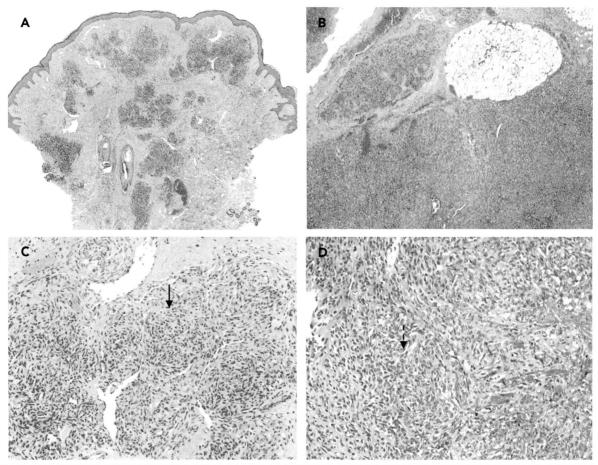

Figure 5.36. SIDE-BY-SIDE COMPARISON: TUFTED ANGIOMA AND KAPOSIFORM HEMANGIOENDOTHELIOMA.
Both tufted angioma and KHE demonstrate lobules of capillary-sized blood vessels. Tufted angioma is a well-circumscribed proliferation in the dermis characterized by capillary tufts. KHE is a poorly circumscribed proliferation in the subcutis characterized by spindle cell fascicles with intervening slit-like vascular spaces. A and C, Tufted angioma. Solid arrow: capillary tuft ("cannonball"). B and D, KHE. Dashed arrow: slit-like vascular space between spindle cells. HHV-8, human herpesvirus 8; KHE, Kaposiform hemangioendothelioma; KS, Kaposi sarcoma; IHC, immunohistochemistry; LNA, latent nuclear antigen.

(Histology images B and D reprinted with permission from Elder DE, Elenitsas R, Rosenbach M, et al. *Lever's Histopathology of the Skin.* 11th ed. Wolters Kluwer; 2015.)

Capillary tufts resemble "cannonballs."
HHV-8 (LNA-1) IHC is negative..

The two most common causes of death include thrombocytopenia and direct tumor infiltration. KHE is treated with WLE. **Embolization, compression, and radiation therapy** may be considered. For suspected Kasabach-Merritt syndrome in either tufted angioma or KHE, **vincristine plus prednisone or sirolimus** are first line. Despite thrombocytopenia, platelets should not be transfused as this may increase clotting. For active bleeding or symptomatic anemia, administer packed red blood cells (PRBCs) and low-molecular-weight heparin (LMWH).

KAPOSI SARCOMA
→ Diagnosis Group 2

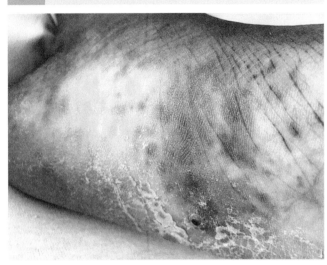

Epidemiology

- Kaposi sarcoma (KS) is a **borderline and low-grade malignant vascular neoplasm.** The causative organism is **HHV-8.** HHV-8 is not believed to be readily transmitted through blood, but likely is transmitted through other bodily substances (saliva, semen). Of note, **20% of men with KS in the US have HHV-8 in their semen.**
  - HHV-8 is also known as Kaposi sarcoma-associated herpesvirus (KSHV).
- KS is classified into **four types: classic (Mediterranean), endemic (African), epidemic (AIDS-associated), and iatrogenic (transplant-related).**

Clinicopathological Features

- **KS types** are summarized in Table 5.28. Cutaneous KS can be found in various stages of regression and progression. Complications include ulceration and superinfection.
  - The lymphadenopathic variant of endemic (African) KS primarily affects children.
- KS may also demonstrate **red patches, plaques, and nodules in the oral cavity.**
- Systemic organ involvement includes the gastrointestinal tract, lymph nodes, and lungs.
  - Figure 5.37.

Evaluation

- The differential diagnosis of KS includes bacillary angiomatosis, CM, PG, KHE, and angiosarcoma.
- Inspect the oral cavity. If visceral involvement is suspected, obtain FOBT to evaluate for gastrointestinal involvement and CT to evaluate for lymph node and lung involvement.

Management

- The 5-year relative survival rate of localized KS is 81%; however, this decreases to 41% with distant disease (eg, hepatic or pulmonary involvement).
- For epidemic (AIDS-associated) KS, **initiation of ART can lead to resolution.** ART should be continued if KS flares in the setting of IRIS.
- For iatrogenic (transplant-associated) KS, cessation of immunosuppressive therapy (articularly cyclosporine) can lead to resolution.

Table 5.28. KAPOSI SARCOMA TYPES

Diagnosis[a]	Classic Description	Notes
Classic (Mediterranean)	Reddish-purple macules, plaques, or tumors on the distal lower extremities.	Elderly (>50 years of age) men (15:1 male:female ratio) of Mediterranean or Ashkenazi Jewish descent.
Endemic (African)	May be nodular, florid, infiltrative, and lymphadenopathic.	Black Africans with a male predominance.
Epidemic (AIDS-associated)	May be solitary or widely disseminated along cleavage lines on the trunk and midface.	Typical CD4 T-cell count <500 cells/mm³. Primarily occurs in MSM (up to 40% of MSM with AIDS develop KS). May flare with IRIS.
Iatrogenic (transplant-associated)	Similar to classic KS.	Cyclosporine is associated with the highest rate.

AIDS, acquired immunodeficiency syndrome; CD, cluster of differentiation; IRIS, immune reconstitution inflammatory syndrome; MSM, men who have sex with men.
[a]Illustrative examples provided.

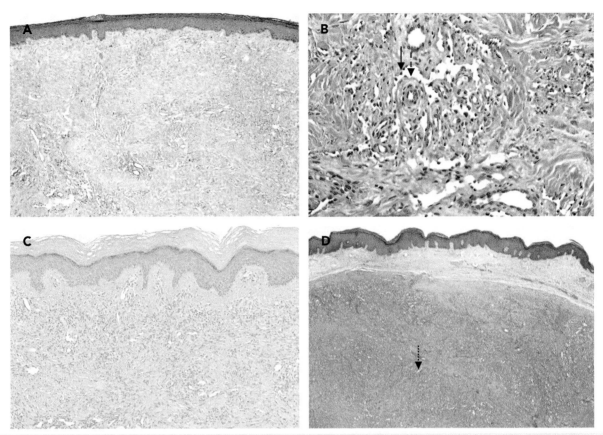

Figure 5.37. CLINICOPATHOLOGICAL CORRELATION: KAPOSI SARCOMA. Patch-stage KS is characterized by endothelial cells with minimal cytologic atypia around stag-horn vascular spaces between collagen bundles. There is a sparse lymphoplasmacytic dermal infiltrate, erythrocyte extravasation, and hemosiderin deposition. Spindle cells appear in plaque-stage KS and form fascicles in nodular-stage KS with intervening slit-like vascular spaces. Hyaline globules (PAS positive, diastase resistant) are observed in plaque- and nodular-stage KS. HHV-8 (LNA-1) IHC is positive in all stages. Other stains include CD31, CD34, factor VIII, podoplanin (D2-40), and ulex europaeus lectin. A, Patch-stage KS low-power view. B, Patch-stage KS high-power view. Solid arrow: endothelial cells around a stag-horn vascular space between collagen bundles. Dashed arrow: "promontory sign." C, Plaque-stage KS. D, Nodular-stage KS. Dotted area: slit-like vascular space between spindle cells. CD, cluster of differentiation; HHV-8, human herpesvirus 8; IHC, immunohistochemistry; KS, Kaposi sarcoma; LNA, latent nuclear antigen; PAS, periodic acid-Schiff.

(A, Histology image reprinted with permission from Elder DE, Elenitsas R, Rosenbach M, et al. *Lever's Histopathology of the Skin.* 11th ed. Wolters Kluwer; 2015. B, Histology image reprinted with permission from Elder DE, Elenitsas R, Rosenbach M, et al. *Lever's Histopathology of the Skin.* 11th ed. Wolters Kluwer; 2015. C, Histology image courtesy of Noel Turner, MD, MHS and Christine J. Ko, MD. D, Histology image reprinted with permission from Elder DE, Elenitsas R, Rosenbach M, et al. *Lever's Histopathology of the Skin.* 11th ed. Wolters Kluwer; 2015.)

The "promontory sign" refers to protrusion of preexisting blood vessels and normal adnexal structures into newly formed blood vessels. Hyaline globules are called "dorfballs."

- **Cryotherapy or surgical excision** may be considered for localized cutaneous KS. Currently for systemic involvement, **radiation therapy** or targeted antineoplastics (eg, **bevacizumab, imatinib, sorafenib, bortezomib**) may be considered.

"Real World" Advice

- KS can be stigmatizing for patients as it is a readily recognizable manifestation of HIV/AIDS. Sensitivity when diagnosing and discussing this diagnosis should be exercised.

ANGIOSARCOMA

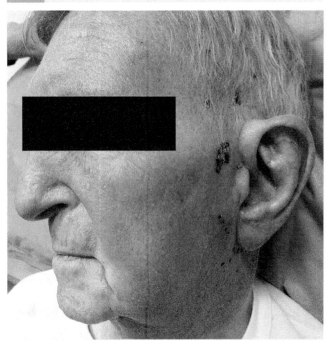

- Angiosarcoma is a malignant vascular neoplasm caused by an upregulation of vascular specific receptor tyrosine kinases (*TIE1, KDR, FLT1, TEK*). It is most common in older or middle-aged adults, particularly **Caucasian men over 70 years of age.** Associations include **lymphedema (Stewart-Treves syndrome) and radiation therapy. Secondary angiosarcoma may have *MYC* amplification** (uncommon in primary angiosarcoma) leading to upregulation of miR-17 to 92 cluster, which can promote angiogenesis.

- Angiosarcoma classically presents with **ecchymoses-like lesions favoring the scalp and face.** It may lead to **bleeding, edema, and pain.** Stewart-Treves variant is most common on the inner aspect of the upper arm. Angiosarcoma **initially metastasizes to regional lymph nodes,** and can spread to distant organs.
  - ◆ Figure 5.38.
  - ◆ Histopathological features of other malignant vascular neoplasms not discussed elsewhere are summarized in Table 5.29.

- **Rosacea is an important mimic of angiosarcoma.** Skin biopsy should be performed when there is expansion of facial papules/nodule refractory to topical treatments or rapidly progressive facial edema. CT or MRI of the affected area will help to determine regional lymph node, soft-tissue, or bone involvement.

- **Angiosarcoma has a poor prognosis with a 5-year survival <15%.** Standard treatment is WLE with adjuvant radiotherapy.

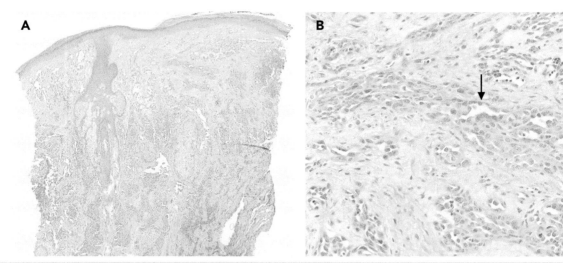

Figure 5.38. CLINICOPATHOLOGICAL CORRELATION: ANGIOSARCOMA. Angiosarcoma is characterized by an infiltrative growth pattern of endothelial cells with cytologic atypia, mitotic activity, and necrosis. Multilayering of endothelial cells occurs around crack-like vascular spaces between collagen bundles. Stains include CD31 (specific), CD34 (not specific), ERG (most sensitive and specific), factor VIII (±), FLI1, and ulex europeus lectin. Podoplanin (D2-40) is positive in cases with lymphatic differentiation. FISH can detect *MYC* amplification in secondary angiosarcoma. A, Low-power view. B, High-power view. Solid arrow: multilayering of endothelial cells around a crack-like vascular space between collagen bundles. AVL, atypical vascular lesion; CD, cluster of differentiation; FISH, fluorescence in situ hybridization; FLI1, friend leukemia integration 1.

(Histology images courtesy of Noel Turner, MD, MHS and Christine J. Ko, MD.)

• Epithelioid angiosarcoma variant: nodular growth pattern of epithelioid endothelial cells.

MYC amplification is helpful to differentiate post-radiation angiosarcoma from postradiation AVL.

Table 5.29. HISTOPATHOLOGICAL FEATURES OF OTHER MALIGNANT VASCULAR NEOPLASMS

Diagnosis[a]	Histopathological Features	Notes
Borderline and Low-Grade		
PILA	Thin, dilated vessels lined by hobnail endothelial cells and papillary strands extending into vessel lumens.	
Retiform hemangioendothelioma	Arborizing vessels with hobnail endothelial cells often associated with a perivascular lymphocytic infiltrate.	Local recurrence is common after surgical excision.
High-Grade		
Epithelioid hemangioendothelioma	Spindle-shaped or epithelioid endothelial cells arranged in nests and cords admixed in myxohyaline stroma.	Associated with t(1;3) translocation leading to *WWTR1-CAMTA1* fusion, which is detectable by FISH. <50% of patients with metastases die from the disease.

FISH, fluorescence in situ hybridization; PILA, papillary intralymphatic angioendothelioma.
[a]Illustrative examples provided.

GLOMUS TUMOR AND GLOMUVENOUS MALFORMATION

Glomus tumor synonym: solid glomus tumor
Glomuvenous malformation synonym: glomangioma

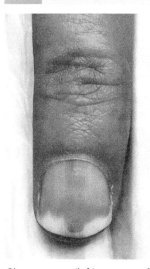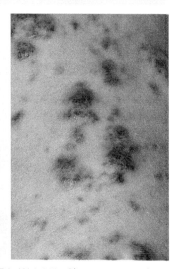

Glomus tumor (left) courtesy of Erin Wei, MD. Glomuvenous malformation (right) reprinted with permission from Gru AA, Wick MR, Mir A, et al. *Pediatric Dermatopathology and Dermatology*. Wolters Kluwer; 2018.

- **Glomus tumor** is a **perivascular neoplasm** derived from **glomus cells.** It occurs most often in **young adults.**
    - **Infantile myofibromatosis (infantile hemangiopericytoma)** is a **perivascular neoplasm** derived from **pericytes** (see Chapter 2: Neurocutaneous and Psychocutaneous Disorders).
    - **Glomuvenous malformation (GVM)** may be due to **AD** mutation of *glomulin.* It occurs most often in **infants and children.**
- Glomus tumor classically presents as a **solitary red-bluish subungual macule** visible through the nail plate **or a discrete blue-red papule on distal extremities.** It may be **painful to touch** and **sensitive to temperature or pressure** leading to paroxysmal pain. There is a small risk of malignant degeneration into malignant glomus tumor (glomangiosarcoma).
    - **GVM** classically presents as **multiple soft pink to deep blue papules with a cobblestone appearance.** It is generally **asymptomatic.**
    - Figure 5.39.
- Glomus tumor is treated with elective surgical excision.
    - Surgical excision is typically not beneficial for GVM. CO_2, KTP, Nd:YAG, or PDL laser treatment may be considered.

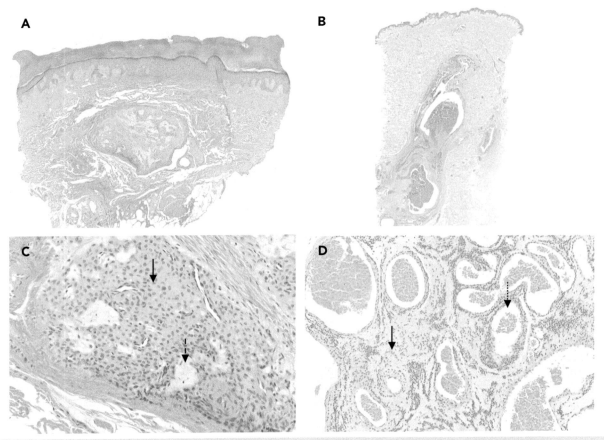

Figure 5.39. SIDE-BY-SIDE COMPARISON: GLOMUS TUMOR AND GLOMUVENOUS MALFORMATION. Both glomus tumor and GVM demonstrate rows of glomus cells, which have round dark nuclei and scant cytoplasm. Glomus cells are positive for collagen IV, SMA, and vimentin (negative for desmin). Glomus tumor contains small blood vessels. GVM contains prominent ectatic veins. Glomus tumor contains small blood vessels. GVM contains prominent ectatic veins. A and C, Glomus tumor. B and D, GVM. Solid arrows: row of glomus cells ("string of black pearls"). Dashed arrow: blood vessel. Dotted arrow: ectatic vein. GVM, glomuvenous malformation; SMA, smooth muscle actin.

(Histology images courtesy of Noel Turner, MD, MHS and Christine J. Ko, MD.)

A row of glomus cells may resemble a "string of black pearls."

- Glomangiomyoma: transition from glomus cells to elongated well-differentiated smooth muscle cells.
- Malignant glomus tumor: cytologic atypia, mitotic activity, and necrosis.

Neural Malformations and Neoplasms

Basic Concepts

- Neural malformations occur due to improper embryogenesis.
- Neural neoplasms are derived from various neural-derived cells.

APLASIA CUTIS CONGENITA
Synonyms: congenital absence of skin, cutis aplasia

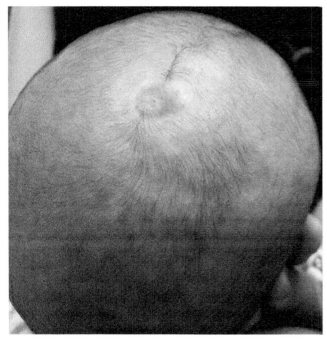

Reprinted with permission from Krakowski AC. *Procedural Pediatric Dermatology.* Wolters Kluwer; 2020.

- Aplasia cutis congenita (ACC) refers to congenital absence of skin. The pathogenesis is unknown. Midline ACC may be due to embryologic arrest or incomplete closure of the neural tube. **Neural tube defects** are summarized in Table 5.30. Nonmidline ACC may be due to a vascular abnormality of the placenta leading to tissue degeneration. Associations include **Adams-Oliver syndrome (ACC of the scalp, CMTC, cardiac abnormalities, transverse limb defects, CNS abnormalities)**, **Bart syndrome (coexistence of ACC and EB)**, and **Setleis syndrome (bilateral temporal ACC, leonine facies, upward-slanting eyebrows, abnormal eyelashes)**. Drug associations include **methimazole.**
- ACC can be solitary or multiple and have a variable presentation including an **(1) erosion or ulceration, (2) membranous lesion, or (3) atrophic scar**. The majority of ACC is on the **scalp**, particularly near the hair whorl. A ring of long dark course hair termed a **"hair collar"** may surround a patch of alopecia over **ectopic brain tissue** (congenital herniation through skull). Complications include hemorrhage, sagittal sinus thrombosis, and meningitis.
  - ACC demonstrates absent or thinned epidermis, dermis, and/or subcutis ± absent or rudimentary skin appendages.
- As opposed to wooly hair nevus, associated with *HRAS* mutation, a "hair collar" in ACC surrounds alopecia. In such cases, **MRI** is typically recommended to assess for intracranial pathology.
- Most ACC do not require treatment. Larger ACC (>4 cm) may require skin grafting.

Table 5.30. NEURAL TUBE DEFECTS

Diagnosis[a]	Classic Description	Notes
Cephalocele	Compressible, pulsatile bluish nodules that transilluminate.	Cephalocele is a general term for congenital herniations of intracranial tissue through a bony defect. Encephalocele (meninges and brain tissue) is more common than meningocele (meninges and CSF). Lesion may expand with increased ICP (i.e. crying, Valsalva, etc.)
Dermoid cyst/sinus	Noncompressible, nonpulsatile mass often near the lateral brow (and less likely nasal area).	MRI is recommended to assess for intracranial pathology. Presence of sinus ostium, tufts of hair, or sebaceous discharge increases risk of intracranial extension. Surgical excision should be performed by neurosurgery and/or otolaryngology.
Dimple	Small depression (>0.5 cm) above the gluteal cleft or >2.5 cm from anal verge in neonates.	
Hypertrichosis	V-shaped patch of long, silky hair ("faun tail") on the lumbosacral area.	Cutaneous marker of spinal dysraphism evident at birth.
Lipoma	Soft, subcutaneous mass located above the gluteal cleft and/or extending to one buttock, leading to a curved gluteal cleft.	Underlying defect may be intraspinal lipoma or lipomyelomeningocele.
Nasal glioma	Firm, noncompressible, sometimes blue-red nodule at the glabella or nasal root.	Represents ectopic neuroectoderm tissue. While the fibrous stalk may connect to the intracranial space, there is no extension with the leptomeninges or CSF.
Nasolacrimal duct cyst	Small, bluish round mass near the medial canthus.	Cystic dilatation of the nasolacrimal apparatus, which can lead to nasal obstruction.
Occult spinal dysraphism	Mass overlying the spine (neural tissue covered in skin).	Abnormal fusion of dorsal midline structures leading to spinal defects.
Tail	Vestigial remnant comprised of mature bone, subcutis, muscle, vessels, and nerves.	
Spina bifida	Tuft of hair, dimple, or subcutaneous mass the overlying spinal column.	

CSF, cerebrospinal fluid; ICP, intracranial pressure; MRI, magnetic resonance imaging.
[a]Illustrative examples provided.

NEUROFIBROMA

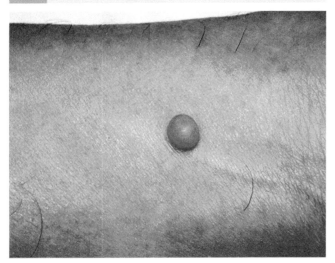

Reprinted with permission from Requena L, Kutzner H. *Cutaneous Soft Tissue Tumors.* Wolters Kluwer Health; 2014.

- Neurofibroma is a benign nerve sheath tumor comprised of neuromesenchymal tissue.
  - Multiple neurofibromas are associated with **NF-1 and NF-2.**
- Neurofibroma classically presents as a **solitary, soft, skin-colored, pedunculated papule ± hyperpigmentation or hypertrichosis.** The diffuse neurofibroma variant classically presents as an **ill-defined subcutaneous mass.** The **plexiform neurofibroma variant (pathognomonic for NF-1)** classically presents as a **boggy subcutaneous mass.** There is an ~10% risk of malignant degeneration of plexiform NF into **malignant peripheral nerve sheath tumor (MPNST; neurofibrosarcoma).**
  - Invagination of neurofibroma into itself is called the "buttonhole sign." The texture of plexiform neurofibroma is often described as a "bag of worms."
  - Figure 5.40.
- Solitary neurofibroma can be treated with simple surgical excision.

SCHWANNOMA

Synonyms: acoustic neuroma, neurilemmoma, neurolemmoma, Schwann cell tumor

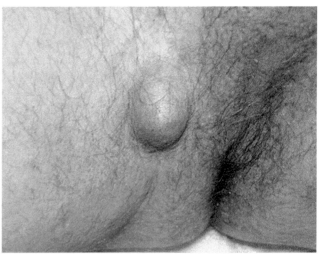

Reprinted with permission from Requena L, Kutzner H. *Cutaneous Soft Tissue Tumors.* Wolters Kluwer Health; 2014.

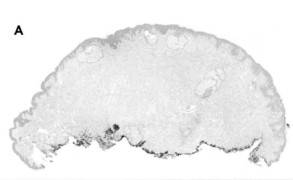

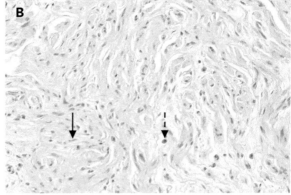

Figure 5.40. CLINICOPATHOLOGICAL CORRELATION: NEUROFIBROMA. Neurofibroma is characterized by a well-circumscribed but nonencapsulated proliferation of spindle cells loosely arranged in pale myxoid stroma. Mast cells are numerous. Positive IHC stains include neurofilament, S100, and SOX-10. A, Low-power view. B, High-power view. Solid arrow: spindle cell with "S-shaped" or "wavy" nucleus. Dashed arrow: mast cell. IHC, immunohistochemistry; MPNST, malignant peripheral nerve sheath tumor; NF, neurofibroma.

(Histology images courtesy of Noel Turner, MD, MHS and Christine J. Ko, MD.)

Spindle cells in neurofibroma have "S-shaped" or "wavy" nuclei.

- **Diffuse neurofibroma:** diffuse replacement of the dermis ± infiltration into the subcutis.
- **Plexiform neurofibroma:** large fascicles of neurofibroma surrounded by perineurium, often coursing through a diffuse neurofibroma.
- **MPNST:** resembles plexiform neurofibroma with hypercellularity ± cytologic atypia and mitotic activity.

- Schwannoma is a benign Schwann cell tumor. Schwann cells are glial cells that form the myelin sheaths of the peripheral nervous system (PNS). Schwannoma may occur after mechanical injury.

  Schwannoma is associated with **NF-2.** Psammomatous melanotic schwannoma is associated with the **Carney complex.**

- Schwannoma presents as a **solitary papule or nodule along a nerve on the flexural aspect of the extremity.** Schwannomas arise within nerves and push axons to the periphery, resulting in **pain.**
  - Figure 5.41.
- No treatment is necessary for asymptomatic schwannoma. Surgical excision is otherwise curative.

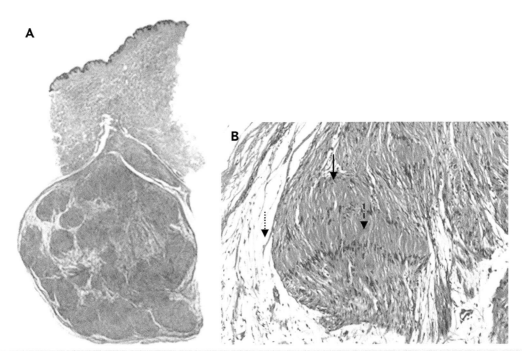

Figure 5.41. CLINICOPATHOLOGICAL CORRELATION: SCHWANNOMA. Schwannoma is characterized by a well-circumscribed encapsulated spindle cell proliferation arising within a nerve in the deep dermis or subcutis. The tumor is biphasic. Antoni A tissue is hypercellular with parallel rows of nuclei separated by acellular areas (Verocay bodies). Antoni B tissue is hypocellular with edematous stroma. S100 is positive; neurofilament is negative. EMA stains the perineural capsule. A, Low-power view. B, High-power view. Solid arrow: Antoni A tissue. Dashed arrow: Verocay body. Dotted arrow: Antoni B tissue. EMA, epithelial membrane antigen.

(Histology images reprinted with permission from Requena L, Kutzner H. *Cutaneous Soft Tissue Tumors.* Wolters Kluwer Health; 2014.)

Parallel rows of nuclei separated by acellular areas (Verocay bodies) give Antoni A tissue the appearance of zebra stripes. Antoni B tissue represents a degenerative change and is often located just below the capsule.

- Ancient schwannoma: spindle cells with large hyperchromatic nuclei.
- Psammomatous melanotic schwannoma: psammoma bodies (concentric calcifications) and melanin.

SPOTLIGHT ON NEUROFIBROMATOSIS
→ Diagnosis Group 2

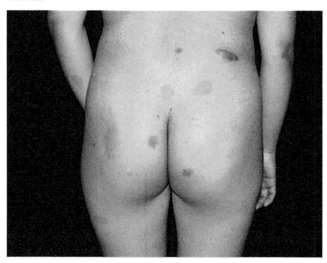

Café-au-lait macules and neurofibromas in neurofibromatosis type 1 reprinted with permission from Requena L, Kutzner H. *Cutaneous Soft Tissue Tumors*. Wolters Kluwer Health; 2014.

Epidemiology

- NF is a group of hereditary neurocutaneous disorders manifesting with dermatologic, CNS, ocular, and other organ system abnormalities. The two main types are:
  - **NF-1 (von Recklinghausen disease): AD or sporadic** mutation in *NF-1*, which encodes **neurofibromin**, a tumor suppressor protein regulating the MAPK signaling pathway. NF-1 has incomplete penetrance and variable expressivity. In patients with **NF-1 and JXG**, there is a **triple association with a 20-fold increased risk of JMML** (controversial).

- **NF-2: AD** mutation in *NF-2*, which encodes **merlin** (also called neurofibromin 2 or schwannomin), a tumor suppressor protein regulating multiple signaling pathways including MAPK and p21-activated kinase signaling.

Clinicopathological Features

- Clinical features of **NF-1** are summarized in the **diagnostic criteria** (Table 5.31). Nevus anemicus was recently associated with NF1 and added as a diagnostic criterion.
- NF-2 also presents with **CALMs (rarer than NF-1), neurofibromas, and schwannomas.** The pathognomonic finding is **bilateral vestibular schwannomas. Juvenile posterior subcapsular lenticular opacity** is an ocular finding found in ~80% of patients.
  - ◆ The histopathology of neurofibroma demonstrates CALMs, neurofibromas, and schwannomas.

Evaluation

- The differential diagnosis of NF includes **hereditary disorders associated with CALMs** (Table 5.32).
- Evaluation in patients with suspected NF-1 should include **genetic testing, ophthalmologic examination yearly until 20 years of age, orbital and brain MRI to visualize undetermined bright objects in basal ganglia, brainstem, and cerebellum on T2-weighted imaging,** and neurology referral.

Management

- Management of NF1 requires a multidisciplinary team that includes dermatology, cardiology, orthopedic surgery, neurology, and ophthalmology. Yearly TBSE is recommended to detect MPNSTs.

Table 5.31. DIAGNOSTIC CRITERIA FOR NEUROFIBROMATOSIS TYPE 1

Neurofibromatosis Type 1

Diagnosis of NF-1 requires ≥ 2 of the following:

Diagnostic Criteria	*Onset of Findings*
• ≥6 CALMs >5 mm in prepubescent individuals and >15 mm in postpubescent individuals	Earliest sign presenting within 2 years of life (prior to development of neurofibromas).
• ≥2 neurofibromas of any type or 1 plexiform neurofibroma	Usually appear in children older than 7 years of age. Diffuse plexiform neurofibroma occurs in early childhood whereas deep, nodular plexiform neurofibroma occurs in adolescence.
• Axillary or inguinal freckling	Appears by 4-6 years of age.
• Optic nerve glioma	Occurs in 15% of children; occurs by school-age.
• ≥2 iris Lisch nodules	Develop as early as age 3; 90% of patients develop by 20 years of age.
• Distinctive osseous lesion (sphenoid wing dysplasia, long bone cortical thinning ± pseudoarthrosis)	Usually present at birth (earliest sign).
• First-degree relative with NF-1	

Other findings include:
- Lipomas, MPNST, cutaneous meningioma, hypertension, pheochromocytoma (~1%)

CALMs, café-au-lait macules; MPNST, malignant peripheral nerve sheath tumor; NF-1, neurofibromatosis type 1.

Table 5.32. HEREDITARY DISORDRS ASSOCIATED WITH CAFÉ-AU-LAIT MACULES

Diagnosis[a]	Inheritance Pattern	Gene(s)	Classic Description
A-T	See Chapter 4: Photodermatoses.		
Bloom syndrome	See Chapter 4: Photodermatoses.		
Cardio-facio-cutaneous syndrome	AD	*BRAF > MEK1, MEK2, KRAS*	CALMs, melanocytic nevi, and xerosis to ichthyosiform eruption. The characteristic hair shaft abnormality without increased fragility is woolly hair. Systemic features include short stature, low-set ears, and coarse facies.
Fanconi anemia	See Chapter 4: Photodermatoses.		
Legius syndrome	AD	*SPRED1*	CALMs and axillary freckling (NO neurofibromas). Systemic features include macrocephaly, intellectual disability, Lish nodule, optic gliomas.
McCune-Albright syndrome	Sporadic, postzygotic	*GNAS*	Large CALM with geographic borders that end at the midline (CALMs can overly bony changes). Systemic features include precocious puberty, hyperthyroidism, hypophosphatemic rickets, Cushing syndrome, and polyostotic fibrous dysplasia.
Do NOT confuse McCune-Albright syndrome with Albright hereditary osteodystrophy.			CALMs in McCune-Albright syndrome resemble the "Coast of Maine."
MEN 1/MEN 2B	See Chapter 5: Fibrous Neoplasms.		
NF-1/NF-2	See above.		
Russell-Silver syndrome	Sporadic	Epigenetic changes or uniparental disomy of chromosomes 7 and 11	CALMs. Systemic features include prominent forehead, triangular face, growth hemihypertrophy, clinodactyly of the fifth digit.

AD, autosomal dominant; A-T, ataxia-telangiectasia; CALMs, café au lait macules; MEN, multiple endocrine neoplasia; NF, neurofibromatosis.
[a]Illustrative examples provided.

- For symptomatic cutaneous neurofibromas, surgical excision is the recommended treatment.
- The first FDA-approved, targeted medical treatment for patients with inoperable plexiform neurofibroma is **selumetinib.** Other potential targeted therapies include **imatinib and sirolimus.**

"Real World" Advice

- Solitary CALMs and neurofibromas are common. Reassurance should be provided to parents unless the above criteria are met.

NEUROMA

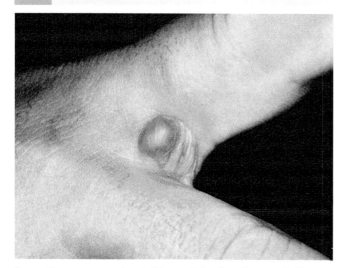

Traumatic neuroma reprinted with permission from Requena L, Kutzner H. *Cutaneous Soft Tissue Tumors.* Wolters Kluwer Health; 2014.

- Neuroma is a benign nerve sheath tumor comprised of **axons and Schwann cells in an ~1:1 ratio.** The two main types are **traumatic neuroma and palisaded encapsulated neuroma (PEN).** Traumatic neuroma is likely caused by abnormal nerve regeneration in the setting of inflammation and fibrosis. PEN has no clear etiology; however, "encapsulated" refers to the proliferation of nerve fibers of the perineurium.
     Multiple mucosal neuromas are associated with **MEN2B and Cowden syndrome.**
- Neuroma presents as a **solitary papule or nodule. Traumatic neuroma** favors the **extremities** (at a site of prior mechanical injury), while **PEN** favors the **lower central face**, especially at **mucocutaneous junctions. Pain** is characteristic of **traumatic neuroma**, but not PEN.
     ◆ Figure 5.42.
- For symptomatic neuroma, surgical excision is curative.

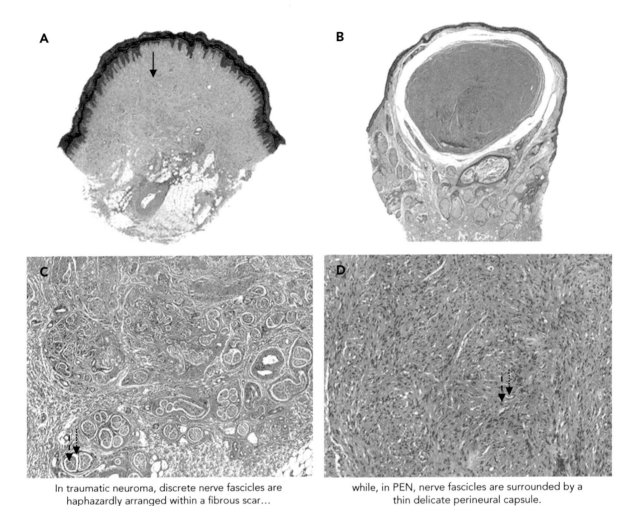

In traumatic neuroma, discrete nerve fascicles are haphazardly arranged within a fibrous scar…

while, in PEN, nerve fascicles are surrounded by a thin delicate perineural capsule.

Figure 5.42. SIDE-BY-SIDE COMPARISON: TRAUMATIC NEUROMA AND PALISADED ENCAPSULATED NEUROMA. Both traumatic neuroma and PEN are characterized by nerve fascicles separated by clefts. In traumatic neuroma, discrete nerve fascicles are haphazardly arranged within a fibrous scar. In PEN, nerve fascicles are surrounded by a thin delicate perineural capsule. A and C, Traumatic neuroma. B and D, PEN. PEN, palisaded encapsulated neuroma.

(Histology images reprinted with permission from Requena L, Kutzner H. *Cutaneous Soft Tissue Tumors*. Wolters Kluwer Health; 2014.)

GRANULAR CELL TUMOR

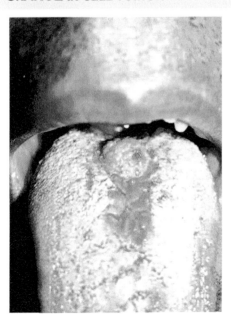

- Granular cell tumor (GCT) represents a rare group of heterogenous tumors **derived from neural tissues.** GCT is most common in females of African descent.
    GCT is associated with **Noonan syndrome.**
- GCT classically presents as a **solitary red-brown papule** favoring the head and neck (up to 40% on the **tongue**). There is a low risk of malignant degeneration (<2%), higher for deep or visceral GCTs.
    ◆ Figure 5.43.
- Surgical excision is the treatment of choice for benign GCT, though recurrence is possible.

Reprinted with permission from Requena L, Kutzner H. *Cutaneous Soft Tissue Tumors*. Wolters Kluwer Health; 2014.

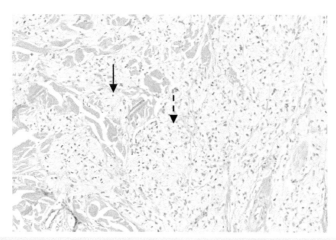

Figure 5.43. CLINICOPATHOLOGICAL CORRELATION: GRANULAR CELL TUMOR. GCT is characterized by large polygonal cells with granular eosinophilic cytoplasm (PAS positive, diastase resistant) and central nuclei. Pustulo-ovoid bodies of Milian are large eosinophilic lysosomal granules surrounded by a clear halo. PEH may occur. Positive IHC stains include CD68 and S100. Solid arrow: large polygonal cell with granular eosinophilic cytoplasm and central nucleus. Dashed arrow: pustulo-ovoid body of Milian. CD, cluster of differentiation; GCT, granular cell tumor; IHC, immunohistochemistry; PAS, periodic acid-Schiff; PEH, pseudoepitheliomatous hyperplasia.

(Histology image courtesy of Noel Turner, MD, MHS and Christine J. Ko, MD.)

- **Malignant GST**: large GST with variable cytologic atypia, mitotic activity, and necrosis.

MERKEL CELL CARCINOMA

Synonyms: primary neuroendocrine carcinoma of the skin, primary small cell carcinoma of the skin, trabecular carcinoma of the skin

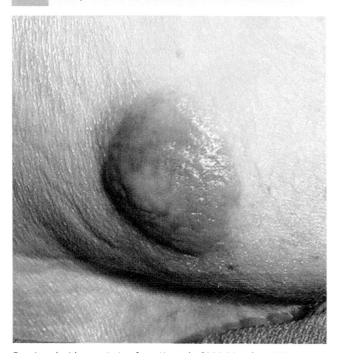

Reprinted with permission from Kransdorf MJ, Murphey MD. *Imaging of Soft Tissue Tumors*. 3rd ed. Wolters Kluwer Health/Lippincott Williams & Wilkins; 2013.

- MCC is a rare and aggressive **neuroendocrine carcinoma of the skin.** The etiology is thought to be multifactorial with **UVR exposure** as one of the major risk factors. Additional risk factors include **age > 50 years, fair skin, and immunosuppression. Merkel cell polyomavirus (MCPyV)** is detected in 80% of tumor tissue samples, suggesting a viral role in the pathogenesis of MCC. **L-MYC gene amplification** has also been implicated. Drug associations include **rituximab.**
- MCC classically presents as an **asymptomatic, solitary, rapidly growing violaceous papulonodule favoring the head and neck.**
    - Figure 5.44.
    - Histopathological features of other neural neoplasms not discussed elsewhere are summarized in Table 5.33.
- **SLNB** is recommended for all patients with MCC.
- MCC has an all-stage mortality of 37% (compared to 8% for melanoma); prognosis is dependent on staging at the time of diagnosis. Detection of anti-MCV antibodies is a positive prognostic factor. Immunosuppression and p63 positivity are negative prognostic factors. Treatment of MCC is challenging. The gold standard is **WLE with 1 to 2 cm margins or MMS.** Those with positive SLNB are often treated with complete lymph node dissection and adjuvant chemotherapy/radiation therapy. MCC responds to ICIs independent of PD-1, PD-L1, or MCV status. **Pembrolizumab and avelumab** are FDA-approved.

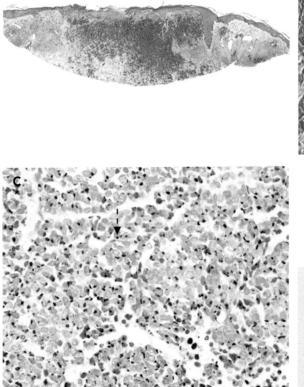

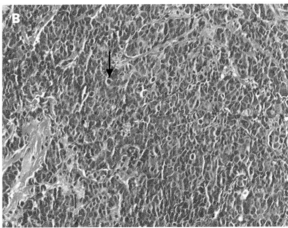

Small blue cell tumors are <u>LEMONS</u>:
- <u>L</u>ymphoma
- <u>E</u>wing sarcoma
- <u>M</u>CC / <u>M</u>elanoma
- <u>O</u>at cell carcinoma (SCLC)
- <u>N</u>euroblastoma
- <u>S</u>mall cell endocrine neoplasia

Figure 5.44. CLINICOPATHOLOGICAL CORRELATION: MERKEL CELL CARCINOMA. MCC is characterized by small blue cells with scant cytoplasm and round nuclei with speckled chromatin. The three primary patterns are trabecular (pseudorosettes), intermediate, or small cell. Cytologic atypia, mitotic activity, and necrosis are frequently observed. CK20 is positive in a perinuclear dot pattern. Other positive IHC stains in MCC include CD56, neuroendocrine markers (eg, bombesin, chromograinin, synaptophysin), neurofilament, neuron-specific enolase, and p63. CK7 and TTF-1 are negative. Electron microscopy demonstrates membrane-bound dense core granules. A, Low-power view. B, High-power view. Solid arrow: small blue cell with scant cytoplasm and round nucleus with speckled chromatin. C, CK20. Dashed arrow: perinuclear dot pattern. CD, cluster of differentiation; CK, cytokeratin; IHC, immunohistochemistry; MCC, Merkel cell carcinoma; SCLC, small cell lung cancer; TTF-1, thyroid transcription factor 1.

(A, Histology image reprinted with permission from Elder DE, Elenitsas R, Rubin AI, et al. *Atlas of Dermatopathology: Synopsis and Atlas of Lever's Histopathology of the Skin.* 4th ed. Wolters Kluwer; 2020. B, Histology image reprinted with permission from Elder DE, Elenitsas R, Rubin AI, et al. *Atlas of Dermatopathology: Synopsis and Atlas of Lever's Histopathology of the Skin.* 4th ed. Wolters Kluwer; 2020. C. Histology image reprinted with permission from Edward S, Yung A. *Essential Dermatopathology.* Wolters Kluwer Health/Lippincott Williams & Wilkins; 2011. Illustration by Caroline A. Nelson, MD.)

IHC is helpful to differentiate MCC from oat cell carcinoma (CK7 and TTF-1 positive, CK20 negative). Neuron-specific enolase is the most consistent MCC stain but is nonspecific ("nonspecific enolase").

Table 5.33. HISTOPATHOLOGICAL FEATURES OF OTHER NEURAL NEOPLASMS

Diagnosis[a]	Histopathological Features	Notes
Benign		
Ganglioneuroma	Large cells with amphophilic cytoplasm, large nuclei, and prominent nucleoli (ganglion cells) admixed in a background of neurofibroma-like tissue.	Asymptomatic skin-colored papules often on the trunk.
Neurothekeoma	Myxoid: S100 positive. Cellular: NKIC3, PGP9.5, and S100A6 (but not S100) positive.	Myxoid: Hands and fingers of middle-aged adults. Cellular: Face of young adult women.
Perineurioma	Well-circumscribed dermal tumor with spindle cells with elongate, bipolar cytoplasmic processes arranged in fascicles or whirls.	Variants include intraneural, soft tissue, sclerosing, and cutaneous. The sclerosing variant has prominent hyalinized stroma and is most often seen on the hands of young men. Others are solitary, nondescript, skin-colored soft tissue masses on the trunk or extremities.

Table 5.33. HISTOPATHOLOGICAL FEATURES OF OTHER NEURAL NEOPLASMS (CONTINUED)

Diagnosis[a]	Histopathological Features	Notes
Malignant		
Neuroblastoma	Small round blue cell tumor with salt and pepper chromatin. Cells can be elongated, have little cytoplasm, and form rosettes.	75% of patients present with metastases at diagnosis, most commonly to the adrenal gland and retroperitoneum. Skin biopsy and urinary catecholamines are important for diagnosis.

[a]Illustrative examples provided.

Neoplasms of Sebaceous, Apocrine, and Eccrine Glands

Basic Concepts

- Adnexal neoplasms can have **sebaceous, apocrine, eccrine, or follicular** differentiation.
- Looking for specific signs of differentiation on histopathology (eg, decapitation secretion in neoplasms of apocrine differentiation) can help narrow down the differential diagnosis.

Adnexal Neoplasms and Proliferations With Sebaceous Differentiation

NEVUS SEBACEOUS
→ **Diagnosis Group 2**
Synonym: organoid nevus, nevus sebaceous of Jadassohn

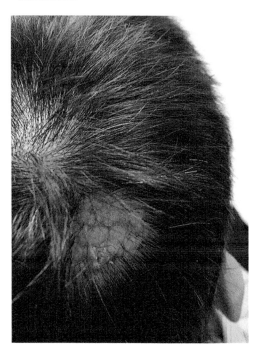

Epidemiology

- Nevus sebaceous is a nonneoplastic malformation that includes sebaceous, apocrine, and follicular elements along with epidermal hyperplasia. It arises due to postzygotic mutation in **HRAS** (95%) and *KRAS* (5%). These mutations primarily lead to activation of the MAPK signaling pathway.

Clinicopathological Features

- Nevus sebaceous classically presents **at birth** with a **yellow-to-brown verrucous papule or plaque following lines of Blaschko** that favors the **scalp (most common)**, face, and eyelid. The lesion often becomes more verrucous during puberty in response to hormone signaling.
- Secondary neoplasms that can develop in a nevus sebaceous include **trichoblastoma (most common)**, poroma, **syringocystadenoma papilliferum (SPAP)**, desmoplastic trichollemmoma, tubular apocrine adenoma, and BCC (<1%).
  - Figure 5.45.

Evaluation

- The differential diagnosis of nevus sebaceous includes epidermal nevus, BCC, and SGH.
- If a patient has extensive involvement with nevus sebaceous, consider associations with **phakomatosis pigmentokeratotica** and **Schimmelpenning syndrome** (nevus sebaceous in conjunction with cardiovascular, skeletal, neurologic, and genitourinary anomalies).

Management

- Historically, nevus sebaceous was excised due to concern for secondary malignant neoplasms. However, while benign secondary tumors are common, secondary malignancies are rare. Therefore, clinical monitoring is now the favored approach.

"Real World" Advice

- Removal by shave biopsy or laser ablation is usually not successful as these techniques often do not remove the malformed deeper sebaceous and apocrine glands, leading to high rates of recurrence.

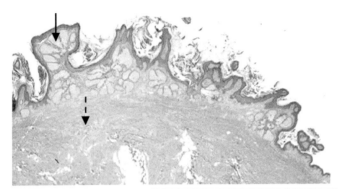

Figure 5.45. CLINICOPATHOLOGICAL CORRELATION: NEVUS SEBACEOUS. Nevus sebaceous is characterized by hyperkeratosis, acanthosis, papillomatosis, fibroplasia of the papillary dermis, enlarged sebaceous lobules contiguous with the DEJ, dilated apocrine glands in the reticular dermis, and absence of normal terminal hairs. Solid arrow: enlarged sebaceous lobules. Dashed arrow: dilated apocrine glands. DEJ, dermo-epidermal junction.

(Histology image reprinted with permission from Gru AA, Wick MR, Mir A, et al. *Pediatric Dermatopathology and Dermatology.* Wolters Kluwer; 2018.)

• **Prepubertal nevus sebaceous:** immature abnormal pilosebaceous units.

Nevus sebaceous is often described as "broad," "bald" (absence of normal terminal hairs), "bumpy" (acanthosis, papillomatosis), and "bubbly" (enlarged sebaceous lobules). A prepubertal nevus sebaceous is "broad" and "bald" but not "bumpy" or "bubbly."

SEBACEOUS GLAND HYPERPLASIA
→ **Diagnosis Group 1**

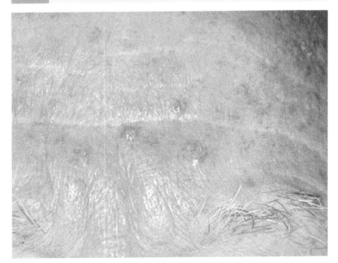

Reprinted with permission from Craft N, Fox LP, Goldsmith LA, et al. *VisualDx: Essential Adult Dermatology.* Wolters Kluwer Health/ Lippincott Williams & Wilkins; 2010.

Epidemiology

- SGH is a benign overgrowth of normal sebaceous glands.
- The prevalence of SGH increases with **age.**
- Eruptive SGH is associated with immunosuppression.
- Drug associations include **corticosteroids** and **cyclosporine.**

Clinicopathological Features

- SGH classically presents with **white-yellow papules with a central dell on the face.** SGH can sometimes also present in a linear configuration on the neck and clavicle.
  - ◆ Figure 5.46.

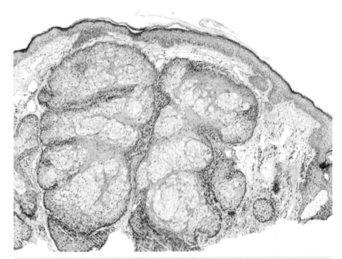

Figure 5.46. CLINICOPATHOLOGICAL CORRELATION: SEBACEOUS GLAND HYPERPLASIA. SGH is characterized by hyperplasia of a single sebaceous gland that is often multilobulated. SGH, sebaceous gland hyperplasia.

(Histology image reprinted with permission from Elder DE, Elenitsas R, Rosenbach M, et al. *Lever's Histopathology of the Skin.* 11th ed. Wolters Kluwer; 2015.)

Evaluation

- The differential diagnosis of SGH includes BCC, nevus sebaceous, and other benign adnexal tumors.
- **Dermoscopy** reveals **white-yellow lobular structures, crown vessels, and central dell.**
  - White-yellow lobular structures are called "popcorn structures."

Management

- Treatment of SGH is solely for cosmetic purposes. If treatment is desired, cryotherapy, laser ablation, and shave removal can be helpful. Long-term topical retinoid application and short courses of isotretinoin have demonstrated mild success in patients with extensive disease.

"Real World" Advice

- Given the presence of arborizing vessels and a shiny appearance, SGH often clinically mimics BCC. Dermoscopy can be helpful in identifying a "crown" vascular pattern in SGH, and thus avoiding an unnecessary biopsy.

SEBACEOUS ADENOMA AND SEBACEOMA
Sebaceoma synonym: sebaceous epithelioma (historical)

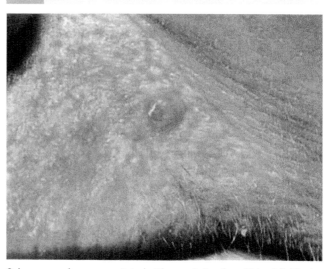

Sebaceous adenoma reprinted with permission from Elder DE, Elenitsas R, Rubin AI, et al. *Atlas of Dermatopathology: Synopsis and Atlas of Lever's Histopathology of the Skin.* 4th ed. Wolters Kluwer; 2020.

- Sebaceous adenoma and sebaceoma are benign sebaceous gland neoplasms. Prevalence increases with **age.**
  - Sebaceous adenomas and sebaceomas are associated with **MTS.**
- Both sebaceous adenoma and sebaceoma classically present as **pink-to-yellow papulonodules on the face.** There is a small risk of malignant transformation to sebaceous carcinoma.
  - Figure 5.47.

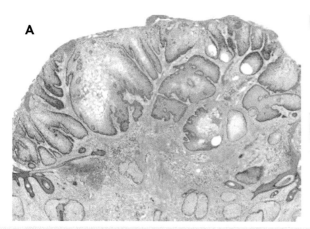

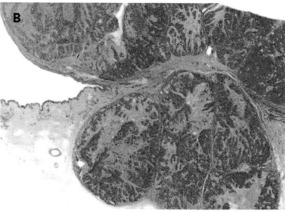

Figure 5.47. SIDE-BY-SIDE COMPARISON: SEBACEOUS ADENOMA AND SEBACEOMA. Both sebaceous adenoma and sebaceoma are composed of basophilic seboblasts and mature sebocytes. Sebaceous adenoma has < 50% seboblasts and typically opens to the surface. Sebaceoma has > 50% seboblasts and is typically located in the deep reticular dermis or superficial subcutis. Stains for sebaceous differentiation include EMA (mature sebocytes), adipophilin (multivacuolated lipid-containing cells), and androgen receptors. Loss of expression of DNA mismatch repair proteins (MLH1, MSH2, MSH6, PMS2) is a screening tool for MTS, but should be confirmed with genetic testing. A, Sebaceous adenoma. B, Sebaceoma. DNA, deoxyribonucleic acid; EMA, epithelial membrane antigen; MTS, Muir-Torre syndrome.

(Histology images reprinted with permission from Edward S, Yung A. *Essential Dermatopathology.* Wolters Kluwer Health/Lippincott Williams & Wilkins; 2011.)

- Treatment is not necessary as sebaceous adenoma and sebaceoma are benign. However, excisional biopsy or surgical excision is curative.

SEBACEOUS CARCINOMA

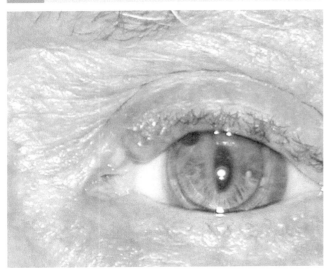

Reprinted with permission from Penne RB. *Oculoplastics*. 3rd ed. Wolters Kluwer; 2018.

- Sebaceous carcinoma is a sebaceous gland malignancy with **significant metastatic potential.**
    Sebaceous carcinomas are associated with **MTS.**
- Sebaceous carcinoma classically presents with a **red, painless, subcutaneous nodule.** Seventy-five percent occur on the **periocular skin.**
    - Figure 5.48.
- Given the periocular location, sebaceous carcinoma is often **confused for a chalazion or blepharitis.** Skin biopsy is important for diagnostic confirmation. Lesions occurring on the trunk tend to be more nodular and thus a superficial shave biopsy can miss the diagnosis.

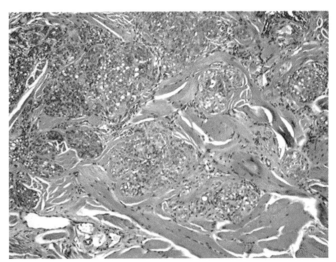

Figure 5.48. CLINICOPATHOLOGICAL CORRELATION: SEBACEOUS CARCINOMA. Sebaceous carcinoma is characterized by a nodular or infiltrative growth pattern of cells with variable sebaceous differentiation (typically >50% seboblasts), cytologic atypia, mitotic activity, and necrosis. Cells often extend deep into the dermis and subcutis ± pagetoid spread in the epidermis and conjunctiva. Androgen receptor staining may be preferred over EMA and adipophilin, particularly in poorly differentiated and pagetoid sebaceous carcinoma. Loss of expression of DNA mismatch repair proteins (MLH1, MSH2, MSH6, PMS2) is a screening tool for MTS, but should be confirmed with genetic testing. DNA, deoxyribonucleic acid; EMA, epithelial membrane antigen; MTS, Muir-Torre syndrome.

(Histology image reprinted with permission from Crowson N, Magro CM, Mihm MC Jr. *Biopsy Interpretation of the Skin: Primary Non-Lymphoid Cutaneous Neoplasia.* Wolters Kluwer Health/Lippincott Williams & Wilkins; 2010.)

- The 5-year survival rate of sebaceous carcinoma is 80%. Treatment is surgical with MMS having the best outcomes (11% recurrence rate vs 30% with standard surgical excision).

SPOTLIGHT ON MUIR-TORRE SYNDROME

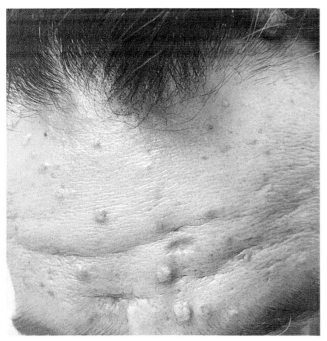

Multiple sebaceous adenomas in Muir-Torre syndrome courtesy of Michael Gowen, MD

- MTS is an **AD** disorder due to mutations in genes encoding **DNA mismatch repair proteins** *MLH1*, *MSH2* (90%), *MSH6*, and *PMS2* leading to **microsatellite instability.** MTS is a subtype of **Lynch syndrome (hereditary nonpolyposis colorectal cancer [HNPCC] syndrome).**
- MTS is associated with **sebaceous adenomas, sebaceomas, and sebaceous carcinomas,** along with **BCCs with sebaceous differentiation and KAs.** The most common internal malignancies are **colon adenocarcinomas** (47%) and **endometrial/ovarian/urinary tract carcinomas** (22%). The **Turcot variant** is associated with **brain neoplasms.**
    - The histopathology of MTS demonstrates cutaneous sebaceous adenomas, sebaceomas, sebaceous carcinomas, BCCs with sebaceous differentiation, and KAs.
- There is a higher likelihood of MTS in patients with ≥2 **sebaceous neoplasms (especially if located outside of the head and neck region),** age < 60 years, personal or family history of colon adenocarcinoma (or other Lynch syndrome-related malignancies), and loss of mismatch repair proteins on IHC staining of sebaceous neoplasm biopsies. The diagnosis should be confirmed with **genetic testing.**
- In addition to age-appropriate malignancy screening, patients need **yearly colonoscopy** starting at 20 to 25 years of age, **yearly pelvic examination/transvaginal US** starting at 30 to 35 years of age, **yearly UA** starting at age 25 to 30 years of age, and esophagogastroduodenoscopy every 2 to 3 years starting at age 30 to 35 years of age.

Adnexal Neoplasms and Proliferations With Primarily Apocrine Differentiation

CYLINDROMA AND SPIRADENOMA

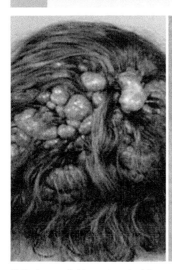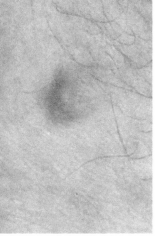

Cylindroma (left) reprinted with permission from Kransdorf MJ, Murphey MD. *Imaging of Soft Tissue Tumors.* 3rd ed. Wolters Kluwer Health/Lippincott Williams & Wilkins; 2013. Spiradenoma (right) reprinted with permission from Elder DE, Elenitsas R, Rubin AI, et al. *Atlas of Dermatopathology: Synopsis and Atlas of Lever's Histopathology of the Skin.* 4th ed. Wolters Kluwer; 2020.

- Cylindroma and spiradenoma are closely related benign sweat gland neoplasms of **apocrine differentiation.**
    - **Cylindromas and spiradenomas,** along with **trichoepitheliomas,** are associated with **Brooke-Spiegler syndrome.** This syndrome is due to **AD mutation in** *CYLD* **leading to increased NFκB signaling** and thus resistance to apoptosis.
- Cylindromas classically present as **solitary or multiple nodules** on the head and neck. The **scalp** is the most common site. Spiradenomas classically present as a **solitary, painful bluish nodule,** most commonly found on the **scalp or upper body.** Spiradenomas have never been observed on acral skin, supporting that they are of apocrine origin. There is a small risk of malignant transformation to cylindrocarcinoma and spiradenocarcinoma, respectively.
    - Figure 5.49.
- Complete surgical excision is curative.

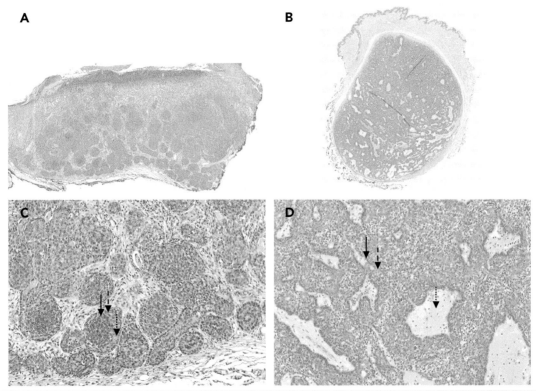

Figure 5.49. SIDE-BY-SIDE COMPARISON: CYLINDROMA AND SPIRADENOMA. Both cylindroma and spiradenoma consist of islands of blue cells with scant cytoplasm and biphasic (dark-pale) nuclei. Hyaline droplets are derived from the basement membrane (PAS positive, diastase resistant). Cylindroma islands have a hyaine sheath. Spiradenoma islands contain lymphocytes. A and C, Cylindroma. B and D, Spiradenoma. Solid arrows: blue cells with dark nuclei (undifferentiated). Dashed arrows: blue cells with pale nuclei (differentiated toward ductal or secretory cells). Dotted arrows: hyaline droplets. PAS, periodic acid-Schiff.

(Histology images courtesy of Noel Turner, MD, MHS and Christine J. Ko, MD.)

- Cylindrocarcinorma: loss of biphasic nature, cytologic atypia, mitotic activity, and necrosis.
- Spiradenocarcinoma: loss of biphasic nature, cytologic atypia, mitotic activity, and necrosis.

Cylindroma islands form a "jigsaw puzzle."
Spiradenoma islands form "blue balls."

SYRINGOCYSTADENOMA PAPILLIFERUM AND HIDRADENOMA PAPILLIFERUM

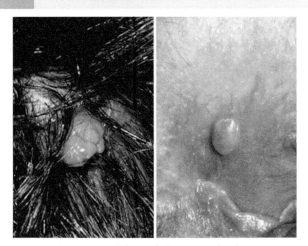

Syringocystadenoma papilliferum (left) reprinted with permission from Craft N, Fox LP, Goldsmith LA, et al. *VisualDx: Essential Adult Dermatology.* Wolters Kluwer Health/Lippincott Williams & Wilkins;

2010. Hidradenoma papilliferum (right) reprinted with permission from Edwards L, Lynch P. Genital *Dermatology Atlas and Manual.* 3rd ed. Wolters Kluwer; 2017.

- SPAP and hidradenoma papilliferum (HPAP) are closely related benign sweat gland neoplasms of **apocrine differentiation. SPAP associated with nevus sebaceous** is often due to mutations in *HRAS.* Sporadic SPAP can also harbor *BRAF* (V600E) mutations. **SPAP** typically occurs **at birth or in early childhood**, while **HPAP** typically occurs in **young adult women.**
- **SPAP** classically presents as a **warty papule or plaque** on the **head and neck**, often within a nevus sebaceous. The surface may be crusted with serosanguinous drainage. **HPAP** classically presents as a **smooth nodule** on the **vulva.** Unlike SPAP, HPAP has little to no epidermal changes.
  - ⬧ Figure 5.50.
- Complete surgical excision is curative as SPAP and HPAP are benign neoplasms.

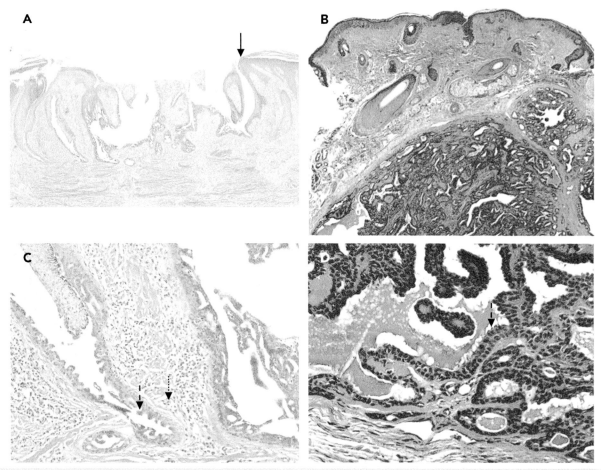

**Figure 5.50. SIDE-BY-SIDE COMPARISON: SYRINGOCYSTADENOMA PAPILLIFERUM AND HIDRADENOMA PAPIL-
LIFERUM.** Both SPAP and HPAP consist of papillary projections of blue cells that demonstrate decapitation secretion. SPAP
connects to the epidermis, and the dermal cores of papillae contain plasma cells. HPAP is a well circumscribed dermal
nodule without an epidermal connection or plasma cells. A and C, SPAP. B and D, HPAP. Solid arrow: epidermal connection. Dashed arrows: papillary projections of blue cells that demonstrate decapitation secretion. Dotted arrow: plasma cell.
HPAP, hidradenoma papilliferum; SPAP, syringocystadenoma papilliferum.

(A, Histology images courtesy of Noel Turner, MD, MHS and Christine J. Ko, MD. B, Histology images reprinted with permission from Elder
DE, Elenitsas R, Rosenbach M, et al. *Lever's Histopathology of the Skin.* 11th ed. Wolters Kluwer; 2015.)

You can slide from the skin surface into an SPAP.
You can hide in the "maze" of HPAP in the dermis.

HIDRADENOMA

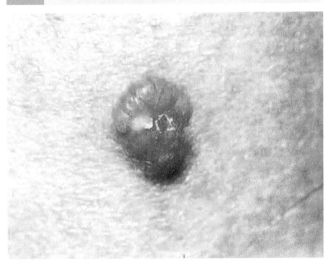

Reprinted with permission from Elder DE, Elenitsas R, Rubin AI, et al. *Atlas of Dermatopathology: Synopsis and Atlas of Lever's Histopathology of the Skin*. 4th ed. Wolters Kluwer; 2020.

- Hidradenoma is a benign sweat gland neoplasm. While primarily of **apocrine differentiation**, hidradenoma can have eccrine differentiation. Some authorities use the broader designation "**acrospiroma**" to refer to hidradenoma, poroma, hidroacanthoma simplex, and dermal duct tumor. t(11;19) translocation is associated with hidradenoma resulting in *CRTC1/MAML2* fusion.
- Hidradenoma lacks distinctive clinical features, but classically presents as a **solitary, red-to-violaceous nodule** on the **head and neck**. There is a small risk of malignant degeneration to hidradenocarcinoma, which is an aggressive tumor.
  - ◆ Figure 5.51.
- Complete surgical excision is curative.

Adnexal Neoplasms and Proliferations With Primarily Eccrine Differentiation

POROMA

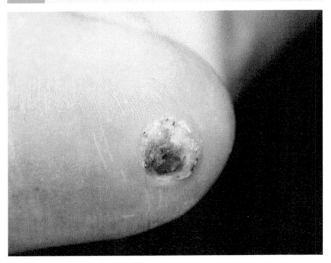

Reprinted with permission Elder DE, Elenitsas R, Rubin AI, et al. *Atlas of Dermatopathology: Synopsis and Atlas of Lever's Histopathology of the Skin*. 4th ed. Wolters Kluwer; 2020.

- Poroma is the **most common benign sweat gland neoplasm.** While primarily of **eccrine differentiation**, poroma can have apocrine differentiation (eg, when arising in a nevus sebaceous). As mentioned above, poroma is sometimes more broadly referred to as "**acrospiroma**." Multiple eruptive eccrine poromas have been associated with cytotoxic chemotherapies, radiation therapy, and pregnancy.
- Poroma classically presents as a **vascular-appearing papulonodule with a thin moat on the palms and soles**, but can occur anywhere on the body. There is a small risk of malignant degeneration to **porocarcinoma**, which is the **most common sweat gland malignancy.** Porocarcinoma favors the **head and neck and lower extremities.** It is **often metastatic** at presentation (despite subtle histopathology).
  - ◆ Figure 5.52.
- Complete surgical excision is curative.

SYRINGOMA
→ Diagnosis Group 2

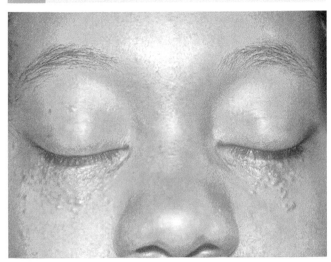

Reprinted with permission from Goodheart HP, Gonzalez ME. *Goodheart's Same-Site Differential Diagnosis: Dermatology for the Primary Health Care Provider*. 2nd ed. Wolters Kluwer; 2022.

Epidemiology

- Syringoma is a benign sweat gland neoplasm with primarily **eccrine ductal differentiation.**
- There is an increased incidence in **females, skin phototypes IV and V, and Asians.**
- A histopathological variant—**clear cell syringoma**—is associated with **diabetes mellitus.**
  - Syringomas along with **atrophoderma vermiculatum and milia**, are associated with **Nicolau-Balus syndrome.**
  - **Eruptive syringomas** are associated with **Down syndrome.**

Clinicopathological Features

- Syringoma classically presents as a **skin-colored papule** on **periocular skin.**

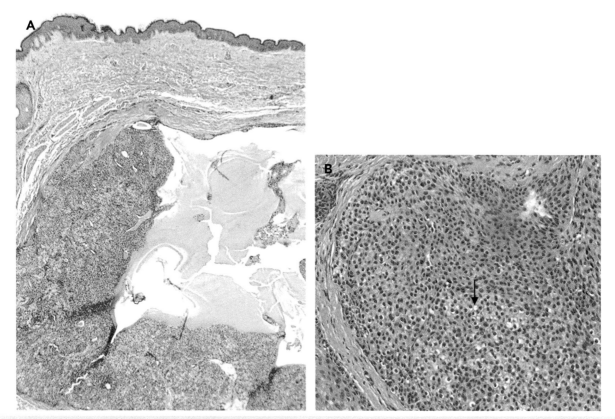

Figure 5.51. CLINICOPATHOLOGICAL CORRELATION: HIDRADENOMA. Hidradenoma is characterized by a well circumscribed cystic dermal nodule focally connected to the epidermis. The nodule contains three cell types—clear cells, "poroid" cells, and squamous cells—and ducts with hyaline sheath (PAS-positive, diastase resistant) ± pink sweat. The stroma is sclerotic with keloidal collagen. IHC may demonstrate the CRTC1 / MAML2 fusion product. A, Low-power view. B, High-power view. Solid arrow: duct. CRTC1, CREB regulated transcription coactivator; MAML2, mastermind like transcriptional coactivator 2; PAS, periodic acid-Schiff.

(Histology images reprinted with permission from Elder DE, Elenitsas R, Rosenbach M, et al. *Lever's Histopathology of the Skin*. 11th ed. Wolters Kluwer; 2015.)

- **Clear cell hidradenoma:** hidradenoma with prominent clear cell degeneration.
- **Hidradenocarcinoma:** infiltrative growth pattern with cytologic atypia, mitotic activity, and necrosis.

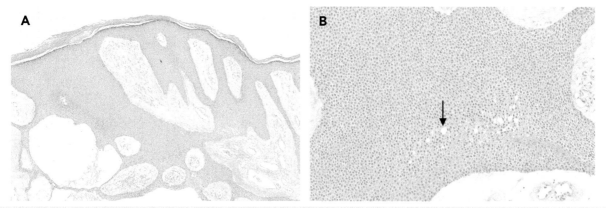

Figure 5.52. CLINICOPATHOLOGICAL CORRELATION: POROMA. Poroma is characterized by inter-anastomosing cords broadly connected to the epidermis. Cords contain pink cuboidal ("poroid") cells with cytoplasmic clearing due to glycogen (PAS positive, diastase sensitive) and ducts with hyaline sheath (PAS-positive, diastase resistant) ± pink sweat. The stroma is highly vascular. A, Low-power view. B, High-power view. Solid arrow: duct. PAS, periodic acid-Schiff; SK, seborrheic keratosis.

(Histology images courtesy of Noel Turner, MD, MHS and Christine J. Ko, MD.)

- **Hidroacanthoma simplex:** intraepidermal poroma.
- **Dermal duct tumor:** intradermal poroma.
- **Porocarcinoma:** infiltrative growth pattern with cytologic atypia, mitotic activity, and necrosis (subtle). Intraepithelial porocarcinoma demonstrates pagetoid spread.

Presence of ducts helps distinguish hidroacanthoma simplex from clonal SK.

- **Eruptive syringomas** are most commonly located on the **anterior chest.**
  - ◆ Figure 5.53.
  - ◆ The histopathological differential diagnosis of syringoma is summarized in Table 5.34.

Evaluation

- The differential diagnosis of syringoma includes comedone, xanthelasma, SGH, milia, and hidrocystoma.

Management

- Treatment of syringomas is purely cosmetic since they are benign and have negligent proliferative capacity. Treatment options include cryotherapy, electrosurgical destruction, punch excision, TCA application, and ablative laser. Topical atropine may be helpful in pruritic eruptive syringomas.

"Real World" Advice

- Since there is an increased incidence of syringomas in skin types IV and V, it is important to counsel these patients on the risk of hypopigmentation and scarring prior to treatment.

Other Adnexal Neoplasms and Proliferations

MICROCYSTIC ADNEXAL CARCINOMA

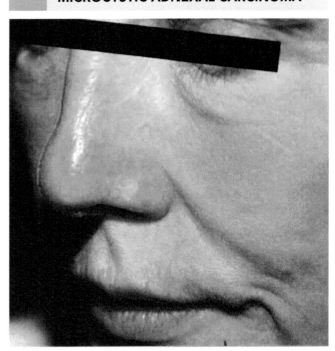

Reprinted with permission from Elder DE, Elenitsas R, Rubin AI, et al. *Atlas of Dermatopathology: Synopsis and Atlas of Lever's Histopathology of the Skin.* 4th ed. Wolters Kluwer; 2020.

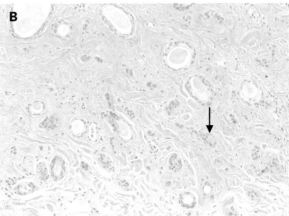

Figure 5.53. CLINICOPATHOLOGICAL CORRELATION: SYRINGOMA. Syringoma is characterized by a well circumscribed superficial dermal proliferation of ducts with hyaline sheath (PAS positive, diastase resistant) ± pink sweat. The stroma is sclerotic. A, Low-power view. B, High-power view. Solid arrow: "tadpole-shaped" duct. PAS, periodic acid-Schiff. (Histology images courtesy of Noel Turner, MD, MHS and Christine J. Ko, MD.)

The ducts in syringoma have been described as "tadpole-shaped" with a "paisley-tie pattern."

- **Clear cell syringoma:** clear cells filled with glycogen (PAS positive, diastase sensitive).

- Microcystic adnexal carcinoma (MAC) is a low-grade **adnexal carcinoma** that most commonly occurs in **young-to-middle-aged females.** Left-sided predominance on the face has led to the hypothesis that UVR exposure (from driving) may be contributory.
- MAC classically presents as a **slow growing, ill-defined, skin-colored-to-pink plaque on the face.** It favors the **cutaneous lip, especially the upper cutaneous lip at the base of the nasal ala.**

- Figure 5.54.
- For the histopathological differential diagnosis of MAC, see Table 5.34. **A superficial shave biopsy may incorrectly be interpreted as a syringoma** if the infiltrative nature of the lesion is not captured. As such, excisional/incisional biopsy is preferred.
- MMS is the preferred treatment as it has been shown to have lower rates of recurrence compared to WLE.

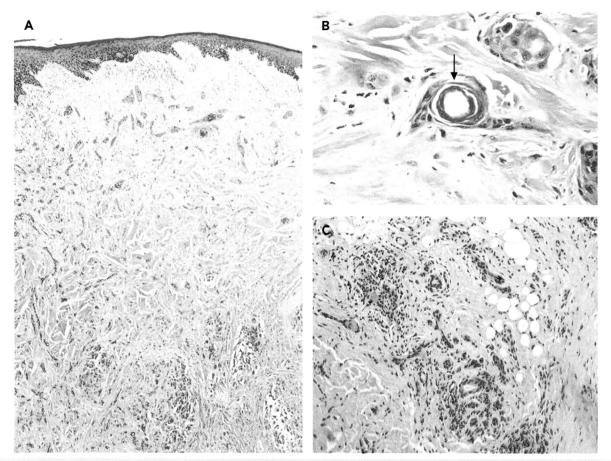

Figure 5.54. CLINICOPATHOLOGICAL CORRELATION: MICROCYSTIC ADNEXAL CARCINOMA. MAC is a deeply infiltrative carcinoma with biphasic or multiphasic differentiation (ductal, follicular, ± sebaceous). Ductal differentiation often resembles syringoma and follicular differentiation often consists of microcysts with infundibular keratinization. Perineural invasion and lymphoid aggregates are common. The stroma is sclerotic. A, Low-power view. B, High-power view of the superficial dermis. Solid arrow: "tadpole-shaped" duct. C, High-power view of the deep dermis. CEA, carcinoembryonic antigen; MAC, microcystic adnexal carcinoma.

(Histology images reprinted with permission from Elder DE, Elenitsas R, Rosenbach M, et al. *Lever's Histopathology of the Skin.* 11th ed. Wolters Kluwer; 2015.)

- **Sclerosing sweat duct carcinoma:** monophasic differentiation (absent follicular component).

The ducts in MAC have been described as "tadpole-shaped" with a "paisley-tie pattern."

Table 5.34. HISTOPATHOLOGICAL DIFFERENTIAL DIAGNOSIS OF SYRINGOMA

Diagnosis[a]	Histopathological Features	Positive IHC Staining	Negative IHC Staining
Syringoma	Well-circumscribed superficial dermal (upper 1/3 of dermis) proliferation of ducts with hyaline sheath (PAS-positive, diastase resistant) ± pink sweat. The stroma is sclerotic.	CEA, EMA	CK20
Morpheaform BCC	Thin strands and small nests of basophilic cells with limited peripheral palisading and minimal retractions around epithelial cells. The stroma is sclerotic. Perineural invasion is common.	Androgen receptor, BCL2 (diffuse), BerEP4, toluidine blue (stroma)	CEA, CK20, EMA, PHLDA1
MAC	Deeply infiltrative (lower half of dermis) carcinoma with biphasic or multiphasic differentiation (ductal, follicular, ± sebaceous). Ductal differentiation often resembles syringoma and follicular differentiation often consists of microcysts with infundibular keratinization. Perineural invasion and lymphoid aggregates are common. The stroma is sclerotic.	CEA, EMA	BerEP4
Desmoplastic trichoepithelioma	Chords of basophilic cells, dystrophic calcification within keratin-filled microcysts, and keratin granulomas. The stroma is sclerotic.	BCL2 (periphery), BerEP4, CK20, PHLDA1	Androgen receptor.

BCC, basal cell carcinoma; BCL2, B-cell lymphoma 2; CEA, carcinoembryonic antigen; CK, cytokeratin; EMA, epithelial membrane antigen; IHC, immunohistochemistry; MAC, microcystic adnexal carcinoma; PAS, periodic acid-Schiff; PHLDA1, Pleckstrin homology-like domain family A member 1.
[a]Illustrative examples provided.

MUCINOUS CARCINOMA

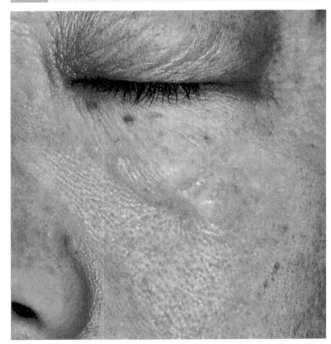

Reprinted with permission from Elder DE, Elenitsas R, Rubin AI, et al. *Atlas of Dermatopathology: Synopsis and Atlas of Lever's Histopathology of the Skin.* 4th ed. Wolters Kluwer; 2020.

- Mucinous carcinoma is a rare **sweat duct carcinoma** that is associated with older age.
- Mucinous carcinoma classically presents as a **solitary papule on the periocular skin (40% eyelid).** Mucinous carci-noma has a high rate of recurrence after treatment, but a relatively low rate of metastasis.
  - ◆ Figure 5.55.
  - ◆ Other adnexal neoplasms and proliferations not discussed elsewhere are summarized in Table 5.35.
- **Multiple lesions or lesions outside the periocular skin** should raise suspicion for **metastatic mucinous carcinoma** from another primary source (eg, breast adenocarcinoma, colon adenocarcinoma).
- There is growing evidence supporting the use of MMS for the treatment of mucinous carcinomas given the higher rate of recurrence with WLE.

Neoplasms of the Hair and Nails

Basic Concepts

- **Neoplasms of the hair** are adnexal neoplasms that recapitulate different parts of the hair follicle. They may be classified according to **superficial follicular (infundibular or isthmic), follicular sheath,** and **follicular matrical differentiation.**
- **Neoplasms of the nails** are adnexal neoplasms that arise in the nail matrix.

Adnexal Neoplasms and Proliferations With Superficial Follicular Differentiation

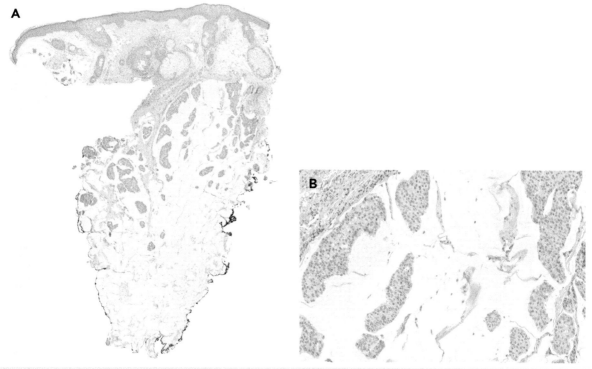

Figure 5.55. CLINICOPATHOLOGICAL CORRELATION: MUCINOUS CARCINOMA. Mucinous carcinoma is characterized by islands of blue cells in a cribriform configuration surrounded by sialomucin (mucicarmine positive; PAS positive, diastase resistant). CK7 is positive and CK20 is negative. A, Low-power view. B, High-power view. CK, cytokeratin; PAS, periodic acid-Schiff.

(Histology image courtesy of Noel Turner, MD, MHS and Christine J. Ko, MD.)

Mucinous carcinoma if often described as "blue islands floating in a sea of mucin."

Table 5.35. OTHER ADNEXAL NEOPLASMS AND PROLIFERATIONS

Diagnosis[a]	Clinical Features	Histopathological Features	Notes
Apocrine			
Tubular apocrine adenoma	Pink papule, often within a nevus sebaceous.	Well-circumscribed lobular proliferation of tubular apocrine structures with pseudopapillae extending into the lumens. Displays decapitation secretion.	
Eccrine			
Eccrine angiomatous hamartoma	Red-purple nodule favoring the extremities.	Proliferation of mature eccrine ducts admixed with blood vessels	Occurs most often in children.
Papillary eccrine adenoma	Papule favoring the lower extremities.	Well-circumscribed proliferation of eccrine ducts with papillary projections extending into the lumens.	Occurs most often in black women.
Mixed/Other			
Mixed tumor (chondroid syringoma)	Papule favoring the nose > cheek and upper lip.	Ducts and tubules embedded in a myxoid or chondroid stroma. The small tubular type demonstrates small tubules, while the branching alveolar type demonstrates long tubules ± decapitation secretion. Sialomucin (mucicarmine+; PAS+, diastase resistant) is present in the stroma.	Small risk of malignant degeneration to malignant mixed tumor. Called "pleomorphic adenoma" when located in the salivary gland.

(Continued)

Table 5.35. OTHER ADNEXAL NEOPLASMS AND PROLIFERATIONS (CONTINUED)

Diagnosis[a]	Clinical Features	Histopathological Features	Notes
Syringofibroadenoma (of Mascaro)	Pink papulonodule favoring the lower extremities.	Thin anastomosing, reticulated strands of cuboidal cells extending from the epidermis to the dermis. Loose fibrovascular stroma surrounds the tumor.	Most commonly reactive (eg, in association with chronic venous stasis dermatitis). Associations include hidrotic ectodermal dysplasia and Schöpf-Schultz-Passarge syndrome.
Adenoid cystic carcinoma	Pink papulonodule, often on the scalp with associated alopecia.	Poorly circumscribed proliferation of cribriform-like glandular structures with a paucity of myxoid stroma. Pools of sialomucin (mucicarmine+; PAS+, diastase resistant) can be seen. Can display perineural invasion and extension into the subcutaneous fat.	Two types: primary cutaneous (indolent, high recurrence rate) and salivary gland (highly aggressive, high metastatic rate).
Aggressive digital papillary adenocarcinoma	Skin-colored to blue nodule favoring the volar digit.	Partly cystic, irregular proliferation with papillary projections. Many mitotic figures.	Strong male predominance. Treatment is usually amputation.

PAS, periodic acid-Schiff.
[a]Illustrative examples provided.

NEVUS COMEDONICUS

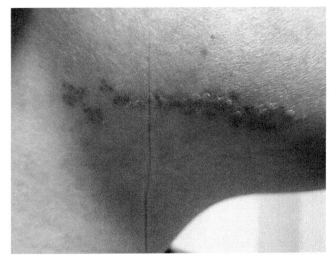

Reprinted with permission from Gru AA, Wick MR, Mir A, et al. *Pediatric Dermatopathology and Dermatology.* Wolters Kluwer; 2018.

- Nevus comedonicus is a **benign adnexal hamartoma with follicular infundibular differentiation** due to **mosaicism of** *FGFR2*. Patients with **Apert syndrome** (sporadic or AD mutation in *FGFR2*) can have generalized comedones. Nevus comedonicus is present at birth in about half of patients, and develops in childhood in the other half. Rarely, nevus comedonicus has been associated with **Alagille syndrome** (AD disorder that primarily affects the heart and liver).
- Nevus comedonicus classically presents with a **cluster of dilated follicular ostia that contain dark, cornified mate-**

rial. The most common location is the **face, followed by the neck and upper trunk.** Nevus comedonicus may have a linear configuration.
  - ◆ Figure 5.56.
- Treatment of nevus comedonicus is challenging. Surgical excision is the most definitive treatment; however, many lesions are too large. Keratolytic agents such as salicylic acid and ammonium lactate may be mildly helpful but are not curative.

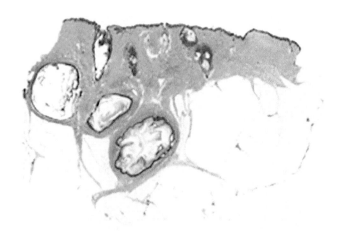

Figure 5.56. CLINICOPATHOLOGICAL CORRELATION: NEVUS COMEDONICUS. Nevus comedonicus is characterized by grouped underdeveloped hair follicles that lack hair shafts that are instead filled with keratin debris.

(Histology images reprinted with permission from Elder DE, Elenitsas R, Rosenbach M, et al. *Lever's Histopathology of the Skin.* 11th ed. Wolters Kluwer; 2015.)

TRICHOEPITHELIOMA

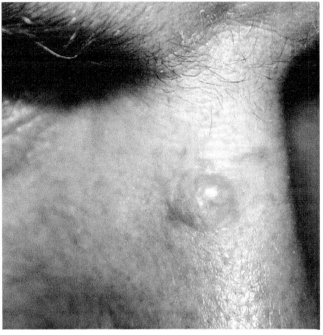

Reprinted with permission from Edward S, Yung A. *Essential Dermato-pathology*. Wolters Kluwer Health/Lippincott Williams & Wilkins; 2011.

- Trichoepithelioma is a **benign** adnexal neoplasm with **follicular infundibular differentiation.** The most commonly affected demographic is **middle-aged women.**
  - Multiple trichoepitheliomas are associated with **Bazex-Christol-Dupré syndrome, Rombo syndrome, Brooke-Spiegler syndrome**, and multiple familial trichoepitheliomas (*CYLD* mutation).
- Trichoepithelioma classically presents as a **skin-colored-to-pink papule favoring the face.** The most common location is the **upper cheek.** The **desmoplastic** variant classically presents as a **skin-colored-to-pink papule with a central dell.** There is a small risk of malignant degeneration to malignant trichoepithelioma.
  - Trichoepithelioma is "dome-shaped." Desmoplastic trichoepithelioma is "donut-shaped."
  - Figure 5.57. For the histopathological differential diagnosis of desmoplastic trichoepithelioma, see Table 5.34.
  - Adnexal neoplasms and proliferations with follicular sheath differentiation are summarized in Table 5.36.
- Given the lack of distinct clinical features, skin biopsy is required for diagnosis.
- Trichoepithelioma is a benign neoplasm and thus does not require treatment. If treatment for cosmetic reasons is desired, spot electrodesiccation and laser ablation can be helpful.

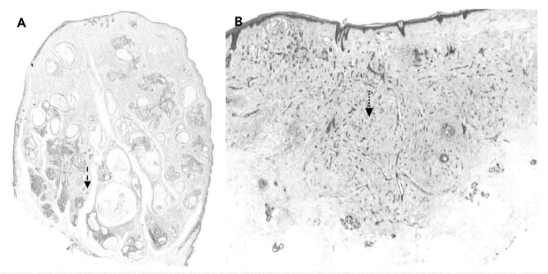

Figure 5.57. CLINICOPATHOLOGICAL CORRELATION: TRICHOEPITHELIOMA. Trichoepithelioma is characterized by proliferations of basophilic cells, sometimes with a cribriform configuration, with minimal to no epidermal connection. Papillary mesenchymal bodies (dense round or oval aggregates of fibroblastic cells) are often prominent. A, Trichoepithelioma. Solid arrow: "finger-like" proliferation of basophilic cells with a cribriform configuration creating a "swiss cheese" appearance. Dashed arrow: papillary mesenchymal body. B, Desmoplastic trichoepithelioma. Dotted arrow: sclerotic stroma. BCC, basal cell carcinoma.

(A, Histology image courtesy of Noel Turner, MD, MHS and Christine J. Ko, MD. B, Histology image reprinted with permission from Edward S, Yung A. *Essential Dermatopathology*. Wolters Kluwer Health/Lippincott Williams & Wilkins; 2011.)

Absence of clefting between basophilic cells and stroma helps distinguish trichoepithelioma from BCC.

- **Desmoplastic trichoepithelioma**: trichoepithelioma with chords of basophilic cells dystrophic calcification within keratin-filled microcysts, and keratin granulomas. The stroma is sclerotic.
- **Malignant trichoepithelioma**: infiltrative growth pattern with cytologic atypia, mitotic activity, and necrosis.
- Proliferations are "finger-like" and the cribriform

Proliferations are "finger-like" and the cribriform configuration creates a "swiss cheese" appearance.
Chords in desmoplastic trichoepithelioma have been described as "tadpole-shaped" with a "paisley-tie pattern." The clinical lesion is "donut-shaped," and "donuts" (microcysts) are observed on histopathology.

Table 5.36. ADNEXAL NEOPLASMS AND PROLIFERATIONS WITH SUPERFICIAL FOLLICULAR DIFFERENTIATION

Diagnosis[a]	Clinical Features	Histopathological Features	Notes
Infundibulum			
IFK	Solitary skin-colored smooth or verrucous papule favoring the cheek and upper lip.	Discrete endophytic growth of keratinocytes demonstrating squamous eddies (keratin pearls).	
Trichoadenoma	Solitary skin-colored-to-pink papule favoring the face.	Proliferation of keratin-filled microcysts in the upper dermis with sclerotic stroma.	Similar to desmoplastic trichoepithelioma on histopathology, but with more microcysts.
		Trichoadenoma has "donuts" (microcysts) on histopathology.	
Trichoepithelioma	See above.		
Trichofolliculoma	Skin-colored papule with emanating vellus hairs from a central punctum favoring the scalp, face, and upper trunk.	Central dilated follicle with numerous connections to multiple surrounding smaller follicles.	
		Trichofolliculoma has a "momma and babies" configuration.	
Isthmus			
Fibrofolliculoma/ trichodiscoma	Skin-colored to hypopigmented papule favoring the face, usually in multiplicity.	Numerous thin strands of follicular epithelium radiating from a central follicle surrounded by fibromyxoid stroma. Trichodiscoma has more stroma and less epithelial cells.	Trichodiscoma is thought to represent a fibrofolliculoma with variable histologic sectioning. Associated with BHD syndrome.
		Epithelial cells form "mitt-like" structures in fibrofolliculoma vs collarettes in trichodiscoma.	
Tumor of the follicular infundibulum	Skin-colored papule favoring the head and neck.	Proliferation of basophilic epithelial cells emanating from the epidermis that form dermal anastomosing chords running parallel to the epidermis.	The name is a misnomer; it has isthmic differentiation, not infundibular.
		Dermal anastomosing chords running parallel to the epidermis are "plate-like."	

BHD, Birt-Hogg-Dubé; IFK, inverted follicular keratosis.
[a]Illustrative examples provided.

SPOTLIGHT ON BIRT-HOGG-DUBÉ SYNDROME

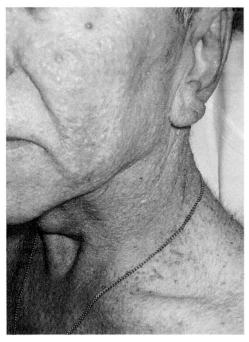

- Birt-Hogg-Dubé (BHD) syndrome is an **AD** disorder due to a mutation in *FLCN* encoding **folliculin.**
- BHD syndrome is characterized by the **classic cutaneous triad of acrochordons, fibrofolliculomas, and trichodis-**

comas favoring the scalp, face, neck, and upper trunk. Systemic findings in BHD syndrome include **medullary thyroid carcinoma, renal tumors (chromophobe, oncocytic, and hybrid), and multiple pulmonary cysts complicated by spontaneous pneumothorax and bullous emphysema.**
  - ◈ The histopathology of BHD syndrome demonstrates cutaneous acrochordons, fibrofolliculomas, and trichodiscomas.
- **Genetic testing** is recommended if patients have:
  - ○ ≥5 facial papules, at least one of which is a fibrofolliculoma.
  - ○ Facial angiofibroma.
  - ○ Family history of spontaneous pneumothoraces without history of smoking or chronic obstructive pulmonary disease (COPD).
  - ○ Family history of renal tumors.
- Management of BHD requires a multidisciplinary approach with endocrine, renal, and pulmonary specialty care. In addition to age-appropriate malignancy screening, patients need:
  - ○ Baseline TBSE.
  - ○ Renal MRI or CT scan to detect renal tumors every 1 to 2 years.
  - ○ Baseline high resolution chest CT to detect pulmonary cysts.
  - ○ Counseling on smoking cessation if applicable.
  - ○ Judicious use of general anesthesia to reduce the risk of spontaneous pneumothorax.

Adnexal Neoplasms and Proliferations With Follicular Sheath Differentiation

TRICHOLEMMOMA
Synonym: trichilemmoma

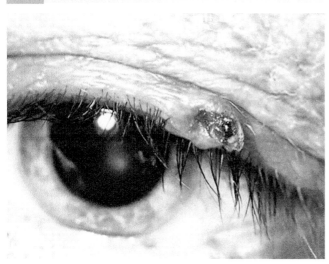

Reprinted with permission from Shields JA, Shields CL. *Eyelid, Conjunctival, and Orbital Tumors: An Atlas and Textbook.* 3rd ed. Wolters Kluwer; 2015.

- **Tricholemmoma** is a **benign** adnexal neoplasm with **follicular sheath differentiation.**
  - Multiple tricholemmomas are associated with Cowden syndrome.
  - ◈ "Tricholemooma" is associated with Cowden syndrome.
- Tricholemmoma classically presents as a **solitary verrucous skin-colored papule.** The most common location is the **face,** followed by the **genital area.** The **desmoplastic** variant presents as a **solitary lesion on the face or within nevus sebaceous.** There is a small risk of malignant degeneration to tricholemmal carcinoma.
  - ◈ Figure 5.58.
  - ◈ Adnexal neoplasms and proliferations with follicular sheath differentiation are summarized in Table 5.37.
- Given the lack of distinct clinical features, skin biopsy is required for diagnosis.
- Tricholemmoma is a benign neoplasm and thus does not require treatment. If treatment for cosmetic reasons is desired, spot electrodesiccation and laser ablation can be helpful.

Adnexal Neoplasms and Proliferations With Follicular Matrical Differentiation

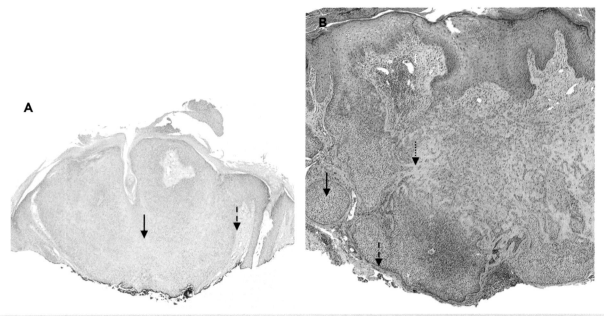

Figure 5.58. CLINICOPATHOLOGICAL CORRELATION: TRICHOLEMMOMA. Tricholemmoma is characterized by lobules of clear cells filled with glycogen (PAS positive, diastase sensitive) that connect to the epidermis. Lobules are outlined by palisading keratinocytes and a thick basement membrane (PAS positive, diastase resistant). CD34 positivity is indicative of ORS differentiation. Loss of expression of PTEN is a screening tool for Cowden syndrome but should be confirmed with genetic testing. A, Tricholemmoma. B, Desmoplastic tricholemmoma. Solid arrows: cells with cytoplasmic clearing due to glycogen (PAS-positive, diastase sensitive). Dashed arrows: thick basement membrane (PAS-positive, diastase resistant). Dotted arrow: sclerotic stroma. CD, cluster of differentiation; ORS, outer root sheath; PAS, periodic acid-Schiff; PTEN, phosphatase and tensin homolog.

(A, Histology image courtesy of Noel Turner, MD, MHS and Christine J. Ko, MD. B, Histology image reprinted with permission from Elder DE, Elenitsas R, Rosenbach M, et al. *Lever's Histopathology of the Skin.* 11th ed. Wolters Kluwer; 2015.)

- **Desmoplastic tricholemmoma:** tricholemmoma with sclerotic stroma.
- **Tricholemmal carcinoma:** infiltrative growth pattern with cytologic atypia, mitotic activity, and necrosis.

Table 5.37. ADNEXAL NEOPLASMS AND PROLIFERATIONS WITH FOLLICULAR SHEATH DIFFERENTIATION

Diagnosis[a]	Clinical Features	Histopathological Features	Notes
Pilar sheath acanthoma	Papule with a central comedone-like opening.	Cystically dilated follicle that opens to the surface. Epithelial lining is acanthotic with lobules that emanate from the centrally dilated follicle.	Histopathology is similar to dilated pore of Winer (lacks lobules) and trichofolliculoma (forms full follicular structures).
Tricholemmoma	See above.		

[a]Illustrative examples provided.

PILOMATRICOMA

Synonyms: calcifying epithelioma (of Malherbe), pilomatrixoma, trichomatrioma

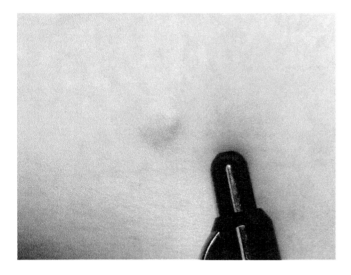

- Pilomatricomas are **benign** adnexal neoplasms with **follicular matrical differentiation.** They are associated with mutations in *CTNNB1* encoding **β-catenin**, an armadillo family protein that plays an important role in adherens junctions and cellular differentiation. **Children** are most commonly affected. Multiple pilomatricomas are associated with **Rubinstein-Taybi syndrome, Turner syndrome, Edwards syndrome, Gardner syndrome, and myotonic dystrophy.**

  ◈ Pilomatricoma has follicular matrical differentiation.
- Pilomatricoma classically presents as a **solitary, skin-colored to bluish papulonodule** that is firm and well circumscribed. The most common locations are the **head and upper trunk.** There is a small risk of malignant degeneration to **pilomatrical carcinoma.**

  ◈ Figure 5.59.
  ◈ Adnexal neoplasms and proliferations with follicular matrical differentiation are summarized in Table 5.38.
- Although there can be a high suspicion for pilomatricoma from the clinical exam, skin biopsy is required to confirm the diagnosis.
- Pilomatricomas are treated with simple enucleation.

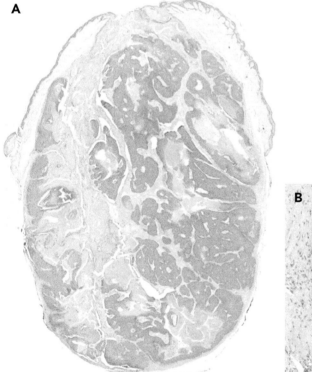

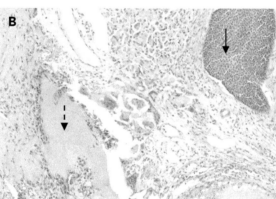

Figure 5.59. CLINICOPATHOLOGICAL CORRELATION: PILOMATRICOMA. Pilomatricoma is characterized by a well circumscribed nodule with internal trabeculae. Basophilic matrical cells keratinize to form eosinophilic anuclear matrical cells, delineated by a transition zone. The stroma often contains multinucleated giant cells adjacent to dystrophic calcification ± ossification. A, Low-power view. B, High-power view. Solid arrow: basophilic matrical cell. Dashed arrow: eosinophilic anuclear matrical cell ("shadow cell").

(Histology images courtesy of Noel Turner, MD, MHS and Christine J. Ko, MD.)

Eosinophilic anuclear matrical cells are called "shadow cells" in reference to the central unstained shadow of the lost nucleus.

- **Pilomatrical carcinoma:** infiltrative growth pattern with cytologic atypia, mitotic activity, and necrosis.

Table 5.38. ADNEXAL NEOPLASMS AND PROLIFERATIONS WITH FOLLICULAR MATRICAL DIFFERENTIATION

Diagnosis[a]	Clinical Features	Histopathological Features	Notes
BCC	See Chapter 5: Epidermal Neoplasms.		
Pilomatricoma	See above.		
Trichoblastoma	Skin-colored to bluish papule favoring the scalp and face.	Primarily dermal basophilic epithelial cells in nests with peripheral palisading. Clefting occurs between the stroma and the dermis (unlike BCC where clefting occurs between epithelial cells and the stroma). Prominent papillary mesenchymal bodies (dense round or oval aggregates of fibroblastic cells).	Some dermatopathologists consider trichoblastoma a variant of trichoepithelioma.

BCC, basal cell carcinoma.
[a]Illustrative examples provided.

Neoplasms of the Nails

ONYCHOMATRICOMA

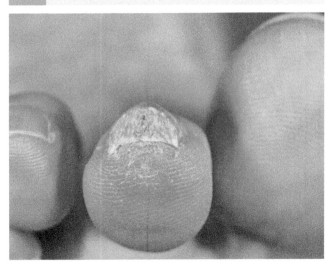

Courtesy of Adam Rubin, MD.

- Onychomatricoma is a rare tumor of the **nail matrix**. The most commonly affected demographic is **adult Caucasian women.**
- Onychomatricoma classically presents with **localized, yellow-white thickening of the nail plate with multiple longitudinal cavities** (appreciated with *en face* examination). **Splinter hemorrhages** and longitudinal melanonychia may also be observed, as well as **longitudinal curvature** of the nail plate.
    - ◆ Figure 5.60.
- Histopathological examination of a **nail plate biopsy (clipping)** is sufficient for the diagnosis of onychopapilloma. Imaging with MRI or US can be helpful if the diagnosis

is unclear, but is usually not needed. **Onychopapilloma** is often included in the differential diagnosis but the clinical appearance with **longitudinal erythronychia** is distinct.
- The definitive treatment of onychomatricoma is complete surgical excision. This involves nail avulsion to visualize the tumor followed by excision of the nail matrix (matricectomy) proximal to the tumor.

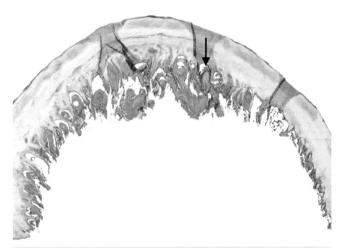

Figure 5.60. CLINICOPATHOLOGICAL CORRELATION: ONYCHOMATRICOMA. Onychomatricoma is characterized by a thick keratogenous zone forming multiple invaginations at the level of epithelial ridges and distal fibroepithelial projections that perforate the attached thick nail plate. Nail plate biopsy (clipping) demonstrates cavities lined with a thin layer of epithelium and filled with serous material. Solid arrow: "glove-finger" projection perforating the attached thick nail plate.

Invaginations are "V-shaped." Projections are often described as "glove-finger" projections.

Other Malformations and Neoplasms

Basic Concepts

- **Accessory malformation** refers to a congenital anomaly that produces an "extra" unit of an otherwise normal ana-tomic structure. The term "accessory" is sometimes inter-changed with "supernumerary."
- **Hamartomas** refer to mostly benign neoplasms **caused by an overgrowth of local cells.** The cell of origin determines the clinical and histopathological features.

ACCESSORY TRAGUS

Synonyms: cartilaginous rest, preauricular ap-pendage, preauricular tag

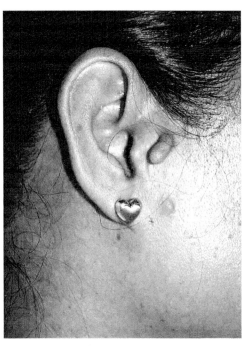

Reprinted with permission from Requena L, Kutzner H. *Cutaneous Soft Tissue Tumors.* Wolters Kluwer Health; 2014.

- Accessory tragus occurs due to **abnormal development** of the **first branchial arch.** While it is a benign, relatively common (3-6 per 1000 live births), normally isolated congenital defect, accessory tragus may be associated with other **branchial arch syndromes and anomalies** (Table 5.39). **Goldenhar syn-drome** is the association of accessory tragus with ipsilateral facial hypoplasia, epibulbar dermoids, ear deformities, and vertebral defects.
- Accessory tragus classically presents as an **exophytic, fleshy papule** that may contain cartilage and epidermal adnexal structures such as vellus hairs. It is usually **unilateral** and **sol-itary**, but can be bilateral and multiple. Because it forms from the first branchial arch, accessory tragus is located along the embryonic migration line extending from the **preauricular cheek to the angle of the mouth**, but can rarely occur on the anterior neck along the sternocleidomastoid (SCM) muscle.
    - ◈ Figure 5.61.

Table 5.39. BRANCHIAL ARCH SYNDROMES AND ANOMALIES

Anomaly[a]	Embryonic Structure	Classic Description
Accessory tragus	1st branchial arch	See above.
Branchial cleft cyst	1st-4th branchial clefts (2nd branchial cleft most common)	See Chapter 5: Cysts and Pseudocysts.
Bronchogenic cyst	Foregut endoderm and mesoderm	See Chapter 5: Cysts and Pseudocysts.
Cleft lip/palate	1st branchial arch	Separation or opening of the lip/palate.
Congenital rests of the neck (wattles)	Branchial arches	Fleshy appendages that hang along arch fusion lines.
Lip pits	1st branchial arches	Depressions of the lip (most commonly the vermilion lip).
Ear pit (preauricular cyst)	1st-2nd branchial arches	See Chapter 5: Cysts and Pseudocysts.
Midline cervical cleft	1st-2nd branchial arches	Suprasternal vertical erythematous band with nipple-like projection.
Nasal glioma	Neuroectoderm (neural tube + neural crest)	Firm, noncompressible papule or nodule at the root of the nose.
Thyroglossal duct cyst	1st and 2nd pharyngeal pouches	See Chapter 5: Cysts and Pseudocysts.

[a]Illustrative examples provided.

- The diagnosis of accessory tragus is often clinical but skin biopsy is definitive. Several studies report **associated hear-ing defects** with preauricular pits/accessory tragus; there-fore, **hearing evaluation** is recommended.
- Generally, **no treatment is required** for accessory tragus, though **surgical excision is definitive.** If the latter is to be performed, referral to otolaryngology is recommended due to the potential for contiguous growth or a fistula with the external ear canal.

RUDIMENTARY SUPERNUMERARY DIGIT

Synonym: rudimentary polydactyly

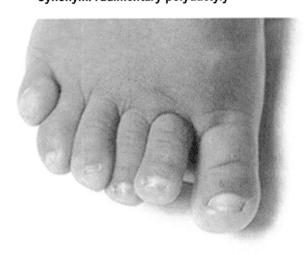

Reprinted with permission from Ricci SS. *Essentials of Maternity, Newborn, and Women's Health Nursing.* 5th ed. Wolters Kluwer; 2020.

- Rudimentary supernumerary digit is a redundancy of the soft tissue of the digit. It may be caused by an AD mutation in *GLI3* (GLI family zinc finger 3).
- Rudimentary supernumerary digits are commonly **bilateral** and favor the **ulnar side of the fifth digit or radial side of the thumb.** The appearance can range from a small papule to a large cartilaginous nodule with concurrent nail formation.
    - ◆ Figure 5.62.

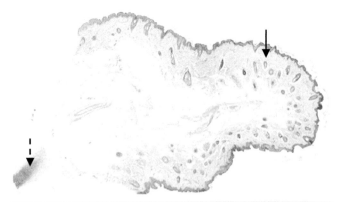

Figure 5.61. CLINICOPATHOLOGICAL CORRELATION: ACCESSORY TRAGUS. Accessory tragus is characterized by the presence of numerous vellus hair follicles in a fibrovascular polyp. A central core of adipose tissue and cartilage may be observed. Solid arrow: vellus hair follicle. Dashed arrow: cartilage.

(Histology image reprinted with permission from Kazakov DV, Michal M, Kacerovska D, et al. *Cutaneous Adnexal Tumors.* Wolters Kluwer Health/Lippincott Williams & Wilkins; 2012.)

- Clinically, **acral fibrokeratoma (AFK)** may be mistaken for rudimentary supernumerary digit. However, AFK is usually located on the finger, including the periungual region, and has a **surrounding collarette of elevated skin.**
- **Complete surgical excision** is the only definitive treatment for rudimentary supernumerary digit. Removal via suture ligation is not recommended due to the risk of complications such as infection and development of a painful neuroma.

A

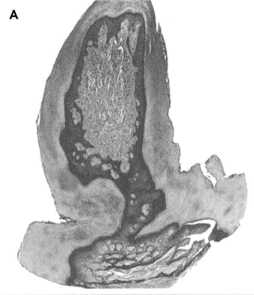

B

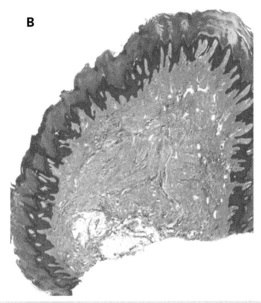

Figure 5.62. SIDE-BY-SIDE COMPARISON: RUDIMENTARY SUPERNUMERARY DIGIT AND ACRAL FIBROKERATOMA. Both rudimentary supernumerary digit and AFK are exophytic papules. Rudimentary supernumerary digit contains fascicles of nerve fibers. AFK contains vertically oriented thick collagen bundles and blood vessels. A, Rudimentary supernumerary digit. B, AFK. AFK, acral fibrokeratoma.

(Reprinted with permission from Requena L, Kutzner H. *Cutaneous Soft Tissue Tumors.* Wolters Kluwer Health; 2014. B, Reprinted with permission from Elder DE, Elenitsas R, Rubin AI, et al. *Atlas of Dermatopathology: Synopsis and Atlas of Lever's Histopathology of the Skin.* 4th ed. Wolters Kluwer; 2020.)

In both rudimentary supernumerary digit and AFK, acral skin is a helpful diagnostic clue.

LEIOMYOMA
Synonym: superficial benign smooth muscle tumor

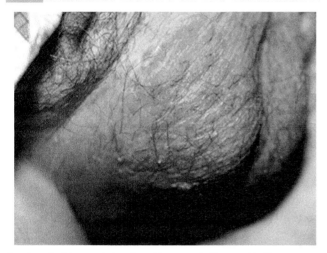

Reprinted with permission from Requena L, Kutzner H. *Cutaneous Soft Tissue Tumors*. Wolters Kluwer Health; 2014.

- Leiomyoma is an uncommon benign **smooth muscle hamartoma.** The following three types of leiomyomas are differentiated by anatomic location and smooth muscle origin:
  - **Piloleiomyoma**: arises from the **arrector pili muscle** of the pilosebaceous unit. Associations include hereditary **leiomyomatosis and renal cell cancer (HLRCC).**
  - **Genital leiomyoma**: arises from the smooth muscle of the **external genitalia, areola, or nipple.**
  - **Angioleiomyoma**: arises from smooth muscle **within vessel walls.**
- The classic presentation of leiomyoma varies based on type:
  - **Piloleiomyoma: solitary or multiple red-brown papules or nodules favoring the trunk and extremities.** Multiple piloleiomyomas often occur in clusters or in a Blaschko-linear distribution. Piloleiomyoma can be **painful**, particularly with palpation or cold exposure.
  - **Genital leiomyoma: solitary papule or nodule favoring the nipple/areola, vulva, penis, and scrotum.** Genital leiomyoma is typically **painless.**
  - **Angioleiomyoma: solitary, subcutaneous nodule favoring the lower extremities.** Angioleiomyoma can be spontaneously **painful.**

  Rarely, malignant degeneration into **leiomyosarcoma** can occur. ◈ Figure 5.63.
- In contrast to leiomyoma, rhabdomyoma is a rare, benign tumor of **striated muscle.** It presents as a **deep-seated lesion** on the head and neck. Rarely, malignant degeneration into rhabdomyosarcoma can occur.
- Though no treatment is necessary, **surgical excision** may be pursued for painful leiomyomas. Special attention should be paid when anesthetizing lesions with local anesthesia

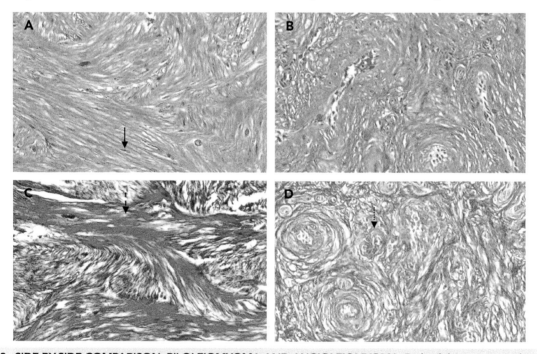

Figure 5.63. SIDE-BY-SIDE COMPARISON: PILOLEIOMYOMA AND ANGIOLEIOMYOMA. Both piloleiomyoma and angioleiomyoma contain smooth muscle fibers that stain with Masson-Trichrome (red), desmin, SMA, and vimentin. Loss of fumarate hydratase is a screening tool for HLRCC. Piloleiomyoma is poorly circumscribed and non-encapsulated with a haphazard array of interlacing fascicles of smooth muscle fibers. Angioleiomyoma is well-circumscribed and encapsulated with a circular array of smooth muscle fibers around vascular spaces. A, Piloleiomyoma. H&E. Solid arrow: "cigar-shaped" nucleus with blunt ends and a paranuclear vacuole representing a glycogen "snack" for the muscle. B, Angioleiomyoma. H&E. C, Piloleiomyoma. Masson-Trichrome. Dashed arrow: red smooth muscle. D, Angioleiomyoma. Masson-Trichrome. Dotted arrow: red smooth muscle and blue-green collagen outlining vessel walls. H&E, hematoxylin & eosin; HLRCC, hereditary leiomyomatosis and renal cell cancer; SMA, smooth muscle actin.

(Figure 5.63. Continued)

(Histology images reprinted with permission from Elder DE, Elenitsas R, Rosenbach M, et al. *Lever's Histopathology of the Skin.* 11th ed. Wolters Kluwer; 2015.)

- Genital leiomyoma: resembles piloleiomyoma but is typically larger on the scrotum or vulva.
- Leiomyosarcoma: resembles piloleiomyoma with hypercellularity, cytologic atypia, and mitotic activity.

The smooth muscle cell has "hot pink" cytoplasm, a "cigar-shaped" nucleus with blunt ends, and a paranuclear vacuole representing a glycogen "snack" for the muscle.

as injection directly into the lesion, particularly piloleiomyoma, may lead to severe pain. If surgery is not feasible, medications to counteract smooth muscle contraction (eg, nifedipine, gabapentin) or ablative techniques (eg, cryo-therapy, CO_2 laser) can be considered. In case of malignant degeneration, **superficial leiomyosarcoma carries a good prognosis, while subcutaneous leiomyosarcoma carries a poor prognosis.**

SPOTLIGHT ON HEREDITARY LEIOMYOMATOSIS AND RENAL CELL CANCER
Synonym: Reed syndrome

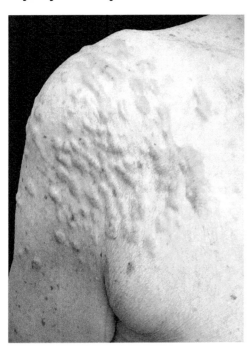

- HLRCC is an **AD** disorder caused by a **mutation in fumarate hydratase,** an enzyme in the Krebs cycle.
- This syndrome is characterized by **numerous cutaneous leiomyomas** (occurring as early as the second decade of life), **uterine leiomyomas** (>90% of women), and **RCC** (10%-16% of patients).
  - ◆ The histopathology of HLRCC demonstrates cutaneous leiomyoma.
- Diagnosis can be established by the following:
  - ○ 1. Identification of germline mutations in the *fumarate hydratase* gene (definitive diagnosis).
  - ○ 2. Major criteria: (a) multiple cutaneous leiomyomas with characteristic pain AND (b) one or more piloleiomyomas with characteristic pain (likely diagnosis).
  - ○ 3. Minor criteria: (a) solitary cutaneous leiomyoma plus family history of HLRCC, (b) early onset renal tumors of type 2 papillary histology, (c) multiple early onset (<40 years) symptomatic uterine fibroids, and (d) first-degree relative with one of the aforementioned criteria (≥2 minor criteria suggests suspected diagnosis).
- In addition to age-appropriate malignancy screening, patients require **yearly abdominal MRI (starting at age 10), yearly pelvic exam (women), and screening of first-degree relatives (offered as early as 8-10 years of age).**

BECKER NEVUS
→ Diagnosis Group 2
Synonym: Becker melanosis

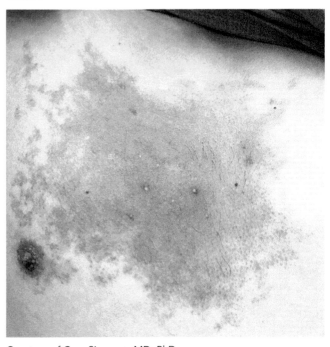

Courtesy of Cory Simpson, MD, PhD.

Epidemiology

- Becker nevus is often classified within the spectrum of **smooth muscle hamartoma.**
- Recently, **a postzygotic mutation in actin gene (ACTB)** was discovered in Becker nevi, suggesting a possible genetic linkage to the condition.
- The prevalence is estimated to be approximately 0.5%. Becker nevus is most common in **adolescent boys.**
- In **Becker nevus syndrome,** Becker nevus is associated with muscular abnormalities (eg, ipsilateral hypoplasia of the underlying musculature) and skeletal defects (eg, hemivertebra, rib and chest wall abnormalities, scoliosis). **Poland syndrome** is a subtype of Becker nevus syndrome particularly characterized by **ipsilateral breast hypoplasia.**

Clinicopathological Features

- Becker nevus classically presents as a **circumscribed hyperpigmented patch with slight acanthosis and hypertrichosis favoring the upper quadrant of anterior/posterior trunk.** Acanthosis and hypertrichosis are androgen-dependent and can therefore become more prominent during puberty.

◆ Figure 5.64.

Evaluation

- The differential diagnosis of Becker nevus includes CALM, giant congenital melanocytic nevus, plexiform neurofibroma, and congenital smooth muscle hamartoma.

Management

- Generally, treatment is not recommended for Becker nevus.
- Laser treatments can be considered though **recurrence is high.**
- At times, Becker nevus can be complicated by pruritus and eruption of acneiform lesions such as comedones, pustules, and cysts, which may require symptom-directed treatment.

"Real World" Advice

- If Becker nevus is present in younger patients, hair may not be visible. Therefore, the absence of hypertrichosis does not exclude the diagnosis.

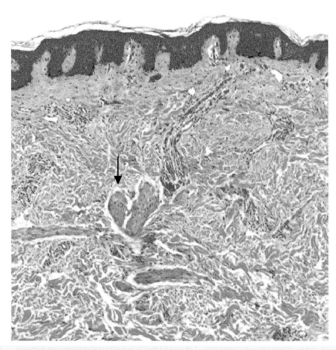

Figure 5.64. CLINICOPATHOLOGICAL CORRELATION: BECKER NEVUS. In Becker nevus, the epidermis demonstrates variable hyperkeratosis, acanthosis with elongated rite ridges, and basal layer hyperpigmentation. The dermis demonstrates increased smooth muscle bundles and variable hypertrichosis. Solid arrow: smooth muscle bundle.

(Histology image reprinted with permission from Elder DE, Elenitsas R, Rubin AI, et al. *Atlas and Synopsis of Lever's Histopathology of the Skin.* 3rd ed. Wolters Kluwer Health/Lippincott Williams & Wilkins; 2012.)

Cysts and Pseudocysts

Basic Concepts

- **Cysts** are nodules with an **epithelial lining** that may consist of stratified squamous epithelium or nonstratified squamous epithelium.
- **Pseudocysts** are nodules that **lack an epithelial lining**.

Cysts Lined With Stratified Squamous Epithelium

EPIDERMOID CYST
Synonyms: epidermal cyst, epidermal inclusion cyst, infundibular cyst

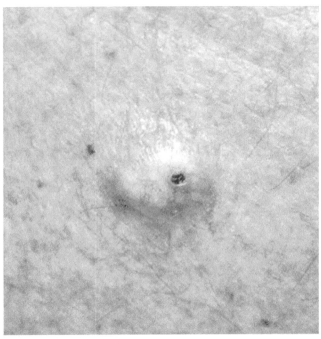

Reprinted with permission from Craft N, Fox LP, Goldsmith LA, et al. *VisualDx: Essential Adult Dermatology*. Wolters Kluwer Health/ Lippincott Williams & Wilkins; 2010.

- Epidermoid cyst is a benign cyst derived from the **follicular infundibulum**. It may arise spontaneously or due to traumatic implantation of the epidermis. Drug associations include **BRAF inhibitors**.

    Multiple epidermoid cysts are associated with **Gardner syndrome**. Associations with **milia (small epidermoid cysts)** include **Bazex-Dupre-Christol syndrome, Nicolau-Balus syndrome, and Rombo syndrome**.

- Epidermoid cyst classically presents as a **skin-colored nodule**, often with a **central punctum**. There is a small risk of transformation to proliferating epidermoid cyst, particularly in men. **Milia** classically present as **white papules around the eyes**.

    ◆ Cysts lined with stratified squamous epithelium are summarized in Table 5.40.

    ◆ Figure 5.65.

- Identification of a central punctum helps distinguish epidermoid cyst from lipoma.
- Complete surgical excision is curative. However, care must be taken to excise all of the cyst lining or it will recur. To accurately identify the cyst lining, it is preferable to excise an epidermoid cyst when it is not inflamed. ILK can help speed the resolution of an inflamed epidermoid cyst. Milia can be treated with extraction, typically using a comedone extractor or a sterile needle.

Table 5.40. CYSTS LINED WITH STRATIFIED SQUAMOUS EPITHELIUM

Diagnosis[a]	Clinical Features	Histopathological Features	Notes
Congenital inclusion cyst	Small nodules in the oral cavity located on the alveolar ridge (Bohn nodules) or palate (Epstein pearls).	Small cysts lined with attenuated stratified squamous epithelium.	Arise from epithelial remnants of dental lamina.
Dermoid cyst	Skin-colored to bluish nodule on the face, most commonly on the lateral eyebrow or nasal root (along embryonic fusion lines).	Resembles an epidermoid cyst with adnexal structures. The cyst may contain terminal hair shafts.	Arise due to entrapment of the epidermis during embryogenesis. CT or MRI should be performed to rule out connection to the CNS prior to surgical excision, especially for midline lesions.
Dilated pore of Winer	Single dilated comedo, usually occurring on the face.	Dilated hair follicle filled with keratin debris. The epithelial lining is acanthotic.	
		The acanthotic epithelial lining has "finger-like" projections.	
Ear pit (preauricular cyst)	Unilateral depressed papules on preauricular skin	Cyst lines with stratified squamous epithelium including a granular layer.	Arises from 1st-2nd branchial arches. Rarely associated with deafness (branchio-otic syndrome).
Epidermoid cyst/milium	See above.	Cyst lined with a stratified squamous epithelium similar to the epidermis but lacking adnexal structures. The cyst is filled with loose lamellar keratin.	The cyst may become inflamed and rupture, with infiltration of neutrophils, histiocytes, and foreign-body giant cells. Giant cells often contain keratin (birefringent material).
		Loose lamellar keratin in an epidermoid cyst resembles "onion skin."	
Pilar cyst (tricholemmal cyst, isthmus catagen cyst)	Nodule most commonly found on the scalp.	Cyst lined with a stratified squamous epithelium that has abrupt keratinization without a granular layer (tricholemmal keratinization similar to the hair follicle ORS). The cyst is filled with homogenous, eosinophilic keratin ± focal calcification.	Multiple pilar cysts can have AD inheritance. Small risk of transformation to proliferating pilar cyst (broad anastomosing nodules resembling small pilar cysts within the cyst), particularly in women. Small risk of malignant degeneration to pilar carcinoma (infiltrative growth pattern, cytologic atypia, mitotic activity).
		The architecture of proliferating pilar cyst resembles "rolls and scrolls."	
Steatocystoma	Small papulonodules favoring the chest that can drain oily material.	Cyst lined with a stratified squamous epithelium without a granular layer but with associated sebaceous glands. The innermost layer of the epithelium is a wavy eosinophilic cuticle (similar to the sebaceous duct). The cyst may overlap with vellus hair cyst and contain vellus hair shafts.	Derived from the follicular isthmus. Associated with PC-K17. A wavy eosinophilic cuticle is rarely present in dermoid cysts; however, dermoid cysts demonstrate apocrine and eccrine glands and may contain terminal hair shafts.
		The wavy eosinophilic cuticle of a steatocystoma resembles "shark teeth."	
Vellus hair cyst	Small dome-shaped pigmented papules favoring the trunk.	Resembles an epidermoid cyst. The cyst contains vellus hair shafts.	Derived from the follicular infundibulum. Often arise in an eruptive pattern. Associated with PC-K17.

AD, autosomal dominant; CNS, central nervous system; CT, computed tomography; K, keratin; ORS, outer root sheath; MRI, magnetic resonance imaging; PC, pachyonychia congenita.
[a]Illustrative examples provided.

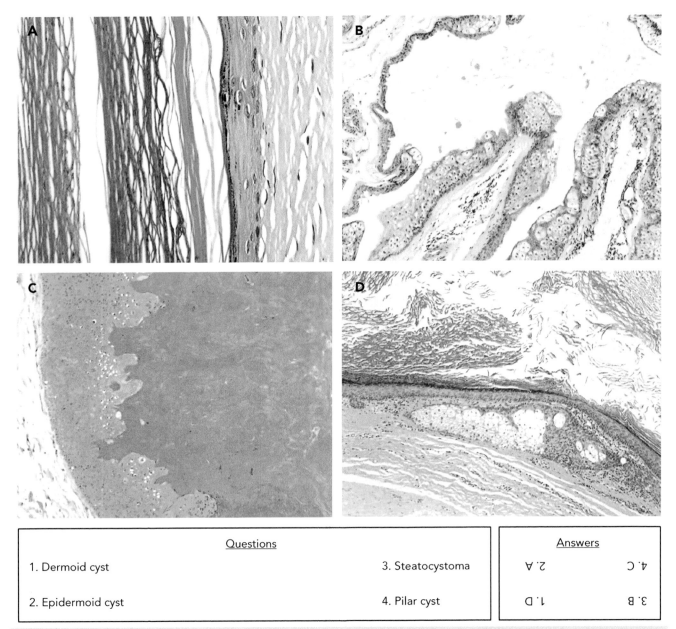

Questions		Answers	
1. Dermoid cyst	3. Steatocystoma	2. A	4. C
2. Epidermoid cyst	4. Pilar cyst	1. D	3. B

Figure 5.65. MATCHING EXERCISE: CYSTS LINED WITH STRATIFIED SQUAMOUS EPITHELIUM. A, Epidermoid cyst. Note the stratified squamous epithelium similar to the epidermis but lacking adnexal structures. The cyst is filled with loose lamellar "onion skin" keratin. B, Steatocystoma. Note the stratified squamous epithelium without a granular layer but with associated sebaceous glands. The innermost layer of the epithelium is a wavy eosinophilic "shark tooth" cuticle. C, Pilar cyst. Note the stratified squamous epithelium that has abrupt keratinization without a granular layer. The cyst is filled with homogenous, eosinophilic keratin. D, Dermoid cyst. Note the stratified squamous epithelium similar to the epidermis with adnexal structures.

(Histology images reprinted with permission from Elder DE, Elenitsas R, Rosenbach M, et al. *Lever's Histopathology of the Skin*. 11th ed. Wolters Kluwer; 2015.)

SPOTLIGHT ON GARDNER SYNDROME
Synonym: familial polyposis of the colon

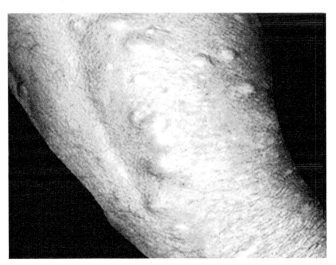

Multiple epidermoid cysts reprinted with permission from Gru AA, Wick MR, Mir A, et al. *Pediatric Dermatopathology and Dermatology*. Wolters Kluwer; 2018.

- Gardner syndrome is an **AD** syndrome due to mutations in *APC*, which normally suppresses **β-catenin.**
- **Clinical features of Gardner syndrome** are summarized in Table 5.41. A clinical subtype called **Turcot syndrome** is associated with development of **glioblastoma and medulloblastoma.**
  - The histopathology of Gardner syndrome demonstrates desmoid tumors, lipomas, pilomatricomas, and epidermoid cysts.

Table 5.41. CLINICAL FEATURES OF GARDNER SYNDROME

Mucocutaneous Features

- Desmoid tumors (female predominance)
- Lipomas
- Pilomatricomas
- Epidermoid cysts (30%-50% of patients)

Systemic Features

- Endocrine: papillary thyroid carcinoma (~1-2% of patients)
- Gastrointestinal: colon adenocarcinoma (100% incidence by 40 years of age)
- Dental: supernumerary teeth
- Orthopedic: odontogenic cysts, osteomas (most commonly on maxilla and mandible)
- Ocular: CHRPE

To remember <u>CHRPE</u> in <u>Gardner</u> syndrome, remember that "birds <u>chirp</u> in the <u>Garden</u>."

CHRPE, congenital hypertrophy of the retinal pigment epithelium.

- **Genetic testing** to confirm the diagnosis should be considered in patients who have multiple epidermoid cysts, osteomas, and colon polyps.
- In addition to age-appropriate malignancy screening, patients need **yearly colonoscopies starting at age 10** and upper endoscopies every 1 to 3 years starting at age 10. Given the inevitable risk of colon adenocarcinoma, **prophylactic colectomy** is required and is usually performed between 15 and 25 years of age.

Cysts Lined With Nonstratified Squamous Epithelium

HIDROCYSTOMA
Synonyms: cystadenoma, Moll gland cyst, sudoriferous cyst

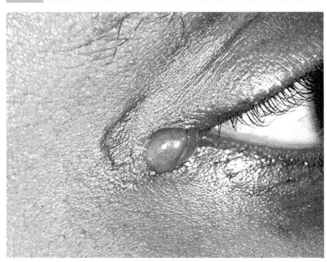

Reprinted with permission from Craft N, Fox LP, Goldsmith LA, et al. *VisualDx: Essential Adult Dermatology*. Wolters Kluwer Health/Lippincott Williams & Wilkins; 2010.

- Hidrocystoma is a benign cyst divided into 2 subtypes: **apocrine and eccrine.**
  - Multiple periocular/eyelid hidrocystomas are associated with **Schöpf-Schulz-Passarge syndrome.**
- Hidrocystoma classically presents as a **translucent skin-colored to bluish papule or papulonodule on the face, especially on the eyelid or cheek.**
  - Cysts lined with nonstratified squamous epithelium are summarized in Table 5.42.
  - Figure 5.66.
- Hidrocystoma can be removed with electrodesiccation, snip excision, or complete surgical excision.

Table 5.42. CYSTS LINED WITH NONSTRATIFIED SQUAMOUS EPITHELIUM

Diagnosis[a]	Clinical Features	Histopathological Features	Notes
Branchial cleft cyst	Nodule most commonly found on the lateral neck anterior to the SCM.	Cyst lined with epidermoid or pseudostratified epithelium and associated lymphoid tissue with germinal centers.	Arises from the 1st-4th branchial clefts (2nd most common). Characterize with CT or MRI prior to surgical excision.
Bronchogenic cyst	Midline nodule most commonly found on the suprasternal notch.	Cyst lined with ciliated pseudostratified columnar epithelium with goblet cells ± concentric smooth muscle and cartilage.	Arises from foregut endoderm and mesoderm.
Cutaneous ciliated cyst	Nodule most commonly on found on the lower extremity of a woman.	Cyst lined with stratified cuboidal or columnar cells with papillary projections into the cyst lumen.	Origin is controversial. Possible arises from metaplasia of eccrine glands.
Ciliated cyst of the vulva	Nodule on vulva.	Cyst lines with stratified cuboidal or columnar cells with papillary projections into cyst lumen.	Arises from Müllerian duct remnants.
Hidrocystoma	See above.	Cyst lined with two layers of cuboidal or columnar cells ± decapitation secretion.	
Median raphe cyst	Midline papulonodules most commonly found on the ventral penis (anogenital raphe).	Cyst with variable lining and amorphous debris. Amorphous debris inside a median raphe cyst is often called "dirty debris."	Arises due to an abnormality in the formation of the urethra.
Omphalomesenteric duct cyst	Umbilical pink papule.	Ectopic intestinal epithelium with villi, crypts, and goblet cells.	Arises due to incomplete degeneration of the intestinal end of the yolk stalk. Meckel diverticulum is the internal equivalent.
Thyroglossal duct cyst	Nodule on the anterior midline neck. Cyst moves upwards with protrusion of the tongue.	Cyst lined with ciliated columnar epithelium ± associated thyroid follicles.	Arises from the 1st-2nd pharyngeal pouches.
Urachal cyst	Pink papule on the umbilicus. Can have urine leakage. Often painful due to infection.	Cyst with cuboidal and transitional epithelium (similar to the urothelium).	Arises when a pocket of air or fluid develops in the urachus.

CT, computed tomography; MRI, magnetic resonance imaging; SCM, sternocleidomastoid.
[a]Illustrative examples provided.

Pseudocysts

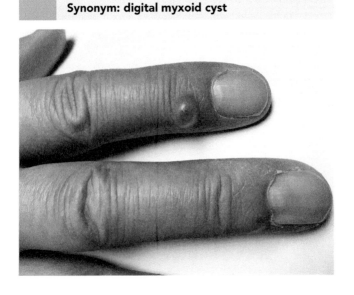

DIGITAL MUCOUS CYST
Synonym: digital myxoid cyst

- Digital mucous cyst is a benign pseudocyst. The content is thought to be **produced by fibroblasts** and is associated with **osteoarthritis.**
- Digital mucous cyst classically presents as a **soft skin-colored to bluish papulonodule on the proximal nail fold with spontaneous viscous drainage and nail plate depression.** There is often a **connection to the joint space.**
  - The histopathological features of pseudocysts are summarized in Table 5.43.
  - Figure 5.67.
- Complete surgical excision has a high cure rate (>90%). **Surgical excision is best done by orthopedic surgery** given the connection to the joint space and risk for infection. Cryotherapy and CO_2 laser are alternative therapies with lower treatment success rates.

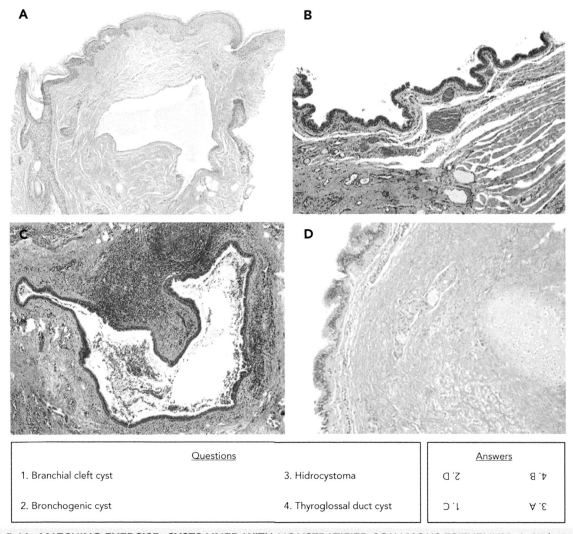

Questions	
1. Branchial cleft cyst	3. Hidrocystoma
2. Bronchogenic cyst	4. Thyroglossal duct cyst

Answers	
2. D	4. B
1. C	3. A

Figure 5.66. MATCHING EXERCISE: CYSTS LINED WITH NONSTRATIFIED SQUAMOUS EPITHELIUM. A, Hidrocystoma. Note the cuboidal or columnar cells and decapitation secretion. B, Thyroglossal duct cyst. Note the ciliated columnar epithelium and associated thyroid follicles in this case. C, Branchial cleft cyst. Note the epidermoid or pseudostratified epithelium in this case and associated lymphoid tissue with a germinal center. D, Bronchogenic cyst. Note the ciliated pseudostratified columnar epithelium with goblet cells.

(A, Histology image courtesy of Noel Turner, MD, MHS and Christine J. Ko, MD. B, Histology image reprinted with permission from Robinson RA. *Head and Neck Pathology: Atlas for Histologic and Cytologic Diagnosis.* Wolters Kluwer Health/Lippincott Williams & Wilkins; 2009. C, Histology image reprinted with permission from Robinson RA. *Head and Neck Pathology: Atlas for Histologic and Cytologic Diagnosis.* Wolters Kluwer Health/Lippincott Williams & Wilkins; 2009. D, Histology image reprinted with permission from Husain AN, Stocker JT, Dehner LP. *Stocker and Dehner's Pediatric Pathology.* 4th ed. Wolters Kluwer; 2015.)

Table 5.43. HISTOPATHOLOGICAL FEATURES OF PSEUDOCYSTS

Diagnosis[a]	Clinical Features	Histopathological Features	Notes
Digital mucous cyst	See above.	Cystic cavity containing mucin. Acral skin is a helpful diagnostic clue.	Often connected to the joint space.
Ganglion cyst	Soft nodule most commonly found on the dorsal aspect of the wrist.	Cystic cavity containing dense layers of fibrillated connective tissue.	Rarely connected to the joint space.
Mucocele (mucous cyst of the oral mucosa)	Pink to bluish papulonodule favoring the lower labial and buccal mucosa.	Cystic cavity containing sialomucin (mucicarmine+; PAS+, diastase resistant) ± surrounding muciphages and granulation tissue within the mucosa.	Arises due to disruption of the excretory duct of a minor salivary gland. A ranula is a mucocele on the floor of the mouth.
Pseudocyst of the auricle	Unilateral nodule most commonly found on the scaphoid fossa of the ear.	Cystic cavity within the cartilage.	Arises due to low-grade mechanical injury (ie, cellphone use).

PAS, periodic acid-Schiff.
[a]Illustrative examples provided.

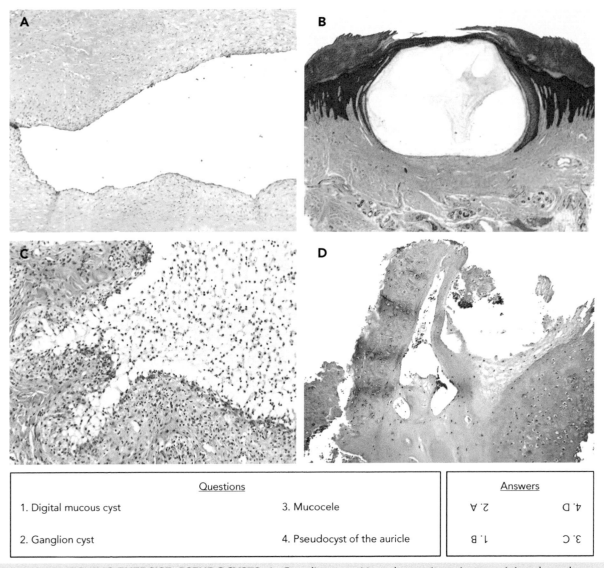

Questions		Answers	
1. Digital mucous cyst	3. Mucocele	2. A	4. D
2. Ganglion cyst	4. Pseudocyst of the auricle	1. B	3. C

Figure 5.67. MATCHING EXERCISE: PSEUDOCYSTS. A, Ganglion cyst. Note the cystic cavity containing dense layers of fibrillated connective tissue. B, Digital mucous cyst. Note the cystic cavity containing mucin on acral skin. C, Mucocele. Note the cystic cavity containing mucin and surrounding muciphages and granulation tissue within the mucosa. D, Pseudocyst of the auricle. Note the cystic cavity within the cartilage.

(A, Histology image courtesy of William E. Damsky, MD, PhD. B, Histology image reprinted with permission from Elder DE, Elenitsas R, Rosenbach M, et al. *Lever's Histopathology of the Skin.* 11th ed. Wolters Kluwer; 2015. C, Histology image reprinted with permission from Robinson RA. *Head and Neck Pathology: Atlas for Histologic and Cytologic Diagnosis.* Wolters Kluwer Health/Lippincott Williams & Wilkins; 2009. D, Histology image reprinted with permission from Elder DE, Elenitsas R, Rosenbach M, et al. *Lever's Histopathology of the Skin.* 11th ed. Wolters Kluwer; 2015.)

Hematolymphoid Neoplasms and Solid Organ Metastases

Basic Concepts

- **Hematolymphoid neoplasms** can be primary cutaneous or secondary cutaneous due to underlying lymphoma or leukemia. Primary cutaneous lymphoma encompasses **CTCL (75%-80%)** and **cutaneous B-cell lymphoma (CBCL) (20%-25%)**. In general, **primary cutaneous** hematolymphoid neoplasms have a **more favorable prognosis.**
- **Solid organ metastases** rarely involve the skin.

CUTANEOUS T-CELL LYMPHOMA
→ Diagnosis Group 1
Mycosis fungoides

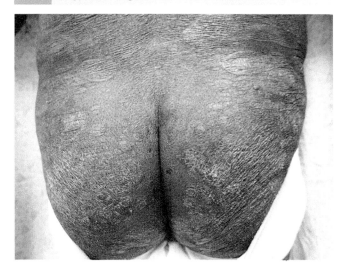

Epidemiology

- CTCL is a heterogenous group of T-cell neoplasms of the skin that vary in clinical phenotype and prognosis. Associations include the overlapping clonal T-cell-related dermatoses **parapsoriasis, PL, and LyP** and **secondary follicular mucinosis.** Drug associations include **pimecrolimus/tacrolimus (controversial).**
- The most common form of CTCL is **MF**, which accounts for ~50% of CTCL. MF may onset at any age, but primarily occurs in adults.
- A rare distinct form of CTCL is **Sézary syndrome**, which accounts for ~5% of CTCL. Sézary syndrome occurs almost exclusively in adults.
- The neoplastic cells in early patch-stage MF are **CD4⁺ T-cells** with a **Th1 cytokine profile.** In tumor-stage MF and Sézary syndrome, the neoplastic cells are derived from **CD8⁺ T-cells** with a **Th2 cytokine profile.**

Clinicopathological Features

- **MF** classically presents with **erythematous scaling patches (patch-stage MF) favoring the buttocks and non–sun-exposed areas of the trunk and extremities.** Pruritus is variable. MF can progress to **plaques (plaque-stage MF) and nodules (tumor-stage MF). MF and other CTCL variants** are summarized in Table 5.44. Clinical variants, such as **bullous and hyper- or hypopigmented MF,** behave similarly to classical MF and therefore are not considered separately. Though included in the 2018 update of the WHO-European Organization for Research and Treatment of Cancer (EORTC) classification for primary cutaneous lymphomas, chronic EBV infection; the rare and provisional subtypes of primary cutaneous peripheral T-cell lymphoma (primary cutaneous aggressive epidermotropic CD8⁺ cytotoxic T-cell lymphoma (CD8⁺AECTCL), primary cutaneous CD4⁺ small/medium T-cell lymphoproliferative disorder, primary cutaneous acral CD8⁺ T-cell lymphoma); and primary cutaneous peripheral T-cell lymphoma, not otherwise specified (NOS) are beyond the scope of this chapter.

  > Do NOT get confused! MF "patches" are in fact thin plaques; however, the thickness should not exceed that of a "necktie." The distribution of MF is commonly referred to as the "bathing trunk distribution" or "double-covered areas."
  >
  > Hypopigmented MF is the **most common clinical variant in children.**

- **Sézary syndrome** classically presents with **erythroderma and intense pruritus at onset. Diagnostic criteria for Sézary syndrome** are presented in Table 5.45.
  - Figure 5.68.

Evaluation

- The differential diagnosis of MF includes psoriasis, nummular dermatitis, and tinea corporis.
- The differential diagnosis of Sézary syndrome includes other etiologies of erythroderma (see Chapter 2: Papulosquamous Disorders and Palmoplantar Keratodermas).
- **Broad shave biopsy** is preferred for diagnosing **patch- or plaque-stage MF**; however, **punch biopsy** is preferred for **folliculotropic MF.**
- The **International Society for Cutaneous Lymphomas (ISCL)/EORTC TNMB classification and staging for MF** is summarized in Table 5.46. **Evaluation for blood involvement is recommended for stage IB or greater (>10% BSA).** This includes assessing for T-cell clonality with **flow cytometry and TCR gene rearrangement.**

Management

- Overall, MF has an **88% 5-year disease-specific survival.** Stage IA, IB, IIB, and III have 5-year disease-specific survivals of 98%, 89%, 56%, and 54%, respectively. **Pagetoid reticulosis and granulomatous slack skin have a better prognosis** than classical MF.
- **For Sézary syndrome, 5-year disease-specific survival ranges from 10% to 20%.**
- In early stages, the goal of CTCL treatment is to improve symptoms and limit toxicity. According to NCCN guidelines, skin-directed therapies including **topicals (eg, corticosteroids, carmustine, mechlorethamine), phototherapy,** and **total skin electron beam therapy (TSEBT)** are first line for stages IA or IB-IIA. For more advanced stages, other medical treatments include **alemtuzumab, bexarotene, brentuximab vedotin, denileukin diftitox (discontinued), liposomal doxorubicin, gemcitabine, IFN, methotrexate/pralatrexate, mogamulizumab, romidepsin/vorinostat, and vinblastine,** while other physical treatments include **ECP** and **localized radiation therapy. Allogeneic HSCT** or clinical trial may be considered for refractory disease.

"Real World" Advice

- **If a patient presents with erythroderma of unclear etiology, always assess for erythrodermic MF or Sézary syndrome with flow cytometry and TCR gene rearrangement.**
- If a patient presents with erythroderma at onset, the diagnosis is Sézary syndrome, not erythrodermic MF.

Table 5.44. MYCOSIS FUNGOIDES AND OTHER CUTANEOUS T-CELL LYMPHOMA VARIANTS

Diagnosis	Classic Description	Notes
MF Variants		
Folliculotropic MF	Acneiform follicular-based papules on the head and neck.	~10% of MF patients. 80% 5-year survival.
Pagetoid reticulosis	Red, scaly patch on an acral surface.	Extremely rare. 100% 5-year survival.
Granulomatous slack skin	Lax skin favoring the axillae, groin, and waist; can be pendulous.	Extremely rare. ~33% associated with Hodgkin lymphoma. 100% 5-year survival.
Sézary Syndrome[a]		
Other CTCL Variants		
ATLL	Skin lesions resembling MF, leukemia, lymphadenopathy, and organomegaly.	Associated with HTLV-1 (endemic to areas with a high prevalence of HTLV-1). Complications include hypercalcemia due to bone resorption. Overall poor prognosis, which depends on the clinical variant (acute ATLL has the lowest 4-year overall survival at 11% whereas smoldering ATLL has the highest at 52%).
Primary cutaneous CD30+ LPDs: C-ALCL[b]	Solitary or localized, often ulcerated, nodules or tumors that may self-resolve.	Predominantly affects adults with a male predominance. ≥90% 5-year survival (primary C-ALCL).
SPTCL	Solitary and deep-seated erythematous nodules and plaques, often on the extremities.	Median age of diagnosis is 36 years of age. ~80% 5-year survival.
Extranodal NK/T-cell lymphoma, nasal type (includes HV-like CTCL)	Destructive tumors of the central face (especially the nasal cavity).	Associated with EBV. Complications include cytophagic histiocytic panniculitis. <5% 5-year survival.
Primary cutaneous peripheral T-cell lymphoma, rare subtypes: PCGD-TCL	Widespread ulcerated plaques and nodules.	Composed of mature, activated, cytotoxic γ/δ T-cells that produce IL-10. Complications include cytophagic histiocytic panniculitis. <5% 5-year survival.

ATLL, adult T-cell leukemia/lymphoma; C-ALCL, cutaneous anaplastic large cell lymphoma; CD, cluster of differentiation; CTCL, cutaneous T-cell lymphoma; EBV, Epstein-Barr virus; HTLV-1, human T-cell lymphotropic virus-1; HV, hydroa vacciniforme; IL, interleukin; LPDs, lymphoproliferative disorders; LyP, lymphomatoid papulosis; MF, mycosis fungoides; NK, natural killer; PCGD-TCL, primary cutaneous γ/δ T-cell lymphoma; SPTCL, subcutaneous panniculitis-like T-cell lymphoma.
[a]For Sézary syndrome, see below.
[b]For LyP, see below.

Table 5.45. DIAGNOSTIC CRITERIA FOR SEZARY SYNDROME

Diagnostic Criteria for Sézary Syndrome[a]

1. **Genotypic analysis**
    a. Detection of T-cell clonality in peripheral blood (and preferably within skin biopsy)
2. **Flow cytometry**
    a. CD4:CD8 ratio >10
    OR
    b. Loss of T-cell antigens
        i. CD7 loss of CD4+ T-cells > 40%
        ii. CD26 loss of CD4+ T-cells > 30%
3. **Sézary cell count (absolute)**
    a. ≥ 1000/μL Sézary cells in blood

CD, cluster of differentiation.
[a]All 3 of the criteria are required for diagnosis.

LYMPHOMATOID PAPULOSIS

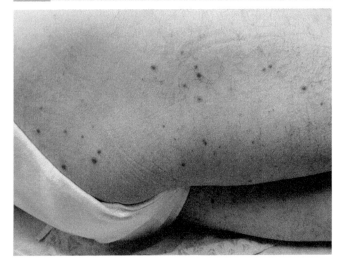

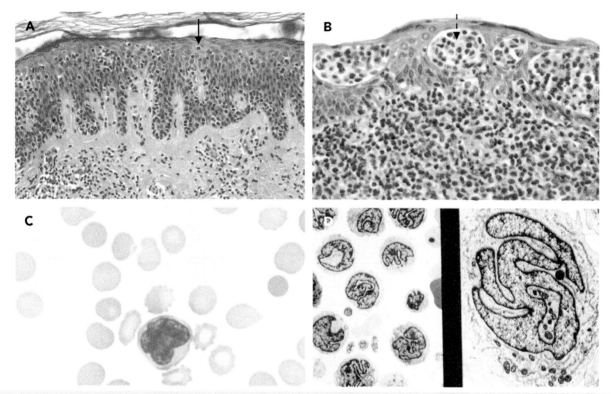

Figure 5.68. CLINICOPATHOLOGICAL CORRELATION: CUTANEOUS T-CELL LYMPHOMA. A, Plaque-stage MF, low-power view. B, Plaque-stage MF, high-power view. Solid arrow: atypical large hyperchromatic lymphocyte with a perinuclear halo ("lump of coal on a pillow") in the epidermis (prominent epidermotropism). Dashed arrow: Pautrier microabscess. C, Sézary cell in the peripheral blood. D, Ultrastructural examination of peripheral blood buffy coat revealing numerous Sézary cells. ALK-1, anaplastic lymphoma-related tyrosine kinase; ATLL, adult T-cell leukemia/lymphoma; C-ALCL, cutaneous anaplastic large cell lymphoma; CD, cluster of differentiation; CTCL, cutaneous T-cell lymphoma; EBV, Epstein-Barr virus; FISH, fluorescence in situ hybridization; HV, hydroa vacciniforme; IHC, immunohistochemistry; LE, lupus erythematosus; LyP, lymphomatoid papulosis; MF, mycosis fungoides; NK, natural killer; PCGD-TCL, primary cutaneous γ/δ T-cell lymphoma; RNA, ribonucleic acid; SPTCL, subcutaneous panniculitis-like T-cell lymphoma; TCR, T-cell receptor; TIA-1, cytotoxic granule associated ribonucleic acid binding protein.

(Histology and electron microscopy images reprinted with permission from Elder DE, Elenitsas R, Rosenbach M, et al. *Lever's Histopathology of the Skin.* 11th ed. Wolters Kluwer; 2015.)

- **MF:** Patch-stage MF is characterized by vacuolar interface dermatitis. In the epidermis, large hyperchromatic atypical T cells with perinuclear haloes (epidermotropism) tend to aggregate and form (Pautrier microabscesses) and there is mild adjacent spongiosis. In the dermis, the superficial perivascular T-cell infiltrate predominates above vessels and there is papillary dermal fibrosis. As MF progresses to plaque and tumor stages, epidermotropism becomes less prominent. The typical IHC pattern is CD2$^+$, CD3$^+$, CD4$^+$, CD8$^-$, CD30$^\pm$, with loss of CD7 > CD5. In tumor stage MF, CD30$^+$ large cell transformation (≥25% of atypical lymphocytes 4 times larger than normal) may occur.

MF Variants:
- **Folliculotropic MF:** minimal to no epidermotropism, atypical T cells in the follicular epithelium, and follicular mucinosis.
- **Pagetoid reticulosis:** prominent epidermotropism. CD4$^-$ and CD8$^+$.
- **Granulomatous slack skin:** variable epidermotropism, numerous atypical T cells in the dermis and/or subcutis with associated edema or fibrosis and admixed large multinucleated giant cells with phagocytosis of atypical T cells and elastic tissue fibers.
- **Sézary syndrome:** minimal to no epidermotropism, atypical Sézary cells with cerebriform nuclei in the superficial perivascular plexus. CD3$^+$, CD4$^+$, CD5$^+$, CD7$^-$, CD30$^\pm$, CD45RO$^+$.

Other CTCL variants:
- **ATLL:** variable epidermotropism, atypical T cells with multilobed nuclei in the dermis and / or subcutis. CD3$^+$, CD4$^+$, CD8$^-$, CD25$^+$.
- **C-ALCL***: numerous large Reed-Sternberg-like cells in the dermis and/or subcutis. CD30$^+$ (>75%). ALK-1 negativity helps distinguish primary C-ALCL from secondary C-ALCL (nodal).
- **LyP:** see below.
- **SPTCL:** resembles LE panniculitis. α/β T-cell phenotype; βF1$^+$, CD4$^-$, CD8$^+$.
- **Extranodal NK/T-cell lymphoma, nasal type** (includes HV-like CTCL): variable epidermotropism, angiocentric atypical T cells in the dermis and / or subcutis with angiodestruction and necrosis. βF1$^+$, CD2$^+$, CD3$^\pm$, CD4$^-$, CD8$^\pm$, CD56$^+$. Cytotoxic phenotype: granzyme B+, perforin+, TIA-1+. FISH for EBV RNA is positive.
- **PCGD-TCL:** variable epidermotropism, atypical T-cells in the dermis and / or subcutis. γ/δ T-cell phenotype; βF1$^-$, CD3$^+$, CD4$^-$, CD8$^-$, CD56$^+$. Cytotoxic phenotype: granzyme B+, perforin+, TIA-1+.

* For LyP, see below.

For all CTCL, TCR gene rearrangement may detect T-cell clonality.

(Figure 5.68 Continued)

The appearance of a hyperchromatic T-cell with a perinuclear halo has been compared to a "lump of coal on a pillow." The "bare underbelly sign" refers to T-cells predominating above vessels.

In pagetoid reticulosis, acral skin is a helpful diagnostic clue.

In ATLL, atypical lymphocytes with multilobed nuclei are called "flower cells."

TCR gene rearrangement is more likely to detect T-cell clonality in SPTCL than LE panniculitis.

The CTCL variants with the poorest prognosis (<5% 5-year survival) have overlapping IHC patterns: CD4- and CD8- (variable for extranodal NK/T-cell lymphoma, nasal type), CD56$^+$, and a cytotoxic phenotype. Remember that "double-negative" is "double trouble."

Table 5.46. INTERNATIONAL SOCIETY FOR CUTANEOUS LYMPHOMAS/EUROPEAN ORGANIZATION OF RESEARCH AND TREATMENT OF CANCER TNMB CLASSIFICATION AND STAGING FOR MYCOSIS FUNGOIDES

T (Skin)

T_1	Patches and plaques covering <10% BSA; may stratify into T_{1a} (patch only) vs T_{1b} (plaque ± patch)
T_2	Patches and plaques covering >10% BSA; may stratify into T_{2a} (patch only) vs T_{2b} (plaque ± patch)
T_3	One or more tumors (≥1 cm)
T_4	Confluent erythema covering >80% BSA

N (Lymph Node)[a]

N_0	No clinically abnormal peripheral lymph nodes; biopsy not required
N_1	Clinically abnormal peripheral lymph nodes, histopathology Dutch grade 1 or NCI LN_{0-2}
N_2	Clinically abnormal peripheral lymph nodes, histopathology Dutch grade 2 or NCI LN_3
N_3	Clinically abnormal peripheral nodes, histopathology Dutch grade 3-4 or NCI LN_4
N_X	Clinically abnormal peripheral lymph nodes; no histologic confirmation

M (Metastasis)

M_0	No visceral metastasis
M_1	Presence of visceral metastasis

B (Blood)

B_0	Absence of significant blood involvement: ≤ 5% peripheral blood lymphocytes are atypical (Sézary) cells
B_1	Low blood tumor burden: >5% peripheral blood lymphocytes are atypical (Sézary) cells, but does not meet B_2 criteria
B_2	High blood tumor burden: ≥1000/μL Sézary cells with positive clone

MF Staging

Stage	T	N	M	B
IA	1	0	0	0,1
IB	2	0	0	0,1
II	1,2	1,2	0	0,1
IIB	3	0-2	0	0,1
III	4	0-2	0	0,1
IIIA	4	0-2	0	0
IIIB	4	0-2	0	1
IVA_1	1-4	0-2	0	2
IVA_2	1-4	3	0	0-2
IVB	1-4	0-3	1	0-2

BSA, body surface area; MF, mycosis fungoides; TNMB, tumor-node-metastasis-blood.
[a]Based on architecture of the node.

- LyP is classified as a **CD30-positive LPD**, and best regarded as a low-grade CTCL. The exact pathogenesis is unclear; however, CD30 is a cytokine receptor belonging to the TNF receptor super-family and is a marker on activated B- and T-cells. LyP is **most common in the fourth decade** but can occur at any age. Parapsoriasis, PL, and LyP are overlapping **clonal T-cell related dermatoses associated with CTCL.** An **antecedent, concomitant, or subsequent lymphoma** may develop in 10% to 20% of patients with LyP, most commonly MF, ALCL, or Hodgkin lymphoma.
- LyP classically presents with **recurrent crops of red-brown papules or nodules favoring the trunk and extremi**ties that ulcerate and spontaneously resolve within 3 to 8 weeks. Lesions can often be found in various stages of healing. They may heal with dyspigmentation or **varioliform scarring.** LyP types are distinguished on histopathology and overlap in the same patients. **Type A is the most common (75%).** Type E is clinically distinctive based on **relatively fewer but larger (up to 4 cm) lesions.**
  - Figure 5.69.
- LyP has an **excellent prognosis.** However, given association with other lymphomas, patients require regular follow-up. Treatment of LyP is difficult. **Phototherapy (nbUVB, UVA1, PUVA, ECP) or methotrexate** can be considered in widespread disease.

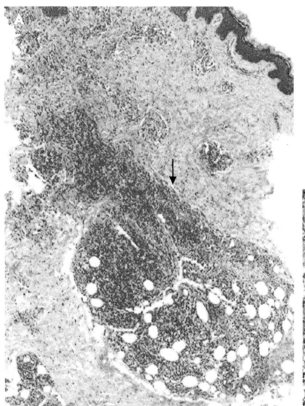

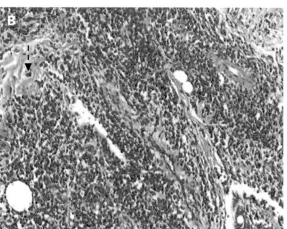

Figure 5.69. CLINICOPATHOLOGICAL CORRELATION: LYMPHOMATOID PAPULOSIS. The histopathology of LyP depends on the type; however, all types may demonstrate CD30 positivity (variable in type B). TCR gene rearrangement may detect T-cell clonality. A, LyP (type A), low-power view. Solid arrow: wedge-shaped dermal infiltrate. B, LyP (type A), high-power view. Dashed arrow: large Reed-Sternberg-like cell. ALCL, anaplastic large cell lymphoma; CD, cluster of differentiation; CD8+ AECTCL, primary cutaneous aggressive epidermotropic CD8+ cytotoxic T-cell lymphoma; LyP, lymphomatoid papulosis; MF, mycosis fungoides; NK, natural killer; TCR, T-cell receptor.

(Histology images reprinted with permission from Edward S, Yung A. *Essential Dermatopathology*. Wolters Kluwer Health/Lippincott Williams & Wilkins; 2011.)

- **Type A:** wedge-shaped dermal infiltrate of large Reed-Sternberg-like cells with admixed neutrophils, eosinophils, and small lymphocytes.
- **Type B:** resembles MF.
- **Type C:** resembles ALCL.
- **Type D:** resembles CD8+ AECTCL.
- **Type E:** resembles extranodal NK / T-cell lymphoma, nasal type.
- **Type 6p25:** 6p25 translocation (*MUM1/IRF4*).

CUTANEOUS B-CELL LYMPHOMA
Diffuse large B-cell lymphoma

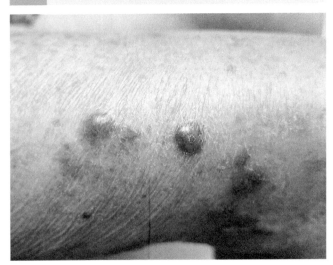

- CBCL is a heterogeneous group of B-cell neoplasms of the skin that vary in clinical phenotype and prognosis. Extra-nodal NHL may occur in the oral cavity, classically as a nonhealing painless ulcer, especially in HIV-infected patients.
- CBCL classically presents with **solitary or grouped, red-purple or plum-colored nodules.** Distribution depends on the variant:
  ○ **Primary cutaneous marginal zone lymphoma (PCMZL)** favors the trunk and extremities.
  ○ **Primary cutaneous follicle center lymphoma (PCFCL)** favors the scalp, forehead, and neck.
  ○ **Primary cutaneous diffuse large B-cell lymphoma, leg type (PCDLBL, LT)** favors the legs.
  ○ **Intravascular large B-cell lymphoma** is a rare CBCL variant that classically presents with noninflammatory retiform purpura favoring the trunk and thighs and neurologic deficits due to CNS involvement at onset.
  Though included in the 2018 update of the WHO-EORTC classification for primary cutaneous lymphomas, the provisional EBV mucocutaneous ulcer is beyond the scope of this chapter. Adenopathy and extensive skin patch overlying a plasmacytoma (AESOP) syndrome refers to a large red to violet-brown patch overlying a plasmacytoma.
  ◆ Figure 5.70.
- Skin biopsy with IHC and clonality analysis is required to diagnose CBCL. Systemic evaluation to rule out secondary CBCL includes LFTs, CBC, LDH, and CT or PET/CT ± bone marrow biopsy.

- The prognosis of CBCL depends on the variant. PCMZL and PCFCL have an indolent course, while PCDLBCL, LT has an intermediate/poor prognosis. Clinical monitoring for low-grade primary CBCL is appropriate. ILK, local radiation therapy, or surgical excision can be considered for low-grade localized disease. Anti-CD20 therapy (rituximab) ± cytotoxic chemotherapy is only necessary for aggressive tumors.

CUTANEOUS LYMPHOID HYPERPLASIA
Synonym: pseudolymphoma of the skin

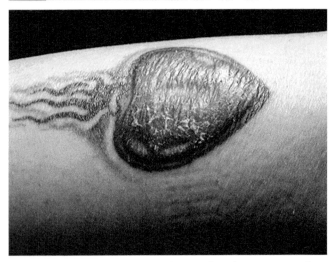

Cutaneous lymphoid hyperplasia at the site of a red tattoo reprinted with permission from Gru AA, Schaffer A. *Hematopathology of the Skin.*

- CLH is a benign lymphoid hyperplasia. Associations include **tattoos, arthropod bites, and mechanical injury.** Drug associations include **aromatic anticonvulsants, lamotrigine, and valproic acid. In Europe, CLH with B-cell predominance** has been associated with ***Borrelia burgdorferi*** infection.
- CLH is clinically indistinguishable from CBCL. It commonly occurs on the face or chest.
  ◆ Figure 5.71.
- **Lymphocytic infiltrate of Jessner,** like CLH, is a benign lymphocytic infiltrate characterized by **annular plaques with central clearing.** It may overlap with LE tumidus and reticular erythematous mucinosis. Skin biopsy with IHC and clonality analysis is required to diagnosis CLH.
- CLH may resolve spontaneously without treatment. Topical or intralesional corticosteroids may be offered as initial treatment. In patients with *B. burgdorferi*-associated CLH, treatment for early Lyme disease should be completed.

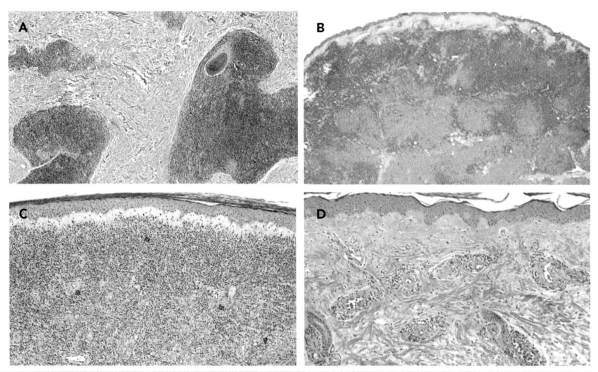

Figure 5.70. CLINICOPATHOLOGICAL CORRELATION: CUTANEOUS B-CELL LYMPHOMA. A, PCMZL. B, PCFCL. C, PCDLCL, LT. D, Intravascular large B-cell lymphoma. BCL2, B-cell lymphoma 2; BCL6, B-cell lymphoma 6; CBCL, cutaneous B-cell lymphoma; CD, cluster of differentiation; CLH, cutaneous lymphoid hyperplasia; IgH, immunoglobulin heavy locus; MUM1, multiple myeloma oncogene 1; PCFCL, primary cutaneous follicle center lymphoma; PCDLCL, LT, primary cutaneous diffuse large B-cell lymphoma, leg-type; PCMZL, primary cutaneous marginal zone lymphoma.

(Histology images reprinted with permission from Elder DE, Elenitsas R, Rosenbach M, et al. *Lever's Histopathology of the Skin*. 11th ed. Wolters Kluwer; 2015.)

- **PCMZL:** pale atypical B cells surrounding dark begin reactive B cells in the dermis and subcutis with a Grenz zone. BCL2+, BCL6−, CD20+, CD79a+. κ or λ restriction.
- **PCFCL:** follicular and / or diffuse pattern of atypical B cells in the dermis and subcutis with a Grenz zone. BCL2−, BCL6+, CD10+ (follicular), CD10− (diffuse), CD20+, CD79a+.
- **PCDLCL, LT:** large atypical B cells in the dermis and subcutis with a Grenz zone. CD20+, CD79a+, MUM1+.
- **Intravascular large B-cell lymphoma:** large atypical B-cells within small vessel lumens. CD20+, CD79a+.

For all CBCL, IgH or Igκ gene rearrangement may detect B-cell clonality.

A "bottom-heavy" architecture suggests CBCL over CLH with B-cell predominance. BCL2 positivity in follicle cell lymphoma should raise suspicion for secondary cutaneous involvement.

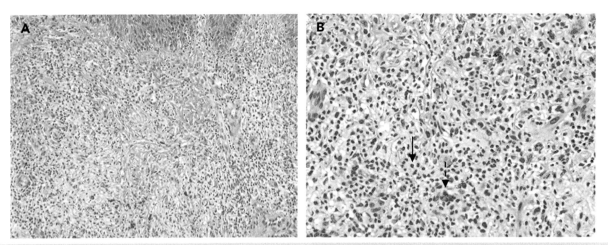

Figure 5.71. CLINICOPATHOLOGICAL CORRELATION: CUTANEOUS LYMPHOID HYPERPLASIA. A, CLH at the site of a red tattoo, low-power view. B, CLH at the site of a red tattoo, high-power view. Solid arrow: lymphohistiocytic infiltrate. Dashed arrow: macrophage containing red tattoo pigment. CBCL, cutaneous B-cell lymphoma; CLH, cutaneous lymphoid hyperplasia; DNA, deoxyribonucleic acid; IgH, immunoglobulin heavy locus; MF, mycosis fungoides; PCR, polymerase chain reaction.

(Histology images courtesy of Michael T. Tetzlaff, MD. From Gru AA, Schaffer A. *Hematopathology of the Skin: A Clinical and Pathologic Approach.* Wolters Kluwer; 2016.)

- CLH with T-cell predominance: resembles CTCL with admixed CD8⁺ cytotoxic/suppressor T cells.
- CLH with B-cell predominance: resembles low-grade CBCL. *Borrelia burgdorferi* DNA PCR is positive in pseudolymphomatous acrodermatitis chronica atrophicans and borrelial lymphocytoma.

TCR gene rearrangement is more likely to detect T-cell clonality in CTCL than CLH with T-cell predominance. IgH or Igκ gene rearrangement is more likely to detect B-cell clonality in CBCL than CLH with B-cell predominance. A "top-heavy" architecture suggests CLH with B-cell predominance over CBCL.

LEUKEMIA CUTIS

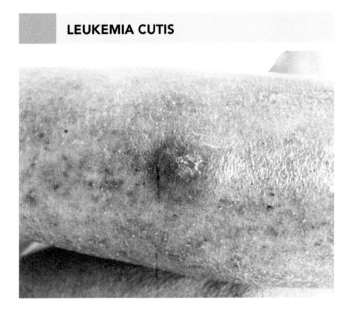

- Leukemia cutis is caused by cutaneous infiltration of malignant leukocytes in patients with preexisting leukemia. It is **most common in CLL and AML, especially acute monocytic leukemia (M5) and acute myelomonocytic leukemia (M4),** and least common in chronic myelogenous leukemia (CML) and acute lymphoblastic leukemia (ALL). **Blastic plasmacytoid dendritic cell neoplasm (BPDCN)** is a precursor hematologic neoplasm **related to AML (~10%-20% of patients).** The cell of origin is a precursor of the CD123⁺ plasmacytoid dendritic cell.
- Leukemia cutis is polymorphic but most commonly presents as a **hemorrhagic, sometimes rubbery, papule, plaque, or nodule.** Myeloid leukemia (**chloroma**) often appears **green due to high MPO levels.** Infiltration of the gingival connective tissue may rarely occur.
  - Figure 5.72.
- Treatment should be directed toward the underlying leukemia.

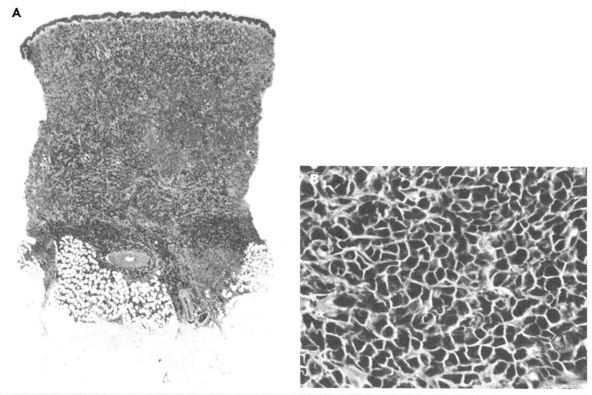

Figure 5.72. CLINICOPATHOLOGICAL CORRELATION: LEUKEMIA CUTIS. Leukemia cutis is characterized by a dense infiltrate of blasts in the dermis and subcutis with a Grenz zone. In AML, blasts have hyperchromatic nuclei and eosinophilic cytoplasm. In ALL, blasts have round or convoluted nuclei with fine chromatin and inconspicuous nucleoli and scant basophilic cytoplasm. Mitoses are frequent. The IHC pattern can be helpful to identify the underlying leukemia. A, Leukemia cutis (AML), low-power view. B, Leukemia cutis (AML), high-power view. ALL, acute lymphoblastic leukemia; AML, acute myeloid leukemia; BPDCN, blastic plasmacytoid dendritic cell neoplasm; CD, cluster of differentiation; CLL, chronic lymphocytic leukemia; CML, chronic myelogenous leukemia; Ig, immunoglobulin; MPO, myeloperoxidase; TdT, terminal deoxynucleotidyl transferase.

(Histology images reprinted with permission from Elder DE, Elenitsas R, Rubin AI, et al. *Atlas of Dermatopathology: Synopsis and Atlas of Lever's Histopathology of the Skin.* 4th ed. Wolters Kluwer; 2020.)

IHC patterns*:
- AML: CD3$^-$, CD20$^-$, CD45$^+$, CD117$^+$ (c-kit), chloroacetate esterase+ (Leder stain), lysozyme+, MPO+.
- ALL: CD10$^+$, CD20$^\pm$, CD22$^+$, CD34$^+$, CD79a$^+$, TdT$^+$.
- BPDCN (precursor hematologic neoplasm related to AML): CD3$^-$, CD4$^+$, CD56$^+$, CD123$^+$, MPO$^-$.

* Flow cytometry and genetic testing are more accurate than skin biopsy IHC in the classification of leukemia cutis.

In AML, blasts often line up in "single file." In ALL, tingible body macrophages create a "starry sky."

SPOTLIGHT ON MASTOCYTOSIS

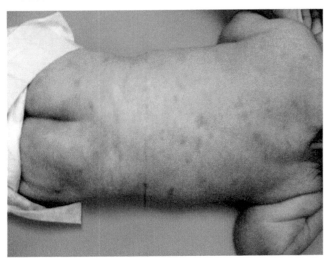

Urticaria pigmentosa reprinted with permission from Gru AA, Wick MR, Mir A, et al. *Pediatric Dermatopathology and Dermatology.* Wolters Kluwer; 2018.

Table 5.47. MASTOCYTOSIS VARIANTS

Diagnosis	Classic Description	Notes
Solitary mastocytoma	Solitary or few tan or yellow-tan papules or nodules with a *peau d'orange* appearance favoring the dorsal hands.	Common in children. May appear as early as 3 months of age and often spontaneously involutes by 10 years of age.
Urticaria pigmentosa	Numerous urticarial, pigmented papules or nodules, which may vesiculate in early disease.	Most common variant in children (60%-90% of childhood cases) and adults. Usually presents within the first few weeks of life.
Diffuse cutaneous mastocytosis	Thick skin with generalized, doughy or leathery texture and hyperpigmentation.	Rare childhood variant. Often presents in the first few months of life.
TMEP	Telangiectatic macules and patches without hyperpigmentation; difficult to elicit the Darier sign.	Rare adult variant.

TMEP, telangiectasia macularis eruptive perstans.

- Mastocytosis refers to the local or systemic proliferation of mast cells. Cutaneous mastocytosis more commonly affects children. Activating mutations in *c-KIT* **proto-oncogene** have been implicated in sporadic adult cases and in children with extensive or persistent disease.
- The characteristic presentation of **mastocytosis variants** is summarized in Table 5.47. **Darier sign**, **urtication with stroking,** is suggestive of the diagnosis of mastocytosis. Symptoms of systemic involvement depend on release of mast cell mediators and particularly affect the vessels, lymph nodes, bone marrow, gastrointestinal tract, liver, spleen, and respiratory tract. These symptoms include pruritus, urticaria, angioedema, anaphylaxis, flushing, abdominal cramps, nausea, vomiting, and respiratory distress.
  - ◆ **Urticaria pigmentosa is the most common mastocytosis variant in adults.** Systemic involvement is more common in adults than children. **Telangiectasia macularis eruptiva perstans (TMEP)** is a rare mastocytosis variant in adults associated with systemic involvement.
  - ◇ Do NOT confuse the "<u>Darier</u> sign" of mastocytosis with <u>Darier</u> disease.
  - ◆ Figure 5.73.
- Evaluation of suspected mastocytosis includes CBC and **tryptase.**
- Avoidance of mast cell degranulators is recommended. There is a risk of mast cell degranulation with certain general anesthetics (ie, atracurium/mivacurium, thiopental); **propofol is a safe choice.** Treatment of mastocytosis is only necessary if symptomatic (topical corticosteroids, oral antihistamines). **Imatinib** is appropriate in select cases of systemic mastocytosis.

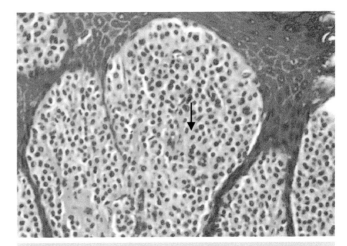

Figure 5.73. CLINICOPATHOLOGICAL CORRELATION: MASTOCYTOSIS. Macular mastocytosis and TMEP are characterized by a superficial perivascular mast cell infiltrate (≥5 mast cells around each vessel). Some mast cells are hyperchromatic and spindle-shaped. Nodular mastocytosis is characterized by mast cell aggregates in the papillary ± reticular dermis and subcutis. Subepidermal bullae, basal layer hyperpigmentation, and eosinophils are variable. CD117 (c-kit)+, chloroacetate esterase (Leder stain)+, and tryptase+. Metachromatic staining of granules with Giemsa or toluidine blue may identify mast cells that have not degranulated. Urticaria pigmentosa. Solid arrow: mast cells with a "fried egg" appearance. CD, cluster of differentiation; IHC, immunohistochemistry; TMEP, telangiectasia macularis eruptiva perstans. (Histology image reprinted with permission from Elder DE, Elenitsas R, Rosenbach M, et al. *Lever's Histopathology of the Skin.* 11th ed. Wolters Kluwer; 2015.)

Mast cells have a "fried egg" appearance.

SOLID ORGAN METASTASIS

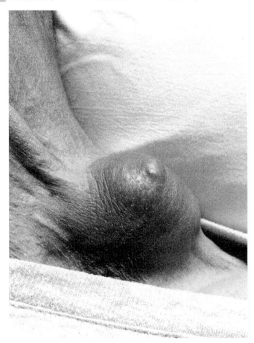

Hepatocellular carcinoma metastasis to Virchow's node courtesy of Megan Noe, MD, MPH, MSCE.

- Solid organ metastases to the skin are rare. For **women**, the most common underlying malignancy is **breast adenocarcinoma;** for **men** the most common underlying malignancy is **lung carcinoma (>40 years of age) or melanoma (<40 years of age).**
- Cutaneous solid organ metastases classically present as **rapidly growing, firm nodules** with various shades of colors. They often arise in the anatomic vicinity of the primary cancer. ***Carcinoma en cuirasse*** is a rare and striking form of cutaneous metastasis (most commonly breast adenocarcinoma) involving the chest wall, which presents as **induration with a *peau d'orange* appearance.** Solid organ metastases to the scalp may be associated with secondary **scarring alopecia (alopecia neoplastica).**
  - Histopathological features of solid organ metastases are summarized in Table 5.48. Of note, endometriosis may mimic a solid organ metastasis on histopathology but shows glandular spaces and a loose concentric fibromyxoid stroma with erythrocytes ± hemosiderin and large polygonal decidual cells (decidualized endometriosis).
  - Figure 5.74.
- Cutaneous solid organ metastases often portend a poor prognosis. Treatment options include antineoplastics, palliative radiation therapy, and surgical excision.

Table 5.48. HISTOPATHOLOGICAL FEATURES OF SOLID ORGAN METASTASES

Diagnosis[a]	Histopathological Features	Notes
SCC	Atypical keratinocytes in the dermis (usually lacks epidermal connection). Pan-CK+, EMA+.	Most commonly originates from oral cavity, esophagus, or lung.
Colon adenocarcinoma	Irregular but relatively well-formed glands. CEA⁺, CDX2⁺, CK7⁻, CK20⁺. CK7 is variably positive in rectal adenocarcinoma. Contains sialomucin (mucicarmine+; PAS+ diastase resistant).	Gastric > colon adenocarcinoma may cause a signet-ring pattern: atypical cells with central pale mucin compressing the nucleus to the periphery.
Thyroid carcinoma	Papillary: fronds of atypical cells ± psammoma bodies (concentric calcifications) and large nuclei with pale centers and pseudoinclusions. Follicular: Thyroid follicles with colloid. Medullary: Sheets of atypical cells with amyloid. Thyroglobulin+, TTF-1+. Calcitonin+ (medullary).	Frequency: papillary > follicular > medullary.
	Large nuclei with pale centers are called "Orphan Annie" nuclei.	
RCC	Atypical cells, often clear due to glycogen (PAS positive, diastase sensitive), with prominent capillaries in the stroma. CD10⁺, RCC⁺.	Due to prominent capillaries in the stroma, RCC may clinically masquerade as a PG.
Breast adenocarcinoma	Highly variable architecture, often with atypical cells infiltrating through dermal collagen bundles with ill-defined attempts at acinus formation. CEA⁺, CK7⁺, CK20⁻, EMA⁺, ER/PR ±, GCDFP-15⁺.	Breast adenocarcinoma may cause a signet-ring pattern.
	Atypical cells often line up in "single file."	
Ovarian adenocarcinoma	Atypical cells with papillary fronding ± psammoma bodies (concentric calcifications). CA-125⁺. Mucinous ovarian adenocarcinoma: CK7⁺ and CK20⁺. Contains sialomucin (mucicarmine+; PAS⁺ diastase resistant).	

(Continued)

Table 5.48. HISTOPATHOLOGICAL FEATURES OF SOLID ORGAN METASTASES CONTINUED

Diagnosis[a]	Histopathological Features	Notes
Prostate adenocarcinoma	Atypical cells infiltrating through dermal collagen bundles. PSA[+].	
Lung carcinoma	NSCLC (lung adenocarcinoma): irregular but relatively well-formed glands. SCLC (oat cell carcinoma): small blue cells with scant cytoplasm and round nuclei. SCC of the lung: see above. CEA[+], CK7[+], CK20[−]. TTF-1[+] (SCLC).	

As a general rule, CK7 is positive above the diaphragm and CK20 is positive below the diaphragm.

CA-125, cancer antigen 125; CD, cluster of differentiation; CDX2, caudal-type homeobox 2; CEA, carcinoembryonic antigen; CK, cytokeratin; EMA, epithelial membrane antigen; ER, estrogen receptor; GCDFP-15, gross cystic disease fluid protein 15; NSCLC, non–small cell lung carcinoma; PAS, periodic acid-Schiff; PG, pyogenic granuloma; PR, progesterone receptor; PSA, prostate specific antigen; RCC, renal cell carcinoma; SCC, squamous cell carcinoma; SCLC, small cell lung carcinoma; TTF-1, thyroid transcription factor 1.
[a]Illustrative examples provided.

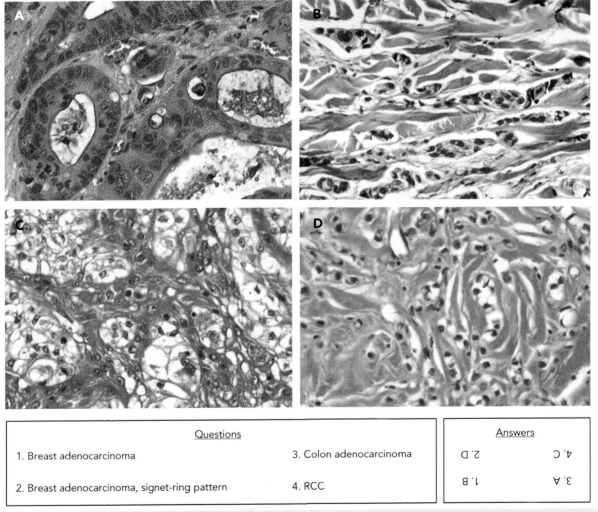

Questions		Answers	
1. Breast adenocarcinoma	3. Colon adenocarcinoma	2. D	4. C
2. Breast adenocarcinoma, signet-ring pattern	4. RCC	1. B	3. A

Figure 5.74. MATCHING EXERCISE: SOLID ORGAN METASTASES. A, Colon adenocarcinoma. Note the irregular but relatively well-formed glands. B, Breast adenocarcinoma. Note the cords of atypical cells with ill-defined attempts at acinus formation ("single filing"). C, RCC. Note the clear glycogenated cells (PAS positive, diastase resistant) with prominent capillaries in the stroma. D, Breast adenocarcinoma, signet-ring pattern. Note the atypical cells with central pale mucin compressing the nucleus to the periphery. PAS, periodic acid-Schiff; RCC, renal cell carcinoma.

(Histology images reprinted with permission from Elder DE, Elenitsas R, Rosenbach M, et al. *Lever's Histopathology of the Skin.* 11th ed. Wolters Kluwer; 2015.)

FURTHER READING

Adefusika et al., 2015 Adefusika JA, Pimentel JD, Chavan RN, Brewer JD. Primary mucinous carcinoma of the skin: the Mayo Clinic experience over the past 2 decades. *Dermatol Surg.* 2015;41(2):201-208. doi:10.1097/dss.0000000000000198

Al Ghazal P, Grönemeyer LL, Schön MP. Lipomatoses. *J Dtsch Dermatol Ges.* 2018;16(3):313-327. doi:10.1111/ddg.13460

Alikhan A, Ibrahimi OA, Eisen DB. Congenital melanocytic nevi: where are we now? Part I. Clinical presentation, epidemiology, pathogenesis, histology, malignant transformation, and neurocutaneous melanosis. *J Am Acad Dermatol.* 2012;67(4):495.e1-17. quiz 512-4. doi:10.1016/j.jaad.2012.06.023

Allen A, Ahn C, Sangüeza OP. Dermatofibrosarcoma protuberans. *Dermatol Clin.* 2019;37(4):483-488. doi:10.1016/j.det.2019.05.006

Ansai SI. Topics in histopathology of sweat gland and sebaceous neoplasms. *J Dermatol.* 2017;44(3):315-326. doi:10.1111/1346-8138.13555

Atzmony L, Lim YH, Hamilton C, et al. Topical cholesterol/lovastatin for the treatment of porokeratosis: a pathogenesis-directed therapy. *J Am Acad Dermatol.* 2020;82(1):123-131. doi:10.1016/j.jaad.2019.08.043

Barrios DM, Do MH, Phillips GS, et al. Immune checkpoint inhibitors to treat cutaneous malignancies. *J Am Acad Dermatol.* 2020;83(5):1239-1253. doi:10.1016/j.jaad.2020.03.131

Bartsch O, Labonté J, Albrecht B, et al. Two patients with EP300 mutations and facial dysmorphism different from the classic Rubinstein-Taybi syndrome. *Am J Med Genet.* 2010;152a(1):181-184. doi:10.1002/ajmg.a.33153

Bayer-Garner IB, Givens V, Smoller B. Immunohistochemical staining for androgen receptors: a sensitive marker of sebaceous differentiation. *Am J Dermatopathol.* 1999;21(5):426-431. doi:10.1097/00000372-199910000-00004

Bayrak-Toydemir P, McDonald J, Akarsu N, et al. A fourth locus for hereditary hemorrhagic telangiectasia maps to chromosome 7. *Am J Med Genet.* 2006;140(20):2155-2162. doi:10.1002/ajmg.a.31450

Bennett KL, Mester J, Eng C. Germline epigenetic regulation of KILLIN in Cowden and Cowden-like syndrome. *JAMA.* 2010;304(24):2724-2731. doi:10.1001/jama.2010.1877.

Betti M, Aspesi A, Biasi A, et al. CDKN2A and BAP1 germline mutations predispose to melanoma and mesothelioma. *Cancer Lett.* 2016;378(2):120-130. doi:10.1016/j.canlet.2016.05.011

Bichakjian CK, Olencki T, Aasi SZ, et al. Basal cell skin cancer, version 1.2016, NCCN clinical practice guidelines in oncology. *J Natl Compr Canc Netw.* 2016;14(5):574-597. doi:10.6004/jnccn.2016.0065

Bieber AK, Martires KJ, Driscoll MS, Grant-Kels JM, Pomeranz MK, Stein JA. Nevi and pregnancy. *J Am Acad Dermatol.* 2016;75(4):661-666. doi:10.1016/j.jaad.2016.01.060

Bolognia JL, Schaffer JV, Cerroni L. *Dermatology.* 4th ed. Elsevier Saunders; 2018.

Cai ED, Sun BK, Chiang A, et al. Postzygotic mutations in Beta-actin are associated with Becker's nevus and Becker's nevus syndrome. *J Invest Dermatol.* 2017;137(8):1795-1798. doi:10.1016/j.jid.2017.03.017

Cameron MC, Lee E, Hibler BP, et al. Basal cell carcinoma: epidemiology; pathophysiology; clinical and histological subtypes; and disease associations. *J Am Acad Dermatol.* 2019;80(2):303-317. doi:10.1016/j.jaad.2018.03.060

Cameron MC, Lee E, Hibler BP, et al. Basal cell carcinoma: contemporary approaches to diagnosis, treatment, and prevention. *J Am Acad Dermatol.* 2019;80(2):321-339. doi:10.1016/j.jaad.2018.02.083

Cetta F, Curia MC, Montalto G, et al. Thyroid carcinoma usually occurs in patients with familial adenomatous polyposis in the absence of biallelic inactivation of the adenomatous polyposis coli gene. *J Clin Endocrinol Metab.* 2001;86(1):427-432. doi:10.1210/jcem.86.1.7095

Chen LL, Jaimes N, Barker CA, Busam KJ, Marghoob AA. Desmoplastic melanoma: a review. *J Am Acad Dermatol.* 2013;68(5):825-833. doi:10.1016/j.jaad.2012.10.041

Chen AC, Martin AJ, Choy B, et al. A phase 3 Randomized trial of nicotinamide for skin-cancer chemoprevention. *N Engl J Med.* 2015;373(17):1618-1626. doi:10.1056/NEJMoa1506197

Cinotti E, Veronesi G, Labeille B, et al. Imaging technique for the diagnosis of onychomatricoma. *J Eur Acad Dermatol Venereol.* 2018;32(11):1874-1878. doi:10.1111/jdv.15108

Clarke CA, Robbins HA, Tatalovich Z, et al. Risk of merkel cell carcinoma after solid organ transplantation. *J Natl Cancer Inst.* 2015;107(2):dju382. doi:10.1093/jnci/dju382

Claudia M, Astrid H, Cozzani E, Cabiddu F, Guadagno A, Parodi A. Unilateral nevoid telangiectasia: a rare and underdiagnosed skin disease. *Eur J Dermatol.* 2020;30(5):601-602. doi:10.1684/ejd.2020.3867

Coggshall K, Tello TL, North JP, Yu SS. Merkel cell carcinoma: an update and review – pathogenesis, diagnosis, and staging. *J Am Acad Dermatol.* 2018;78(3):433-442. doi:10.1016/j.jaad.2017.12.001

Compton LA, Murphy GF, Lian CG. Diagnostic immunohistochemistry in cutaneous neoplasia: an update. *Dermatopathology (Basel).* 2015;2(1):15-42. doi:10.1159/000377698

Cornejo CM, Jambusaria-Pahlajani A, Willenbrink TJ, Schmults CD, Arron ST, Ruiz ES. Field cancerization: treatment. *J Am Acad Dermatol.* 2020;83(3):719-730. doi:10.1016/j.jaad.2020.03.127

Crane JS, Rutt V, Oakley AM. *Birt Hogg Dube Syndrome.* StatPearls Publishing LLC.; 2021. StatPearls. StatPearls Publishing Copyright © 2021.

Cribier B, Scrivener Y, Grosshans E. Tumors arising in nevus sebaceus: a study of 596 cases. *J Am Acad Dermatol.* 2000;42(2 pt 1):263-268. doi:10.1016/s0190-9622(00)90136-1

Cunningham TJ, Tabacchi M, Eliane JP, et al. Randomized trial of calcipotriol combined with 5-fluorouracil for skin cancer precursor immunotherapy. *J Clin Invest.* 2017;127(1):106-116. doi:10.1172/jci89820

Curry JL, Torres-Cabala CA, Kim KB, et al. Dermatologic toxicities to targeted cancer therapy: shared clinical and histologic adverse skin reactions. *Int J Dermatol.* 2014;53(3):376-384. doi:10.1111/ijd.12205

Davis LE, Shalin SC, Tackett AJ. Current state of melanoma diagnosis and treatment. *Cancer Biol Ther.* 2019;20(11):1366-1379. doi:10.1080/15384047.2019.1640032

Dika E, Ravaioli GM, Fanti PA, Neri I, Patrizi A. Spitz nevi and other spitzoid neoplasms in children: overview of incidence data and diagnostic criteria. *Pediatr Dermatol.* 2017;34(1):25-32. doi:10.1111/pde.13025

Driscoll MS, Martires K, Bieber AK, Pomeranz MK, Grant-Kels JM, Stein JA. Pregnancy and melanoma. *J Am Acad Dermatol.* 2016;75(4):669-678. doi:10.1016/j.jaad.2016.01.061

Duffy K, Grossman D. The dysplastic nevus: from historical perspective to management in the modern era – part II. Molecular aspects and clinical management. *J Am Acad Dermatol.* 2012;67(1):19.e1-12. quiz 31-2. doi:10.1016/j.jaad.2012.03.013

Duffy K, Grossman D. The dysplastic nevus: from historical perspective to management in the modern era – part I. Historical, histologic, and clinical aspects. *J Am Acad Dermatol.* 2012;67(1):1.e1-16. quiz 17-8. doi:10.1016/j.jaad.2012.02.047

Durgin JS, Weiner DM, Wysocka M, Rook AH. The immunopathogenesis and immunotherapy of cutaneous T cell lymphoma: pathways and targets for immune restoration and tumor eradication. *J Am Acad Dermatol.* 2021;84(3):587-595. doi:10.1016/j.jaad.2020.12.027

Eisen DB, Michael DJ. Sebaceous lesions and their associated syndromes: part II. *J Am Acad Dermatol.* 2009;61(4):563-578. quiz 579-80. doi:10.1016/j.jaad.2009.04.059

Eisen DB, Michael DJ. Sebaceous lesions and their associated syndromes: part I. *J Am Acad Dermatol.* 2009;61(4):549-560. quiz 561-2. doi:10.1016/j.jaad.2009.04.058

Elder DE. *Lever's Histopathology of the Skin.* 11th ed. Wolters Kluwer; 2015.

Elston DM, Ferringer T. *Dermatopathology.* 2nd ed. Elsevier Saunders; 2014.

Eng C. Will the real Cowden syndrome please stand up: revised diagnostic criteria. *J Med Genet.* 2000;37(11):828-830. doi:10.1136/jmg.37.11.828

Ferrara G, Gianotti R, Cavicchini S, Salviato T, Zalaudek I, Argenziano G. Spitz nevus, Spitz tumor, and spitzoid melanoma: a comprehensive clinicopathologic overview. *Dermatol Clin.* 2013;31(4):589-598. viii. doi:10.1016/j.det.2013.06.012

Firsowicz M, Boyd M, Jacks SK. Follicular occlusion disorders in Down syndrome patients. *Pediatr Dermatol.* 2020;37(1):219-221. doi:10.1111/pde.14012

Fox MC, Lao CD, Schwartz JL, Frohm ML, Bichakjian CK, Johnson TM. Management options for metastatic melanoma in the era of novel therapies—a primer for the practicing dermatologist—part II: management of stage IV disease. *J Am Acad Dermatol.* 2013;68(1):13.e1-13. quiz 26-8. doi:10.1016/j.jaad.2012.09.041

Fox MC, Lao CD, Schwartz JL, Frohm ML, Bichakjian CK, Johnson TM. Management options for metastatic melanoma in the era of novel therapies: a primer for the practicing dermatologist—part I—management of stage III disease. *J Am Acad Dermatol.* 2013;68(1):1.e1-9. quiz 10-12. doi:doi:10.1016/j.jaad.2012.09.040.

Gardner LJ, Strunck JL, Wu YP, Grossman D. Current controversies in early-stage melanoma: questions on incidence, screening, and histologic regression. *J Am Acad Dermatol.* 2019;80(1):1-12. doi:10.1016/j.jaad.2018.03.053

Garzon MC, Epstein LG, Heyer GL, et al. PHACE syndrome: consensus-derived diagnosis and care recommendations. *J Pediatr.* 2016;178:24-33. e2. doi:10.1016/j.jpeds.2016.07.054

Gibney GT, Messina JL, Fedorenko IV, Sondak VK, Smalley KSM. Paradoxical oncogenesis—the long-term effects of BRAF inhibition in melanoma. *Nat Rev Clin Oncol.* 2013;10(7):390-399. doi:10.1038/nrclinonc.2013.83

Giordano CN, Yew YW, Spivak G, Lim HW. Understanding photodermatoses associated with defective DNA repair: syndromes with cancer predisposition. *J Am Acad Dermatol.* 2016;75(5):855-870. doi:10.1016/j.jaad.2016.03.045

Higgins HW II, Lee KC, Galan A, Leffell DJ. Melanoma in situ: Part II. Histopathology, treatment, and clinical management. *J Am Acad Dermatol.* 2015;73(2):193-203. quiz 203-204. doi:10.1016/j.jaad.2015.03.057

Higgins HW II, Lee KC, Galan A, Leffell DJ. Melanoma in situ: part I. Epidemiology, screening, and clinical features. *J Am Acad Dermatol.* 2015;73(2):181-190. quiz 191-2. doi:10.1016/j.jaad.2015.04.014

Humphrey SR, Hu X, Adamson K, Schaus A, Jensen JN, Drolet B. A practical approach to the evaluation and treatment of an infant with aplasia cutis congenita. *J Perinatol.* 2018;38(2):110-117. doi:10.1038/jp.2017.142

Humphreys TR, Nemeth A, McCrevey S, Baer SC, Goldberg LH. A pilot study comparing toluidine blue and hematoxylin and eosin staining of basal cell and squamous cell carcinoma during Mohs surgery. *Dermatol Surg.* 1996;22(8):693-697. doi:10.1111/j.1524-4725.1996.tb00619.x

Humphreys TR, Shah K, Wysong A, Lexa F, MacFarlane D. The role of imaging in the management of patients with nonmelanoma skin cancer: when is imaging necessary? *J Am Acad Dermatol.* 2017;76(4):591-607. doi:10.1016/j.jaad.2015.10.009

Ibrahimi OA, Alikhan A, Eisen DB. Congenital melanocytic nevi: where are we now? Part II. Treatment options and approach to treatment. *J Am Acad Dermatol.* 2012;67(4):515.e1-515.e13. quiz 528-30. doi:10.1016/j.jaad.2012.06.022

Jabbour S, Kechichian E, Haber R, Tomb R, Nasr M. Management of digital mucous cysts: a systematic review and treatment algorithm. *Int J Dermatol.* 2017;56(7):701-708. doi:10.1111/ijd.13583

Jacks SK, Witman PM. Tuberous sclerosis complex: an update for dermatologists. *Pediatr Dermatol.* 2015;32(5):563-570. doi:10.1111/pde.12567

Jackson JM, Alexis A, Berman B, Berson DS, Taylor S, Weiss JS. Current understanding of seborrheic keratosis: prevalence, etiology, clinical presentation, diagnosis, and management. *J Drugs Dermatol.* 2015;14(10):1119-1125.

Jaju PD, Ransohoff KJ, Tang JY, Sarin KY. Familial skin cancer syndromes: increased risk of nonmelanotic skin cancers and extracutaneous tumors. *J Am Acad Dermatol.* 2016;74(3):437-451. quiz 452-4. doi:10.1016/j.jaad.2015.08.073

Jakobiec FA, Werdich X. Androgen receptor identification in the diagnosis of eyelid sebaceous carcinomas. *Am J Ophthalmol.* 2014;157(3):687-696. e1-2. doi:10.1016/j.ajo.2013.12.009

James WD, Elston DM, Treat JR, Rosenbach MA, Neuhaus IM. *Andrews' Diseases of the Skin: Clinical Dermatology.* 13th ed. Elsevier; 2020.

Jawed SI, Myskowski PL, Horwitz S, Moskowitz A, Querfeld C. Primary cutaneous T-cell lymphoma (mycosis fungoides and Sezary syndrome): part II. Prognosis, management, and future directions. *J Am Acad Dermatol.* 2014;70(2):223.e1-17. quiz 240-2. doi:10.1016/j.jaad.2013.08.033

Jawed SI, Myskowski PL, Horwitz S, Moskowitz A, Querfeld C. Primary cutaneous T-cell lymphoma (mycosis fungoides and Sezary syndrome): part I. Diagnosis—clinical and histopathologic features and new molecular and biologic markers. *J Am Acad Dermatol.* 2014;70(2):205.e1-205.e16. quiz 221-2. doi:10.1016/j.jaad.2013.07.049

Jensen DK, Villumsen A, Skytte AB, Madsen MG, Sommerlund M, Bendstrup E. Birt-Hogg-Dubé syndrome: a case report and a review of the literature. *Eur Clin Respir J.* 2017;4(1):1292378. doi:10.1080/20018525.2017.1292378

John AM, Schwartz RA. Muir-Torre syndrome (MTS): an update and approach to diagnosis and management. *J Am Acad Dermatol.* 2016;74(3):558-566. doi:10.1016/j.jaad.2015.09.074

John AM, Schwartz RA. Basal cell naevus syndrome: an update on genetics and treatment. *Br J Dermatol.* 2016;174(1):68-76. doi:10.1111/bjd.14206

Juhn E, Khachemoune A. Gardner syndrome: skin manifestations, differential diagnosis and management. *Am J Clin Dermatol.* 2010;11(2):117-122. doi:10.2165/11311180-000000000-00000

Kankkunen A, Thiringer K. Hearing impairment in connection with pre-auricular tags. *Acta Paediatr Scand.* 1987;76(1):143-146. doi:10.1111/j.1651-2227.1987.tb10431.x

Katsuya H, Ishitsuka K, Utsunomiya A, et al. Treatment and survival among 1594 patients with ATL. *Blood.* 2015;126(24):2570-2577. doi:10.1182/blood-2015-03-632489

Keung EZ, Gershenwald JE. The eighth edition American Joint Committee on Cancer (AJCC) melanoma staging system: implications for melanoma treatment and care. *Expert Rev Anticancer Ther.* 2018;18(8):775-784. doi:10.1080/14737140.2018.1489246

Kim SJ, Thompson AK, Zubair AS, et al. Surgical treatment and outcomes of patients with extramammary Paget disease: a cohort study. *Dermatol Surg.* 2017;43(5):708-714. doi:10.1097/dss.0000000000001051

Kim CC, Berry EG, Marchetti MA, et al. Risk of subsequent cutaneous melanoma in moderately dysplastic nevi excisionally biopsied but with positive histologic margins. *JAMA Dermatol.* 2018;154(12):1401-1408. doi:10.1001/jamadermatol.2018.3359.

Klapperich ME, Bowen GM, Grossman D. Current controversies in early-stage melanoma: questions on management and surveillance. *J Am Acad Dermatol.* 2019;80(1):15-25. doi:10.1016/j.jaad.2018.03.054

Krooks J, Minkov M, Weatherall AG. Langerhans cell histiocytosis in children: history, classification, pathobiology, clinical manifestations, and prognosis. *J Am Acad Dermatol.* 2018;78(6):1035-1044. doi:10.1016/j.jaad.2017.05.059

Krooks J, Minkov M, Weatherall AG. Langerhans cell histiocytosis in children: diagnosis, differential diagnosis, treatment, sequelae, and standardized follow-up. *J Am Acad Dermatol.* 2018;78(6):1047-1056. doi:10.1016/j.jaad.2017.05.060

Krowchuk DP, Frieden IJ, Mancini AJ, et al. Clinical practice guideline for the management of infantile hemangiomas. *Pediatrics.* 2019;143(1):e20183475. doi:10.1542/peds.2018-3475

Kugelman A, Hadad B, Ben-David J, Podoshin L, Borochowitz Z, Bader D. Preauricular tags and pits in the newborn: the role of hearing tests. *Acta Paediatr.* 1997;86(2):170-172. doi:10.1111/j.1651-2227.1997.tb08860.x

Lazar AJF, Lyle S, Calonje E. Sebaceous neoplasia and Torre-Muir syndrome. *Curr Diagn Pathol.* 2007;13(4):301-319. doi:10.1016/j.cdip.2007.05.001

Luo S, Sepehr A, Tsao H. Spitz nevi and other Spitzoid lesions part II. Natural history and management. *J Am Acad Dermatol.* 2011;65(6):1087-1092. doi:10.1016/j.jaad.2011.06.045

Luo S, Sepehr A, Tsao H. Spitz nevi and other Spitzoid lesions part I. Background and diagnoses. *J Am Acad Dermatol.* 2011;65(6):1073-1084. doi:10.1016/j.jaad.2011.04.040

MacFarlane D, Shah K, Wysong A, Wortsman X, Humphreys TR. The role of imaging in the management of patients with nonmelanoma skin cancer: diagnostic modalities and applications. *J Am Acad Dermatol.* 2017;76(4):579-588. doi:10.1016/j.jaad.2015.10.010

Mantri MD, Pradeep MM, Kalpesh PO, Pranavsinh RJ. Hyaline fibromatosis syndrome: a rare inherited disorder. *Indian J Dermatol.* 2016;61(5):580. doi:10.4103/0019-5154.190129

March J, Hand M, Grossman D. Practical application of new technologies for melanoma diagnosis: part I. Noninvasive approaches. *J Am Acad Dermatol.* 2015;72(6):929-941. quiz 941-2. doi:10.1016/j.jaad.2015.02.1138

March J, Hand M, Truong A, Grossman D. Practical application of new technologies for melanoma diagnosis: part II. Molecular approaches.

J Am Acad Dermatol. 2015;72(6):943-958. quiz 959-60. doi:10.1016/j.jaad.2015.02.1140

Marque M, Roubertie A, Jaussent A, et al. Nevus anemicus in neurofibromatosis type 1: a potential new diagnostic criterion. *J Am Acad Dermatol.* 2013;69(5):768-775. doi:10.1016/j.jaad.2013.06.039

Mayer JE, Swetter SM, Fu T, Geller AC. Screening, early detection, education, and trends for melanoma: current status (2007-2013) and future directions—part II. Screening, education, and future directions. *J Am Acad Dermatol.* 2014;71(4):611.e1-611.e10. quiz 621-622. doi:10.1016/j.jaad.2014.05.045

Mayer JE, Swetter SM, Fu T, Geller AC. Screening, early detection, education, and trends for melanoma: current status (2007-2013) and future directions—part I. Epidemiology, high-risk groups, clinical strategies, and diagnostic technology. *J Am Acad Dermatol.* 2014;71(4):599.e1-599.e12. quiz 610, 599.e12. doi:10.1016/j.jaad.2014.05.046

McDonald NM, Ramos GP, Sweetser S. SMAD4 mutation and the combined juvenile polyposis and hereditary hemorrhage telangiectasia syndrome: a single center experience. *Int J Colorectal Dis.* 2020;35(10):1963-1965. doi:10.1007/s00384-020-03670-3

McGinty S, Siddiqui WJ. *Keloid.* StatPearls Publishing LLC; 2021. StatPearls Publishing Copyright © 2021.

Mehta-Shah N, Horwitz SM, Ansell S, et al. NCCN guidelines insights: primary cutaneous lymphomas, version 2.2020. *J Natl Compr Canc Netw.* 2020;18(5):522-536. doi:10.6004/jnccn.2020.0022

Micali G, Lacarrubba F, Nasca MR, Ferraro S, Schwartz RA. Topical pharmacotherapy for skin cancer: part II. Clinical applications. *J Am Acad Dermatol.* 2014;70(6):979.e1-12. quiz 9912. doi:10.1016/j.jaad.2013.12.037

Morris CR, Hurst EA. Extramammary Paget's disease: a review of the literature part II—treatment and prognosis. *Dermatol Surg.* 2020;46(3):305-311. doi:10.1097/dss.0000000000002240

Moshiri AS, Doumani R, Yelistratova L, et al. Polyomavirus-negative merkel cell carcinoma: a more aggressive subtype based on analysis of 282 cases using multimodal tumor virus detection. *J Invest Dermatol.* 2017;137(4):819-827. doi:10.1016/j.jid.2016.10.028

Olsen E, Vonderheid E, Pimpinelli N, et al. Revisions to the staging and classification of mycosis fungoides and Sezary syndrome: a proposal of the International Society for Cutaneous Lymphomas (ISCL) and the cutaneous lymphoma task force of the European Organization of Research and Treatment of Cancer (EORTC). *Blood.* 2007;110(6):1713-1722. doi:10.1182/blood-2007-03-055749

O'Reilly Zwald F, Brown M. Skin cancer in solid organ transplant recipients: advances in therapy and management—part II. Management of skin cancer in solid organ transplant recipients. *J Am Acad Dermatol.* 2011;65(2):263-279. doi:10.1016/j.jaad.2010.11.063

O'Reilly Zwald F, Brown M. Skin cancer in solid organ transplant recipients: advances in therapy and management – part I. Epidemiology of skin cancer in solid organ transplant recipients. *J Am Acad Dermatol.* 2011;65(2):253-261. doi:10.1016/j.jaad.2010.11.062

Paradisi A, Abeni D, Rusciani A, et al. Dermatofibrosarcoma protuberans: wide local excision vs. Mohs micrographic surgery. *Cancer Treat Rev.* 2008;34(8):728-736. doi:10.1016/j.ctrv.2008.06.002

Patel VM, Handler MZ, Schwartz RA, Lambert WC. Hereditary leiomyomatosis and renal cell cancer syndrome: an update and review. *J Am Acad Dermatol.* 2017;77(1):149-158. doi:10.1016/j.jaad.2017.01.023

Paulson KG, Iyer JG, Blom A, et al. Systemic immune suppression predicts diminished Merkel cell carcinoma-specific survival independent of stage. *J Invest Dermatol.* 2013;133(3):642-646. doi:10.1038/jid.2012.388

Perrin C, Baran R, Pisani A, Ortonne JP, Michiels JF. The onychomatricoma: additional histologic criteria and immunohistochemical study. *Am J Dermatopathol.* 2002;24(3):199-203. doi:10.1097/00000372-200206000-00002

Phan GQ, Messina JL, Sondak VK, Zager JS. Sentinel lymph node biopsy for melanoma: indications and rationale. *Cancer Control.* 2009;16(3):234-239. doi:10.1177/107327480901600305

Que SKT, Zwald FO, Schmults CD. Cutaneous squamous cell carcinoma: incidence, risk factors, diagnosis, and staging. *J Am Acad Dermatol.* 2018;78(2):237-247. doi:10.1016/j.jaad.2017.08.059

Que SKT, Zwald FO, Schmults CD. Cutaneous squamous cell carcinoma: management of advanced and high-stage tumors. *J Am Acad Dermatol.* 2018;78(2):249-261. doi:10.1016/j.jaad.2017.08.058

Rambhia KD, Kharkar V, Mahajan S, Khopkar US. Schopf-schulz-passarge syndrome. *Indian Dermatol Online J.* 2018;9(6):448-451. doi:10.4103/idoj.IDOJ_26_18

Ransohoff KJ, Jaju PD, Jaju PD, et al. Familial skin cancer syndromes: increased melanoma risk. *J Am Acad Dermatol.* 2016;74(3):423-434. quiz 435-6. doi:10.1016/j.jaad.2015.09.070

Rastrelli M, Tropea S, Rossi CR, Alaibac M. Melanoma: epidemiology, risk factors, pathogenesis, diagnosis and classification. *In Vivo.* 2014;28(6):1005-1011.

Redondo P, Aguado L, Martinez-Cuesta A. Diagnosis and management of extensive vascular malformations of the lower limb: part II. Systemic repercussions [corrected], diagnosis, and treatment. *J Am Acad Dermatol.* 2011;65(5):909-923. quiz 924. doi:10.1016/j.jaad.2011.03.009

Redondo P, Aguado L, Martinez-Cuesta A. Diagnosis and management of extensive vascular malformations of the lower limb: part I. Clinical diagnosis. *J Am Acad Dermatol.* 2011;65(5):893-906. quiz 907-8. doi:10.1016/j.jaad.2010.12.047

Richard G, De Laurenzi V, Didona B, Bale SJ, Compton JG. Keratin 13 point mutation underlies the hereditary mucosal epithelial disorder white sponge nevus. *Nat Genet.* 1995;11(4):453-455. doi:10.1038/ng1295-453

Roh MR, Eliades P, Gupta S, Tsao H. Genetics of melanocytic nevi. *Pigment Cell Melanoma Res.* 2015;28(6):661-672. doi:10.1111/pcmr.12412

Rugg EL, McLean WH, Allison WE, et al. A mutation in the mucosal keratin K4 is associated with oral white sponge nevus. *Nat Genet.* 1995;11(4):450-452. doi:10.1038/ng1295-450

Sakamoto A. Atypical fibroxanthoma. *Clin Med Oncol.* 2008;2:117-127. doi:10.4137/cmo.s506

Sánchez TS, Daudén E, Casas AP, García-Díez A. Eruptive pruritic syringomas: treatment with topical atropine. *J Am Acad Dermatol.* 2001;44(1):148-149. doi:10.1067/mjd.2001.109854

Anonymous, 2021 *SEER Cancer Statistics Review, 1975-2017.* Accessed August 6, 2021. https://seer.cancer.gov/csr/1975_2017

Sharma AN, Foulad DP, Doan L, Lee PK, Atanaskova Mesinkovska N. Mohs surgery for the treatment of lentigo maligna and lentigo maligna melanoma: a systematic review. *J Dermatolog Treat.* 2021;32(2):157-163. doi:10.1080/09546634.2019.1690624

Shoag JE, Nyame YA, Hu JC. Reconsidering the trade-offs of prostate cancer screening. Reply. *N Engl J Med.* 2020;383(13):1290. doi:10.1056/NEJMx200013

Shustef E, Kazlouskaya V, Prieto VG, Ivan D, Aung PP. Cutaneous angiosarcoma: a current update. *J Clin Pathol.* 2017;70(11):917-925. doi:10.1136/jclinpath-2017-204601

Sloot S, Fedorenko IV, Smalley KSM, Gibney GT. Long-term effects of BRAF inhibitors in melanoma treatment: friend or foe? *Expert Opin Pharmacother.* 2014;15(5):589-592. doi:10.1517/14656566.2014.881471

Sobanko JF, Dagum AB, Davis IC, Kriegel DA. Soft tissue tumors of the hand. 1. Benign. *Dermatol Surg.* 2007;33(6):651-667. doi:10.1111/j.1524-4725.2007.33140.x

Somoano B, Tsao H. Genodermatoses with cutaneous tumors and internal malignancies. *Dermatol Clin.* 2008;26(1):69-87. viii. doi:10.1016/j.det.2007.08.011

Soura E, Eliades PJ, Shannon K, Stratigos AJ, Tsao H. Hereditary melanoma: update on syndromes and management—emerging melanoma cancer complexes and genetic counseling. *J Am Acad Dermatol.* 2016;74(3):411-420. quiz 421-2. doi:10.1016/j.jaad.2015.08.037

Soura E, Eliades PJ, Shannon K, Stratigos AJ, Tsao H. Hereditary melanoma: update on syndromes and management—genetics of familial atypical multiple mole melanoma syndrome. *J Am Acad Dermatol.* 2016;74(3):395-407. quiz 408-10. doi:10.1016/j.jaad.2015.08.038

Spiteri BS, Stafrace Y, Calleja-Agius J. Silver-russell syndrome: a review. *Neonatal Netw.* 2017;36(4):206-212. doi:10.1891/0730-0832.36.4.206

Stanienda-Sokół K, Salwowska N, Sławińska M, et al. Primary locations of malignant melanoma lesions depending on patients' gender and age. *Asian Pac J Cancer Prev.* 2017;18(11):3081-3086. doi:10.22034/apjcp.2017.18.11.3081

Suarez AL, Pulitzer M, Horwitz S, Moskowitz A, Querfeld C, Myskowski PL. Primary cutaneous B-cell lymphomas: part I. Clinical features, diagnosis, and classification. *J Am Acad Dermatol*. 2013;69(3):329.e1-13. quiz 341-2. doi:10.1016/j.jaad.2013.06.012

Suarez AL, Querfeld C, Horwitz S, Pulitzer M, Moskowitz A, Myskowski PL. Primary cutaneous B-cell lymphomas: part II. Therapy and future directions. *J Am Acad Dermatol*. 2013;69(3):343.e1-11. quiz 355-6. doi:10.1016/j.jaad.2013.06.011

Suh KY, Frieden IJ. Infantile hemangiomas with minimal or arrested growth: a retrospective case series. *Arch Dermatol*. 2010;146(9):971-976. doi:10.1001/archdermatol.2010.197

Swetter SM, Tsao H, Bichakjian CK, et al. Guidelines of care for the management of primary cutaneous melanoma. *J Am Acad Dermatol*. 2019;80(1):208-250. doi:10.1016/j.jaad.2018.08.055

Tellechea O, Cardoso JC, Reis JP, et al. Benign follicular tumors. *An Bras Dermatol*. 2015;90(6):780-796. quiz 797-798. doi:doi:10.1590/abd1806-4841.20154114.

Tello TL, Coggshall K, Yom SS, Yu SS. Merkel cell carcinoma: an update and review – current and future therapy. *J Am Acad Dermatol*. 2018;78(3):445-454. doi:10.1016/j.jaad.2017.12.004

Torrelo A, Colmenero I, Kristal L, et al. Papular epidermal nevus with "skyline" basal cell layer (PENS). *J Am Acad Dermatol*. 2011;64(5):888-892. doi:10.1016/j.jaad.2010.02.054

Vaidya DC, Schwartz RA, Janniger CK. Nevus spilus. *Cutis*. 2007;80(6):465-468.

Valdebran MA, Hong C, Cha J. Multiple eruptive eccrine poromas associated with chemotherapy and autologous bone marrow transplantation. *Indian Dermatol Online J*. 2018;9(4):259-261. doi:10.4103/idoj.IDOJ_242_17

van der Horst MPJ, Brenn T. Update on malignant sweat gland tumors. *Surg Pathol Clin*. 2017;10(2):383-397. doi:10.1016/j.path.2017.01.010

Vargas-Mora P, Morgado-Carrasco D, Fustà-Novell X. Porokeratosis: a review of its pathophysiology, clinical manifestations, diagnosis, and treatment. *Actas Dermosifiliogr*. 2020;111(7):545-560. Poroqueratosis. Revisión de su etiopatogenia, manifestaciones clínicas, diagnóstico y tratamiento. doi:10.1016/j.ad.2020.03.005

Vega-Ruiz A, Cortes JE, Sever M, et al. Phase II study of imatinib mesylate as therapy for patients with systemic mastocytosis. *Leuk Res*. 2009;33(11):1481-1484. doi:10.1016/j.leukres.2008.12.020

Wang CX, Pusic I, Anadkat MJ. Association of leukemia cutis with survival in acute myeloid leukemia. *JAMA Dermatol*. 2019;155(7):826-832. doi:10.1001/jamadermatol.2019.0052

Weiner DM, Durgin JS, Wysocka M, Rook AH. The immunopathogenesis and immunotherapy of cutaneous T cell lymphoma: current and future approaches. *J Am Acad Dermatol*. 2021;84(3):597-604. doi:10.1016/j.jaad.2020.12.026

Wilder EG, Frieder J, Sulhan S, et al. Spectrum of orocutaneous disease associations: genodermatoses and inflammatory conditions. *J Am Acad Dermatol*. 2017;77(5):809-830. doi:10.1016/j.jaad.2017.02.017

Willemze R, Jansen PM, Cerroni L, et al. Subcutaneous panniculitis-like T-cell lymphoma: definition, classification, and prognostic factors – an EORTC Cutaneous Lymphoma Group Study of 83 cases. *Blood*. 2008;111(2):838-845. doi:10.1182/blood-2007-04-087288

Willenbrink TJ, Ruiz ES, Cornejo CM, Schmults CD, Arron ST, Jambusaria-Pahlajani A. Field cancerization: definition, epidemiology, risk factors, and outcomes. *J Am Acad Dermatol*. 2020;83(3):709-717. doi:10.1016/j.jaad.2020.03.126

Williams K, Shinkai K. Evaluation and management of the patient with multiple syringomas: a systematic review of the literature. *J Am Acad Dermatol*. 2016;74(6):1234-1240.e9. doi:10.1016/j.jaad.2015.12.006

Wilson BN, John AM, Handler MZ, Schwartz RA. Neurofibromatosis type 1: new developments in genetics and treatment. *J Am Acad Dermatol*. 2021;84(6):1667-1676. doi:10.1016/j.jaad.2020.07.105

Wollina U, Langner D, Tchernev G, França K, Lotti T. Epidermoid cysts: a wide spectrum of clinical presentation and successful treatment by surgery—a retrospective 10-year analysis and literature review. *Open Access Maced J Med Sci*. 2018;6(1):28-30. doi:10.3889/oamjms.2018.027

Work Group Invited Reviewers; Kim JYS, Kozlow JH, Mittal B, Moyer J, Olencki T, Rodgers P. Guidelines of care for the management of basal cell carcinoma. *J Am Acad Dermatol*. 2018;78(3):540-559. doi:10.1016/j.jaad.2017.10.006

Work Group Invited Reviewers; Kim JYS, Kozlow JH, Mittal B, Moyer J, Olenecki T, Rodgers P. Guidelines of care for the management of cutaneous squamous cell carcinoma. *J Am Acad Dermatol*. 2018;78(3):560-578. doi:10.1016/j.jaad.2017.10.007

Yamaguchi Y, Coelho SG, Zmudzka BZ, et al. Cyclobutane pyrimidine dimer formation and p53 production in human skin after repeated UV irradiation. *Exp Dermatol*. 2008;17(11):916-924. doi:10.1111/j.1600-0625.2008.00722.x

Yelamos O, Braun RP, Liopyris K, et al. Usefulness of dermoscopy to improve the clinical and histopathologic diagnosis of skin cancers. *J Am Acad Dermatol*. 2019;80(2):365-377. doi:10.1016/j.jaad.2018.07.072

Yelamos O, Braun RP, Liopyris K, et al. Dermoscopy and dermatopathology correlates of cutaneous neoplasms. *J Am Acad Dermatol*. 2019;80(2):341-363. doi:10.1016/j.jaad.2018.07.073

Yew YW, Giordano CN, Spivak G, Lim HW. Understanding photodermatoses associated with defective DNA repair: photosensitive syndromes without associated cancer predisposition. *J Am Acad Dermatol*. 2016;75(5):873-882. doi:10.1016/j.jaad.2016.03.044

Zhou H, Lu K, Zheng L, et al. Prognostic significance of mammary Paget's disease in Chinese women: a 10-year, population-based, matched cohort study. *OncoTargets Ther*. 2018;11:8319-8326. doi:10.2147/ott.S171710

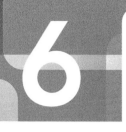

6 Medical Treatments

John S. Barbieri, MD, MBA and Caroline A. Nelson, MD

Immunosuppressants and Immunomodulators

Basic Concepts

- Immunosuppressants and immunomodulators include corticosteroids and steroid-sparing therapies.
- Conventional steroid-sparing therapies include antimalarials, antimetabolites, calcineurin inhibitors, colchicine, cyclophosphamide, PDE4 inhibitors, SSKI, and thalidomide.
- Biologic and small molecule inhibitors are designed to target specific components of the immune system.
- IVIG is a sterile solution of globulins extracted from pooled plasma with immunomodulatory activity.

Corticosteroids

- Selected drugs:
  - Group 1 (formerly A, D2, and budesonide): **cortisone, hydrocortisone, methylprednisolone, prednisolone, prednisone.**
  - Group 2 (formerly B): **desonide, fluocinolone, fluocinonide, flurandrenolide, triamcinolone (acetonide).**
  - Group 3 (formerly C, D1): **alclometasone, betamethasone, clobetasol, desoximetasone, dexamethasone, halobetasol, mometasone.**
- Mechanism:
  - The **hypothalamic-pituitary-adrenal (HPA) axis** involves hypothalamic production of **corticotropin-releasing hormone (CRH)**, which stimulates the anterior pituitary to synthesize **ACTH**, which stimulates the middle layer of the adrenal cortex to synthesize ~**20 to 30 mg cortisol (5-7.5 mg prednisone equivalent) daily.** Cortisol synthesis may increase up to 10-fold under maximal stress. In contrast, mineralocorticoid production is controlled by the renin-angiotensin system and serum potassium levels.
  - The free (unbound) fraction of exogenous glucocorticoids enters cells and binds to a **cytoplasmic glucocorticoid receptor**, which leads to **translocation into the nucleus.** Glucocorticoids bind **glucocorticoid response elements** in the promoter region of certain genes and interact with other transcription factors (eg, **inhibition of activator protein 1 (AP1) and NF-κB**).
  - Anti-inflammatory effects include **downregulation** of pro-inflammatory molecules (eg, **IL-1**), **upregulation** of anti-inflammatory molecules (eg, **IL-10**), and diverse

effects on inflammatory cells (eg, **neutrophilia** due to release of neutrophils from the bone marrow with decreased infiltration into sites of inflammation and decreased apoptosis).
  - Other effects include decreased bone production (**inhibit osteoblasts and stimulate osteoclasts [direct], induce hypocalcemia that leads to secondary hyperparathyroidism [indirect]**), decreased collagen production (**inhibit fibroblasts**), and hair growth (**stimulate ODC**).
- FDA-approved dermatology indications:
  - Systemic: **anaphylaxis, angioedema, dermatomyositis, gout, systemic rheumatic disorders (eg, ANCA vasculitis, mixed cryoglobulinemia, PAN, RA, SLE), temporal arteritis.**
  - Topical: **AD, aphthous stomatitis, ACD, psoriasis, pruritus (anal, genital), seborrheic dermatitis.**
- Mucocutaneous adverse events include **acneiform eruption/rosacea/periorificial dermatitis, AN, contact dermatitis (eg, ACD to group 1 corticosteroid, ACD and/or ICD to propylene glycol)**, and **skin atrophy, lipodystrophy, pigmentary changes, plethora, purpura, striae, and/or telangiectasia. Rapid tapering of systemic corticosteroids** may trigger GPP. In terms of hair, corticosteroids may cause **hypertrichosis (hirsutism)/trichomegaly.**

  > Lipodystrophy associated with corticosteroids may manifest with "moon facies" (buccal fat pads), a "buffalo hump" (dorsocervical fat pad), and central obesity. These are collectively known as "Cushingoid features." **Rapid tapering of systemic corticosteroids** may trigger **poststeroid panniculitis**, most often in **children.**

- Other adverse events include:
  - Circulatory: **atherosclerosis, hypertension, peripheral edema.**
  - Digestive: **pancreatitis, peptic ulcer disease (PUD).**
    - Prevention pearl: Consider **H2 receptor antagonist antihistamines or proton pump inhibitors (PPIs)** for patients at risk for PUD (eg, on NSAIDs).
  - Endocrine: **hyperglycemia, hyperlipidemia, obesity. HPA axis suppression**, which typically occurs after **3 to 4 weeks of ≥20 mg/d prednisone equivalent**, may result in **withdrawal syndrome or adrenal crisis.**
    - Management pearl: If HPA axis suppression is suspected, order **AM plasma cortisol,** urine cortisol, or ACTH stimulation test.
    - Management pearl: **Stress-dose corticosteroids** may be required for patients taking systemic corticosteroids (eg, prior to a major surgical procedure).

* Do NOT confuse the ACTH stimulation test to diagnose adrenal insufficiency with the dexamethasone suppression test to diagnose Cushing syndrome.

○ Lymphatic/immune: **immunosuppression.**
  * Prevention pearl: Ensure vaccines are up to date (see below). **Live or live-attenuated vaccines are contraindicated** during systemic corticosteroid therapy.
  * Prevention pearl: Patients with **untreated latent TB infection** should receive a **9-month course of INH.**
  * Prevention pearl: *Pneumocystis jirovecii* pneumonia **(PCP) prophylaxis** should be given to **high-risk patients** (eg, additional immunosuppression, lymphopenia, pulmonary disease) **receiving ≥20 mg/d prednisone equivalent ≥1 month.**

○ Musculoskeletal: **muscle atrophy/myopathy, osteonecrosis, osteoporosis. Young men have the greatest degree of bone loss, but postmenopausal Caucasian women have the highest risk of fracture.**
  * Prevention pearl: To prevent osteoporosis, initiate **calcium/vitamin D.** Initiate a **bisphosphonate (eg, alendronate, pamidronate, risedronate) in postmenopausal women and men ≥ 50 to 65 years.**
  * Management pearl: If osteonecrosis is suspected (eg, **hip pain**), order **MRI.**
    * Systemic corticosteroids may cause **growth retardation.**

○ Nervous: **pseudotumor cerebri, psychiatric disturbances, seizures.**
○ Ocular: **cataracts, glaucoma.**
○ Renal/urinary/excretory: **fluid/sodium retention, hypocalcemia, hypokalemic alkalosis.**
○ Reproductive: **amenorrhea.**

* Monitoring parameters for systemic corticosteroids include:
  ○ Labs: CMP. **TB history** and, if negative or uncertain, **PPD or IFN-γ release assay.**
  ○ Imaging: **CXR** for patients with **positive PPD or IFN-γ release assay,** history of TB, or other risk factors (eg, preexisting immunosuppression) **receiving ≥15 mg/d prednisone equivalent ≥ 1 month. Dual-energy X-ray absorptiometry (DEXA)** of the hip and lumbar spine.
  ○ Other: blood pressure. Weight. **Ophthalmologic examination.**
    * **Monitor growth** in pediatric patients on systemic corticosteroids.

* Dosing notes:
  ○ Oral: **Physiologic dosing is 5 to 7.5 mg prednisone equivalent daily, while pharmacologic dosing is >7.5 mg prednisone equivalent daily. Split-day dosing increases efficacy and toxicity. With the exception of cataracts and osteoporosis, alternate-day dosing decreases toxicity and allows HPA axis recovery** but is often not feasible in patients with diabetes mellitus.
    * As a rule of thumb, taper prednisone in 20 mg increments above 60 mg/d, 10 mg increments between 30 and 60 mg/d, and 5 mg increments between 30 and 5 to 7.5 mg/d. In case of adrenal insufficiency, taper prednisone in 1 to 2.5 mg increments below physiologic dosing.

○ Topical: **Steroid acne risk** is highest on the **face. Atrophy risk** is highest on the **face and body folds.** Avoid application of potent topical corticosteroids to these areas, if possible.
○ Intralesional: 2 to 40 mg/mL triamcinolone acetonide. Advantages include decreased risk of epidermal atrophy. Disadvantages include **increased risk of dermal or SC atrophy.**
○ IM: Advantages include **guaranteed compliance and steady release.** Disadvantages include **less physiologic/precise dosing, HPA axis suppression,** and risk of lipoatrophy or sterile abscess.
○ IV: ≥2 mg/kg/d methylprednisolone divided every 6 to 8 hours or pulse 0.5 to 1 g methylprednisolone for 1 to 5 days. **Acute electrolyte shifts** may lead to **arrhythmias.**
  * Prevention pearl: Strategies to prevent arrhythmias include **slow infusion over 2 hours and potassium coadministration.**

* Pharmacodynamics notes:
  ○ Efficacy: Topical corticosteroids may exhibit **tachyphylaxis,** defined as rapidly diminishing response to successive doses of a drug (controversial).
  ○ Potency: Steroids differ in relative glucocorticoid and mineralocorticoid potencies. For example, **hydrocortisone has significant mineralocorticoid potency, while methylprednisolone has none.** Topical corticosteroids are classified into **four major WHO potency groups and seven classes** (Table 6.1). Beyond creams and ointments, vehicles include **foams, gels, lotions, oils, shampoos, solutions, sprays,** and even **tape (flurandrenolide 4 µg/cm²).**
    * The potency of hydrocortisone (acetate < butyrate < valerate) follows the order of the alphabet, while the potency of betamethasone (dipropionate > valerate) is the reverse.

* Pharmacokinetics notes:
  ○ Absorption: The *stratum corneum* **acts as the rate-limiting barrier** to percutaneous absorption.
    Topical corticosteroid absorption is increased in patients with severe skin barrier dysfunction (eg, **Netherton syndrome).**
  ○ Distribution: The free fraction of exogenous glucocorticoids is increased when binding proteins in the plasma are decreased (eg, hepatic or renal disease).
  ○ Metabolism: Corticosteroids may be **short-acting (8-12 hours, eg, cortisone, hydrocortisone), intermediate-acting (24-36 hours, eg, methylprednisolone, prednisolone, prednisone, triamcinolone),** or **long-acting (36-54 hours, eg, betamethasone, dexamethasone).** Cortisone and prednisone require **activation** via **hepatic conversion into hydrocortisone and prednisolone,** respectively, and are **not preferred in patients with severe hepatic disease.**

* Historical pregnancy risk category: **C.** Topical corticosteroids do not increase risk of malformations or preterm delivery but potent topical corticosteroids increase risk of fetal growth restriction. Low-to-moderate potency topical corticosteroids are preferred. If a potent topical corticoste-

Table 6.1. TOPICAL CORTICOSTEROIDS

WHO Potency Group	Class	Selected Drugs[a]
Ultrahigh	1	Betamethasone dipropionate 0.05% (O[b]), clobetasol propionate 0.05% (C, O), fluocinonide 0.1% (C), halobetasol propionate 0.05% (C, O)
High	2	Betamethasone dipropionate 0.05% (C[b], O), desoximetasone 0.25% (C, O), fluocinonide 0.05% (C, O), mometasone furoate 0.1% (O), triamcinolone acetonide 0.5% (O)
	3	Betamethasone dipropionate 0.05% (C), triamcinolone acetonide 0.1% (O)/0.5% (C)
Moderate	4	Desoximetasone 0.05% (C), fluocinolone acetonide 0.025% (O), hydrocortisone valerate 0.2% (O), mometasone furoate 0.1% (C), triamcinolone acetonide 0.1% (C, O)
	5	Betamethasone valerate 0.1% (C), fluocinolone acetonide 0.025% (C), hydrocortisone butyrate 0.1% (C, O), hydrocortisone valerate 0.2% (C), triamcinolone acetonide 0.025% (O)
Low	6	Alclometasone dipropionate 0.05% (C, O), desonide 0.05% (C, O), fluocinolone acetonide 0.01% (C), triamcinolone acetonide 0.025% (C)
	7	Hydrocortisone acetate 0.5%-2.5% (C, O)

C, cream; O, ointment; WHO, World Health Organization.
[a]Illustrative examples are provided.
[b]Optimized vehicle.

roid is required, the treatment duration should be limited. Systemic corticosteroids increase risk of cleft lip/palate (controversial), preterm delivery, fetal growth restriction, and adrenal insufficiency in the newborn. If a systemic corticosteroid is required, prednisolone is preferred as it is largely inactivated in the placenta.

Other Immunosuppressants and Immunomodulators

Antimalarials

- Selected drugs: **chloroquine, hydroxychloroquine, quinacrine.**
- Mechanism: inhibit UVR-induced cutaneous reactions by **inhibiting ROS.**
- FDA-approved dermatology indications: **LE (hydroxychloroquine).** Quinacrine is no longer marketed in the US.
- Mucocutaneous adverse events include **lichenoid drug reaction, morbilliform eruption (DM > LE), pigmentation (blue-gray—chloroquine and hydroxychloroquine, yellow—quinacrine), and porphyria flare.**
  - ◆ On histopathology, antimalarial pigmentation may stain positive for hemosiderin (Perls Prussian blue) and melanin (Fontana-Masson).
- Other adverse events include:
  - ○ Circulatory: **arrhythmias (eg, QT prolongation, ventricular tachycardia) [US Safety Alert].**
  - ○ Digestive: hepatotoxicity.
  - ○ Endocrine: hypoglycemia.
  - ○ Lymphatic/immune: bone marrow suppression, **hemolytic anemia, methemoglobinemia** (see below).

- ○ Ocular (chloroquine > hydroxychloroquine, additive): **corneal opacity (reversible) or retinopathy (irreversible), transient scotoma.**
  - ☀ "Bull's-eye" maculopathy results in central visual field defects.
- Monitoring parameters include:
  - ○ Labs: CMP. CBC.
  - ○ Imaging: ECG.
  - ○ Other: **Ophthalmologic examination.**
- Dosing notes:
  - ○ Oral: The dose of hydroxychloroquine is typically 200 to 400 mg daily. Due to retinopathy risk, the **maximum dose** for most patients is **5 mg/kg/d** (actual body weight) or 400 mg, whichever is lower. **Lower doses** (eg, hydroxychloroquine 100 mg twice weekly) are used off-label in **PCT.**
- Pharmacodynamics:
  - ○ Efficacy: **Smoking decreases antimalarial therapy efficacy.**
- Historical pregnancy risk category: **C.**

Antimetabolites

Azathioprine

- Mechanism: **purine analogue** that interferes with DNA synthesis. Azathioprine is **converted into 6 mercaptopurine (6-MP), which is converted by hypoxanthine-guanine phosphoribosyltransferase (HGPRT) into active metabolites (6-thioguanine). 6-MP may alternatively be converted into inactive metabolites by thiopurine S-methyltransferase (TPMT) or xanthine oxidase (XO)** (Figure 6.1).

- ○ Related drugs include **6-MP** (see Chapter 6: Antineoplastics).
- Mucocutaneous adverse events include **DRESS, SCCs, and Sweet syndrome.**
- Other adverse events include:
  - ○ Digestive: **hepatotoxicity, nausea/vomiting.**
  - ○ Lymphatic/immune: **bone marrow suppression, immunosuppression, malignancy [US Boxed Warning].**
- Monitoring parameters include:
  - ○ Labs: CMP. **CBC.** UA. HBV/HCV/HIV/TB screening. human chorionic gonadotropin (HCG). **TPMT.**
  - ○ Other: **TBSE.**
- Pharmacokinetics notes:
  - ○ **TPMT genotyping or phenotyping** may assist in identifying poor metabolizers at risk for bone marrow suppression. **Avoidance or dose reduction** is also recommended for poor NUDT15 metabolizers and patients on concomitant XO inhibitor therapy (eg, **allopurinol**, febuxostat).
- Historical pregnancy risk category: **D.**

Methotrexate

- Mechanism: **interferes with folic acid synthesis** needed for nucleic acid synthesis through **competitive inhibition of dihydrofolate reductase (DHFR)** (Figure 6.2).
  - ○ Related drugs include **pemetrexed** (see Chapter 6: Antineoplastics) and **TMP** (see Chapter 6: Antimicrobials).

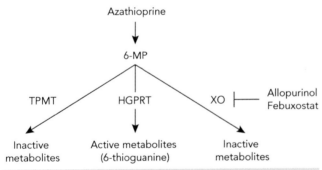

Figure 6.1. AZATHIOPRINE METABOLISM. HGPRT, hypoxanthine-guanine phosphoribosyltransferase; 6-MP, 6-mercaptopurine; TPMT, thiopurine methyltransferase; XO, xanthine oxidase.

- FDA-approved dermatology indications: **CTCL, psoriasis.**
- Mucocutaneous adverse events [US Boxed Warning] include **accelerated rheumatoid nodulosis, hyperpigmentation (sun-exposed), necrosis of psoriasis plaques, oral ulcers, phototoxic eruption, recall reactions, and vitamin B$_9$ deficiency.** In terms of hair, methotrexate may cause **alopecia and hyperpigmentation.**
  - The "flag sign" refers to alternating horizontal bands of hyperpigmented and normal hair.
- Other adverse events include:
  - ○ Digestive: **diarrhea/ulcerative stomatitis with risk of hemorrhagic enteritis/intestinal perforation [US Boxed Warning]; nausea/vomiting; hepatotoxicity, fibrosis, cirrhosis [US Boxed Warning].**
    - Prevention pearl: To decrease risk of hepatotoxicity, patients should **avoid alcohol.**
  - ○ Lymphatic/immune: **bone marrow suppression [US Boxed Warning], immunosuppression [US Boxed Warning], secondary malignancy [US Boxed Warning],** tumor lysis syndrome [US Boxed Warning].
  - ○ Musculoskeletal: osteonecrosis (increased risk with radiation therapy [US Boxed Warning]).
  - ○ Renal/urinary/excretory: **nephrotoxicity.**
  - ○ Respiratory: **chronic interstitial pneumonitis [US Boxed Warning].**
- Monitoring parameters include:
  - ○ Labs: **CMP. CBC.** HBV/HCV/HIV/TB screening. **HCG.**
  - ○ Other: In patients without risk factors for hepatotoxicity, **liver biopsy** should be considered in patients with persistent transaminitis or low albumin despite normal nutrition. Liver biopsy **after cumulative dose of 3.5 to 4 g** is controversial. Alternative screening tests for liver fibrosis include amino terminal levels of **type III procollagen and transient elastography (Fibroscan).**
- Dosing notes:
  - ○ Oral/SC/IM/IV: The typical dose of methotrexate for psoriasis is **10 to 25 mg weekly.** An initial **test dose** of 2.5 to 5 mg is recommended for patient with risk factors for hematologic toxicity or renal impairment. Concomitant **folic acid** decreases toxicity without decreasing efficacy. **Folinic acid (leucovorin) and thymidine** are used for high-dose methotrexate overexposure.

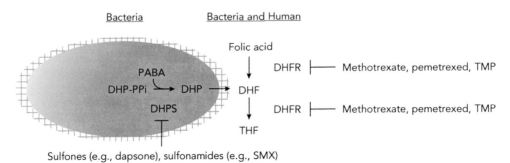

Figure 6.2. FOLIC ACID PATHWAY. DHF, dihydrofolate; DHFR, dihydrofolate reductase; DHP, dihydropteroate; DHP-PPi, dihydropteroate pyrophosphate; DHPS, dihydropteroate synthetase; PABA, p-aminobenzoic acid; SMX, sulfamethoxazole; THF, tetrahydrofolate; TMP, trimethoprim.

For high-dose methotrexate overexposure, folinic acid administration is called a "leucovorin rescue" and thymidine administration is called a "thymidine rescue."

- Pharmacodynamics notes:
  - Efficacy: **SC** as compared to oral methotrexate may have **increased efficacy and decreased gastrointestinal toxicity.**
- Pharmacokinetics notes:
  - Distribution: **NSAIDs displace methotrexate from plasma protein-binding sites**, increasing its free serum concentration.
  - Metabolism: Risk of methotrexate toxicity is increased with **concomitant dapsone, NSAIDs, tetracyclines, and TMP-SMX.**
  - Excretion: **Renal impairment reduces methotrexate elimination [US Boxed Warning].**
- Historical pregnancy risk category: **X [US Boxed Warning].**

Mycophenolate

- Mechanism: **inhibits *de novo* purine (guanine nucleotide) synthesis** through **noncompetitive inhibition of inosine monophosphate dehydrogenase (IMPDH).**
- Adverse events include:
  - Digestive: hepatotoxicity, **nausea/vomiting.**
  - Lymphatic/immune: **bone marrow suppression, immunosuppression [US Boxed Warning], malignancies [US Boxed Warning].**
  - Renal/urinary/excretory: nephrotoxicity.
- Monitoring parameters include:
  - Labs: CMP. CBC. HBV/HCV/HIV/TB screening. **HCG.**
- Dosing notes:
  - Oral: Formulations include mycophenolate mofetil and mycophenolate sodium (enteric-coated).
- Historical pregnancy risk category: **D [US Boxed Warning, US Risk Evaluation and Mitigation Strategy (REMS) program].** Mycophenolate is associated with increased risks of **first trimester pregnancy loss and congenital malformations. Females of reproductive potential should avoid pregnancy** and **males must use condoms** during sexual contact with females of reproductive potential. Patients should **avoid blood and sperm donation.**

Calcineurin Inhibitors

- Selected drugs: **cyclosporine, pimecrolimus, tacrolimus.**
- Mechanism:
  - Under normal circumstances, **TCR activation** causes release of intracellular **Ca^{2+} that binds calmodulin and activates calcineurin.** This calcineurin complex **dephosphorylates the nuclear factor of activated T cells (NFAT$_c$)** in the cytoplasm, which translocates into the nucleus, **binds NFAT$_n$**, and upregulates transcription of pro-inflammatory molecules (eg, **IL-2, IL-2Rs**).
  - **Cyclosporine** inhibits calcineurin by binding **cyclophilin. Pimecrolimus and tacrolimus** inhibit calcineurin by binding **FK506-binding protein (FKBP).**
  - Calcineurin inhibitors **reduce CD4$^+$ and CD8$^+$ (cytotoxic) T cells** in the epidermis.

- FDA-approved dermatology indications:
  - Oral (cyclosporine): psoriasis.
  - Topical (pimecrolimus, tacrolimus): AD.
- Mucocutaneous adverse events of cyclosporine include **gingival hyperplasia and malignancy** in psoriasis patients previously treated with **PUVA** > methotrexate, other immunosuppressive agents, coal tar preparations, or radiation therapy [**US Boxed Warning**]. In terms of hair, cyclosporine may cause **hypertrichosis and trichomegaly.**
- Other adverse events of cyclosporine include:
  - Circulatory: **hypertension [US Boxed Warning].**
    - Management pearl: **Dihydropyridine CCBs (eg, amlodipine, nifedipine)** are first line for cyclosporine-induced hypertension.
  - Endocrine: **hyperlipidemia.**
  - Lymphatic/immune: **immunosuppression [US Boxed Warning].**
  - Nervous: **paresthesias, seizures.**
  - Renal/urinary/excretory: **hyperkalemia, hyperuricemia, hypomagnesemia, nephrotoxicity [US Boxed Warning]. Treatment longer than 1 year is not recommended** (up to 2 years may be safe at lower "dermatologic" doses).
    - Prevention pearl: **If Cr rises by >25% over baseline, recheck in 2 weeks. If Cr returns to <25% over baseline, continue therapy. If Cr remains elevated, decrease the dose by 25% to 50%** and then recheck in 1 month. If Cr remains elevated, discontinue therapy until Cr is within 10% of the baseline value, then consider restarting at a significantly lower dose.
- Monitoring parameters for cyclosporine include:
  - Labs: CMP including **potassium, uric acid, and magnesium.** Fasting lipid panel. CBC. HBV/HCV/HIV/TB screening.
  - Other: **blood pressure.**
- Mucocutaneous adverse events of pimecrolimus and tacrolimus include **burning/stinging/sensation of warmth and malignancy [US Boxed Warning (controversial)].**
- Dosing notes:
  - Oral: The **initial dose of cyclosporine (microemulsion formulation) for psoriasis is 2.5 mg/kg/d divided twice daily**; the **maximum dose is 4 mg/kg/d.**
  - Topical: Pimecrolimus 1% cream, tacrolimus 0.03%, or 0.1% ointment twice daily.

    Pimecrolimus and tacrolimus are **not approved for use in children < 2 years.** Only tacrolimus 0.03% ointment is indicated for use in children 2 to 15 years of age [**US Boxed Warning**]. However, AAD guidelines recommend off-label use of pimecrolimus 1% cream and tacrolimus 0.03% ointment <2 years of age.
- Pharmacokinetics notes:
  - Absorption: The *stratum corneum* acts as the **rate-limiting barrier** to percutaneous absorption.

    Topical calcineurin inhibitor absorption is increased in patients with severe skin barrier dysfunction (eg, **Netherton syndrome**).
  - Metabolism: Cyclosporine is a **CYP3A4 inhibitor.**
- Historical pregnancy risk category: **C.**

Colchicine

- Mechanism: **downregulates IL-1β** by inhibiting inflammasome assembly; **prevents activation, degranulation, and migration of neutrophils** by inhibiting β-tubulin polymerization into microtubules.
- FDA-approved dermatology indications: **FMF, gout.**
- Adverse events include:
  - Digestive: **diarrhea, nausea/vomiting.**

Cyclophosphamide

- Mechanism: **alkylating agent** that **cross-links with DNA molecules.**
- For mucocutaneous adverse events, see Chapter 6: Anti-Neoplastics.
- Other adverse events include:
  - Digestive: diarrhea, nausea/vomiting.
  - Lymphatic/immune: **bone marrow suppression, immunosuppression.**
  - Renal/urinary/excretory: **hemorrhagic cystitis, transitional cell bladder cancer.**
    - Prevention pearl: **Hydration and mesna** reduce risk of hemorrhagic cystitis.
  - Reproductive: **amenorrhea, infertility.**
- Historical pregnancy risk category: **D.**

Dapsone

- Mechanism: **sulfone** antibacterial that **interferes with bacterial folic acid synthesis** needed for nucleic acid synthesis through **competitive inhibition of bacterial dihydropteroate synthetase (DHPS). Anti-inflammatory** properties derive from **inhibition of neutrophil chemotaxis, the neutrophil MPO, and eosinophil peroxidase (EPO).**
  - Related drugs include the sulfonamide antibacterials **SMX, sulfacetamide, sulfadiazine, and sulfapyridine** (see Chapter 6: Antimicrobials). Use with caution in patients with sulfonamide allergy.
- FDA-approved dermatology indications:
  - Systemic: **DH, leprosy.**
  - Topical: **acne** (see Chapter 6: Antimicrobials).
- Mucocutaneous adverse events include **morbilliform eruption/DRESS and SJS/TEN. HLA-B1301** is associated with SCAR to dapsone in **Asian** populations.
- Other adverse events include:
  - Digestive: cholestatic jaundice, hepatitis, superinfection (eg, *Clostridium difficile*).
  - Lymphatic/immune: **leukopenia, agranulocytosis, hemolytic anemia, methemoglobinemia.**
    - Management pearl: Due to risk of hemolytic anemia and methemoglobinemia, use with caution in patients with anemia, **glucose-6-phosphate dehydrogenase (G6PD) deficiency**, hemoglobin M deficiency, and methemoglobin reductase deficiency. **Antimalarials, topical anesthetics (eg, benzocaine spray), and inhaled nitrous oxide** may also induce methemoglobinemia. **Routine pulse oximetry cannot detect methemoglobin.** A high concentration of methemoglobin causes the oxygen saturation to display as ~85%, regardless of the true value, and to fail to improve with administration of supplemental oxygen. Check **co-oximetry** (multiple wavelength oximetry). **Methylene blue** is first line for methemoglobinemia. **Cimetidine and vitamins C and E** may increase dapsone tolerance by chronically lowering methemoglobin but are not appropriate for acute management. **Sulfapyridine produces less hemolytic anemia.**
  - Nervous: **lower motor neuron toxicity > peripheral neuropathy** (typically prolonged therapy).
  - Renal/urinary/excretory: nephrotic syndrome.
- Monitoring parameters:
  - Labs: CMP. **CBC. Reticulocyte count. G6PD.**

Phosphodiesterase 4 Inhibitors

- Selected drugs: **apremilast, crisaborole, roflumilast.**
- Mechanism: **inhibits PDE4.**
- FDA-approved dermatology indications:
  - Oral (apremilast): **Behçet disease, psoriasis, psoriatic arthritis.**
  - Topical (crisaborole, roflumilast): **AD (crisaborole), psoriasis (roflumilast).**
- Mucocutaneous adverse events of crisaborole and roflumilast include **ACD and pain.**
- Adverse events of apremilast include:
  - Digestive: **diarrhea, nausea/vomiting.**
  - Endocrine: **weight loss.**
  - Nervous: **depression, SI.**
- Historical pregnancy risk category (apremilast): **C.**

Saturated Solution of Potassium Iodide

- Mechanism: unknown; however, suppression of neutrophil chemotaxis and ROS production likely contributes to immunomodulation.
- Mucocutaneous adverse events include **iododerma.**
- Other adverse events include:
  - Endocrine: **hyperthyroidism, hypothyroidism.** The **Wolff-Chaikoff effect** describes the **inhibition of organic binding of iodide in the thyroid gland by excess iodide**, resulting in the cessation of thyroid hormone synthesis.
- Monitoring parameters include:
  - Labs: **TFTs.**
- Historical pregnancy risk category: **D.**

Thalidomide

- Mechanism: unknown; however, **TNFα inhibition** likely contributes to immunomodulation.
  - Related drugs include **lenalidomide.**
- FDA-approved dermatology indications: erythema nodosum leprosum.
- Adverse events include:
  - Circulatory: **thromboembolism [US Boxed Warning].**
  - Endocrine: hypothyroidism.
  - Lymphatic/immune: **bone marrow suppression [US Boxed Warning—lenalidomide].**

- ○ Nervous: **peripheral neuropathy, somnolence** (thalidomide > lenalidomide).
- Monitoring parameters include:
  - ○ Labs: LFTs. **CBC.** TFTs. HIV viral load (if applicable). **HCG.**
- Historical pregnancy risk category: **X [US Boxed Warning, US REMS Program]. A single dose of thalidomide during 21 to 36 days of gestation yields a 100% incidence of birth defects**, most notably **phocomelia** (severe extremity under-development). **Females of reproductive potential must avoid pregnancy** and **males must use condoms** during sexual contact with females of reproductive potential. Patients should **avoid blood and sperm donation.**

Biologic and Small Molecule Inhibitors

TNFα Inhibitors

- Selected drugs:
  - ○ **Fusion protein (TNFαR/Fc-IgG1): etanercept (human).**
  - ○ **Monoclonal antibodies: adalimumab (human), certolizumab (humanized), golimumab (human), infliximab (chimeric).**
    For monoclonal antibodies and fusion proteins, the generic name holds the clue to the source system and inhibitor type (Table 6.2).
- Mechanism: **inhibit TNFα.** The **fusion protein** etanercept binds only **soluble** TNFα. **Monoclonal antibodies** bind **soluble and membrane** bound TNFα.
  - ○ Related drugs include the **biologic and small molecule inhibitors for psoriasis** summarized in Table 6.3.
- FDA-approved dermatology indications: **HS (adalimumab), psoriasis/psoriatic arthritis.**
- Mucocutaneous adverse events include **accelerated rheumatoid nodulosis, anaphylaxis/infusion/injection site reactions, CSVV, DM, eczematous eruptions, EN, lichenoid drug reaction, SLE, psoriasis (paradoxical), sarcoidal/GA/interstitial granulomatous eruptions, and serum sickness–like eruption.**
- Other adverse events include:
  - ○ Circulatory: **CHF.**
  - ○ Digestive: autoimmune hepatitis.
  - ○ Lymphatic/immune: bone marrow suppression, **serious infections [US Boxed Warning], lymphoma, and other malignancies (controversial) [US Boxed Warning].**

Table 6.2. NOMENCLATURE PEARLS: MONOCLONAL ANTIBODIES AND FUSION PROTEINS

Source System (Substem B)		Inhibitor Type (Suffix)	
-u-	Human	-cept	Receptor
-xi-	Chimeric	-mab	Immunoglobulin variable domain
-zu-	Humanized	-nib	Tyrosine kinase inhibitor

- Ensure vaccines are up to date (Table 6.4). **Live or live attenuated vaccines are contraindicated** during TNFα inhibitor therapy.
  - Prevention pearl: Patients with **untreated latent TB infection** should receive a **9-month course of INH. Treat for 1 to 2 months** prior to initiating TNFα inhibitor therapy.
  - ○ Nervous: **demyelinating disease.**
- Monitoring parameters include:
  - ○ Labs: CMP. CBC. **HBV/HCV/HIV/TB** screening. Consider screening for coccidioidomycosis, histoplasmosis, and strongyloidiasis if appropriate epidemiologic history.
  - ○ Other: **cervical Papanicolaou smear/HPV DNA testing.**
- Dosing notes:
  - ○ SC: **adalimumab, certolizumab, golimumab, etanercept.**
  - ○ IV: **infliximab.**
- Pharmacodynamics notes:
  - ○ Efficacy: **Immunogenicity** may reduce the efficacy of TNFα inhibitors (eg, infliximab).
    - Prevention pearl: **Infliximab and methotrexate coadministration may reduce risk of antichimeric antibody development.**
- Historical pregnancy risk category: **B.**
  - ○ Management pearl: The category B designation considers teratogenic risk only. While the AAD considers TNFα inhibitors for the treatment of psoriasis to be compatible with pregnancy, **risk of maternal and fetal immunosuppression** remains an important factor when weighing risks and benefits of TNFα inhibitors during pregnancy.

Anifrolumab

- Mechanism: monoclonal antibody (human) that **inhibits the type I IFN receptor.**
- FDA-approved dermatology indications: **SLE.**
- Mucocutaneous adverse events include **anaphylaxis/infusion reactions.**
- Adverse events include:
  - ○ Lymphatic/immune: infection.

Dupilumab

- Mechanism: monoclonal antibody (human) that blocks the IL-4Rα subunit to **inhibit IL-4 and IL-13.**
- FDA-approved dermatology indications: **AD.**
- Mucocutaneous adverse events include **anaphylaxis/injection site reactions, CTCL progression, EGPA, psoriasis flare, and serum sickness–like eruption.**
- Other adverse events include:
  - ○ Lymphatic/immune: helminth infection (possible).
  - ○ Ocular: **conjunctivitis, keratitis.**

Omalizumab

- Mechanism: monoclonal antibody (humanized) that **inhibits IgE.**
- FDA-approved dermatology indications: **chronic idiopathic urticaria.**

Table 6.3. BIOLOGIC AND SMALL MOLECULE INHIBITORS FOR PSORIASIS

Target	Selected Drugs	FDA-Approved Dermatology Indications	Notes[a]
B7-1	Abatacept	Psoriatic arthritis	CTLA-4/Fc-IgG1 fusion protein.
CD2	Alefacept	Psoriasis	LFA-3/Fc-IgG1 fusion protein. IM. Required monitoring of CD4+ T-cell count. Discontinued.
CD11	Efalizumab	Psoriasis	Discontinued due to risk of PML. Historical pregnancy risk category C.
GM-CSF	Namilumab	Psoriasis/psoriatic arthritis[b]	
IL-12, IL-23	Ustekinumab	Psoriasis/psoriatic arthritis	Ustekinumab targets the p40 subunit of IL-12 and IL-23. Other adverse events include malignancy including SCC (controversial), nasopharyngitis, and reversible posterior leukoencephalopathy syndrome.
IL-17	Brodalumab, ixekizumab, secukinumab	Psoriasis/psoriatic arthritis	Brodalumab targets the IL-17RA, while ixekizumab and secukinumab target IL-17A. Other adverse events include IBD, nasopharyngitis, and SI [US Boxed Warning, US REMS Program—Brodalumab].
IL-23	Guselkumab, risankizumab, tildrakizumab	Psoriasis/psoriatic arthritis	Guselkumab, risankizumab, and tildrakizumab target the p19 subunit of IL-23.
JAK	Baricitinib, ruxolitinib, tofacitinib	GVHD (ruxolitinib), psoriatic arthritis (tofacitinib)	Baricitinib and ruxolitinib target JAK1/2, while tofacitinib targets JAK1/3. Adverse events include serious infections/malignancies/mortality/thrombosis [US Boxed Warning].
TNFα	Adalimumab, certolizumab, etanercept, golimumab, infliximab	See above.	

CD, cluster of differentiation; CTLA, cytotoxic T-lymphocyte–associated protein; Fc, fragment crystallizable; FDA, Food and Drug Administration; GVHD, graft-versus-host disease; IBD, inflammatory bowel disease; Ig, immunoglobulin; IL, interleukin; IM, intramuscular; JAK, Janus kinase; LFA, lymphocyte function–associated antigen; PML, progressive multifocal leukoencephalopathy; SCC, squamous cell carcinoma; US, United States.
[a]Infections and anaphylaxis/injection site/infusion reactions may be associated with all of the above biologic and small molecule inhibitors.
[b]Under investigation.

Table 6.4. ADVISORY COMMITTEE ON IMMUNIZATION PRACTICES–RECOMMENDED IMMUNIZATION SCHEDULE FOR PATIENTS >19 YEARS OF AGE (2020)

Vaccine	Dosing Schedule	Notes for Immunocompromised Patients[a]	Mucocutaneous Adverse Events[b]
Influenza inactivated (IIV), influenza recombinant (RIV)	1 dose annually		LP, LABD, serum sickness–like reaction, Sweet syndrome.
Influenza live attenuated (ILAV)	1 dose annually ≤50 years	Contraindicated (live).	
Tetanus, diphtheria, pertussis (Tdap or Td)	1 dose Tdap, then Td or Tdap booster every 10 years		
Measles, mumps, and rubella (MMR)	1 dose if no evidence of immunity	Contraindicated (live).	Vaccination may result in reduced severity disease after exposure to natural measles (modified measles).
Varicella (VAR)	2 doses in adults if no evidence of immunity	Contraindicated (live).	
Zoster recombinant (RZV) (Shingrix)	2 doses ≥ age 50 years		

(Continued)

Table 6.4. ADVISORY COMMITTEE ON IMMUNIZATION PRACTICES–RECOMMENDED IMMUNIZATION SCHEDULE FOR PATIENTS >19 YEARS OF AGE (2020) (CONTINUED)

Vaccine	Dosing Schedule	Notes for Immunocompromised Patients[a]	Mucocutaneous Adverse Events[b]
Zoster live (ZVL) (Zostavax)	1 dose ≥ age 60 years	Contraindicated (live).	Varicella-like eruption. Vaccination may result in reduced severity disease after exposure to natural varicella (modified varicella–like syndrome).
Human papillomavirus (HPV)	2-3 doses through age 26 years[c]		
Pneumococcal conjugate (PCV13)	1 dose	1 dose PCV13 followed by 1 dose PPSV23 at least 8 weeks later, then another dose PPSV23 at least 5 years after previous PPSV23. ≥65 years, administer 1 dose PPSV23 at least 5 years after most recent PPSV23 (only 1 dose PPSV23 recommended ≥ age 65 years).	
Pneumococcal polysaccharide (PPSV23)	1 or 2 doses		
Hepatitis A (HepA)	2 or 3 doses		
Hepatitis B (HepB)	2 or 3 doses		LP, PAN, GA, Gianotti-Crosti syndrome.
Meningococcal A, C, W, Y (MenACWY)	1 or 2 doses		
Meningococcal B (MenB)	1 or 2 doses		
Haemophilus influenzae type b (Hib)	1 or 3 doses		
Miscellaneous Vaccines			
Variola (vaccinia)	N/A	Contraindicated (live).	Adequate immunity requires formation of a vesicular ulcer with 4 cm of erythema (>10 cm is a robust take). Mucocutaneous adverse events include EM, SJS/TEN, superinfection including autoinoculation, contact transmission, eczema vaccinatum, and vaccinia necrosum/gangrenosum (progressive vaccinia). Generalized vaccinia in an immunocompromised host, eczema vaccinatum, progressive vaccinia, and ocular implants are indications for vaccinia Ig.
Monkeypox (JYNNEOS)	2 doses		
SARS-CoV-2	1 or 2 doses ≥ age 12 years	3 doses.	Delayed localized hypersensitivity reactions (COVID arm).
TB (BCG strain of *Mycobacterium bovis*)	N/A	Contraindicated (live). CGD patients have a high risk of disseminated infection.	DM, Sweet syndrome, GA, enlarging granulomatous plaque at the injection site (BCGitis) and superinfection/tuberculids. May result in a false-positive PPD.

ACD, allergic contact dermatitis; BCG, bacille Calmette-Guérin; CGD, chronic granulomatous disease; DM, dermatomyositis; EM, erythema multiforme; GA, granuloma annulare; Ig, immunoglobulin; IM, intramuscular; LABD, linear IgA bullous dermatosis; LP, lichen planus; PAN, polyarteritis nodosa; PPD, purified protein derivative; SARS-CoV-2, severe acute respiratory syndrome coronavirus 2; SJS, Stevens-Johnson syndrome; TB, tuberculosis; TEN, toxic epidermal necrolysis.

[a]Patients already receiving TNFα inhibitor therapy are considered "immunocompromised." See full Advisory Committee on Immunization Practices recommendations for other at-risk populations.

[b]Illustrative examples provided. Anaphylaxis/injection site/infusion reactions may be associated with all of the above vaccines. Nicolau syndrome may occur after IM vaccinations. Aluminum-containing vaccines may cause foreign body reactions. Thimerosal-containing vaccines (a mercury-based preservative) may cause ACD.

[c]Age 27 to 45 years based on shared clinical decision-making.

- Mucocutaneous adverse events include **anaphylaxis (may be delayed-onset) [US Boxed Warning]/infusion reactions, EGPA, injection site reactions, and serum sickness–like eruption.**
  - Management pearl: Patients should receive omalizumab only under **direct medical supervision** and be closely observed afterward for signs or symptoms of anaphylaxis. Healthcare providers should be prepared to administer appropriate therapy and should prescribe an **epinephrine autoinjector** for all patients.
- Other adverse events include:
  - Circulatory: cerebrovascular events.
  - Lymphatic/immune: helminth infection (possible), malignancies (possible).

Rituximab

- Mechanism: monoclonal antibody (chimeric) that inhibits **CD20.**
- FDA-approved dermatology indications: **GPA, MPA, PV.**
- Mucocutaneous adverse events include **anaphylaxis/infusion reactions [US Boxed Warning], mucocutaneous reactions (eg, PNP, SJS/TEN) [US Boxed Warning], malignancy (MCCs, SCCs), and serum sickness–like eruption.**
- Other adverse events include:
  - Circulatory: cardiovascular events (eg, **angina, arrhythmias**).
  - Digestive: **bowel obstructions/perforation.**

- Lymphatic/immune: **bone marrow suppression, HBV reactivation [US Boxed Warning], infections, progressive multifocal leukoencephalopathy (PML) [US Boxed Warning].**
  - Prevention pearl: **Screen all patients for HBV.** Monitor HBsAg negative/anti-HBc positive patients with HBV DNA and alanine aminotransferase (ALT) every ~3 months during therapy. Consider antiviral prophylaxis (eg, **entecavir**).
  - Prevention pearl: **PCP prophylaxis** should be given to all patients with GPA or MPA and should be considered in high-risk patients with PV.
- Monitoring parameters include:
  - Labs: **CBC. HBV**/HCV/HIV/TB screening.
  - Other: vital signs including **blood pressure** ± cardiac monitoring. Fluid/hydration status.
- Dosing notes:
  - IV: Standard dosing regimens are 375 mg/m^2 once weekly for 4 weeks ("lymphoma dosing") and 1 g initially then at 2 weeks ("RA dosing").
- Pharmacodynamics notes:
  - Efficacy: **Immunogenicity** may reduce the efficacy of rituximab.
    - Prevention pearl: **Rituximab and methotrexate coadministration may reduce risk of antichimeric antibody development.**

Other Biologic and Small Molecule Inhibitors (Table 6.5)

Table 6.5. OTHER BIOLOGIC AND SMALL MOLECULE INHIBITORS

Target	Selected Drugs	FDA-Approved Dermatology Indications	Mucocutaneous Adverse Events[a,b]	Notes[b]
BLyS	Belimumab	SLE		
C5	Eculizumab	PNH		Adverse events include serious meningococcal infection [US Boxed Warning, US REMS Program].
IL-1	Anakinra, canakinumab, rilonacept	Adult Still disease, CAPS, FMF (canakinumab), HIDS (canakinumab), TRAPS (canakinumab)		Anakinra targets IL-1R, while canakinumab and rilonacept target IL-1β.
IL-2	Basiliximab			
IL-5	Mepolizumab, reslizumab	EGPA (mepolizumab)	Anaphylaxis [US Boxed Warning—reslizumab].	
IL-6	Sarilumab, siltuximab, tocilizumab	GCA (tocilizumab)		Adverse events include serious infections [US Boxed Warning—tocilizumab].
IL-31	Nemolizumab	Pruritus associated with AD[c]		

AD, atopic dermatitis; BLyS, B lymphocyte stimulator; C, complement; CAPS, cryopyrin-associated periodic syndromes; EGPA, eosinophilic granulomatosis with polyangiitis; FDA, Food and Drug Administration; FMF, familial Mediterranean fever; GCA, giant cell arteritis; GVHD, graft-versus-host disease; HIDS, hyperimmunoglobulin D syndrome; Ig, immunoglobulin; IL, interleukin; PML, progressive multifocal leukoencephalopathy; PNH, paroxysmal nocturnal hemoglobinuria; R, receptor; REMS, Risk Evaluation and Mitigation Strategy; SLE, systemic lupus erythematosus; TRAPS, TNF receptor-associated periodic syndrome; US, United States.

[a]Illustrative examples are provided.

[b]Infections and anaphylaxis/injection site/infusion reactions may be associated with all of the above biologic and small molecule inhibitors. US Boxed Warning labels are omitted for non-mucocutaneous adverse events of drugs without FDA-approved dermatology indications.

[c]Under investigation.

Intravenous Immunoglobulin

- Mechanism: The immunomodulatory activity of IVIG may be mediated by functional blockade of Fc receptors, inhibition of complement-mediated damage, alteration of cytokine and cytokine antagonist profiles, reduction of circulating antibodies, neutralization of toxins that trigger autoantibody production, and (in SJS/TEN) inhibition of Fas/Fas-ligand interactions.
- FDA-approved dermatology indications: **Kawasaki disease, primary humoral immunodeficiency syndromes, measles/rubella/varicella prophylaxis.**
- Mucocutaneous adverse events include **anaphylaxis/infusion reactions and dyshidrotic eczema.** Patients with **IgA deficiency are at higher risk of anaphylaxis.**
- Other adverse events include:
  - Circulatory: **fluid overload,** hyperproteinemia, hypertension, **thrombosis [US Boxed Warning].**
  - Lymphatic/immune: hemolytic anemia.
  - Nervous: **aseptic meningitis.**
  - Renal/urinary/excretory: hyponatremia, **nephrotoxicity [US Boxed Warning]. Acute renal failure** is more common after administration of IVIG containing **sucrose.**
  - Respiratory: pulmonary edema.
- Dosing notes:
  - IV: The typical dose is 2 g/kg/mo for chronic disorders and 3 g/kg/mo for acute disorders. Do not administer IVIG containing **sorbitol** to patients with **hereditary fructose intolerance.**

Antihistamines and Related Drugs

Basic Concepts

- Histamine is a **preformed mast cell mediator** synthesized via the enzyme histamine decarboxylase. Histamine acts on a wide range of target cells including **endothelial cells, nerves (histaminergic C-type fibers),** and cellular effectors of the **immune system:**
  - Histamine-induced **vasodilation** is mediated by **both H_1 and H_2 receptors.**
  - Histamine-induced **pruritus** is mediated by H_1 **receptors.**
  - Histamine suppresses T-cell proliferation and cytotoxicity via H_2 receptors.
- Antihistamines are inverse agonists that downregulate the constitutive activated state of the corresponding receptor. Antihistamines are classified into first generation H_1, second generation H_1, and H_2. Other drugs (eg, TCAs) may also inhibit H_1 and H_2 receptors.
- Related drugs include mast cell stabilizers and leukotriene inhibitors.

Antihistamines (Table 6.6)

Cromolyn Sodium

- Mechanism: **mast cell stabilizer.**
- FDA-approved dermatology indications: **systemic mastocytosis.**

Leukotriene Inhibitors

- Selected drugs: **montelukast, zafirlukast.**
- Mechanism: selective **leukotriene receptor antagonist.**
  - Related drugs include **zileuton,** which blocks leukotriene synthesis by **inhibiting 5-lipoxygenase.**
- Mucocutaneous adverse events include **EGPA.**
- Other adverse events include:
  - Nervous: **serious neuropsychiatric events including SI [US Boxed Warning—montelukast].**

Retinoids

Basic Concepts

- Retinoids bind to **retinoid acid receptors (RARs) and retinoid X receptors (RXRs) in the nucleus.** RARs are always paired with an RXR, whereas RXRs can exist as a homodimer or heterodimer with several other families of receptors. Retinoids are classified into first, second, third, and fourth generations.
- Diverse effects of retinoids include:
  - **Downregulating proliferative keratins,** particularly **K6 and K16;**
  - **Promoting keratinocyte differentiation;**
  - **Upregulating** collagen synthesis, particularly **collagens I and VII;**
  - **Inducing sebaceous gland atrophy;**
  - **Inhibiting ODC;**
  - **Downregulating TLRs** (particularly **TLR2**) and antagonizing transcription factors such as **IL-6 and AP1,** which result in **anti-inflammatory and antiproliferative effects.**

Systemic Retinoids (Table 6.7)

- Mucocutaneous adverse events include **eruptive xanthomas, PGs, phototoxic eruption, pseudoporphyria, sticky skin syndrome, and xerosis/xerophthalmia/xerostomia.** In terms of hair, systemic retinoids may cause TE. The characteristic hair shaft abnormality with **increased fragility** is **pili torti,** while the characteristic hair shaft abnormality without increased fragility is **acquired progressive kinking of the hair.** In terms of nails, systemic retinoids may cause **median canaliform dystrophy.**
  - Management pearl: **1 g/d omega-3** has been reported to reduce mucocutaneous adverse events associated with isotretinoin.
  Tretinoin (ATRA) is associated with **Sweet syndrome and scrotal ulcers.**
- Other adverse events include:
  - Digestive: **hepatotoxicity [US Boxed Warning—acitretin], IBD** (controversial), **pancreatitis.**
  - Endocrine: **hyperlipidemia (hypertriglyceridemia** is the most common laboratory abnormality). **Bexarotene** is associated with **central hypothyroidism.**
  - Lymphatic/immune: **nasal colonization with *Staphylococcus aureus.* Tretinoin (ATRA) degrades the**

Table 6.6. ANTIHISTAMINES

Selected Drugs	Mechanism	FDA-Approved Dermatology Indications	Mucocutaneous Adverse Events[a]	Notes
First-generation H_1 antihistamines (eg chlorpheniramine, cyproheptadine, diphenhydramine, hydroxyzine, promethazine)	Inhibit H_1.	Anaphylaxis, pruritus, urticaria. For topical diphenhydramine, see Chapter 6: Miscellaneous Drugs.	Photoallergic/phototoxic eruption, severe tissue injury [US Boxed Warning—promethazine (injection)].	Other adverse events include anticholinergic toxicity, sedation, and respiratory depression [US Boxed Warning—promethazine (<2 y)]. Cetirizine is a metabolite of hydroxyzine. First-generation H_1 antihistamines are preferred in pregnancy (historical pregnancy risk category B).
Second-generation H_1 antihistamines (eg cetirizine, fexofenadine, loratadine, terfenadine)	Inhibit H_1.	Urticaria.	Photoallergic/phototoxic eruption.	Second-generation H_1 antihistamines are less likely to cross the BBB due to minimal lipophilicity, thus reducing anticholinergic toxicity and sedation. Terfenadine, a CYP3A4 substrate, was discontinued due to cardiotoxic potential when combined with CYP3A4 inhibitors. Fexofenadine is a metabolite of terfenadine. If a second-generation H_1 antihistamine is required in pregnancy, loratadine > cetirizine are preferred.
H_2 antihistamines (eg cimetidine, famotidine, ranitidine)	Inhibit H_2.		Ichthyosis vulgaris (cimetidine).	Adverse events include bone marrow suppression. Cimetidine is an antiandrogen. Ranitidine was discontinued due to contamination by NDMA, a probable human carcinogen.
TCAs (eg amitriptyline, doxepin, imipramine, nortriptyline)	Inhibit H_1 and H_2.	For topical doxepin, see Chapter 6: Miscellaneous Drugs.	Blue-gray pigmentation, photoallergic/phototoxic eruption.	Other adverse events include anticholinergic toxicity, QT prolongation, sedation, seizures, and SI [US Boxed Warning]. TCAs are CYP2D6 substrates.

[a]Illustrative examples are provided.
BBB, blood-brain barrier; CYP, cytochrome P450; FDA, Food and Drug Administration; H, histamine; NDMA, N-nitrosodimethylamine; SI, suicidal ideation; TCAs, tricyclic antidepressants; US, United States.

Table 6.7. SYSTEMIC RETINOIDS

Selected Drugs	Ligand-Receptor Binding	FDA-Approved Dermatology Indications	Half-Life (Excretion)
First Generation			
Isotretinoin (13-*cis*-retinoic acid)	Converted to metabolites that bind RAR/RXR	Acne.	10-20 hours (hepatic/renal)
Tretinoin (all-*trans* retinoic acid)	RAR ($\beta > \gamma >> \alpha$)		40-60 minutes (hepatic/renal)
Second Generation			
Etretinate	RAR	Psoriasis.	80-160 days (hepatic/renal)
Acitretin	RAR	Psoriasis.	50 hours (hepatic/renal)
Third Generation			
Bexarotene	RXR	CTCL.	7-9 hours (hepatic)

ATRA, all-*trans* retinoic acid; CTCL, cutaneous T-cell lymphoma; FDA, Food and Drug Administration; RAR, retinoid acid receptor; RXR, retinoid X receptor.

promyelocytic leukemia-RARα (PML-RAR) fusion pro-tein, which may induce **APL differentiation syndrome and leukocytosis [US Boxed Warning]. Bexarotene** is associated with **bone marrow suppression.**

- ○ Musculoskeletal: **arthralgias, myalgias, skeletal hyperostosis.** Isotretinoin may cause **premature epiphyseal closure.**
- ○ Nervous: **pseudotumor cerebri, psychiatric effects including SI.**
  - Management pearl: Due to risk of pseudotumor cere-bri, **avoid coadministration of systemic retinoids and tetracyclines.**
- ○ Ocular: decreased visual acuity (eg, **night blindness**).
- Monitoring parameters include:
  - ○ Labs: **LFTs. Fasting lipid panel. HCG.** For **bexarotene,** monitor **CBC and free T4 (not TSH).**
- Dosing notes:
  - ○ Oral: The goal **cumulative dose** of isotretinoin is typically **120 to 150 mg/kg (0.5-2 mg/kg/d).**
- Pharmacokinetics notes:
  - ○ Metabolism: **Isotretinoin absorption is improved with a fatty meal** (not required for Lidose preparations). **Bexar-otene is a CYP3A4 inducer.**
    - Management pearl: **Coadministration of bexarotene and gemfibrozil, a CYP3A4 inhibitor, may increase toxicity.** For hyperlipidemia, statins and fibrates are preferred.
- Historical pregnancy risk category: **X** (except ATRA, which is category D) **[US Boxed Warning, US iPLEDGE REMS program—isotretinoin]. Retinoid embryopathy** is charac-terized by cardiovascular, parathyroid, thymic, **craniofacial,** and CNS abnormalities.
  - ○ Isotretinoin: **Females of reproductive potential must avoid pregnancy beginning 1 month prior to therapy,**

during therapy, and for at least 1 month after therapy. Use of **two forms of contraception or total abstinence** is required along with **negative pregnancy tests 30 days and immediately prior to therapy, every month during therapy, and 1 month after therapy.** All except the first pregnancy test must be performed at a **Clinical Labora-tory Improvement Amendments (CLIA)-certified lab-oratory.** Females have a **7-day "window"** to pick up the prescription and **no more than a 30-day supply** can be dispensed. Patients should **avoid blood donation for at least 1 month** after therapy.

- ○ Acitretin: **Etretinate, which is 50× more lipophilic than its metabolite acitretin,** was discontinued due to terato-genicity. **Alcohol indirectly enhances reesterification of acitretin to etretinate.** As a result, despite its relatively short half-life, **females of reproductive potential must avoid pregnancy for at least 3 years after acitretin therapy.**

Topical Retinoids (Table 6.8)

- Mucocutaneous adverse events include **desquamation and exfoliation, erythema, hypopigmentation, ICD, photo-toxic eruption, and xerosis.**
- Pharmacodynamics note:
  - ○ Efficacy: Adapalene may be combined with benzoyl per-oxide. **Tretinoin is degraded by benzoyl peroxide and sunlight** but may be combined with clindamycin.
- Historical pregnancy risk category:
  - ○ Adapalene, tretinoin (ATRA): **C.**
  - ○ Bexarotene, tazarotene: **X.**
    - Bexarotene binds RXR and is category X. Tazarotene is a topical teratogen.

Table 6.8. TOPICAL RETINOIDS

Selected Drugs	Ligand-Receptor Binding	FDA-Approved Dermatology Indications
First Generation		
Tretinoin (ATRA)	RAR (β>γ>>α)	Acne; palliation of fine wrinkles, mottled hyperpigmentation, and tactile roughness of facial skin.
Third Generation		
Adapalene	RAR (β,γ>α)	Acne.
Tazarotene	RAR (β,γ>α)	Acne; palliation of fine facial wrinkles, facial mottled hyper-/hypopigmentation, benign facial lentigines; psoriasis.
Bexarotene	RXR	CTCL.
Fourth Generation		
Trifarotene	Potent and selective agonist RAR-γ	Acne.

ATRA, all-*trans* retinoic acid; CTCL, cutaneous T-cell lymphoma; FDA, Food and Drug Administration; RAR, retinoid acid receptor; RXR, retinoid X receptor.

Hormonal Drugs

Basic Concepts

- Hormonal drugs include androgens, antiandrogens, and combined (estrogen-progestin) OCPs.
- **Androgens stimulate sebaceous glands** and, depending on location, either **terminal hair development (eg, face) or reversion to vellus hair follicles (eg, scalp).**
- **Estrogens decrease androgen production and free testosterone by increasing sex hormone binding globulin (SHBG). Estrogens also delay or prevent skin aging and prolong anagen while reducing the hair growth rate.**

Androgens

- Selected drugs: **danazol, stanozolol.**
- Mechanism: **anabolic steroids derived from testosterone; increase C4.**
- FDA-approved dermatology indications: **hereditary angioedema.**
- Mucocutaneous adverse events include **acneiform eruption.** In terms of hair, androgens may cause **hirsutism.**
- Other adverse events include:
  - Circulatory: **thromboembolic events [US Boxed Warning].**
  - Digestive: **peliosis hepatis and benign hepatic adenoma [US Boxed Warning].**
  - Nervous: **intracranial hypertension [US Boxed Warning].**
- Historical pregnancy risk category: **X.**

Antiandrogens

- Selected drugs/mechanism:
  - **Steroidal androgen receptor antagonists: clascoterone, drospirenone, spironolactone;**
  - **Nonsteroidal androgen receptor antagonists: flutamide;**
  - **5α-reductase inhibitors: dutasteride (types 1 and 2), finasteride (type 1);**
    - Dutasteride has dual action on 5α-reductase types 1 and 2.
  - Antihistamine: cimetidine (see above).
- FDA-approved dermatology indications:
  - Systemic: **AGA (finasteride, men).**
  - Topical: **acne (clascoterone).**
- Adverse events include:
  - Circulatory: **hypovolemia (spironolactone).**
    - It is easy to remember that hypovolemia is an adverse event of spironolactone since it was originally developed as a potassium-sparing diuretic.
  - Digestive: **hepatic injury [US Boxed Warning—flutamide].**
  - Renal/urinary/excretory: **hyperkalemia (spironolactone).**
    - Management pearl: **Routine potassium monitoring is unnecessary for healthy young women (18-45 years) taking spironolactone for acne.** Exercise caution with **drugs (eg, ACEIs, angiotensin II receptor blockers [ARBs], NSAIDs), excessive potassium intake, and renal impairment.**

- Reproductive: **breast tenderness, gynecomastia, irregular menses, sexual dysfunction. Breast cancer** has been reported in patients taking **spironolactone, which has been shown to be a tumorigen in rats [US Boxed Warning]; however, a cause-and-effect relationship has not been established. High-grade prostate cancer** has been reported in patients taking **5α-reductase inhibitors** (controversial).
    - Sexual dysfunction after discontinuation of finasteride is sometimes called "post-finasteride syndrome."
- Dosing notes:
  - Oral: The **initial dose of spironolactone for acne is 25 to 50 mg/d in 1 to 2 divided doses**; the **maximum dose is 200 mg/d.**
- Pharmacodynamics notes:
  - Efficacy: **Dutasteride may be more efficacious than finasteride** but may also lead to longer-lasting adverse events including potentially irreversible drop in sperm count and motility.
- Historical pregnancy risk category:
  - Spironolactone: **C. Feminization of the male fetus is a theoretical risk** (not reported in humans).
  - Flutamide: **D.**
  - Dutasteride, finasteride: **X.**

Combined Oral Contraceptive Pills

- Selected drugs: **ethinyl estradiol and drospirenone (Yaz); ethinyl estradiol and norethindrone (Estrostep Fe); ethinyl estradiol and norgestimate (Ortho Tri-Cyclen).**
- Mechanism: inhibit ovulation. Drospirenone is a steroidal androgen receptor antagonist.
- FDA-approved dermatology indications: **acne.**
- Mucocutaneous adverse events include **AN, EN, eruptive xanthomas, melasma, porphyria flare, pruritus, and Sweet syndrome.** In terms of hair, OCP discontinuation may lead to **TE.**
- Other adverse events include:
  - Circulatory: **venous thromboembolism** (~6-9/10,000 person-years relative to ~30/10,000 person-years in pregnancy), **arterial thromboembolism, cardiovascular disease [US Boxed Warning].** Combined OCPs are **contraindicated** in high-risk patients including **women >35 years who smoke [US Boxed Warning].**
  - Digestive: nausea/vomiting.
  - Endocrine: weight changes.
  - Reproductive: **breakthrough bleeding; breast tenderness; increased risk for breast, cervical, and endometrial cancer [US Boxed Warning].** Overall **~30% decreased risk for gynecologic malignancies.**
  - Nervous: **dementia [US Boxed Warning]**, headache, migraine, mood changes.
  For adverse events of drospirenone, see above.
- Dosing notes:
  - Sunday starter: start the first Sunday after onset of menstruation (backup contraception should be used for the first 7 days).

- Day 1 starter: start the first day of the menstrual cycle.
- The **"quick start" method**: **start any time during the menstrual cycle** if reasonably sure the woman is not pregnant (backup contraception should be used for the first 7 days unless initiated within the first 5 days of menstrual bleeding or the woman abstains from sexual intercourse).
- Pharmacodynamics notes:
  - Efficacy: Combined OCPs containing progestins with greater intrinsic antiandrogen activity (eg, drospirenone) may have greater efficacy for acne.
- Historical pregnancy risk category: **X.**

Antimicrobials

Basic Concepts

- Antimicrobials have antiviral, antibacterial, antifungal, and/ or antiparasitic activity.
    The term "antibiotic" technically refers to all antimicrobials but is colloquially used as a synonym for antibacterial.
- Antimicrobial **spectrum of activity** (coverage) depends not only on the antimicrobial but also on **local resistance patterns.** In most circumstances, **a culture should be performed prior to initiating empiric therapy** so that antimicrobial(s) may be adjusted according to **sensitivity testing.**
- Indiscriminate use of broad-spectrum antimicrobials fosters the emergence of resistant microbes.

Antivirals

Systemic Antivirals

Amantadine

- Mechanism: unknown; however, primarily prevents release of infectious viral nucleic acid into the host cell by **interfering with the transmembrane domain of the viral matrix 2 protein.**
- FDA-approved dermatology indications: **influenza A treatment/prophylaxis.**
- Mucocutaneous adverse events include **livedo reticularis.**
- Other adverse events include:
  - Circulatory: **anticholinergic toxicity.**

Antiretrovirals (Table 6.9)

Purine Analogues

- Selected drugs: **acyclovir/valacyclovir (prodrug), ganciclovir/valganciclovir (prodrug), penciclovir/famciclovir (prodrug), remdesivir (prodrug).**
- Mechanism (acyclovir example): **phosphorylated by viral thymidine kinase** to acyclovir monophosphate, which is then twice phosphorylated by cellular kinases to acyclovir triphosphate, a guanine analogue that interferes with viral DNA synthesis through **competitive inhibition of viral DNA polymerase.**

Table 6.9. ANTIRETROVIRALS

Selected Drugs[a]	Mucocutaneous Adverse Events[b]	Notes[c]
NRTIs/NtRTIs	Hyperpigmentation, lipodystrophy, morbilliform drug eruption/DRESS [US Boxed Warning—abacavir]; hypertrichosis/trichomegaly (eg zidovudine); mucocutaneous hyperpigmentation and blue lunulae/longitudinal melanonychia (eg zidovudine), paronychia/excessive periungual granulation tissue (eg lamivudine).	HLA-B5701 is associated with SCAR to abacavir. All patients should be screened prior to initiating abacavir.
NNRTIs	Lipodystrophy, morbilliform drug eruption/DRESS, and SJS/TEN [US Boxed Warning—nevirapine].	
Protease inhibitors	Angiolipomas/lipodystrophy, morbilliform drug eruption/DRESS, xerosis, paronychia/excessive periungual granulation tissue (eg indinavir).	Protease inhibitors are CYP3A4 inhibitors.
	Lipodystrophy associated with protease inhibitors may manifest with "cheek hollowing" (buccal fat pads), a "buffalo hump" (dorsocervical fat pad), and "protease pouch" (central obesity).	Ritonavir, a potent CYP4A4 inhibitor, can "boost" other protease inhibitors.
Integrase inhibitors		
CCR5 inhibitors		
Fusion inhibitors	Injection site reactions.	

CCR5, cysteine-cysteine chemokine receptor 5; DRESS, drug reaction with eosinophilia and systemic symptoms; FDA, Food and Drug Administration; HIV, human immunodeficiency virus; HLA, human leukocyte antigen; NNRTIs, nonnucleoside reverse transcriptase inhibitors; NRTIs, nucleoside reverse transcriptase inhibitors; NtRTIs, nucleotide reverse transcriptase inhibitors; SCAR, severe cutaneous adverse reaction; SJS/TEN, Stevens-Johnson syndrome/toxic epidermal necrolysis; US, United States.

[a]FDA approved for HIV infection.
[b]Illustrative examples are provided.
[c]US Boxed Warning labels are omitted for non-mucocutaneous adverse events.

- FDA-approved dermatology indications: **HSV (acyclovir/valacyclovir, penciclovir/famciclovir), VZV (acyclovir/valacyclovir, famciclovir), CMV (ganciclovir/valganciclovir), COVID-19 (remdesivir).**
- Adverse events include:
  - Lymphatic/immune: **bone marrow suppression [US Boxed Warning—ganciclovir/valganciclovir],** mutagenesis and carcinogenesis [US Boxed Warning—ganciclovir/valganciclovir], **thrombotic thrombocytopenic purpura (TTP)/hemolytic uremic syndrome (HUS) (valacyclovir, immunocompromised).**
  - Renal/urinary/excretory: **reversible crystalluria-induced nephropathy (acyclovir, IV).**
    - Prevention pearl: To prevent crystalluria-induced nephropathy, maintain adequate hydration during high-dose IV acyclovir therapy.
  - Reproductive: impairment of fertility [US Boxed Warning—ganciclovir/valganciclovir].
- Historical pregnancy risk category:
  - Acyclovir/valacyclovir, penciclovir/famciclovir: **B.**
  - Ganciclovir/valganciclovir: **C [US Boxed Warning].**
    - Ganciclovir/valganciclovir for C̲MV are category C̲.

Pyrimidine Analogues

- Selected drugs: **cidofovir.**
- Mechanism: phosphorylated by cellular kinases into a diphosphate that interferes with viral DNA synthesis through **competitive inhibition of viral DNA polymerase.**
  - C̲idofovir is self-c̲ontained (functions independent of viral thymidine kinase activation).
- FDA-approved dermatology indications: **CMV.**
- Adverse events include:
  - Lymphatic/immune: carcinogenic [US Boxed Warning], neutropenia [US Boxed Warning].
  - Renal/urinary/excretory: nephrotoxicity [US Boxed Warning].
- Historical pregnancy risk category: **C [US Boxed Warning].**
  - Cidofovir for C̲MV is category C̲.

Pyrophosphate Analogues

- Selected drugs: **foscarnet.**
- Mechanism: interferes with viral DNA synthesis through **noncompetitive inhibition of viral DNA polymerase.**
  - F̲oscarnet is f̲ree spirited (functions independent of viral thymidine kinase activation).
- FDA-approved dermatology indications: **HSV (acyclovir-resistant), CMV.**
- Mucocutaneous adverse events include **penile ulcers.**
- Other adverse events include:
  - Nervous: seizures [US Boxed Warning].
  - Renal/urinary/excretory: renal impairment [US Boxed Warning].
- Historical pregnancy risk category: **C.**
  - Foscarnet for C̲MV is category C̲.

Topical Antivirals (Table 6.10)

Table 6.10. TOPICAL ANTIVIRALS

Selected Drugs	Mechanism	FDA-Approved Dermatology Indications	Mucocutaneous Adverse Events[a]	Notes
Acyclovir, penciclovir	See above.	HSV.	Burning.	
Cantharidin	Releases neutral serine proteases that cause desmosomal plaque degeneration.	Molluscum contagiosum, warts.	Blister formation, ring wart. / Clearance in the center but not the periphery is called a "doughnut wart."	Derived from the "blister beetle" also known as the Spanish fly (*Lytta vesicatoria*). Painless application. Intraepidermal acantholysis is nonscarring.
Docosanol	Prevents viral entry and replication at the cellular level.	Cold sore/fever blister.	Burning.	
Immunotherapies (IFNα, IFNβ, IFNγ, imiquimod, SADBE)	See Chapter 6: Antineoplastics.			
Podophyllin, Podofilox	Disrupt microtubule function (M phase).	Condyloma acuminata.	Local inflammation.	Crude extract from the may apple plant. Podophyllin is historical pregnancy risk category X.
Salicylic acid, sinecatechins, urea	See Chapter 9: Cosmetics and Cosmeceuticals.			

FDA, Food and Drug Administration; HSV, herpes simplex virus; IFN, interferon; SADBE, squaric acid dibutyl ester; ROS, reactive oxygen species.
[a]Illustrative examples are provided.

Antibacterials

- **Antibacterials** may be **bacteriostatic (inhibit growth and replication of bacteria)** or **bactericidal (kill bacteria).** Example antibacterial classes include:
  - Bacteriostatic: **macrolides, lincomycins, sulfonamides, tetracyclines.**
  - Bactericidal: **aminoglycosides, β-lactams, quinolones, glycopeptides.**
  Factors such as bacterial susceptibility and antibacterial concentration may influence whether an antibacterial is bacteriostatic or bactericidal (eg, clindamycin at low vs high concentration).
- Figure 6.3 illustrates the **antibacterial spectrum of activity against GP bacteria, GN bacteria, and mycobacteria.** Given substantial overlap, FDA-approved dermatology indications are omitted from the discussion of systemic antibacterials.

Systemic Antibacterials

Aminoglycosides

- Selected drugs: **gentamicin, neomycin, streptomycin.**
- Mechanism: interfere with bacterial protein synthesis by **binding the 30S ribosomal subunit.**
  - Figure 6.4.
- Adverse events include:
  - Nervous: **neurotoxicity (eg, ototoxicity) [US Boxed Warning].**
  - Renal/urinary/excretory: **nephrotoxicity [US Boxed Warning].**
- Pharmacokinetics notes:
  - Absorption: **Efflux by brush border cells of the small intestine limits efficacy of oral aminoglycoside administration.**
- Historical pregnancy risk category: **D.**

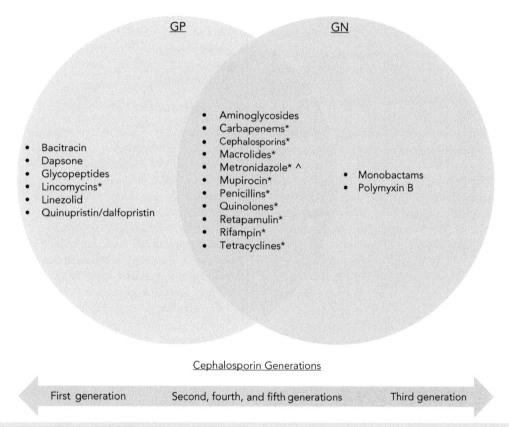

GP

GN

- Bacitracin
- Dapsone
- Glycopeptides
- Lincomycins*
- Linezolid
- Quinupristin/dalfopristin

- Aminoglycosides
- Carbapenems*
- Cephalosporins*
- Macrolides*
- Metronidazole* ^
- Mupirocin*
- Penicillins*
- Quinolones*
- Retapamulin*
- Rifampin*
- Tetracyclines*

- Monobactams
- Polymyxin B

Cephalosporin Generations

First generation   Second, fourth, and fifth generations   Third generation

Figure 6.3. ANTIBACTERIAL SPECTRUM OF ACTIVITY. Illustrative examples provided. Antibacterial spectrum of activity depends not only on the antibacterial but also on local resistance patterns.

GN, gram-negative; GP, gram-positive; INH, isoniazid.

Mycobacteria
- *Mycobacterium tuberculosis:* ethambutol, INH, pyrazinamide, rifampin.
- *Mycobacterium leprae:* clofazimine, dapsone, minocycline, ofloxacin, rifampin.
- **Nontuberculous mycobacterioses:** clarithromycin.^^

* Activity against anaerobes.
^ Activity against protozoa.
^^ May be considered for empiric therapy. Antibacterial selection varies based on the causative organism.

Clindamycin (clinda-<u>mighty</u>-cin) and <u>macro</u>lides bind the 50S ribosomal subunit.

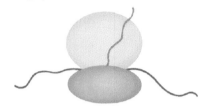

Aminoglycosides (a-<u>mini</u>-glycosides) and tetracyclines (<u>teeny</u>-cyclines) bind the 30S ribosomal subunit.

Figure 6.4. ANTIBACTERIALS AND THE RIBOSOME. Chloramphenicol, oxazolidinones, quinupristin/dalfopristin, and retapamulin are other antibiotics that bind the 50S ribosomal subunit.
(Illustration by Caroline A. Nelson, MD.)

β-lactams

- Selected drugs:
  - Penicillins: **penicillin G, penicillin V** (natural); **dicloxacillin, methicillin, nafcillin** (penicillinase-resistant); **amoxicillin, ampicillin** (aminopenicillins); **piperacillin, ticarcillin** (antipseudomonal).
  - Cephalosporins: **cefadroxil, cefazolin, cephalexin** (first generation); **cefaclor, cefuroxime** (second generation); **cefdinir, cefixime, cefpodoxime, ceftazidime, ceftriaxone** (third generation); **cefepime** (fourth generation); **ceftaroline** (fifth generation); **cefotetan, cefoxitin** (cephamycins).
  - Carbapenems: **ertapenem, imipenem, meropenem.**
  - Monobactams: **aztreonam.**
- Mechanism: **interfere with bacterial cell wall synthesis by inhibiting the transpeptidase cross-linking of peptidoglycan chains.**
- Mucocutaneous adverse events include AGEP, CSVV, LABD, morbilliform drug eruption, PV, SDRIFE, serum sickness–like reaction (especially cefaclor), urticaria/anaphylaxis. **Ampicillin and amoxicillin** almost invariably cause **morbilliform eruption** in patients with **infectious mononucleosis.** Of note, only 10% to 20% of patients who report a history of penicillin allergy have an allergy identified upon skin testing. **The potential for penicillin-cephalosporin cross-reactivity is related to the structural R1 side chain.**
- Other adverse events include:
  - Digestive: diarrhea.
  - Renal/urinary/excretory: acute interstitial nephritis.
- Pharmacodynamics notes:
  - Efficacy: Addition of a **β-lactamase inhibitor (avibactam, clavulanic acid, sulbactam, tazobactam)** can extend the spectrum of a β-lactam against **β-lactamase–producing bacteria (most notably staphylococci).**
- Pharmacokinetics notes:
  - Excretion: **Probenecid may decrease renal tubular excretion of β-lactams.**
- Historical pregnancy risk category: **B.**
  - β-lactams are category <u>B</u>.

Chloramphenicol

- Mechanism: interferes with bacterial protein synthesis by **binding the 50S ribosomal subunit.**

- Adverse events include:
  - Lymphatic/immune: **blood dyscrasias [US Boxed Warning]. Gray baby syndrome, circulatory collapse characterized by an ashen-gray color,** may occur in premature and newborn infants with chloramphenicol overexposure.

Clofazimine

- Mechanism: unknown.
- Mucocutaneous adverse events include **ichthyosis vulgaris, phototoxic eruption, red-brown hyperpigmentation/chromhidrosis.**

Glycopeptides

- Selected drugs: **vancomycin.**
- Mechanism: **interferes with bacterial cell wall synthesis** by blocking glycopeptide polymerization through binding tightly to **D-alanyl-D-alanine** portion of cell wall precursor.
  - Related drugs include lipoglycopeptides (eg, **dalbavancin, oritavancin, telavancin**) and lipopeptides (eg, **daptomycin**).
- Mucocutaneous adverse events include **extravasation and thrombophlebitis, infusion reactions/"red man syndrome," LABD, urticaria/anaphylaxis, and DRESS.**
  - Management pearl: "**Red man syndrome**" is a rate-dependent infusion reaction, not a true allergic reaction. **Slow the infusion rate** to >1.5 to 2 hours and increase the dilution volume. Consider pretreatment with **antihistamines.**
    - Do NOT get confused! "Red man syndrome" may refer to idiopathic erythroderma OR a rate-dependent infusion reaction to vancomycin.
    - Vancomycin is a mast cell degranulator.
- Other adverse events include:
  - Nervous: **ototoxicity.**
  - Renal/urinary/excretory: **nephrotoxicity.**
- Historical pregnancy risk category: C. Risk of embryo-fetal toxicity due to excipients [US Boxed Warning].

Isoniazid

- Mechanism: **inhibits synthesis of mycoloic acids**, an essential component of the bacterial cell wall.
- Mucocutaneous adverse events include **acneiform eruption, drug-induced LE, vitamin B$_3$ deficiency, and vitamin B$_6$ deficiency.**

- Other adverse events include:
  - Digestive: **hepatitis [US Boxed Warning]**.
  - Nervous: **peripheral neuropathy**.
    - Prevention pearl: **Vitamin B$_6$ supplementation** is recommended for individuals at-risk for **INH-induced peripheral neuropathy** (eg, alcoholics).

Lincomycins

- Selected drugs: **clindamycin**.
- Mechanism: interferes with bacterial protein synthesis by **binding the 50S ribosomal subunit**.
- Adverse events include:
  - Digestive: **superinfection (eg, C. difficile) [US Boxed Warning]**.
- Pharmacodynamics notes:
  - Efficacy: Staphylococci and β-hemolytic streptococci that are **sensitive to clindamycin but resistant to erythromycin on initial susceptibility testing** should be evaluated with the **D (double-disk diffusion)-test for inducible clindamycin resistance**.
- Historical pregnancy risk category: **B**.

Linezolid

- Mechanism: interferes with bacterial protein synthesis by **binding the 50S ribosomal subunit**.
- Adverse events include:
  - Lymphatic/immune: **bone marrow suppression**.
  - Nervous: **serotonin syndrome**.

Macrolides

- Selected drugs: **azithromycin, clarithromycin, erythromycin**.
- Mechanism: interfere with bacterial protein synthesis by **binding the 50S ribosomal subunit. Anti-inflammatory** properties derive from **inhibition of MMPs, pro-inflammatory cytokines, and leukocyte migration and adhesion**.
- Mucocutaneous adverse events include **AGEP**.
- Other adverse events include:
  - Circulatory: **QT prolongation**.
  - Digestive: **nausea/vomiting**.
    Macrolides may lead to **pyloric stenosis** in exposed infants.
- Pharmacokinetics notes:
  - Metabolism: Macrolides are **CYP3A4 inhibitors**.
- Historical pregnancy risk category: **B** (except **erythromycin estolate**, which is category C due to risk of **cholestatic hepatitis**).
    Erythromycin estolate can escalate bilirubin.

Metronidazole

- Mechanism: diffuses into the organism and causes a **loss of helical DNA structure and strand breakage**, resulting in inhibition of protein synthesis and death.
- Adverse events include:
  - Circulatory: **disulfiram-like reaction**.
  - Lymphatic/immune: **carcinogenic in rats [US Boxed Warning]**.

Quinolones

- Selected Drugs: **ciprofloxacin, ofloxacin** (second generation), **levofloxacin** (third generation), **moxifloxacin** (fourth generation).
- Mechanism: **inhibit bacterial DNA gyrase (topoisomerase II)**.
- Mucocutaneous adverse events include CSVV, **photoallergic/phototoxic eruption, and pseudoporphyria**. In terms of nails, quinolones may cause **photoonycholysis**.
- Other adverse events include:
  - Circulatory: aortic aneurysm and dissection, **QT prolongation**.
  - Digestive: hepatotoxicity, **superinfection (eg, C. difficile)**.
  - Musculoskeletal: **tendinitis and tendon rupture [US Boxed Warning]**.
  - Nervous: **CNS effects/peripheral neuropathy/psychiatric reactions [US Boxed Warning], exacerbation of myasthenia gravis [US Boxed Warning]**.
- Pharmacokinetics notes:
  - Absorption: **Antacids and multivalent cations may reduce quinolone absorption**.
  - Metabolism: Ciprofloxacin is a **CYP1A2 inhibitor**.
- Historical pregnancy risk category: **C**.

Rifampin

- Mechanism: interfere with bacterial RNA synthesis by **inhibiting DNA-dependent RNA polymerase**.
- Mucocutaneous adverse events include **porphyria flare**.
- Other adverse events include:
  - Renal/urinary/excretory: **yellow, orange, red, or brown discoloration of secretions (eg, urine)**.
- Pharmacokinetics notes:
  - Metabolism: Rifampin is a **CYP3A4 inducer (decreases the efficacy of OCPs by accelerating metabolism and by reducing the bacterial population of the small intestine, thereby interfering with enterohepatic cycling of ethinylestradiol)**.

Quinupristin/Dalfopristin

- Mechanism: interfere with bacterial protein synthesis by **binding the 50S ribosomal subunit**.

Sulfonamides

- Selected drugs: **SMX, sulfadiazine, sulfapyridine**.
  - **Sulfasalazine** consists of sulfapyridine linked to mesalamine by an azo chemical linker.
- Mechanism: **interfere with bacterial folic acid synthesis** needed for nucleic acid synthesis through **competitive inhibition of bacterial DHPS**.
  - **TMP-SMX (cotrimoxazole)** combines SMX with TMP, an antibacterial that **interferes with bacterial folic acid synthesis** needed for nucleic acid synthesis by **inhibiting DHFR**.
  - Related drugs include **dapsone** (see Chapter 6: Immunosuppressants and Immunomodulators).
    The sulfone dapsone has the same mechanism as the sulfonamides.
- Mucocutaneous adverse events include CSVV, EN, FDE, **morbilliform drug eruption/DRESS, photoallergic/**

phototoxic eruption, porphyria flare, SJS/TEN, and Sweet syndrome.

  ◦ TMP-SMX is the leading cause of cutaneous drug eruptions in HIV-infected patients.
- Other adverse events of TMP-SMX resemble methotrexate (eg, gastrointestinal toxicity, hepatotoxicity, bone marrow suppression, nephrotoxicity).
- Pharmacokinetics notes:
  ◦ Metabolism: **Slow acetylation** is associated with sulfonamide reactions.
- Historical pregnancy risk category:
  ◦ Sulfadiazine: **C.**
  ◦ TMP-SMX: **D.**

Tetracyclines

- Selected drugs: **demeclocycline, doxycycline, minocycline, sarecycline, tetracycline, tigecycline.**
- Mechanism: interfere with bacterial protein synthesis by **binding the 30S ribosomal subunit. Anti-inflammatory** properties are similar to macrolides.
- Mucocutaneous adverse events include **ANCA vasculitis (anti-MPO p-ANCA positive) (minocycline), EN, FDE**

(especially tetracycline), **blue-black hyperpigmentation, black hairy tongue (minocycline), drug-induced LE (minocycline), morbilliform drug eruption/DRESS (minocycline), PAN (minocycline), phototoxic eruption (demeclocycline >>>> minocycline), porphyria flare, pseudoporphyria, and Sweet syndrome.** In terms of nails, tetracyclines may cause **blue lunulae/longitudinal melanonychia (minocycline) and photoonycholysis.**

Minocycline pigmentation is divided into three types:
  ◦ **Type 1: focal blue-black pigmentation in areas of previous inflammation or scarring;**
  ◦ **Type 2: blue-gray pigmentation favoring the legs;**
  ◦ **Type 3: diffuse brown pigmentation favoring the sunexposed skin.**
    ◦ Type 3 minocycline pigmentation may be described as "muddy."
    ◦ Figure 6.5.
- Other adverse events include:
  ◦ Digestive: **autoimmune hepatitis** (minocycline), **gastrointestinal upset, pill esophagitis.**
  ◦ Musculoskeletal: **tooth staining (doxycycline gingival third, minocycline midportion).**

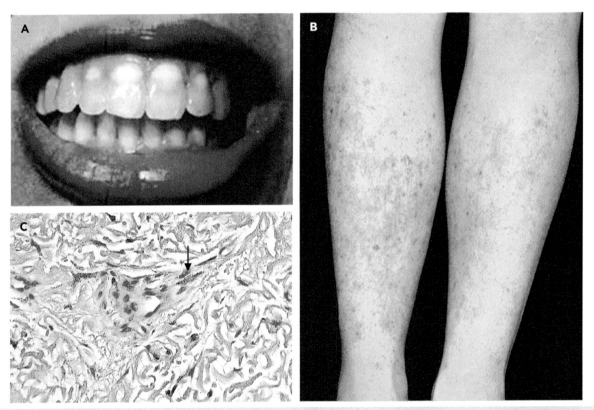

Figure 6.5. CLINICOPATHOLOGICAL CORRELATION: MINOCYCLINE PIGMENTATION. Histopathological features of minocycline pigmentation vary based on type. A, Minocycline pigmentation of the mucosa and midportion of the teeth. B, Minocycline pigmentation of the legs. C, Minocycline pigmentation. Solid arrow: pigment within a dermal melanophage.

(A, Reprinted with permission from Bobonich MA, Nolen ME, Honaker J, et al. *Dermatology for Advanced Practice Clinicians: A Comprehensive Guide to Diagnosis and Treatment.* 2nd ed. Wolters Kluwer; 2021. B, Reprinted with permission from Craft N, Fox LP, Goldsmith LA, et al. *VisualDx: Essential Adult Dermatology.* Wolters Kluwer Health/Lippincott Williams & Wilkins; 2010. C, Histology image reprinted with permission from Elder DE, Elenitsas R, Rosenbach M, et al. *Lever's Histopathology of the Skin.* 11th ed. Wolters Kluwer; 2015.)

- **Type 1:** hemosiderin (Perls Prussian blue)
- **Type 2:** hemosiderin (Perls Prussian blue) and melanin (Fontana-Masson)
- **Type 3:** melanin (Fontana-Masson)

Use of tetracyclines in children < 8 years should be reserved for severe, potentially life-threatening infections or when better alternatives are unavailable.
- Nervous: **pseudotumor cerebri.**
  - Management pearl: Due to risk of pseudotumor cerebri, **avoid coadministration of systemic retinoids and tetracyclines.**

Tigecycline is associated with an increase in all-cause mortality [US Boxed Warning].
- Pharmacokinetics notes:
  - Absorption: **Antacids and multivalent cations may reduce the absorption of tetracyclines.** Food impairs tetracycline absorption, but not doxycycline or minocycline absorption.
  - Excretion: **Doxycycline and tigecycline are primarily excreted in the feces and are therefore preferred in patients with renal dysfunction.**
- Historical pregnancy risk category: **D.** Teratogenic effects include **staining of the deciduous teeth,** enamel hypoplasia, and impaired skeletal growth.

Topical Antibacterials and Other Antimicrobials (Table 6.11)

◆ Figure 6.6.

Antifungals (Figure 6.7)

- **Antifungals** may be **fungistatic (inhibit growth and replication of fungus)** or **fungicidal (kill fungus).** Examples antifungal classes include:
  - Fungistatic: **echinocandins (mold), imidazoles and triazoles, polyenes.**
  - Fungicidal: **allylamines, echinocandins (yeast).**

Factors such as fungal susceptibility and antifungal concentration may influence whether an antifungal is fungistatic or fungicidal (eg, amphotericin B at low vs high concentration).
- **Spectrum of activity against superficial** versus **deep mycoses** depends on the antifungal.

Systemic Antifungals

Allylamines

- Selected drugs: **terbinafine.**
- Mechanism: **interferes with fungal cell membrane synthesis by inhibiting squalene epoxidase.**
- FDA-approved dermatology indications: **onychomycosis.**
- Mucocutaneous adverse events include **SCLE.**
- Other adverse events include:
  - Digestive: **smell and/or taste disturbances, hepatic failure.**
    - Management pearl: Continuous dosing of terbinafine is 250 mg daily for 6 weeks (fingernail) or 12 weeks (toenail). Due to hepatotoxicity, **check LFTs at baseline and during treatment > 6 weeks** or in at-risk patients. **Pulsed dosing is less effective but may reduce the risk of adverse events,** reduce cost, and improve patient compliance.
  - Lymphatic/immune: lymphopenia (transient), neutropenia (immunocompromised).

- Pharmacokinetics notes:
  - Absorption: terbinafine should not be taken with apple sauce as it becomes inactivated.
  - Metabolism: terbinafine is a **CYP2D6 inhibitor.**
- Historical pregnancy risk category: **B.**

Imidazoles and Triazoles

- Selected drugs:
  - Imidazoles: **ketoconazole.**
  - Triazoles: **fluconazole, isavuconazole, itraconazole, posaconazole, voriconazole.**
- Mechanism: **interfere with fungal cell membrane synthesis by inhibiting 14α-demethylase.**
- FDA-approved dermatology indications: **aspergillosis** (isavuconazole, itraconazole, posaconazole, voriconazole), **blastomycosis** (itraconazole), **candida** (all except isavuconazole), **cryptococcal meningitis** (fluconazole), **histoplasmosis** (itraconazole), **mucormycosis** (isavuconazole), **onychomycosis** (itraconazole), **scedosporiosis/fusariosis** (voriconazole), **sporotrichosis** (itraconazole). Ketoconazole is FDA approved for systemic fungal infections but is rarely used due to its adverse event profile.
- Mucocutaneous adverse events include **phototoxic eruption/photocarcinogenesis (voriconazole) and pseudoporphyria (voriconazole). Sticky skin syndrome** may occur when **ketoconazole is combined with doxorubicin.**
- Other adverse events include:
  - Circulatory: **CHF [US Boxed Warning—itraconazole], QT prolongation [US Boxed Warning—ketoconazole].**
  - Digestive: **hepatotoxicity [US Boxed Warning—ketoconazole].**
  - Ocular: **visual disturbances (voriconazole).**
  - Reproductive: **gynecomastia (ketoconazole), sexual dysfunction (ketoconazole).**
- Pharmacokinetics notes:
  - Absorption: **Antacids may reduce azole absorption.**
  - Metabolism: Azoles are **CYP3A4 inhibitors [US Boxed Warning—itraconazole].** Fluconazole is a **CYP2C19 and CYP2C9 inhibitor.**
- Historical pregnancy risk category: C (except **voriconazole,** which is category **D**).

Echinocandins

- Selected drugs: **anidulafungin, caspofungin, micafungin.**
- Mechanism: **interfere with fungal cell wall synthesis by inhibiting 1,3-beta-D-glucan synthase.**
- FDA-approved dermatology indications: **aspergillosis** (caspofungin), **candida.**
- Mucocutaneous adverse events include **infusion reactions.**
- Historical pregnancy risk category: **C.**

Flucytosine

- Mechanism: **cytosine analogue** that selectively interferes with DNA synthesis in fungi.

Table 6.11. TOPICAL ANTIBACTERIALS AND OTHER ANTIMICROBIALS

Selected Drugs	Mechanism	FDA-Approved Dermatology Indications	Mucocutaneous Adverse Events[a]	Notes
Azelaic acid	Dicarboxylic acid with unknown antibacterial mechanism. Inhibits tyrosinase (competitive).	Acne, rosacea.	ICD.	Produced by *Malassezia* species. Preferred acne therapy in pregnancy (historical pregnancy risk category B).
Bacitracin Do NOT confuse bacitracin with Bactroban, a brand name of mupirocin.	Inhibits bacterial cell wall synthesis by complexing with C55-prenol pyrophosphatase.	Topical infection prevention.	ACD (bacitracin coreacts with neomycin), contact urticaria/anaphylaxis.	Double antibiotic (Polysporin) combines bacitracin and polymyxin B. Triple antibiotic (Neosporin) combines bacitracin, neomycin, and polymyxin B.
Benzoyl peroxide	Oxidizes *Cutibacterium acnes* proteins (no resistance reported).	Acne.	ICD. Bleaches hair and colored fabrics.	Degrades tretinoin. May be combined with adapalene, clindamycin, and erythromycin. Historical pregnancy risk category C.
Clindamycin	See above.	Acne.	GN folliculitis.	May be combined with tretinoin or benzoyl peroxide (reduces bacterial resistance).
Dapsone	Sulfone (see Chapter 6: Immunosuppressants and Immunomodulators).	Acne.	ICD.	Hemolytic anemia (G6PD deficiency), methemoglobinemia.
Erythromycin	Macrolide (see above).	Acne.	GN folliculitis.	May be combined with benzoyl peroxide (reduces bacterial resistance).
Iodoquinol	Unknown antibacterial and antifungal mechanism.	Dermatological conditions.		High iodine content.
Gentamicin, neomycin	Aminoglycosides (see above).	Dermatologic infections, topical infection prevention.	ACD (neomycin coreacts with bacitracin), contact urticaria/anaphylaxis.	Triple antibiotic (Neosporin) combines bacitracin, neomycin, and polymyxin B.
Metronidazole	See above.	Rosacea.		
Minocycline	Tetracycline (see above).	Acne.		
Mupirocin Do NOT confuse Bactroban, a brand name of mupirocin, with bacitracin.	Interferes with bacterial protein synthesis by reversibly binding bacterial isoleucyl-tRNA synthetase.	*Staphylococcus aureus* decolonization, superficial skin infection (impetigo, secondary).		Naturally occurring antibiotic produced by fermentation using the organism *Pseudomonas fluorescens*. Mupirocin is made by *Pseudomonas* so it does NOT kill *Pseudomonas*.
Retapamulin	Interferes with bacterial protein synthesis by binding the L3 protein on the 50S ribosomal subunit.	Impetigo.	ACD.	
Polymyxin B	Interacts with phospholipids of the bacterial cell membranes, increasing permeability.	Topical infection prevention.	Contact urticaria/anaphylaxis.	Double antibiotic (Polysporin) combines bacitracin and polymyxin B. Triple antibiotic (Neosporin) combines bacitracin, neomycin, and polymyxin B.
	Polymyxin B mixes up membranes.	Polymyxin B is NOT a treatment for impetigo.	Polymyxin B is a mast cell degranulator.	

(Continued)

Selected Drugs	Mechanism	FDA-Approved Dermatology Indications	Mucocutaneous Adverse Events[a]	Notes
Mafenide, silver sulfadiazine, sulfacetamide, sulfur and sulfacetamide	Sulfonamides (see above).	Mafenide, silver sulfadiazine: burn treatment. Sulfacetamide: acne, bacterial infections, scaling dermatoses. Sulfur and sulfacetamide: acne, rosacea, seborrheic dermatitis.	ICD. Silver sulfadiazine: argyria.	Hemolytic anemia (G6PD deficiency), methemoglobinemia. Avoid in pregnant women, nursing mothers, infants > kernicterus. Topical medications often seem innocuous but remember that topical sulfonamides can cross-react in patients allergic to oral sulfonamides.

ACD, allergic contact dermatitis; DNA, deoxyribonucleic acid; DHPS, dihydropteroate synthetase; FDA, Food and Drug Administration; G6PD, glucose-6-phosphate dehydrogenase; GN, gram-negative; ICD, irritant contact dermatitis; RNA, ribonucleic acid; tRNA, transfer RNA.
[a]Illustrative examples are provided.

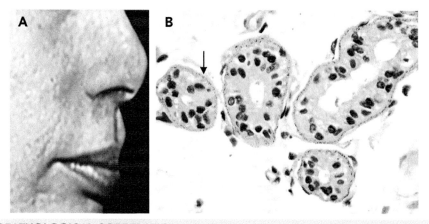

Figure 6.6. CLINICOPATHOLOGICAL CORRELATION: ARGYRIA. Argyria is characterized by silver granules in the basement membrane surrounding eccrine sweat glands. A, Argyria. Note the slate-gray skin discoloration. B, Argyria. Solid arrow: silver granule.

(A, Reprinted with permission from Gru AA, Wick MR, Mir A, et al. Pediatric Dermatopathology and Dermatology. Philadelphia: Wolters Kluwer; 2018. B, Histology image reprinted with permission from Elder DE, Elenitsas R, Rosenbach M, et al. *Lever's Histopathology of the Skin.* 11 ed. Wolters Kluwer; 2015.)

Do NOT confuse flucytosine with <u>flu</u>darabine. Flucytosine is an antimetabolite in fungi, while fludarabine is an antimetabolite in humans.

- FDA-approved dermatology indications: **cryptococcal meningitis.**
- Adverse events include:
  - Renal/urinary/excretory: **renal failure [US Boxed Warning].**

Griseofulvin

- Mechanism: **inhibits dermatophyte mitosis by disrupting microtubule function.**
- FDA-approved dermatology indications: **dermatophyte infections.**
- Mucocutaneous adverse events include **photoallergic eruption and porphyria flare.**

- Pharmacokinetics notes:
  - Metabolism: Griseofulvin is a **CYP3A4 inducer.** Griseofulvin increases the metabolism of estrogen derivatives (eg, combined OCPs) and may lead to **contraceptive failure.**

Polyenes

- Selected drugs: **amphotericin B.**
- Mechanism: **increases fungal cell membrane permeability by binding irreversibly to sterols.**
- FDA-approved dermatology indications: **aspergillus, blastomycosis, candidiasis, coccidioidomycosis, cryptococcosis, histoplasmosis, leishmaniasis, sporotrichosis.**
- Mucocutaneous adverse events include **infusion reactions.**
  Rigors and fever have inspired the nicknames "shake and bake" and "amphoterrible."

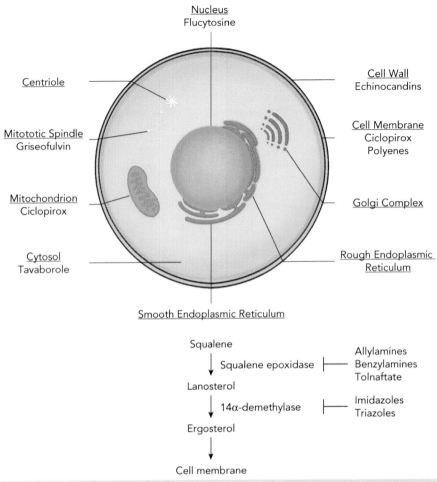

Nucleus
Flucytosine

Centriole

Cell Wall
Echinocandins

Mitototic Spindle
Griseofulvin

Cell Membrane
Ciclopirox
Polyenes

Mitochondrion
Ciclopirox

Golgi Complex

Cytosol
Tavaborole

Rough Endoplasmic
Reticulum

Smooth Endoplasmic Reticulum

Squalene

$\downarrow$ Squalene epoxidase —— Allylamines
Benzylamines
Tolnaftate

Lanosterol

$\downarrow$ 14α-demethylase —— Imidazoles
Triazoles

Ergosterol

$\downarrow$

Cell membrane

Figure 6.7. ANTIFUNGALS. Antifungal mechanisms. Antifungals may also have anti-inflammatory properties. (Illustration by Caroline A. Nelson, MD).

- Other adverse events include:
  - Renal/urinary/excretory: **nephrotoxicity.**
    - Management pearl: **Lipid formulations** of amphotericin B have been shown to **reduce nephrotoxicity** without compromising efficacy.
- Historical pregnancy risk category: **B (first-choice parenteral antifungal during pregnancy).**
  - Prescribing "amphoterrible" to a pregnant woman is not intuitive. It may help to remember that amphotericin <u>B</u> is category <u>B</u>.

Topical Antifungals (Table 6.12)

Antiparasitics

Systemic Antiparasitics

Antimony Compounds

- Selected drugs: **meglumine antimonate, sodium stibogluconate.**
- Mechanism: unknown.
- FDA-approved dermatology indications: **leishmaniasis (sodium stibogluconate).**

- Other drugs for leishmaniasis include miltefosine and pentamidine.
- Adverse events include:
  - Circulatory: ECG changes (eg, **QT prolongation**).

Albendazole

- Mechanism: **disrupts microtubules and inhibits fumarate reductase,** reducing energy production by the Krebs cycle and **impairing glucose uptake.**
- FDA-approved dermatology indications: **hydatid disease, neurocysticercosis.**
  - Related drugs include **mebendazole, thiabendazole, and triclabendazole.** Other antihelminthic drugs include benznidazole, bithionol, eflornithine, levamisole, nifurtimox, pyrantel pamoate, praziquantel, and suramin.

Diethylcarbamazine

- Mechanism: unknown.
- FDA-approved dermatology indications: **loiasis, lymphatic filariasis.**
- Mucocutaneous adverse events include the **Mazzotti reaction** (pruritus, fever, arthralgia) ± cornea/retina inflammation

Table 6.12. TOPICAL ANTIFUNGALS

Selected Drugs	Mechanism	FDA-Approved Dermatology Indications
Butenafine, naftifine, terbinafine, tolnaftate	Benzylamine (butenafine), allylamines (naftifine, terbinafine), and tolnaftate share the same mechanism (see above).	Tinea corporis, tinea cruris (butenafine, naftifine), tinea pedis, tinea versicolor (butenafine).
Ciclopirox	Interferes with fungal respiration and amino acid transport and alters cell membrane permeability by chelating polyvalent cations (eg Fe^{3+}) that function in cytochromes, catalases, and peroxidases.	Cutaneous candidiasis, onychomycosis, seborrheic dermatitis, tinea corporis, tinea cruris, tinea pedis, tinea versicolor.
Clotrimazole, econazole, ketoconazole	Imidazoles (see above).	Cutaneous candidiasis, dandruff/seborrheic dermatitis (ketoconazole), tinea corporis, tinea cruris, tinea pedis, tinea versicolor. Oral clotrimazole (lozenge or troche): oropharyngeal candidiasis (historical pregnancy category B).
Efinaconazole	Triazole (see above).	Onychomycosis.
Nystatin	Polyene (see above).	Fungal infections. Oral nystatin (suspension): oral candidiasis (historical pregnancy category C).
Selenium sulfide	Antimitotic, facilitates shedding of fungi by reducing cellular adhesion in the stratum corneum.	Dandruff/scalp seborrhea, tinea versicolor.
Tavaborole	Interferes with fungal protein synthesis by inhibiting leucyl-tRNA synthetase.	Onychomycosis.
Undecylenic acid	Fungistatic fatty acid ± zinc that acts as an astringent, reducing rawness and irritation.	Tinea corporis, tinea cruris, tinea pedis.

FDA, Food and Drug Administration, RNA, ribonucleic acid; tRNA, transfer RNA.

leading to permanent visual damage in patients with **onchocerciasis (contraindicated).**

Ivermectin

- Mechanism: **binds glutamate-gated chloride ion channels in nerve and muscle cells** resulting in increased chloride permeability, hyperpolarization of the nerve or muscle cell, and parasite death.
- FDA-approved dermatology indications: **onchocerciasis, strongyloidiasis.**

Topical Antiparasitics (Table 6.13)

Antineoplastics

Basic Concepts

- Antineoplastics include cytotoxic chemotherapies, targeted antineoplastics, and immunotherapies.
- The most widely used severity grading scale for adverse events related to antineoplastics is the National Cancer Institute's **Common Terminology Criteria for Adverse Events (CTCAE).**

- A five-point grading scale is customized for each adverse event term as follows: grade 1 mild, grade 2 moderate, grade 3 severe, grade 4 life-threatening, and grade 5 death.
- BSA and psychosocial impact are key determinants of severity for many mucocutaneous adverse event terms. BSA cutoffs vary; however, a common designation is grade 1 < 10%, grade 2 10% to 30%, and grade 3 > 30%. BSA calculation only includes affected skin.
- Management of mucocutaneous adverse events relies on common principles of dermatologic therapy. Specific pearls are highlighted below.
- **In general, drug interruption is recommended for grade ≥ 3 and intolerable grade 2 eruptions** with a decision to reinstate, dose reduce, or discontinue the drug based on response to dermatologic therapy.

Cytotoxic Chemotherapies (Table 6.14, Figure 6.8)

- Cytotoxic chemotherapies are associated with diverse mucocutaneous adverse events (Figure 6.9, Figure 6.10) including **TEC** (Chapter 2: Interface Dermatoses and Other Connective Tissue Disorders), multiple eruptive eccrine poromas (Chapter 5: Neoplasms of Sebaceous, Apocrine, and Eccrine

Table 6.13. TOPICAL ANTIPARASITICS

Selected Drugs	Mechanism	FDA-Approved Dermatology Indications	Notes
Benzyl benzoate	Unknown.		Adverse events include disulfiram-like reaction. Discontinued.
Crotamiton	Unknown.	Pruritus, scabies.	
Ivermectin	See above.	Head lice, rosacea.	
Lindane	Stimulates the nervous system resulting in parasite seizures and death (GABAergic).	Head/crab lice, scabies.	Adverse events include neurologic toxicity (seizures and death)/contraindicated in premature infants and individuals with known uncontrolled seizure disorders [US Boxed Warning].
			Lindane induces seizures and death in parasites AND people.
Malathion	Organophosphate anticholinesterase.	Head lice.	Flammable.
Permethrin, pyrethrins	Inhibit nerve cell membrane sodium channels resulting in delayed repolarization and parasite paralysis and death.	Permethrin: head lice, scabies. Pyrethrins: *Pediculus humanus*.	Permethrin is man-made, while pyrethrins are derived from flowers in the Asteraceae (Compositae) family. Avoid in patients with ACD to chrysanthemums or other members of this family. Permethrin is historical pregnancy risk category B.
Spinosad	CNS excitation and involuntary muscle contractions resulting in parasite paralysis.	Head lice.	
	Spinosad induces parasite tetanus.		
Sulfur	See above.		

ACD, allergic contact dermatitis; CNS, central nervous system; FDA, Food and Drug Administration; GABA, gamma-aminobutyric acid; US, United States.

Table 6.14. CYTOTOXIC CHEMOTHERAPIES

Selected Drugs	Mechanism	FDA-Approved Dermatology Indications	Mucocutaneous Adverse Events[a]	Notes[b]
Alkylating agents (eg, bendamustine, busulfan, carmustine, cisplatin, chlorambucil, cyclophosphamide, ifosfamide, mechlorethamine, thiotepa)	Cross-link with DNA molecules (cell cycle nonspecific).	For cyclophosphamide, see Chapter 6: Immunosuppressants and Immunomodulators.	AE, hyperpigmentation, TEC. Bendamustine: PNP. Cisplatin: hyperpigmentation at sites of pressure. Cyclophosphamide: DM. Mechlorethamine (systemic): extravasation [US Boxed Warning]; mechlorethamine (topical): ACD (aqueous > ointment), SCCs. Platinum alkylating agents: relatively higher risk of type I hypersensitivity reactions. • Management pearl: Consider pretreatment with antihistamines/systemic corticosteroids and desensitization. Ifosfamide, thiotepa: hyperpigmentation at sites of occlusion.	Other adverse events of alkylating agents include bone marrow suppression and seizures (chlorambucil). Topical carmustine: check CBC weekly for at least 6 weeks.

Table 6.14. CYTOTOXIC CHEMOTHERAPIES (CONTINUED)

Selected Drugs	Mechanism	FDA-Approved Dermatology Indications	Mucocutaneous Adverse Events[a]	Notes[b]
Antibiotics (eg, bleomycin, doxorubicin)	Bleomycin: induces DNA strand breaks (G$_2$ phase). Doxorubicin: intercalates with DNA base pairs and interferes with topoisomerase II (cell cycle nonspecific).	Doxorubicin: AIDS-related Kaposi sarcoma.	Bleomycin: flagellate hyperpigmentation, Raynaud phenomenon (periungual wart treatment), sclerodermoid reaction, sclerosis at injection sites. Doxorubicin: extravasation [US Boxed Warning], longitudinal melanonychia, recall reactions, sticky skin syndrome,[c] TEC. • Management pearl: In case of extravasation, stop the infusion, attempt aspiration, elevate the limb, and apply heat packs. Cold compresses may reduce pain, inflammation, and vesicant spread. Dexrazoxane is an antidote.	Other adverse events of bleomycin include pulmonary toxicity. Other adverse events of doxorubicin include bone marrow suppression/ cardiomyopathy/secondary malignancy [US Boxed Warning]. Bleomycin impairs breathing; doxorubicin dilates the heart.
Antimetabolites (eg, 5-FU, 6-MP, capecitabine, cytarabine, fludarabine, gemcitabine, methotrexate, pemetrexed) Do NOT confuse fludarabine with flucytosine. Fludarabine is an antimetabolite in humans, while flucytosine is an antimetabolite in fungi.	Interfere with DNA synthesis (S phase). 5-FU: binds thymidylate synthase (capecitabine is a prodrug of 5-FU).	5-FU (topical): AK, superficial BCC. For methotrexate, see Chapter 6: Immunosuppressants and Immunomodulators.	AE, hyperpigmentation, TEC. 5-FU: inflammation of AKs/ DSAP, serpentine supravenous and sun-exposed hyperpigmentation, phototoxic eruption. 6-MP: phototoxic eruption/ photoonycholysis. Capecitabine: paronychia, pseudopyogenic granulomas. • Management pearl: For paronychia and pseudopyogenic granulomas, consider topical β-blockers (eg, topical timolol 0.5% gel BID under occlusion for 1 month). Cytarabine: inflammation of SKs, NEH, Sweet syndrome. Fludarabine: PNP. Gemcitabine: pseudocellulitis in patients with lower extremity edema. Pemetrexed: edema, recall reactions.	5-FU is historical pregnancy risk category X.
Antimicrotubule taxanes (eg, docetaxel, paclitaxel) and vinca alkaloids derived from the periwinkle plant (eg, vinblastine, vincristine)	Disrupt microtubule function (M phase).	Paclitaxel: AIDS-related Kaposi sarcoma. Vinblastine: CTCL, Kaposi sarcoma, LCH.	Taxanes: bullous FDE, SCLE, sclerodermoid reaction, TEC (dorsal HFS); hemorrhagic onycholysis. Vinka alkaloids: extravasation [US Boxed Warning—vinblastine]. • Management pearl: In case of extravasation, consider hyaluronidase. Cold compresses may worsen vinca alkaloid necrosis.	Other adverse events of antimicrotubular taxanes include bone marrow suppression/ hypersensitivity [US Boxed Warning—paclitaxel]. Other adverse events of vinca alkaloids include peripheral neuropathy.
Arsenic	Induces apoptosis and differentiation of leukemic promyelocytes by degrading the fusion protein PML-RAR.		AE, guttate hypopigmentation superimposed on hyperpigmentation, arsenical keratoses on the palms and soles/SCCs.	Other adverse events include differentiation syndrome.
Hypomethylaters (eg, azacitidine)	Hypomethylate DNA.		Sweet syndrome	
L-asparaginase	Inhibits protein synthesis.		Flushing	

(Continued)

Table 6.14. CYTOTOXIC CHEMOTHERAPIES (CONTINUED)

Selected Drugs	Mechanism	FDA-Approved Dermatology Indications	Mucocutaneous Adverse Events[a]	Notes[b]
Ribonucleotide reductase inhibitors (eg, hydroxyurea)	Interfere with conversion of RNA to DNA (S phase).	Sickle cell disease.	DM, leg ulcers (malleolar).	Other adverse events include bone marrow suppression, hepatotoxicity, nephrotoxicity.
Topoisomerase inhibitors (eg, irinotecan)	Interfere with topoisomerase I or II during DNA replication.			

ACD, allergic contact dermatitis; AE, anagen effluvium; AIDS, acquired immune deficiency syndrome; AK, actinic keratosis; APL, acute promyelocytic leukemia; ATRA, all-trans retinoic acid; BCC, basal cell carcinoma; BID, twice daily; CBC, complete blood count; CTCL, cutaneous T-cell lymphoma; DM, dermatomyositis; DNA, deoxyribonucleic acid; DSAP, disseminated superficial actinic porokeratosis; FDA, Food and Drug Administration; FDE, fixed drug eruption; 5-FU, 5-fluorouracil; G$_2$, gap 2 phase; HFS, hand-foot syndrome; LCH, Langerhans cell histiocytosis; M, mitosis phase; 6-MP, 6-mercaptopurine; NEH, neutrophilic eccrine hidradenitis; PML-RAR; promyelocytic leukemia–retinoic acid receptor α; PNP, paraneoplastic pemphigus; RNA, ribonucleic acid; S phase, deoxyribonucleic acid synthesis phase; SCC, squamous cell carcinoma; SCLE, subacute cutaneous lupus erythematosus; SK, seborrheic keratosis; TEC, toxic erythema of chemotherapy; US, United States.

[a]Illustrative examples are provided.

[b]US Boxed Warning labels are omitted for non-mucocutaneous adverse events of drugs without FDA-approved dermatology indications.

[c]Sticky skin syndrome may occur when doxorubicin is combined with ketoconazole.

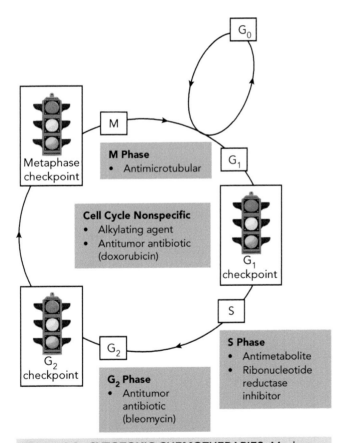

Figure 6.8. CYTOTOXIC CHEMOTHERAPIES. Mechanism in the cell cycle. Illustrative examples provided. G0, resting phase; G1, gap 1 phase; G2, gap 2 phase; M, mitosis phase; S, deoxyribonucleic acid synthesis phase. (Illustration by Caroline A. Nelson, MD.)

Glands), **mucositis, AE** (see Chapter 2: Disorders of the Hair and Nails) and nail changes such as **Beau lines** (see Chapter 2: Disorders of the Hair and Nails), **leukonychia (Mees lines, Muehrcke lines)**, onycholysis, and paronychia.

○ Prevention pearl: Analogous to TEC, **cooling** before, during, and after chemotherapy infusions may reduce **mucositis (ice chips), AE (cold caps), and nail changes (ice packs).** Other preventative measures for mucositis include antifungals, antivirals, early use of colony stimulating factors, and oral hygiene.

○ Management pearl: **Palifermin, a keratinocyte growth factor,** may be considered for mucositis; adverse events include **benign leukoplakia.**

Targeted Antineoplastics (Table 6.15, Figure 6.11)

• Targeted antineoplastics cause a diverse array of mucocutaneous adverse events (Figure 6.12).

⸙ Figure 6.13.

Immunotherapies (Table 6.16, Figure 6.14)

• Immunotherapies cause a diverse array of mucocutaneous adverse events (Figure 6.15).

Topical Antineoplastics for Actinic Keratosis (Table 6.17)

Antineoplastics for Cutaneous T-Cell Lymphoma (Table 6.18)

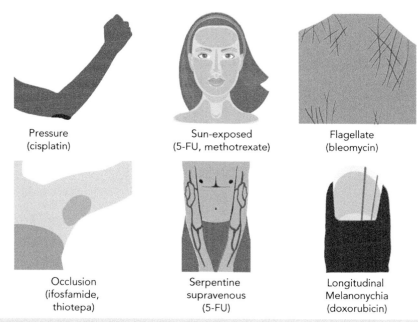

Pressure
(cisplatin)

Sun-exposed
(5-FU, methotrexate)

Flagellate
(bleomycin)

Occlusion
(ifosfamide,
thiotepa)

Serpentine
supravenous
(5-FU)

Longitudinal
Melanonychia
(doxorubicin)

Figure 6.9. HYPERPIGMENTATION PATTERNS. Given overlap between antineoplastics, illustrative examples are provided. Shiitake mushrooms are an alternative etiology of flagellate hyperpigmentation. 5-FU, 5-fluorouracil.
(Illustration by Caroline A. Nelson, MD.)

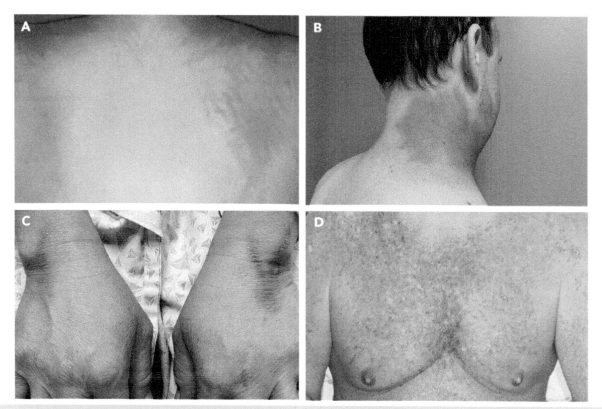

Figure 6.10. MUCOCUTANEOUS ADVERSE EVENTS OF CYTOTOXIC CHEMOTHERAPIES. A, Flagellate hyperpigmentation due to bleomycin. B, Radiation recall, most classically due to doxorubicin and pemetrexed. C, Serpentine supravenous hyperpigmentation, most classically due to 5-FU. D, Inflammation of AKs, most classically due to 5-FU. E, Pseudocellulitis due to gemcitabine in a patient with lower extremity edema. F, Sclerodermoid reaction due to docetaxel. AK, actinic keratosis; 5-FU, 5-fluorouracil.
(A, Courtesy of William James, MD.)

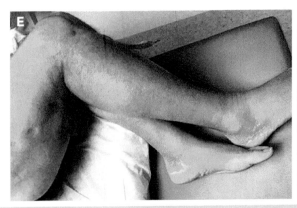
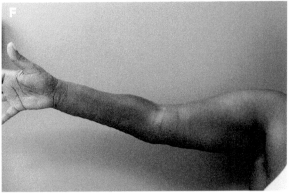

Figure 6.10. Continued

Table 6.15. TARGETED ANTINEOPLASTICS				
Selected Drugs	Mechanism	FDA-Approved Dermatology Indications	Mucocutaneous Adverse Events[a]	Notes[b]
Inhibitors at the Cellular Membrane				
EGFR inhibitors (eg, cetuximab, erlotinib, gefitinib)	Inhibit EGFR signaling.		Fissures, hair changes (eg, hypertrichosis/ trichomegaly), mucositis, nail changes (eg, paronychia, pseudopyogenic granulomas), papulopustular eruption,[c] phototoxic eruption, *Staphylococcus aureus* overgrowth, xerosis. • Management pearl: For papulopustular eruption, topical steroids and antibiotics are preferable to benzoyl peroxide and topical retinoids to avoid xerosis. Treat grade 2-3 eruptions with tetracyclines; consider low-dose oral isotretinoin in refractory cases. Counsel regarding sun protection.	
			PRIDE syndrome—papulopustules and/or paronychia, regulatory abnormalities of hair growth, itching, and dryness due to EGFR inhibitors.	
BCR-ABL/KIT/PDGFR inhibitors (eg imatinib)	Inhibit BCR-ABL/KIT/PDGFR signaling.	Imatinib: DFSP, HES, mastocytosis	Morbilliform eruption, periorbital edema, hypopigmentation > hyperpigmentation.	
			KIT mutation causes piebaldism.	
VEGF inhibitors (eg, bevacizumab)	Inhibit angiogenesis.		Disturbed wound healing, ulcers (often in *striae distensae*). • Management pearl: Consider delaying angiogenesis inhibitors for 28 days after surgery.	
Multikinase inhibitors (eg, sorafenib, sunitinib)	Inhibit multikinase signaling.		Hand-foot skin reaction. • Management pearl: Consider orthopedic shoe inserts. Sunitinib—yellow skin discoloration.	
			Sorafenib makes hands and feet sore.	

Table 6.15. TARGETED ANTINEOPLASTICS (CONTINUED)

Selected Drugs	Mechanism	FDA-Approved Dermatology Indications	Mucocutaneous Adverse Events[a]	Notes[b]
Inhibitors of Intracellular Molecular Signaling Pathways				
BRAF (V600E) inhibitors (eg, dabrafenib, vemurafenib)	Inhibit Ras-Raf-MEK-ERK (MAPK) pathway.	Melanoma. Vemurafenib: Erdheim-Chester disease.	Epidermoid cysts/milia, exanthematous eruption, hand-foot skin reaction, keratotic squamoproliferative lesions (benign VKs > malignant KAs/SCCs), KP-like reaction, melanocytic nevi/melanoma, panniculitis, phototoxic eruption, sarcoidal granulomatous eruptions, seborrheic dermatitis–like reaction, Sweet syndrome.	Concurrent BRAF and MEK inhibition reduces mucocutaneous adverse events.
MEK 1/2 inhibitors (eg, trametinib)	Inhibit Ras-Raf-MEK-ERK (MAPK) pathway.	Melanoma.	Fissures, morbilliform eruption, papulopustular eruption, paronychia, xerosis. Mucocutaneous adverse events of EGFR inhibitors and MEK inhibitors overlap.	Other adverse events include cardiomyopathy, edema, fever, and retinal vein occlusion.
mTOR inhibitors (eg, everolimus, sirolimus)	Inhibit PI3K-Akt-mTOR pathway.		Nummular dermatitis, papulopustular eruption, stomatitis (discrete aphthae on nonkeratinizing epithelium).	Other adverse events include immunosuppression [US Boxed Warning].
SMO inhibitors (eg, vismodegib) Vismodegib inhibits SMO.	Inhibit hedgehog signaling pathway.	BCC.	Dysgeusia, TE.	Other adverse events include muscle spasms and teratogenicity [US Boxed Warning].
Proteosome inhibitors (eg, bortezomib)	Inhibit ubiquitin proteasome pathway.		SJS/TEN-like eruption, Sweet syndrome.	

BCC, basal cell carcinoma; DFSP, dermatofibrosarcoma protuberans; EGFR, epidermal growth factor receptor; ERK, extracellular signal–regulated kinases; FDA, Food and Drug Administration; HES, hypereosinophilic syndrome; KA, keratoacanthoma; KIT/BCR-ABL, kinase receptor/breakpoint cluster region-Abelson; KP, keratosis pilaris; MAPK, mitogen-activated protein kinase; MEK, mitogen-activated protein kinase; mTOR, mammalian target of rapamycin; PDGFR, platelet-derived growth factor receptor; PI3K, phosphatidylinositol 3-kinase; SCC, squamous cell carcinoma; SJS/TEN, Stevens-Johnson syndrome/toxic epidermal necrolysis; SMO, smoothened; TBSE, total body skin examination; TE, anagen effluvium; US, United States; V600E, substitution of valine (V) for glutamic acid (E) at amino acid position number 600; VEGF, vascular endothelial growth factor; VK, verrucous keratosis.
[a]Illustrative examples are provided.
[b]US Boxed Warning labels are omitted for non-mucocutaneous adverse events of drugs without FDA-approved dermatology indications.
[c]Presence or severity may correlate with efficacy.

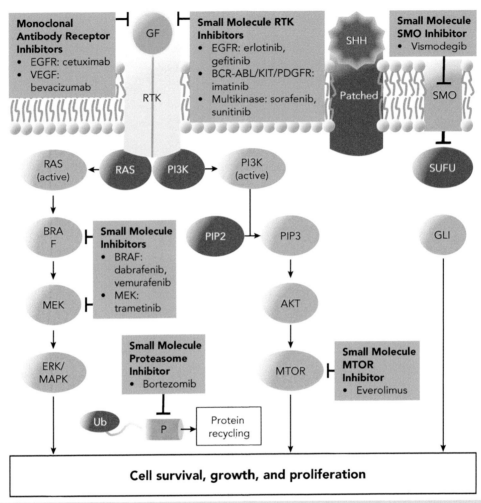

Figure 6.11. TARGETED ANTINEOPLASTICS. Mechanism in molecular signaling pathways. Illustrative examples provided. EGFR, epidermal growth factor receptor; GF, growth factor; KIT/BCR-ABL, kinase receptor/breakpoint cluster region-Abelson; MAPK, mitogen-activated protein kinase; MTOR, mammalian target of rapamycin; P, proteasome; PI3K, phosphoinositide 3-kinase; PIP2, phosphatidylinositol 4,5-bisphosphate; PIP3, phosphatidylinositol (3,4,5)-trisphosphate; RTK, receptor tyrosine kinase; SHH, sonic hedgehog; SMO, smoothened; SUFU, suppressor of fused; Ub, ubiquitin; VEGF, vascular endothelial growth factor.

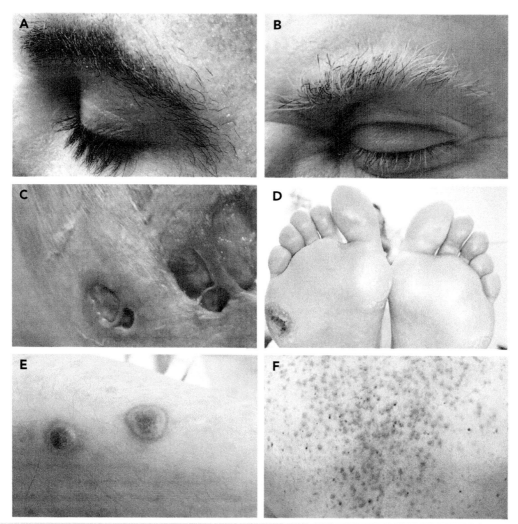

Figure 6.12. MUCOCUTANEOUS ADVERSE EVENTS OF TARGETED ANTINEOPLASTICS. A, Trichomegaly due to EGFR inhibition. B, Hair depigmentation due to BCR-ABL/KIT/PDGFR inhibition. C, Deep ulcers localizing to *striae distensae* on the breast due to VEGF inhibition. D, Hand-foot skin reaction due to multikinase inhibition. E, Keratoacanthomas due to BRAF inhibition. F, Papulopustular eruption due to MEK inhibition. EGFR, epidermal growth factor receptor; KIT/BCR-ABL, kinase receptor/breakpoint cluster region-Abelson; MEK, mitogen-activated protein kinase; PDGFR, platelet-derived growth factor receptor; VEGF, vascular endothelial growth factor.

(C, Courtesy of Robert G. Micheletti, MD.)

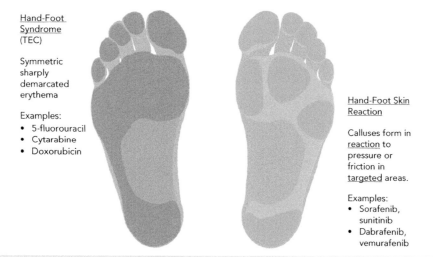

Hand-Foot Syndrome (TEC)

Symmetric sharply demarcated erythema

Examples:
- 5-fluorouracil
- Cytarabine
- Doxorubicin

Hand-Foot Skin Reaction

Calluses form in reaction to pressure or friction in targeted areas.

Examples:
- Sorafenib, sunitinib
- Dabrafenib, vemurafenib

Figure 6.13. HAND-FOOT ADVERSE EVENTS OF ANTINEOPLASTICS TEC, toxic erythema of chemotherapy.

(Illustration by Caroline A. Nelson, MD.)

Table 6.16. IMMUNOTHERAPIES

Selected Drugs	Mechanism	FDA-Approved Dermatology Indications	Mucocutaneous Adverse Events[a]	Notes
IFNα, IFNβ, IFNγ	See Chapter 1: Immunology and Inflammation.	IFNα, IFNβ: AIDS-associated Kaposi sarcoma, condyloma acuminata, melanoma. IFNγ: CGD.	LE, psoriasis flare, sarcoidal granulomatous eruptions, sclerosis at injection sites, TE, hypertrichosis/trichomegaly.	Other adverse events include autoimmune/ischemic/infectious/neuropsychiatric disorders [US Boxed Warning—IFNα].
IL-2	See Chapter 1: Immunology and Inflammation.	Melanoma.	Granulomas, lobular panniculitis, pruritus.	Other adverse events include capillary leak syndrome/CNS toxicity/infections [US Boxed Warning].
Imiquimod	Increase TLR7 ± TLR8 signaling.	AK, condyloma acuminata, superficial BCC.	Local inflammation, hypopigmentation, psoriasis flare.	Other adverse events include flu-like symptoms.
ICIs: CTLA4 inhibitors (eg, ipilimumab) PD-1 inhibitors (eg, cemiplimab, nivolumab, pembrolizumab) PD-L1 inhibitors (eg, avelumab)	Inhibit the immune checkpoint.	Ipilimumab: melanoma. Cemiplimab: BCC, SCC. Nivolumab: melanoma. Pembrolizumab: MCC, melanoma. Avelumab: MCC.	AA; AGEP; BP; DM; DRESS; eczematous, lichenoid, and morbilliform eruptions; KA; SLE; panniculitis; pruritus; psoriasis flare; repigmentation of gray hair; sarcoidal granulomatous eruptions; SJS/TEN-like eruption; Sweet syndrome; vasculitis; vitiligo-like leukoderma/poliosis. • Management pearl: For pruritus, consider aprepitant, a substance P/NK1 receptor antagonist. ICIs cause "dermatology."	Perform a thorough ROS to exclude systemic IRAEs (eg colitis, pneumonitis) [US Boxed Warning—ipilimumab]. • Management pearl: Use systemic corticosteroids with caution, but do not delay in case of a life-threatening IRAE.[b]
T-VEC	Oncolytic virus.[c]	Melanoma.	Cellulitis, Sweet syndrome–like infiltrate.	Other adverse events include flu-like symptoms.

AA, alopecia areata; AGEP, acute generalized exanthematous pustulosis; AIDS, acquired immune deficiency syndrome; AK, actinic keratosis; BCC, basal cell carcinoma; BP, bullous pemphigoid; CGD, chronic granulomatous disease; CTLA4, cytotoxic T lymphocyte–associated antigen 4; DM, dermatomyositis; DRESS, drug reaction with eosinophilia and systemic symptoms; FDA, Food and Drug Administration; GM-CSF, granulocyte-macrophage colony-stimulating factor; HSV, herpes simplex virus; ICIs, immune checkpoint inhibitors; IFN, interferon; Ig, immunoglobulin; IL, interleukin; IRAEs, immune-related adverse events; KA, keratoacanthoma; LE, lupus erythematosus; MCC, Merkel cell carcinoma; NK1, neurokinin-1; PD-1, programmed death 1; ROS, review of systems; SCC, squamous cell carcinoma; SJS/TEN, Stevens-Johnson syndrome/toxic epidermal necrolysis; SLE, systemic lupus erythematosus; TE, telogen effluvium; TNF, tumor necrosis factor; T-VEC, talimogene laherparepvec; US, United States.

[a]Illustrative examples are provided.

[b]Presence or severity of systemic IRAEs may correlate with efficacy. There is conflicting evidence on the potential for systemic corticosteroids to attenuate the antitumor immune response; however, timing and dose may be important factors. Consider early introduction of targeted steroid-sparing therapies to minimize high-dose systemic corticosteroid exposure, when possible (eg, omalizumab for patients with BP and elevated IgE).

[c]Attenuated HSV-1 engineered to express GM-CSF.

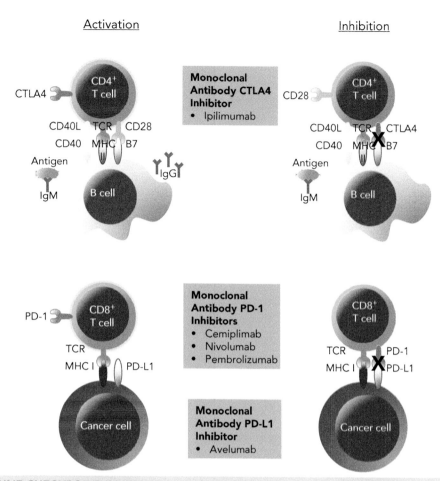

Activation   Inhibition

Figure 6.14. IMMUNE CHECKPOINT INHIBITORS. Mechanism at immune checkpoints. Illustrative examples provided. CD, cluster of differentiation; CTLA4, cytotoxic T lymphocyte–associated protein 4; Ig, immunoglobulin; L, ligand; MHC, major histocompatibility complex; PD, programmed death; TCR, T-cell receptor.

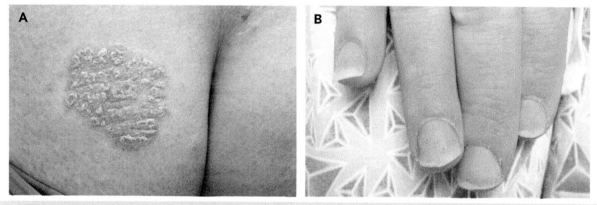

Figure 6.15. MUCOCUTANEOUS ADVERSE EVENTS OF IMMUNOTHERAPIES. A and B, Psoriasis in the setting of PD-1 inhibition. C, Vitiligo in the setting of PD-1 inhibition. D, Bullous pemphigoid in the setting of PD-1 inhibition. E, Lichenoid dermatitis in the setting of PD-1 inhibition. F, Sweet syndrome in the setting of CTLA4 inhibition. CTLA4, cytotoxic T lymphocyte–associated antigen 4; PD-1, programmed death 1.

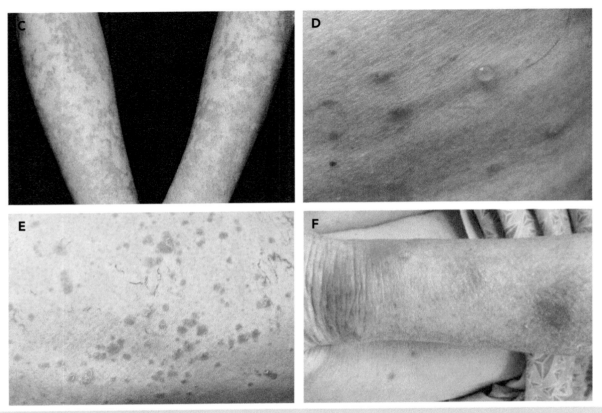

Figure 6.15. Continued

Table 6.17. TOPICAL ANTINEOPLASTICS FOR ACTINIC KERATOSIS

Selected Drugs	Mechanism	FDA-Approved Dermatology Indications	Mucocutaneous Adverse Events[a]	Notes
5-FU	See above.			
Diclofenac	Reversibly inhibits COX-2 > COX-1.	AK	Local inflammation.	Adverse events of NSAIDs include serious cardiovascular thrombotic events/serious gastrointestinal bleeding, ulceration, and perforation [US Boxed Warning].
Imiquimod	See above.			
Ingenol mebutate	Induces cell death by disrupting plasma membranes and mitochondria and triggers inflammation.	AK	Local inflammation.	
Tirbanibulin	Microtubule inhibitor	AK	Local inflammation.	

AK, actinic keratosis; COX, cyclooxygenase; FDA, Food and Drug Administration; 5-FU, 5-fluorouracil; NSAID, nonsteroidal anti-inflammatory drug; SCC, squamous cell carcinoma; US, United States.
[a]Illustrative examples are provided.

Table 6.18. ANTINEOPLASTICS FOR CUTANEOUS T-CELL LYMPHOMA

Selected Drugs	Mechanism	FDA-Approved Dermatology Indications	Mucocutaneous Adverse Events[a]	Notes
Alemtuzumab	Inhibits CD52.	CTCL, GVHD.	Infusion reactions [US Boxed Warning, US REMS program], sarcoidal granulomatous eruptions.	Other adverse events include autoimmune conditions/ bone marrow suppression/ malignancies, stroke [US Boxed Warning, US REMS Program].
Bexarotene	See Chapter 6: Retinoids.			
Brentuximab vedotin	Inhibits CD30.	CTCL.		Adverse events include neuropathy and PML [US Boxed Warning].
Carmustine, mechlorethamine	See above.			
Denileukin diftitox	Kills cells expressing IL-2 through introduction of diphtheria toxin.	CTCL.		Discontinued. Adverse events include capillary leak syndrome.
Methotrexate	See Chapter 6: Immunosuppressants and Immunomodulators.			
Mogamulizumab	Inhibits CCR4.	CTCL.	Infusion reactions, cutaneous eruptions (eg granulomatous, psoriasiform).	Other adverse events include autoimmune toxicity, bone marrow suppression, infections.
Romidepsin, vorinostat	Inhibit histone deacetylase.	CTCL.		Adverse events include weight loss.
Vinblastine	See above.			

CD, cluster of differentiation; CCR4, CC chemokine receptor 4; CTCL, cutaneous T-cell lymphoma; FDA, Food and Drug Administration; GVHD, graft-versus-host disease; IL, interleukin; PML, progressive multifocal leukoencephalopathy; REMS, Risk Evaluation and Mitigation Strategy; US, United States.
[a]Illustrative examples are provided.

Miscellaneous Drugs

Basic Concepts

- This section covers other medical treatments commonly prescribed by dermatologists.
- **Complementary and alternative medicines** (eg, herbals, dietary supplements, homeopathy, acupuncture), while commonly used by dermatology patients, are beyond the scope of this chapter.

Topical Antipsoriatic Drugs (Table 6.19)

Topical Antipruritic Drugs (Table 6.20)

Other Drugs

Hydroquinone

- Mechanism: **competitive inhibition of tyrosinase.**
  - Related drugs include **azelaic acid, monobenzyl ether of hydroquinone, and mequinol.**

Azelaic acid is produced by *Malassezia* species, which is also responsible for skin hypopigmentation often observed in tinea versicolor.
- FDA-approved dermatology indications: **skin bleaching.**
- Mucocutaneous adverse events include **exogenous ochronosis.**
  - Figure 6.16.

Afamelanotide

- Mechanism: **α-MSH analogue.**
- FDA-approved dermatology indications: **EPP.**
- Mucocutaneous adverse events include **hyperpigmentation, darkening of preexisting nevi.**

Pentoxifylline

- Mechanism: **increases blood flow** through decreased blood viscosity, erythrocyte flexibility, and leukocyte deformability. Decreases neutrophil adhesion and activation.

Table 6.19. TOPICAL ANTIPSORIATIC DRUGS

Selected Drugs	Mechanism	FDA-Approved Dermatology Indications	Mucocutaneous Adverse Events[a]	Notes
Anthralin	Inhibits epidermal cell proliferation by interfering with DNA synthesis.	Psoriasis.	ACD.	
Calcipotriene	Vitamin D analogue that downregulates pro-inflammatory molecules (eg IL-2) and upregulates anti-inflammatory molecules (eg IL-10).	Psoriasis.	ICD, phototoxic eruption.	Other adverse events include hypercalcemia. Calcipotriene is inactivated by acidic pH (eg, coapplication with lactic acid) and UVR (eg phototherapy).
Coal tar	Antiseptic, antibacterial, antiseborrheic.	Psoriasis, seborrheic dermatitis.	ICD, phototoxic eruption.	
Corticosteroids	See Chapter 6: Immunosuppressants and Immunomodulators.			
Tazarotene	See Chapter 6: Retinoids.			

ACD, allergic contact dermatitis; DNA, deoxyribonucleic acid; ICD, irritant contact dermatitis; FDA, Food and Drug Administration; IL, interleukin; UVR, ultraviolet radiation.
[a]Illustrative examples are provided.

Table 6.20. TOPICAL ANTIPRURITIC DRUGS

Selected Drugs	Mechanism	FDA-Approved Dermatology Indications	Mucocutaneous Adverse Events[a]	Notes
Camphor	Local anesthetic effect ("cooling sensation").	Pain, pruritus.	ICD.	
Capsaicin	Releases and depletes substance P from C-type fibers.	Neuropathic pain.	Erythema, edema, and burning for ~1 week, followed by relief of pruritus.	Found in chili peppers and other nightshades (*Solanaceae*).
Diphenhydramine	See Chapter 6: Antihistamines and Related Drugs.	Pain, pruritus.	ACD.	Not recommended.
Doxepin	See Chapter 6: Antihistamines and Related Drugs.	Pruritus.	ACD or ICD.	Other adverse events include sedation (systemic absorption). Contraindicated in patients with untreated narrow-angle glaucoma.
Menthol, phenol	Activate cold receptors ("cooling sensation").	Pain, pruritus.	ACD (rare), ICD.	Found in throat sprays and lozenges.
				Topical menthol and phenol preparations behave like "cough drops for the skin."
Pramoxine	Ester anesthetic.	Minor skin irritation.	ACD (rare).	

ACD, allergic contact dermatitis; DNA, deoxyribonucleic acid; ICD, irritant contact dermatitis; FDA, Food and Drug Administration; IL, interleukin; UVR, ultraviolet radiation.
[a]Illustrative examples are provided.

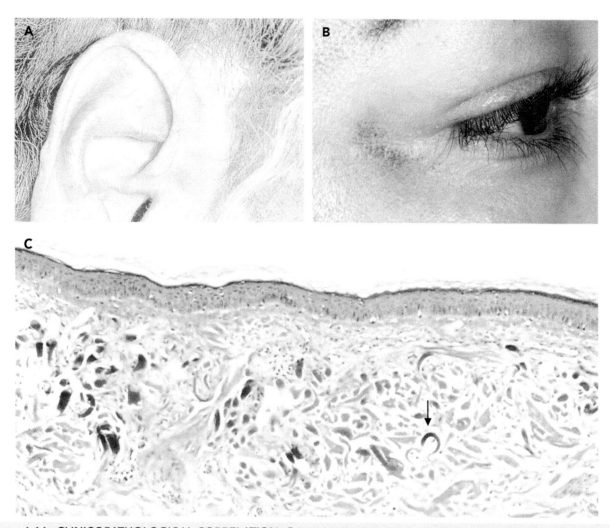

Figure 6.16. CLINICOPATHOLOGICAL CORRELATION: OCHRONOSIS. Ochronosis, both endogenous and exogenous, is characterized by yellow-brown deposits in the dermis. A, Endogenous ochronosis. B, Exogenous ochronosis. C, Exogenous ochronosis. Solid arrow: yellow-brown banana-shaped deposit.

(A, Reprinted with permission from Gold DH, Weingeist TA. *Color Atlas of the Eye in Systemic Disease.* Lippincott Williams & Wilkins; 2000. B, Reprinted with permission from Elder DE, Elenitsas R, Rosenbach M, et al. *Lever's Histopathology of the Skin.* 11th ed. Wolters Kluwer; 2015. C, Histology image reprinted with permission from Elder DE, et al. *Lever's Histopathology of the Skin*, 11 ed. Wolters Kluwer; 2015.)

Deposits in <u>och</u>ronosis are <u>ocher</u> in color and often resemble "bananas."

Pimozide

- Mechanism: dopamine receptor antagonist (first-generation antipsychotic).
  - Related drugs include **chlorpromazine and haloperidol.**
- Mucocutaneous adverse events include **drug-induced LE (chlorpromazine), lichenoid drug reaction, photoallergic/phototoxic eruption (chlorpromazine), slate gray pigmentation (chlorpromazine), and xerosis/xerophthalmia/ xerostomia.**
- Other adverse events include:
  - Circulatory: **anticholinergic toxicity**, QT prolongation.
  - Endocrine: **hyperprolactinemia, weight gain.**
  - Nervous: extrapyramidal effects (eg, **tardive dyskinesia**), **sedation.**
- Pharmacokinetics notes:
  - Pimozide is a **CYP2D6 and CYP3A4 substrate.**

Risperidone

- Mechanism: serotonin and dopamine receptor antagonist (second-generation antipsychotic).
  - Related drugs include **aripiprazole, clozapine, olanzapine, quetiapine, and ziprasidone.**
- Adverse event profile is similar to pimozide with a **relatively higher risk of metabolic effects and lower risk of anticholinergic toxicity, QT prolongation, extrapyramidal effects, and sedation.** Olanzapine is associated with postinjection delirium/sedation syndrome [US REMS Program].

α-Adrenergic Agonists

- Selected drugs: **brimonidine, oxymetazoline.**
- Mechanism: **adrenergic agonists (brimonidine is selective for α_2, oxymetazoline is selective for α_{1A})** that reduce erythema through direct **vasoconstriction.**

- FDA-approved dermatology indications: **rosacea.**
- Mucocutaneous adverse events include burning and **rebound redness.**
- Other adverse events include:
  - Ocular: **angle closure glaucoma** in patients with narrow-angle glaucoma (oxymetazoline).

Glycopyrrolate

- Mechanism: **anticholinergic** that **inhibits perspiration** by blocking acetylcholine.
- FDA-approved dermatology indications:
  - Topical: **primary axillary hyperhidrosis.**
- Mucocutaneous adverse events include **xerosis/ xerophthalmia/xerostomia.**
    - "Dry as a bone."
- Other adverse events include:
  - Circulatory: **flushing, tachycardia.**
    - "Red as a beet."
  - Nervous: **altered mental status, fever.**
    - "Mad as a hatter." "Hot as a hare."
  - Ocular: **mydriasis.**
    - "Blind as a bat."
  - Renal/urinary/excretory: **urinary retention.**
    - "Full as a flask."

Bimatoprost

- Mechanism: **prostaglandin analogue.**
  - Related drugs include **latanoprost.**
- FDA-approved dermatology indications:
  - Topical: **hypotrichosis of the eyelashes.**
- Other systemic adverse events include:
  - Ocular: **iris hyperpigmentation.**

Minoxidil

- Mechanism: stimulates hair growth through **vasodilation** (relaxes arteriolar smooth muscle), increased cutaneous blood flow, and **stimulation of resting hair follicles** (prolongs the anagen phase).
- FDA-approved dermatology indications:
  - Topical: **alopecia.** 2% solution (men, women), 5% solution (men), 5% foam (men, women).
    - It is important to be aware of gender-based pricing. One study reported that minoxidil 5% foams with identical active and inactive ingredients were priced significantly more per volume when sold to women compared with men.
- Mucocutaneous adverse events include **contact dermatitis** (eg, **ACD and/or ICD to propylene glycol in the solution vehicle**). In terms of hair, minoxidil may cause **unwanted hypertrichosis** (eg, forehead, cheeks) and **paradoxical worsening of hair loss** due to self-limited TE ~4 to 6 weeks after initiation.
    - Minoxidil use during pregnancy may result in **fetal hypertrichosis.**
- Other adverse events of oral minoxidil include:
  - Cardiovascular: **pericardial effusion, angina pectoris exacerbation [US Boxed Warning].**
- Dosing notes:
  - Oral: low dose minoxidil 2.5 to 5 mg/d may be used off label for alopecia.
- Pharmacodynamics notes:
  - Efficacy: **minoxidil must be continued indefinitely to maintain response.**

Platelet-Rich Plasma

- Mechanism: supernatant of platelet-enriched plasma isolated from autologous blood hypothesized to **stimulate collagenesis, wound healing, and hair growth.**
- Dosing notes:
  - Topical: Gel systems encompass platelet-rich fibrin matrix and platelet-rich fibrin membrane that may be delivered in combination with controlled skin injury techniques such as **microneedling.**
  - Intralesional: Typical initial regimen is three sessions at 1-month intervals.

Eflornithine

- Mechanism: **slows hair growth by inhibiting ODC (irreversible).**
- FDA-approved dermatology indications: **facial hair reduction.**

FURTHER READING

Administration USFaD, Administration USFaD. *Risk Evaluation and Mitigation Strategies (REMS).* Accessed May 26, 2019. https://www.fda.gov/drugs/drug-safety-and-availability/risk-evaluation-and-mitigation-strategies-rems

Al-Lamki Z, Pearson P, Jaffe N. Localized cisplatin hyperpigmentation induced by pressure. A case report. *Cancer.* 1996;77(8):1578-1581. doi:10.1002/(sici)1097-0142(19960415)77:8<1578::Aid-cncr23>3.0.Co;2-w

Amor KT, Ryan C, Menter A. The use of cyclosporine in dermatology: part I. *J Am Acad Dermatol.* 2010;63(6):925-946. quiz 947-948. doi:10.1016/j.jaad.2010.02.063

Arbour KC, Mezquita L, Long N, et al. Impact of baseline steroids on efficacy of programmed cell death-1 and programmed death-ligand 1 blockade in patients with non-small-cell lung cancer. *J Clin Oncol.* 2018;36(28):2872-2878. doi:10.1200/jco.2018.79.0006

Bartra J, Valero AL, del Cuvillo A, et al. Interactions of the H1 antihistamines. *J Investig Allergol Clin Immunol.* 2006;16(suppl 1):29-36.

Bolognia et al., 2018 Bolognia JL, Schaffer JV, Cerroni L. *Dermatology.* 4 ed. Elsevier Saunders; 2018.

Butler et al., 2014 Butler DC, Heller MM, Murase JE. Safety of dermatologic medications in pregnancy and lactation: Part II. Lactation. *J Am Acad Dermatol.* 2014;70(3):417.e1-10; quiz 427. doi:10.1016/j.jaad.2013.09.009

Caplan A, Fett N, Rosenbach M, Werth VP, Micheletti RG. Prevention and management of glucocorticoid-induced side effects: a comprehensive review – infectious complications and vaccination recommendations. *J Am Acad Dermatol.* 2017;76(2):191-198. doi:10.1016/j.jaad.2016.02.1240

Caplan A, Fett N, Rosenbach M, Werth VP, Micheletti RG. Prevention and management of glucocorticoid-induced side effects: a comprehensive review – gastrointestinal and endocrinologic side effects. *J Am Acad Dermatol.* 2017;76(1):11-16. doi:10.1016/j.jaad.2016.02.1239

Caplan A, Fett N, Rosenbach M, Werth VP, Micheletti RG. Prevention and management of glucocorticoid-induced side effects: a comprehensive review – a review of glucocorticoid pharmacology and bone health. *J Am Acad Dermatol.* 2017;76(1):1-9. doi:10.1016/j.jaad.2016.01.062

Chirch LM, Cataline PR, Dieckhaus KD, Grant-Kels JM. Proactive infectious disease approach to dermatologic patients who are taking tumor necrosis factor-alfa antagonists: Part II. Screening for patients on tumor necrosis factor-alfa antagonists. *J Am Acad Dermatol.* 2014;71(1):11.e1-7. quiz 18-20. doi:10.1016/j.jaad.2014.01.879

Chirch LM, Cataline PR, Dieckhaus KD, Grant-Kels JM. Proactive infectious disease approach to dermatologic patients who are taking tumor necrosis factor-alfa antagonists: Part I. Risks associated with tumor necrosis factor-alfa antagonists. *J Am Acad Dermatol.* 2014;71(1):1.e1-8. quiz 1.e8-9, 10. doi:10.1016/j.jaad.2014.01.875

Costa RO, Macedo PM, Carvalhal A, Bernardes-Engemann AR. Use of potassium iodide in dermatology: updates on an old drug. *An Bras Dermatol.* 2013;88(3):396-402. doi:10.1590/abd1806-4841.20132377

Damsky W, Kole L, Tomayko MM. Development of bullous pemphigoid during nivolumab therapy. *JAAD Case Rep.* 2016;2(6):442-444. doi:10.1016/j.jdcr.2016.05.009

de Medeiros SF. Risks, benefits size and clinical implications of combined oral contraceptive use in women with polycystic ovary syndrome. *Reprod Biol Endocrinol.* 2017;15(1):93. doi:10.1186/s12958-017-0313-y

Ebede TL, Arch EL, Berson D. Hormonal treatment of acne in women. *J Clin Aesthet Dermatol.* 2009;2(12):16-22.

Elder DE. *Lever's Histopathology of the Skin.* 11th ed. Wolters Kluwer; 2015.

Elston DM, Ferringer T. *Dermatopathology.* 2nd ed. Elsevier Saunders; 2014.

Epstein E. Persisting Raynaud's phenomenon following intralesional bleomycin treatment of finger warts. *J Am Acad Dermatol.* 1985;13(3):468-471.

Espinosa ML, Nguyen MT, Aguirre AS, et al. Progression of cutaneous T-cell lymphoma after dupilumab: case review of 7 patients. *J Am Acad Dermatol.* 2020;83(1):197-199. doi:10.1016/j.jaad.2020.03.050

Faje AT, Lawrence D, Flaherty K, et al. High-dose glucocorticoids for the treatment of ipilimumab-induced hypophysitis is associated with reduced survival in patients with melanoma. *Cancer.* 2018;124(18):3706-3714. doi:10.1002/cncr.31629

Fernandez-Villa D, Aguilar MR, Rojo L. Folic acid antagonists: antimicrobial and immunomodulating mechanisms and applications. *Int J Mol Sci.* 2019;20(20):E4996. doi:10.3390/ijms20204996

Freites-Martinez A, Shapiro J, Goldfarb S, et al. Hair disorders in patients with cancer. *J Am Acad Dermatol.* 2019;80(5):1179-1196. doi:10.1016/j.jaad.2018.03.055

Freites-Martinez A, Shapiro J, van den Hurk C, et al. Hair disorders in cancer survivors. *J Am Acad Dermatol.* 2019;80(5):1199-1213. doi:10.1016/j.jaad.2018.03.056

Geisler AN, Phillips GS, Barrios DM, et al. Immune checkpoint inhibitor–related dermatologic adverse events. *J Am Acad Dermatol.* 2020;83(5):1255-1268. doi:10.1016/j.jaad.2020.03.132

Heymann WR. Potassium iodide and the Wolff-Chaikoff effect: relevance for the dermatologist. *J Am Acad Dermatol.* 2000;42(3):490-492. doi:10.1016/S0190-9622(00)90224-X

Horn TD, Beveridge RA, Egorin MJ, Abeloff MD, Hood AF. Observations and proposed mechanism of N, N', N"-triethylenethiophosphoramide (thiotepa)-induced hyperpigmentation. *Arch Dermatol.* 1989;125(4):524-527.

Horvat TZ, Adel NG, Dang TO, et al. Immune-related adverse events, need for systemic immunosuppression, and effects on survival and time to treatment failure in patients with melanoma treated with ipilimumab at memorial sloan kettering cancer center. *J Clin Oncol.* 2015;33(28):3193-3198. doi:10.1200/jco.2015.60.8448

Introcaso CE, Hines JM, Kovarik CL. Cutaneous toxicities of antiretroviral therapy for HIV: part II. Nonnucleoside reverse transcriptase inhibitors, entry and fusion inhibitors, integrase inhibitors, and immune reconstitution syndrome. *J Am Acad Dermatol.* 2010;63(4):563-569. quiz 569-570. doi:10.1016/j.jaad.2010.02.059

Introcaso CE, Hines JM, Kovarik CL. Cutaneous toxicities of antiretroviral therapy for HIV: part I. Lipodystrophy syndrome, nucleoside reverse transcriptase inhibitors, and protease inhibitors. *J Am Acad Dermatol.* 2010;63(4):549-561. quiz 561-562. doi:10.1016/j.jaad.2010.01.061

James WD, Elston DM, Treat JR, Rosenbach MA, Neuhaus IM. *Andrews' Diseases of the Skin: Clinical Dermatology.* 13 ed. Elsevier; 2020.

Jhaj R, Sivagnanam G. Concomitant prescription of oral fluoroquinolones with an antacid preparation. *J Pharmacol Pharmacother.* 2013;4(2):140-142. doi:10.4103/0976-500x.110898

Johnston MS, Galan A, Watsky KL, Little AJ. Delayed localized hypersensitivity reactions to the moderna COVID-19 vaccine: a case series. *JAMA Dermatol.* 2021;157(6):716-720. doi:10.1001/jamadermatol.2021.1214

Kar S, Krishnan A, Preetha K, Mohankar A. A review of antihistamines used during pregnancy. *J Pharmacol Pharmacother.* 2012;3(2):105-108. doi:10.4103/0976-500X.95503

Kreidieh FY, Moukadem HA, El Saghir NS. Overview, prevention and management of chemotherapy extravasation. *World J Clin Oncol.* 2016;7(1):87-97. doi:10.5306/wjco.v7.i1.87

Lacouture ME. *Dermatologic Principles and Practice in Oncology: Conditions of the Skin, Hair, and Nails in Cancer Patients.* John Wiley & Sons, Inc.; 2014.

Layton AM, Eady EA, Whitehouse H, Del Rosso JQ, Fedorowicz Z, van Zuuren EJ. Oral spironolactone for acne vulgaris in adult females: a hybrid systematic review. *Am J Clin Dermatol.* 2017;18(2):169-191. doi:10.1007/s40257-016-0245-x

Lebwohl MG, Papp KA, Stein Gold L, et al. Trial of roflumilast cream for chronic plaque psoriasis. *N Engl J Med.* 2020;383(3):229-239. doi:10.1056/NEJMoa2000073

Leurs R, Church MK, Taglialatela M. H1-antihistamines: inverse agonism, anti-inflammatory actions and cardiac effects. *Clin Exp Allergy.* 2002;32(4):489-498. doi:10.1046/j.0954-7894.2002.01314.x

Liszewski W, Boull C. Lack of evidence for feminization of males exposed to spironolactone in utero: a systematic review. *J Am Acad Dermatol.* 2019;80(4):1147-1148. doi:10.1016/j.jaad.2018.10.023

Macdonald JB, Macdonald B, Golitz LE, LoRusso P, Sekulic A. Cutaneous adverse effects of targeted therapies: part I – inhibitors of the cellular membrane. *J Am Acad Dermatol.* 2015;72(2):203-218. quiz 219-220. doi:10.1016/j.jaad.2014.07.032

Macdonald JB, Macdonald B, Golitz LE, LoRusso P, Sekulic A. Cutaneous adverse effects of targeted therapies: part II—inhibitors of intracellular molecular signaling pathways. *J Am Acad Dermatol.* 2015;72(2):221-236. quiz 237-238. doi:10.1016/j.jaad.2014.07.033

Mackenzie IS, Morant SV, Wei L, Thompson AM, MacDonald TM. Spironolactone use and risk of incident cancers: a retrospective, matched cohort study. *Br J Clin Pharmacol.* 2017;83(3):653-663. doi:10.1111/bcp.13152

Makrantonaki E, Ganceviciene R, Zouboulis C. An update on the role of the sebaceous gland in the pathogenesis of acne. *Dermatoendocrinol.* 2011;3(1):41-49. doi:10.4161/derm.3.1.13900

Micali G, Lacarrubba F, Nasca MR, Schwartz RA. Topical pharmacotherapy for skin cancer: part I. Pharmacology. *J Am Acad Dermatol.* 2014;70(6):965. e1-12. quiz 977-978. doi:10.1016/j.jaad.2013.12.045

Micali G, Lacarrubba F, Nasca MR, Ferraro S, Schwartz RA. Topical pharmacotherapy for skin cancer: part II. Clinical applications. *J Am Acad Dermatol.* 2014;70(6):979.e1-12. quiz 9912. doi:10.1016/j.jaad.2013.12.037

Mirnezami M, Rahimi H. Is oral omega-3 effective in reducing mucocutaneous side effects of isotretinoin in patients with acne vulgaris? *Dermatol Res Pract.* 2018;2018:6974045. doi:10.1155/2018/6974045

Mori A, Tamura S, Katsuno T, et al. Scrotal ulcer occurring in patients with acute promyelocytic leukemia during treatment with all-trans retinoic acid. *Oncol Rep.* 1999;6(1):55-58.

Murase JE, Heller MM, Butler DC. Safety of dermatologic medications in pregnancy and lactation: Part I. Pregnancy. *J Am Acad Dermatol.* 2014;70(3):401.e1-14. quiz 415. doi:10.1016/j.jaad.2013.09.010

Opel D, Kramer ON, Chevalier M, Bigby M, Albrecht J. Not every patient needs a triglyceride check, but all can get pancreatitis: a systematic review and clinical characterization of isotretinoin-associated pancreatitis. *Br J Dermatol.* 2017;177(4):960-966. doi:10.1111/bjd.15207

Orvis AK, Wesson SK, Breza TS, Jr. Church AA, Mitchell CL, Watkins SW. Mycophenolate mofetil in dermatology. *J Am Acad Dermatol.* 2009;60(2):183-199. quiz 200-2. doi:10.1016/j.jaad.2008.08.049

Overbosch D, Van Gulpen C, Hermans J, Mattie H. The effect of probenecid on the renal tubular excretion of benzylpenicillin. *Br J Clin Pharmacol.* 1988;25(1):51-58.

Parekh V, Gangadhar T, Kreider KL, Elenitsas R, Chu EY. Complete response of advanced melanoma treated with talimogene laherparepvec and subsequent sweet's-like infiltrate. *JAMA Dermatol.* 2017;153(7):719-721. doi:10.1001/jamadermatol.2017.0466

Payette M, Grant-Kels JM. Generic drugs in dermatology: part I. *J Am Acad Dermatol.* 2012;66(3):343.e1-8. quiz 351-352. doi:10.1016/j.jaad.2011.11.944

Payette M, Grant-Kels JM. Generic drugs in dermatology: part II. *J Am Acad Dermatol.* 2012;66(3):353.e1-15. quiz 367-368. doi:10.1016/j.jaad.2011.11.945

Pelle MT, Callen JP. Adverse cutaneous reactions to hydroxychloroquine are more common in patients with dermatomyositis than in patients with cutaneous lupus erythematosus. *Arch Dermatol.* 2002;138(9):1231-1233; discussion 1233. %J Archives of Dermatology. doi:10.1001/archderm.138.9.1231

Piette WW, Trapp JF, O'Donnell MJ, Argenyi Z, Talbot EA, Burns CP. Acute neutrophilic dermatosis with myeloblastic infiltrate in a leukemia patient receiving all-trans-retinoic acid therapy. *J Am Acad Dermatol.* 1994;30(2 pt 2):293-297.

Pilmis B, Jullien V, Sobel J, Lecuit M, Lortholary O, Charlier C. Antifungal drugs during pregnancy: an updated review. *J Antimicrob Chemother.* 2015;70(1):14-22. doi:10.1093/jac/dku355

Plovanich M, Weng QY, Mostaghimi A. Low usefulness of potassium monitoring among healthy young women taking spironolactone for acne. *JAMA Dermatol.* 2015;151(9):941-944. doi:10.1001/jamadermatol.2015.34

Prevention CfDCa. *Recommended Adult Immunization Schedule for Ages 19 Years or Older, United States,* 2020. Accessed June 1, 2020. https://www.cdc.gov/vaccines/schedules/hcp/imz/adult.html

Prussick R, Ali MA, Rosenthal D, Guyatt G. The protective effect of vitamin E on the hemolysis associated with dapsone treatment in patients with dermatitis herpetiformis. *Arch Dermatol.* 1992;128(2):210-213.

Ramjan KA, Williams AJ, Isbister GK, Elliott EJ. "Red as a beet and blind as a bat" Anticholinergic delirium in adolescents: lessons for the paediatrician. *J Paediatr Child Health.* 2007;43(11):779-780. doi:10.1111/j.1440--1754.2007.01220.x

Resende C, Araujo C, Gomes J, Brito C. Bleomycin-induced flagellate hyperpigmentation. *BMJ Case Rep.* 2013;2013:bcr2013009745. doi:10.1136/bcr-2013-009745

Reyes-Habito CM, Roh EK. Cutaneous reactions to chemotherapeutic drugs and targeted therapy for cancer: part II. Targeted therapy. *J Am Acad Dermatol.* 2014;71(2):217.e1-217.e11. quiz 227-228. doi:10.1016/j.jaad.2014.04.013

Reyes-Habito CM, Roh EK. Cutaneous reactions to chemotherapeutic drugs and targeted therapies for cancer: part I. Conventional chemotherapeutic drugs. *J Am Acad Dermatol.* 2014;71(2):203.e1-203.e12. quiz 215-216. doi:10.1016/j.jaad.2014.04.014

Ryan C, Amor KT, Menter A. The use of cyclosporine in dermatology: part II. *J Am Acad Dermatol.* 2010;63(6):949-972. quiz 973-974. doi:10.1016/j.jaad.2010.02.062

Schutte RJ, Sun Y, Li D, Zhang F, Ostrov DA. Human leukocyte antigen associations in drug hypersensitivity reactions. *Clin Lab Med.* 2018;38(4):669-677. doi:10.1016/j.cll.2018.08.002

Sewell WAC, Jolles S. Immunomodulatory action of intravenous immunoglobulin. *Immunology.* 2002;107(4):387-393. doi:10.1046/j.1365--2567.2002.01545.x

Siegel J, Totonchy M, Damsky W, et al. Bullous disorders associated with anti-PD-1 and anti-PD-L1 therapy: a retrospective analysis evaluating the clinical and histopathologic features, frequency, and impact on cancer therapy. *J Am Acad Dermatol.* 2018;79(6):1081-1088. doi:10.1016/j.jaad.2018.07.008

Sowerby L, Dewan AK, Granter S, Gandhi L, LeBoeuf NR. Rituximab treatment of nivolumab-induced bullous pemphigoid. *JAMA Dermatol.* 2017;153(6):603-605. doi:10.1001/jamadermatol.2017.0091

Thornton MJ. Estrogens and aging skin. *Dermatoendocrinol.* 2013;5(2):264-270. doi:10.4161/derm.23872

Tintle S, Patel V, Ruskin A, Halasz C. Azacitidine: a new medication associated with Sweet syndrome. *J Am Acad Dermatol.* 2011;64(5):e77-e79. doi:10.1016/j.jaad.2010.06.032

Tracey EH, Modi B, Micheletti RG. Pemetrexed-induced pseudocellulitis reaction with eosinophilic infiltrate on skin biopsy. *Am J Dermatopathol.* 2017;39(1):e1-e2. doi:10.1097/dad.0000000000000645

Wehner MR, Nead KT, Lipoff JB. Association between gender and drug cost for over-the-counter minoxidil. *JAMA Dermatol.* 2017;153(8):825-826. doi:10.1001/jamadermatol.2017.1394

Wei SC, Duffy CR, Allison JP. Fundamental mechanisms of immune checkpoint blockade therapy. *Cancer Discov.* 2018;8(9):1069-1086. doi:10.1158/2159-8290.Cd-18-0367

Wolkenstein P, Carriere V, Charue D, et al. A slow acetylator genotype is a risk factor for sulphonamide-induced toxic epidermal necrolysis and Stevens-Johnson syndrome. *Pharmacogenetics.* 1995;5(4):255-258.

Zhanel GG, Siemens S, Slayter K, Mandell L. Antibiotic and oral contraceptive drug interactions: is there a need for concern? *Can J Infect Dis.* 1999;10(6):429-433.

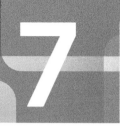

Physical Treatments

John S. Barbieri, MD, MBA and Sherry H. Yu, MD

Phototherapy

Basic Concepts

- In **phototherapy**, UVR is used to induce a therapeutic effect. Methods include:
  - **bbUVB: 290 to 320 nm.**
  - **nbUVB: 311 to 313 nm.**
  - **Excimer laser: 308 nm.**
  - **UVA: 320 to 400 nm.**
  - **UVA1: 340 to 400 nm.**
  - **PUVA:** Psoralens such as **8-methoxsalen (8-MOP) (peak erythema action spectrum 330-335 nm)** are applied topically or taken orally and then the patient is exposed to **UVA radiation (peak 352 nm).**
  - **ECP:** WBCs are extracted from the body and treated with UVA irradiation after exposure to 8-MOP.
- To review the electromagnetic spectrum, see Figure 1.19.
- The most important **chromophore for nbUVB is nuclear DNA, causing cyclobutane-pyrimidine dimers.** In **PUVA, psoralens cross-link with pyrimidine bases in nuclear DNA.** nbUVB and PUVA each **reduce cellular proliferation and suppress the immune system (adaptive > innate)** through release of anti-inflammatory cytokines, which is helpful in the treatment of inflammatory dermatoses.

Clinical Applications

- **nbUVB** is commonly used for the management of **psoriasis, parapsoriasis, pityriasis lichenoides, PR, AD, vitiligo, LP, pigmented purpura, pruritus, GA, CTCL, and LyP.**
- **UVA1 and PUVA** are commonly used for the management of **psoriasis, GVHD, morphea, SSc, scleredema, and CTCL.**
  - Calcipotriene should not be applied prior to phototherapy, since it will both block UVR and be broken down by UVR.
- **ECP** is commonly used for the management of **GVHD and CTCL.**

Safety Considerations

- **Short-term complications from phototherapy include sunburn and increased risk of HSV reactivation.** PUVA can be complicated by **phototoxic eruption/photoonycholysis and transient pruritus.** UVB erythema appears after 4 to 6 hours and peaks 12 to 24 hours after exposure, whereas PUVA erythema appears after 24 to 36 hours and peaks 72 to 96 hours after exposure.
- **Long-term complications from nbUVB include photoaging** and skin cancer, although the **increased risk of skin cancer with nbUVB is minimal to nonexistent.**
- **Long-term complications from PUVA include hyperpigmentation and lentigines, photoaging, skin cancer, cataracts, and hepatotoxicity.** It is important for patients being treated with oral PUVA to wear eye protection following treatment.
- Phototherapy dosing can be determined by skin type or by checking the **MED/minimal phototoxic dose (MPD), which is the lowest dose resulting in erythema 48 hours after exposure to UVR.**
  - While the solar simulator is used for MED/MPD testing, the spot size is too small for use in phototherapy.
- **ECP is contraindicated in severe cardiac disease** due to fluid shifts from the apheresis procedure.

Photodynamic Therapy

Basic Concepts

- In PDT, a photosensitizer, commonly **ALA or methyl aminolevulinate (MAL), is activated by light** to induce a therapeutic effect.
- The **penetration of these photosensitizers is limited by the thickness of the *stratum corneum*.** Thus, acetone scrubs and superficial chemical peels can reduce incubation times. In addition, the methyl group in MAL makes it more lipophilic, allowing for deeper penetration.
- ALA and MAL are metabolized along the heme pathway into porphyrins, notably **protoporphyrin IX.**
  - PDT generates protoporphyrin IX.
- Protoporphyrin IX has **excitation peaks at the Soret band (400-410 nm), which can be activated by blue light, and ~625 nm, which can be activated by red light.** Following excitation, porphyrins generate **ROS** resulting in cellular damage.

- ALA is typically used with blue light and MAL is typically used with red light. Since red light has deeper penetration, it may be more appropriate for dermal processes, whereas blue light may be more appropriate for epidermal processes.

Clinical Applications

- PDT is primarily used for **field treatment of AKs** and treatment of some superficial keratinocyte skin cancers.

The **abnormal epidermis** of these lesions is thought to **facilitate increased penetration by ALA and MAL**, leading to selective destruction.

- *Cutibacterium acnes* naturally accumulates porphyrins. **Blue or red light alone can act as a potential treatment for acne**; however, the evidence is limited.

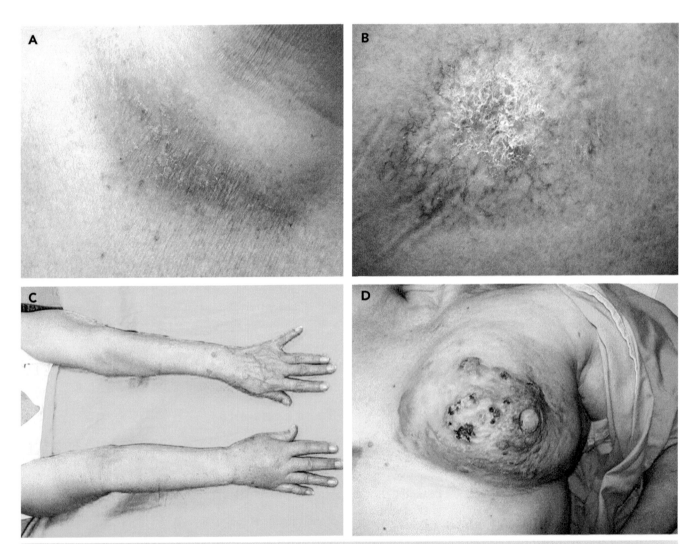

Figure 7.1. MUCOCUTANEOUS ADVERSE EVENTS OF RADIATION THERAPY. A, Acute radiation dermatitis. B, Chronic radiation dermatitis (fluoroscopy-induced). C, Lymphedema of the right upper extremity secondary to modified radical mastectomy, lymph node dissection, and radiation therapy for breast cancer. D, Radiation therapy-induced angiosarcoma.

(A, Reprinted with permission from Elder DE, Elenitsas R, Rosenbach M, et al. *Lever's Histopathology of the Skin.* 11th ed. Wolters Kluwer; 2015. C, Reprinted with permission from Strauch B, Vasconez LO, Herman CK, et al. *Grabb's Encyclopedia of Flaps: Head and Neck.* 4th ed. Wolters Kluwer; 2015. D, Reprinted with permission from Mulholland MW, Lillemoe KD, Doherty GM, et al. *Greenfield's Surgery: Scientific Principles and Practice.* 6th ed. Wolters Kluwer; 2016.)

Safety Considerations

- After PDT, patients should not expose themselves to sunlight or other intense light for at least 48 hours. Since the porphyrins are excited by light in the visible spectrum, **sunscreen will not be effective in preventing complications such as phototoxic eruption.**
- Daylight PDT, in which ALA or MAL is applied and then sunlight is used for photoexcitation, may have similar effectiveness to conventional blue light or red light PDT with fewer complications.

Radiation Therapy

Basic Concepts

- In **radiation therapy**, **ionizing radiation** is used to induce a therapeutic effect. Methods include:
  - Low-energy photons.
  - Electrons.
  - Brachytherapy: direct application of a radioactive source to involved tissues (eg, radioactive molds and implants).
  - Office-based radiation therapy.
- X-rays produce double-stranded deoxyribonucleic acid (dsDNA) breaks that cause cell death in more rapidly dividing malignant cells out of proportion to normal adjacent tissues.

Clinical Applications

- Radiation therapy may be used for definitive, adjuvant, or palliative treatment for skin cancer, such as **patients with BCC or SCC who refuse surgery, are not optimal surgical candidates, or who have microscopic involvement of the surgical margins.** Cure rates for primary BCC can exceed 90%. **CTCL** lesions can be treated with **either localized radiation therapy or TSEBT.**
- Radiation therapy can be used to **prevent recurrence of keloids following excision.**

Safety Considerations

- Complications of ionizing radiation exposure include **radiation acne, radiation dermatitis, radiation stomatitis, induction of skin diseases (eg, BP, morphea, Sweet syndrome), lymphedema, and induction of malignancies such as BCC, SCC, atypical vascular lesions (AVL), and angiosarcoma** (Figure 7.1). Radiation dermatitis may be associated with secondary **scarring alopecia.** The **left upper back** is a characteristic location for patients with **fluoroscopy-induced radiation dermatitis** in patients with cardiovascular disease following cardiac catheterizations with attempted revascularization (eg, angioplasty, stent placement).
  - Figure 7.2.
- Low-energy (superficial) radiation therapy has less penetration than high-energy radiation therapy and therefore may have reduced risk of complications.

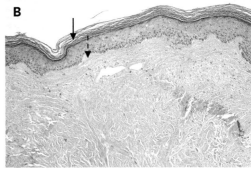

Figure 7.2. CLINICOPATHOLOGICAL CORRELATION: RADIATION DERMATITIS. Acute radiation dermatitis is characterized by apoptotic keratinocytes. Chronic radiation dermatitis is characterized by compact hyperorthokeratosis ± epidermal atrophy and papillary dermal pallor. Other features include dermal sclerosis resulting in a square punch, elastosis, superficial vascular ectasia, absent appendages, and large stellate radiation fibroblasts. Chronic radiation dermatitis. A, Low-power view. B, Medium-power view. Solid arrow: Compact hyperorthokeratosis (red). Dashed arrow: Papillary dermal pallor (white). LS, lichen sclerosus. (Illustration by Caroline A. Nelson, MD.)

The flag of Indonesia, like chronic radiation dermatitis, has two horizontal stripes: red (compact hyperorthokeratosis) and white (papillary dermal pallor). Absence of a blue horizontal stripe (lymphocytic infiltrate) helps distinguish chronic radiation dermatitis from LS.

Cryosurgery

Basic Concepts

- In **cryosurgery, low temperatures** are used to destroy tissue via heat transfer from hot to cold. Conductors of cold include metal > ice > water > air. The rate of heat transfer is a function of the temperature difference. **Liquid nitrogen is the most common cryogen used in dermatology** due to the low temperatures achieved (**boiling point −196°C**). Methods include:
  - **Open (spray)**: handheld spray unit with an adjustable nozzle.
  - **Semi-open (confined spray)**: instrument (eg, polycarbonate plate with holes, neoprene cone, or otoscope speculum) restricts spray to a limited area.
  - **Semi-closed (chamber)**: rubber-protected metal cylinder against the skin connected to a cryogen unit for potent freezing.
  - **Closed (contact)**: pressure and duration of contact with either an instrument (eg, cotton tip applicator or metal probe) control depth of freeze.
- Table 7.1 summarizes **mechanisms of injury in cryosurgery**. Necrosis is achieved through **damage to cellular membranes and organelles due to extracellular then intracellular ice crystal formation**. During thaw, increased solute gradients result in cell membrane shrinkage and **recrystallization patterns** result in further damage.

- **Rapid freezing with a slow thaw is desirable.** Longer freeze times (5-12 seconds) and multiple freeze-thaw cycles (≥2) are associated with higher rates of clearance.
- The response can be augmented by:
  - Ice injury (glycine).
  - Inducers of apoptosis (5-FU).
  - Immunomodulators (imiquimod).
- Table 7.2 summarizes **cell specific sensitivities to cold. Cellular components are more susceptible than stromal components.** Preservation of collagen bundles minimizes scarring. Cartilage and bone are relatively insensitive to cold.

Clinical Applications

- Cryosurgery is a common treatment modality for a **spectrum of benign, premalignant, and malignant skin lesions** (Table 7.3). Advantages include ease of use, versatility, low cost, and minimal scarring.

Safety Considerations

- Complications of cryotherapy include **blistering, pain, and pigmentary changes**, along with scarring and superficial nerve injury.
  - Melanocyte sensitivity to cold explains pigmentary changes observed after cryotherapy.

Table 7.1. MECHANISMS OF INJURY IN CRYOSURGERY

Type of Injury	Mechanism of Cell Death	Phase	Location	Type of Response
Direct	Necrosis (−20 °C for most cells; −50 °C for malignant cells)	Freeze	Central	Significant inflammation, innate immune response
Vascular	Ischemia due to secondary damage of vascular endothelium	Thaw (~1 h after freeze)	Periphery	Mild/moderate inflammation
Apoptosis	Due to sublethal temperatures (approximately −20 °C for malignant cells)	Thaw (4-8 h after thaw)	Periphery	Little inflammation
Immunologic	Due to stimulation of immune response by antigen released from damaged cells	Late	Lymph nodes	Acquired immune response

Table 7.2. CELL-SPECIFIC SENSITIVITIES TO COLD

Cell Type	Target Temperature for Cell Damage
Melanocyte	−4°C
Vascular endothelium	−15 to −40°C
Benign keratinocyte	−35°C
Malignant keratinocyte	−50°C
Sarcoma	−60°C

Table 7.3. SPECTRUM OF SKIN LESIONS AMENABLE TO CRYOSURGERY

Benign	Premalignant/Malignant
Wart	BCC
Molluscum contagiosum	AK
SK	SCCis
Spider angioma	SCC
Digital mucous cyst	Lentigo maligna

AK, actinic keratosis; BCC, basal cell carcinoma; SCC, squamous cell carcinoma; SCCis, SCC in situ; SK, seborrheic keratosis.

Electrocautery and Electrosurgery

Basic Concepts

- In **electrocautery, direct current (DC) produces thermal energy.** No heat is generated in deeper tissue. **Electrocautery works in a wet field.**
- In **electrosurgery,** passage of **high-frequency alternating current (AC)** from the active electrode through tissue to the return electrode leads to heat production due to tissue resistance. In order to minimize complications, lateral heat spread should be kept to a minimum by using the appropriate waveform, power setting, and electrode size. **Methods** are summarized in Table 7.4.
- **Damping the waveform** (eg, electrodessication, electrofulguration > electrocoagulation) **increases hemostasis but may delay wound healing.**
- The terms **"monopolar" vs "bipolar"** refer to the **number of tissue-contacting tips (electrodes). A pointed electrode is monopolar,** while **electrosurgical forceps are bipolar** (eg, electrocoagulation).
- The terms **"monoterminal" vs "biterminal"** refer to the presence of a **dispersive electrode.** In a **monoterminal** setup (eg, electrodessication, electrofulguration), the **patient's body** and/or earth **acts as the dispersive electrode.** In a **biterminal** setup (eg, electrocoagulation, electrosection), **a dispersive electrode (ground plate) is attached to the patient.** Biterminal setups can use higher power and are generally safer.
- Electrocautery and electrosurgery are illustrated in Figure 7.3.

Clinical Applications

- Electrosurgery is a common treatment modality in dermatology. **Electrodessication and electrofulguration are preferable for superficial skin ablation (eg, SK), electrocoagulation is preferable for deep skin ablation (eg, SCCis), and electrosection is preferable for skin incision/excision (eg, surgical excision of benign or malignant neoplasms).**
  - An advantage of electrosurgery over scalpel surgery is use of a blended cutting and coagulating current to achieve hemostasis immediately as the incision is made.
  - Figure 7.4.

Safety Considerations

- Although most modern implantable devices have shielding and are resistant to external electromagnetic signals, there is a risk of **electromagnetic interference from monopolar electrosurgery.** Factors include:
  - Device: **implantable cardioverter-defibrillators (ICDs)** are higher risk than pacemakers.
  - Method: **electrosection** is the highest risk.
    - Electrocautery is safe to use with an implantable device.
  - Location: **use above the umbilicus** is higher risk than use below the umbilicus.

Table 7.4. METHODS OF ELECTROSURGERY

Method	Definition	Depth	Voltage	Amperage	Electrical Current	Circuit
Electrocoagulation	Tissue heated below boiling point leading to thermal denaturation	Deep skin ablation	Low	High	Continuous current (moderately damped)	Biterminal
Electrodessication	Vaporization of water content	Superficial skin ablation	High	Low	Continuous current (damped)	Monoterminal
Electrofulguration	Active electrode held slightly above tissue and current bridges the air gap	Very superficial skin ablation	High	Low	Interrupted current (damped)	Monoterminal
Electrosection	Sudden increase in tissue temperature above boiling point leads to tissue fragmentation and cutting with little coagulation	Skin incision/ excision while achieving hemostasis	Low	High	Continuous current (undamped)	Biterminal (pure cutting)

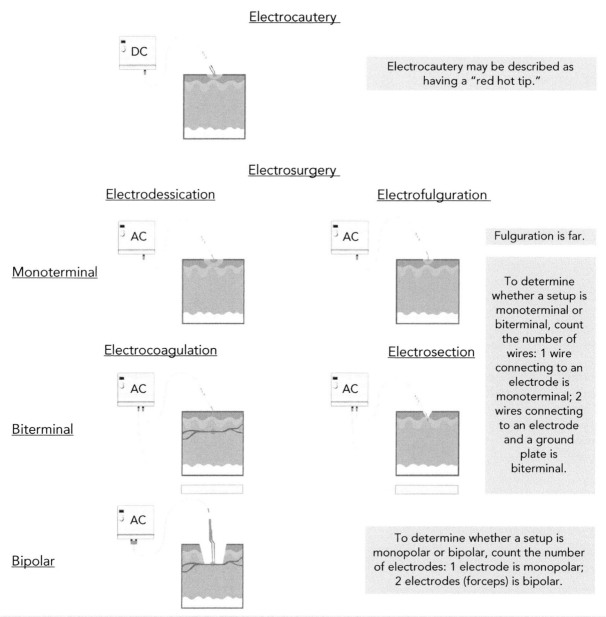

Figure 7.3. ELECTROCAUTERY AND ELECTROSURGERY. AC, alternating current; DC, direct current.
(Illustration by Caroline A. Nelson, MD.)

Depending on the device, **magnets can convert pacemakers into an asynchronous mode. For ICDs, magnets can prevent both antitachycardic pacing and defibrillation.**
- Electrosurgery is a potential **fire hazard.** It is important to **avoid fire risks such as alochol-based preps, aluminum chloride, and high oxygen concentrations.**

- **Surgical smoke** from electrosurgery can contain **harmful pathogens (eg, HPV) or carcinogens**; therefore, smoke evacuators should be considered.

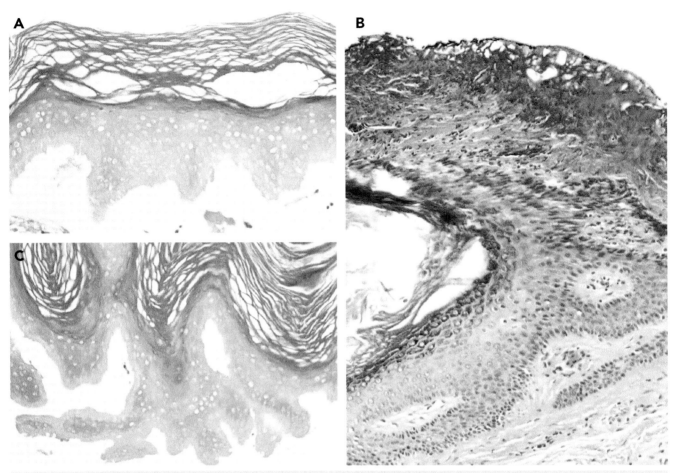

Figure 7.4. SIDE-BY-SCOMPARISON: CRYOTHERAPY AND ELECTROSURGERY. Both cryotherapy and electrosurgery result in detachment of the epidermis from the dermis. Cryotherapy is characterized by keratinocyte pallor with loss of the cellular outline (homogenization) along with dermal edema or coagulation (homogenization) depending on its intensity. Electrosurgery is characterized by keratinocyte elongation with nuclear pyknosis and cytoplasmic eosinophilia along with dermal coagulation (homogenization). A and C, Cryotherapy. B, Electrodessication.

(Histology images reprinted with permission from Elder DE, Elenitsas R, Rosenbach M, et al. *Lever's Histopathology of the Skin.* 11th ed. Wolters Kluwer; 2015.)

FURTHER READING

Anolik R, Brauer JA, Soter NA. An unusual bullous eruption in a patient with psoriasis: calcipotriene phototoxicity. *J Am Acad Dermatol.* 2010;62(6):1081-1082.

Berman B, Shabbir AQ, MacNeil T, Knudsen KM. Variables in cryosurgery technique associated with clearance of actinic keratosis. *Dermatol Surg.* 2017;43(3):424-430.

Bhatnagar A. Nonmelanoma skin cancer treated with electronic brachytherapy: results at 1 year. *Brachytherapy.* 2013;12(2):134-140.

Boen M, Brownell J, Patel P, Tsoukas MM. The role of photodynamic therapy in acne: an evidence-based review. *Am J Clin Dermatol.* 2017;18(3):311-321.

Bolderston A, Lloyd NS, Wong RKS, Holden L, Robb-Blenderman L; Supportive Care Guidelines Group of Cancer Care Ontario Program in Evidence-Based Care. The prevention and management of acute skin reactions related to radiation therapy: a systematic review and practice guideline. *Support Care Cancer.* 2006;14(8):802-817.

Bolognia JL, Schaffer JV, Cerroni L. *Dermatology.* 4th ed. Elsevier Saunders; 2018.

Cooper SM, Dawber RP. The history of cryosurgery. *J R Soc Med.* 2001; 94(4):196-201.

Dawber RP. Cryosurgery: complications and contraindications. *Clin Dermatol.* 1990;8(1):108-114.

Elder DE. *Lever's Histopathology of the Skin.* 11th ed. Wolters Kluwer; 2015.

Elston DM, Ferringer T. *Dermatopathology.* 2nd ed. Elsevier Saunders; 2014.

Farhangian ME, Snyder A, Huang KE, Doerfler L, Huang WW, Feldman SR. Cutaneous cryosurgery in the United States. *J Dermatolog Treat.* 2016;27(1):91-94.

James WD, Elston DM, Treat JR, Rosenbach MA, Neuhaus IM. *Andrews' Diseases of the Skin: Clinical Dermatology.* 13th ed. Elsevier; 2020.

Kuflik EG. Cryosurgery updated. *J Am Acad Dermatol.* 1994;31(6):925-944. quiz 944-926.

Laughlin SA, Dudley DK. Electrosurgery. *Clin Dermatol.* 1992;10(3): 285-290.

Neelankavil JPT, Thompson A, Mahajan A. Managing Cardiovascular Implantable Electronic Devices (CIEDs) During Perioperative Care. Accessed January 4, 2022. https://www.apsf.org/article/managing-cardiovascular-implantable-electronic-devices-cieds-during-perioperative-care/

Price ML, Lim HW. Narrow-band UVB: is it carcinogenic? *Psoriasis Forum.* 2009;15:41-49.

Schulman PM, Treggiari MM, Yanez ND, et al. Electromagnetic interference with protocolized electrosurgery dispersive electrode positioning in patients with implantable cardioverter defibrillators. *Anesthesiology.* 2019;130(4):530-540.

Sruthi K, Chelakkot PG, Madhavan R, Nair RR, Dinesh M. Single-fraction radiation: a promising adjuvant therapy to prevent keloid recurrence. *J Cancer Res Ther.* 2018;14(6):1251-1255.

Taheri A, Mansoori P, Sandoval LF, Feldman SR, Pearce D, Williford PM. Electrosurgery: part II. Technology, applications, and safety of electrosurgical devices. *J Am Acad Dermatol.* 2014;70(4):607.e601-607.e612.

Taheri A, Mansoori P, Sandoval LF, Feldman SR, Pearce D, Williford PM. Electrosurgery: part I. Basics and principles. *J Am Acad Dermatol.* 2014;70(4):591.e1-591.e14.

Zhu L, Wang P, Zhang G, et al. Conventional versus daylight photodynamic therapy for actinic keratosis: a randomized and prospective study in China. *Photodiagnosis Photodyn Ther.* 2018;24:366-371.

8 Surgery

Sherry H. Yu, MD

Surgical Anatomy

Basic Concepts

- In-depth knowledge of surgical anatomy is fundamental to the safe execution of dermatologic procedures.
- The face is divided into **eight major cosmetic subunits** (Figure 8.1): **forehead, temples, eyelids, nose, cheeks, ears, lips, and chin.** Cosmetic subunits are delineated based on similarities in **topographic anatomy, texture and color, solar exposure, sebaceous features, and hair density.**
- Important landmarks of the face include the **midline** and the **mid-pupillary line**, on which the **supraorbital foramen, infraorbital foramen, and mental foramen** are located.

Topography of the eyelids, nose, lips, and ears is illustrated in Figure 8.2, Figure 8.3, Figure 8.4, and Figure 8.5.
- The scalp and face have distinct **layers** (Figure 8.6):
  - **Scalp:** epidermis/dermis, subcutaneous fat, **galea aponeurotica**, loose subaponeurotic tissue, periosteum.
  - **Face:** epidermis/dermis, subcutaneous fat, **superficial musculoaponeurotic system (SMAS)**, periosteum.

Muscles

Muscles

- **Muscles of the head and neck** are illustrated in Figure 8.7.
  - **Muscles of mastication** arise from the **first branchial arch.**

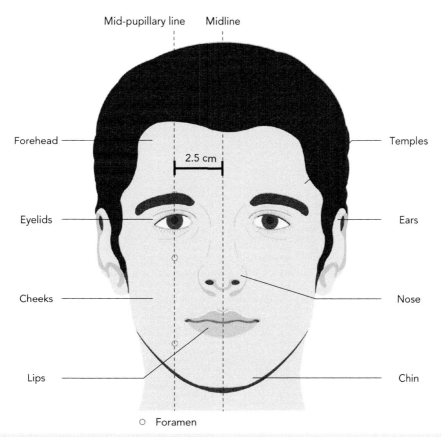

Figure 8.1. MAJOR COSMETIC SUBUNITS OF THE FACE.
(Illustration by Caroline A. Nelson, MD.)

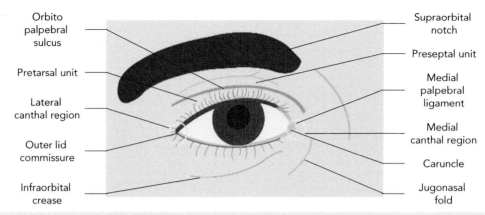

Figure 8.2. TOPOGRAPHY OF THE EYELIDS.
(Illustration by Caroline A. Nelson, MD.)

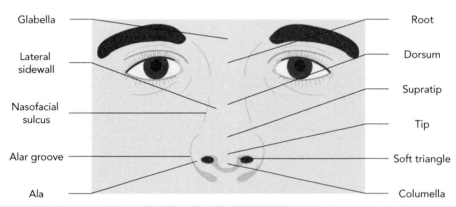

Figure 8.3. TOPOGRAPHY OF THE NOSE.
(Illustration by Caroline A. Nelson, MD.)

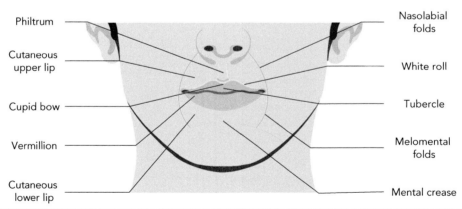

Figure 8.4. TOPOGRAPHY OF THE LIPS.
(Illustration by Caroline A. Nelson, MD.)

- ○ **Muscles of facial expression** arise from the **second branchial arch.**
- **The SMAS, extending from the frontalis to the platysma, allows organized movement of muscles of facial expression.** As a general rule, **blood vessels and sensory nerves lie within or superficial to the SMAS,** while **motor nerves lie deep to the SMAS.**
  - The SMAS is pulled tight during a face-lift.

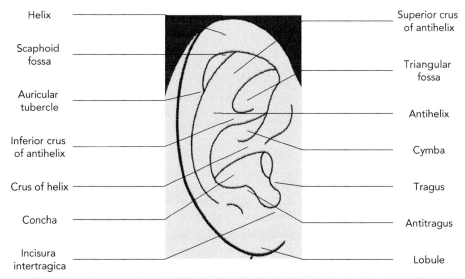

Figure 8.5. TOPOGRAPHY OF THE EARS.
(Illustration by Caroline A. Nelson, MD.)

Scalp

1. Epidermis/dermis
2. Subcutaneous fat
3. Galea aponeurotica
4. Loose subaponeurotic tissue
5. Periosteum

Face

1. Epidermis/dermis
2. Subcutaneous fat
3. SMAS
4. Periosteum

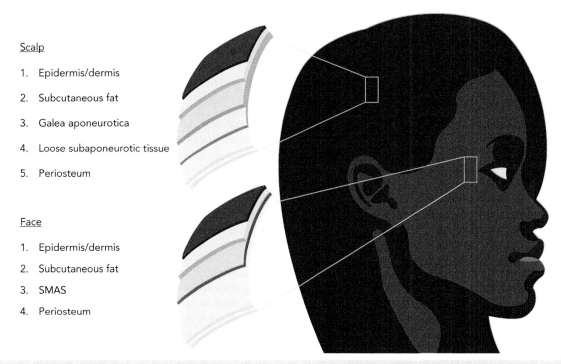

Figure 8.6. LAYERS OF THE SCALP AND FACE. The SMAS extends from the galea aponeurotica of the scalp to the playtsma of the neck. Layers of the scalp and face are illustrated. Layers of the face vary based on location, with the addition of deep fascia, fat, muscle, and/or retaining ligaments below the SMAS. SMAS, superficial musculoaponeurotic system.
(Illustration by Caroline A. Nelson, MD.)

<u>SCALP</u> layers: <u>S</u>kin (epidermis/dermis), <u>C</u>onnective tissue (subcutaneous fat), <u>A</u>poneurosis (galea aponeurotica), <u>L</u>oose subaponeurotic tissue, and <u>P</u>eriosteum.

Skin Lines

- **Langer lines run parallel to underlying muscles.**
    If pierced, the skin will naturally gape open along Langer lines.

- **Skin tension lines** (Kraissl and Borges lines) **run perpendicular to underlying muscles** (Figure 8.8).
    Incision or excision should be oriented parallel to skin tension lines.

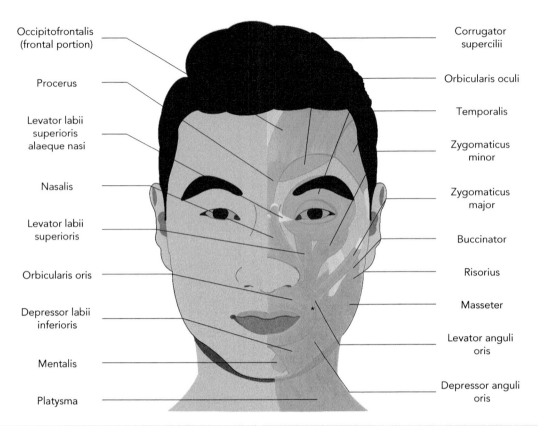

Occipitofrontalis (frontal portion)

Procerus

Levator labii superioris alaeque nasi

Nasalis

Levator labii superioris

Orbicularis oris

Depressor labii inferioris

Mentalis

Platysma

Corrugator supercilii

Orbicularis oculi

Temporalis

Zygomaticus minor

Zygomaticus major

Buccinator

Risorius

Masseter

Levator anguli oris

Depressor anguli oris

Figure 8.7. MUSCLES OF THE HEAD AND NECK. * Modiolus anguli oris is a chiasma of facial muscles (buccinator, depressor anguli oris, levator anguli oris, levator labii superioris, orbicularis oris, platysma, risorius, zygomaticus major) held together by fibrous tissue that is important for mouth movement.

(Illustration by Caroline A. Nelson, MD.)

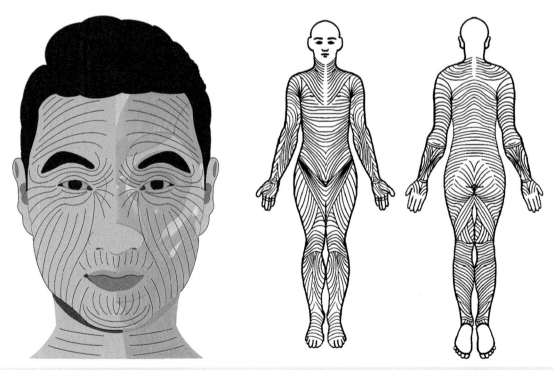

Figure 8.8. SKIN TENSION LINES.

(Illustration by Caroline A. Nelson, MD.)

Blood Vessels

- **Arteries of the head and neck,** consisting of anastomosing branches of the **internal carotid artery (ICA)** and the **external carotid artery (ECA),** are illustrated in Figure 8.9.
- **Veins of the head and neck** follow the arterial supply. The **ophthalmic veins** drain through the orbit into the **cavernous sinus,** which also drains blood from the anterior part of the base of the brain.
  Figure 8.10.
- The **lymphatic drainage of the head and neck** varies, but generally flows in a **downward diagonal** direction. The **parotid nodes** (forehead and eyelids), **submandibular nodes** (lower and medial face), and **submental nodes** (central lower lip and chin) drain into the **lateral cervical nodes.**

Nerves

Sensory Innervation

- Sensory nerves of the head and neck are illustrated in Figure 8.11.

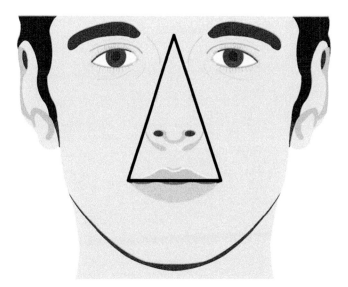

Figure 8.10. DANGER TRIANGLE OF THE FACE. Retrograde spread of infection from the nasal area to the brain may lead to cavernous sinus thrombosis, meningitis, or brain abscesses. The area from the oral commissures to the nasal bridge is called the "danger triangle" of the face. (Illustration by Caroline A. Nelson, MD.)

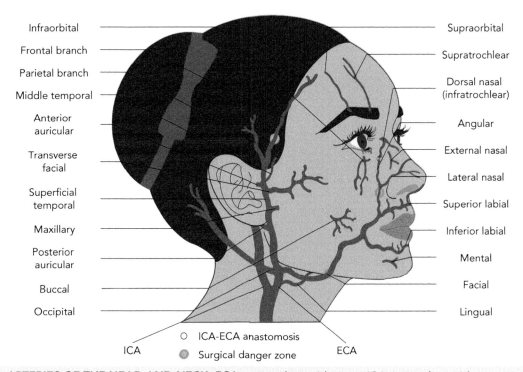

Figure 8.9. ARTERIES OF THE HEAD AND NECK. ECA, external carotid artery; ICA, internal carotid artery. (Illustration by Caroline A. Nelson, MD.)

Selected Arteries of the Head and Neck
- ICA → ophthalmic → central retinal, lacrimal, posterior ciliary, muscular branches, supraorbital, posterior ethmoidal, anterior ethmoidal → external nasal, medial palpebral, supratrochlear, dorsal nasal (infratrochlear)
- ECA → lingual; facial → angular, inferior labial, superior labial, lateral nasal; occipital; posterior auricular; maxillary → inferior alveolar → mental, buccal, infraorbital; superficial temporal → transverse facial, middle temporal, anterior auricular, frontal branch, parietal branch

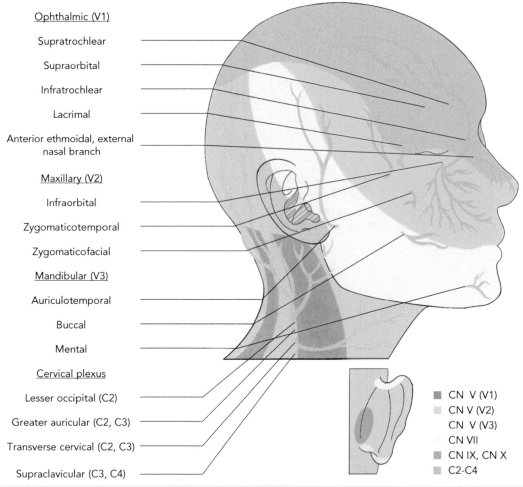

Ophthalmic (V1)
Supratrochlear
Supraorbital
Infratrochlear
Lacrimal
Anterior ethmoidal, external nasal branch
Maxillary (V2)
Infraorbital
Zygomaticotemporal
Zygomaticofacial
Mandibular (V3)
Auriculotemporal
Buccal
Mental
Cervical plexus
Lesser occipital (C2)
Greater auricular (C2, C3)
Transverse cervical (C2, C3)
Supraclavicular (C3, C4)

■ CN V (V1)
▫ CN V (V2)
  CN V (V3)
▫ CN VII
■ CN IX, CN X
▪ C2-C4

Figure 8.11. SENSORY NERVES OF THE HEAD AND NECK. CN, cranial nerve.
(Illustration by Caroline A. Nelson, MD.)

○ The **trigeminal nerve (cranial nerve [CN] V)** arises from **gasserian ganglion** to provide **sensory innervation to the face and anterior 2/3 of the tongue (somatic).**
  ◦ Trigeminal trophic syndrome may develop after surgical trigeminal ablation by rhizotomy or alcohol injection into the gasserian ganglion.
○ The **facial nerve (CN VII)** arises from the **geniculate ganglion** to provide **sensory innervation to the conchal bowl** (with glossopharyngeal and vagus nerves), **external auditory meatus, and anterior 2/3 of the tongue (taste, chorda tympani nerve).**

  ◦ Ramsay Hunt syndrome occurs when VZV reactivates from the geniculate ganglion.
○ The **glossopharyngeal nerve (CN IX)** innervates the **conchal bowl** (with facial and vagus nerves) and **posterior 1/3 of the tongue (somatic and taste).**
○ The **vagus nerve (CN X)** innervates the **conchal bowl** (with facial and glossopharyngeal nerves).
  ◦ A ring block around the ear will NOT anesthetize the conchal bowl or external auditory meatus.
• Sensory nerves of the hands and feet are illustrated in Figure 8.12.

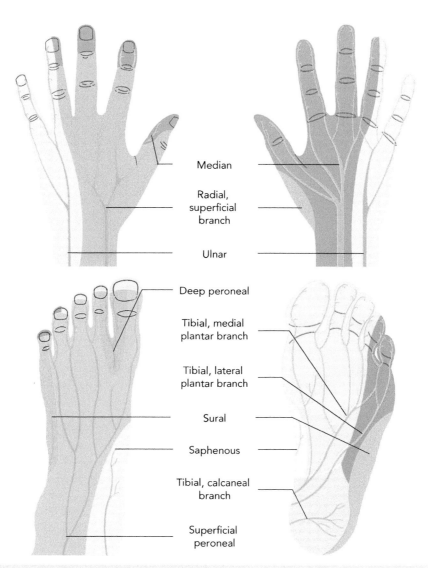

Figure 8.12. SENSORY NERVES OF THE HANDS AND FEET.
(Illustration by Caroline A. Nelson, MD.)

Remember that the u̲lnar nerve and the su̲ral nerve innervate the 5th digits because both have u̲ in the name.

Motor Innervation

- Motor nerves of the head and neck are illustrated in Figure 8.13.
  - ○ The **trigeminal nerve (CN V)** provides **motor innervation to the muscles of mastication.**
  - ○ The **facial nerve (CN VII)** provides **motor innervation to the muscles of facial expression.** It exits the stylomas-toid foramen, enters the parotid gland, and divides into branches (Table 8.1).

Surgical Danger Zones of the Head and Neck

- Surgical danger zones of the head and neck are summarized in Table 8.2.

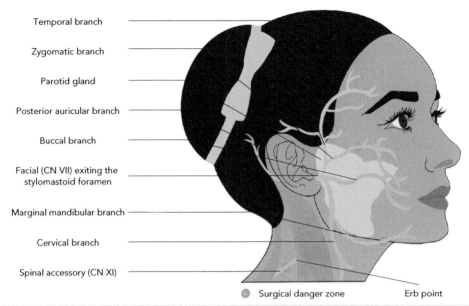

Temporal branch

Zygomatic branch

Parotid gland

Posterior auricular branch

Buccal branch

Facial (CN VII) exiting the
stylomastoid foramen

Marginal mandibular branch

Cervical branch

Spinal accessory (CN XI)

Surgical danger zone   Erb point

Figure 8.13. MOTOR NERVES OF THE HEAD AND NECK. CN, cranial nerve.
(Illustration by Caroline A. Nelson, MD.)

Remember the Temporal, Zygomatic, Buccal, Marginal mandibular, and Cervical branches of the facial nerve (CNVII)
with the mnemonic "To Zanzibar By Motor Car."

Table 8.1. FACIAL NERVE (CN VII) BRANCHES

Branch	Innervated Muscle(s)	Function	Notes
Temporal	Frontalis	Elevates eyebrows and wrinkles forehead.	Responsible for horizontal forehead rhytides.
	Corrugator supercilii	Pulls eyebrows medially and downward.	Responsible for vertical glabellar rhytides.
Temporal and zygomatic	Orbicularis oculi	Blinking and tight closure of eyelids. Lesser role as brow depressor.	Responsible for lateral canthal rhytides.
Zygomatic and buccal	Procerus	Pulls medial eyebrows and glabellar skin downward.	Responsible for horizontal glabellar rhytides.
	Nasalis	Alar flaring and compression.	Responsible for nasalis rhytides.
Buccal	Levator labii superioris	Elevates upper lip.	
	Levator labii superioris alaeque nasi	Elevates upper lip and dilates nostrils.	
	Levator anguli oris	Elevates corners of mouth.	
	Zygomaticus major	Elevates and draws corner of mouth laterally.	Main contributor to smiling (nasolabial folds).
	Zygomaticus minor	Elevates upper lip.	
	Buccinator	Presses cheek against teeth.	Allows blowing of cheeks. The buccinator is innervated on its surface, increasing risk of paralysis. The parotid duct is at risk of injury posterior to the buccinator.
Marginal mandibular	Risorius	Draws back corners of mouth.	
	Orbicularis oris	Closes and purses lips.	Responsible for perioral rhytides.
	Depressor anguli oris	Depresses corners of mouth.	Responsible for melomental folds.
	Depressor labii inferioris	Depresses lower lip.	
	Mentalis	Protrudes lower lip.	Responsible for mental crease and *peau d'orange* skin.
Cervical	Platysma	Depresses corners of mouth and tenses neck.	Responsible for platysma bands.
Posterior auricular	Occipitalis	Pulls scalp posteriorly.	

Table 8.2. SURGICAL DANGER ZONES OF THE HEAD AND NECK

Structure	Location	Function	Complication(s)
Artery[a]			
Superficial temporal artery, frontal branch	Temple	Supplies blood to forehead.	Hemorrhage.
Facial artery	Mandibular rim	Supplies blood to face.	Hemorrhage.
Angular artery	Base of nasal ala	Supplies blood to nose and eyelids.	Hemorrhage.
Posterior auricular artery	Sulcus between ear and mastoid	Supplies blood to external ear and posterior auricular scalp.	Hemorrhage.
Motor Nerve			
Facial nerve (CN VII), temporal branch	Between two lines: earlobe to lateral edge of eyebrow and tragus to lateral edge of highest horizontal forehead line.	Innervates frontalis.	Inability to raise ipsilateral eyebrow (loss of forehead furrows) and drooping (ptosis).
Facial nerve (CN VII), zygomatic branch	Inferomedial to the upper masseteric retaining ligament. Nerve is most superficial over bony prominence (zygomatic arch).	Innervates orbicularis oculi.	Inability to completely appose ipsilateral upper and lower eyelids and corneal desiccation.
Facial nerve (CN VII), marginal mandibular branch	Anterior to angle of mandible. Nerve is most superficial over bony prominence.	Innervates lip depressors.	Asymmetric smile or grimace and ipsilateral drooling. Highest risk of permanent motor deficit.
Spinal accessory nerve (CN XI)	Posterior triangle of neck within 2 cm of Erb point, located at the mid-posterior margin of the SCM where the cervical plexus emerges.	Innervates trapezius.	Ipsilateral winged scapula and difficulty with arm abduction.

CN, cranial nerve; SCM, sternocleidomastoid.
[a]For danger zones related to vascular occlusion after soft-tissue dermal filler injection, see Chapter 9: Soft Tissue Dermal Fillers.

Preoperative Considerations

Basic Concepts

- Preoperative considerations include evaluating surgical options based on indication and cure rate, patient preference, medical comorbidities, and cost-effectiveness.
- It is important to assess and minimize **risk factors for poor wound healing such as medications** (eg, systemic corticosteroids, isotretinoin, VEGF inhibitors, sorafenib) and **cigarette smoking.**
- There is considerable practice variation in the management of anticoagulation and antibiotic prophylaxis.

Anticoagulation Management

- **Risk factors for bleeding** include medications and supplements with **anticoagulant** effects, significant **alcohol** use, and **hypertension.**
  - Medications include **ASA, NSAIDs, clopidogrel/ticlopidine, enoxaparin, warfarin, direct oral anticoagulants**

(DOACs), new oral anticoagulants (NOACs), and ibrutinib.
  - Supplements include **bilberry, chondroitin, danshen, devil's claw, dong quai, fish oil, feverfew, garlic, ginger, gingko, ginseng, licorice, and vitamin E.**
- **ASA may be held** for 10 days prior to and 5 to 7 days after surgery as long as doing so does not increase risk of MI or stroke. **NSAIDs may be held** 2 to 3 days prior to surgery. **Other anticoagulant medications should not be discontinued in most patients;** however, **ensure INR < 3 for patients on warfarin.**

Antibiotic Prophylaxis

- There exists considerable practice variation in the use of prophylactic antibiotics.
- Dermatologic surgery wounds are typically classified as **clean** and have **low infection rates (1%-2%).**
- **Recommendations for antibiotic prophylaxis in dermatologic surgery** are shown in Figure 8.14.
- Sterile technique and minimizing wound tension are other measures to reduce infection risk.

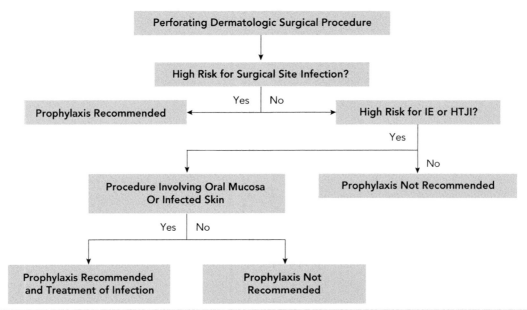

Figure 8.14. RECOMMENDATIONS FOR ANTIBIOTIC PROPHYLAXIS IN DERMATOLOGIC SURGERY. * Dicloxacillin 2 g PO is an alternative to cephalexin (nonoral surgical site). If PCN allergic, clindamycin 600 mg PO or azithromycin/clarithromycin 500 mg PO. If unable to take PO, cefazolin/ceftriaxone 1 g IV/IM or ampicillin 2 g IV/IM (oral surgical site). If unable to take PO and PCN allergic, clindamycin 600 mg IV/IM. AAOS, American Academy of Orthopaedic Surgeons; ADA, American Dental Association; AHA, American Heart Association; CHD, congenital heart disease; DS, double strength; HIV, human immunodeficiency virus; HTJI, hematogenous total joint infection; IE, infective endocarditis; PCN, penicillin; PO, per os; TMP-SMX, trimethoprim-sulfamethoxazole.

(Adapted from Wright TI, Baddour LM, Berbari EF, et al. Antibiotic prophylaxis in dermatologic surgery: advisory statement 2008. *J Am Acad Dermatol.* 2008;59(3):464-473. Copyright © 2008 American Academy of Dermatology, Inc. With permission. An alternative prophylaxis algorithm for dermatologic surgery has been proposed Bae-Harboe YS, Liang CA. Perioperative antibiotic use of dermatologic surgeons in 2012. *Dermatol Surg.* 2013;39(11):1592-1601.)

Antibiotic Regimens
• Prevention of surgical site infection:Wedge excisions of the lip and ear, skin flaps on the nose, and skin grafts: cephalexin 2 g PO*Lesions in the groin and lower extremity: cephalexin 2 g PO^
• Prevention of IE, HTJI: Nonoral surgical site: cephalexin 2 g PO*Oral surgical site: amoxicillin 2 g PO*

^ If PCN allergic, TMP-SMX DS PO or levofloxacin 500 mg PO (lesions in the groin and lower extremity).

AHA recommends 30-60 minutes/ADA-AAOS recommends 60 minutes preoperative dosing.

High-risk Indications:
• Surgical site infection: lower extremity (especially leg), groin, wedge excision of lip or ear, skin flaps on nose, skin grafting, extensive inflammatory skin disease.
• IE: prosthetic cardiac valve, previous IE, CHD^^, cardiac transplantation recipients who develop cardiac valvulopathy.
• HTJI: first 2 years following joint replacement, previous prosthetic joint infections, immunocompromised/immunosuppressed patients, insulin-dependent (type 1) diabetes mellitus, HIV infection, malignancy, malnourishment, hemophilia.

^^ Unrepaired cyanotic CHD, including palliative shunts and conduits; completely repaired congenital heart defects with prosthetic material or device whether placed by surgery or catheter intervention, during the first 6 months after the procedure; repaired CHD with residual defects at the site or adjacent to the site of a prosthetic patch or prosthetic device (which inhibits endothelialization).

Anesthetics and Antiseptics

Basic Concepts

• **Anesthetics** may be delivered via **topical application, local injection, nerve block, or tumescent anesthesia** (see Chap-ter 9: Body Contouring). Systemic anesthetics are beyond the scope of this chapter. In addition to anesthesia, **anxiolytics** may be considered (eg, **benzodiazepines**, reverse with **flumazenil**).

• **Antiseptics** prevent the growth of disease-causing microorganisms.

Anesthetics

- **Local anesthetics temporarily interfere with sodium influx across the cell membrane**, thereby inhibiting depolarization and nerve conduction.
- Loss of sensation occurs in the following temporal order: **temperature → pain (C-type fibers) → touch → pressure → vibration → proprioception → motor function.**
- Local anesthetics possess a basic chemical structure: **aromatic end (lipophilic), intermediate chain (amide or ester), amine end (hydrophilic).**
  - **Amides (eg, bupivacaine, etidocaine, lidocaine, mepivacaine, prilocaine, ropivacaine)**: metabolized by **CYP3A4 (contraindicated in ESRD), excreted by kidneys.** Less cross-reactivity and sensitization than esters; however, **methylparaben preservative** (metabolized to PABA) may cause allergy (switch to preservative-free lidocaine).
    - Amides have 2 "I"s in the name.
  - **Esters (eg, chloroprocaine, procaine, tetracaine)**: metabolized by **plasma pseudocholinesterases (contraindicated in pseudocholinesterase deficiency), excreted by kidneys.** Contraindicated in **PABA** sensitivity—may cross-react (see Chapter 2: Eczematous Dermatoses and Related Disorders).
    - Esters have 1 "I" in the name.
    - The most well-known local anesthetic in each class provides a clue to its metabolism: lidocaine is metabolized by the liver; procaine is metabolized by plasma pseudocholinesterases.
- Properties of local anesthetics:
  - **Onset of action (amine end): lower pKa** correlates with more rapid onset. **Lidocaine has the fastest onset of action** (<1 minute).
  - **Duration of action (aromatic end): increased protein binding** correlates with increased duration of action (lesser role for lipid solubility). **Prilocaine has the shortest duration of action, while bupivacaine has the longest duration of action** (up to 8 hours with epinephrine).
  - **Potency (aromatic end)**: lipid solubility correlates with increased potency (ease of diffusion across cell membranes).
- Adverse effects of local anesthetics include:
  - Local reactions (most commonly related to improper injection technique): bleeding, pain, infection, nerve injury, and tissue necrosis (rare).
  - Systemic reactions: **allergy (amides do not cross-react with esters)** and **cardiovascular toxicity (bupivacaine has the highest risk**.
    - Bupivacaine may cause **fetal bradycardia.**
- **Safe adult dosing of lidocaine: 4.5 to 5 mg/kg (without epinephrine), 7 mg/kg (with epinephrine). 1% lidocaine is 10 mg/mL.**

- **Safe pediatric dosing of lidocaine: 1.2 to 2 mg/kg (without epinephrine), 3 to 4.5 mg/kg (with epinephrine).**
- **β-Blockers increase lidocaine levels.**
- **Lidocaine** is the anesthetic of choice in pregnancy (**historical pregnancy risk category B**).
- Local anesthetics are **vasodilatory except for cocaine.** Adding **epinephrine improves hemostasis, prolongs duration, and decreases systemic toxicity risk due to decreased absorption. 1:200,000 compared to 1:100,000 has equivalent efficacy with decreased toxicity. Maximal vasoconstriction is achieved 15 minutes after injection.** Epinephrine should be used with caution in patients with preexisting conditions (eg, ischemic heart disease, narrow-angle glaucoma, **pheochromocytoma [absolute contraindication]**, uncontrolled hypertension or hyperthyroidism), **pregnancy (decreases uterine blood flow, historical pregnancy risk category C**), and select medications (eg, β-blockers, MAOIs, and TCAs).
- Adding **hyaluronidase** increases anesthetic diffusion and decreases tissue distortion but decreases duration of action and toxicity and may contain the **contact allergen thimerosal.**
- Adding **sodium bicarbonate (8.5%, 1 mL to 9 mL of 1% lidocaine) increases onset of action and decreases injection pain but decreases shelf life.** Other methods to decrease injection pain include pretreating with ice packs or topical anesthetics, warming the anesthetic to body temperature, using small diameter needles (eg, 30 gauge), injecting with a slow fanning motion, reintroducing the needle at previously anesthetized sites, music and mental distraction, and **pinching or rubbing surrounding skin (based on "gate theory" of pain).**
  - Preservatives prevent pain.

Topical Anesthetics

- Topical anesthetics are more effective on **mucosal** surfaces because the *stratum corneum* of nonmucosal surfaces limits efficacy.
- Preparations include:
  - **Eutectic mixture of local anesthesia (EMLA): 2.5% lidocaine and 2.5% prilocaine.** Requires **occlusion**, cannot be used near the eye due to **risk of corneal injury.**
    - Do NOT use **prilocaine** in **infants or patients with G6PD deficiency** due to risk of **methemoglobinemia.**
    - EMLA causes artifactual swelling and vacuolization of the upper epidermis and a basal layer split.
  - **LMX4: 4% lidocaine.** Does not require occlusion.
  - Other: benzocaine (mucosal), cocaine (illicit drug), proparacaine/tetracaine (ocular).

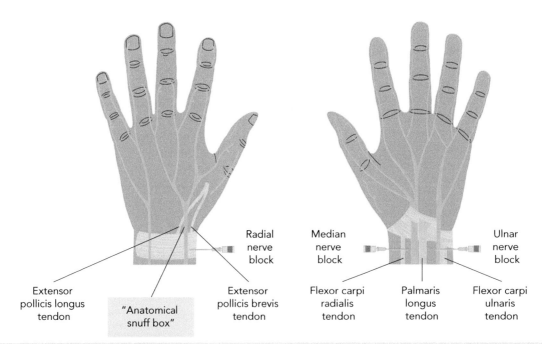

Figure 8.15. NERVE BLOCKS OF THE HAND.
(Illustration by Caroline A. Nelson, MD.)

Labels:
- Radial nerve block
- Extensor pollicis longus tendon
- "Anatomical snuff box"
- Extensor pollicis brevis tendon
- Median nerve block
- Flexor carpi radialis tendon
- Palmaris longus tendon
- Ulnar nerve block
- Flexor carpi ulnaris tendon

Nerve Blocks

- **Face: supraorbital, supratrochlear, infraorbital, and mental nerve blocks.** Injection into these foramina leads to prolonged anesthesia. The nose and oral commissures are relatively resistant to nerve blocks.
- **Hand** (Figure 8.15):
  - **Median nerve block**: inject at proximal wrist crease **between palmaris longus and flexor carpi radialis tendons.**
  - **Radial nerve block**: inject along proximal wrist crease just lateral to radial artery.
  - **Ulnar nerve block**: inject at proximal wrist crease radial to flexor carpi ulnaris.
- **Foot**:
  - **Posterior tibial block (sole numbness)**: inject in groove between medial malleolus and Achilles tendon, posterior to the posterior tibial artery.
  - **Sural nerve block (lateral foot numbness)**: inject in groove between lateral malleolus and Achilles tendon.
  - **Deep peroneal block (first interdigital webspace numbness)**: inject lateral to hallucis longus tendon or inject between the first and second toe in the interdigital cleft.
  - **Saphenous and superficial peroneal block (dorsal foot numbness)**: inject just anterior to the lateral malleolus.
- For nail unit anesthetic considerations, see Chapter 8: Nail Unit Surgery.
- Advantages: immediate pain relief, allow damaged nerve time to heal.
- Disadvantages: **lack of epinephrine hemostasis**, risk of neurovascular injury or infiltration.

Antiseptics

- **Hand hygiene** is fundamental to eliminating the **superficial (transient, nonresident)** pathogens responsible for most healthcare worker–transmitted infections. **Hand sanitizer with alcohol (70% optimal) works by denaturing proteins.** Cleaning with **soap and water** is preferable for **soiled hands** (eg, Norwalk virus, *Clostridium difficile*).
- **Clippers or chemical depilatories are preferable to shaving**, which creates microscopic abrasions that may serve as a portal of entry for pathogens.
- Antiseptics are summarized in Table 8.3.

Table 8.3. ANTISEPTICS

Name[a]	Spectrum	Advantages	Disadvantages
Benzalkonium (Zephiran)	GP and GN bacteria	Not irritating, stable, strong antimicrobial	Slow onset of action, short duration of action, inactivated by anionic compounds (eg, soaps)
Chlorhexidine (Hibiclens)	Broad (viruses, bacteria, fungi)	Rapid onset of action, long duration of action, additive effect with repetitive use, low absorption	Corneal injury, ototoxicity (use with caution around eye or ear), does not cover *Serratia* or spores
Hexachlorophene (pHisoHex)	GPCs	Sustained activity	Teratogenic, neurotoxic (avoid in pregnant women and children)
Hydrogen peroxide	Bacteria, fungi (at high concentrations)	Rapid onset of action	Corrosive to normal skin, bleaching potential
Isopropyl alcohol	GP bacteria	Rapid onset of action, inexpensive	Flammable, skin irritant, inactive against spores
Povidone-iodine (Betadine)	Broad (bacterial, viral, fungal)	Fast acting	Short onset of action, efficacious when dry, inactivated by blood or sputum, may stain skin/fabrics, risk of contact dermatitis, cross-reacts with iodides in medication/radiopaque isotopes
Silver sulfadiazine (Silvadene)	See Chapter 6: Antimicrobials.		

FDA, Food and Drug Administration; GN, gram-negative; GP, gram-positive; GPCs, gram-positive cocci.
[a]Triclosan, a previously popular antiseptic, is now banned by the FDA.

Surgical Instruments and Materials

Basic Concepts

- **Surgical instruments** include forceps, needles, needle drivers, scalpels, and scissors.
- **Surgical materials** include topical hemostasis materials, wound closure materials, and wound dressings.

Surgical Instruments

- Most surgical instruments are a blend of stainless steel admixed with carbon alloy, chromium, nickel, and/or **tungsten carbide (gold handles). Steam autoclave can dull sharp instruments.**
- **Scalpel handles and blades** (Figure 8.16) are used for incising tissue.
  - **Scalpel handle:** holds the blade. **Bard-Parker (most common) is flat.** Siegel is a thin, round, knurled handle that makes it well suited for MMS. **Beaver is round/hexagonal** and holds smaller and sharper blades used in delicate areas (eg, **eyelid, conchal bowl**).
  - **Scalpel blades** (in order of decreasing popularity): **#15, #10, and #11.** The #10 blade is larger than the #15 blade and is preferred in sites with thick dermis (eg, back). The #11 blade is tapered to a sharp point and is used for cutting and stabbing incisions. The #67 blade (smaller ver-

sion of #15 blade) and #65 blade (smaller version of #11 blade) are used in delicate areas (eg, eyelid, conchal bowl).
  - **The Shaw hemostatic scalpel is an electronically heated metal cutting blade.**
- **Forceps** (Figure 8.17) are used for grasping the tissue and the needle.
  - **Serrated forceps facilitate gripping the needle** but **increase risk of damage to tissue compared to toothed forceps.**
  - **Adson forceps** are relatively large. They are commonly used on the **trunk and extremities.**
  - **Bishop-Harmon forceps** are fine tipped and small with **three holes** on the handle to decrease overall weight. They are commonly used on delicate tissue (eg, **eyelids**).
  - **Jewelers forceps** are pointy tipped. They are commonly used for **suture removal.**
- **Needles and needle drivers** (Figure 8.18):
  - **Needle tip:** distal portion. **A round tip is less likely to cut or tear tissue. A cutting (triangular-shaped) tip** is preferred for skin. Conventional cutting needles have a cutting surface along the inner arc. **Reverse cutting needles** have cutting surface on outer arc, which **minimizes risk of sutures tearing through wound edge.** Frequent grasping of the tip will quickly dull it.
  - **Needle body:** middle and **strongest** portion. **3/8 circle** is most common shape.
  - **Needle shank (swage):** weakest portion that attaches to suture. **Determines suture tract size.**

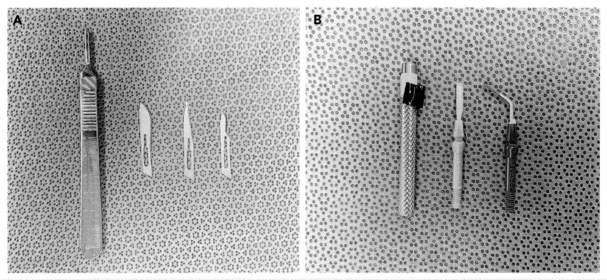

Figure 8.16. SCALPEL HANDLES AND BLADES. A, Bard-Parker scalpel handle with #10, #11, and #15 blades. B, Beaver scalpel handle with straight and curved blades.

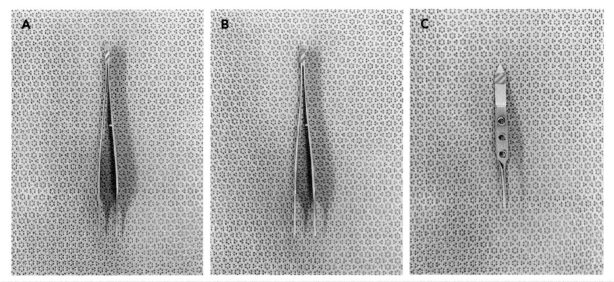

Figure 8.17. SELECTED FORCEPS. A, Adson forceps (serrated). B, Adson forceps (toothed). C, Bishop-Harmon forceps. Jewelers forceps (not shown) are pointy tipped.

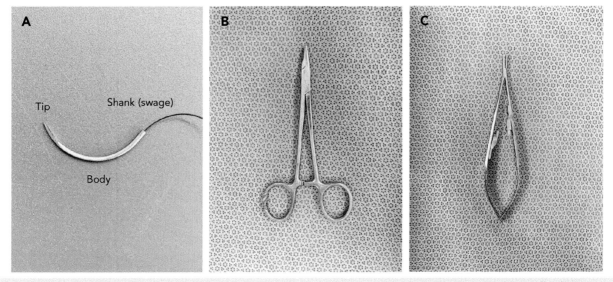

Figure 8.18. NEEDLES AND NEEDLE DRIVERS. A, Needle. B, Webster needle driver. C, Castroviejo needle driver.

Table 8.4. SCISSOR TYPES

Type	Handle	Tip	Notes
Gradle	Short	Sharp	Curved and tapered tip, used for sharp dissection of delicate tissue (eg, periorbital skin) and snip biopsy
Iris	Short	Sharp	Curved or straight blade, used for sharp dissection and snip biopsy
Mayo	Long	Blunt	1:1 handle:blade length, used for blunt dissection
Metzenbaum	Long	Blunt	Long handles used for blunt dissection in areas requiring long reach
O'Brien	Short	Sharp	Fine-angled tip, used for suture removal
Spencer	Short	Blunt	Hook-shaped tip on one blade, used for suture cutting
Westcott	Short	Sharp	Spring loaded, used for dissection of delicate tissue (eg, eyelid)

- **Needle driver**: holds the needle. **Serrated jaws minimize twisting of needles** during suturing but **increase risk of damage to delicate needles** (P3 and smaller) **and suture** (6-0 and smaller) **as compared to smooth jaws.** Use of large needles with small needle drivers (eg, **Webster**) will ruin them. The **Castroviejo needle driver** has spring handles and an optional self-locking device, which provides increased control for surgery near the eye.
- **Scissors** (Table 8.4, Figure 8.19) are used for cutting tissue, suture material, and wound dressings.
  - Tip: sharp scissors are used for sharp dissection; blunt scissors are used for blunt dissection. **Supercuts (one blade with a razor edge, black handle)** are available for multiple scissor types.
  - Shape: curved scissors are helpful for undermining cysts; straight scissors are helpful for trimming tissue and cutting suture. **Serrated** scissors are helpful for **grabbing the tissue.**
  - Handle: **shorter handles** are used for **delicate work**; longer handles are used for undermining.
- Miscellaneous surgical instruments (Figure 8.20):
  - **Hemostats are used to clamp bleeding vessels prior to ligation.** They are available in different lengths and tips and may be straight or curved.
  - **Chalazion clamps** are useful when operating on **mobile surfaces** (eg, eyelid, lip, earlobe).
  - **Curettes** are commonly used to treat or debulk skin tumors. Curettes are available in different sizes and head shapes (Fox = round, Cannon = oval).
  - **Skin hooks enable tissue handling with minimal trauma** and are useful for reflecting skin edges during undermining and suturing. Skin hooks may be single, double, or multiple pronged. Skin hooks are a **sharps hazard** and should be handled with caution.
  - For nail unit surgical instruments, see Chapter 8: Nail Unit Surgery.

Topical Hemostasis Materials

- Chemical: **aluminum chloride, Monsel solution** (adverse events include dermal fibrosis, dyspigmentation, infection,

and inflammation), **silver nitrate** (adverse events include impaired wound healing and pain), **zinc paste** (adverse events include irritation and pain).
  - ◈ Figure 8.21.
- Mechanical: **adhesives, bone wax** (physical barrier tamponades vessels), **Ostene** (alkylene oxide copolymer similar to bone wax), **pressure.**
- Physical: **cellulose, gelatin, hydrophilic polyurethane gel foams, microfibrillar collagen.**
  - ◈ Figure 8.22.
- Physiologic: biologics (eg, **fibrin sealants** [act independent of coagulation cascade]), **hemostatic matrix** (thrombin and gelatin), **thrombin, cocaine, epinephrine, hydrogen peroxide** (adverse events include impaired wound healing), **tranexamic acid** (patients with hemophilia, inhibits activation of plasminogen).

Wound Closure Materials

- **Suture:**
  - **Properties of suture** are summarized in Table 8.5.
  - **Absorbable sutures** are summarized in Table 8.6.
    - Pearl: Poliglecaprone 25 (Monocryl) has the highest tensile strength.
    - Pearl: Plain gut has the shortest absorption time (70 days), while polydioxanone (PDS) and glycolic acid (Maxon) have the longest absorption time (180 days).
    - Pearl: Plain gut has the highest tissue reactivity, while glycolic acid (Maxon) and poliglecaprone 25 (Monocryl) have the lowest tissue reactivity.
  - **Nonabsorbable sutures** are summarized in Table 8.7.
    - Pearl: Silk has the lowest tensile strength, while polyester (Ethibond) has the highest tensile strength.
    - Pearl: Silk is the gold standard for handling.
    - Pearl: Silk has the highest tissue reactivity, while polypropylene (Prolene) has the lowest tissue reactivity.
  - Coating suture with **triclosan** has been shown to **decrease infection**; however, triclosan is now banned by US FDA.

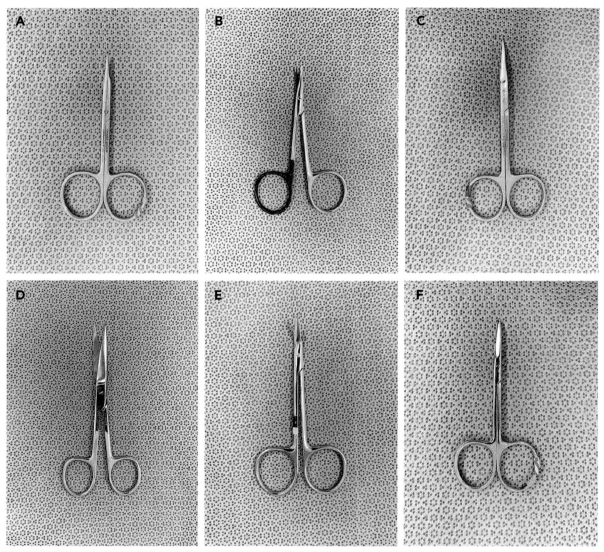

Figure 8.19. SCISSORS. A, Gradle scissors. B, Gradle supercut scissors. C, Iris scissors. D, Mayo scissors. E, O'Brien scissors. F, Spencer scissors. Metzenbaum scissors (not shown) have long handles. Westcott scissors (not shown) are spring loaded (resemble Castroviejo).

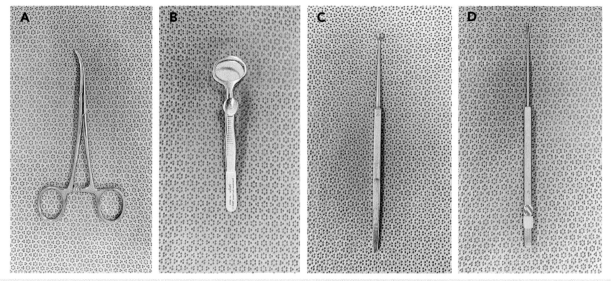

Figure 8.20. MISCELLANEOUS SURGICAL INSTRUMENTS. A, Hemostat (curved). B, Chalazion clamp. C, Curette (oval). D, Skin hook (double prong).

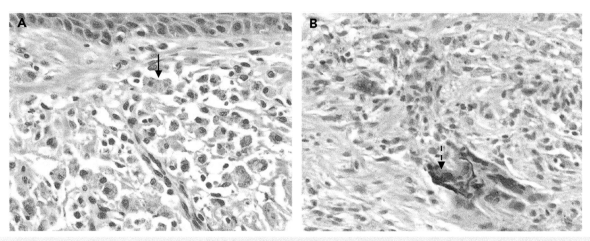

Figure 8.21. SIDE-BY-SIDE COMPARISON: ALUMINUM CHLORIDE AND MONSEL SOLUTION. Both aluminum chloride and Monsel solution may induce a granulomatous response. Aluminum chloride leaves purplish granules. Monsel solution leaves gray-brown pigment. A, Aluminum chloride. Solid arrow: purplish granules. B, Monsel solution. Dashed arrow: gray-brown pigment.

(Histology images reprinted with permission from Elder DE, Elenitsas R, Rosenbach M, et al. *Lever's Histopathology of the Skin.* 11th ed. Wolters Kluwer; 2015.)

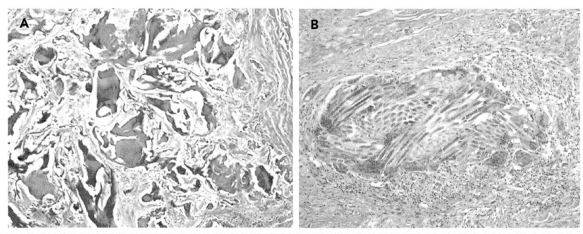

Figure 8.22. SIDE-BY-SIDE COMPARISON: GEL FOAM AND SUTURE. Both gel foam and suture may induce a granulomatous response. Gel foam is a blue-purple material. Suture is a birefringent material. A, Gel foam. B, Suture (nylon).

(A, Histology image reprinted with permission from Rosen PP, Hoda SA. *Breast Pathology: Diagnosis by Needle Core Biopsy.* 3th ed. Wolters Kluwer Health/Lippincott Williams & Wilkins; 2010. B, Histology image reprinted with permission from Elder DE, Elenitsas R, Rosenbach M, et al. *Lever's Histopathology of the Skin.* 11th ed. Wolters Kluwer; 2015.)

Gel foam has an "arabesque netlinke" pattern.
Suture is linear.

○ **Suture techniques** are summarized in Table 8.8 and Figure 8.23. Simple closure involves superficial sutures; layered closure involves more than one layer of sutures.

○ **Knots**: The **surgeon's knot (most common)** is a **square knot** that is first thrown as a double knot to prevent slipping. The **Aberdeen hitch knot** (used to tie the end of a running subcuticular suture) is relatively **more compact, is more secure, and uses less material.**

○ **Suture removal** is typically ≤ **7 days (head and neck)** and **10 to 14 days (trunk and extremities).**

• **Staples:**
○ Nonabsorbable: advantages include **decreased time needed for skin closure and infection (controversial).** Disadvantages include **increased pain.**
○ Absorbable: advantages (relative to nonabsorbable) are decreased pain and improved cosmesis.
• **Tissue adhesives:**
○ Advantages include **improved cosmesis of scars not under tension.**
○ Disadvantages include **increased risk of wound dehiscence.**

Table 8.5. PROPERTIES OF SUTURE

Property	Definition	Notes
Structural Properties		
Composition	Natural or synthetic	Natural fibers are digested via proteolysis. They are highly inflammatory and rapidly degraded. Synthetic fibers are broken down by hydrolysis. They are less inflammatory and slowly degraded.
Configuration	Monofilament, multifilament, or pseudomonofilament	In a coated or pseudo-monofilament suture, a bundle of parallel filaments is embedded in a coating that provides a smooth cover.
Texture	Barbed or smooth	Barbed sutures redistribute tension evenly for large, high-tension wounds.
USP designation	Diameter	A higher USP designation indicates a smaller diameter.
Physical Properties		
Capillarity	Ability to absorb fluid	Multifilament > monofilament, associated with increased infection risk.
COF	Degree of friction when trying to pull suture through tissue	Multifilament > monofilament (eg, polypropylene), associated with increased knot stability.
Ease of handling	Ability to adjust and use suture material	Multifilament > monofilament, associated with increased pliability and decreased memory.
Elasticity	Ability to return to original length after being stretched	Ideal suture property (eg, poliglecaprone 25, polybutester), allows wound edge approximation after edema resolves.
Degradation	Absorbable or nonabsorbable	Absorption is faster in moist areas and in febrile or protein-deficient patients.
Knot security	Likelihood that a knot will hold without slipping	Multifilament > monofilament, associated with increased COF and decreased memory.
Memory	Tendency to retain original shape (determined by elasticity and plasticity)	Monofilament > multifilament, associated with decreased knot security and decreased ease of handling.
Plasticity	Ability to retain tensile strength after being stretched	Allows accommodating of postoperative swelling, associated with increased knot security and increased ease of handling.
Pliability	Stiffness of suture; ease with which suture can be bent into knot	Multifilament > monofilament.
Tensile strength	Force required to break suture	Synthetic > natural, lower > higher USP designation.
Tissue reactivity	Foreign body reaction	Natural > synthetic, multifilament > monofilament, lower > higher USP designation.

COF, coefficient of friction; USP, United States Pharmacopeia.

○ **Butyl tissue adhesives** (eg, butyl cyanoacrylate [LiquiBand] or *N*-butyl-2-cyanoacrylate [GluSeal]) **are more rigid and dry faster than the octyl tissue adhesives** (eg, octyl cyanoacrylate [Dermabond]).

○ **Adhesive strips (Steri-Strips)** are often applied in combination with subcuticular sutures and used with skin adhesive (Mastisol).

Wound Dressings

- Wound healing may occur via three processes:
  ○ **Primary intention**: wound closure is accomplished by approximating the wound edges. Preferable for wounds on **convex** surfaces (eg, malar cheek, nasal tip, vermilion border of lip).
  ○ **Secondary intention**: wound heals without approximating the edges. Consider for wounds on **concave** surfaces (eg, temple, medial canthus, nasal alar crease, conchal bowl).
  ○ **Tertiary intention**: dehiscence following primary intention, which results in wound healing by secondary intention.
- Wound dressings (Table 8.9) substitute for the native epithelium. **The most important role is to immobilize the wound to provide hemostasis.** Other roles include enabling gaseous exchange without leakage, maintaining a moist environment while removing excess exudate, preventing infection, and providing mechanical protection. The ideal dressing should be **nonadherent.**
- **Least to most absorbent dressings: films < hydrocolloids < hydrogels < foams < alginates.**

Table 8.6. ABSORBABLE SUTURES

Suture	Configuration	Tensile Strength	Absorption (Days)	Knot Security	Handling	Tissue Reactivity	Notes
Plain gut (collagen)	Multifilament (twisted)	Low	70	Poor	Poor	High	Fast absorbing plain gut absorbs in 14-28 d
Chromic gut (collagen)	Multifilament (twisted)	Low	90-120	Poor	Poor	High	Can have true allergy
Polyglycolic acid (Dexon)	Multifilament (braided)	Good 30% at 3 wk	60-90	Good	Good	Low	Suture spitting
Polyglactin 910 (Vicryl) (copolymer of glycolide + L-lactide)	Multifilament (braided)	High 50% at 3 wk	40-70	Good	Good	Low	High COF
Polydioxanone (PDS) (polyester polymer)	Monofilament	High 50% at 4 wk	180	Poor	Poor	Low	High-tension areas
Glycolic acid (Maxon) (polytrimethylene carbonate)	Monofilament	High 60% at 4 wk	180	Good	Good	Low	High-tension areas
Poliglecaprone 25 (Monocryl) (copolymer of glycolide + ε-caprolactone)	Monofilament	High 70% at 1 wk 30% at 2 wk	90-120	Good	Good	Low	
Glycomer 631 (Biosyn)	Monofilament	Good 40% at 3 wk	90-110	Good	Good	Low	

COF, coefficient of friction.

Table 8.7. NONABSORBABLE SUTURES

Suture	Configuration	Tensile Strength	Memory	Knot Security	Handling	Tissue Reactivity	Notes
Silk (fibroin protein)	Braided	Low	Low	Excellent	Excellent	High	Mucosa, folds, high capillarity (infection risk)
Nylon (Ethilon, Monosof) (long chain of aliphatic polymers)	Monofilament	High	High	Poor	Poor	Poor	
Nylon (Surgilon, Nurolon) (long chain of aliphatic polymers)	Multifilament (braided)	High	Medium to high	Fair	Good	Low	
Polypropylene (Surgipro, Prolene) (isotactic crystalline stereoisomer of polypropylene + polyethylene)	Monofilament	Moderate	High	Poor	Good	Least	Running subcuticular sutures, antiptosis subdermal suspension sutures in facial rejuvenation, low COF
Polyester (Ethibond) (polyethylene terephthalate coated with polybutylene)	Braided	High	Good	Good	Good	Low	Mucosa
Polybutester (Novofil) (copolymer of butylenes terephthalate and polytetramethylene ether glycol)	Monofilament	High	Low	Fair to good	Good	Low	

COF, coefficient of friction.

Table 8.8. SUTURE TECHNIQUES

Repair	Advantages	Disadvantages	Use
Superficial			
Simple interrupted	Wound edge eversion, high-low correction ("step-off" stitch), individual (selective) suture removal	Increased time, more prominent track marks, skin irritation	Moderate to high tension
Simple running	Fast, suture bulk spread over entire wound (running locked stitches may help with hemostasis)	Integrity dependent on knots on either end, therefore increased risk of wound dehiscence (running locked stitches increase tissue ischemia)	Wounds with minimal tension
Vertical mattress	Reduces tension, wound edge eversion, eliminates dead space	Tram tracking	High-tension areas A pulley stitch is a modified vertical mattress that reduces tension but increases tissue ischemia
			Vertical mattress: "Far-Far Near-Near." Pulley: "Far-Near-Near-Far."
Horizontal mattress	Hemostasis, wound edge eversion, eliminates dead space (running horizontal mattress is faster)	Increased tissue ischemia (decreased with running horizontal mattress), tram tracking	High-tension areas where vertical mattress not possible A tip stitch is a half-buried horizontal mattress used for M-plasty and flap tips
Deep			
Simple buried	Simple to execute	Minimal wound eversion, risk of spitting suture	Most commonly used dermal suture
Buried vertical mattress	Wound edge eversion (most successful sources say "set-back" suture)		
	To achieve symmetric wound eversion with a buried vertical mattress, imagine tracing a "heart" under the skin.		
Running subcuticular	No suture marks along skin surface	Slow, increased tissue reactivity, risk of spitting suture	Minimal tension and mobility
Purse string	Decreases wound size and decreases healing time		Wounds healing by secondary intention
Subcuticular pulley	Reduces tension	Increased tissue ischemia	High-tension areas
"Figure-of-eight"			Hemostasis
Suspension	Reduces tension, prevents distortion of free margin, prevents flap tenting		Anchor tissue to periosteum

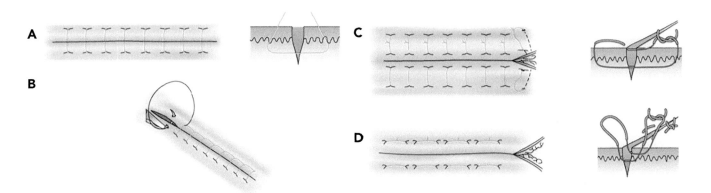

Figure 8.23. SUPERFICIAL SUTURE TECHNIQUES. A, Simple interrupted suture. B, Simple running suture. C, Vertical mattress suture. D, Horizontal mattress suture.

(Illustration reprinted with permission from Jarrell BE, Kavic SM. *NMS Surgery.* 6th ed. Wolters Kluwer; 2016.)

Table 8.9. WOUND DRESSINGS

Wound Type	Recommended Dressing (Commercially Available Product)	Composition	Advantage	Disadvantage
Need moisture	Hydrogel (Nu-Gel, 2nd skin, Vigilon)	Hydrophilic polymer gel	Semitransparent, semipermeable, semiadherent (↓pain), highly absorbent, hydrating	Frequent dressing changes, allows GP organism growth
Maintain moisture	Film (Tegaderm, Bioclusive, Blisterfilm, Carrafilm, Kendall Polyskin, Opsite)	Sheets of polyurethane or copolyester	Permeable, barrier to bacteria, comfortable, flexible, transparent, promotes autolytic debridement, can be left in place up to 7 d	May adhere to wound, nonabsorbent
	Hydrocolloid (Duoderm, Hydrocol, NuDerm, Tegasorb)	Sheets of starch, gelatin, pectin, elastomer, and adhesive (gel formed with exudate)	Semipermeable, waterproof, cut to shape, cushioning, autolytic debridement, stimulates angiogenesis, painless	Surrounding maceration, allergic or irritant contact dermatitis, excess granulation tissue, opaque, expensive
Absorb/remove moisture	Foam (Hydrasorb, Vigifoam, Synthoderm, Flexzan)	Polyurethane or silicone-based polymer	Semipermeable barrier, absorption, nonadherent, molds to wound shape	Opaque, frequent dressing change, drying
	Alginate (Sorbsan, Algisorb, Seasorb)	Calcium alginate (seaweed or kelp derived)	Hemostasis, nonadherent, minimal dressing changes	Desiccation
	Gelling fibers (gelling fibers)	Carboxymethyl cellulose fibers	Similar to alginates, decreased periwound maceration	
Bleeding	Alginate	See above	See above	See above
Painful	Hydrogel	See above	See above	See above
Infected	Silver (Acticoat, Flex 7 Silver, Actisorb, Algicell Ag, Aquacel Ag, SilvaSorb, Silvercel, etc)	Impregnated with antimicrobial agent	Broad spectrum including MRSA and VRE, lasts 3-7 d	Stain local tissue, slows wound healing
	Chlorhexidine or poly-hexamethylene biguanide (PHMB) (Bactigras, Kendall AMD foam)		Broad spectrum, low tissue toxicity, reduces pain	Irritant contact dermatitis, ear/eye toxicity, hypersensitivity
	Honey (Medihoney, Activon Tulle)		Broad spectrum, autolytic debridement, low tissue toxicity	Maceration, ACD to propolis

ACD, allergic contact dermatitis; GP, gram-positive; MRSA, methicillin-resistant *Staphylococcus aureus*; VRE, vancomycin-resistant enterococci.

Basic Surgical Procedures

Basic Concepts

- **Basic surgical procedures** include **I&D, biopsy, and excision.**

Incision and Drainage

- I&D is a common method utilized for the treatment of skin abscesses.
- Technique:
  - Achieve adequate anesthesia.
  - Make a linear incision through the total length of the abscess.
  - Culture the purulent exudate.
  - Probe the cavity to break up loculations, identify foreign bodies, and ensure proper drainage.
  - Irrigate the cavity.
  - Allow to heal by secondary intention to permit any residual exudate to drain from the cavity.

Biopsy (Table 8.10)

Excision

- Excision is a common procedure utilized for the treatment of skin tumors. Margins:
  - BCC: **4 mm** (high risk 0.6-1 cm or MMS).
  - SCC: **4 mm** (high risk 0.6 cm or MMS).
  - **Melanoma: in situ (0.5-1 cm margin), Breslow depth < 1 mm (1 cm margin), Breslow depth 1 to 2 mm (1-2 cm margin), Breslow depth > 2 mm (2 cm margin).**
  - **DFSP: 2 to 3 cm (but MMS is the gold standard).**
- Design: The **elliptical (fusiform) excision** has a **3:1 length:width ratio. To minimize tension** and improve cosmesis, excisions should be oriented **parallel to skin tension lines. Excision variants** are summarized in Table 8.11. The **elliptical excision and M-plasty** are illustrated in Figure 8.24.
- Technique: **incision, excision, undermining, placement of deep and superficial sutures.**

Table 8.10. BIOPSY TYPES

Type	Lesion-Specific Indications	Specimen Obtained	Technique
Shave	Epidermis and superficial dermis, broad, elevated	Epidermis, papillary dermis ± reticular dermis	Wheal of anesthesia, #15 blade or razor blade with smooth sawing motion, heals by secondary intention
Punch	Dermal process, depressed/atrophic lesion	Epidermis, dermis ± subcutaneous fat or fascia	Rotate disposable instrument, closure by simple epidermal suture
Snip	Pedunculated	Tissue above connection to epidermis	Wheal of anesthesia, fine iris or sharp Gradle scissors, heals by secondary intention
Saucerization	Epidermis and dermis, pigmented lesions	Deeper than shave (contains reticular dermis)	Wheal of anesthesia, #15 blade or razor blade with smooth sawing motion, heals by secondary intention
Incisional	Deeper process involving fat or fascia, large size	Epidermis, dermis, subcutaneous fat ± fascia	Infiltration of anesthesia, #15 blade, hemostasis, layered closure
Excisional	High suspicion of malignancy (intent = definitive treatment)	Epidermis, dermis, subcutaneous fat ± fascia	Infiltration of anesthesia, #15 blade, hemostasis, layered closure

Table 8.11. EXCISION VARIANTS

Variant	Common Location	Notes
Crescent	Cheek, chin	Reduces length of scar. Ideal along curved skin tension lines or cosmetic subunit junctions.
M-plasty	Eyebrow, oral commissures	Reduces length of scar. Ideal to avoid encroaching on important structures. Repair option for standing cone ("dog ear").
S-plasty (lazy S repair)	Jaw, forearm, shin	Reduces contraction and buckling by redistributing tension vectors. Ideal along convex surfaces.
V-shaped full-thickness excision	Lip	Lesions <1/3 of the lower lip length can be repaired with primary closure in layers: submucosal, orbicularis oris, dermis/subcutaneous, and epidermis. The vermillion border should be marked prior to excision.

- Excising in the appropriate plane is critical to avoid injury.
  - **Scalp: subgaleal plane** (avascular).
  - **Face: superficial to SMAS** in the mid-fat (ensure **deep to hair bulbs on eyebrow**).
  - **Nose: deep to SMAS**, superficial to periosteum or perichondrium.
  - **Ear: superficial to perichondrium.**
  - **Trunk/extremities: deep fat**, superficial to fascia.
- **Quality control checkpoints** are summarized in Table 8.12.

Mohs Micrographic Surgery

Basic Concepts

- **MMS** is a specialized method of skin tumor excision that enables **circumferential microscopic margin control.**
- MMS **increases cure rates (97%-98% for BCC/SCC), is tissue sparing, and is cost-effective.**
- MMS is safe, with a reported **complication rate of 0.7% to 2.6%** and zero fatalities.

Indications

- **A tumor must grow in a contiguous fashion** to be appropriate for MMS.

- Indication for MMS is defined by the **MMS AUC.**
- Tumor characteristics:
  - Recurrent.
  - **High-risk anatomic location** (Figure 8.25).
  - Aggressive histologic subtypes (eg, **morpheaform/micronodular/infiltrating BCC**, high-grade/poorly differentiated/deeply penetrating SCC, infiltrating/spindle cell SCC, perineural invasion).
  - **Large size (≥1 cm face, ≥2 cm trunk and extremities).**
  - Poorly-defined clinical borders (lateral and/or deep).
  - Rapid growth.
- Background skin characteristics:
  - Prior exposure to ionizing radiation.
  - Chronic scar (Marjolin ulcer).
  - **Site of positive margins on prior excision.**
- Patient characteristics:
  - **Immunocompromised.**
  - Underlying genetic syndrome (eg, XP, Gorlin, Bazex-Dupré-Christol).

Technique

- The MMS technique is illustrated in Figure 8.26. MMS involves a **small (1-2 mm) margin** and a beveled excision **(scalpel held at 45° angle).**

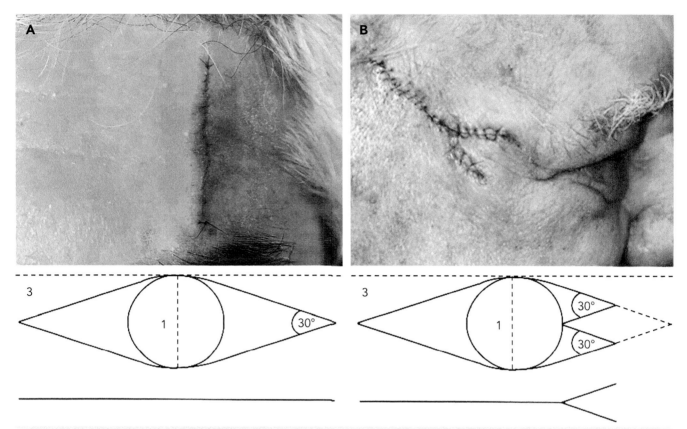

Figure 8.24. PRINCIPLES OF EXCISION DESIGN: ELLIPTICAL EXCISION AND M-PLASTY A, Elliptical excision. B, M-plasty designed to prevent the incision from crossing the lateral canthus.

(Image reported with permission from Kaufman AJ. *Practical Facial Reconstruction: Theory and Practice.* Wolters Kluwer; 2016. Illustration by Caroline A. Nelson, MD.)

Table 8.12. QUALITY CONTROL CHECKPOINTS

Stage	Goal(s)	Checkpoints
Incision	To achieve a uniform release along the entire skin edge to the desired anatomic depth. To create smooth and perpendicular wound edges with no bevel.	Has the incision achieved uniform release to the desired anatomic plane? Are the incised wound edges perpendicular without a bevel of the dermis or fat? Are the wound edges cut cleanly without jagged edges?
Excision	To remove the skin in a uniform and efficient anatomic plane with minimal morbidity to the underlying structures.	Is the excision effortless and does it cause minimal bleeding? Does the excision specimen have a uniform thickness? Does the base of the wound have a uniform depth at the desired anatomic plane?
Undermining	To facilitate advancement of skin edges by releasing the skin edges from underlying adhesions. To facilitate eversion of the wound edges during suturing.	Is undermining effortless, and does it cause minimal bleeding? Can the incised skin edge be retracted in an everted position? Are the wound edges sharply perpendicular from the epidermis to the plane of undermining?
Placement of deep sutures	To transfer tension to the reticular dermis and evert the wound edges, allowing for precise and tension-free approximation of the papillary dermis and epidermis.	Is there blood between the wound edges?[a] Are both wound edges clearly visible?
Placement of superficial sutures	To align the papillary dermis and epidermis with precision.	Is there blood between the wound edges?[a] Are both wound edges clearly visible?

[a]Blood between the wound edges is undesirable because it indicates incomplete wound edge approximation.
Adapted from Miller CJ, Antunes MB, Sobanko JF. Surgical technique for optimal outcomes: Part I. Cutting tissue—incising, excising, and undermining. *J Am Acad Dermatol.* 2015;72(3):377-387 and Miller CJ, Antunes MB, Sobanko JF. Surgical technique for optimal outcomes: Part II. Repairing tissue: suturing. *J Am Acad Dermatol.* 2015;72(3):389-402. Copyright © 2014 American Academy of Dermatology, Inc. With permission.

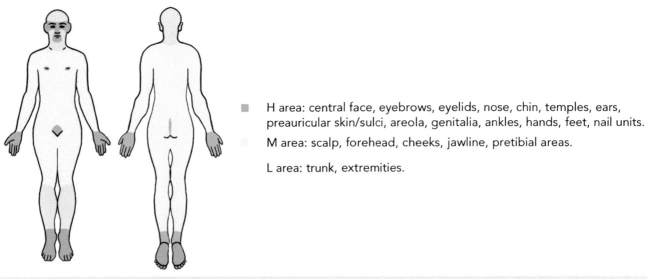

H area: central face, eyebrows, eyelids, nose, chin, temples, ears, preauricular skin/sulci, areola, genitalia, ankles, hands, feet, nail units.

M area: scalp, forehead, cheeks, jawline, pretibial areas.

L area: trunk, extremities.

Figure 8.25. MOHS MICROGRAPHIC SURGERY AREAS.
(Illustration by Caroline A. Nelson, MD.)

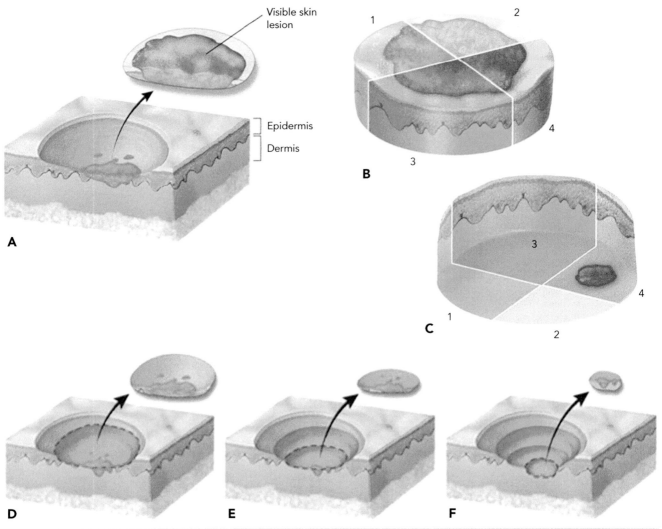

Figure 8.26. MOHS MICROGRAPHIC SURGERY. A, Gross tumor with a thin margin is excised. B, The sample is divided and mapped with color to help pinpoint any areas of residual tumor with frozen section analysis. C, Microscopic evaluation reveals that there is residual tumor in segment 4. D-F, The process is repeated, focusing on re-excision of the involved quadrant until all clear margins are obtained.

(Illustration reprinted with permission from Chung KC. *Operative Techniques in Hand and Wrist Surgery.* Wolters Kluwer; 2019.)

- To enable circumferential evaluation of the microscopic margin, it is essential for the histotechnician to flatten the tissue such that the **epidermis lies in the same plane as the deep tissue.** Often, four radial incisions are visible and stained with four different colors of ink for orientation. Stains include **H&E and toluidine blue.**

Flaps and Grafts

Basic Concepts

- **Flaps** involve the **movement of adjacent skin and subcutaneous tissue with an intact vascular supply into a defect.**

- **Grafts** involve the **movement of skin from a donor site into a defect.**

Flaps

- **Flap nomenclature** is summarized in Table 8.13.
- There are three basic **flap types:**
  - **Advancement: unidirectional advancement of adjacent tissue into the primary defect** (Table 8.14, Figure 8.27). The goal is to **redistribute Burow triangle away from free margins,** but this flap design is **limited by elasticity of adjacent tissue.**
  - **Rotation: curvilinear movement of adjacent tissue into the primary defect** (Table 8.15, Figure 8.28). **Maximum**

Table 8.13. FLAP NOMENCLATURE

Term	Definition
Primary defect	Initial wound that requires reconstruction
Secondary defect	Wound created by mobilization of flap from adjacent tissue
Primary movement	Motion of flap toward primary defect (creates primary tension vector opposite the direction of flap movement)
Secondary movement	Motion of tissue surrounding secondary defect to close it (creates secondary tension vector)
Pedicle	Vascular base of flap, supplies blood to the body and the tip (highest risk for necrosis)
Pivot point	Flap rotation point, critical to undermine this area for flap movement
Key stitch	Initial stitch to move the flap into the primary defect
Random pattern flap	Flaps supplied by anastomotic subdermal and dermal vascular plexuses
Axial flap	Flaps supplied by named vessel

Table 8.14. ADVANCEMENT FLAPS

Type	Technique	Notes
Unilateral O→U advancement (U-plasty, helical rim advancement)	Excise defect as square and extend incision along two parallel sides with Burow triangle at the end of each extension, then advance into defect.	Hyper-evert helical rim flaps to prevent notching.
Unilateral Burow advancement (A→L, O→L)	Excise defect as equilateral triangle with one arm extended to displace Burow triangle to a more cosmetically desired location.	
Unilateral crescentic advancement	Variant of A→L in which a crescentic standing cone is removed within flap body.	Often used for cheek-to-nose advancement.
Bilateral O→H advancement (H-plasty)	Double (mirror image) O→U flaps.	Forehead numbness is a complication.
Bilateral A→T advancement (O→T, T-plasty)	Divide one of two standing cones into two smaller Burow triangles, advance two opposing flaps into defect.	
V→Y advancement (island pedicle, kite)	Advance V-shaped island with pedicle into defect.	Length:width ≤4:1. Ensure ≥40% of pedicle remains intact. Triangular scar and trapdooring may worsen cosmesis.
Mucosal advancement	Undermine to gingival sulcus (deep to minor salivary glands but superficial to orbicularis muscle) and advance flap into defect.	Used on vermillion lip. Lip numbness is a complication.

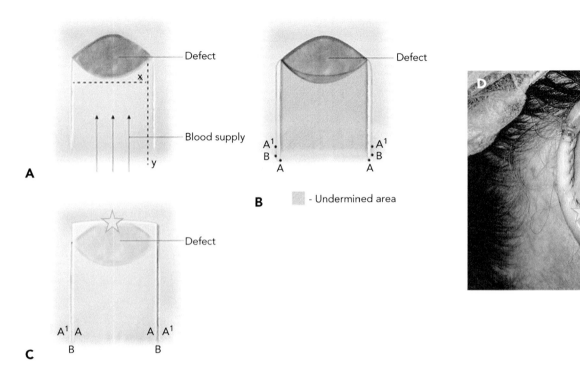

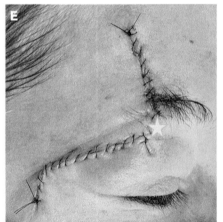

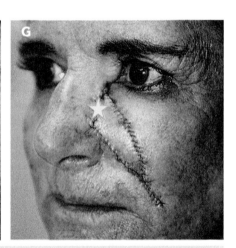

Selected Variants

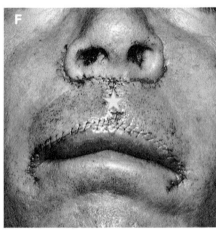

Figure 8.27. PRINCIPLES OF FLAP DESIGN: ADVANCEMENT FLAPS. The design of an advancement flap is based on subdermal blood supply from the base of the flap. The initial parallel incisions are drawn from the wound edges (A). The advancement flap is undermined toward the base, leaving only the subdermal blood supply to vascularize the distal tip (B). The flap is then advanced forward and pushed into the defect. The previous base corner of the flap (point A) has been pushed forward and is approximated to point A[1] (C). D, Unilateral O→U advancement flap (U-plasty) (helical rim advancement). E, Unilateral Burow advancement flap (A→L, O→L). F, Bilateral O→H advancement flap (H-plasty). G, V→Y advancement flap (island pedicle/kite). Noteworthy key stitches are indicated by stars.

(C, Illustration reprinted with permission from Mulholland MW, Hawn MT, Hughes SJ, et al. *Operative Techniques in Surgery.* Wolters Kluwer Health; 2014. D, Reprinted with permission from Kaufman AJ. *Practical Facial Reconstruction: Theory and Practice.* Wolters Kluwer; 2016. E, Reprinted with permission from Kaufman AJ. *Practical Facial Reconstruction: Theory and Practice.* Wolters Kluwer; 2016. G, Reprinted with permission from Kaufman AJ. *Practical Facial Reconstruction: Theory and Practice.* Wolters Kluwer; 2016.)

tension occurs at the pivot point. The goal is to **recruit distant tissue laxity to avoid distorting free margins**, but this flap design is **heavy** and rotation leads to **loss of length and height and secondary tension vectors** that can undesirably distort free margins.

○ **Transposition: pivotal and rotational movement of tissue from nonadjacent areas across intervening islands of unaffected skin** (Table 8.16, Figure 8.29). The goal is to **recruit distant tissue laxity to areas with minimal**

inherent tissue laxity, but this flap design is prone to **pincushioning/trapdooring.** An **interpolation** flap is a **two-stage** transposition flap (the second stage of pedicle division takes place **3 weeks** after the first stage) that enables **increased flap length:width ratio (>4:1).**

- All flaps **recruit tissue laxity.** Only rotation and transposition flaps **redirect wound tension vectors.**
- Flap size (for billing purposes) includes the surface area of flap elevation and the primary defect.

Table 8.15. ROTATION FLAPS

Type	Technique	Notes
Unilateral rotation	Make a curvilinear incision, undermine pivot point, rotate flap into defect.	Back cuts increase mobility but decrease blood flow.
Unilateral rotation, Rieger variant (dorsal nasal rotation, Hatchet flap, glabellar turn-down flap)	Make curvilinear incision, undermine at perichondrium/periosteum and pivot point (medial canthal tendon), back cut in glabella, rotate flap (glabella) into defect.	The dorsal nasal flap is a variant of the glabellar flap. Axial: angular artery. Poor cosmesis may result from transposition of thick glabellar skin onto the medial canthus and "pig-nose" deformity from inadequate undermining.
Unilateral rotation, Mustardé/Tenzel variant	Make curvilinear incision, undermine pivot point, rotate flap (cheek or temple reservoir) into defect.	Mustardé = entire cheek for larger lower lid defects (≥50%). Tenzel = partial cheek for smaller lower lid defects (<50%). Tacking suture to lateral orbital rim periosteum can decrease ectropion risk.
Bilateral rotation (O→Z)	Double rotation flap with Z shape.	Often used on scalp.

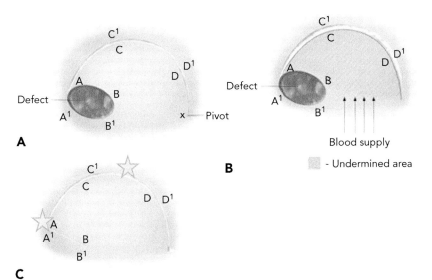

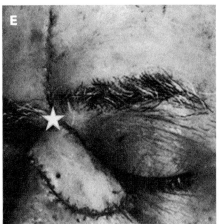

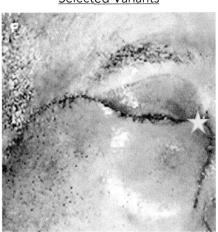

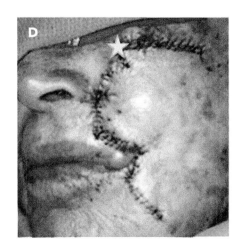

Selected Variants

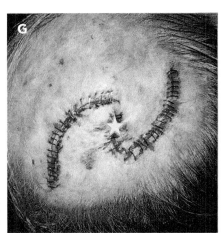

Figure 8.28. PRINCIPLES OF FLAP DESIGN: ROTATION FLAPS. The semicircular markings for a rotation flap are demonstrated. The subsequent advancement of the flap is demonstrated by the movement of points A, B, C, and D to A^1, B^1, C^1, and D^1, respectively (A). The rotation flap is undermined back toward the base, leaving the distal portion of the tissue perfused through the subdermal plexus. Additional back cuts across the base should be done judicious to not compromise vascularity of the flap (B). The rotation flap is rotated into the defect for closure. The movement of the flap relative to the adjacent skin is noted by the changed alignment of the C and D marks to the C^1 and D^1 marks, respectively. C, A small standing cutaneous deformity at the base of the flap may require excision. D, Unilateral rotation flap. E, Glabellar rotation flap. F, Unilateral rotation (Mustardé variant). G, Bilateral rotation flap (O→Z). Noteworthy key stitches are indicated by stars.

(C, Illustration reprinted with permission from Mulholland MW, Hawn MT, Hughes SJ, et al. *Operative Techniques in Surgery.* Wolters Kluwer Health; 2014. D, Reprinted with permission from Chung KC. *Grabb and Smith's Plastic Surgery.* 8th ed. Wolters Kluwer; 2019. E, Reprinted with permission from Chung KC. *Grabb and Smith's Plastic Surgery.* 8th ed. Wolters Kluwer; 2019. F, Reprinted with permission from Chung KC. *Grabb and Smith's Plastic Surgery.* 8th ed. Wolters Kluwer; 2019.)

Table 8.16. TRANSPOSITION FLAPS		
Type	Technique	Notes
One Stage		
Bilobed (Zitelli modification)	Raise a bilobed flap (proximal nasal dorsum), undermine in submuscular plane to nasofacial sulcus, close tertiary defect, then secondary defect, then primary defect (distal 1/3 of nose).	Primary defect diameter = primary lobe diameter = secondary lobe diameter (or slightly smaller). Overall angle of rotation is 90°. Use as many lobes as necessary (eg, trilobe) to reach area of tissue laxity. Risk of pincushioning/trapdooring.
Rhombic	Raise a rhombic flap, undermine, close secondary defect first, then primary defect. Final suture line looks like a question mark.	The classic Limburg flap is a parallelogram with 60° angles x2 and 120° angles x2. By decreasing the angle of the flap tip, the Dufourmentel and Webster modifications decrease the arc of rotation (increase tension sharing between primary and secondary defects).
Banner	Long narrow flap.	Length:width ratio 3-5:1. Risk of ischemia, pincushioning/trapdooring.
Nasolabial/melolabial (transposition)	Raise flap from medial cheek and transpose into defect (nasal ala) (variant of banner transposition flap).	Pivot point should be the piriform aperture. Risks are blunting of the nasal crease and pincushioning/trapdooring. The Spear flap variant folds in on itself to provide internal nasal lining.
Z-plasty	Lengthen contracted scar.	Increased angle size leads to increased length gain and tension reorientation (eg, 65° angle leads to 75% increase in length and 90° tension reorientation).
Two Stage (Interpolation)		
Paramedian forehead	Raise flap from paramedian forehead and suture onto large distal nasal defect on contralateral side. Divide pedicle after 3 wk.	Axial: supratrochlear artery. Ideal pedicle width = 1-1.5 cm (too narrow or too wide increases ischemia risk). Maximum length of flap is distance from orbital rim to hairline or hair will be transplanted onto the nose.
Abbé lip-switch	Raise lip flap containing both mucosa and orbicularis oris and suture onto opposing lip. Divide pedicle after 3 wk.	Axial: labial artery.
Nasolabial/melolabial (interpolation)	Similar to single-stage nasolabial/melolabial transposition flap but retains vascular pedicle, which is divided after 3 wk.	
Mastoid interpolation/retroauricular ("book")	Raise a rectangular-shaped flap from retroauricular sulcus to hairline, thin tip, and suture onto helix. Divide pedicle after 3 wk.	

Grafts

- There are four basic **graft types** (Table 8.17).
- Grafts may be harvested using specialized surgical instruments:
  - **Dermatome**: a dermatome may be manual or electric (eg, **Zimmer**).
  - **Mesher**: flat bed with roller that compresses STSG on plastic template that creates fine **fenestrations** in a gridlike pattern. Fenestrations enlarge graft and allow serosanguinous drainage but **worsen cosmesis.**
- **Stages of graft survival:**
  - **Imbibition: first 24 to 48 hours (ischemic period).** Fibrin attaches graft to wound bed. Graft sustained by plasma exudate of wound bed. Graft edema with **dusky blue** (venous congestion).

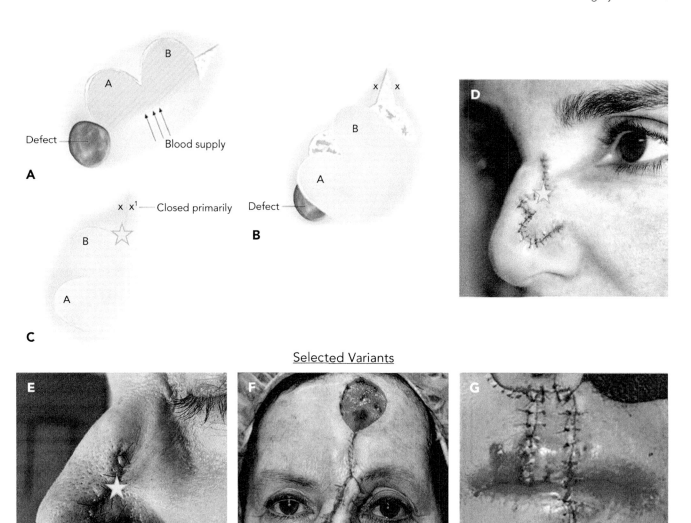

Selected Variants

Figure 8.29. PRINCIPLES OF FLAP DESIGN: TRANSPOSITION FLAPS. The bilobed flap uses two rotation-transposition flaps for closure of a defect. A, Flap A is used to close the primary defect and flap B is used to close the donor site from flap A. B, The flap is elevated in the subcutaneous tissues leaving blood supply from the subdermal plexus at the base of the both "lobes" of the flap. C, The flaps are then transposed with primary closure of the donor site for flap B by reapproximation of x to x¹. D, Bilobed transposition flap. E, Rhombic transposition flap. F, Paramedian forehead interpolation flap. G, Abbé ,ip-switch interpolation flap. Noteworthy key stitches are indicated by stars.

(C, Illustration reprinted with permission from Mulholland MW, Hawn MT, Hughes SJ, et al. *Operative Techniques in Surgery*. Wolters Kluwer Health; 2014. D, Reprinted with permission from Kaufman AJ. *Practical Facial Reconstruction: Theory and Practice*. Wolters Kluwer; 2016. E and F, Reprinted with permission from Kaufman AJ. *Practical Facial Reconstruction: Theory and Practice*. Wolters Kluwer; 2016. Reprinted with permission from Myers JN, Hanna EYN, Myers EN. *Cancer of the Head and Neck*. 5th ed. Wolters Kluwer; 2016.)

- **Inosculation: starts 48 to 72 hours, lasts 7 to 10 days.** Revascularization of graft dermal vessels and wound bed (anastomosis). Pink seen around day 7 = graft survival (**recheck graft at 7 days postoperatively**). **Delayed grafting over sites without perichondrium or periosteum allows granulation tissue to form, thereby increasing survival rate.**

- **Neovascularization**: concurrent with inosculation. Capillary ingrowth from wound bed and sidewalls to the graft. **Full circulation reestablished within 7 days.** Edema starts to resolve.
- **Reinnervation/maturation: starts at 2 months.** Reinnervation of graft months to years later with potential that full sensation never returns.

Table 8.17. GRAFT TYPES

Type	Description	Advantages	Disadvantages	Donor Sites	Recipient Sites
FTSG	Epidermis and full-thickness dermis	Improved cosmesis, decreased graft contraction (oversize graft 10%-20% to account for contracture), retention of appendages, amenable to delayed grafting after granulating deep defects	Increased metabolic demand → increased graft failure (cigarette smoking is the leading cause, trimming fat increases chances of graft survival [controversial])	Eyelid, preauricular, postauricular, conchal bowl, nasolabial fold, supraclavicular, lateral neck, inner upper arm, Burrow graft	Convex and concave sites (scalp, forehead, lower eyelid/medial canthus, ear, nasal ala, dorsum/sidewalls/tip)
STSG	Epidermis and partial-thickness dermis Thin: 0.005-0.012 in Medium: 0.012-0.018 in Thick: 0.018-0.030 in	Can be fenestrated to cover large defects (>5 cm), decreased metabolic demand = increased chance of graft survival, allows for detection of tumor recurrence	Worse cosmesis, increased graft contraction, bullae, no adnexal structures	Arms, abdomen, buttocks, thighs	
Composite	Epidermis, dermis, one more component (cartilage > fat)	Restores missing cartilage, maintains tissue architecture and function	Highest metabolic demand → increased graft failure, limited size due to vascular supply	Helix of ear, conchal bowl	Nose (ala to prevent alar collapse)
Xenograft	Tissue from different species	Protects underlying structure	Can be malodorous, must be replaced every 1-2 wk, porcine grafts are contraindicated in patients with pork-related allergies	N/A	Biologic dressing

FTSG, full-thickness skin graft; N/A, not applicable; STSG, split-thickness skin graft.

Surgical Emergencies and Complications

Basic Concepts

- Serious errors related to dermatologic surgery in descending order of frequency: **wrong-site procedures** > technical error > inaccurate quality/quantity of specimen > incorrect information on sample bottle/request form > laser procedure.
- **Biopsy site photography** may reduce wrong-site procedures (see Chapter 1: Epidemiology and Statistics). **If the surgeon and patient cannot identify the biopsy site, the surgeon should contact the primary dermatologist to obtain photographs or diagrams.**
- Common surgical safety threats and precautions include:
  - **Needle sticks:** educational training, double gloving.
  - **Splashes with bodily fluids:** eye protection.
  - **Broken glass:** sharps containers.
  - For **electromagnetic interference** and **fire risk**, see Chapter 7: Electrocautery and Electrosurgery.
- In addition to taking safety precautions, it is important to have a thorough understanding of surgical emergencies and complications.

Surgical Emergencies (Table 8.18)

Table 8.18. SURGICAL EMERGENCIES

Emergency Situations	Signs/Symptoms	Management	Prevention
Air embolism	Headache, CVA, TIA, seizures, visual disturbance	Alert EMS/CPR if necessary, transcranial doppler or head CT	Position prone or recumbent, seal bone with bone wax or petrolatum-impregnated gauze (most common scenario is excision of large scalp tumor with calvarial invasion)
Anaphylaxis	Angioedema ± inspiratory stridor/bronchospasm, hypotension, urticaria	Alert EMS/CPR if necessary, position supine CPR, supplemental fluids/oxygen, antihistamines/corticosteroids/IM epinephrine	Thorough preoperative drug (allergy) history
Expanding hematoma with risk of blindness or airway compromise	Enlarging ecchymotic fluctuant to firm mass with new pain ± throbbing in periorbital region or neck	See below	See Chapter 8: Preoperative Considerations
Hypertensive urgency/emergency	Elevated BP (hypertensive emergency BP > 180/120 mm Hg with impending or progressive cardiopulmonary, CNS, and/or renal organ dysfunction)	Alert EMS/CPR if necessary, anxiolytic/relaxation exercises	Epinephrine reaction leads to tachycardia and hypertension
Local anesthetic (lidocaine) toxicity	Mild: circumoral numbness/paresthesia, euphoria, light-headedness, metallic taste, restlessness, talkativeness Moderate: blurred vision, confusion/psychosis, muscle tremors/twitching, nausea/vomiting, slurred speech, tinnitus Severe: cardiopulmonary depression (bradycardia, low BP), seizures Life threatening: cardiopulmonary arrest, coma The stages of lidocaine toxicity mimic alcohol overdose: "buzzed" → "hammered" → alcohol poisoning → death.	Mild: observe Moderate: diazepam Severe or life threatening: alert EMS/CPR if necessary	Nerve blocks, safe dosing (see Chapter 8: Anesthetics and Antiseptics)
Motor nerve injury	Motor deficit (see Chapter 8: Surgical Anatomy)	Nerve reconstruction ± graft (label ends of severed nerve with nonabsorbable colored suture)	Undermine more superficially in danger zones (see Chapter 8: Surgical Anatomy)
MI	Chest/extremity pain, cold perspiration, dizziness, nausea/vomiting, sense of impending doom, shortness of breath, weakness	Alert EMS/CPR if necessary	See Chapter 8: Preoperative Considerations
Stroke/CVA	Headache, nausea/vomiting, neurologic deficits	Alert EMS/CPR if necessary	See Chapter 8: Preoperative Considerations
Vasovagal reaction	Anxiety, diaphoresis, nausea, skin pallor, tachycardia, tachypnea	Anxiolytic/relaxation exercises, cold compresses, restore BP with recumbency (Trendelenburg)	Adequate hydration, exercises (supine position)
Venous thromboembolism	DVT: lower limb pain or swelling, Homan sign PE: low grade fever, chest pain, cough, dyspnea, hemoptysis, tachycardia, tachypnea	Alert EMS/CPR if necessary	See Chapter 8: Preoperative Considerations

Heart rate and BP are important to distinguishing anaphylaxis (tachycardia/hypotension), epinephrine reaction (tachycardia/hypertension), local anesthetic toxicity (bradycardia, hypotension), and vasovagal reaction (bradycardia and hypotension).

BP, blood pressure; CNS, central nervous system; CPR, cardiopulmonary resuscitation; CT, computed tomography; CVA, cerebrovascular accident; DVT, deep venous thrombosis; EMS, emergency medical services; IM, intramuscular; MI, myocardial infarction; PE, pulmonary embolism; TIA, transient ischemic attack.

Surgical Complications

Early Complications (Table 8.19)

Table 8.19. EARLY COMPLICATIONS			
Complication	Description	Appearance	Management
Contact dermatitis	Dermatitis most often induced by topical antimicrobial or adhesive	See Chapter 2: Eczematous Dermatoses and Related Disorders	
Hematoma	Bleeding (risk highest 48 hours postoperatively), increases risk of infection, ischemia/necrosis, wound dehiscence	Stable: ecchymotic fluctuant to firm mass with a pressure sensation	Stable: Small = observation ± warm compresses Larger/older = aspiration, bromelain (organized hematomas ≥1 wk postoperatively cannot be aspirated until undergoing liquefaction ~2 wk postoperatively)
		Expanding: enlarging ecchymotic fluctuant to firm mass with pain ± throbbing	Expanding: open part/entire wound and evacuate hematoma, stop bleeding, irrigation
Infection	Infection (risk highest 4-8 d postoperatively), increases risk of ischemia/necrosis, wound dehiscence *Staphylococcus* is the leading pathogen Chondritis (after any ear procedure involving cartilage) may be associated with *Pseudomonas*	*Calor, dolor, rubor, tumor* ± purulent discharge, lymphangitic streaks, constitutional symptoms	Culture and topical/systemic antimicrobials ± drainage/irrigation, packing vs resuturing (controversial) Treat chondritis with NSAIDs and quinolone (if infected)
Ischemia/necrosis	Inadequate arterial supply or excessive tension	Venous congestion (cyanosis) Arterial insufficiency (pallor) evolving into a black/brown eschar	Venous congestion: observe Arterial insufficiency: conservative management, use hydrogen peroxide to cleanse (superficial eschar can act as a biological dressing as long as no evidence of hematoma/infection)
Pain	Pain at surgical site (or graft donor site)	Discomfort (maximal on night of surgery)	Rest, ice, compression, and elevation (RICE), NSAIDs + acetaminophen (maximum dose 4 g/d <60 y, 3 g/d >60 y) ± opioids Limit acetaminophen to 2 g/d and avoid NSAIDs/opioids in case of liver failure
Nerve injury	Motor or sensory deficit	Motor: paralysis Sensory: numbness, pain, tingling	Motor: see Table 8.18 Sensory: improves with time (avoid transection of multiple sensory nerve branches, eg, horizontal forehead incision)
Shearing	Graft separation from the wound bed, increases risk of hematoma, ischemia/necrosis	Graft displacement	Prevention is key: bolster dressing
Wound dehiscence	Separation of wound edges due to excessive tension (risk highest at suture removal), increases risk of ischemia/necrosis	Separation of wound edges	Early (<24 h) or without signs of hematoma, infection, ischemia/necrosis: resuture

NSAIDS, non-steroidal anti-inflammatory drugs.

Late Complications (Table 8.20)

Table 8.20. LATE COMPLICATIONS

Complication	Description	Appearance	Management
Eyebrow elevation/ ectropion/eclabium	Scar retraction on eyebrow, eyelid, or lip	Eyebrow asymmetry, inability to close eye fully/dry eye, or lip eversion	Prevention is key: tension vectors should be oriented parallel to free margins (perpendicular scar); the "snap test" should be performed before eyelid surgery and tacking/suspension sutures should be considered; secondary intension healing should be avoided (increases risk of scar contraction)
Excess granulation tissue	Reaction mainly in wounds healing by secondary intention, which inhibits wound healing	Beefy, red friable tissue	Destruction with silver nitrate, TCA, cautery, curettage, shave removal
Suture reactions	Suture spitting (1-3 mo after surgery)	Exposed suture	Prevention is key: avoid placing sutures too high in the dermis; remove spitting sutures
	Suture granuloma (1-3 mo after surgery)	Erythematous papule/sterile pustule	Consider intralesional corticosteroid (risk factors include multifilament suture with low USP designation and more knots)
	Suture track marks	Railroad appearance of puncture scars on either side of wound	Prevention is key: do not tie sutures too tightly or leave sutures in too long
Unsatisfactory scar cosmesis	Contour irregularity	Spread scar, depressed scar	Consider dermabrasion (6 wk postoperatively), ablative laser, scar revision
	Contraction/webbing	Fixed rigid scar (maximal in first 2 mo postoperatively)	Consider intralesional corticosteroid, massage, scar revision (eg, Z-plasty)
	Hypertrophic scar/keloid	See Chapter 5: Fibrous Neoplasms	
	Pincushioning/trapdooring	Elevation of tissue above surrounding tissue	Prevention is key: careful flap sizing, incision (remove bevel), undermining (remove excessive subcutaneous fat), and positioning Consider intralesional corticosteroid, scar revision
	Telangiectasias	See Chapter 5: Vascular Malformations and Neoplasms	

TCA, trichloroacetic acid; USP, United States Pharmacopeia.

Nail Unit Surgery

Basic Concepts

- Nail unit surgery has unique anesthetic considerations, surgical instruments, surgical techniques, and complications.

Nail Unit Anesthetic Considerations

- Anesthetic choice depends on expected level of postoperative pain. **1% to 2% plain lidocaine** is a common selection. **0.5% bupivacaine has a slower onset but longer duration of action.**
    - Ignore outdated dogma regarding the digits. It is safe to inject lidocaine with epinephrine into the digits provided there is no history of peripheral vascular compromise and the recommended volume is injected. However, use of a tourniquet often renders epinephrine unnecessary.

- **Proximal digital block (ring block): 1 to 1.5 mL of 1% to 2% plain lidocaine** is injected superficially into the **lateral aspects of the base of the digit (2-3 mL total).**
- **Distal digital block (wing block): 0.5 mL of 1% to 2% plain lidocaine** is injected vertically **1 cm lateral and proximal to the junction of the proximal and lateral folds.** After advancing the needle, an **additional 0.5 mL** is injected on each side **(2 mL total).**
- Advantages of wing block relative to ring block include quicker onset of action, less volume, and less pain.

Nail Unit Surgical Instruments (Figure 8.30)

- **Nail elevator**: atraumatically detaches the nail plate from the nail bed.
- **Nail nipper**: cuts the nail plate.
- **Tourniquet**: applies pressure to limit blood flow. It should be applied for a **maximum of 30 minutes.**

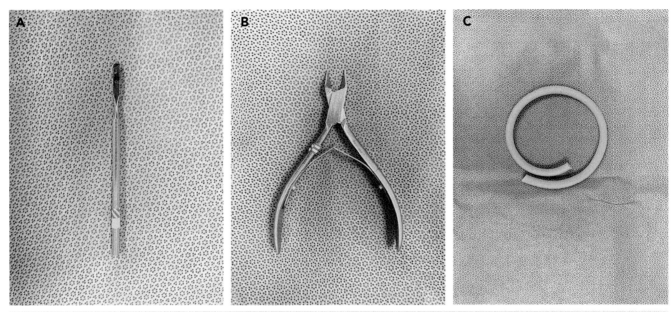

Figure 8.30. NAIL UNIT SURGICAL INSTRUMENTS. A, Nail elevator. B, Nail nipper. C, Tourniquet.

The finger of an undersized sterile glove, cut and rolled back to the base of the proximal phalanx, makes a "handy" tourniquet.

Nail Unit Surgical Techniques

- **Trephination of a subungual hematoma** involves placing hole(s) in the nail plate to permit drainage of blood. Given potential association with **distal phalanx fracture, obtain x-ray.**

- **Nail avulsion** may be **partial (preferred) or total** and **distal or proximal** (rarely used except when **subungual hyperkeratosis** is prominent).
- **Lateral matricectomy** via **chemical cautery (eg, 88% phenol)** is the primary technique for permanently treating an ingrown toenail.
- **Nail unit biopsy** techniques are illustrated in Figure 8.31.
- Nail unit excisions include **matricectomy, MMS, and en-bloc excision.**

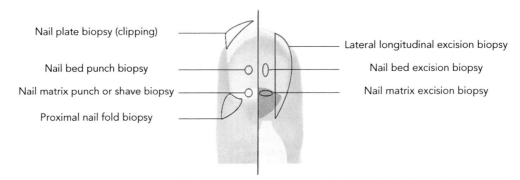

Nail plate biopsy (clipping)
Nail bed punch biopsy
Nail matrix punch or shave biopsy
Proximal nail fold biopsy

Lateral longitudinal excision biopsy
Nail bed excision biopsy
Nail matrix excision biopsy

Figure 8.31. NAIL UNIT BIOPSY TECHNIQUES.
(Illustration by Caroline A. Nelson, MD.)

Key Points
- Excision biopsies, as opposed to punch biopsies, require prior avulsion of the nail plate.
- To allow visualization, the proximal nail fold should be reflected prior to nail matrix biopsy (5 mm).
- Nail bed excision biopsies should be oriented longitudinally. Since the thickness of the nail plate is proportional to the length of the nail matrix, nail matrix excision biopsies should be oriented transversely to minimize nail plate thinning.
- Nail bed and matrix biopsies extend to bone (there is no subcutis in the nail unit).
- During proximal nail fold biopsy, a Freer elevator may be inserted to shield the underlying nail matrix.
- Suturing a defect ≤ 3 mm is not required.

Remember that the nail grows out like a "rainbow." The distal matrix synthesizes the ventral aspect of the plate; the proximal matrix synthesizes the dorsal aspect of the plate. Therefore, biopsy of the proximal matrix is more likely to result in visible nail dystrophy than biopsy of the distal matrix.

Nail Unit Surgical Complications

- Short-term complications include bleeding, pain, infection (eg, septic arthritis, osteomyelitis), and PG.

- Long-term complications include neurologic deficits, **dystrophy**, distal embedding, **spicule (due to incomplete removal of the lateral horns of the matrix)**, tumor recurrence, **implantation cyst**, and hypertrophic scars and keloids.

FURTHER READING

Asgari MM, Olson JM, Alam M. Needs assessment for Mohs micrographic surgery. *Dermatol Clin.* 2012;30(1):167-175. x. doi:10.1016/j.det.2011.08.010

Bae-Harboe YSC, Liang CA. Perioperative antibiotic use of dermatologic surgeons in 2012. *Dermatol Surg.* 2013;39(11):1592-1601. doi:10.1111/dsu.12272

Bolognia JL, Schaffer JV, Cerroni L. *Dermatology.* 4th ed. Elsevier Saunders; 2018.

Dennis C, Sethu S, Nayak S, Mohan L, Morsi YY, Manivasagam G. Suture materials: current and emerging trends. *J Biomed Mater Res A.* 2016;104(6):1544-1559. doi:10.1002/jbm.a.35683

Elder DE. *Lever's Histopathology of the Skin.* 11th ed. Wolters Kluwer; 2015.

Elston DM, Ferringer T. *Dermatopathology.* 2nd ed. Elsevier Saunders; 2014.

Elston DM, Stratman EJ, Miller SJ. Skin biopsy: biopsy issues in specific diseases. *J Am Acad Dermatol.* 2016;74(1):1-16. quiz 17-18. doi:10.1016/j.jaad.2015.06.033

Goldsmith LAK, Stephen I, Gilchrest BA, Paller AS, Leffell DJ, Wolff K. *Fitzpatrick's Dermatology in General Medicine.* 8th ed. The McGraw-Hill Companies, Inc; 2012.

Haneke E. Nail surgery. *Clin Dermatol.* 2013;31(5):516-525. doi:10.1016/j.clindermatol.2013.06.012

Hansen TJ, Lolis M, Goldberg DJ, MacFarlane DF. Patient safety in dermatologic surgery: Part I. Safety related to surgical procedures. *J Am Acad Dermatol.* 2015;73(1):1-12; quiz 13-4. doi:10.1016/j.jaad.2014.10.047

Howe N, Cherpelis B. Obtaining rapid and effective hemostasis: Part II. Electrosurgery in patients with implantable cardiac devices. *J Am Acad Dermatol.* 2013;69(5):677.e1-677.e9. doi:10.1016/j.jaad.2013.07.013

Howe N, Cherpelis B. Obtaining rapid and effective hemostasis: Part I. Update and review of topical hemostatic agents. *J Am Acad Dermatol.* 2013;69(5):659.e1-659.e17. doi:10.1016/j.jaad.2013.07.014

Iavazzo C, Gkegkes ID, Vouloumanou EK, Mamais I, Peppas G, Falagas ME. Sutures versus staples for the management of surgical wounds: a meta-analysis of randomized controlled trials. *Am Surg.* 2011;77(9):1206-1221.

James WD, Elston DM, Treat JR, Rosenbach MA, Neuhaus IM. *Andrews' Diseases of the Skin: Clinical Dermatology.* 13th ed. Elsevier; 2020.

Koay J, Orengo I. Application of local anesthetics in dermatologic surgery. *Dermatol Surg.* 2002;28(2):143-148. doi:10.1046/j.1524-4725.2002.01126.x

Kouba DJ, LoPiccolo MC, Alam M, et al. Guidelines for the use of local anesthesia in office-based dermatologic surgery. *J Am Acad Dermatol.* 2016;74(6):1201-1219. doi:10.1016/j.jaad.2016.01.022

Miller CJ, Antunes MB, Sobanko JF. Surgical technique for optimal outcomes—Part II. Repairing tissue: suturing. *J Am Acad Dermatol.* 2015;72(3):389-402. doi:10.1016/j.jaad.2014.08.006.

Miller CJ, Antunes MB, Sobanko JF. Surgical technique for optimal outcomes—Part I. Cutting tissue: incising, excising, and undermining. *J Am Acad Dermatol.* 2015;72(3):377-387. doi:10.1016/j.jaad.2014.06.048

Minkis K, Whittington A, Alam M. Dermatologic surgery emergencies: complications caused by systemic reactions, high-energy systems, and trauma. *J Am Acad Dermatol.* 2016;75(2):265-284. doi:10.1016/j.jaad.2015.11.054

Minkis K, Whittington A, Alam M. Dermatologic surgery emergencies: complications caused by occlusion and blood pressure. *J Am Acad Dermatol.* 2016;75(2):243-262. doi:10.1016/j.jaad.2015.11.013

Regula CG, Yag-Howard C. Suture products and techniques: what to use, where, and why. *Dermatol Surg.* 2015;41(suppl 10):S187-S200. doi:10.1097/dss.0000000000000492

Russo F, Linares M, Iglesias ME, et al. Reconstruction techniques of choice for the facial cosmetic units. *Actas Dermosifiliogr.* 2017;108(8):729-737. Técnicas reconstructivas de elección por unidades estéticas faciales. doi:10.1016/j.ad.2017.02.017.

Stratman EJ, Elston DM, Miller SJ. Skin biopsy: identifying and overcoming errors in the skin biopsy pathway. *J Am Acad Dermatol.* 2016;74(1):19-25. quiz 25-6. doi:10.1016/j.jaad.2015.06.034

Strickler AG, Shah P, Bajaj S, et al. Preventing and managing complications in dermatologic surgery: procedural and postsurgical concerns. *J Am Acad Dermatol.* 2021;84(4):895-903. doi:10.1016/j.jaad.2021.01.037

Strickler AG, Shah P, Bajaj S, et al. Preventing complications in dermatologic surgery: presurgical concerns. *J Am Acad Dermatol.* 2021;84(4):883-892. doi:10.1016/j.jaad.2020.10.099

Tziotzios C, Profyris C, Sterling J. Cutaneous scarring: pathophysiology, molecular mechanisms, and scar reduction therapeutics Part II. Strategies to reduce scar formation after dermatologic procedures. *J Am Acad Dermatol.* 2012;66(1):13-24. quiz 25-26. doi:10.1016/j.jaad.2011.08.035

Wright TI, Baddour LM, Berbari EF, et al. Antibiotic prophylaxis in dermatologic surgery: advisory statement 2008. *J Am Acad Dermatol.* 2008;59(3):464-473. doi:10.1016/j.jaad.2008.04.031

Yang L, Mullan B. Reducing needle stick injuries in healthcare occupations: an integrative review of the literature. *ISRN Nurs.* 2011;2011:315432. doi:10.5402/2011/315432

Ad Hoc Task Force; Connolly SM, Baker DR, et al. AAD/ACMS/ASDSA/ASMS 2012 appropriate use criteria for Mohs micrographic surgery: a report of the American Academy of Dermatology, American College of Mohs Surgery, American Society for Dermatologic Surgery Association, and the American Society for Mohs Surgery. *J Am Acad Dermatol.* 2012;67(4):531-550. doi:10.1016/j.jaad.2012.06.009

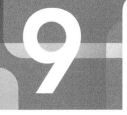

Cosmetics

John S. Barbieri, MD, MBA, Caroline A. Nelson, MD, and Sherry H. Yu, MD

Cosmetics and Cosmeceuticals

Basic Concepts

- **Chronologic aging and photoaging** each contribute to change in human physical appearance over time. A simple systematic tool is the **Glogau photoaging classification—wrinkle scale** (Table 9.1).
- **Cosmetics and cosmeceuticals are topicals with desirable aesthetic effects. Cosmeceuticals are scientifically designed** and meet rigid chemical, physical, and medical standards.

Clinical Applications

Cosmetics

- **Cleansers, moisturizers, and astringents** are the three primary categories of skin care products.
- **Cleansers** remove sebum, desquamating corneocytes, pathogens, and dirt while leaving the intercellular lipid barrier intact.
  - **Soap**: long-chain fatty acid alkali salts in a bar that **alkalinize the skin**, leading to disruption of the *stratum corneum* and the feeling of tightness after washing.
  - **Syndet** (synthetic detergent): "beauty cleanser" in a bar or liquid that contains <10% soap and has a pH of 5.5 to 7.0.
  - **Combar**: combination of soap and syndet in a bar.
  - Body wash: combination of syndet and moisturizer in an emulsion system applied with a puff.
  - Lipid-free cleanser: may contain cetyl alcohol, glycerin, propylene glycol, sodium lauryl sulfate, or stearyl alcohol.
  - Cleansing cream: waxes and mineral oil with detergent action from borax.
  - Exfoliant cleanser: contains glycolic acid or salicylic acid.
  - Abrasive cleanser: syndet with small particles (eg, polyethylene beads).
- **Gentle cleansers** (eg, syndets, lipid-free cleansers, and cleansing creams) that are **fragrance-free** may be preferred by patients with **eczematous dermatitis or xerosis**. **Exfoliant cleansers** may be preferred by patients with **acne**.
- **Moisturizers** retard TEWL and facilitate restoration of the *stratum corneum* barrier through occlusion and humectancy. **Petrolatum, the most effective occlusive moisturizer**, reduces TEWL by 99%. Other types of moisturizers include cream, polymer-based, vegetable oil and wax, dimethicone and ceramides. **Humectants (eg, glycerin, HA, propylene glycol, urea) attract moisture.** Urea is a keratolytic FDA-approved for **hyperkeratotic conditions.**
  - Occlusion and humectancy work hand in hand, since water drawn by a humectant to the *stratum corneum* will be lost to the atmosphere unless trapped by an occlusive.
- **Astringents (toners)** are applied after cleanser and before moisturizer. **Oily complexion** astringents are formulated to **remove sebum or deliver keratolytics. Dry complexion** astringents are formulated to **deliver humectants or skin-soothing agents**.
  - Toners "tone down" deficiencies in cleansers and moisturizers.

Table 9.1. GLOGAU PHOTOAGING CLASSIFICATION—WRINKLE SCALE

Type	Photoaging Characteristics	Rhytides	Patient Age
I—"No wrinkles"	Uniform in color to mild pigmentary changes, no keratoses	None	20-30s
II—"Wrinkles in motion"	Early solar lentigines, keratoses palpable but not visible	None at rest, but rhytides appear with facial expression at the corners of mouth, melolabial folds, corners of the eyes, and malar cheeks	Late 30-40s
III—"Wrinkles at rest"	Dyschromia, telangiectasias, keratoses	Present at rest	50s or older
IV—"Only wrinkles"	Yellow-gray color of skin, prior skin malignancies	Wrinkled throughout, most obvious in the perioral area	60-70s or older

- Facial foundations can add or blend color, camouflage pigmentation irregularities, normalize facial skin tone, provide photoprotection, and act as a treatment product.
- Facial powders can be used to prevent migration of foundation, add photoprotection, and absorb oil. Facial blushes and eye shadow can be used to add color.
- Mascaras are designed to color, camouflage, elongate, and thicken the eyelashes.
- Lipsticks are designed to add color. "Lip plumpers" cause transient edema due to irritants (eg, capsaicin).
- **Pigmentation defects** can be camouflaged with a cosmetic that is opaque or complementary in color (eg, **green undercover foundation for patients with rosacea**).
- **Contour defects** can be camouflaged with artistic shading based on the principle that dark colors make protuberances appear to recede and light colors make depressions appear more shallow.
- Hair care products include shampoos that cleanse the hair and conditioners that reverse hair damage.
- Nail care products include nail polish and nail sculptures (artificial nails).

Cosmeceuticals

- **α-Hydroxy acids** include monocarboxylic acids (**glycolic, lactic, mandelic**), dicarboxylic acids (**malic, tartaric**), and tricarboxylic acids (**citric**). These acids **thin the *stratum corneum* and decrease melanogenesis** in the epidermis as well as **stimulate synthesis of GAGs and collagen** in the dermis. They are commonly used in the management of **acne and photodamage.**
- **β-Hydroxy acids include salicylic acid, which enters the pilosebaceous unit and is comedolytic and keratolytic** (possibly by disrupting desmosomes). Salicylic acid is FDA-approved for **acne, calluses and corns, dermatitis, hyperkeratotic skin disorders, psoriasis, seborrheic dermatitis, and warts.**
- **Antioxidants** include carotenoids (eg, **retinol**), flavonoids (eg, **silymarin**), polyphenols (eg, **green tea**), and endogenous antioxidants (eg, **vitamins B3, C, and E**). Epigallocatechin gallate, a green tea polyphenol, is the major ingredient of **sinecatechins**, which are FDA-approved for **condyloma acuminata.**
- **Anti-inflammatories** include **aloe vera.**
- **Pigment lighteners** include **kojic acid** (inhibits tyrosinase activity) **and vitamin C.**
- Cosmeceuticals used to **diminish ecchymoses** include **arnica, bromelain, and vitamin K.**

Safety Considerations

- Cosmetics and cosmeceuticals (eg, **urea, propylene glycol, α-hydroxy acids, β-hydroxy acids, sinecatechins**) may cause **ICD.**
  - **Salicylism** has been reported after topical salicylic acid use in **infants.**
- Cosmetics and cosmeceuticals may also cause **ACD.** Common culprits include **triclosan,** a previously popular antiseptic in cleansers now banned by the FDA,

paraphenylenediamine (PPD) in permanent hair dyes, and **tosylamide formaldehyde resin** in nail polish.
- **Polyethylene beads** in abrasive cleansers may contribute to the **microplastics** detected in human stool and, ultimately, to environmental pollution.
  - Globally, humans ingest ~5 g of plastic every week, the equivalent of a credit card.
- Facial powders typically contain predominantly **talc.** Application of talc to the genital area has been associated with **ovarian cancer;** however, data are inconclusive.
- **Liquid mascara** contaminated with bacteria can lead to **infection.** Tubes should be discarded after 3 months and should not be shared. Mascara may also cause **conjunctival pigmentation.**

Chemical and Mechanical Skin Resurfacing

Basic Concepts

- Ablative skin resurfacing involves **controlled injury of the skin to a specific depth to promote the growth of new skin with improved surface characteristics.** The three primary categories are **chemical, mechanical, and laser** resurfacing. For laser resurfacing, see Chapter 9: Lasers.
- **Chemical resurfacing** is accomplished with **chemical peels** (Table 9.2). **The degree of frosting correlates with depth:**
  - Level I: Erythema with blotchy frosting;
  - Level II: White-coated frosting with patchy erythema showing through;
  - Level III: Solid white enamel frosting.
- **Mechanical resurfacing** may be superficial (eg, microdermabrasion, microneedling), medium-depth (eg, conservative manual dermasanding), or deep (eg, aggressive manual dermasanding, wire-brush or diamond-fraise dermabrasion). **Microdermabrasion** propels a rough substance (eg, aluminum oxide crystals) at the skin while simultaneously removing it with suction. **Microneedling** uses multiple fine needles to cause a superficial injury to the skin.
- Cleaning and degreasing the face is important prior to resurfacing to create a smoother and more regular surface that will enable better control over depth of the procedure.

Clinical Applications

- Indications for skin resurfacing include **melasma, acne** (limited evidence), **multiple pre-neoplastic or neoplastic epidermal lesions, scarring, and photoaging.**
- Skin resurfacing for melasma is **more effective for epidermal than dermal melanin** and is often combined with **hydroquinone.**
- Medium but particularly deep peels can **stimulate new collagen production.**
- While TCA concentrations ≥40% are not recommended, **high TCA concentrations (>70%)** can be used for **focal** chemical reconstruction of **acne scars** via the TCA Chemical Reconstruction Of Skin Scars (TCA CROSS) technique.

Table 9.2. CHEMICAL PEELS

Peel	Endpoint	Neutralization	Notes
Superficial (Epidermis ± Papillary Dermis)			
50%-70% Glycolic Acid (other α-hydroxy Acids)	Erythema or 2-4 min (No Frosting)	Sodium Bicarbonate or Washed off with Water	Water Soluble
20%-30% salicylic acid (β-hydroxy acid)	Pseudofrosting	Self-neutralizing	Lipid soluble. Since the crystals formed during treatment (pseudofrost) cannot penetrate the skin, the peel is self-limited. Including polyethylene glycol in the vehicle reduces overpenetration.
Jessner solution: 14 g each of resorcinol, salicylic acid, and lactic acid per 100 mL of 95% ethanol	Frosting	Self-neutralizing	Resorcinol has similar effects to hydroquinone and can cause cross-sensitivity.
10%-30% TCA	Frosting	Self-neutralizing[a]	
Tretinoin	See Chapter 6: Retinoids.		
Medium-depth (papillary dermis ± upper reticular dermis)			
Solid CO_2 + TCA 35% (Brody and Hailey)	Frosting with residual erythema	Self-neutralizing[a]	
70% glycolic acid + 35% TCA (Coleman and Futrell)	Frosting	Sodium bicarbonate or washed off with water	
Jessner solution + 35% TCA (Monheit)	Frosting	Self-neutralizing[a]	
40% TCA peel	Frosting	Self-neutralizing[a]	
88% phenol peel	Erythema and frosting	Self-neutralizing	Rarely used as high concentration of phenol causes rapid keratocoagulation, inhibiting further peeling.
Deep (mid reticular dermis)			
Baker-Gordon phenol peel: 3 mL phenol, 2 mL tap water, 8 drops of Septisol liquid soap, 3 drops of croton oil	Solid frosting to fine gray cast	Self-neutralizing	Croton oil enhances phenol absorption and is the primary determinant of efficacy. Occlusion with tape can increase penetration.
TCA > 50%	Solid frosting	Self-neutralizing[a]	

CO_2, carbon dioxide; TCA, trichloroacetic acid.
[a]Although TCA peels are technically self-neutralizing, they are often neutralized once the depth of ablation is achieved to prevent unwanted deeper injury.

Safety Considerations

- **Complications** from chemical peels include:
  - **Ocular exposure:** Sodium bicarbonate is used to neutralize glycolic acid, saline is used to dilute TCA, and mineral oil is used to dilute Baker-Gordon phenol solutions.
  - **Pigmentary changes: Postoperative photoprotection** is critical. **Salicylic acid has the lowest risk of postinflammatory hyperpigmentation and is safe in all skin phototypes.** Phenol may cause permanent hypopigmentation. Phenol peels may result in an "alabaster" or "plastic" appearance.
  - **Persistent erythema (>2 months):** Consider massage, corticosteroids, silicone gel sheeting, and PDL therapy.
  - **Delayed wound healing: Postoperative tobacco avoidance** is critical. Abnormal healing may also occur in patients without intact pilosebaceous units (eg, **history of radiation therapy**). **Pretreatment with topical tretinoin** (2-4 weeks prior to resurfacing) **improves penetration and decreases healing time;** however, tretinoin should be held in the postoperative period until re-epithelialization is complete and erythema is diminished.
  - **Scarring: Mechanical and laser resurfacing** may be delayed for patients exposed to **isotretinoin** during the prior 6 months due to risk of abnormal scarring (controversial).
  - **Infection: HSV prophylaxis for 10 to 14 days** starting on the day of the procedure should be considered for superficial resurfacing in patients with a history of HSV and is required for medium-depth or deep resurfacing. **Acetic acid soaks** can decrease bacterial infections.

- **Phenol peels may cause cardiotoxicity** (7% of patients will exhibit transient arrhythmias). History of cardiac arrhythmias or taking a medication known to precipitate arrhythmias are absolute contraindications; hepatic or renal disease are relative contraindications. **IV hydration and monitoring (continuous ECG, pulse oximetry, blood pressure)** are required.

Lasers

Basic Concepts

- **LASERs (Light Amplification by Stimulated Emission of Radiation)** emit light that is **monochromatic (single wavelength), spatially coherent (wavelengths are aligned in phase), and collimated (moves in parallel fashion).**
  - The 3Cs of lasers are mono<u>c</u>hromatic, <u>c</u>oherent, and <u>c</u>ollimated.
- Laser parameters include:
  - **Fluence:** How **much** energy is delivered (typical units: J/cm²).
  - **Spot size:** Over what **area** is the energy delivered.
  - **Pulse duration:** How **quickly** is the energy delivered.

- The wavelength of a laser is determined by the **lasing medium**: liquid (dye), gas (for example argon, krypton, carbon dioxide [CO_2]), solid (eg, alexandrite crystal).
- Major interactions between laser light and skin include **absorption, reflection, scatter, and transmission.**
  - Radiation is NOT a major interaction between laser light and skin.
- At the interface between air and the *stratum corneum* (skin surface), **4% to 7% of light is reflected** because of the difference in the refractive index between air ($n = 0$) and the *stratum corneum* ($n = 1.45$): **Fresnel reflectance.**
- Between 308 nm (excimer) and 1064 nm (long-pulsed [Nd:YAG]), **the depth of penetration increases as the wavelength increases.** However, for longer wavelengths (for example, 10,600 nm [CO_2]), energy is absorbed primarily by the epidermis.
- **Larger spot sizes result in deeper energy penetration** due to decreased scattering.
- By targeting specific **chromophores** in the skin that absorb the energy (Figure 9.1), it is possible to selectively damage structures of interest while minimizing damage to surrounding tissue (**selective photothermolysis**). It is import-

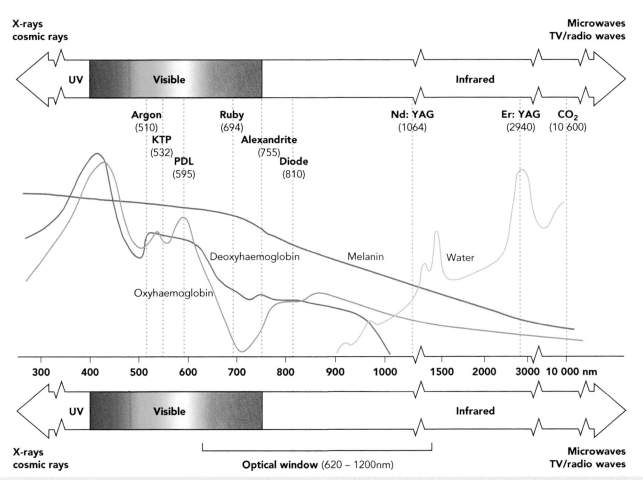

Figure 9.1. CHROMOPHORE ABSORPTION SPECTRUM THE ACTION OF EACH LASER DEPENDS ON THE ABSORPTION SPECTRUM OF THE TARGETED CHROMOPHORE. CO_2, carbon dioxide; Er:YAG, erbium-doped yttrium aluminum garnet; KTP, potassium-titanyl-phosphate; Nd:YAG, neodymium-doped yttrium aluminum garnet; PDL, pulsed dye laser.
(Reprinted with permission from Chung KC. *Grabb and Smith's Plastic Surgery.* 8th ed. Wolters Kluwer; 2019.)

ant for the chromophore to have **high absorption relative to other chromophores at that particular wavelength to prevent off-target damage.** For example, melanin has a strong absorption at 595 nm, but so does oxyhemoglobin. The PDL is therefore not ideal for hair removal because it will also target blood vessels. In contrast, melanin has strong relative absorption at 755 and 810 nm, which is why the alexandrite and diode lasers are preferable for hair removal.

- **The pulse duration should be less than or equal to the target chromophore's thermal relaxation time (cooling time to lose 50% of heat), which is proportional to the square of the diameter of the target.** Large targets such as a leg vein or hair follicle require a long pulse duration (ms), while small targets such as tattoo pigment granules are best targeted with a short pulse duration (ns, ps).

- **IPL** uses a flash lamp and subsequent filtering to deliver a narrow **range of wavelengths of light** to the skin. Since it can output multiple wavelengths, it can target multiple chromophores simultaneously.

    IPL is NOT a laser.

Clinical Applications

- Table 9.3 summarizes clinical applications of lasers in dermatology.

Table 9.3. CLINICAL APPLICATIONS OF LASERS IN DERMATOLOGY

Laser	Wavelength	Medium	Mode	Target Chromophore	Indications[a]
Excimer	308	Xenon chloride (gas)	Pulsed	Proteins	Inflammatory disorders (eg, psoriasis, vitiligo)
Argon	510	Argon (gas)	CW	Hemoglobin, melanin	Vascular lesions, diabetic retinopathy
KTP	532	KTP (crystal)	Quasi-CW	Hemoglobin, melanin	Vascular lesions (superficial), rosacea, poikiloderma
Q-switched, frequency doubled Nd:YAG	532	Nd:YAG (crystal)	Pulsed	Melanin, red pigments	Purple, red, orange, yellow, tan, and white tattoos
PDL	595	Rhodamine dye (liquid)	Pulsed	Hemoglobin	Vascular lesions (superficial), striae (red), acne (limited evidence), rosacea, poikiloderma
Ruby	694	Ruby (crystal)	Pulsed	Melanin	Pigmented lesions
Q-switched Ruby	694	Ruby (crystal)	Pulsed	Melanin, tattoo pigments	Black, brown, green, and red tattoos
Alexandrite	755	Alexandrite (crystal)	Pulsed	Melanin, deoxyhemoglobin	Hair removal, lentigines and pigmented lesions
Q-switched Alexandrite	755	Alexandrite (crystal)	Pulsed	Melanin, tattoo pigments	Black, brown, and green tattoos
Diode	~810	AlGaAs (semiconductor)	CW/pulsed	Melanin, hemoglobin	Hair removal
Long-pulsed Nd:YAG	1064	Nd:YAG (crystal)	Pulsed	Hemoglobin	Vascular lesions (deeper), leg veins, hair removal, acne scars
Q-switched Nd:YAG	1064	Nd:YAG (crystal)	Pulsed	Melanin, tattoo pigments	Black and brown tattoos, lentigines and pigmented lesions
Er:YAG	2940	Er:YAG (crystal)	Pulsed	Water	Scars, laser resurfacing
CO_2	10,600	CO_2 (gas)	CW/pulsed	Water	Scars, laser resurfacing, actinic cheilitis, drug delivery (fractional)
IPL	515-1200	N/A (light is from flash lamp)	N/A	Variable	Telangiectasia, poikiloderma, hair removal, lentigines

AlGaAs, aluminum gallium arsenide; CO_2, carbon dioxide; CW, continuous wave; Er:YAG, erbium-doped yttrium aluminum garnet; IPL, intense pulsed light; KTP, potassium-titanyl-phosphate; N/A, not applicable; ND:YAG, neodymium-doped yttrium aluminum garnet; PDL, pulsed dye laser; Q, quality.
[a]Illustrative examples provided.

- **Vascular lesions**
  - The target is **oxyhemoglobin.**
  - The desired clinical endpoint depends on treatment goals and lesion type (in general, settings that cause purpura will be more efficacious but have more downtime). Typically, the desired clinical endpoint for **port wine stains and angiomas is immediate purpura.** The desired clinical endpoint for **telangiectasia is immediate vessel disappearance or darkening.**
  - Longer wavelengths will be helpful for deeper lesions (better penetration). Longer pulse durations will be helpful for larger lesions that have longer thermal relaxation times (eg, leg veins).
  - Use of topical vitamin K before vascular lesion treatment (eg, PDL) may reduce purpura.
- **Hair removal**
  - The target is **melanin** in the hair follicle with the goal of destroying nearby hair stem cells in the **bulge** region. As a result, it is **difficult to treat vellus, blonde, or white hairs.**
  - The desired immediate clinical endpoint is **perifollicular erythema.**
  - Complications include pigmentary changes (long-pulsed **Nd:YAG is safer for skin of color**) and "stamping" (epidermal burn from presence of hair residue on the skin contact cooling window).
- **Pigmented lesions**
  - The target is **melanin.**
  - The desired clinical endpoint depends on device. **Q-switched lasers will cause immediate whitening,** which corresponds to cavitation and rupture of melanosomes. Long-pulsed lasers and light sources (ie, IPL), will cause subtle darkening that will gradually fade over minutes to days, which corresponds to necrotic pigmented cells in the epidermis.
  - **Nevus of Ota responds well to Q-switched lasers** (eg, ruby, alexandrite, Nd:YAG).
- **Tattoos**
  - The target is **tattoo pigment particles.** Shorter pulse durations are optimal (ie, picosecond is preferable to nanosecond laser) given the small size of these particles.
  - The desired clinical endpoint is **immediate whitening,** which corresponds to **small gas bubbles in the dermis.**
  - Complications include **anaphylaxis. Tattoos with white pigment can undergo paradoxical darkening** after treatment due to reduction of titanium dioxide or ferric oxide (classically reported after treatment of red/pink "lip liner"). A test spot is recommended when treating tattoos that may include a component of white pigment.
- **Scars and laser resurfacing**
  - With erbium-doped yttrium aluminum garnet (Er:YAG) and CO_2 lasers, the target is **water,** resulting in heating of the targeted tissue.
  - Proper dosimetry (fluence) is crucial for successful outcomes. **Ablative laser settings cause vaporization of the tissue,** which can be used for destruction of lesions, treatment of scars, and laser resurfacing. In **fractional photo-**thermolysis (ie, Fraxel), the laser beam is split into small microthermal zones (MTZs) to reduce overall damage to the tissue, which can decrease downtime associated with the procedure.

Safety Considerations

- When operating lasers it is important to protect the eyes of the patient and clinicians in the room. The effectiveness of protective eyewear is defined by the logarithmic measure of light that can be transmitted through the material—the **optical density (OD)** —at a particular wavelength. Eye damage from lasers is related to the wavelength of the device. **Visible light devices (eg, PDL, Nd:YAG)** can damage the **retina and iris. Ablative lasers (eg, Er:YAG, CO_2)** can cause **corneal and scleral injury.**
- Nonablative lasers will often use **cooling** (eg, spray, contact) to protect the superficial epidermis from off-target injury. This cooling can be parallel to the laser pulse, prepulse, or postpulse. **Cooling can decrease treatment-associated pain, erythema, and edema. Misaligned cooling can result in crescent-shaped burns.**
- For lasers and **fire risk (particularly the ablative Er:YAG and CO_2 lasers),** see Chapter 7: Electrocautery and Electrosurgery.
- When treating potentially contagious lesions (eg, **warts**) with lasers using ablative settings, use a **smoke evacuator and appropriate ventilation.**
- For safety considerations when resurfacing, see Chapter 9: Chemical and Mechanical Skin Resurfacing

Botulinum Neurotoxins

Basic Concepts

- *Clostridium botulinum* strains produce seven serotypes (A-G) of **BoNTs.**
- BoNTs cause **chemodenervation of muscles by inhibiting acetylcholine release.** Specifically, BoNTs **cleave proteins in the SNARE protein complex** at the neuromuscular junction:
  - **BoNT-A** cleaves **synaptosome-associated protein 25 (SNAP25);**
  - **BoNT-B** cleaves **synaptobrevin,** a vesicle-associated membrane protein (VAMP).
    - To release acetylcholine from the SNARE, BoNT-A cleaves SNAP25 and BoNT-B cleaves synaptobrevin.
- Neurogenesis, formation of axonal sprouts and new motor end plates, followed by absorption of dysfunctional neurons leads to the temporary nature of BoNT effects.

Clinical Applications

- BoNTs are most effective for **reducing dynamic facial rhytides** but can also change face and neck contour. From a medical standpoint, BoNTs also denervate sweat glands in **hyperhidrosis** and improve **Raynaud phenomenon. BoNTs** are summarized in Table 9.4 and Figure 9.2. FDA-approved indications outside of dermatology include chronic migraine, blepharospasm, and cervical dystonia.

Table 9.4. BOTULINUM NEUROTOXINS

Trade Name	Formulationª	FDA-Approved Dermatology Indications	OnaA Dose Ratio	Notes
BOTOX/BOTOX cosmetic	OnaA	Glabellar lines, axillary hyperhidrosis	N/A	
Dysport, Azzalure	AboA	Glabellar lines	1:2.5	Greatest diffusion area.
Xeomin/Bocouture	IncoA		1:1	Stable at room temperature. No complexing proteins.
MYOBLOC/NeuroBloc	RimaB		1:100	More rapid onset, shorter duration of action.

AboA, abobotulinumtoxinA; BoNT, botulinum neurotoxin; DaxiA, daxibotulinumtoxinA; FDA, Food and Drug Administration; IncoA, incobotulinumtoxinA; OnaA, onabotulinumtoxinA; RimaB, rimabotulinumtoxinB.
ªTopical BoNT-A formulations are under investigation, as is injectable DaxiA.

- BoNT effects may take 1 week, commonly last **3 to 4 months**, and may increase with subsequent injections.
- Combination use with soft tissue augmentation and/or lasers can lead to superior, longer lasting results.
- BoNTs require cold storage for 4 weeks postreconstitution. No difference in efficacy has been observed between refrigeration and freezing.

Safety Considerations

- **Immediate complications** include **erythema, bruising, injection site pain, and temporary headache.** Methods to **reduce injection site pain** include ice, topical anesthetic, vibration, nerve blocks, ultra-fine needles, and **reconstitution in preservative-containing bacteriostatic saline with benzoyl alcohol.**

  Preservatives Prevent Pain.
- **Functional complications** are summarized in Table 9.5.
- Rare complications include formation of neutralizing antibodies, granulomas, and anaphylaxis.
- Absolute contraindications:
  - Hypersensitivity;
  - Infection of the proposed injection site.
- **Relative contraindications:**
  - Breathing/swallowing difficulties;
  - **Neuromuscular disorders (eg, myasthenia gravis);**

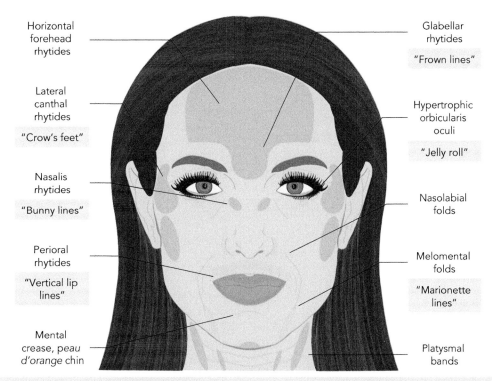

Figure 9.2. BOTULINUM NEUROTOXINS. Common injection locations for chemodenervation are shaded. Lightly shaded locations are safe to inject if appropriate precautions are observed.
(Illustration by Caroline A. Nelson, MD.)

Table 9.5. FUNCTIONAL COMPLICATIONS OF BOTULINUM NEUROTOXIN

Rhytides	Associated Muscle(s)	Functional Complications	Notes
Horizontal forehead rhytides	Frontalis	Brow ptosis, quizzical appearance	Need concomitant treatment of eyebrow depressors to prevent angry expression.
Glabellar rhytides	Corrugator supercilii and orbicularis oculi; procerus and depressor supercilii	Brow and upper eyelid ptosis	Stay 1 cm above orbital rim. Apraclonidine, an α-adrenergic agonist that causes Müller muscle to contract, is a potential treatment for ptosis.
Lateral canthal rhytides Hypertrophic orbicularis oculi	Orbicularis oculi	Eyelid ptosis; diplopia, ectropion, drooping lateral lower eyelid, asymmetric smile	Inject lateral to the orbital rim. Inject while patient is not smiling to avoid ipsilateral zygomaticus complex.
Nasalis rhytides	Nasalis		Avoid angular vein.
Nasolabial folds	Lip elevator complex	Asymmetric smile, flaccid cheek, incompetent mouth	Use caution.
Perioral rhytides	Orbicularis oris		
Melomental folds	Lip depressor complex		
Mental crease, *peau d'orange* chin	Mentalis		
Masseteric hypertrophy	Masseter		May improve symptoms of bruxism.
Platysmal bands	Platysma	Neck flexor weakness, dysphagia, hoarseness	

○ Medications that may potentiate BoNT effects including **aminoglycoside antibiotics**, CCBs, cholinesterase inhibitors, lincosamides, $MgSO_4$, polymyxins, and quinidine;

○ Pregnancy/planned pregnancy (historical pregnancy risk category C), breastfeeding.

Age < 12 years is a relative contraindication to BoNT injection.

Soft-Tissue Dermal Fillers

Basic Concepts

- **Facial aging is a combination of decreased thickness and elasticity of skin, absorption of fat, and resorption of craniofacial skeleton.** Decreased concentration of naturally occurring HA leads to decreased ability to retain water leading to volume loss and rhytides. Subcutaneous facial fat is highly compartmentalized and there is a change in volume and position of compartments over time.
- **Soft-tissue augmentation** provides a more youthful appearance.

Clinical Applications

- **Bovine collagen (Zyderm I, Zyderm II, and Zyplast)** was the first FDA-approved xenogeneic agent for soft-tissue augmentation. **Glabellar injection was contraindicated due to risk of necrosis. Pretesting with two tests, 2 to 4 weeks apart was mandatory due to risk of hypersensitivity in 3% of patients.** Human ingenuity led to derivation of historical fillers from a wide variety of sources ranging from **neonatal**

foreskin **(CosmoDerm 1, CosmoDerm 2, CosmoPlast)** to rooster comb HA **(Hylaform, Hylaform Plus).**

- **Soft-tissue dermal fillers currently available in the United States** are summarized in Table 9.6 and Figure 9.3. **HA derived from bacterial (*Streptococcus*) fermentation** is now the most commonly used material; **cross-linking increases durability.**
- Pretreatment evaluation includes medical history, defect parameters, and patient goals.
- Injection techniques include:
  ○ Serial puncture: sequential deposition of filler along wrinkle/fold with postinjection massage.
  ○ Linear threading: full length of needle inserted in proper plane and filler injected as the needle is withdrawn.
  ○ Fanning: multiple passes in different, evenly spaced directions while needle remains at initial insertion point.
  ○ Cross-hatching (radial injections): evenly spaced, linear injections in a grid-like pattern for filling large areas.
  ○ Depot injections: injection immediately followed by massage for blending.

Safety Considerations

- **Immediate complications** include **edema, erythema, bruising, and pain.** Methods to **reduce injection site pain** include use of fillers premixed with lidocaine, ice, topical anesthetic, vibration, nerve blocks, and ultra-fine needles and **microcannulas.** Cannula use may also minimize bruising.
- Rare complications include:
  ○ **Hypersensitivity reactions: Bellafill** has the highest risk; **pretreatment skin testing for bovine collagen** is

Table 9.6. SOFT-TISSUE DERMAL FILLERS

Trade Name	Material	FDA-Approved Dermatology Indications	Volume	Injection Level	Duration of Effect
Bacteria-Derived					
Restylane, Restylane-L,[a] Restylane Refyne,[a] Restylane Defyne[a]	HA	Moderate to severe facial wrinkles and folds, lip augmentation.		Subdermal	6-12 months
Restylane Silk[a]		Lip augmentation, correction of perioral rhytides		Subdermal	
Restylane Lyft[a]		Moderate to severe facial folds and wrinkles, age-related volume loss	Y	Subdermal	
Perlane, Perlane-L[a]		Moderate to severe facial wrinkles and folds	Y	Subdermal	
Belotero Balance		Moderate to severe facial wrinkles and folds	Y	Dermis	
Juvéderm Ultra, Juvéderm Ultra XC[a]		Moderate to severe facial wrinkles and folds, lip augmentation	Y	Subdermal	
Juvéderm Ultra Plus, Juvéderm Ultra Plus XC[a]		Moderate to severe facial wrinkles and folds	Y	Subdermal	
Juvéderm Voluma XC[a]		Age-related fat (volume) loss in the midface	Y	Subcutaneous/ periosteal	
Juvéderm Volbella XC[a]		Lip augmentation, perioral rhytides		Dermis	
Juvéderm Vollure XC[a]		Moderate to severe facial wrinkles and folds		Subdermal	
Synthetic[b]					
Bellafill (previously known as ArteFill)	Polymethylmethacrylate microspheres plus bovine collagen *Acrylic paints are used to make art. Polymethylmethacrylate is used to make ArteFill.*	Correction of nasolabial folds, acne scars	Y	Dermal- subcutaneous junction	Permanent
Sculptra[c]	Poly-L-lactic acid	HIV-associated lipoatrophy, shallow-to-deep nasolabial folds, contour deficiencies, and other facial wrinkles	Y	Subcutaneous	24 months
Radiesse[c], Radiesse +[a]	Calcium hydroxyapatite *Calcium renders Radiesse radio-opaque.*	HIV-associated lipoatrophy, moderate to severe facial wrinkles and folds, dorsal hand augmentation	Y	Dermal- subcutaneous junction	>12 months
Silikon 1000	Silicone		Y		
Autologous					
Autologous fat	Fat	Not regulated as long as not modified			
Azficel-T (LAVIV)	Fibroblasts[d] *Isolagen, a filler that isolated fibroblasts, is no longer available in the US.*	Moderate to severe nasolabial fold wrinkles	Y		

FDA, Food and Drug administration; HA, hyaluronic acid; HIV, human immunodeficiency virus; US, United States; Y, yes.
[a]Contains 0.3% lidocaine.
[b]Bellafill contains bovine collagen.
[c]Contains carboxymethyl-cellulose. Multiple treatments are required for the desired effect of Sculptra, whereas the effect of Radiesse is immediate.
[d]Azficel-T (LAVIV) is high cost and requires pretreatment skin biopsies.

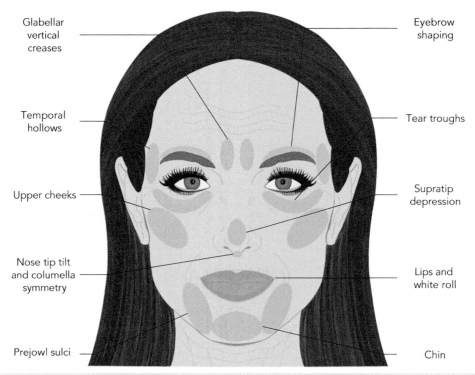

Glabellar vertical creases

Temporal hollows

Upper cheeks

Nose tip tilt and columella symmetry

Prejowl sulci

Eyebrow shaping

Tear troughs

Supratip depression

Lips and white roll

Chin

Figure 9.3. SOFT-TISSUE DERMAL FILLERS. Common injection locations for soft-tissue augmentation, in addition to rhytides and folds, are shaded. FDA, Food and Drug Administration; HIV, human immunodeficiency virus.
(Illustration by Caroline A. Nelson, MD.)

Other FDA-Approved Dermatology Indications:
• Acne scars: Bellafill®™
• Contour deficiencies: Sculptra®™
• HIV-associated lipoatrophy: Sculptra®™; Radiesse®™

required. **Radiesse** is **hypoallergenic** and **safe in all skin phototypes.**
○ **Infections**: cleanse (eg, chlorhexidine, isopropyl alcohol) the skin prior to injection. Treat infection with I&D, culture, and appropriate antimicrobials. Consider HSV prophylaxis.
○ **Contour irregularities: nodules, beading, and the Tyndall effect** may result when HA is injected too superficially into the dermis. Belotero Balance integrates more smoothly into the dermis and is less likely to cause the Tyndall effect.
  ◦ The level of injection for most fillers is subdermal. Belotero Balance and Juvéderm Volbella XC are truly "dermal fillers."
Hyaluronidase may be helpful to address contour irregularities. Pretreatment skin testing is required for patients with severe reactions or anaphylaxis to bee stings.
○ **Persistent papules** may result from **Bellafill, Sculptra, and silicone.** Silicone may migrate far from the site of injection ("silicone drift").
  ◦ Sculptra rule of 5s: massage for 5 minutes 5 times daily for 5 days.
○ **Delayed nodules**: the differential diagnosis includes hypersensitivity, **biofilm-related**, infectious, and **granulomatous (eg, Bellafill, Sculptra, silicone). Radiesse** may cause **mucosal granulomas.**

○ **Vascular occlusion:** ischemic or embolic phenomena from direct injection of filler into the vasculature may result in devastating and irreversible complications. The risk of **tissue necrosis** is highest after injection of the **glabella or medial cheek**. In case of **skin pain, arborizing blanching, duskiness, or reticulated erythema**, stop injecting and consider **warm compresses, vigorous massage, nitropaste under occlusion, and hyaluronidase** (if applicable). The risk of **blindness (central retinal artery occlusion)** is highest after injection of the **glabella, nose, or nasolabial folds**. In case of **ocular pain and visual impairment**, seek **urgent ophthalmology consultation and consider retrobulbar injection of hyaluronidase** (if applicable).

Body Contouring

Basic Concepts

• Body contouring encompasses a variety of modalities to **remove undesired fat.**
• **Liposuction aspirates fat.** In **tumescent** liposuction, **dilute lidocaine (maximum total dose 55 mg/kg) with epinephrine is injected into the affected areas**. Advantages of

tumescent anesthesia include **minimizing blood loss** (due to epinephrine vasoconstriction) and **decreasing anesthetic risk** (compared to IV or general anesthesia). **Liposuction cannulas** connected to a vacuum aspirator are used to aspirate subcutaneous fat (maximum volume 4500-5000 mL).

- Noninvasive modalities:
  - **Injection lipolysis such as deoxycholic acid (Kybella) dissolves** adipocytes.
  - **High-intensity focused ultrasound** leads to **thermal destruction** of adipocytes.
  - **Low-intensity focused ultrasound** leads to **cavitation destruction** of adipocytes.
  - **Cryolipolysis (CoolSculpting)** relies on **relative sensitivity of adipocytes to cold.** A vacuum cooling device applied to the skin causes **selective apoptosis** of adipocytes and panniculitis.
  - **Radiofrequency lipolysis** utilizes an **oscillating electrical field to noninvasively generate heat in the target tissues,** causing **thermal destruction** of adipocytes.
  - **Low-level light therapy (LLLT)** theoretically creates photochemical adipocyte membrane pores.
- As compared to liposuction, noninvasive modalities have less downtime but more modest efficacy.

Clinical Applications

- Liposuction is used for the treatment of **localized subcutaneous fat.** It is **NOT effective** for the treatment of **visceral fat or for weight loss.** In fact, **severe obesity is an absolute contraindication.** Other clinical applications of tumescent liposuction include hyperhidrosis and lipoma removal.
- Noninvasive modalities may also be used for the treatment of localized subcutaneous fat. **Deoxycholic acid** SC injection is FDA-approved for **submental convexity/fullness.**
- **Cellulite (herniation of subcutaneous fat)** occurs in the majority of **postpubertal women.** Severity ranges from slight textural abnormalities to larger irregularities and dimpling. Treatment is challenging.

Safety Considerations

- Complications of body contouring include surface irregularities and asymmetry, swelling, bruising, pain, and sensory changes.
- **Liposuction** may result in hematoma, nerve injury (eg, **marginal mandibular nerve injury during neck liposuction**), **fat embolism, pulmonary embolism, abdominal perforation** (under general anesthesia only), and **bacterial or atypical mycobacterial infection.**
- **Radiofrequency lipolysis** may result in **late-occurring lipoatrophy.**

Sclerotherapy

Basic Concepts

- Sclerotherapy involves injection of a sclerosing solution into a vessel.

- The main categories of sclerosants are:
  - **Hypertonic:** induces endothelial damage by a dehydration effect.
  - **Chemical:** causes corrosive endothelial damage.
  - **Detergent:** draws water into the cell causing an overhydration maceration effect.

Clinical Applications

- The superficial venous systems of the leg include the small and great saphenous veins. The deep venous systems of the leg include the femoral and popliteal veins. Routine sclerotherapy ± ambulatory phlebectomy is indicated for the treatment of **visible telangiectasias, reticular veins, and varicosities** without incompetence of the saphenofemoral junction. **Polidocanol, sodium morrhuate, and sodium tetradecyl sulfate (STS)** are FDA-approved for sclerotherapy.
- **A detergent solution can be foamed** by rapidly agitating it with air or CO_2. This process is **helpful when treating larger varicosities** as it allows for increased quantity to be injected and for the solution to have greater potency (sclerosant is present on the outer micelle of each microbubble).
- Alternative techniques include endovenous radiofrequency or laser ablation.

Safety Considerations

- **Complications** of sclerotherapy include **urticaria/anaphylaxis, pain, nerve damage, superficial thrombophlebitis, hyperpigmentation, telangiectatic matting, ulceration, and arterial injection (highest risk in the popliteal fossa).** Table 9.7 summarizes **complications** of sclerosing solutions.
- **Compression** following sclerotherapy **theoretically decreases the diameter of the treated vein, thereby minimizing the inflammatory reaction and degree of hyperpigmentation, vein recanalization, and telangiectatic matting.** In addition, compression **increases contact between the sclerosant and the vessel wall, thereby increasing the probability of successful treatment.**

Hair Restoration

Basic Concepts

- Hair restoration procedures include hair transplantation and LLLT.
- **Hair transplantation** involves placing follicular unit grafts into recipient sites (Table 9.8). **Each follicular unit contains 1 to 4 terminal hairs.** The **theory of donor dominance** dictates that hair retains characteristics of the donor site. Follicular unit grafts are harvested from the **occipital scalp,** which is relatively unaffected in AGA. Transplanted hair begins to appear in **3 to 6 months** and is fully grown at 9 to 14 months.
- **LLLT** stimulates respiration in mitochondria. The patient **combs light (650-700 nm) through the hair** 2 to 3 times weekly or **wears a laser cap** daily.
- Hair follicle regeneration and cloning are the next frontier in hair restoration.

Table 9.7. COMPLICATIONS OF SCLEROSING SOLUTIONS

Sclerosant	Anaphylaxis	Other Complications
Hyperosmotic		
Hypertonic saline	No risk	Highest risk of pain (can be decreased with addition of dextrose) and ulceration.
Chemical		
Glycerin	Low risk	
Polyiodide iodide	Low risk[a]	Dark brown color makes intravascular placement harder to confirm.
Detergent		
Ethanolamine oleate	High risk	Acute renal failure, hemolytic reactions.
Polidocanol	Low risk	Lowest risk of pain. Disulfiram-like reaction.
		Polidocanol causes a disulfiram-like reaction.
Sodium morrhuate	Highest risk	
	Anaphylaxis due to sodium morrhuate may cause mortality.	
STS	Low risk	

STS, sodium tetradecyl sulfate.
[a]May cause iodine hypersensitivity reactions.

TABLE 9.8 HAIR TRANSPLANTATION METHODS

Characteristic	Elliptical Donor Harvesting (Strip Excision)	Follicular Unit Extraction
Time requirement for harvest	10-20 min	30-90 min
Time requirement to create grafts	Lengthy	Minimal
Follicle density (from donor site)	100 follicular units per cm² (maximum length 30 cm)	Individual follicular units
Advantages	Minimal transection of hair follicles	Less scarring, less distortion of the natural geometry of the donor area, and less reduction of hair mass index while harvesting more follicular units with more targeting and less risk in "unpredictable zones" outside the SDA.

SDA, safe donor area

Clinical Applications

- **Hair transplantation** is commonly used for **AGA and end-stage scarring alopecia** (without evidence of inflammation for 6 months off therapy).
- Recommended candidate selection criteria include:
  - **Age > 25** is preferable.
  - Hair shaft caliber > 70 μm allows for denser coverage.
  - Donor hair shaft density > 80 follicular U/cm² is ideal. Patients with donor hair shaft density < 40 follicular U/cm² are poor candidates.
  - **Frontal scalp > vertex scalp** hair transplantation creates a more dramatic positive change.
  - "Salt-and-pepper," red hair, or blonde hair > jet-black hair transplantation due to less color contrast between hair and skin. Transplanting individual fol-

licular units in the frontal hairline can make a graft less apparent.
- For AGA patients, taking **finasteride for 6 to 12 months may stabilize hair loss prior to hair transplantation.** AGA is an ongoing process and all patients are encouraged to continue topical minoxidil and/or oral finasteride.
- The efficacy of LLLT for AGA has not yet been established.

Safety Considerations

- Patients must be warned about the risk of **posttransplantation TE.**
- Complications are rare. **Strip excision** may lead to **keloid formation. Follicular unit extraction** may lead to **multiple white dots** at the donor site and **cobblestoning** if grafts heal above the surrounding skin.

FURTHER READING

Al Dujaili Z, Karcher C, Henry M, Sadick N. Fat reduction: pathophysiology and treatment strategies. *J Am Acad Dermatol.* 2018;79(2):183-195.

Al Dujaili Z, Karcher C, Henry M, Sadick N. Fat reduction: complications and management. *J Am Acad Dermatol.* 2018;79(2):197-205.

Alam M, Tung R. Injection technique in neurotoxins and fillers: planning and basic technique. *J Am Acad Dermatol.* 2018;79(3):407-419.

Alam M, Tung R. Injection technique in neurotoxins and fillers: indications, products, and outcomes. *J Am Acad Dermatol.* 2018;79(3):423-435.

Alam M, Bolotin D, Carruthers J, et al. Consensus statement regarding storage and reuse of previously reconstituted neuromodulators. *Dermatol Surg.* 2015;41(3):321-326.

Ballin AC, Brandt FS, Cazzaniga A. Dermal fillers: an update. *Am J Clin Dermatol.* 2015;16(4):271-283.

Bolognia JL, Schaffer JV, Cerroni L. *Dermatology.* 4th ed. Elsevier Saunders; 2018.

Carruthers JC. *Alastair. Procedures in Cosmetic Dermatology Series.* Elsevier; 2017.

Creadore A, Watchmaker J, Maymone MBC, Pappas L, Vashi NA, Lam C. Cosmetic treatment in patients with autoimmune connective tissue diseases: best practices for patients with lupus erythematosus. *J Am Acad Dermatol.* 2020;83(2):343-363.

Creadore A, Watchmaker J, Maymone MBC, Pappas L, Lam C, Vashi NA. Cosmetic treatment in patients with autoimmune connective tissue diseases: best practices for patients with morphea/systemic sclerosis. *J Am Acad Dermatol.* 2020;83(2):315-341.

Elder DE. *Lever's Histopathology of the Skin.* 11th ed. Wolters Kluwer; 2015.

Elston DM, Ferringer T. *Dermatopathology.* 2nd ed. Elsevier Saunders; 2014.

Fonda-Pascual P, Moreno-Arrones OM, Saceda-Corralo D, et al. Effectiveness of low-level laser therapy in lichen planopilaris. *J Am Acad Dermatol.* 2018;78(5):1020-1023.

Gibson K, Gunderson K. Liquid and foam sclerotherapy for spider and varicose veins. *Surg Clin.* 2018;98(2):415-429.

Giordano CN, Matarasso SL, Ozog DM. Injectable and topical neurotoxins in dermatology: basic science, anatomy, and therapeutic agents. *J Am Acad Dermatol.* 2017;76(6):1013-1024.

Giordano CN, Matarasso SL, Ozog DM. Injectable and topical neurotoxins in dermatology: indications, adverse events, and controversies. *J Am Acad Dermatol.* 2017;76(6):1027-1042.

Glogau RG, Matarasso SL. Chemical face peeling: patient and peeling agent selection. *Facial Plast Surg.* 1995;11(1):1-8.

Gubelin Harcha W, Barboza Martínez J, Tsai TF, et al. A randomized, active- and placebo-controlled study of the efficacy and safety of different doses of dutasteride versus placebo and finasteride in the treatment of male subjects with androgenetic alopecia. *J Am Acad Dermatol.* 2014;70(3):489-498.e3.

Gupta AK, Cole J, Deutsch DP, et al. Platelet-rich plasma as a treatment for androgenetic alopecia. *Dermatol Surg.* 2019;45(10):1262-1273.

Hamblin MR. Photobiomodulation for the management of alopecia: mechanisms of action, patient selection and perspectives. *Clin Cosmet Investig Dermatol.* 2019;12:669-678.

Humphrey S, Carruthers J, Carruthers A. Clinical experience with 11, 460 mL of a 20-mg/mL, smooth, highly cohesive, viscous hyaluronic acid filler. *Dermatol Surg.* 2015;41(9):1060-1067.

Ibrahim O, Overman J, Arndt KA, Dover JS. Filler nodules: inflammatory or infectious? A review of biofilms and their implications on clinical practice. *Dermatol Surg.* 2018;44(1):53-60.

Ingargiola MJ, Motakef S, Chung MT, Vasconez HC, Sasaki GH. Cryolipolysis for fat reduction and body contouring: safety and efficacy of current treatment paradigms. *Plast Reconstr Surg.* 2015;135(6):1581-1590.

James WD, Elston DM, Treat JR, Rosenbach MA, Neuhaus IM. *Andrews' Diseases of the Skin: Clinical Dermatology.* 13rd ed. Elsevier; 2020.

Lanzafame RJ, Blanche RR, Bodian AB, Chiacchierini RP, Fernandez-Obregon A, Kazmirek ER. The growth of human scalp hair mediated by visible red light laser and LED sources in males. *Laser Surg Med.* 2013;45(8):487-495.

Lee KC, Wambier CG, Soon SL, et al. Basic chemical peeling: superficial and medium-depth peels. *J Am Acad Dermatol.* 2019;81(2):313-324.

Lolis M, Dunbar SW, Goldberg DJ, Hansen TJ, MacFarlane DF. Patient safety in procedural dermatology: Part II. Safety related to cosmetic procedures. *J Am Acad Dermatol.* 2015;73(1):15-24. quiz 25-16.

O'Brien KM, Tworoger SS, Harris HR, et al. Association of powder use in the genital area with risk of ovarian cancer. *JAMA.* 2020;323(1):49-59.

Requena L, Requena C, Christensen L, Zimmermann US, Kutzner H, Cerroni L. Adverse reactions to injectable soft tissue fillers. *J Am Acad Dermatol.* 2011;64(1):1-34. quiz 35-36.

Santos JI, Swensen P, Glasgow LA. Potentiation of Clostridium botulinum toxin aminoglycoside antibiotics: clinical and laboratory observations. *Pediatrics.* 1981;68(1):50-54.

Scaglione F. Conversion ratio between Botox*, Dysport*, and Xeomin* in clinical practice. *Toxins.* 2016;8(3):E65.

Schwabl P, Köppel S, Königshofer P, et al. Detection of various microplastics in human stool: a prospective case series. *Ann Intern Med.* 2019;171(7):453-457.

Small R. Botulinum toxin injection for facial wrinkles. *Am Fam Physician.* 2014;90(3):168-175.

Soleymani T, Lanoue J, Rahman Z. A practical approach to chemical peels: a review of fundamentals and step-by-step algorithmic protocol for treatment. *J Clin Aesthet Dermatol.* 2018;11(8):21-28.

Spring LK, Krakowski AC, Alam M, et al. Isotretinoin and timing of procedural interventions: a systematic review with consensus recommendations. *JAMA Dermatol.* 2017;153(8):802-809.

Urdiales-Gálvez F, Delgado NE, Figueiredo V, et al. Treatment of soft tissue filler complications: expert consensus recommendations. *Aesthetic Plast Surg.* 2018;42(2):498-510.

Waldman A, Bolotin D, Arndt KA, et al. ASDS guidelines task force: consensus recommendations regarding the safety of lasers, dermabrasion, chemical peels, energy devices, and skin surgery during and after isotretinoin use. *Dermatol Surg.* 2017;43(10):1249-1262.

Wambier CG, Lee KC, Soon SL, et al. Advanced chemical peels: phenol-croton oil peel. *J Am Acad Dermatol.* 2019;81(2):327-336.

Wanner M, Sakamoto FH, Avram MM, Anderson RR. Immediate skin responses to laser and light treatments: warning endpoints—how to avoid side effects. *J Am Acad Dermatol.* 2016;74(5):807-819. quiz 819-820.

Wanner M, Sakamoto FH, Avram MM, et al. Immediate skin responses to laser and light treatments: therapeutic endpoints—how to obtain efficacy. *J Am Acad Dermatol.* 2016;74(5):821-833. quiz 834, 833.

Appendix 1: Mucosal and Adnexal Disorders

Caroline A. Nelson, MD

Basic Concepts

- This appendix provides an overview of mucosal and adnexal disorders.
- Mucosal disorders are organized into normal findings of the oral cavity and mucocutaneous disorders.
- Adnexal disorders are organized into disorders of glands, hair, and nails with a focus on topography.

Mucosal Disorders

Normal Findings of the Oral Cavity (Table A1.1, Figure A1.1)

Table A1.1. NORMAL FINDINGS OF THE ORAL CAVITY		
Normal Finding[a]	Classic Description	Notes
Tongue		
Fissured tongue (furrowed tongue, plicated tongue, scrotal tongue)	Multiple asymptomatic 2-3 mm fissures on the dorsal tongue.	Associated with Melkersson-Rosenthal syndrome.
Geographic tongue	Asymptomatic sharply demarcated erythematous patches with yellow-white serpiginous borders favoring the lateral and dorsal tongue.	Associated with psoriasis.
Hairy tongue (black hairy tongue)	Confluent hairlike projections on the middorsal tongue ± bad breath, bad taste, gagging sensation when the tongue touches the palate.	Retention of keratin on the tips of filiform papillae. Associated with HIV infection, minocycline use, tobacco use, and poor oral hygiene. Treat with tongue scraper.
Pigmented papillae of the tongue	Multiple, uniformly spaced, tiny brown papules (normal fungiform papillae) on the tip and lateral tongue.	More common in skin phototypes IV-VI.
Miscellaneous		
Leukoedema	Gray-white discoloration of the buccal mucosa.	Becomes less apparent when stretched.
Physiologic pigmentation	Multifocal or diffuse melanin pigmentation of the oral mucosa.	More common in skin phototypes IV-VI.
Fordyce granules	Multiple asymptomatic yellow to white papules on the buccal mucosa/vermilion upper lip.	Ectopic free sebaceous glands.
Congenital inclusion cysts	Small nodules in the oral cavity located on the alveolar ridge (Bohn nodules) or palate (Epstein pearls).	Arise from epithelial remnants of dental lamina.
Torus palatinus/mandibularis	Bony prominence of the midline hard palate/lingual side of the mandible.	The prevalence of tori varies widely in different populations.

HIV, human immunodeficiency virus.
[a]Illustrative examples provided. Central papillary atrophy (median rhomboid glossitis) was previously considered a normal finding of the oral cavity but is now considered a candidiasis variant. Of note, vestibular papillomatosis is a normal finding of the vulva.

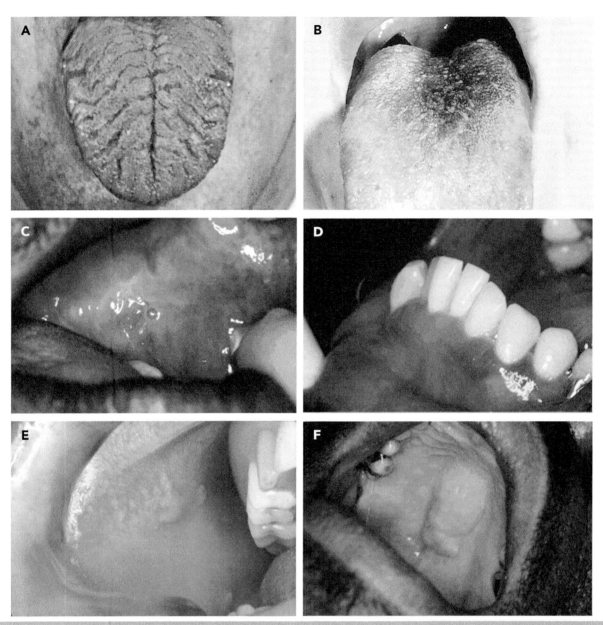

Figure A1.1. NORMAL FINDINGS OF THE ORAL CAVITY. A, Fissured tongue. B, Hairy tongue. C, Leukoedema. D, Physiologic pigmentation. E, Fordyce granules. F, Torus palatinus.

(A, Reprinted with permission from Robinson HBG, Miller AS. *Colby, Kerr, and Robinson's Color Atlas of Oral Pathology*. JB Lippincott; 1990. B, Reprinted with permission from Bickley LS. *Bates' Guide to Physical Examination and History Taking*. 8th ed. Lippincott Williams & Wilkins; 2002. C, Reprinted with permission from DeLong L, Burkhart NW. *General and Oral Pathology for the Dental Hygienist*. 2nd ed. Wolters Kluwer Health/Lippincott Williams & Wilkins; 2012. D, Reprinted with permission from DeLong L, Burkhart NW. *General and Oral Pathology for the Dental Hygienist*. 2nd ed. Wolters Kluwer Health/Lippincott Williams & Wilkins; 2012. E, Reprinted with permission from DeLong L, Burkhart NW. *General and Oral Pathology for the Dental Hygienist*. 3rd ed. Wolters Kluwer; 2018. F, Reprinted with permission from DeLong L, Burkhart NW. *General and Oral Pathology for the Dental Hygienist*. 2nd ed. Wolters Kluwer Health/Lippincott Williams & Wilkins; 2012.)

Mucocutaneous and Other Anogenital Disorders (Table A1.2)

Table A1.2. MUCOCUTANEOUS AND OTHER ANOGENITAL DISORDERS	
Disorder	Mucosal Sign(s)[a]
Nonneoplastic Disorders	
Psoriasis	Sharply demarcated erythematous plaques in the anogenital area (inverse psoriasis); annulus migrans (GPP/acrodermatitis continua of Hallopeau).
Reactive arthritis	Conjunctivitis, mucosal erosions/ulcers, balanitis circinata.
Febrile ulceronecrotic Mucha-Habermann disease	Mucosal erosions/ulcers.
Mal de Meleda nonepidermolytic PPK	Angular cheilitis.
Howel-Evans syndrome	Leukoplakia (premalignant/malignant).
AD	Conjunctivitis.
Seborrheic dermatitis	Pink-yellow to red-brown patches or thin plaques with scale in the anogenital area.
Contact dermatitis	Cheilitis, mucosal erosions/ulcers.
ARCI	Ectropion, eclabium.
Vitiligo	Mucosal depigmentation.
Heavy metal exposure (eg, amalgam, bismuth, lead, silver)	Deposition in mucous membranes.
Goltz syndrome	"Raspberry-like" papillomas.
DKC	Leukoplakia (premalignant/malignant).
PV	Mucosal erosions/ulcers, desquamative gingivitis.
PNP	Mucosal erosions/ulcers.
Hailey-Hailey disease	Mucosal erosions/ulcers (rare).
Darier disease	Cobblestoning.
BP/pemphigoid gestationis	Mucosal erosions/ulcers.
Anti-p105 pemphigoid	Mucosal erosions/ulcers.
Anti-p200 pemphigoid	Mucosal erosions/ulcers.
LABD	Mucosal erosions/ulcers.
MMP	Mucosal erosions/ulcers, desquamative gingivitis; ankyloblepharon, entropion, symblepharon, trichiasis (ocular).
EBA	Mucosal erosions/ulcers.
EB/Kindler syndrome	Mucosal erosions/ulcers.
LP	Desquamative gingivitis, Wickham striae (oral LP); annular pruritic, flat-topped, polygonal, violaceous papules (penile LP); erosions/ulcerations ± scarring with dyspareunia and postcoital bleeding (vulvovaginal LP).
EM/MIRM	Mucosal erosions/ulcers.
SJS/TEN	Mucosal erosions/ulcers.
FDE	Mucosal hyperpigmentation; mucosal erosions/ulcers (bullous FDE).
GVHD	Desquamative gingivitis, Wickham striae (chronic nonsclerotic GVHD).

(Continued)

Table A1.2. MUCOCUTANEOUS AND OTHER ANOGENITAL DISORDERS (CONTINUED)

Disorder	Mucosal Sign(s)[a]
SLE	Mucosal erosions/ulcers.
Sjögren syndrome	Xerophthalmia, xerostomia.
DM	Mucosal erosions/ulcers (anti-MDA5 DM).
LS	Phimosis, paraphimosis, or recurrent balanitis (balanitis xerotica obliterans); burying of the clitoris, fusion of the labia minora to the labia majora, and scarring of the vaginal introitus (vulvar LP).
Relapsing polychondritis	Conjunctivitis.
MKD/HIDS	Mucosal erosions/ulcers.
CAPS	Conjunctivitis.
Oral allergy syndrome	Urticaria.
Anaphylaxis/C1-INH deficiency/Ascher syndrome	Angioedema.
Glucagonoma syndrome	Angular cheilitis, glossitis.
Kawasaki disease	Conjunctivitis, cheilitis, "strawberry tongue."
GPA	Gingival hyperplasia ("strawberry gums"), mucosal erosions/ulcers.
Temporal arteritis	Mucosal erosions/ulcers.
LSC	Anogenital skin-colored to erythematous plaques with exaggerated skin lines.
Pruritus ani, pruritus scroti, pruritus vulvae	Anal, scrotal, vulvar pruritus.
Familial dysautonomia	Reduced lingual fungiform papillae.
Burning mouth syndrome/dysesthetic anogenital pain syndromes	Dysesthesia.
Ocular rosacea	Chalazion/hordeolum, conjunctivitis.
PC	Leukoplakia (benign).
Sweet syndrome	Conjunctivitis.
Recurrent aphthous stomatitis	Mucosal erosions/ulcers.
Behçet disease/MAGIC syndrome	Mucosal erosions/ulcers.
Pyostomatitis vegetans	Creamy-yellow tiny pustules arranged in a linear configuration ("snail track") on a background of diffuse intense erythema favoring the labial, gingival, and buccal mucosa.
HES	Mucosal erosions/ulcers.
Sarcoidosis	Deposition in mucous membranes; xerophthalmia, xerostomia (Mikulicz syndrome).
Crohn disease	Deposition in mucous membranes, cobblestoning, mucosal erosions/ulcers.
Granulomatous cheilitis/HPS/Melkersson-Rosenthal syndrome	Deposition in mucous membranes.
LCH	Mucosal erosions/ulcers.
NXG	Deposition in mucous membranes.
Xanthoma disseminatum	Deposition in mucous membranes.
JXG	Deposition in mucous membranes.
Verruciform xanthoma	Deposition in mucous membranes.
Scleromyxedema	Deposition in mucous membranes.

Table A1.2. MUCOCUTANEOUS AND OTHER ANOGENITAL DISORDERS (CONTINUED)

Disorder	Mucosal Sign(s)[a]
Scleredema	Deposition in mucous membranes.
Primary systemic amyloidosis	Macroglossia.
Alkaptonuria	Deposition in mucous membranes.
Lipoid proteinosis	Deposition in mucous membranes, macroglossia.
MPS	Macroglossia.
Kwashiorkor	Xerophthalmia, xerostomia, cheilitis, vulvovaginitis.
Vitamin A deficiency	Gray-white conjunctival patches (Bitot spots), xerophthalmia, xerostomia.
Vitamin A excess	Xerophthalmia, xerostomia.
Vitamin B_1 deficiency	Glossitis.
Vitamin B_2 deficiency/vitamin B_6 deficiency	Conjunctivitis, angular cheilitis, glossitis.
Vitamin B_9 deficiency, vitamin B_{12} deficiency	Glossitis.
Vitamin C deficiency	Spongy gingivae with bleeding and erosions.
Zinc deficiency/cystic fibrosis/biotinidase and holocarboxylase synthetase deficiencies/vitamin B_7 deficiency	Angular cheilitis, anogenital erythema, scale crusts, and erosions ± vesicles, bullae, and psoriasiform plaques.
Hypothyroidism/cretinism	Macroglossia.

Infections, Infestations, and Other Animal Kingdom Encounters

Disorder	Mucosal Sign(s)
Hyper-IgM syndrome	Mucosal erosions/ulcers.
Adenovirus infection	Conjunctivitis.
Herpes simplex	Conjunctivitis, mucosal erosions/ulcers.
Varicella/herpes zoster	Conjunctivitis, mucosal erosions/ulcers.
EBV infection	Palatal petechiae (Forchheimer spots) (infectious mononucleosis); acute anogenital ulcer (Lipschütz ulcer); leukoplakia (benign) (oral hairy leukoplakia).
CMV infection	Perianal ulcer.
Roseola	Red papules on the soft palate and uvula (Nagayama spots).
Wart	Focal epithelial hyperplasia, recurrent respiratory papillomatosis, genital wart.
Molluscum contagiosum	Conjunctivitis, anogenital shiny skin-colored umbilicated papules.
Variola	Mucosal vesiculopustular eruption.
Erythema infectiosum (parvovirus B19 infection)	Erythema of the tonsils and pharynx.
Rubeola	Gray papules on buccal mucosa (Koplik spots).
HFMD/herpangina	Mucosal erosions/ulcers.
HIV infection	Angular cheilitis, lineal gingival erythema, mucosal erosions and ulcers; leukoplakia (benign) (oral hairy leukoplakia).
Rubella	Palatal petechiae (Forchheimer spots).
Staphylococcus aureus infection (especially MRSA)	Hordeolum, anogenital impetigo.
GAS infection	Palatal petechiae (Forchheimer spots), "strawberry tongue" (scarlet fever); perianal erythema (perianal streptococcal infection).
Intraoral dental sinus tract/cutaneous sinus of dental origin	Erosion to oral mucosa/erosion to facial skin.

(Continued)

Table A1.2. MUCOCUTANEOUS AND OTHER ANOGENITAL DISORDERS (CONTINUED)

Disorder	Mucosal Sign(s)[a]
Normal oral flora	Necrotizing ulcerative gingivitis.
Necrotizing fasciitis (Fournier gangrene)	Anogenital rapidly evolving erythema with a poorly defined border that progresses to duskiness, tense edema, crepitus, and a foul-smelling brown exudate. Pain out of proportion to examination.
Cervicofacial actinomycosis	Jawline multiple nodules and sinus tracts with yellow grains.
Infective endocarditis	Conjunctival and palatal petechiae.
Ecthyma gangrenosum	Anogenital erythematous nodules with dusky-gray centers that evolve into eschars.
Syphilis	Primary: oral (endemic) or anogenital (venereal) inoculation site papule that evolves into a painless indurated ulcer (chancre). Early congenital/secondary: mucous patches, split papules at the oral commissures, condyloma lata. Late congenital/tertiary: gummata.
Chancroid	Anogenital papule evolves into painful nonindurated ulcer (soft chancre) with ragged undermined borders.
Gonococcal urethritis/cervicitis	Urethritis/cervicitis with dysuria/purulent discharge.
Granuloma inguinale	Anogenital papule evolves into painful ulcer with red granulation tissue.
LGV	Anogenital painless papule that evolves into an ulcer (stage I).
TB cutis orificialis	Edematous papule on mucosal site that ulcerates.
Candidiasis	Angular cheilitis, leukoplakia (benign), median rhomboid glossitis, balanitis, vulvovaginitis.
Paracoccidioidomycosis	Ulcerative or verrucous plaques in the nasal or oral mucosa.
Histoplasmosis	Molluscum-type central umbilicated papules.
Cryptococcosis	Molluscum-type central umbilicated papules, nodules, plaques.
Mucocutaneous leishmaniasis	Infiltrative and ulcerative plaques of the nasal or oral mucosa ± perforation of the nasal septum ("tapir face").
Entamoeba histolytica infection	Perianal cysts, nodules, or ulcers.
Rhinosporidiosis	Raspberry-like papillomas favoring the nasal mucosa.
American trypanosomiasis	Conjunctivitis (unilateral, Romaña sign).
Loiasis	Conjunctivitis (patient may observe the adult worm migrating across the conjunctiva).
Pinworm infection	Perianal pruritus.
Theraphosidae species exposure	Conjunctivitis (ophthalmia nodosa).
Millipede exposure	Conjunctivitis.
Sea cucumber	Conjunctivitis.
Disorders Due to Physical Agents	
Actinic prurigo	Conjunctivitis, cheilitis.
A-T	Telangiectasias on the bulbar conjunctivae.
Injury	Mechanical: eosinophilic ulcer of the oral mucosa/Riga-Fede disease, necrotizing sialometaplasia. Friction: bite fibroma, *morsicatio buccarum*.
Zoon balanitis/vulvitis	Discrete, erythematous, moist, speckled plaques on the glans penis/vulva.

Table A1.2. MUCOCUTANEOUS AND OTHER ANOGENITAL DISORDERS (CONTINUED)

Disorder	Mucosal Sign(s)[a]
Neoplasms and Cysts	
Melanoacanthoma	Mucosal pigmented lesion (reactive).
White sponge nevus	Soft white plaque on the buccal mucosa.
Glandular cheilitis	Inflammatory hyperplasia of the lower labial salivary glands.
SCCis/SCC	Erythroplakia, leukoplakia (premalignant/malignant), SIL (bowenoid papulosis, erythroplasia of Queyrat)/SCC, CIN/cervical cancer, VIN/vulvar cancer, VAIN/vaginal cancer, PIN/penile cancer, AIN/anal cancer.
Verrucous carcinoma	Florid oral papillomatosis, giant condylomata acuminata.
PVL	Multiple red and white patches on the oral mucosa with variable verrucous change.
Pseudoepitheliomatous keratotic and micaceous balanitis	Thick keratotic plaques on the glans penis.
Salivary gland tumor (eg, benign pleomorphic adenoma, malignant mucoepidermoid carcinoma)	Mucosal nodule.
EMPD	Anogenital well-demarcated, erythematous expanding plaque.
Lentigo (mucosal melanotic macule)	Mucosal pigmented lesion.
Peutz-Jeghers syndrome	Oral lentigines.
Cronkite-Canada syndrome	Oral lentigines.
Laugier-Hunziker syndrome	Oral lentigines, genital lentigines.
Cowden syndrome and other PTEN hamartoma syndromes	Cobblestoning, mucosal sclerotic fibromas, mucosal neuromas, mucosal papillomas, genital lentigines.
Mucosal melanoma	Mucosal pigmented lesion.
Hyaline fibromatosis syndrome	Gingival hyperplasia.
Angiofibroma	Pearly penile papules around the corona of the glans penis.
TSC/MEN1	Gingival/intraoral fibromas.
MEN2	Mucosal neuromas favoring the tongue or lip.
HHT	Mucosal telangiectasias.
Beckwith-Wiedemann syndrome	Macroglossia.
Down syndrome	Macroglossia.
PG	Mucosal bleeding, friable, soft red papulonodule.
KS	Red papules, plaques, and nodules.
GCT	Solitary red-brown papule favoring the tongue.
Leiomyoma (genital)	Genital painless solitary papule or nodule.
Ciliated cyst of the vulva	Nodule on vulva.
Mucocele	Pink to bluish papulonodule favoring the lower labial and buccal mucosa.
Extra-nodal NHL	Nonhealing painless ulcer.
Leukemia	Infiltration of the gingival connective tissue.
Miscellaneous Exposures	
Sun (chronic)	Actinic cheilitis.
Dentures	Angular cheilitis.

(Continued)

Table A1.2. MUCOCUTANEOUS AND OTHER ANOGENITAL DISORDERS (CONTINUED)

Disorder	Mucosal Sign(s)[a]
Alcohol	Leukoplakia (premalignant/malignant).
Tobacco	Deposition in mucous membranes, leukoplakia (premalignant/malignant), nicotinic stomatitis.
Betel nut	Leukoplakia (premalignant/malignant).
Medical Treatments	
Antimalarials	Mucosal hyperpigmentation.
Cyclosporine	Gingival hyperplasia.
Methotrexate	Mucosal erosions/ulcers.
Dupilumab	Conjunctivitis.
Systemic retinoids	Xerophthalmia, xerostomia.
Zidovudine	Mucosal hyperpigmentation.
Minocycline	Mucosal hyperpigmentation.
Cytotoxic chemotherapies	Mucosal erosions/ulcers.
Palifermin	Leukoplakia (benign).
EGFR inhibitors	Mucosal erosions/ulcers.
mTOR inhibitors	Stomatitis (discrete aphthae on nonkeratinizing epithelium).
Pimozide	Xerophthalmia, xerostomia.
Glycopyrrolate	Xerophthalmia, xerostomia.
CCBs	Gingival hyperplasia.
Phenytoin	Gingival hyperplasia.
Physical Treatments	
Radiation therapy	Mucosal erosions/ulcers.

AD, atopic dermatitis or autosomal dominant; AIN, anal intraepithelial neoplasia; ARCI, autosomal recessive congenital ichthyosis; A-T, ataxia-telangiectasia; BP, bullous pemphigoid; BRR, Bannayan-Riley-Ruvalcaba; C, complement; CAPS, cryopyrin-associated periodic syndromes; CCBs, calcium channel blockers; CIN, cervical intraepithelial neoplasia; CMV, cytomegalovirus; DKC, dyskeratosis congenita; DM, dermatomyositis; EB, epidermolysis bullosa; EBA, epidermolysis bullosa acquisita; EBV, Epstein-Barr virus; EGFR, epidermal growth factor receptor; EM, erythema multiforme; EMPD, extramammary Paget disease; FDE, fixed drug eruption; GAS, group A β-hemolytic *Streptococcus*; GCT, granular cell tumor; GPA, granulomatosis with polyangiitis; GPP, generalized pustular psoriasis; GVHD, graft-versus-host disease; HFMD, hand-foot-mouth disease; HES, hypereosinophilic syndrome; HHT, hereditary hemorrhagic telangiectasia; HIDS, hyper-IgD syndrome; HIV, human immunodeficiency virus; HPS, Hermansky-Pudlak syndrome; INH, inhibitor; IBD, inflammatory bowel disease; Ig, immunoglobulin; JXG, juvenile xanthogranuloma; KS, Kaposi sarcoma; LABD, linear IgA bullous dermatosis; LCH, Langerhans cell histiocytosis; LGV, lymphogranuloma venereum; LP, lichen planus; LS, lichen sclerosus; LSC, lichen simplex chronicus; MAGIC, mouth and genital ulcers with inflamed cartilage; MDA5, melanoma differentiation–associated protein 5; MEN, multiple endocrine neoplasia; MIRM, mycoplasma-induced rash and mucositis; MKD, mevalonate kinase deficiency; MMP, mucous membrane pemphigoid; MRSA, methicillin-resistant *Staphylococcus aureus*; MPS, mucopolysaccharidosis; mTOR, mammalian target of rapamycin; NHL, non-Hodgkin lymphoma; NXG, necrobiotic xanthogranuloma; PC, pachyonychia congenita; PG, pyogenic granuloma; PIN, penile intraepithelial neoplasia; PNP, paraneoplastic pemphigus; PPK, palmoplantar keratoderma; PV, pemphigus vulgaris; PVL, proliferative verrucous leukoplakia; SCC, squamous cell carcinoma; SCCis, squamous cell carcinoma *in situ*; SIL, squamous intraepithelial lesion; SJS/TEN, Stevens-Johnson syndrome/toxic epidermal necrolysis; SLE, systemic lupus erythematosus; TB, tuberculosis; TSC, tuberous sclerosis complex; VAIN, vaginal intraepithelial neoplasia; VIN, vulvar intraepithelial neoplasia; XP, xeroderma pigmentosum.

[a]Illustrative examples provided.

Adnexal Disorders

Gland Disorders (Table A1.3, Figure A1.2)

Table A1.3. GLAND DISORDERS		
Disorder	**Classic Description**	**Association(s)[a]**
Acne	Closed and open comedones (non-inflammatory); papules, pustules, nodules, and pseudocysts (inflammatory) favoring the face, upper chest, and back.	Hereditary: nevus comedonicus, Apert syndrome (generalized comedones), Alagille syndrome (nevus comedonicus). Acquired: Neonatal acne: *Malassezia* species. Mid-childhood acne: hyperandrogenism, precocious puberty, XYY karyotype. Acne conglobata: PRP (type VI), follicular occlusion tetrad, syndromic PG, IBD. Acne excoriée: excoriation disorder. Acne fulminans: SAPHO syndrome. Hormonal acne: • Pituitary: Cushing disease, prolactinoma. • Constitutional: SAHA syndrome/HAIR-AN. • Adrenal: CAH, Cushing syndrome. • Ovarian: PCOS, hyperthecosis, tumor (eg, arrhenoblastoma). • Ectopic hormone production: ACTH (eg, small cell lung cancer), HCG (eg, choriocarcinoma). • Iatrogenic: corticosteroids, androgens.
Acneiform eruption	Variable.	Acquired: Acne mechanica: recurrent mechanical obstruction. Occupational acne, acne cosmetica, pomade acne: follicle-occluding substances. Chloracne: halogenated aromatic hydrocarbons. Tropical acne: extreme heat. Iatrogenic: corticosteroids, androgens, INH, lithium, and phenytoin; halogenoderma (eg, iododerma due to SSKI or iodinated radiocontrast media); papulopustular reaction (eg, EGFR inhibitors, MEK 1/2 inhibitors, mTOR inhibitors).
Bromhidrosis	Exaggeration of body odor.	Hereditary: Eccrine: phenylketonuria. Acquired: Eccrine: maceration of the *stratum corneum* and bacterial degradation of keratin, exogenous (eg, garlic). Apocrine: bacterial degradation of apocrine sweat.
Chromhidrosis	Colored sweating.	Acquired: Eccrine: exogenous chemicals that color the sweat. Iatrogenic: clofazimine, rifampin. Apocrine: intrinsic excretion of lipofuscin.
Cyst	Variable.	Hereditary: PC-K17 (steatocystomas), Schöpf-Schulz-Passarge syndrome (hidrocystomas). Acquired: steatocystoma, hidrocystoma.
Erythema	Variable.	Acquired: rosacea, NEH, EMPD.
HS	Boggy, fluctuant, interconnected nodules with purulent drainage favoring the axillae, inframammary area, and anogenital area.	Acquired: PRP (type VI), follicular occlusion tetrad, syndromic PG, obesity, smoking.

(Continued)

Table A1.3. GLAND DISORDERS (CONTINUED)		
Disorder	Classic Description	Association(s)[a]
Hyperhidrosis	Excessive sweating.	Hereditary: Mal de Meleda nonepidermolytic PPK, familial dysautonomia, primary focal hyperhidrosis, granulosis rubra nasi. Acquired: CPRS, VM (blue rubber bleb nevus syndrome). Iatrogenic: acetylcholine, Frey syndrome (parotid surgery, forceps assistance during delivery).
Hypohidrosis/ anhidrosis	Decreased/absent sweating.	Hereditary: IP, ectodermal dysplasia (hypohidrotic, ankyloblepharon–ectodermal defects–cleft lip/palate syndrome), Bazex-Christol-Dupré syndrome. Acquired: tuberculoid leprosy. Iatrogenic: glycopyrrolate.
Miliaria (eccrine)	Miliaria crystallina: clear vesicles. Miliaria rubra: erythematous papules and pustules. Miliaria profunda: white papules.	Acquired: hot humid climates.
Miliaria (apocrine)	Intensely pruritic skin-colored follicular papules in the axillae, periareolar area, and anogenital area. Favoring sites of occlusion and excessive sweating.	Acquired: Fox-Fordyce disease.
Papule/plaque/ nodule	Variable.	Hereditary: nevus sebaceous; phakomatosis pigmentokeratotica, Schimmelpenning syndrome (nevus sebaceous); Muir-Torre syndrome (sebaceous adenomas, sebaceomas, sebaceous carcinomas, BCCs with sebaceous differentiation); Brooke-Spiegler syndrome (cylindromas, spiradenomas); Nicolau-Balus syndrome, Down syndrome (syringomas); hidrotic ectodermal dysplasia, Schöpf-Schulz-Passarge syndrome (syringofibroadenomas). Acquired: SGH, sebaceous adenoma/sebaceoma (sebaceous carcinoma), BCC with sebaceous differentiation, cylindroma (cylindrocarcinoma)/spiradenoma (spiradenocarcinoma), SPAP/HPAP, hidradenoma (hidradenocarcinoma), poroma (porocarcinoma), syringoma, MAC, mucinous carcinoma, tubular apocrine adenoma, eccrine angiomatous hamartoma, papillary eccrine adenoma, mixed tumor (malignant mixed tumor), syringofibroadenoma, adenoid cystic carcinoma, aggressive digital papillary adenocarcinoma.

BCC, basal cell carcinoma; CAH, congenital adrenal hyperplasia; CPRS, complex regional pain syndrome; EGFR, epidermal growth factor receptor; EMPD, extramammary Paget disease; HAIR-AN, hyperandrogenemia, insulin resistance, and acanthosis nigricans; HPAP, hidradenoma papilliferum; HS, hidradenitis suppurativa; IBD, inflammatory bowel disease; IP, incontinentia pigmenti; K, keratin; MAC, microcystic adnexal carcinoma; MEK, mitogen-activated protein kinase; mTOR, mammalian target of rapamycin; NEH, neutrophilic eccrine hidradenitis; PC, pachyonychia congenita; PCOS, polycystic ovary syndrome; PG, pyoderma gangrenosum; PPK, palmoplantar keratoderma; PRP, pityriasis rubra pilaris; SAHA, seborrhea, acne, hirsutism, and alopecia; SAPHO, synovitis, acne, pustulosis, hyperostosis, and osteitis; SGH, sebaceous gland hyperplasia; SPAP, syringocystadenoma papilliferum; SSKI, saturated solution of potassium iodide; VM, venous malformation.

[a]Illustrative examples provided.

Nonneoplastic Disorders   Neoplasms and Cysts

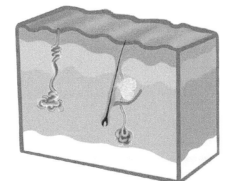

Sebaceous
- Acne
- HS

Sebaceous
- Nevus sebaceous
- SGH
- Sebaceous adenoma /sebaceoma
- BCC with sebaceous differentiation
- Dermoid cyst
- Steatocystoma

Apocrine
- Bromhidrosis (apocrine)
- Chromhidrosis (apocrine)
- Miliaria (apocrine)

Apocrine
- EMPD
- Cylindroma/spiradenoma
- SPAP/HPAP
- Hidradenoma
- Tubular apocrine adenoma
- Hidrocystoma (apocrine)

Eccrine
- Bromhidrosis (eccrine)
- Chromhidrosis (eccrine)
- Hyperhidrosis
- Hypohidrosis/anhidrosis
- Miliaria (crystallina, rubra, profunda)
- NEH

Eccrine
- Poroma
- Syringoma
- Eccrine angiomatous hamartoma
- Papillary eccrine adenoma
- Hidrocystoma (eccrine)

Mixed/Other
- MAC
- Mucinous carcinoma
- Mixed tumor
- Syringofibroadenoma

Figure A1.2. TOPOGRAPHY OF SELECTED GLAND DISORDERS. Neoplasms are sorted according to the most common differentiation. BCC, basal cell carcinoma; EMPD, extramammary Paget disease; HPAP, hidradenoma papilliferum; HS, hidradenitis suppurativa; MAC, microcystic adnexal carcinoma; NEH, neutrophilic eccrine hidradenitis; SGH, sebaceous gland hyperplasia; SPAP, syringocystadenoma papilliferum
(Illustration by Caroline A. Nelson, MD.)

Hair Disorders (Table A1.4, Figure A1.3)

Table A1.4. HAIR DISORDERS		
Disorder	Classic Description	Association(s)[a]
Alopecia (nonscarring)	Circumscribed.	Acquired: psoriasiform alopecia, PRP (type II), AA, trichotillomania, secondary syphilis, tinea capitis (biphasic), pressure alopecia.
	Patterned.	Acquired: AA ophiasis pattern (posterolateral scalp)/sisaipho pattern (spares posterolateral scalp), female pattern alopecia (vertex/midline scalp and widened part line in a "Christmas tree" pattern), male pattern alopecia (frontotemporal and vertex scalp), traction alopecia (frontotemporal scalp and widened part line), temporal triangular alopecia (temporal scalp), pressure alopecia (occipital scalp)/halo scalp ring.
	Diffuse.	Hereditary: SCID (Omenn syndrome). Acquired: SLE, DM, AA, female pattern hair loss, AE, TE.

(Continued)

Table A1.4. HAIR DISORDERS (CONTINUED)

Disorder	Classic Description	Association(s)[a]
Alopecia (scarring)	Circumscribed.	Acquired: DLE, morphea (plaque-type), FFA/LPP, CCCA/folliculitis decalvans, acne keloidalis, dissecting cellulitis of the scalp, tinea capitis (biphasic).
	Patterned.	Acquired: traction alopecia (frontotemporal scalp and widened part line) (biphasic), FFA (frontotemporal scalp ± eyebrows), CCCA (vertex/midline scalp).
	Diffuse.	Acquired: LPP.
Alopecia (madarosis)	Eyebrow/eyelash hair loss.	Hereditary: Rothmund-Thomson syndrome, cardiofaciocutaneous syndrome. Acquired: AD, AA, lepromatous leprosy, hypothyroidism (lateral one third of eyebrows).
Alopecia (miscellaneous)	Variable distribution of hair loss.	Hereditary: Vohwinkel syndrome, ARCI, Conradi-Hünermann-Happle syndrome, VHK, IP, DPR, EB, congenital atrichia with papules, loose anagen hair syndrome, hereditary PCT, progeria/adult progeria. Acquired: MMP, EBA, sarcoidosis, NL, follicular mucinosis (AD, CTCL), acquired PCT, cutaneous TB, tuberculoid leprosy, deep burns, alopecia neoplastica, radiation dermatitis. Nutritional: essential fatty acid deficiency, iron deficiency, vitamin A excess, zinc deficiency/cystic fibrosis/biotinidase and holocarboxylase synthetase deficiencies/vitamin B_7 deficiency. Iatrogenic: AE: colchicine, cytotoxic chemotherapies (eg, alkylating agents, antimetabolites, topoisomerase inhibitors), arsenic, thallium. TE: systemic retinoids, OCP discontinuation, SMO inhibitors, IFNs, minoxidil, anticoagulants (eg, heparin), anticonvulsants, antithyroid drugs, β-blockers.
Brittle hair	Increased fragility of the hair shaft.	Hereditary: trichothiodystrophy with ichthyosis. Acquired: hypothyroidism. Nutritional: Kwashiorkor.
Chlorotrichosis	Green hair.	Acquired: copper or selenium exposure.
Corkscrew hairs	Corkscrew-shaped hair shafts with perifollicular erythema or hemorrhage.	Nutritional: vitamin C deficiency.
Cyst	Variable.	Hereditary: Gardner syndrome (epidermoid cysts); Bazex-Dupré-Christol syndrome, Rombo syndrome, Nicolau-Balus syndrome (milia); PC-K17 (steatocystomas, vellus hair cysts). Acquired: dilated pore of Winer, epidermoid cyst/milium, pilar cyst (proliferating pilar cyst/pilar carcinoma), steatocystoma, vellus hair cyst.
Distichiasis	Double row of eyelashes.	Hereditary: lymphedema-distichiasis syndrome.
Folliculitis	Hair follicle inflammation.	Acquired: disseminate and recurrent infundibulofolliculitis, acne keloidalis, pseudofolliculitis barbae, eosinophilic pustular folliculitis, herpes folliculitis, bacterial folliculitis, *Malassezia* folliculitis, Majocchi granuloma, demodicosis (pityriasis folliculorum).
Follicular atrophoderma	Follicular dimple-like or ice pick depressions favoring the cheeks and dorsal hands/feet.	Hereditary: Conradi-Hünermann-Happle syndrome, Bazex-Dupré-Christol syndrome.
Follicular hyperkeratotic spicules	Follicular hyperkeratotic spicules favoring the face.	Acquired: multiple myeloma.
Follicular keratinization disorder	Prominent plug of keratin within the follicular orifice.	Hereditary: atrophoderma vermiculatum (Nicolau-Balus syndrome, Rombo syndrome), keratosis follicularis spinulosa decalvans, KP atrophicans faciei (cardio-facio-cutaneous syndrome, Noonan syndrome). Acquired: PRP, KP, erythromelanosis follicularis faciei, lichen spinulosus, FFA/LPP. Nutritional: phrynoderma.
Follicular occlusion tetrad	Follicular occlusion.	Acquired: acne conglobata, HS, dissecting cellulitis of the scalp, pilonidal sinus.
Follicular predilection	Eruption favoring the hair follicle.	Acquired: PR (darkly pigmented skin), AD (papular eczema), GVHD.
Furuncle/carbuncle	Walled-off purulent collection centered on a hair follicle/coalescent.	Acquired: *Staphylococcus aureus* infection (especially MRSA).
Hirsutism	Excessive terminal hair growth in androgen-dependent sites of female individuals.	See hormonal acne.

Table A1.4. HAIR DISORDERS (CONTINUED)

Disorder	Classic Description	Association(s)[a]
Hypertrichosis lanuginosa	Excessive lanugo hair growth.	Hereditary: congenital. Acquired: malignancy (eg, breast, lung, colon). Nutritional: marasmus.
Hypertrichosis (miscellaneous)/ trichomegaly	Variable excessive hair growth/ excessively long eyelashes.	Hereditary: Congenital/localized: nevoid hypertrichosis, hypertrichosis of specific anatomic sites, congenital melanocytic nevus, hair collar sign/faun tail nevus, plexiform neurofibroma, Becker nevus, Cornelia de Lange syndrome, Rubinstein-Taybi syndrome, fetal alcohol syndrome/fetal hydantoin syndrome, porphyria (eg, CEP, HEP). Congenital/generalized: universal hypertrichosis, Ambras syndrome, neural tube defect (eg, spina bifida). Neoplastic: congenital melanocytic nevus, neurofibroma, Becker nevus. Acquired: Localized: CPRS, porphyria (eg, PCT), and friction injury (eg, under plaster cast). Generalized; prepubertal hypertrichosis, POEMS syndrome, HIV infection, pregnancy. Iatrogenic: corticosteroids, cyclosporine, zidovudine, EGFR inhibitors, IFN, bimatoprost/latanoprost, minoxidil, phenytoin, PUVA.
Hypotrichosis	Decreased hair growth.	Hereditary: ectodermal dysplasia (hypohidrotic, hidrotic, ankyloblepharon–ectodermal defects–cleft lip/palate syndrome, ectodermal dysplasia-ectrodactyly-clefting syndrome), Bazex-Christol-Dupré syndrome, Rombo syndrome.
Papule/plaque/nodule	Variable.	Hereditary: Bazex-Christol-Dupré syndrome, Rombo syndrome, Brooke-Spiegler syndrome, multiple familial trichoepitheliomas (trichoepitheliomas); BHD syndrome (fibrofolliculomas, trichodiscomas); Cowden syndrome (trichilemmomas); Rubinstein-Taybi syndrome, Turner syndrome, Edwards syndrome, Gardner syndrome, myotonic dystrophy (pilomatricomas). Acquired: follicular mucinosis, nevus comedonicus, IFK, trichoadenoma, trichoepithelioma (malignant trichoepithelioma), trichofolliculoma, fibrofolliculoma/trichodiscoma, tumor of the follicular infundibulum, pilar sheath acanthoma, tricholemmoma (tricholemmal carcinoma, BCC, pilomatricoma (pilomatrical carcinoma), trichoblastoma.
Pigmentary changes	Flag sign.	Nutritional: Kwashiorkor. Iatrogenic: methotrexate.
	Pigmentary dilution.	Hereditary: OCA/HPS/CHS/GS/homocystinuria, phenylketonuria. Nutritional: copper deficiency (Menkes kinky hair disease), selenium deficiency.
	Poliosis.	Hereditary: piebaldism, WS. Acquired: vitiligo, AA (forme fruste).
	Premature canities.	Hereditary: prolidase deficiency, A-T.
	Repigmentation of gray hair.	Iatrogenic: ICIs.
Synophrys	Eyebrow fusion.	Hereditary: WS, Cornelia de Lange syndrome, Rubinstein-Taybi syndrome.
Trichodysplasia spinulosa	Numerous spiny papules favoring the midface and ears.	Iatrogenic: TSPyV (solid organ transplant recipients on immunosuppressive therapy, leukemia/lymphoma patients on chemotherapy).
Trichomycosis axillaris	Concretions along hair shafts.	Acquired: *Corynebacterium tenuis* infection.
Trichostasis spinulosa	Keratin and vellus hair shafts embedded within hair follicles favoring the head and neck.	Acquired: trichostasis spinulosa.

AA, alopecia areata; ACTH, adrenocorticotropic hormone; AD, atopic dermatitis; AE, anagen effluvium; AGA, androgenetic alopecia; ARCI, autosomal recessive congenital ichthyoses; A-T, ataxia-telangiectasia; BCC, basal cell carcinoma; BHD, Birt-Hogg-Dubé; CAH, congenital adrenal hyperplasia; CCCA, central centrifugal cicatricial alopecia; CEP, congenital erythropoietic porphyria; CHS, Chédiak-Higashi syndrome; CPRS, complex regional pain syndrome; CTCL, cutaneous T-cell lymphoma; DLE, discoid lupus erythematosus; DM, dermatomyositis; DPR, dermatopathia pigmentosa reticularis; EB, epidermolysis bullosa; EBA, epidermolysis bullosa acquisita; EGFR, epidermal growth factor receptor; FFA, frontal fibrosing alopecia; GAS, group A *Streptococcus*; GVHD, graft-versus-host disease; HCG, human chorionic gonadotropin; HEP, hepatoerythropoietic porphyria; HIV, human immunodeficiency virus; HPS, Hermansky-Pudlak syndrome; HS, hidradenitis suppurativa; IFK, inverted follicular keratosis; IFNs, interferons; IP, incontinentia pigmenti; K, keratin; KP, keratosis pilaris; LPP, lichen planopilaris; MM, multiple myeloma; MMP, mucous membrane pemphigoid; MRSA, methicillin-resistant *Staphylococcus aureus*; NL, necrobiosis lipoidica; OCA, oculocutaneous albinism; OCP, oral contraceptive pill; PC, pachyonychia congenita; PCOS, polycystic ovarian syndrome; PCT, porphyria cutanea tarda; POEMS, polyneuropathy, organomegaly, endocrinopathy, monoclonal gammopathy, and skin changes; PR, pityriasis rosea; PRP, pityriasis rubra pilaris; PUVA, psoralen ultraviolet A; SCID, severe combined immunodeficiency; SLE, systemic lupus erythematosus; SMO, smoothened; TB, tuberculosis; TE, telogen effluvium; TSPyV, trichodysplasia spinulosa–associated polyomavirus; VHK, Vogt-Koyanagi-Harada; WS, Waardenburg syndrome.
[a]Illustrative examples provided. For hair shaft abnormalities, see Appendix 4.

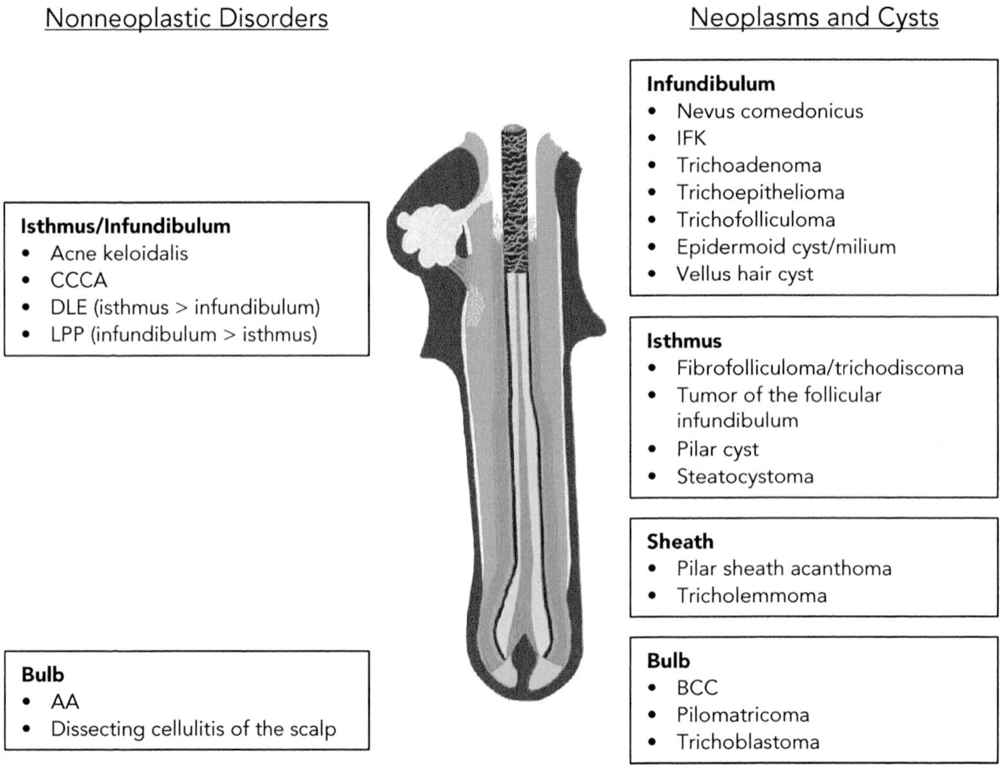

Nonneoplastic Disorders

Neoplasms and Cysts

Infundibulum
- Nevus comedonicus
- IFK
- Trichoadenoma
- Trichoepithelioma
- Trichofolliculoma
- Epidermoid cyst/milium
- Vellus hair cyst

Isthmus/Infundibulum
- Acne keloidalis
- CCCA
- DLE (isthmus > infundibulum)
- LPP (infundibulum > isthmus)

Isthmus
- Fibrofolliculoma/trichodiscoma
- Tumor of the follicular infundibulum
- Pilar cyst
- Steatocystoma

Sheath
- Pilar sheath acanthoma
- Tricholemmoma

Bulb
- AA
- Dissecting cellulitis of the scalp

Bulb
- BCC
- Pilomatricoma
- Trichoblastoma

Figure A1.3. TOPOGRAPHY OF SELECTED HAIR DISORDERS. AA, alopecia areata; BCC, basal cell carcinoma; CCCA, central centrifugal cicatricial alopecia; DLE, discoid lupus erythematosus; IFK, inverted follicular keratosis; LPP, lichen planopilaris.
(Illustration by Caroline A. Nelson, MD.)

Nail Disorders (Table A1.5, Figure A1.4)

Table A1.5. NAIL DISORDERS		
Disorder	Classic Description	Association(s)[a]
Anonychia/micronychia	Absent or small nail.	Hereditary: DPR, ectodermal dysplasia (ankyloblepharon–ectodermal defects–cleft lip/palate syndrome, ectodermal dysplasia-ectrodactyly-clefting syndrome, hidrotic, Witkop tooth, and nail syndrome), Coffin-Siris syndrome (fifth nails), COIF (second fingernails), nail-patella syndrome, DKC.
Beau lines	Transverse depressions in the nail plate.	Acquired: AD, marasmus, mechanical injury. Iatrogenic: cytotoxic chemotherapies.
Beige nail	Beige opacity in the nail plate.	Acquired: proximal subungual onychomycosis, distal subungual onychomycosis, primary total dystrophic onychomycosis.
Black nail	Black pigmentation of the nail plate.	Acquired: black nail syndrome (*Proteus mirabilis* infection).
Blue lunulae	Blue pigmentation of the lunulae.	Hereditary: Wilson disease. Acquired: heavy metals (eg, silver). Iatrogenic: zidovudine, minocycline.
Brachyonychia (racquet nails)/macronychia	Short and wide nail.	Hereditary: Rubinstein-Taybi syndrome.
Brittle nail/hapalonychia	Increased fragility of the nail plate/soft nail plate.	Hereditary: trichothiodystrophy with ichthyosis. Acquired: contact dermatitis, Kwashiorkor, hypothyroidism.

Table A1.5. NAIL DISORDERS (CONTINUED)

Disorder	Classic Description	Association(s)[a]
Bywaters lesions	Nail fold thromboses and purpuric papules on the distal digits (especially the digital pulp)	Acquired: RA.
Clubbing	Enlarged and excessively curved nail plate (>180° angle between proximal nail fold and nail plate) due to enlargement of the soft tissue of the distal digit (bulbous).	Hereditary: pachydermoperiostosis. Acquired: thyroid acropachy, bronchopulmonary diseases (eg, neoplasms), POEMS syndrome.
Cuticular hypertrophy	Ragged hypertrophic cuticles.	Acquired: DM.
Cyst	Soft skin-colored nodule on the proximal nail fold with spontaneous viscous drainage and nail plate depression.	Acquired: digital mucous cyst (pseudocyst).
Dolichonychia	Long and slender nail.	Hereditary: Marfan syndrome.
Green nail	Green pigmentation of the nail plate.	Acquired: green nail syndrome (*Pseudomonas aeruginosa* infection).
Habit tic deformity	Multiple midline Beau lines resembling a washboard.	Acquired: friction injury.
Koilonychia	Hollow or spoon-shaped nail.	Hereditary: Mal de Meleda nonepidermolytic PPK, monilethrix. Acquired: primary systemic amyloidosis, hyperthyroidism. Nutritional: iron deficiency.
Leukonychia (apparent)	White discoloration that fades with pressure due to nail bed edema.	Acquired: renal disease on hemodialysis (Lindsay nails), hypoalbuminemia (Muehrcke lines), liver cirrhosis (Terry nails). Iatrogenic: cytotoxic chemotherapies (Muehrcke lines).
Leukonychia (true)	White discoloration that remains with pressure due to parakeratotic cells within the ventral nail plate.	Hereditary: Bart-Pumphrey syndrome (diffuse), Hailey-Hailey disease/Darier disease (longitudinal, candy cane nails). Acquired: arsenic and thallium poisoning (transverse, Mees lines), mechanical injury (transverse, Mees lines or punctate) Iatrogenic: cytotoxic chemotherapies (transverse, Mees lines).
Longitudinal erythronychia	Longitudinal red coloration of the nail.	Hereditary: Darier disease (candy cane nails). Acquired: onychopapilloma.
Longitudinal melanonychia	Longitudinal brown or black pigmentation of the nail plate. Periungual extension of pigmentation onto the nail folds (Hutchinson sign) is concerning for melanoma.	Normal finding: more common in skin phototypes IV-VI. Hereditary: Peutz-Jeghers syndrome, Laugier-Hunziker syndrome. Acquired: HIV infection, dematiaceous onychomycosis, friction injury (fourth/fifth digits), lentigo, melanocytic nevus, melanoma, Addison disease, pregnancy. Iatrogenic: zidovudine, minocycline, doxorubicin.
Median canaliform dystrophy of Heller	Central longitudinal split resembling an inverted fir tree.	Acquired: friction injury. Iatrogenic: systemic retinoids.
"Oil drop" sign (salmon patches)	Irregular orange discoloration visible through the nail plate.	Acquired: psoriasis.
Onychauxis	Thick nail plate.	Acquired: psoriasis, pressure injury, onychomatricoma (multiple longitudinal cavities).
Onychoatrophy	Thin nail plate.	Hereditary: EB. Acquired: EBA, LP, CPRS.
Onychocryptosis	Ingrown toenail.	Hereditary: congenital malalignment of the great toenails/congenital hypertrophy of the lateral fold of the hallux. Acquired: mechanical/pressure injury.
Onychogryphosis	Hard, thick, and yellow-brown nail plate with ram's horn shape due to asymmetric growth.	Hereditary: Haim-Munk syndrome. Acquired: elder self-neglect.

(Continued)

Table A1.5. NAIL DISORDERS (CONTINUED)		
Disorder	Classic Description	Association(s)[a]
Onycholysis	Detachment of the distal nail plate from the nail bed.	Hereditary: Vohwinkel syndrome. Acquired: psoriasis/acrodermatitis continua of Hallopeau, contact dermatitis, onychomycosis, mechanical/friction injury, water exposure injury (repeated wet dry cycles)/chemical exposure injury (acrylic nails), hyperthyroidism. Iatrogenic: cytotoxic chemotherapies; taxanes (hemorrhagic onycholysis); quinolones, tetracyclines, 6-MP, psoralens (photoonycholysis).
Onychomadesis (nail shedding)	Detachment of the nail plate from the proximal nail fold.	Acquired: HFMD, mechanical/friction injury.
Onychophagia/onychotillomania	Nail biting/pulling.	Hereditary: Lesch-Nyhan syndrome. Acquired: body-focused repetitive behavior disorder.
Onychophosis	Hyperkeratotic tissue between the nail folds and the nail plate.	Normal finding: age-related.
Onychorrhexis	Longitudinal ridging and fissuring of the nail plate.	Normal finding: age-related. Acquired: LP, friction injury, water exposure injury (repeated wet dry cycles)/chemical exposure injury (nail varnish solvents), hypothyroidism.
Onychoschizia	Splitting of the nail plate.	Acquired: LP, friction injury, water exposure injury (repeated wet dry cycles)/chemical exposure injury (nail varnish solvents).
Pachyonychia	Thick nail plate.	Hereditary: PC.
Papule/plaque/nodule	Skin-colored periungual/subungual papule.	Hereditary: IP (keratotic tumors), TSC (Koenen tumors). Acquired: wart, SCC, AFK.
	Coral periungual papule.	Acquired: MRH.
	Red periungual/subungual papule.	Acquired: onychocryptosis (PG), mechanical/pressure/friction injury (PG). Iatrogenic: systemic retinoids (PG).
	Red subungual papule.	Acquired: glomus tumor.
Paronychia (acute)	Red and swollen nail fold associated with pain.	Acquired: herpes simplex (herpetic whitlow variant), *Staphylococcus aureus* infection, GAS infection. Iatrogenic: ± excessive periungual granulation tissue: NRTIs/NtRTIs (eg, lamivudine) and protease inhibitors (eg, indinavir). ± pseudopyogenic granulomas: cytotoxic chemotherapies (eg, capecitabine) and targeted antineoplastic therapies (eg, EGFR inhibitors, MEK 1/2 inhibitors).
Paronychia (chronic)	Red and swollen nail fold associated with absent cuticle and secondary pseudomonal or candidal infection.	Hereditary: PC, CMC (primary total dystrophic onychomycosis). Acquired: psoriasis, contact dermatitis. Nutritional: zinc deficiency/cystic fibrosis/biotinidase and holocarboxylase synthetase deficiencies/vitamin B_7 deficiency.
Pincer nails (trumpet nails)	Increased transverse curvature of the nail plate.	Hereditary: PC. Acquired: pressure injury.
Pitting	Punctate depressions of the nail plate surface. Elkonyxis refers to large pits.	Acquired: psoriasis (large and irregular), AD (large and irregular), AA (small and geographically distributed).
Platonychia	Decreased transverse curvature of the nail plate (flat nails).	Nutritional: iron deficiency.
Proximal nail fold dilated capillaries	Dilated tortuous capillaries.	Acquired: SLE (normal density); DM, SSc (reduced density).
Pseudoleukonychia	Exogenous white discoloration of the nail plate.	Acquired: superficial white onychomycosis.

Table A1.5. NAIL DISORDERS (CONTINUED)		
Disorder	Classic Description	Association(s)[a]
Pterygium (dorsal)	Adhesion of the proximal nail fold to the nail bed, creating a wing-like appearance.	Acquired: MMP, LP.
Pterygium (ventral)	Adhesion of the distal nail plate to the hyponychium.	Acquired: SSc.
Red lunulae	Red coloration of the lunulae.	Acquired: psoriasis, LP, SLE, DM, RA, AA, CO poisoning.
Splinter hemorrhages	Red to black thin longitudinal lines in the nail.	Acquired: psoriasis (distal), APLS (proximal), vasculitis (proximal), endocarditis (proximal), onychomycosis (distal), trichinosis (proximal), mechanical injury (distal).
Subungual hematoma	Blood accumulation under the nail plate.	Acquired: mechanical injury.
Subungual hyperkeratosis	Accumulation of subungual scale leading to thickened appearance of nail plate.	Hereditary: Vohwinkel syndrome. Acquired: psoriasis, onychomycosis.
Subungual exostosis	Hard tender nodule that elevates the nail plate due to bone proliferation.	Acquired: mechanical/friction injury.
Trachyonychia	Diffuse homogenous nail roughness (sandpapered nails).	Acquired: LP.
Triangular lunulae	Triangular shape of the lunulae.	Hereditary: nail-patella syndrome.
V-shaped nicking	Wedge-shaped subungual hyperkeratosis and fissuring of the free margin of the distal nail plate.	Hereditary: Darier disease.
Yellow nail syndrome	Arrested or reduced linear nail growth, absent lunulae and eponychium, thick and yellow nail plate.	Acquired: lymphedema, respiratory tract involvement (eg, chronic bronchitis, bronchiectasis, sinusitis, pleural effusions).

AA, alopecia areata; AD, atopic dermatitis; AFK, acral fibrokeratoma; APLS, antiphospholipid antibody syndrome; CMC, chronic mucocutaneous candidiasis; CO, carbon monoxide; COIF, congenital onychodysplasia of the index fingers; COPD, chronic obstructive pulmonary disease; CPRS, complex regional pain syndrome; DKC, dyskeratosis congenita; DM, dermatomyositis; DPR, dermatopathia pigmentosa reticularis; EB, epidermolysis bullosa; EBA, epidermolysis bullosa acquisita; EGFR, epidermal growth factor receptor; HFMD, hand-foot-mouth disease; HIV, human immunodeficiency virus; IP, incontinentia pigmenti; LP, lichen planus; MEK, mitogen-activated protein kinase; MMP, mucous membrane pemphigoid; 6-MP, 6-mercaptopurine; MRH, multicentric reticulohistiocytosis; NRTIs, nucleoside reverse transcriptase inhibitors; NtRTIs, nucleotide reverse transcriptase inhibitors; OA, osteoarthritis; PC, pachyonychia congenita; PG, pyogenic granuloma; POEMS, polyneuropathy, organomegaly, endocrinopathy, monoclonal gammopathy, and skin changes; PPK, palmoplantar keratoderma; PRP, pityriasis rubra pilaris; RA, rheumatoid arthritis; SCC, squamous cell carcinoma; SLE, systemic lupus erythematosus; SSc, systemic sclerosis; TS, tuberous sclerosis complex.
[a]Illustrative examples provided. Psoriasiform onychodystrophy may also occur in other papulosquamous disorders (eg, acrokeratosis paraneoplastica, reactive arthritis, PRP).

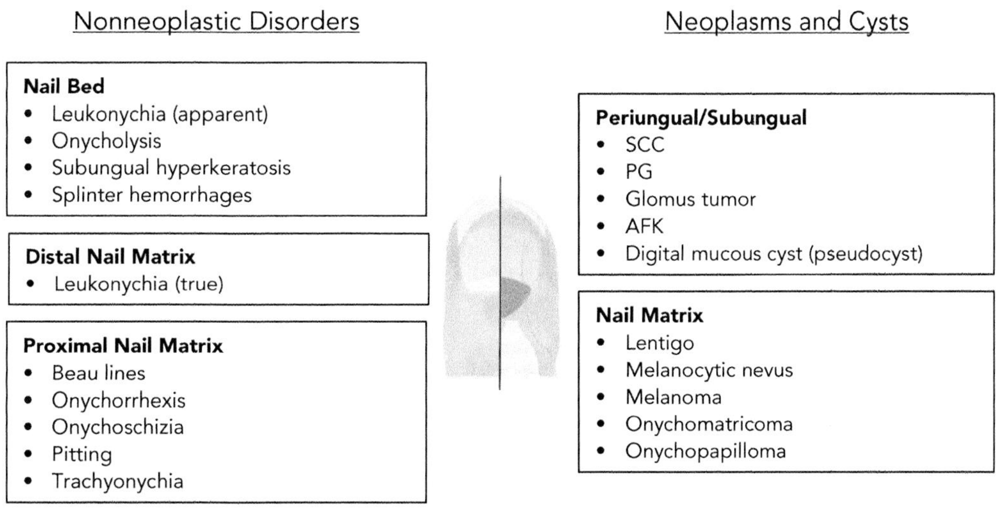

Nonneoplastic Disorders

Nail Bed
- Leukonychia (apparent)
- Onycholysis
- Subungual hyperkeratosis
- Splinter hemorrhages

Distal Nail Matrix
- Leukonychia (true)

Proximal Nail Matrix
- Beau lines
- Onychorrhexis
- Onychoschizia
- Pitting
- Trachyonychia

Neoplasms and Cysts

Periungual/Subungual
- SCC
- PG
- Glomus tumor
- AFK
- Digital mucous cyst (pseudocyst)

Nail Matrix
- Lentigo
- Melanocytic nevus
- Melanoma
- Onychomatricoma
- Onychopapilloma

Figure A1.4. TOPOGRAPHY OF SELECTED NAIL DISORDERS. AFK, acral fibrokeratoma; PG, pyogenic granuloma; SCC, squamous cell carcinoma.
(Illustration by Caroline A. Nelson, MD.)

FURTHER READING

Bolognia JL, Schaffer JV, Cerroni L. *Dermatology*. 4th ed. Elsevier Saunders; 2018.

Cizenski JD, Michel P, Watson IT, et al. Spectrum of orocutaneous disease associations: immune-mediated conditions. *J Am Acad Dermatol.* 2017;77(5):795-806.

Day A, Abramson AK, Patel M, Warren RB, Menter MA. The spectrum of oculocutaneous disease: part II. Neoplastic and drug-related causes of oculocutaneous disease. *J Am Acad Dermatol.* 2014;70(5):821.e1-821.19.

Horner ME, Abramson AK, Warren RB, Swanson S, Menter MA. The spectrum of oculocutaneous disease: part I. Infectious, inflammatory, and genetic causes of oculocutaneous disease. *J Am Acad Dermatol.* 2014;70(5):795.e1-795.25.

James WD, Elston DM, Treat JR, Rosenbach MA, Neuhaus IM. *Andrews' Diseases of the Skin: Clinical Dermatology.* 13th ed. Elsevier; 2020.

Maymone MBC, Greer RO, Burdine LK, et al. Benign oral mucosal lesions: clinical and pathological findings. *J Am Acad Dermatol.* 2019;81(1):43-56.

Maymone MBC, Greer RO, Kesecker J, et al. Premalignant and malignant oral mucosal lesions: clinical and pathological findings. *J Am Acad Dermatol.* 2019;81(1):59-71.

Wilder EG, Frieder J, Sulhan S, et al. Spectrum of orocutaneous disease associations: genodermatoses and inflammatory conditions. *J Am Acad Dermatol.* 2017;77(5):809-830.

Appendix 2: Dermatologic Signs of Internal Malignancy

Caroline A. Nelson, MD

Basic Concepts

- This appendix provides an overview of dermatologic signs of internal malignancy as well as monoclonal gammopathies of cutaneous significance.

Paraneoplastic Syndromes and Other Dermatologic Signs of Internal Malignancy (Table A2.1)

Table A2.1. PARANEOPLASTIC SYNDROMES AND OTHER DERMATOLOGIC SIGNS OF INTERNAL MALIGNANCY	
Internal Malignancy	Association(s)[a]
Circulatory	
Atrial myxoma	Noninflammatory retiform purpura.
Digestive	
Gastric cancer	Pityriasis rotunda, AN ± florid cutaneous papillomatosis ± tripe palms syndrome, anti–laminin-332 MMP, adult-onset DM, papuloerythroderma of Ofuji, sign of Leser-Trélat.
Hepatocellular cancer	Pityriasis rotunda, PCT, eruptive disseminated porokeratosis.
Colon adenocarcinoma	Adult-onset DM, pruritus, acquired hypertrichosis lanuginosa, sign of Leser-Trélat, EMPD.
Endocrine	
Pituitary adenoma	Cushing disease (hormonal acne/AGA/hirsutism ± signs of virilization).
Prolactinoma	Hormonal acne/AGA/hirsutism.
Adrenal adenoma or carcinoma	Cushing syndrome (hormonal acne/AGA/hirsutism ± signs of virilization).
Pheochromocytoma	Flushing.
Pancreatic cancer	Adult-onset DM, pancreatic panniculitis, Trousseau syndrome.
Glucagonoma	Glucagonoma syndrome (necrolytic migratory erythema, angular cheilitis, glossitis).
Carcinoid tumor	Carcinoid syndrome (pruritus, flushing, vitamin B_3 deficiency).
Lymphatic/Immune	
T-cell lymphoma	DH (enteropathy-associated T-cell lymphoma), cytophagic histiocytic panniculitis (extranodal NK/T-cell lymphoma, nasal type, primary cutaneous γ/δ T-cell lymphoma), papuloerythroderma of Ofuji, lymphocytic HES.

(Continued)

Table A2.1. PARANEOPLASTIC SYNDROMES AND OTHER DERMATOLOGIC SIGNS OF INTERNAL MALIGNANCY (CONTINUED)

Internal Malignancy	Association(s)[a]
B-cell lymphoma	Hodgkin disease: acquired ichthyosis vulgaris, pruritus.
	Intravascular large B-cell lymphoma: noninflammatory retiform purpura favoring the trunk and thighs.
	NHL, NOS: PNP, adult-onset DM, acquired angioedema, mixed cryoglobulinemia.
Lymphoma, NOS	Paraneoplastic erythroderma, CSVV, cryoglobulinemia type I, NXG/normolipemic plane xanthoma, sign of Leser-Trélat, lymphoma cutis.
Castleman disease	PNP, glomeruloid hemangiomas.
Hypergammaglobulinemic purpura of Waldenström	Petechiae, ecchymoses, palpable purpura.
Primary systemic amyloidosis	Waxy papulonodules and plaques, ecchymoses > hemorrhagic bullae, macroglossia, alopecia, koilonychia.
Plasma cell dyscrasia, NOS	Pityriasis rotunda, cutis laxa, angioedema, crystalglobulin vasculopathy, CSVV, cryoglobulinemia type I, NXG/normolipemic plane xanthoma, follicular hyperkeratotic spicules.
Plasmacytoma	AESOP syndrome.
MDS	Relapsing polychondritis, CSVV, Sweet syndrome, PG.
Myeloproliferative disorders	EF, CSVV, erythromelalgia type 3, aquagenic pruritus (PV).
AML	Sweet syndrome, NEH, leukemia cutis.
JMML	JXG/NF1 (increased risk).
CML	Leukemia cutis (rare).
ALL	Leukemia cutis (rare).
CLL	PNP, mixed cryoglobulinemia, pruritus, bullous arthropod bites, leukemia cutis.
Hairy cell leukemia	CSVV, PAN.
HES	Pruritus.
Mastocytosis	Flushing.
Hematologic disorders and malignancies, NOS	GA, NXG/normolipemic plane xanthoma, generalized eruptive histiocytoma, HLH, indeterminate cell histiocytosis.
Thymoma	PNP.
Renal/Urinary/Excretory	
Bladder adenocarcinoma	EMPD.
Reproductive	
Breast adenocarcinoma	Adult-onset DM, SSc (diffuse cutaneous, anti-RNA polymerase III), Mondor syndrome of superficial thrombophlebitis, acquired hypertrichosis lanuginosa, sign of Leser-Trélat, MPD/EMPD.
Ovarian adenocarcinoma	Adult-onset DM, hormonal acne/AGA/hirsutism ± signs of virilization.
Cervical carcinoma	Pruritus.
Prostate adenocarcinoma	Pruritus.
Choriocarcinoma	Pemphigoid gestationis, hormonal acne, AGA/hirsutism.
Respiratory	
Upper aerodigestive tract carcinoma	Acrokeratosis paraneoplastica (Bazex sign), adult-onset DM (nasopharyngeal carcinoma, Southeast Asian populations).

Table A2.1. PARANEOPLASTIC SYNDROMES AND OTHER DERMATOLOGIC SIGNS OF INTERNAL MALIGNANCY (CONTINUED)

Internal Malignancy	Association(s)[a]
Lung carcinoma	Tripe palms syndrome, anti–laminin-332 MMP, adult-onset DM, erythema gyratum repens, Trousseau syndrome, IgA vasculitis, hormonal acne/AGA/hirsutism and hyperpigmentation due to ectopic ACTH syndrome (SCLC), acquired hypertrichosis lanuginosa, clubbing.
Miscellaneous	
Solid organ tumors, NOS	Lymphedema (malignant obstruction), GA, MRH, cutis gyrata, solid organ metastases.

ACTH, adrenocorticotropic hormone; AESOP, adenopathy and extensive skin patch overlying a plasmacytoma; AGA, androgenetic alopecia; ALL, acute lymphoblastic leukemia; AML, acute myeloid leukemia; AN, acanthosis nigricans; CLL, chronic lymphocytic leukemia; CML, chronic myelogenous leukemia; CSVV, cutaneous small-vessel vasculitis; DH, dermatitis herpetiformis; DM, dermatomyositis; EBV, Epstein-Barr virus; EF, eosinophilic fasciitis; EMPD, extramammary Paget disease; GA, granuloma annulare; HES, hypereosinophilic syndrome; HLH, hemophagocytic lymphohistiocytosis; JMML, juvenile myelomonocytic leukemia; JXG, juvenile xanthogranuloma; MDS, myelodysplastic syndrome; MMP, mucous membrane pemphigoid; MPD, mammary Paget disease; MRH, multicentric reticulohistiocytosis; NEH, neutrophilic eccrine hidradenitis; NF, neurofibromatosis; NHL; non-Hodgkin lymphoma; NK, natural killer; NOS, not otherwise specified; NXG, necrobiotic xanthogranuloma; PAN, polyarteritis nodosa; PCT, porphyria cutanea tarda; PNP, paraneoplastic pemphigus; PV, polycythemia vera; RNA, ribonucleic acid; SCLC, small-cell lung cancer; SSc, systemic sclerosis; TMEP, telangiectasia macularis eruptiva perstans.
[a]Illustrative examples provided.

Monoclonal Gammopathies of Cutaneous Significance (Table A2.2)

Table A2.2. MONOCLONAL GAMMOPATHIES OF CUTANEOUS SIGNIFICANCE

Paraprotein	Association(s)[a]
IgA	IgA pemphigus, EED, PG, POEMS syndrome ($\lambda > \kappa$).
IgM	Schnitzler syndrome.
IgG	IgG4-RD (ALHE, granuloma faciale, Kimura disease, Rosai-Dorfman disease), NXG/normolipemic plane xanthoma ($\kappa > \lambda$), scleromyxedema ($\lambda > \kappa$), scleredema (type II) ($\kappa > \lambda$), primary systemic amyloidosis ($\lambda > \kappa$), POEMS syndrome ($\lambda > \kappa$).
Multiple	Cutis laxa, cryoglobulinemia type I (monoclonal IgM > IgG > IgA), cryoglobulinemia type II (monoclonal IgM > IgG against polyclonal IgG), cryoglobulinemia type III (polyclonal IgM against polyclonal IgG).

ALHE, angiolymphoid hyperplasia with eosinophilia; EED, erythema elevatum diutinum; Ig, immunoglobulin; IgG4-RD, immunoglobulin G4–related disease; NXG, necrobiotic xanthogranuloma; PG, pyoderma gangrenosum.
[a]Illustrative examples provided.

FURTHER READING

Bolognia JL, Schaffer JV, Cerroni L. *Dermatology*. 4th ed. Elsevier Saunders; 2018.

James WD, Elston DM, Treat JR, Rosenbach MA, Neuhaus IM. *Andrews' Diseases of the Skin: Clinical Dermatology*. 13th ed. Elsevier; 2020.

Pascoe VL, Fenves AZ, Wofford J, Jackson JM, Menter A, Kimball AB. The spectrum of nephrocutaneous diseases and associations: inflammatory and medication-related nephrocutaneous associations. *J Am Acad Dermatol*. 2016;74(2):247-270. quiz 271-242.

Shah KR, Boland CR, Patel M, Thrash B, Menter A. Cutaneous manifestations of gastrointestinal disease: part I. *J Am Acad Dermatol*. 2013;68(2):189. e1-189.e21. quiz 210.

Thrash B, Patel M, Shah KR, Boland CR, Menter A. Cutaneous manifestations of gastrointestinal disease: part II. *J Am Acad Dermatol*. 2013;68(2):211. e211-211.e233. quiz 244-216.

Waldman RA, Finch J, Grant-Kels JM, Stevenson C, Whitaker-Worth D. Skin diseases of the breast and nipple: benign and malignant tumors. *J Am Acad Dermatol*. 2019;80(6):1467-1481.

Waldman RA, Finch J, Grant-Kels JM, Whitaker-Worth D. Skin diseases of the breast and nipple: Inflammatory and infectious diseases. *J Am Acad Dermatol*. 2019;80(6):1483-1494.

Wofford J, Fenves AZ, Jackson JM, Kimball AB, Menter A. The spectrum of nephrocutaneous diseases and associations: genetic causes of nephrocutaneous disease. *J Am Acad Dermatol*. 2016;74(2):231-244. quiz 245-246.

Appendix 3: Dermatologic Signs of Metabolic Disorders and Pregnancy

Caroline A. Nelson, MD

Basic Concepts

- This appendix provides an overview of dermatologic signs of metabolic disorders and pregnancy.
- Dermatologic signs of metabolic disorders are divided into disorders of endocrine glands and other organs involved in metabolism. For hereditary enzyme deficiencies and nutritional deficiencies, see Chapter 2: Depositional Disorders, Porphyrias, and Nutritional Deficiencies.
- Dermatologic signs of pregnancy are divided into pregnancy dermatoses, physiologic changes of pregnancy, and dermatoses influenced by pregnancy.

Dermatologic Signs of Metabolic Disorders (Table A3.1)

Table A3.1. DERMATOLOGIC SIGNS OF METABOLIC DISORDERS	
Metabolic Disorder	Association(s)[a]
Endocrine Disorders	
Cushing disease/Cushing syndrome	"Cushingoid features" (eg, moon facies, buffalo hump, central obesity), hormonal acne/AGA/hirsutism, acquired immunodeficiency.
Diabetes insipidus	LCH, xanthoma disseminatum, benign cephalic histiocytosis.
Thyroid disorders	General: pruritus, GA, and other noninfectious granulomas; TE.
	Hypothyroidism: skin changes (xerotic, coarse, cold, pale), asteatotic dermatitis, acquired ichthyosis vulgaris, carotenemia, ecchymosis, xanthoma (eruptive, tendinous, tuberous/tuberoeruptive), generalized myxedema; macroglossia; brittle hair; madarosis of lateral one third of eyebrows; brittle nails, onychorrhexis.
	Hyperthyroidism: skin changes (moist, smooth, warm, flushed), circumscribed and diffuse hyperpigmentation, urticaria, flushing (thyrotoxicosis), localized (pretibial) myxedema; clubbing (thyroid acropachy), koilonychia, onycholysis.
	Nontoxic thyroid enlargement: Ascher syndrome.
Diabetes mellitus	AN, carotenemia, bullous diabeticorum, RPD/Kyrle disease, palmar erythema, nonuremic calciphylaxis, arterial ulcer (acral dry gangrene), pruritus, neuropathic ulcers, flushing (rubeosis), GA (generalized), NL, xanthoma (eruptive), scleredema (type III), diabetic cheiroarthropathy, diabetic dermopathy, acquired immunodeficiency, syringoma.

(Continued)

Table A3.1. DERMATOLOGIC SIGNS OF METABOLIC DISORDERS (CONTINUED)	
Metabolic Disorder	**Association(s)[a]**
Hypoglycemia	Subcutaneous fat necrosis of the newborn.
Pancreatitis	Pancreatic panniculitis.
Addison disease	Hyperpigmentation; longitudinal melanonychia.
SAHA syndrome	Seborrheic dermatitis, hormonal acne/AGA/hirsutism ± signs of virilization.
HAIR-AN syndrome	AN, hormonal acne/AGA/hirsutism ± signs of virilization.
PCOS	Hormonal acne/AGA/hirsutism.
Ovarian hyperthecosis	Hormonal acne/AGA/hirsutism ± signs of virilization.
Menopause	Flushing.
Other Metabolic Disorders	
Liver disease	General: skin changes (jaundice), pruritus.
	Cirrhosis: pityriasis rotunda, palmar erythema, ecchymoses, non-uremic calciphylaxis, edema blister, spider nevus; hair changes (sparse axillary, pubic, and pectoral hair); Muehrcke nails, Terry nails.
	PBC/ICP: diffuse hyperpigmentation, xanthoma (eruptive, plane).
	Hemochromatosis: diffuse hyperpigmentation.
	α1AT deficiency: α1AT deficiency panniculitis.
	Wilson disease: pretibial hyperpigmentation; blue lunulae.
Renal disease	ESRD: acquired ichthyosis vulgaris ± uremic frost, RPD/Kyrle disease, calciphylaxis, edema blister, pruritus, NSF, PCT, pseudoporphyria; Lindsay nails.
	Nephrotic syndrome: edema blister, lymphedema, acquired essential fatty acid deficiency, acquired immunodeficiency; Muehrcke nails.
Electrolyte imbalances	Hypocalcemia: GPP.
	Hypercalcemia: subcutaneous fat necrosis of the newborn, sarcoidosis.
	Hyperoxaluria: retiform purpura.
	Hyperuricemia: gout.
Dyslipidemia	Cholesterol emboli (following vascular surgery), GA, NL, NXG (low HDL-C), xanthoma (plane, tendinous, tuberous/tuberoeruptive).
Metabolic syndrome/obesity	Psoriasis, lipodystrophy, non-uremic calciphylaxis, lymphedema, NL, xanthoma (eruptive).

AGA, androgenetic alopecia; AN, acanthosis nigricans; APL, acquired partial lipodystrophy; CKD, chronic kidney disease; ESRD, end-stage renal disease; GA, granuloma annulare; GPP, generalized pustular psoriasis; HAIR-AN, hyperandrogenemia, insulin resistance, and acanthosis nigricans; HDL-C, high density lipoprotein cholesterol; LCH, Langerhans cell histiocytosis; NL, necrobiosis lipoidica; NSF, nephrogenic systemic fibrosis; NXG, necrobiotic xanthogranuloma; PCOS, polycystic ovary syndrome; PCT, porphyria cutanea tarda; RPD, reactive perforating dermatosis; SAHA, seborrhea, acne, hirsutism, and androgenetic alopecia; TE, telogen effluvium.
[a]Illustrative examples provided.

Dermatologic Signs of Pregnancy

Pregnancy Dermatoses (Table A3.2)

- Other dermatologic disorders associated with increased fetal risk include:
  - PR: spontaneous abortion (first 15 weeks).
  - Steroid sulfatase deficiency: prolonged labor.
  - PV: transient skin lesions (30%-45%).
  - Maternal anti-Ro (SSA)/La (SSB) > anti-U1-RNP autoantibodies (a minority have identified LE or Sjögren syndrome): neonatal LE.
  - PXE: miscarriage (first trimester).
  - Vascular EDS: uterine rupture.
  - APLS: spontaneous abortion.
  - Congenital infections: herpes simplex, varicella, CMV infection, parvovirus B19 infection, mumps, Zika, HIV infection, rubella, syphilis, toxoplasmosis.

Table A3.2. PREGNANCY DERMATOSES

Pregnancy Dermatosis[a]	Risk Factors	Timing	Classic Description	Complications	Management	Risk of Recurrence
Pustular psoriasis of pregnancy	Psoriasis	Late pregnancy or postpartum	GPP favoring flexural sites	Mother: hypocalcemia Fetus: stillbirth, neonatal demise due to placental insufficiency	Antihistamines, topical corticosteroids, systemic corticosteroids (prednisolone)	High
AEP	Atopy	Early pregnancy	Resembles AD		Antihistamines, topical corticosteroids, nbUVB	High
Pemphigoid gestationis	HLA-DR3 and HLA-DR4	Late pregnancy or postpartum	BP-like skin lesions involving the umbilicus (due to circulating autoantibodies to BPAG2 [NC16A domain])	Mother: Graves disease Fetus: prematurity, SGA, mild and transient skin lesions (~10%)	Antihistamines, topical corticosteroids, systemic corticosteroids (prednisolone)	High
PEP	Primiparous, multiple-gestation pregnancy, increased maternal weight gain	Late pregnancy or postpartum	Urticarial papules and plaques arising in *striae distensae* with periumbilical sparing (polymorphic)		Antihistamines, topical corticosteroids	Low
ICP		Late pregnancy	Pruritus (due to elevated serum bile acid levels)	Fetus: prematurity, intrapartum distress, stillbirth	Ursodeoxycholic acid	Medium

AD, atopic dermatitis; AEP, atopic eruption of pregnancy; BP, bullous pemphigoid; BPAG2, bullous pemphigoid antigen 2; GPP, generalized pustular psoriasis; HLA, human leukocyte antigen; ICP, intrahepatic cholestasis of pregnancy; nbUVB, narrowband ultraviolet B; PEP, polymorphic eruption of pregnancy; SGA, small for gestational age.

[a]Since pustular psoriasis of pregnancy is a GPP variant, some authors do not classify it as a pregnancy dermatosis.

Physiologic Changes During Pregnancy
(Table A3.3)

Category	Association(s)[a]
Table A3.3. PHYSIOLOGIC CHANGES DURING PREGNANCY	
Pigmentary changes	Areolar hyperpigmentation, linea nigra, melasma, melanocytic nevi (darkening); longitudinal melanonychia.
Connective tissue changes	*Striae distensae.*
Vascular changes	Palmar erythema, spider nevus, unilateral nevoid telangiectasia, AVM (worsening), PG, cherry angioma (edema blister, varicosities, vasomotor instability, purpura, gingival hyperemia or hyperplasia, hemorrhoids).
Glandular changes	Increased sebaceous and eccrine function with decreased apocrine function, multiple eruptive eccrine poromas.
Hair changes	Hirsutism (due to hyperandrogenemia during late pregnancy), AGA (postpartum), TE (postpartum), acquired generalized hypertrichosis.
Nail changes	There are no pathognomonic nail changes.

AGA, androgenetic alopecia; AVM, arteriovenous malformation; PG, pyogenic granuloma; TE, telogen effluvium
[a]Illustrative examples provided.

Dermatoses Influenced by Pregnancy
(Table A3.4)

Dermatosis	Association(s)[a]
Table A3.4. DERMATOSES INFLUENCED BY PREGNANCY	
Improved by pregnancy	Psoriasis (except for pustular psoriasis of pregnancy), acne.[b]
Triggered or exacerbated by pregnancy	AD, autoimmune progesterone dermatitis, stasis dermatitis, PV, SLE, acne,[b] rosacea (rosacea fulminans), Sweet syndrome, acquired zinc deficiency, TV, disseminated coccidioidomycosis.

AD, atopic dermatitis; PV, pemphigus vulgaris; SLE, systemic lupus erythematosus; TV, tinea versicolor.
[a]Illustrative examples provided.
[b]Acne typically improves during pregnancy but may flare due to hyperandrogenemia during late pregnancy.

FURTHER READING

Bolognia JL, Schaffer JV, Cerroni L. *Dermatology*. 4th ed. Elsevier Saunders; 2018.

Hirt PA, Castillo DE, Yosipovitch G, Keri JE. Skin changes in the obese patient. *J Am Acad Dermatol*. 2019;81(5):1037-1057.

James WD, Elston DM, Treat JR, Rosenbach MA, Neuhaus IM. *Andrews' Diseases of the Skin: Clinical Dermatology*. 13th ed. Elsevier; 2020.

Pascoe VL, Fenves AZ, Wofford J, Jackson JM, Menter A, Kimball AB. The spectrum of nephrocutaneous diseases and associations: Inflammatory and medication-related nephrocutaneous associations. *J Am Acad Dermatol*. 2016;74(2):247-270. quiz 271-272.

Rosen J, Darwin E, Tuchayi SM, Garibyan L, Yosipovitch G. Skin changes and manifestations associated with the treatment of obesity. *J Am Acad Dermatol*. 2019;81(5):1059-1069.

Wofford J, Fenves AZ, Jackson JM, Kimball AB, Menter A. The spectrum of nephrocutaneous diseases and associations: genetic causes of nephrocutaneous disease. *J Am Acad Dermatol*. 2016;74(2):231-244. quiz 245-246.

Appendix 4: Dermatology Diagnostics

Caroline A. Nelson, MD

Basic Concepts

- **Dermoscopy** refers to visualization of the skin using skin surface microscopy (epiluminoscopy or epiluminescence microscopy). It combines a high-quality magnifying lens with a powerful lighting system. Translucency of the *stratum corneum* is achieved either by placing fluid on the lesion or by using polarized light. Dermoscopy is associated with a significant decrease in the number of excised benign pigmented skin lesions and a significant increase in the number of excised melanomas.
- **Reflectance confocal microscopy (RCM)** refers to noninvasive *in vivo* visualization of the skin. Uses include evaluation of equivocal skin lesions to decrease the number of benign biopsies, presurgical cancer margin mapping, tumor recurrence surveillance, monitoring of ablative and noninvasive therapies, and stratification of inflammatory disorders.
- **Artificial intelligence (AI)** refers to the ability of a machine or computer program to solve problems typically handled by humans. **Augmented intelligence (AuI)**, focusing on AI's assistive role, is designed to enhance human intelligence and the physician-patient relationship rather than replace them. Studies have demonstrated superior skin cancer classification using the combination of dermatologists and AI than either alone, and improved malignancy prediction by dermatologists using AI.
- **Bedside diagnostics** refer to bedside procedures that often enable rapid and low-cost diagnosis.
- **Histopathology** refers to examination of tissue changes under a microscope.
- This appendix summarizes dermoscopy, bedside diagnostics, and histopathology, specifically histopathological bodies, special stains, immunohistochemical stains, molecular tests, and DIF patterns. RCM, AI, and AuI are beyond the scope of this appendix.

Dermoscopy

- Dermoscopy is founded on a **two-step algorithm: (1) classification of a lesion as melanocytic or nonmelanocytic and (2) classification of a melanocytic lesion as nevus, indeterminate, or melanoma.** For step 1, an **eight-level criterion ladder** has been proposed and is presented in Table A4.1. For step 2, **pattern analysis (modified)** is the most specific method and is presented in Table A4.2. **Dermoscopy of melanocytic lesions** is illustrated in Figures A4.1-A4.3. **Dermoscopy of nonmelanocytic lesions** is illustrated in Figure A4.4.
- **Dermoscopy of nonneoplastic disorders** is presented in Table A4.3.
- **Trichoscopy** (dermoscopy of the scalp and hair) is presented in Table A4.4 and illustrated in Figures A4.5, A4.6, and A4.7. Computerized trichometric analysis additionally measures and records density/cm² and average hair shaft diameters.

613

Table A4.1. EIGHT-LEVEL CRITERION LADDER

Level[a]	Dermoscopy Criteria
1. Melanocytic lesions	(a) Pigment network (exception: DF); (b) negative network; (c) angulated lines; (d) streaks; (e) aggregated globules; (f) peripheral globules; (g) homogeneous blue pigmentation; (h) pseudonetwork (facial skin); (i) parallel pigment pattern (palms and soles).
2. BCC	(a) Arborizing blood vessels; (b) spoke wheel-like structures; (c) leaflike areas; (d) large blue-gray ovoid nests; (e) multiple nonaggregated blue-gray globules; (f) ulceration; (g) shiny white blotches and strands.
3. SCC	(a) Focal glomerular vessels; (b) rosettes; (c) keratin pearls (white circles); (d) yellow scale; (e) brown dots aligned radially at the periphery.
4. SK	(a) Multiple (3+) milia-like cysts; (b) comedo-like openings; (c) gyri and sulci (fissures and ridges); (d) fingerprint-like structures[b]; (e) moth-eaten borders.[b]
5. Hemangioma/angioma/angiokeratoma	(a) Red lacunae; (b) blue lacunae; (c) black lacunae.
6. Blood vessels as seen in nonmelanocytic tumors	(a) Arborizing vessels; (b) glomerular vessels; (c) hairpin vessels with white halo; (d) crown vessels; (e) serpiginous or string of pearls; (f) "strawberry" pattern.
7. Blood vessels as seen in melanocytic tumors	(a) Comma-shaped vessels; (b) dotted vessels; (c) serpentine vessels (linear irregular); (d) corkscrew vessels; (e) polymorphous vessels; (f) milky-red areas and milky-red globules.
8. Structureless/featureless lesions or lesions with nonspecific/nondiagnostic features	No vessels noted.

BCC, basal cell carcinoma; DF, dermatofibroma; SCC, squamous cell carcinoma; SK, seborrheic keratosis.
[a]Illustrative examples provided.
[b]Shared features between early SK and solar lentigo.

Table A4.2. PATTERN ANALYSIS (MODIFIED)

Global Features

Pattern	Pigment Distribution/Variant	Association(s)
Reticular pattern	(1) Diffuse; (2) patchy; (3) central hyperpigmentation; (4) central hypopigmentation; (5) central globules.	Acquired melanocytic nevus, congenital melanocytic nevus.
Globular pattern	Cobblestone pattern.	Cobblestone pattern: congenital melanocytic nevus. Noncobblestone pattern: acquired melanocytic nevus, Spitz nevus.
Homogeneous pattern	Gray-blue.	Blue nevus.
	Brown.	Congenital melanocytic nevus (usually).
	Tan-pink.	Nevus in fair skin.
Starburst pattern	Peripheral globules in a tiered distribution.	Spitz/pigmented spindle cell nevus of Reed.
Two-component pattern		Acquired melanocytic nevus, congenital melanocytic nevus.
Multicomponent pattern		Atypical nevus, congenital melanocytic nevus, melanoma.
Parallel pattern		Acral nevus, melanoma.
Nonspecific pattern		Consider melanoma.

Local Features

Criteria	Variants	Association(s)
Pigment network	*Typical*: Light to dark brown. Minimal variation in line color, width, and distribution and hole size.	Benign melanocytic lesion.
	Atypical: Increased variability in line color, width, and distribution and hole size. Gray hues. Abrupt end at the periphery.	Atypical nevus, Spitz nevus, melanoma.

Table A4.2. PATTERN ANALYSIS (MODIFIED) (CONTINUED)		
Negative network	*Regular*: Symmetric.	Congenital melanocytic nevus, Spitz nevus, melanoma.
	Irregular: Diffuse or focal.	Spitz nevus, melanoma.
Dots	*Regular*: Located on top of, in the holes of, or in the center of a typical pigment network.	Benign melanocytic lesion.
	Irregular: Located at the periphery of an atypical pigment network or negative network.	Spitz nevus, melanoma.
Globules	*Regular*: Minimal variation in color, shape, and size; organized or symmetric central or peripheral distribution.	Benign melanocytic lesion.
	Irregular: Increased variability in globule color, shape, and size; asymmetric or focal distribution.	Spitz nevus, melanoma.
Streaks (pseudopods and radial streaming)	*Regular*: Radial projections at the periphery; distribution around the entire perimeter.	Spitz/pigmented spindle cell nevus of Reed.
	Irregular: Radial projections at the periphery; asymmetric, focal, or irregular distribution.	Spitz nevus, melanoma.
Blue-white veil over raised areas	*Regular*: Central location or homogeneous.	Blue nevus, Spitz nevus.
	Irregular: Asymmetric location or diffuse but with different hues.	Melanoma.
Regression structures (granularity and scar-like areas)[a]	*Regular*: Symmetric location (<10% of surface area).	Nevus.
	Irregular: Asymmetric location (>50% of surface area).	Melanoma.
Hypopigmented areas (structureless/homogeneous)	*Regular*: Central location.	Nevus.
	Irregular: Peripheral location (>10% of surface area).	Melanoma.
Blotch	*Regular*: 1 blotch; central location.	Acquired melanocytic nevus.
	Irregular: >1 blotch and/or peripheral location.	Melanoma.
Vascular structures[b]	*Regular*: Comma vessels.	Intradermal nevus, congenital melanocytic nevus.
	Irregular: Dotted vessels (over tan background suggests atypical nevus versus over milky-red background suggests Spitz nevus or amelanotic melanoma); serpentine (linear irregular) vessels; polymorphous vessels; corkscrew vessels (usually nodular melanoma, desmoplastic melanoma, melanoma metastasis).	Atypical nevus, Spitz nevus, melanoma.
Crystalline structures (shiny, white streaks)		Spitz nevus, melanoma.

Site-Related Features		
Site	Variants	Association(s)
Face	Typical pseudonetwork (round, equally sized network holes corresponding to the preexisting follicular ostia).	Benign melanocytic lesion.
	Annular-granular structures (multiple blue-gray dots surrounding the follicular ostia with an annular-granular appearance).	Melanoma.
	Gray pseudonetwork (gray pigmentation surrounding the follicular ostia, formed by the confluence of annular-granular structures).	Melanoma.
	Rhomboidal structures (gray-brown pigmentation surrounding the follicular ostia with a rhomboidal appearance).	Melanoma.
	Asymmetric pigmented follicles (eccentric annular pigmentation around follicular ostia).	Melanoma.

(Continued)

Table A4.2. PATTERN ANALYSIS (MODIFIED) (CONTINUED)

Palms and soles	Parallel furrow pattern (pigmentation following the *sulci superficiales*).	Acral nevus ("furrows are friendly").
	Lattice-like pattern (pigmentation following and crossing the furrows).	Acral nevus.
	Fibrillar pattern (numerous, finely pigmented filaments perpendicular to the furrows and ridges).	Acral nevus.
	Parallel ridge pattern (pigmentation aligned along the *cristae superficiales*).	Melanoma.

BCC, basal cell carcinoma; SCC, squamous cell carcinoma.

[a]Granularity and scar-like areas present together give the appearance of a blue-white veil over macular areas.

[b]The presence of a given vessel morphology is not specific. Dotted vessels can also be seen in nonmelanocytic skin lesions (eg, clear cell acanthoma, BCC, porokeratosis, SCC). Polymorphous vessels can also be seen in nonmelanocytic skin lesions (eg, BCC) and stasis dermatitis.

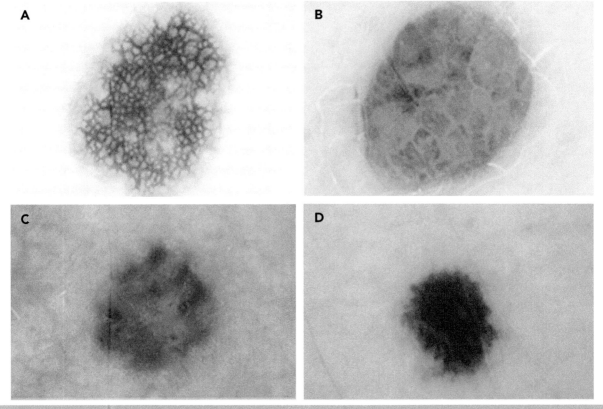

Figure A4.1. DERMOSCOPY OF MELANOCYTIC LESIONS: GLOBAL FEATURES. A, Reticular pattern (diffuse with perifollicular hypopigmentation): junctional nevus. B, Globular pattern (cobblestone): congenital melanocytic nevus. C, Homogeneous pattern (gray-blue): blue nevus. D, Starburst pattern (peripheral globules in a tiered distribution): Spitz nevus (pigmented spindle cell nevus of Reed).

(Images reprinted with permission from Markowitz O. A Practical Guide to Dermoscopy. Wolters Kluwer; 2017.)

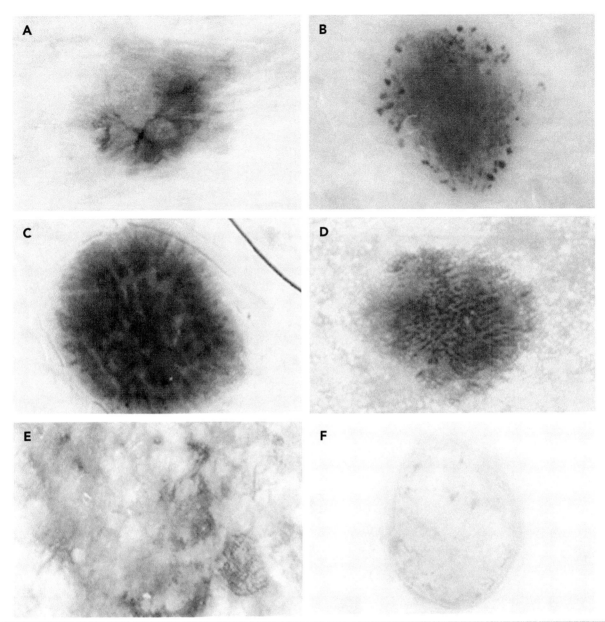

Figure A4.2. DERMOSCOPY OF MELANOCYTIC LESIONS: LOCAL FEATURES. A, Pigment network (atypical): MIS. The global pattern is reticular. B, Dots (irregular): MIS. The global pattern is homogenous. Pigment network (atypical) is another local feature of this lesion. C, Streaks (irregular): melanoma. The global pattern is homogenous. Pigment network (atypical), negative network (focal), and blue-white veil over raised areas (irregular) are other local features of this lesion. D, Blue-white veil over raised areas (regular): congenital melanocytic nevus. The global pattern is reticular. E, Regression structures (irregular): melanoma. The global pattern is reticular. F, Vessel structures (regular, comma): intradermal nevus. The global pattern is homogenous. MIS, melanoma in situ.

(Images reprinted with permission from Markowitz O. A Practical Guide to Dermoscopy. Wolters Kluwer; 2017.)

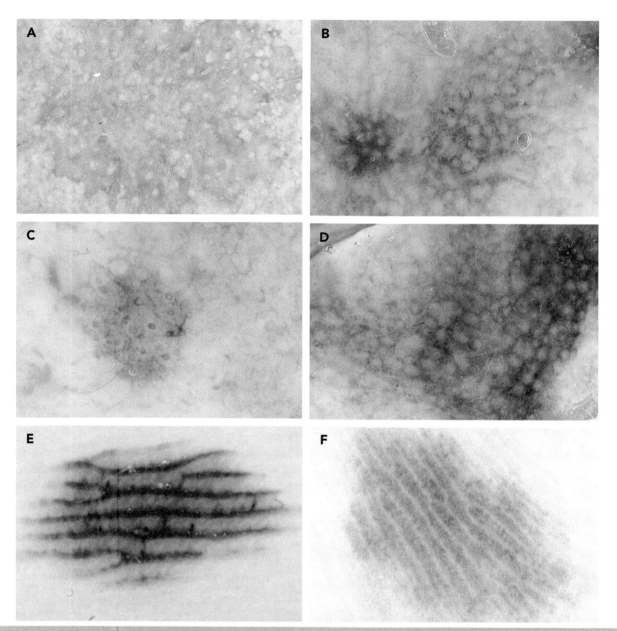

Figure A4.3. DERMOSCOPY OF MELANOCYTIC LESIONS: SITE-RELATED FEATURES. A, Typical pseudonetwork: solar lentigo on the face. B, Annular-granular structures: lentigo maligna on the face. C, Gray pseudonetwork: lentigo maligna on the face. Asymmetric pigmented follicles is another local feature of this lesion. D, Rhomboidal structures: lentigo maligna melanoma on the face. E, Parallel furrow pattern: acral nevus. F, Parallel ridge pattern: acral lentiginous melanoma.

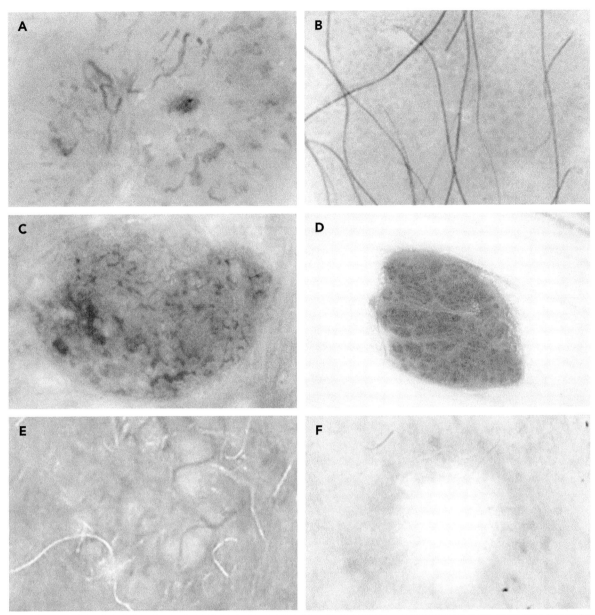

Figure A4.4. DERMOSCOPY OF NONMELANOCYTIC LESIONS. A, BCC. Arborizing blood vessels, large blue-gray ovoid nests, and multiple nonaggregated blue-gray globules are features of this lesion. B, SCC. Focal glomerular vessels is a feature of this lesion. C, SK. Multiple (3+) milia-like cysts, comedo-like openings, and gyri and sulci are features of this lesion. D, Cherry angioma. Red lacunae is a feature of this lesion. E, SGH. White-yellow lobular structures ("popcorn structures"), crown vessels, and central dell are features of this lesion. F, DF. Central crystalline structures with a typical pseudonetwork at the periphery are features of this lesion. BCC, basal cell carcinoma; DF, dermatofibroma; SCC, squamous cell carcinoma; SGH, sebaceous gland hyperplasia; SK, seborrheic keratosis.

(Images reprinted with permission from Markowitz O. A Practical Guide to Dermoscopy. Wolters Kluwer; 2017.)

Table A4.3. DERMOSCOPY OF NONNEOPLASTIC DISORDERS

Diagnosis[a]	Features[a]
Psoriasis (clear cell acanthoma)	White superficial scales and dotted vessels in a uniform distribution against a light red background ± red globular rings.
LP	White crossing streaks (Wickham striae) and dotted or linear vessels at the periphery.
Molluscum contagiosum	Central umbilication with polylobular white-yellow amorphous structures surrounded by arborizing vessels.
Scabies	"Delta-wing jet with contrail" sign: small dark brown triangular structure (corresponding to the anterior part of the mite) located at the end of a white line (corresponding to the burrow).

LP, lichen planus
[a]Illustrative examples provided.

Table A4.4. TRICHOSCOPY

Pattern[a]	Classic Description	Association(s)[a]
Hair Shaft Abnormalities With Increased Fragility		
Bubble hair	Large, unevenly spaced bubbles that enlarge and thin the hair shaft cortex, predisposing to fracture.	Heat styling.
Monilethrix	Uniform elliptical nodes with periodic constrictions of the hair shaft resembling a "regularly bended ribbon" or a "string of beads."	Hereditary.
Pili torti	Twisting and flattening of the hair shaft.	Ankyloblepharon–ectodermal defects–cleft lip/palate syndrome, Björnstad syndrome/Crandall syndrome, Menkes kinky hair disease, argininosuccinic aciduria/citrullinemia, anorexia nervosa, Bazex-Dupré-Christol syndrome. Iatrogenic: systemic retinoids.
Trichorrhexis invaginata	Intussusception of the distal hair shaft (ball) into the proximal hair shaft (socket) resulting in fracture. Before fracture, trichorrhexis invaginata resembles "bamboo." After fracture, the proximal hair shaft resembles a "golf tee."	Netherton syndrome.
Trichorrhexis nodosa	Incomplete transverse fracture of the hair shaft with frayed ends resembling "two paint brushes facing each other."	Most common hair shaft abnormality. Netherton syndrome, Menkes kinky hair disease, argininosuccinic aciduria/citrullinemia, mechanical injury.
Trichoschisis	Clean transverse fracture of the hair shaft.	Trichothiodystrophy with ichthyosis, mechanical injury.
Trichothiodystrophy	Alternating light and dark bands under polarizing light resembling a "tiger tail" under polarizing light.	Trichothiodystrophy with ichthyosis.
Hair Shaft Abnormalities Without Increased Fragility		
Acquired progressive kinking of the hair	Curled hair shaft.	AGA (early), HIV infection. Iatrogenic: systemic retinoids.
Loose anagen hair	Hair shaft with ruffled proximal cuticle, absent root sheath, and bent matrix. The proximal cuticle resembles a "crumpled sock."	Hereditary.
Pili annulati	Alternating bright and dark bands in the hair shaft with reflected light. Bright bands (due to abnormal air-filled cavities) appear paradoxically dark on light microscopy.	Hereditary. Pseudopili annulati is observed in blond hair.

Table A4.4. TRICHOSCOPY (CONTINUED)

Pattern[a]	Classic Description	Association(s)[a]
Pili bifurcati	Hair shaft exits the same follicle, divides into two branches (with individual cuticles), which subsequently fuse.	Hereditary.
Pili multigemini	Hair shafts (with individual IRS but shared ORS) exit the same dermal papilla.	Hereditary (favors beard distribution).
Pili trianguli et canaliculi	Hair shaft with triangular cross section and central linear groove due to premature keratinization of the IRS.	Ankyloblepharon–ectodermal defects–cleft lip/palate syndrome, uncombable hair syndrome.
Trichonodosis	Knots in the hair shaft.	Excessive combing or rustling of curly hair.
Trichoptilosis	Longitudinal splits originating at the free end of the hair shaft ("split ends").	Mechanical injury.
Woolly hair	Hair shaft with elliptical cross section and axial twisting ± trichorrhexis nodosa.	Carvajal syndrome/Naxos disease, cardiofaciocutaneous syndrome/Noonan syndrome, woolly hair nevus.

Miscellaneous Patterns

Black dots	Hair shaft remnants. Hair shafts are of diverse lengths.	Trichotillomania, tinea capitis (endothrix).
Brown halos	Perifollicular brown discoloration. Hair shafts are of diverse diameters.	AGA. In contrast, hair shafts in TE are of equal diameter.
Comma hairs	Ruptured hair shafts filled with hyphae with marked distal angulation.	Tinea capitis (ectothrix and endothrix).
Corkscrew hairs	Corkscrew-shaped hair shafts with perifollicular erythema or hemorrhage.	Vitamin C deficiency.
Exclamation point hairs	Short broken hair shafts that are narrower closer to the scalp.	AA.
Follicular red dots	Erythematous polycyclic, concentric structures regularly distributed in and around follicular ostia.	DLE. Perifollicular erythema is also observed at the periphery of FFA/LPP.
Hair casts	Cylindrical keratin rings (shed IRS) that slide freely along the hair shaft.	DLE, FFA/LPP (periphery). In contrast, nits do not slide freely along the hair shaft.
Pili recurvati	Hair shafts exit and then reenter the skin, causing a foreign body reaction ("ingrown hairs").	Pseudofolliculitis barbae.
Pohl-Pinkus constrictions	Periodic constrictions of the hair shaft that predispose to fracture.	AA, AE.
Rolled hairs	Hair shafts trapped in the *stratum corneum.*	KP, friction.
White dots	Discrete loss of melanin over scarred fibrotic tracts and perifollicular fibrosis.	FFA/LPP.
Yellow dots	Dilated follicular ostia containing keratin plugs.	AA.

AA, alopecia areata; AE, anagen effluvium; AGA, androgenetic alopecia; DLE, discoid lupus erythematosus; FFA, frontal fibrosing alopecia; HIV, human immunodeficiency virus; IRS, inner root sheath; KP, keratosis pilaris; LPP, lichen planopilaris; ORS, outer root sheath.
[a]Illustrative examples provided.

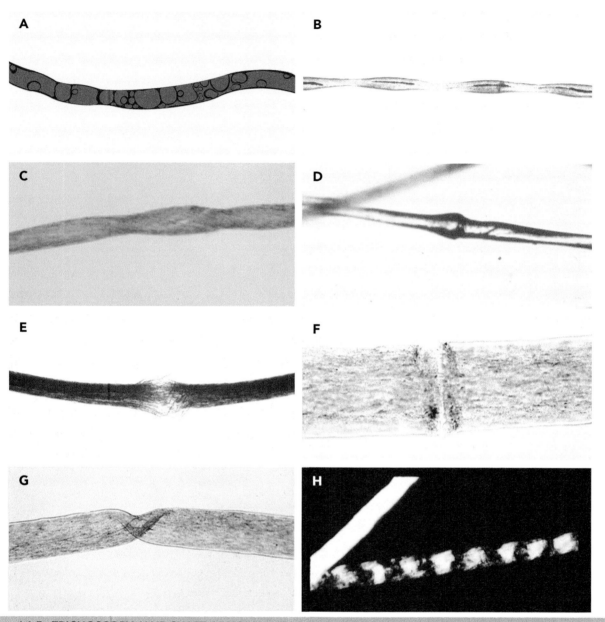

Figure A4.5. TRICHOSCOPY: HAIR SHAFT ABNORMALITIES WITH INCREASED HAIR FRAGILITY. A, Bubble hair. B, Monilethrix. C, Pili torti. D, Trichorrhexis invaginata. E, Trichorrhexis nodosa. F, Trichoschisis. G, Trichothiodystrophy. H, Trichothiodystrophy under polarizing light.

(A, Reprinted with permission from Hall BJ, Hall JC. *Sauer's Manual of Skin Diseases.* 11th ed. Wolters Kluwer; 2017. B and C, From Mirmirani P, Huang KP, Price VH. A practical, algorithmic approach to diagnosing hair shaft disorders. *Int J Dermatol.* 2011;50(1):1-12. Copyright © 2011 The International Society of Dermatology. Reprinted by permission of John Wiley & Sons, Inc. D, Courtesy of Kenneth E. Greer, MD, FAAD. From Gru AA, Wick MR, Mir A, et al. *Pediatric Dermatopathology and Dermatology.* Wolters Kluwer; 2018. E-H, From Mirmirani P, Huang KP, Price VH. A practical, algorithmic approach to diagnosing hair shaft disorders. *Int J Dermatol.* 2011;50(1):1-12. Copyright © 2011 The International Society of Dermatology. Reprinted by permission of John Wiley & Sons, Inc.)

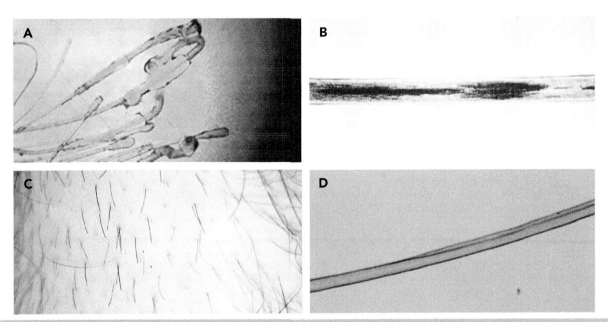

Figure A4.6. TRICHOSCOPY: HAIR SHAFT ABNORMALITIES WITHOUT INCREASED HAIR FRAGILITY. A, Loose anagen hair. B, Pili annulati. C, Pili multigemini. D, Pili trianguli et canaliculi.

(A, Courtesy of Barrett Zlotoff, MD. From Gru AA, Wick MR, Mir A, et al. *Pediatric Dermatopathology and Dermatology.* Wolters Kluwer; 2018. B and D, From Mirmirani P, Huang KP, Price VH. A practical, algorithmic approach to diagnosing hair shaft disorders. *Int J Dermatol.* 2011;50(1):1-12. Copyright © 2011. The International Society of Dermatology. Reprinted by permission of John Wiley & Sons, Inc.)

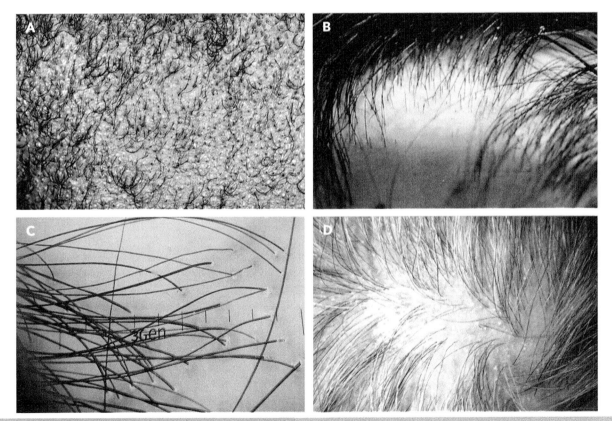

Figure A4.7. TRICHOSCOPY: MISCELLANEOUS PATTERNS. A, Black dots in endothrix tinea capitis. B, Exclamation point hairs in AA. C, Perifollicular erythema and hair casts at the periphery in FFA. D, White dots at the center in LPP. AA, alopecia areata; FFA, frontal fibrosing alopecia; LPP, lichen planopilaris.

(A, Courtesy of Anne W. Lucky, MD. From Marino BS, Fine KS. *Blueprints Pediatrics.* 7th ed. Wolters Kluwer; 2019. B, Reprinted with permission from Elder DE, Elenitsas R, Rubin AI, et al. *Atlas and Synopsis of Lever's Histopathology of the Skin.* 3rd ed. Wolters Kluwer Health/Lippincott Williams & Wilkins; 2012. D, Reprinted with permission from Edward S, Yung A. *Essential Dermatopathology.* Wolters Kluwer Health/Lippincott Williams & Wilkins; 2011.)

Bedside Diagnostics (Table A4.5, Figure A4.8)

Table A4.5. BEDSIDE DIAGNOSTICS			
Bedside Diagnostic[a]	Description	Finding	Associations(s)[a]
Microscopy			
FNA	Fix mass with nondominant hand, cleanse, advance 23-25 gauge needle, apply suction to syringe, move needle tip back and forth, release suction, remove needle, express contents onto glass slide, spread with another glass slide, air-dry, fix with 10% formalin for 15 minutes, stain with AFB stain (eg, Ziehl-Neelsen), apply coverslip.	AFB.	TB.
Gentle hair pull test	Gently pull the hair (unwashed for 24 hours), set onto glass slide, apply coverslip.	≥2 telogen hairs.	TE.
Gram stain (Brown-Brenn)	Cleanse, obtain specimen, smear onto glass slide, air-dry or heat, apply crystal violet then rinse after 30-60 seconds, apply Gram iodine then rinse after 30-60 seconds, apply decolorizer (eg, acetone, alcohol) until runoff is clear, apply safranin (counterstain) then rinse after 30-60 seconds, air-dry, apply coverslip.	GP bacteria (purple).	GP bacterial infections (eg, impetigo).
		GN bacteria (red).	GN bacterial infections (eg, ecthyma gangrenosum).
"Jelly roll" preparation	Peel or scrape off blister roof with blade, wrap around cotton swab and place in sterile saline, process section in cryostat, stain with H&E, apply coverslip.	Intraepidermal split.	SSSS.
		Subepidermal split.	SJS/TEN.
KOH	Wipe with alcohol, scrape scale or unroofed pustule with a #15 scalpel at (perpendicular angle), smear contents onto glass slide, apply one drop of 10%-20% KOH (helps dissolve background keratinocytes), apply coverslip, gently heat (if no other dissolving agents such as dimethyl sulfoxide are present), lower condenser to reduce microscope illumination until epithelial cells are clearly visible. Combination of KOH with chlorazol black E (chitin-specific) turns fungal elements green. Combination of KOH with Parker blue ink (Swartz-Lamkins) turns fungal elements blue. Calcofluor white (binds cellulose and chitin) fluoresces under UVR (most sensitive). KOH "crush preparation" of cut hair shafts can diagnose piedra.	Monomorphic, cuboidal, pathognomonic 30-35 μm virally transformed cells.	Molluscum contagiosum.
		Variable fungi.	Fungal infections (eg, TV, tinea nigra, piedra, tinea, tinea capitis, onychomycosis, candidiasis, dimorphic fungal infections, angioinvasive fungal infections).
		Demodex mites.	Rosacea/pityriasis folliculorum/steroid-induced rosacea, demodicosis.
Mineral oil preparation	Dip #15 scalpel in mineral oil, scrape skin vigorously, smear scale onto glass slide, apply coverslip. To increase diagnostic yield, obtain multiple specimens.	*Demodex* mites.	Rosacea/pityriasis folliculorum/steroid-induced rosacea, demodicosis.
		Sarcoptes scabiei mites, eggs, feces (scybala).	Scabies.
"Scotch tape" test	Press the adhesive side of a piece of transparent tape to the skin around the anus as soon as the patient awakens.	Pinworms, eggs.	Pinworm infection.
Skin snip	Pierce nonlesional skin with needle, tent up, snip off small piece with scalpel, place onto glass slide in one drop of normal saline, incubate at room temperature for 24 hours, apply coverslip.	Elongated, motile round worm.	Onchocerciasis.
Slit-skin	Cleanse, pinch skin, make small linear incision, scrape wound to obtain 5-7-mm sample of dermis and fluid, smear onto glass slide, air-dry, fix with 10% formalin for 15 minutes, stain with AFB stain (eg, Ziehl-Neelsen), apply coverslip. To increase diagnostic yield, obtain multiple specimens.	AFB.	Leprosy.
Touch preparation	Smear base of punch biopsy specimen or tissue scraped from wound base on glass slide, stain, apply coverslip.	Variable bacteria (Gram stain).	Bacterial infections (eg, ecthyma gangrenosum).
		Variable fungi (KOH).	Fungal infections (eg, angioinvasive fungal infections).
		Leishman-Donovan bodies (Wright-Giemsa).	Leishmaniasis.

Table A4.5. BEDSIDE DIAGNOSTICS (CONTINUED)

Bedside Diagnostic[a]	Description	Finding	Associations(s)[a]
Tzanck smear	Cleanse, scrape base of unroofed crust or vesicle with #15 scalpel, smear contents onto glass slide, air-dry, stain with Wright-Giemsa (or other commercially available kit), apply coverslip.	Acantholytic epidermal cells within the blister cavity.	Pemphigus.
		Multinucleated keratinocytes with nuclear molding and margination of basophilic chromatin to the periphery ("eggshell chromatin") ("3 Ms").	HSV, VZV.
		Monomorphic, cuboidal, pathognomonic 30-35 μm virally transformed cells.	Molluscum contagiosum.
		Encapsulated 5-10 μm round, dark-walled, pleomorphic yeast with clear gelatinous capsules (India ink preparation).	Cryptococcosis.
		Demodex mites.	Rosacea/pityriasis folliculorum/steroid-induced rosacea, demodicosis.
	"Thick drop method" (modified Tzanck smear): nick lesional inflamed border with #15 scalpel, drop blood onto glass slide, air-dry, stain with Wright-Giemsa, apply coverslip.	Leishman-Donovan bodies.	Leishmaniasis.
Wright stain	Cleanse, scrape base of unroofed pustule with #15 scalpel, smear contents onto glass slide, air-dry, stain with Wright, apply coverslip.	Neutrophils > eosinophils.	Transient neonatal pustular melanosis.
		Eosinophils > neutrophils.	Erythema toxicum neonatorum.
Miscellaneous			
Diascopy	Apply pressure with glass slide.	Blanching.	Erythema, venous lake.
		Apple jelly color.	LMDF, sarcoidosis, lupus vulgaris, leishmaniasis recidivans.
DTM	Place specimen in Sabouraud dextrose agar with cycloheximide, gentamicin, and chlortetracycline (retard growth of contaminant organisms) and phenol red (pH indicator).	Color change from amber to red.	Dermatophytes (alkaline by-products).
		Color change from amber to yellow.	Nondermatophytes (acid by-products).
Wood's lamp	Illuminate with light source containing nickel oxide–doped glass (365 nm peak).	Enhanced contrast between hypomelanosis and amelanosis.	Vitiligo.
		Coral red fluorescence.	Erythrasma.
		Orange fluorescence.	TV.
		Variable fluorescence, most often blue-green.	Fluorescent ectothrix tinea capitis, favus.

AFB, acid-fast bacilli; DTM, dermatophyte test medium; FNA, fine needle aspiration; GN, gram-negative; GP, gram-positive; H&E, hematoxylin and eosin; HSV, herpes simplex virus; KOH, potassium hydroxide; LMDF, lupus miliaris disseminatus faciei; SJS, Stevens-Johnson syndrome; SSSS, staphylococcal scalded skin syndrome; TB, tuberculosis; TE, telogen effluvium; TEN, toxic epidermal necrolysis; TV, tinea versicolor; UVR, ultraviolet light; VZV, varicella zoster virus.
[a]Illustrative examples provided.

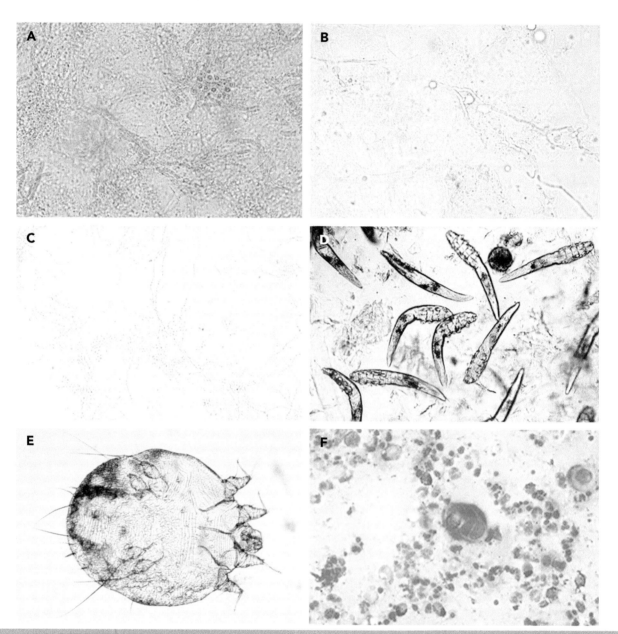

Figure A4.8. BEDSIDE DIAGNOSTICS A, KOH: TV. B, KOH: tinea. C, KOH: candidiasis. D, Mineral oil preparation: *Demodex folliculorum*. E, Mineral oil preparation: *Sarcoptes scabiei* var. *hominis* (itch mite). F, Tzanck smear: viral herpetic infection. KOH, potassium hydroxide; TV, tinea versicolor.

(A, Reprinted with permission from Goodheart HP. *Goodheart's Photoguide to Common Skin Disorders: Diagnosis and Management.* 3rd ed. Wolters Kluwer Health/Lippincott Williams & Wilkins; 2009. B and C, Reprinted with permission from Goodheart HP. *Goodheart's Photoguide of Common Skin Disorders: Diagnosis and Management.* 2nd ed. Lippincott Williams & Wilkins; 2003. D, Courtesy of Margaret Bobonich, DNP, FNP-C, DCNP, FAANP. From Bobonich MA, Nolen ME, Honaker J, et al. *Dermatology for Advanced Practice Clinicians: A Comprehensive Guide to Diagnosis and Treatment.* 2nd ed. Wolters Kluwer; 2021. E, Reprinted with permission from Craft N, Fox LP, Goldsmith LA, et al. *VisualDx: Essential Adult Dermatology.* Wolters Kluwer Health/Lippincott Williams & Wilkins; 2010. F, Reprinted with permission from Hall BJ, Hall JC. *Sauer's Manual of Skin Diseases.* 11th ed. Wolters Kluwer; 2017.)

Histopathology

Histopathological Bodies (Table A4.6)

Table A4.6. HISTOPATHOLOGICAL BODIES

Body[a]	Classic Description	Association(s)[a]
Actin bodies	Round intracytoplasmic inclusion bodies (stain red with H&E and Masson trichrome; stain purple with PTAH; positive for SMA).	Infantile digital fibroma.
Asteroid bodies	Eosinophilic "starburst" inclusions in giant cells.	Sarcoidosis.
	Pleomorphic yeast ± a Splendore-Hoeppli reaction.	Sporotrichosis.
"Caterpillar bodies"	Hyaline globules in the epidermis (PAS positive, diastase resistant).	Porphyria.
Colloid bodies (Civatte bodies, cytoid bodies, hyaline bodies)	Apoptotic keratinocytes (PAS positive, diastase resistant).	Lichenoid interface dermatitis.
Cowdry A bodies	Eosinophilic intranuclear inclusion bodies surrounded by a halo.	HSV, VZV.
Cowdry B bodies	Homogenous amphophilic glassy intranuclear inclusion bodies surrounded by a halo.	CMV ("owl's eyes"), poliovirus.
Donovan bodies	Bipolar ("safety pin"–shaped) intracellular inclusions on Giemsa and Warthin-Starry stains.	Granuloma inguinale.
Gamna-Favre bodies	Large intracytoplasmic basophilic inclusion bodies in endothelial cells.	LGV.
Guarnieri bodies	Eosinophilic cytoplasmic inclusion bodies (± eosinophilic intranuclear inclusion bodies).	Poxvirus infections.
Henderson-Patterson bodies (molluscum bodies)	Eosinophilic-to-basophilic cytoplasmic inclusion bodies.	Molluscum contagiosum.
Kamino bodies	Pink bodies derived from the basement membrane.	Spitz nevus.
Leishman-Donovan bodies	Protozoa randomly spaced within histiocytes or lining the periphery of intracellular histiocyte vacuoles.	Leishmaniasis.
Medlar bodies	Pigmented clumps of dematiaceous organisms ("copper pennies") highlighted by Fontana-Masson stain.	Chromoblastomycosis.
Michaelis-Gutmann bodies	Basophilic inclusions within foamy histiocytes that are round or ovoid and homogenous or targetoid due to concentric laminations. PAS positive, diastase resistant, and von Kossa positive.	Malakoplakia.
Palmoplantar wart bodies	Eosinophilic cytoplasmic and nuclear inclusion bodies.	Palmoplantar warts.
Papillary mesenchymal bodies	Dense round or oval aggregates of fibroblastic cells.	Trichoepithelioma, trichoblastoma.
Russell bodies	Plasma cells containing brightly eosinophilic Ig ("pregnant plasma cells") within foamy histiocytes.	Rhinoscleroma.
Psammoma bodies	Concentric calcifications.	Schwannoma (psammomatous melanotic), thyroid carcinoma (papillary), ovarian adenocarcinoma.
Pustulo-ovoid bodies of Milian	Large eosinophilic lysosomal granules surrounded by a clear halo.	GCT.
Schaumann bodies	Cytoplasmic, laminated calcifications,	Sarcoidosis.
Verocay bodies	Parallel rows of nuclei separated by acellular areas ("zebra stripes").	Schwannoma.

CMV, cytomegalovirus; GCT, granular cell tumor; H&E, hematoxylin and eosin; HSV, herpes simplex virus; Ig, immunoglobulin; LGV, lymphogranuloma venereum; PAS, periodic acid-Schiff; PTAH, phosphotungstic acid hematoxylin; SMA, smooth muscle actin; VZV, varicella zoster virus.
[a]Illustrative examples provided.

Special Stains (Table A4.7)

	Table A4.7. SPECIAL STAINS		
Stain	Color	Target(s)	Association(s)[a]
Alcian blue (pH 2.5)	Light blue	Mucin (acid mucopolysaccharides)	LE, DM, palisading granulomas, mucinoses (eg, NSF/scleromyxedema/scleredema), neoplasms (eg, BCC, pleomorphic fibroma, sclerotic fibroma [±]), digital mucous cyst.
Alcian blue (pH 0.5)	Blue	Mucin (sulfated mucopolysaccharides)	
Alizarin red	Red	Calcium	Calciphylaxis.
Chloroacetate esterase (Leder stain)	Red	Myeloid cells	AML.
		Mast cells	Mastocytosis.
Colloidal iron	Blue	Mucin (acid mucopolysaccharides)	LE, DM, palisading granulomas, mucinoses (eg, NSF/scleromyxedema/scleredema), neoplasms (eg, BCC, pleomorphic fibroma, sclerotic fibroma [±]), digital mucous cyst.
Congo red	"Brick red" with "apple green" birefringence under polarized light	Amyloid	Amyloidosis.
Crystal violet	Metachromatically purple with blue background	Mucin (acid mucopolysaccharides)	LE, DM, palisading granulomas, mucinoses (eg, NSF/scleromyxedema/scleredema), neoplasms (eg, BCC, pleomorphic fibroma, sclerotic fibroma [±]), digital mucous cyst.
		Amyloid	Amyloidosis.
Fite-Faraco	Red	AFB organisms	*Nocardia* species, mycobacterial infections (eg, TB, leprosy).
Fontana-Masson (argentaffin)	Black	Melanin	EDP, antimalarial pigmentation, minocycline pigmentation (types 2 and 3), dematiaceous fungal infections (eg, tinea nigra, chromoblastomycosis, eumycotic mycetoma). In vitiligo, Fontana-Masson may demonstrate a contrast with melanocytes in normal surrounding skin.
Giemsa	Blue	Nuclei of cells, microorganisms	Granuloma inguinale, histoplasmosis, leishmaniasis.
	Metachromatically purple.	Mast cell granules	Mastocytosis.
GMS	Black	Fungal cell walls (primarily)	Actinomycosis, fungal infections (eg, TV, tinea, tinea capitis, onychomycosis, candidiasis, blastomycosis, chromoblastomycosis, paracoccidioidomycosis, coccidioidomycosis, histoplasmosis, penicilliosis, cryptococcosis, lobomycosis, sporotrichosis, aspergillosis, zygomycosis), protothecosis, rhinosporidiosis.
Gram (Brown-Brenn)	Purple	GP bacteria	GP bacterial infections (eg, impetigo).
	Red	GN bacteria	GN bacterial infections (eg, ecthyma gangrenosum).
India ink	Purple yeast surrounded by a clear capsule with a dark background	Yeast	Cryptococcosis.
Masson trichrome	Blue-green	Collagen	RPD.
	Red	Smooth muscle	Infantile digital fibroma (actin bodies), leiomyoma/leiomyosarcoma.
Methyl violet	Metachromatically purple	Amyloid	Amyloidosis.
MPO	Orange	Immature myeloid cells	Histiocytoid Sweet syndrome (granules), AML. Negative in BPDCN.
Mucicarmine	Red	Sialomucin	Cryptococcosis (capsule), neoplasms (eg, MPD/EMPD, mucinous carcinoma, mixed tumor, adenoid cystic carcinoma, colon adenocarcinoma, mucinous ovarian adenocarcinoma), and mucocele.
Oil Red O	Red	Lipids	Neutral lipid storage disease with ichthyosis.
Pagoda red	Red	Amyloid	Amyloidosis.

Table A4.7. SPECIAL STAINS (CONTINUED)

Stain	Color	Target(s)	Association(s)[a]
PAS (diastase sensitive)	Magenta with a green background	Glycogen	SCC (clear cells), clear cell acanthoma, poroma (clear cells), syringoma (clear cell), trichilemmoma, RCC (clear cell).
PAS (diastase resistant)	Magenta with green background	Apoptotic keratinocytes	Lichenoid interface dermatitis (colloid bodies).
		Cryoprecipitates/ paraprotein	Cryoglobulinemia.
		Foreign bodies	Selected foreign body granulomas (eg, starch, wood splinter).
		Amyloid	Amyloidosis.
		Hyaline material (eg, basement membrane)	Lipoid proteinosis, porphyria (caterpillar bodies), malakoplakia (Michaelis-Gutmann bodies), Spitz nevus (Kamino bodies), hyaline fibromatosis syndrome, glomeruloid hemangioma (eosinophilic globules), KS (hyaline globules), cylindroma/spiradenoma (hyaline droplets), hidradenoma (hyaline sheath), poroma (hyaline sheath), syringoma (hyaline sheath), trichilemmoma (basement membrane).
		Organisms	Fungal infections (eg, TV, tinea, tinea capitis, onychomycosis, candidiasis, blastomycosis, chromoblastomycosis, paracoccidioidomycosis, coccidioidomycosis, histoplasmosis, penicilliosis, cryptococcosis (capsule), lobomycosis, sporotrichosis, aspergillosis, zygomycosis), prototheccosis, rhinosporidiosis.
		Granular cells	GCT.
		Sialomucin	Cryptococcosis (capsule), neoplasms (eg, MPD/EMPD, mucinous carcinoma, mixed tumor, adenoid cystic carcinoma, colon adenocarcinoma, mucinous ovarian adenocarcinoma), and mucocele.
Perls Prussian blue	Blue	Iron (hemosiderin, ferric ions)	Pigmented purpura, antimalarial pigmentation, minocycline pigmentation (types 1 and 2). Negative in black heel and palm.
PTAH	Purple	Actin	Infantile digital fibroma (actin bodies).
Sirius red	Red	Amyloid	Amyloidosis.
Sudan black	Black	Lipids	Neutral lipid storage disease with ichthyosis.
Thioflavin T	Yellow-green by fluorescence microscopy	Amyloid	Amyloidosis.
Toluidine blue	Metachromatically purple	Mucin (acid mucopolysaccharides)	LE, DM, palisading granulomas, mucinoses (eg, NSF/ scleromyxedema/scleredema), neoplasms (eg, BCC, pleomorphic fibroma, sclerotic fibroma [±]), digital mucous cyst.
		Mast cell granules	Mastocytosis.
Truant (auramine-rhodamine)	Yellow-green by fluorescence microscopy	AFB organisms	*Nocardia* species, mycobacterial infections (eg, TB, leprosy).
Von Kossa	Black	Calcium salts	PXE, calciphylaxis, malakoplakia (Michaelis-Gutmann bodies), hyaline fibromatosis syndrome.
VVG (Weigert)	Pink-red	Collagen	Morphea/SSc (parallel array), EPS, PXE, dermatomyofibroma.
	Black	Elastin	
	Yellow	Muscle, nerves	
Warthin-Starry (modified Steiner)	Black	Bacteria	Rhinoscleroma, *Bartonella* infections (eg, cat scratch disease), spirochete infections (eg, Lyme disease, syphilis), granuloma inguinale.
Ziehl-Neelsen	Red	AFB organisms	*Nocardia* species, mycobacterial infections (eg, TB, leprosy).

AFB, acid-fast bacillus; AML, acute myeloid leukemia; BCC, basal cell carcinoma; BPDCN, blastic plasmacytoid dendritic cell neoplasm; DM, dermatomyositis; EDP, erythema dyschromicum perstans; EMPD, extramammary Paget disease; EPS, elastosis perforans serpiginosa; GCT, granular cell tumor; GMS, Grocott-Gomori methenamine silver; GN, gram-negative; GP, gram-positive; KS, Kaposi sarcoma; LE, lupus erythematosus; MMS, Mohs micrographic surgery; MPD, mammary Paget disease; MPO, myeloperoxidase; NSF, nephrogenic systemic fibrosis; PAS, periodic acid-Schiff; PTAH, phosphotungstic acid hematoxylin; PXE, pseudoxanthoma elasticum; RPD, reactive perforating dermatosis; SCC, squamous cell carcinoma; SSc, systemic sclerosis; TB, tuberculosis; TV, tinea versicolor; VVG, Verhoeff-van Gieson.
[a]Illustrative examples provided.

Immunohistochemical Stains (Table A4.8)

Table A4.8. IMMUNOHISTOCHEMICAL STAINS	
Stain	Association(s)[a]
Adipophilin	Xanthomas, sebaceous adenoma/sebaceoma/sebaceous carcinoma.
ALK-1	Secondary C-ALCL (nodal). Negative in primary C-ALCL.
Amyloid P protein	Amyloidosis.
Androgen receptor	BCC, sebaceous adenoma/sebaceoma/sebaceous carcinoma. Negative in trichoepithelioma.
BCL2	BCC (diffuse), trichoepithelioma (periphery), PCMZL. Negative in PCFCL (positive in secondary cutaneous involvement).
BCL6	PCFCL. Negative in PCMZL.
BerEP4	BCC, trichoepithelioma. Negative in MAC.
βF1	SPTCL, extranodal NK/T-cell lymphoma, nasal type (includes HV-like CTCL). Negative PCGD-TCL.
CA-125	Ovarian adenocarcinoma.
Calcitonin	Thyroid carcinoma (medullary).
CAM5.2	MPD/EMPD, intraepithelial porocarcinoma (±).
β-catenin	Desmoid tumor.
CD1a	LCH, indeterminate cell histiocytosis, leishmaniasis.
CD2	MF, extranodal NK/T-cell lymphoma, nasal type (includes HV-like CTCL).
CD3	MF, Sézary syndrome, ATLL, extranodal NK/T-cell lymphoma, nasal type (includes HV-like CTCL) (±), PCGD-TCL. Negative in AML and BPDCN.
CD4	Parapsoriasis, PLC, MF, Sézary syndrome, ATLL, extranodal NK/T-cell lymphoma, nasal type (includes HV-like CTCL) (±). Negative in SPTCL and PCGD-TCL.
CD5	Sézary syndrome. Loss in MF.
CD7	Loss in MF. Negative in Sézary syndrome.
CD8	PLEVA, SPTCL, extranodal NK/T-cell lymphoma, nasal type (includes HV-like CTCL) (±), CLH with T-cell predominance. Negative in MF (except pagetoid reticulosis variant), ATLL, and PCGD-TCL.
CD10	AFX, PCFCL (follicular), ALL, RCC. Negative in PCFCL (diffuse).
CD20	PCMZL, PCFCL, PCDLBL-LT, intravascular large B-cell lymphoma. Negative in AML, ALL (±).
CD22	ALL.
CD35	ATLL.
CD30	MF (±, large cell transformation), Sézary syndrome (±), C-ALCL, LyP.
CD31	DDA, KS, angiosarcoma.
CD34	Morphea/SSc (loss), NSF/scleromyxedema, DFSP, epithelioid sarcoma, lipoma (spindle cell, pleomorphic), KS, angiosarcoma, trichilemmoma, ALL. Negative in scar/hypertrophic scar/keloid and DF.
CD45RO	Sézary syndrome, AML.
CD56	MCC, extranodal NK/T-cell lymphoma, nasal type (includes HV-like CTCL), PCGD-TCL, BPDCN.
CD68	Non-LCHs, AFX, GCT.
CD79a	PCMZL, PCFCL, PCDLBL-LT, intravascular large B-cell lymphoma, ALL.
CD117 (c-KIT)	AML, mastocytosis.
CD123	LE, BPDCN.
CD163	Non-LCHs.
CD207 (Langerin)	LCH (Birbeck granules).

Table A4.8. IMMUNOHISTOCHEMICAL STAINS (CONTINUED)

Stain	Association(s)[a]
CDX2	Colon adenocarcinoma.
CEA	MPD (±)/EMPD (±), sebaceous carcinoma, intraepithelial porocarcinoma, syringoma, MAC, colon adenocarcinoma, breast adenocarcinoma, lung carcinoma. Negative in BCC.
CK7	MPD/EMPD (use in MMS), SCCis/SCC, sebaceous carcinoma, mucinous carcinoma (primary cutaneous), breast adenocarcinoma., ovarian adenocarcinoma (mucinous), lung carcinoma. Negative in MCC and colon adenocarcinoma (rectal adenocarcinoma [±]).
CK20	EMPD (secondary), MCC (perinuclear dot pattern), trichoepithelioma, colon adenocarcinoma, ovarian adenocarcinoma (mucinous). Negative in BCC, syringoma, mucinous carcinoma (primary cutaneous), breast adenocarcinoma, and lung carcinoma including SCLC (oat cell carcinoma).
Pan-CK	SCC, epithelioid sarcoma.
CMV	CMV infection.
Collagen IV	Glomus tumor, GVM.
COX-1	Scar < hypertrophic scar < keloid.
CRTC1/MAML2	Hidradenoma.
Cytotoxic phenotype (granzyme B+, perforin+, TIA-1+)	Extranodal NK/T-cell lymphoma, nasal type (includes HV-like CTCL), PCGD-TCL.
Desmin	Leiomyoma/leiomyosarcoma. Negative in glomus tumor and GVM.
DNA mismatch repair proteins (MLH1, MSH2, MSH6, PMS2)	Loss in sebaceous adenoma/sebaceoma/sebaceous carcinoma associated with MTS.
EMA	SCC, MPD/EMPD, schwannoma (perineural capsule), sebaceous adenoma/sebaceoma/sebaceous carcinoma, intraepithelial porocarcinoma, syringoma, MAC, breast adenocarcinoma. Negative in BCC.
ER/PR	Breast adenocarcinoma (±).
ERG	Angiosarcoma.
Factor VIII	KS, angiosarcoma (±).
Factor XIIIa	NSF/scleromyxedema, non-LCHs, angiofibroma, DF. Negative in scar/hypertrophic scar/keloid and DFSP.
FcγRII	IH.
FLI1	Angiosarcoma.
Fumarate hydratase	Loss in leiomyoma/leiomyosarcoma associated with HLRCC.
GCDFP-15	EMPD (primary), breast adenocarcinoma.
GLUT-1	IH. Negative in RICH/PICH/NICH.
HER-2/Neu	MPD/EMPD.
HHV-8 (LNA-1)	KS. Negative in KHE.
HMB-45	Nevocellular nevus (top heavy), atypical nevus, Spitz nevus, melanoma (strong staining throughout). In vitiligo, HMB-45 may demonstrate a contrast with melanocytes in normal surrounding skin.
HSV	Herpes simplex, eczema herpeticum.
INI1	Negative in epithelioid sarcoma.
κ or λ restriction	PCMZL.
Lewis Y antigen	IH.

(Continued)

Table A4.8. IMMUNOHISTOCHEMICAL STAINS (CONTINUED)

Stain	Association(s)[a]
Lysozyme	AML.
Melan-A (MART-1)	Nevocellular nevus, atypical nevus, Spitz nevus, melanoma (use in MMS). In vitiligo, melan-A (MART-1) may demonstrate a contrast with melanocytes in normal surrounding skin.
Merosin	IH.
MITF	Nevocellular nevus, atypical nevus, Spitz nevus, melanoma (including desmoplastic melanoma). In vitiligo, MITF may demonstrate a contrast with melanocytes in normal surrounding skin.
MUM1	PCDLBL-LT.
Neuroendocrine markers (eg, bombesin, chromogranin, synaptophysin)	MCC.
Neurofilament	Neurofibroma, MCC. Negative in schwannoma.
Neuron-specific enolase	MCC.
NKIC3	Neurothekeoma (cellular).
p16 (CDKN2A)	Nevocellular nevus, atypical nevus, Spitz nevus. Negative or diminished in atypical Spitz nevus and negative in melanoma.
p63	MCC.
PGP9.5	Neurothekeoma (cellular).
PHLDA1	Trichoepithelioma. Negative in BCC.
Podoplanin (D2-40)	LM, KS, angiosarcoma (lymphatic differentiation).
PRAME	Melanoma. Negative in nevocellular nevus, atypical nevus, and Spitz nevus.
Procollagen-1	NSF/scleromyxedema, DFSP.
PSA	Prostate adenocarcinoma.
PTEN	Loss in trichilemmoma associated with Cowden syndrome.
S100	LCH, indeterminate cell histiocytosis, Rosai-Dorfman disease, nevocellular nevus, atypical nevus, Spitz nevus, melanoma (including desmoplastic melanoma), neurofibroma, schwannoma, GCT, neurothekeoma (myxoid), intraepithelial porocarcinoma (±). In vitiligo, S100 may demonstrate a contrast with melanocytes in normal surrounding skin. Negative in neurothekeoma (cellular).
S100A6	Neurothekeoma (cellular).
SMA	Myofibroma, dermatomyofibroma, infantile digital fibroma (actin bodies), infantile myofibromatosis, glomus tumor, GVM, leiomyoma/leiomyosarcoma.
SOX10	Nevocellular nevus, atypical nevus, Spitz nevus, melanoma (including desmoplastic melanoma), neurofibroma. In vitiligo, SOX10 may demonstrate a contrast with melanocytes in normal surrounding skin.
Spike glycoprotein	COVID-19.
Stromelysin-3	Angiofibroma, DF. Negative in DFSP.
TdT	ALL.
Thyroglobulin	Thyroid carcinoma.
Treponema pallidum	Syphilis.
Tryptase	Mastocytosis.
TTF-1	Thyroid carcinoma, SCLC (oat cell carcinoma). Negative in MCC.
Ulex europaeus lectin	KS, angiosarcoma.

Table A4.8. IMMUNOHISTOCHEMICAL STAINS (CONTINUED)	
Stain	**Association(s)[a]**
Vimentin	DFSP, AFX, epithelioid sarcoma, glomus tumor, GVM, leiomyoma/leiomyosarcoma.
VZV	Varicella, herpes zoster.

AFX, atypical fibroxanthoma; ALK-1, anaplastic lymphoma–related tyrosine kinase; ALL, acute lymphoblastic leukemia; AML, acute myeloid leukemia; ATLL, adult T-cell leukemia/lymphoma; BCC, basal cell carcinoma; BCL2, B-cell lymphoma 2; BCL6, B-cell lymphoma 6; BPDCN, blastic plasmacytoid dendritic cell neoplasm; CA-125, cancer antigen 125; C-ALCL, cutaneous anaplastic large cell lymphoma; CD, cluster of differentiation; CDKN2A, cyclin-dependent kinase inhibitor 2A; CDX2, caudal-type homeobox 2; CEA, carcinoembryonic antigen; CK, cytokeratin; CLH, cutaneous lymphoid hyperplasia; CMV, cytomegalovirus; COVID-19; coronavirus disease 2019; COX-1, cyclooxygenase 1; CRTC1, CREB-regulated transcription coactivator; CTCL, cutaneous T-cell lymphoma; DDA, diffuse dermal angiomatosis; DF, dermatofibroma; DNA, deoxyribonucleic acid; DFSP, dermatofibrosarcoma protuberans; EMA, epithelial membrane antigen; EMPD, extramammary Paget disease; ER, estrogen receptor; Fc, fragment crystallizable; FLI1, friend leukemia integration 1; GCDFP-15, gross cystic disease fluid protein 15; GCT, granular cell tumor; GLUT-1, glucose transporter 1; GVM, glomuvenous malformation; HHV-8, human herpesvirus 8; HMB, human melanoma black; HLRCC, hereditary leiomyomatosis and renal cell cancer; HSV, herpes simplex virus; HV, hydroa vacciniforme; IH, infantile hemangioma; INI1, integrase interactor 1, KHE, Kaposiform hemangioendothelioma; KS, Kaposi sarcoma; MAC, microcystic adnexal carcinoma; MCC, Merkel cell carcinoma; MF, mycosis fungoides; MPO, myeloperoxidase; LCH, Langerhans cell histiocytosis; LE, lupus erythematosus; LM, lymphatic malformation; LNA, latent nuclear antigen; LyP, lymphomatoid papulosis; MAML2, mastermind-like transcriptional coactivator 2; MART, melanoma antigen recognized by T cells; MITF, microphthalmia-associated transcription factor; MMS, Mohs micrographic surgery; MPD, mammary Paget disease; MTS, Muir-Torre syndrome; MUM1, multiple myeloma oncogene 1; NICH, noninvoluting congenital hemangioma; NK, natural killer; NSF, nephrogenic systemic fibrosis; PCDLBL-LT, primary cutaneous diffuse large B-cell lymphoma, leg type; PCFCL, primary cutaneous follicle center lymphoma; PCGD-TCL, primary cutaneous γ/δ T-cell lymphoma; PCMZL, primary cutaneous marginal zone lymphoma PHLDA1, Pleckstrin homology-like domain family A, member 1; PICH, partially involuting congenital hemangioma; PLEVA, pityriasis lichenoides et varioliformis acuta; PLC, pityriasis lichenoides chronica; PR, progesterone receptor; PRAME, preferentially expressed antigen in melanoma; PSA, prostate-specific antigen; PTEN, phosphatase and tensin homolog; RCC, renal cell carcinoma; RICH, rapidly involuting congenital hemangioma; SCC, squamous cell carcinoma; SCCis, squamous cell carcinoma *in situ*; SCLC, small-cell lung carcinoma; SMA, smooth muscle actin; SOX10, sry-related HMg-box gene 10; SPTCL, subcutaneous panniculitis-like T-cell lymphoma; SSc, systemic sclerosis; TdT, terminal deoxynucleotidyl transferase; TIA-1, cytotoxic granule-associated ribonucleic acid binding protein; TTF-1, thyroid transcription factor 1; VZV, varicella-zoster virus.
[a]Illustrative examples provided.

Molecular Tests (Table A4.9)

Table A4.9. MOLECULAR TESTS		
Molecular Test[a]	**Target(s)**	**Association(s)[a]**
FISH	EBV	HV, extranodal NK/T-cell lymphoma, nasal type (includes HV-like CTCL).
	ALK1 fusions, gain of chromosome 11p	Spitz nevus. Negative in nevocellular nevus, atypical nevus, and melanoma.
	COL1A1-PDGFB fusion, supernumerary ring chromosomes containing sequences of chromosomes 17 and 22	DFSP.
	MDM2 and *CDK4* amplification	Well-differentiated liposarcoma/atypical lipomatous tumor.
	MYC amplification	Angiosarcoma (secondary).
	WWTR1-CAMTA1 fusion	Epithelioid hemangioendothelioma.
	MUM1/IRF4 fusion	LyP type 6p25.
PCR	*Rickettsia* species	Rickettsial infections (eg, RMSF).
	Borrelia species	Borrelia infections (eg, Lyme disease).
	Mycobacterium tuberculosis	Nodular vasculitis, TB.
	Mycobacterium leprae	Leprosy (lepromatous > tuberculoid).
	Leishmania species	Leishmaniasis.
	TCR gene rearrangement (T-cell clonality)	Large plaque parapsoriasis, PL, CTCL (α/β T-cell phenotype in SPTCL; γ/δ T-cell phenotype in PCGD-TCL), LyP, CLH with T-cell predominance (±).
	IgH or Igκ gene rearrangement (B-cell clonality)	CBCL, CLH with B-cell predominance (±).

CBCL, cutaneous B-cell lymphoma; CLH, cutaneous lymphoid hyperplasia; CTCL, cutaneous T-cell lymphoma; DFSP, dermatofibrosarcoma protuberans; EBV, Epstein-Barr virus; FISH, fluorescence *in situ* hybridization; HV, hydroa vacciniforme; LyP, lymphomatoid papulosis; PCR, polymerase chain reaction; PCGD-TCL, primary cutaneous γ/δ T-cell lymphoma; PL, pityriasis lichenoides; RMSF, Rocky Mountain spotted fever; SPTCL, subcutaneous panniculitis-like T-cell lymphoma; TB, tuberculosis; TCR, T-cell receptor.
[a]Illustrative examples provided of molecular tests performed on skin biopsies.

Direct Immunofluorescence Patterns (Table A4.10)

Table A4.10. DIRECT IMMUNOFLUORESCENCE PATTERNS			
Pattern	Location	Immunoreactant(s)	Association(s)[a]
Granular deposition	DEJ	IgM, IgG, IgA, and C3	LP, LE/pemphigus erythematosus, relapsing polychondritis, FFA/LPP.
	DEJ	IgM and C3	EM.
	Dermal papillae tips	IgA	DH.
	Vessels	C3, IgM, IgA, and IgG	CSVV.
		IgA	IgA vasculitis.
		IgM and C3	Cryoglobulinemic vasculitis.
		C3, IgM, and fibrin	PAN.
	DEJ and vessels	Ig, C3, and fibrinogen	Urticarial vasculitis.
Homogenous deposition	DEJ and vessels	IgG, C3, IgA and IgM	PCT.
Intercellular deposition	Upper epidermis	IgG and C3	PF.
		IgA	IgA pemphigus (subcorneal pustular dermatosis variant).
	Lower epidermis	IgG and C3	PV, PNP.
		IgA	IgA pemphigus (intraepidermal neutrophilic variant).
Linear deposition	DEJ	IgG and C3	Roof (*n-serrated*): BP, pemphigoid gestationis, MMP (including ocular). Floor (*u-serrated*): anti-p200 pemphigoid, anti-p105 pemphigoid, MMP (anti-epiligrin). Miscellaneous: PNP.
		IgA	Roof (*n-serrated*): LABD.
		IgG	Floor (*u-serrated*): EBA.
		IgM, IgG, IgA, and C3	Floor (*u-serrated*): bullous SLE.
Shaggy deposition	DEJ	Fibrin	LP, FFA/LPP.

BP, bullous pemphigoid; C, complement; CSVV, cutaneous small vessel vasculitis; DEJ, dermal-epidermal junction; DH, dermatitis herpetiformis; EBA, epidermolysis bullosa acquisita; EM, erythema multiforme; FFA, frontal fibrosing alopecia; Ig, immunoglobulin; LABD, linear IgA bullous dermatosis; LE, lupus erythematosus; LP, lichen planus; LPP, lichen planopilaris; MMP, mucous membrane pemphigoid; PAN, polyarteritis nodosa; PCT, porphyria cutanea tarda; PF, pemphigus foliaceus; PNP, paraneoplastic pemphigus; PV, pemphigus vulgaris; RMSF, Rocky Mountain spotted fever; SLE, systemic lupus erythematosus.
[a]Illustrative examples provided.

FURTHER READING

Argenziano G, Soyer HP, Chimenti S, et al. Dermoscopy of pigmented skin lesions: results of a consensus meeting via the Internet. *J Am Acad Dermatol.* 2003;48(5):679-93. doi:10.1067/mjd.2003.281

Blum A, Clemens J, Argenziano G. Modified dermoscopic algorithm for the differentiation between melanocytic and nonmelanocytic skin tumors. *J Cutan Med Surg.* 2006;10(2):73-78. doi:10.2310/7750.2006.00021.

Bolognia JL, Schaffer JV, Cerroni L. *Dermatology.* 4th ed. Elsevier Saunders; 2018.

Elder DE. *Lever's Histopathology of the Skin.* 11th ed. Wolters Kluwer; 2015.

Elston DM, Ferringer T. *Dermatopathology.* 2nd ed. Elsevier Saunders; 2014.

Han SS, Park I, Eun Chang S, et al. Augmented intelligence dermatology: deep neural networks empower medical professionals in diagnosing skin cancer and predicting treatment options for 134 skin disorders. *J Invest Dermatol.* 2020;140(9):1753-1761. doi:10.1016/j.jid.2020.01.019

Hekler A, Utikal JS, Enk AH, et al. Superior skin cancer classification by the combination of human and artificial intelligence. *Eur J Cancer.* 2019;120:114-121. doi:10.1016/j.ejca.2019.07.019

James WD, Elston DM, Treat JR, Rosenbach MA, Neuhaus IM. *Andrews' Diseases of the Skin: Clinical Dermatology.* 13th ed. Elsevier; 2020.

Kovarik C, Lee I, Ko J, Ad Hoc Task Force on Augmented Intelligence. Commentary: position statement on augmented intelligence (AuI). *J Am Acad Dermatol.* 2019;81(4):998-1000. doi:10.1016/j.jaad.2019.06.032

Marghoob AA, Braun R. Proposal for a revised 2-step algorithm for the classification of lesions of the skin using dermoscopy. *Arch Dermatol.* 2010;146(4):426-428. doi:10.1001/archdermatol.2010.41

Mathur M, Acharya P, Karki A, Shah J, Kc N. Tubular hair casts in trichoscopy of hair and scalp disorders. *Int J Trichology.* 2019;11(1):14-19. doi:10.4103/ijt.ijt_77_18

Micheletti RG, Dominguez AR, Wanat KA. Bedside diagnostics in dermatology: Parasitic and noninfectious diseases. *J Am Acad Dermatol.* 2017;77(2):221-230. doi:10.1016/j.jaad.2016.06.035

Nusbaum KB, Korman AM, Tyler K, Kaffenberger J, Trinidad J, Kaffenberger BH. In vitro diagnostics for the medical dermatologist. Part I: autoimmune tests. *J Am Acad Dermatol.* 2021;85(2):287-298. doi:10.1016/j.jaad.2021.02.090

Nusbaum KB, Korman AM, Tyler KH, et al. In vitro diagnostics for the medical dermatologist. Part II: hypercoagulability tests. *J Am Acad Dermatol.* 2021;85(2):301-310. doi:10.1016/j.jaad.2021.03.108

Shahriari N, Grant-Kels JM, Rabinovitz H, Oliviero M, Scope A. Reflectance confocal microscopy: giagnostic criteria of common benign and malignant neoplasms, dermoscopic and histopathologic correlates of key confocal criteria, and diagnostic algorithms. *J Am Acad Dermatol.* 2021;84(1):17-31. doi:10.1016/j.jaad.2020.05.154

Shahriari N, Grant-Kels JM, Rabinovitz H, Oliviero M, Scope A. Reflectance confocal microscopy: principles, basic terminology, clinical indica-tions, limitations, and practical considerations. *J Am Acad Dermatol.* 2021;84(1):1-14. doi:10.1016/j.jaad.2020.05.153

Wanat KA, Dominguez AR, Carter Z, Legua P, Bustamante B, Micheletti RG. Bedside diagnostics in dermatology: viral, bacterial, and fungal infections. *J Am Acad Dermatol.* 2017;77(2):197-218. doi:10.1016/j.jaad.2016.06.034

Yelamos O, Braun RP, Liopyris K, et al. Dermoscopy and dermatopathology correlates of cutaneous neoplasms. *J Am Acad Dermatol.* 2019;80(2):341-363. doi:10.1016/j.jaad.2018.07.073

Yelamos O, Braun RP, Liopyris K, et al. Usefulness of dermoscopy to improve the clinical and histopathologic diagnosis of skin cancers. *J Am Acad Dermatol.* 2019;80(2):365-377. doi:10.1016/j.jaad.2018.07.072

Appendix 5: Billing

Caroline A. Nelson, MD

Basic Concepts

- Coding correctly requires understanding International Classification of Diseases, Tenth Revision, Clinical Modification (ICD-10-CM) diagnosis codes and Current Procedural Terminology (CPT) codes.
- This appendix reviews common CPT codes encountered in dermatologic practice, which can be divided into evaluation and management (E/M) codes, procedure codes, and modifiers. Inpatient E/M codes are beyond the scope of this appendix.
- It is important to note that guidelines are continually evolving. Please refer to www.cms.gov for updates.

Evaluation and Management Codes

- A **new patient** is an individual who did not receive any professional services from the physician/nonphysician practitioner (NPP) or another physician of the same specialty who belongs to the same group practice within the previous **3 years**. In order to qualify for a **consultation**, three documentation elements are required: **a request, a reason, and a report.**
- Historically, all E/M codes were determined by documentation of EITHER three key components—history, examination, and medical decision making (MDM)—OR face-to-face time with the patient (counseling and coordination of care ≥50%).
- **History:**
  - **Chief complaint.**
  - **History of present illness (HPI):** eight elements are location, quality, severity, duration, timing, context, modifying factors, and associated signs and symptoms.
  - **Review of systems (ROS):** 14 body systems are constitutional symptoms; eyes; ear, nose, mouth, throat; cardiovascular; respiratory; gastrointestinal; genitourinary; musculoskeletal; integumentary; neurological; psychiatric; endocrine; hematologic/lymphatic; and allergic/immunologic.
  - **Personal, family, and social history (PFSH).**
- **Examination:** The skin examination is summarized in Table A5.1.
- **MDM**: Types are summarized in Table A5.2.
- **E/M codes for outpatient consultations (99241-99245)** are summarized in Table A5.3.
- On January 1, 2021, the Centers for Medicare & Medicaid Services changed guidelines so that **E/M codes for new and established outpatient encounters are determined by documentation of EITHER MDM OR total time on the day of the encounter.** Activities that count toward **total time on the day of the encounter** include:
  - Preparing to see the patient;
  - Obtaining and/or reviewing separately obtained history;
  - Performing a medically appropriate examination and/or evaluation;
  - Counseling and educating the patient/family/caregiver;
  - Ordering medications, tests, or procedures;
  - Referring and communicating with other healthcare professionals;
  - Documenting clinical information in the electronic or other health record;
  - Independently interpreting results and communicating results to the patient/family/caregiver;
  - Care coordination.
    The 2021 guidelines for calculating total time on the day of the encounter emphasize "who" not "where." While time spent by ancillary staff and trainees does not count, time spent by the practitioner at home ("pajama time") does count.
- **E/M codes for new (99202-99205) and established (99211-99215) outpatient encounters** are summarized in Tables A5.4 and A5.5.

Table A5.1. SKIN EXAMINATION

System/Body Area[a]	Elements of Examination
Constitutional	• Vital signs (at least three) • General appearance of patient
Eyes	• Inspection of conjunctivae and lids
Ear, nose, mouth, and throat	• Inspection of teeth and gums • Examination of oropharynx
Neck	• Examination of thyroid
Cardiovascular	• Examination of peripheral vascular system by observation and palpation
Gastrointestinal (abdomen)	• Examination of liver and spleen • Examination of anus
Lymphatic	• Palpation of lymph nodes in neck, axillae, groin, and/or other location
Extremities	• Inspection and palpation of digits and nails

Skin	• Palpation of scalp and inspection of hair of scalp, eyebrows, face, chest, pubic area (when indicated), and extremities
	• Inspection and/or palpation of skin and subcutaneous tissue in 8/10 body areas:
	  ○ Head, including the face
	  ○ Neck
	  ○ Chest, including breasts and axillae
	  ○ Abdomen
	  ○ Genitalia, groin, buttocks
	  ○ Back
	  ○ Right upper extremity
	  ○ Left upper extremity
	  ○ Right lower extremity
	  ○ Left upper extremity
	• Inspection of eccrine and apocrine glands

Neurological/psychiatric	• Orientation to time, place, and person • Mood and affect

[a]A comprehensive examination requires performing all elements identified by a bullet and documenting every element in each shaded box and at least one element in each unshaded box. For noncomprehensive examinations, each body area is counted separately.

Table A5.2. MEDICAL DECISION-MAKING TYPES

MDM Type[a]	Number and Complexity of Problems Addressed	Amount and/or Complexity of Data to be Reviewed and Analyzed[b]	Risk of Complications and/or Morbidity or Mortality of Patient Management
Straightforward	Minimal	Minimal or none	Minimal
Low complexity	Low	Limited	Low
Moderate complexity	Moderate	Moderate	Moderate
High complexity	High	Extensive	High

[a]2021 guidelines. To qualify for a given MDM type, 2/3 elements must either be met or exceeded.
[b]Data are divided into three categories: tests, documents, orders, or independent historian(s); independent interpretation of tests; discussion of management or test interpretation with external physician or other qualified healthcare professional or appropriate source.
MDM, medical decision making.

Table A5.3. EVALUATION AND MANAGEMENT CODES FOR OUTPATIENT CONSULTATIONS

Code[a]		99241	99242	99243	99244	99245
History	CC	Required	Required	Required	Required	Required
	HPI	1-3 elements	1-3 elements	≥4 elements or status of ≥3 chronic or inactive conditions	≥4 elements or status of ≥3 chronic or inactive conditions	≥4 elements or status of 3 chronic conditions
	ROS	None	Pertinent	2-9 body systems	≥10 body systems	≥10 body systems
	PFSH	None	None	1 history area	3 history areas	Complete
Examination		1-5 elements	6-11 elements	≥12 elements	Comprehensive	Comprehensive
MDM		Straightforward	Straightforward	Low complexity	Moderate complexity	High complexity
Time (minutes)		15	30	40	60	80

CC, chief complaint; HPI, history of present illness; MDM, medical decision making, PFSH, personal, family, and social history; ROS, review of systems.
[a]3/3 components at or above the level of complexity of the E/M code.

Table A5.4. EVALUATION AND MANAGEMENT CODES FOR NEW OUTPATIENT ENCOUNTERS

Code[a]	99202	99203	99204	99205
MDM	Straightforward	Low complexity	Moderate complexity	High complexity
Time (minutes)	15-29	30-44	45-59	60-74

MDM, medical decision making.
[a]99201 has been deleted.

Table A5.5. EVALUATION AND MANAGEMENT CODES FOR ESTABLISHED OUTPATIENT ENCOUNTERS

Code[a]	99211	99212	99213	99214	99215
MDM	N/A	Straightforward	Low complexity	Moderate complexity	High complexity
Time (minutes)	N/A	10-19	20-29	30-39	40-54

MDM, medical decision making; N/A, not applicable.
[a]99211 may not require the presence of a physician or other qualified healthcare professional.

Procedure Codes (Table A5.6)

Table A5.6. PROCEDURE CODES
0-Day Postoperative Period
Remember modifier "-25!" Otherwise the E/M service will be included in the global package.

• Intralesional injection
• Skin biopsy[a]
  ○ Tangential (shave, scoop, saucerize, curette): 11102
  ○ Tangential (shave, scoop, saucerize, curette), additional: 11103
  ○ Punch: 11104
  ○ Punch, additional: 11105
  ○ Incisional: 11106
  ○ Incisional, additional: 11107
• Shave removal (therapeutic)
• Mohs micrographic surgery

10-Day Postoperative Period
Global period is 11 days (count day of the surgery).
• Benign, premalignant, or malignant destruction (curettage, electrosurgery, cryosurgery, laser treatment, or chemical treatment) • Benign or malignant excision (full-thickness removal to the subcutis, including margins) • Simple, intermediate, or complex repair
90-Day Postoperative Period
Global period is 92 days (count day before and day of surgery).
• Flap or graft

E/M, evaluation and management.

[a]When performing multiple skin biopsies, code the primary biopsy based on hierarchy (incisional > punch > tangential), followed by additional biopsies. These biopsy codes do not replace site-specific biopsy codes (nail unit, lip, penis, vulva or perineum, excisional biopsy of eyelid skin including lid margin, and external ear).

Modifiers (Table A5.7)

Table A5.7. MODIFIERS	
Modifier	Description
24	Unrelated E/M service by the same physician during a postoperative period.
25	Significant, separately identifiable E/M service by the same physician on the same day of the procedure.
50	Bilateral procedure (eg, Unna boot).
57	Decision for surgery.
58	Staged or related procedure or service (eg, re-excision after positive margins) by the same physician during the postoperative period.
59	Distinct procedural service.
79	Unrelated procedure or service by the same physician during a postoperative period.
91	Repeat clinical diagnostic laboratory test.

E/M, evaluation and management

FURTHER READING

American Academy of Dermatology. *Coding Resource Center*. Accessed August 13, 2019. https://www.aad.org/practicecenter/coding-and-reimbursement/coding-resource-center

Centers for Medicare and Medicaid Services. Accessed August 18, 2019. https://www.cms.gov/

Abbreviations

A

AA, alopecia areata
AAD, American Academy of Dermatology
ABD, American Board of Dermatology
ABI, ankle-brachial index
ABSIS, Autoimmune Bullous Skin Disorder Intensity Score
AC, alternating current
ACC, aplasia cutis congenita
ACD, allergic contact dermatitis
ACE, angiotensin-converting enzyme
ACEI, angiotensin-converting enzyme inhibitor
ACGME, Accreditation Council for Graduate Medical Education
ACTH, adrenocorticotropic hormone
AD, atopic dermatitis OR autosomal dominant
ADA, adenosine deaminase
AE, anagen effluvium
AEP, atopic eruption of pregnancy
AESOP, adenopathy and extensive skin patch overlying a plasmacytoma
AFB, acid-fast bacilli
AFK, acral fibrokeratoma
AFX, atypical fibroxanthoma
AGA, androgenetic alopecia
AGEP, acute generalized exanthematous pustulosis
AHEI, acute hemorrhagic edema of infancy
AI-CTD, autoimmune connective tissue disorder
AJCC, American Joint Committee on Cancer
AK, actinic keratosis
AKI, acute kidney injury
ALA, aminolevulinic acid
ALL, acute lymphoblastic leukemia
ALT, alanine transaminase
AML, acute myeloid leukemia
AN, acanthosis nigricans
ANA, antinuclear antibody
ANCA, antineutrophil cytoplasmic antibody
AoSD, adult-onset Still disease
AP-1, activator protein 1
APC, antigen-presenting cell
APD, acquired perforating dermatosis
APECED, autoimmune polyendocrinopathy–candidiasis–ectodermal dystrophy
APL, acute promyelocytic leukemia
APLS, antiphospholipid antibody syndrome
AR, autosomal recessive
ARB, angiotensin II receptor blocker
ARF, alternative reading frame
ARI, absolute risk increase
ARR, absolute risk reduction
ART, antiretroviral therapy
ASA, aspirin
ASAP, acute syndrome of apoptotic pan-epidermolysis
ASO, antistreptolysin O
A-T, ataxia-telangiectasia
ATRA, all-trans retinoic acid
ATTR, amyloid transthyretin
AUC, appropriate use criteria
AVL, atypical vascular lesion
AVM, arteriovenous malformation
$\alpha 1$AT, α-1 antitrypsin

B

BADAS, bowel-associated dermatosis-arthritis syndrome
BB, mid-borderline leprosy
bbUVB, broadband ultraviolet B
BCC, basal cell carcinoma
BCG, bacille Calmette-Guérin
BCL2, B-cell lymphoma 2
BCNS, basal cell nevus syndrome
BHD, Birt-Hogg-Dubé
BID, twice daily
BL, borderline lepromatous leprosy
BLyS, B lymphocyte stimulator
BMI, body mass index
BMP, bone morphogenic protein
BMZ, basement membrane zone
BoNT, botulinum neurotoxin
BP, bullous pemphigoid
BPAG1, bullous pemphigoid antigen 1
BPAG2, bullous pemphigoid antigen 2
BPDAI, BP Disease Area Index
BPDCN, blastic plasmacytoid dendritic cell neoplasm
BRR, Bannayan-Riley-Ruvalcaba
BSA, body surface area
BT, borderline tuberculoid leprosy
BUN, blood urea nitrogen

C

C, complement OR cytoplasmic
CA, cancer antigen
CAD, chronic actinic dermatitis
CALM, café-au-lait macule

cAMP, cyclic adenosine monophosphate

CANDLE, chronic atypical neutrophilic dermatosis with lipodystrophy and elevated temperature

CAPS, cryopyrin-associated periodic syndromes

CAR, chimeric autoantibody receptor

CARP, confluent and reticulated papillomatosis

CBC, complete blood count

CBCL, cutaneous B-cell lymphoma

CCB, calcium channel blocker

CCCA, central centrifugal cicatricial alopecia

CCP, cyclic citrullinated peptide

CD, cluster of differentiation

CD8$^+$ AECTCL, primary cutaneous aggressive epidermotropic CD8$^+$ cytotoxic T-cell lymphoma

CDASI, Cutaneous Dermatomyositis Disease Area and Severity Index

CDK, cyclin-dependent kinase

CDKN2A, cyclin-dependent kinase inhibitor 2A

CDR, complementarity-determining region

CF, cystic fibrosis

CGD, chronic granulomatous disease

CH, congenital hemangioma

CH50, total hemolytic complement

CHF, congestive heart failure

CHILD, congenital hemidysplasia with ichthyosiform erythroderma and limb defects

C1-inh, C1-inhibitor

CI, confidence interval

CINCA, chronic infantile neurological cutaneous and articular syndrome

CK, creatine kinase

CKD, chronic kidney disease

CKI, cyclin-dependent kinase inhibitor

CLH, cutaneous lymphoid hyperplasia

CLIA, Clinical Laboratory Improvement Amendments

CLL, chronic lymphocytic leukemia

CM, capillary malformation

CML, chronic myelogenous leukemia

CMP, comprehensive metabolic panel

CMTC, cutis marmorata telangiectatica congenita

CMV, cytomegalovirus

CN, cranial nerve

CNH, chondrodermatitis nodularis helicis

CNS, central nervous system

CO$_2$, carbon dioxide

CONSORT, Consolidated Standards of Reporting Trials

COPD, chronic obstructive pulmonary disease

COVID-19, coronavirus disease 2019

CP, cicatricial pemphigoid

CPPD, calcium pyrophosphate dihydrate

CPRS, complex regional pain syndrome

Cr, creatinine

CR1, complement receptor type 1

CREST, Calcinosis, Raynaud phenomenon, Esophageal dysmotility, Sclerodactyly, and Telangiectasia

CRH, corticotropin-releasing hormone

CRP, C-reactive protein

CSVV, cutaneous small-vessel vasculitis

CT, computed tomography

CTA, computed tomography angiogram

CTCAE, Common Terminology Criteria for Adverse Events

CTCL, cutaneous T-cell lymphoma

CTD, connective tissue disorder

CVID, common variable immunodeficiency

CXCL, CXC chemokine ligand

CXR, chest x-ray

CYP, cytochrome P450

D

DAMP, damage-associated molecular pattern

DC, dendritic cell OR direct current

DDA, diffuse dermal angiomatosis

DEET, N,N-diethyl-3-methylbenzamide

DEJ, dermal-epidermal junction

DEXA, dual-energy x-ray absorptiometry

DF, dermatofibroma

DFA, direct fluorescent antibody

DFSP, dermatofibrosarcoma protuberans

DH, dermatitis herpetiformis

DHEAS, dehydroepiandrosterone sulfate

DHFR, dihydrofolate reductase

DHPS, dihydropteroate synthetase

DHT, dihydrotestosterone

DIC, disseminated intravascular coagulation

DIF, direct immunofluorescence

DIRA, deficiency of the interleukin-1 receptor antagonist

DITRA, deficiency of the interleukin-36 receptor antagonist

DKC, dyskeratosis congenita

DLCO, diffusing capacity for carbon monoxide

DLE, discoid lupus erythematosus

DM, dermatomyositis

DMARD, disease-modifying antirheumatic drug

DNA, deoxyribonucleic acid

DOAC, direct oral anticoagulant

DOPA, dihydroxyphenylalanine

DPN, dermatosis papulosa nigra

DPP-4, dipeptidyl peptidase-4

DRESS, drug reaction with eosinophilia and systemic symptoms

DSAP, disseminated superficial actinic porokeratosis

dsDNA, double-stranded deoxyribonucleic acid

DSM, *Diagnostic and Statistical Manual of Mental Disorders*

DSSI, Dermatomyositis Skin Severity Index

DTM, dermatophyte test medium

E

EAC, erythema annulare centrifugum

EAI, erythema ab igne

EB, epidermolysis bullosa

EBA, epidermolysis bullosa acquisita

EBNA1, Epstein-Barr nuclear antigen 1

EBV, Epstein-Barr virus

ECA, external carotid artery

ECG, electrocardiogram
ECM, extracellular matrix
ECP, extracorporeal photopheresis
ED&C, electrodessication and curettage
EDA, ectodysplasin A
EDP, erythema dyschromicum perstans
EDS, Ehlers-Danlos syndrome
EDV, epidermodysplasia verruciformis
EED, erythema elevatum diutinum
EF, eosinophilic fasciitis
EGA, estimated gestational age
EGFR, epidermal growth factor receptor
EGPA, eosinophilic granulomatosis with polyangiitis
EHK, epidermolytic hyperkeratosis
EI, epidermolytic ichthyosis OR erythema induratum
ELISA, enzyme-linked immunosorbent assay
EM, erythema multiforme
EMG, electromyography
EMLA, eutectic mixture of local anesthetics
EMPD, extramammary Paget disease
EN, erythema nodosum
EORTC, European Organization for Research and Treatment of Cancer
EPF, eosinophilic pustular folliculitis
EPO, eosinophil peroxidase
EPP, erythropoietic protoporphyria
EPS, elastosis perforans serpiginosa
Er:YAG, erbium-doped yttrium aluminum garnet
ESR, erythrocyte sedimentation rate
ESRD, end-stage renal disease
ET, exfoliative toxin
ETTR, erythematotelangiectatic rosacea
EULAR, European League Against Rheumatism

F

5-FU, 5-fluorouracil
Fab, fragment antigen-binding
FAMMM, familial atypical multiple mole melanoma
Fc, fragment crystallizable
FCAS, familial cold autoinflammatory syndrome
FDA, Food and Drug Administration
FDE, fixed drug eruption
FFA, free fatty acid OR frontal fibrosing alopecia
FFP, fresh frozen plasma
FGF, fibroblast growth factor
FGFR, fibroblast growth factor receptor
FISH, fluorescence *in situ* hybridization
FKBP, FK506-binding protein
FLT3, FMS-like tyrosine kinase 3
FMF, familial Mediterranean fever
FNA, fine needle aspiration
FOBT, fecal occult blood test
FOP, fibrodysplasia ossificans progressiva
FSH, follicle-stimulating hormone
FTA-ABS, fluorescent treponemal antibody absorption test

G

G6PD, glucose-6-phosphate dehydrogenase
GA, granuloma annulare
GAG, glycosaminoglycan
GAS, group A β-hemolytic *Streptococcus*
GBFDE, generalized bullous fixed drug eruption
GBS, group B *Streptococcus*
GCA, giant cell arteritis
G-CSF, granulocyte colony-stimulating factor
GCT, granular cell tumor
GD, Grover disease
GERD, gastroesophageal reflux disease
GM-CSF, granulocyte-monocyte colony-stimulating factor
GN, gram-negative
GP, gram-positive
GPA, granulomatosis with polyangiitis
GPC, gram-positive cocci
GPP, generalized pustular psoriasis
GPR, gram-positive rod
GVHD, graft-versus-host disease
GVM, glomuvenous malformation

H

H, histamine
HA, hyaluronic acid
HAIR-AN, hyperandrogenism, insulin resistance, and acanthosis nigricans
Hb, hemoglobin
HbS, sickle hemoglobin
HBV, hepatitis B virus
HCG, human chorionic gonadotropin
HCV, hepatitis C virus
HDL-C, high-density lipoprotein cholesterol
H&E, hematoxylin and eosin
HEP, hepatoerythropoietic porphyria
HES, hypereosinophilic syndrome
HFMD, hand-foot-mouth disease
HFS, hand-foot syndrome
HGH, human growth hormone
HGPRT, hypoxanthine-guanine phosphoribosyltransferase
HHT, hereditary hemorrhagic telangiectasia
HHV, human herpesvirus
HIAA, hydroxyindoleacetic acid
HIV, human immunodeficiency virus
HLA, human leukocyte antigen
HLRCC, hereditary leiomyomatosis and renal cell cancer
HMFD, hand-foot-mouth disease
HNPCC, hereditary nonpolyposis colorectal cancer
HPA, hypothalamic-pituitary-adrenal
HPV, human papillomavirus
HS, hidradenitis suppurativa
HSCT, hematopoietic stem cell transplantation
HSV, herpes simplex virus
HTLV, human T-lymphotropic virus
HTS, high-throughput TCR sequencing

HUS, hemolytic uremic syndrome
HUVS, hypocomplementemic urticarial vasculitis syndrome
HV, hydroa vacciniforme

I

I, intermediate leprosy
IBD, inflammatory bowel disease
ICA, internal carotid artery
ICD, implantable cardioverter-defibrillator OR irritant contact dermatitis
ICI, immune checkpoint inhibitor
I&D, incision and drainage
IEN, intraepidermal neutrophilic
IFAG, idiopathic facial aseptic granuloma
IFE, immunofixation
IFN, interferon
Ig, immunoglobulin
IGD, interstitial granulomatous dermatitis
IgG4-RD, immunoglobulin G4–related disease
IGH, idiopathic guttate hypomelanosis
IH, infantile hemangioma
IHC, immunohistochemistry
IIF, indirect immunofluorescence
IL, interleukin
ILD, interstitial lung disease
ILK, intralesional Kenalog
ILVEN, inflammatory linear verrucous epidermal nevus
IM, intramuscular
IMPDH, inosine monophosphate dehydrogenase
INH, isoniazid
IP, incontinentia pigmenti
IPEH, intravascular papillary endothelial hyperplasia
IPEX, immune dysregulation, polyendocrinopathy, enteropathy, X-linked
IPL, intense pulsed light
IRIS, immune reconstitution inflammatory syndrome
IRS, inner route sheath
ISCL, International Society for Cutaneous Lymphomas
ITP, idiopathic thrombocytopenic purpura
IV, intravenous
IVDU, intravenous drug use
IVIG, intravenous immune globulin

J

JAK, Janus kinase

K

K, keratin
KA, keratoacanthoma
KHE, Kaposiform hemangioendothelioma
KIT/BCR-ABL, kinase receptor/breakpoint cluster region-Abelson
KOH, potassium hydroxide
KP, keratosis pilaris
KPR, keratosis pilaris rubra
KS, Kaposi sarcoma

KSHV, Kaposi sarcoma–associated herpesvirus

L

LABD, linear IgA bullous dermatosis
LAD, leukocyte adhesion deficiency
LASER, Light Amplification by Stimulated Emission of Radiation
LC, Langerhans cell
LCH, Langerhans cell histiocytosis
LDH, lactate dehydrogenase
LE, lupus erythematosus
LFT, liver function test
LGBT, Lesbian, gay, bisexual, and transgender
LGV, lymphogranuloma venereum
LH, luteinizing hormone
LK, lichenoid keratosis
LL, lepromatous leprosy
LLLT, low-level light therapy
LM, lymphatic malformation
LMDF, lupus miliaris disseminatus faciei
LMP2, latent membrane protein 2
LMWH, low-molecular-weight heparin
LP, lichen planus
LPD, lymphoproliferative disorder
LPP, lichen planopilaris
LS, lichen sclerosus
LSC, lichen simplex chronicus
LyP, lymphomatoid papulosis

M

MAC, microcystic adnexal carcinoma
MAGIC, mouth and genital ulcers with inflamed cartilage
MAL, methyl aminolevulinate
MAPK, mitogen-activated protein kinase
MB, multibacillary
MBL, mannose-binding lectin
MBP, major basic protein
MC1R, melanocortin 1 receptor
MCC, Merkel cell carcinoma
MCI/MI, methylchloroisothiazolinone/methylisothiazolinone
MCP, metacarpophalangeal
MCPyV, Merkel cell polyomavirus
MCTD, mixed connective tissue disease
MCV, molluscum contagiosum virus
MDM2, mouse double minute 2
MDS, myelodysplastic syndrome
MED, minimal erythema dose
MEK, mitogen-activated protein kinase
MELTUMP, melanocytic tumor of unknown malignant potential
MEN, multiple endocrine neoplasia
MF, mycosis fungoides
MHC, major histocompatibility complex
MI, myocardial infarction
MIRM, *Mycoplasma pneumoniae*-induced rash and mucositis

MKD/HIDS, mevalonate kinase deficiency/hyper-IgD syndrome
MMP, matrix metalloproteinase OR mucous membrane pemphigoid
MMR, measles, mumps, and rubella
MMS, Mohs micrographic surgery
MOC, maintenance of certification
8-MOP, 8-methoxypsoralen
6-MP, 6-mercaptopurine
MPA, microscopic polyangiitis
MPD, mammary Paget disease
MPNST, malignant peripheral nerve sheath tumor
MPO, myeloperoxidase
MRA, magnetic resonance angiogram
MRI, magnetic resonance imaging
MRSA, methicillin-resistant *Staphylococcus aureus*
MSH, melanocyte-stimulating hormone
MSM, men who have sex with men
MSSA, methicillin-sensitive *Staphylococcus aureus*
MSU, monosodium urate
MTOR, mammalian target of rapamycin
MTP, metatarsophalangeal
MTS, Muir-Torre syndrome
MTZ, microthermal zone
MVP, mitral valve prolapse
MWS, Muckle-Wells syndrome
MyD88, myeloid differentiation factor 88

N

NADPH, nicotinamide adenine dinucleotide phosphate hydrogen
nbUVB, narrowband ultraviolet B
NCCN, National Comprehensive Cancer Network
NCM, neurocutaneous melanosis
Nd:YAG, neodymium-doped yttrium aluminum garnet
NEH, neutrophilic eccrine hidradenitis
NER, nucleotide excision repair
NET, neutrophil extracellular trap
NF, neurofibromatosis
NFAT, nuclear factor of activated T cells
NF-κB, nuclear factor κ-light-chain-enhancer of activated B cells
NHL, non-Hodgkin lymphoma
NIH, National Institutes of Health
NK, natural killer
NL, necrobiosis lipoidica
NLD, necrobiosis lipoidica diabeticorum
NLRP3, nucleotide-binding domain leucine-rich repeat-containing receptor protein 3
NMF, natural moisturizing factor
NMSC, nonmelanoma skin cancer
NNH, number needed to harm
NNRTI, nonnucleoside reverse transcriptase inhibitor
NNT, number needed to treat
NOAC, new oral anticoagulant
NOMID, neonatal-onset multisystem inflammatory disease
NOS, not otherwise specified

NPF, National Psoriasis Foundation
NPV, negative predictive value
NRTI, nucleoside reverse transcriptase inhibitor
NSAID, nonsteroidal anti-inflammatory drug
NSF, nephrogenic systemic fibrosis
NT-proBNP, N-terminal prohormone of brain natriuretic peptide
NtRTI, nucleotide reverse transcriptase inhibitor
NXG, necrobiotic xanthogranuloma

O

OCA, oculocutaneous albinism
OCP, oral contraceptive pill
OD, optimal density
ODC, ornithine decarboxylase
OHP, hydroxyprogesterone
OMIM, Online Mendelian Inheritance in Man™
OR, odds ratio
ORS, outer route sheath

P

P, perinuclear
PABA, para-aminobenzoic acid
PAD, peripheral arterial disease
PAH, pulmonary arterial hypertension
PAMP, pathogen-associated molecular pattern
PAN, polyarteritis nodosa
Pap, Papanicolaou
PAPA, pyogenic arthritis, pyoderma gangrenosum, and acne
PAPASH, pyogenic arthritis, acne, pyoderma gangrenosum, and suppurative hidradenitis
PAS, periodic acid-Schiff
PASH, pyoderma gangrenosum, acne, and suppurative hidradenitis
PASI, Psoriasis Area and Severity Index
PB, paucibacillary
PBC, primary biliary cirrhosis
PBP, penicillin-binding protein
PC, pachyonychia congenita OR pseudoatrophoderma colli
PCDLBL-LT, primary cutaneous diffuse large B-cell lymphoma, leg type
PCFCL, primary cutaneous follicle center lymphoma
PCMZL, primary cutaneous marginal zone lymphoma
PCOS, polycystic ovarian syndrome
PCP, *Pneumocystis jirovecii* pneumonia
PCR, polymerase chain reaction
PCT, porphyria cutanea tarda
PDAI, Pemphigus Disease Area Index
pDC, plasmacytoid dendritic cell
PDE, phosphodiesterase
PDGFR, platelet-derived growth factor receptor
PDL, pulsed dye laser
PDT, photodynamic therapy
PEH, pseudoepitheliomatous hyperplasia
PEN, palisaded encapsulated neuroma
PENS, palisaded epidermal nevus with "skyline" basal cell layer

PEP, polymorphic eruption of pregnancy
PET, positron emission tomography
PF, pemphigus foliaceus
PFT, pulmonary function test
PG, pyoderma gangrenosum OR pyogenic granuloma
PHN, postherpetic neuralgia
PI3K, phosphoinositide 3-kinase
PIP, proximal interphalangeal
PIP2, phosphatidylinositol 4,5-bisphosphate
PIP3, phosphatidylinositol (3,4,5)-trisphosphate
PL, pityriasis lichenoides
PLC, pityriasis lichenoides chronica
PLEVA, pityriasis lichenoides et varioliformis acuta
PM, polymyositis
PMH, progressive macular hypomelanosis
PML, progressive multifocal leukoencephalopathy
PMLE, polymorphous light eruption
PML-RAR, promyelocytic leukemia–retinoic acid receptor
PMR, polymyalgia rheumatica
PNS, peripheral nervous system
POEMS, polyneuropathy, organomegaly, endocrinopathy, monoclonal gammopathy, and skin changes
POMC, proopiomelanocortin
PNGD, palisaded neutrophilic granulomatous dermatitis
PNP, paraneoplastic pemphigus
PPAR, peroxisome proliferator–activated receptor
PPD, paraphenylenediamine OR purified protein derivative
PPE, pruritic papular eruption
PPI, proton pump inhibitor
PPK, palmoplantar keratoderma
PPR, papulopustular rosacea
PPV, positive predictive value
PR, pityriasis rosea
PR3, proteinase 3
PRBCs, packed red blood cells
PRP, pityriasis rubra pilaris
PSA, prostate-specific antigen
PSORS1, psoriasis susceptibility region 1
PSTPIP1, proline-serine-threonine phosphatase-interacting protein 1
PTH, parathyroid hormone
PTLD, posttransplant lymphoproliferative disorder
PTT, partial thromboplastin time
PUD, peptic ulcer disease
PUMA, p53 upregulated modulator of apoptosis
PUPPP, pruritic urticarial papules and plaques of pregnancy
PUVA, psoralen ultraviolet A
PV, pemphigus vulgaris
p-value, probability value
PVL, Panton-Valentine leukocidin
PWS, port-wine stain
PXE, pseudoxanthoma elasticum

R

RA, rheumatoid arthritis
RAR, retinoid acid receptor

RAST, radioallergosorbent test
RB, retinoblastoma protein
RCC, renal cell carcinoma
RCM, reflectance confocal microscopy
RCT, randomized control trial
RegiSCAR, European Registry of Severe Cutaneous Adverse [Drug] Reactions
REMS, Risk Evaluation and Mitigation Strategy
RF, rheumatoid factor
RMSF, Rocky Mountain spotted fever
RNA, ribonucleic acid
RND, rheumatoid neutrophilic dermatosis
RNP, ribonucleoprotein
ROM, range-of-motion
ROS, reactive oxygen species
RPD, reactive perforating dermatosis
RPR, rapid plasma reagin
RR, relative risk
RT, reverse transcriptase
RTK, receptor tyrosine kinase
RXR, retinoid X receptor

S

SADBE, squaric acid dibutyl ester
SAHA, seborrhea, acne, hirsutism, and androgenetic alopecia
SAPHO, synovitis, acne, pustulosis, hyperostosis, and osteitis
SARS-CoV-2, severe acute respiratory syndrome coronavirus 2
SAVI, STING-associated vasculopathy with onset in infancy
SC, subcutaneous
SCAR, severe cutaneous adverse reaction
SCC, squamous cell carcinoma or staphylococcal chromosome cassette
SCCis, squamous cell carcinoma *in situ*
SCID, severe combined immunodeficiency
SCLE, subacute cutaneous lupus erythematosus
SCM, sternocleidomastoid
SD, standard deviation
SDRIFE, symmetrical drug-related intertriginous and flexural exanthema
SE, standard error
SEM, skin, eye, and mouth
SGH, sebaceous gland hyperplasia
SHBG, sex hormone binding globulin
SHH, sonic hedgehog
SI, suicidal ideation
SIADH, syndrome of inappropriate antidiuretic hormone secretion
SJS, Stevens-Johnson syndrome
SK, seborrheic keratosis
SLE, systemic lupus erythematosus
SLNB, sentinel lymph node biopsy
SMAS, superficial musculoaponeurotic system
SMO, smoothened
SNAP-25, synaptosome-associated protein, 25kDa
SNRI, serotonin–norepinephrine reuptake inhibitor

SPAP, syringocystadenoma papilliferum
SPD, subcorneal pustular dermatosis
SPE, streptococcal pyrogenic exotoxin
SPEP, serum protein electrophoresis
SPF, sun protection factor
SSc, systemic sclerosis
SSKI, saturated solution of potassium iodide
SSRI, selective serotonin reuptake inhibitor
SSSS, staphylococcal scalded skin syndrome
STD, sexually-transmitted disease
STROBE, Strengthening the Reporting of Observational
    studies in Epidemiology
STS, sodium tetradecyl sulfate OR sodium thiosulfate
SUFU, suppressor of fused
SVC, superior vena cava

T

T4, thyroxine
TB, tuberculosis
TBSE, total body skin examination
TCA, trichloroacetic acid OR tricyclic antidepressant
TCA-CROSS, trichloroacetic acid chemical reconstruction of
    skin scars
TCR, T-cell receptor
TE, telogen effluvium
TEC, toxic erythema of chemotherapy
TEN, toxic epidermal necrolysis
TEWL, transepidermal water loss
TFT, thyroid function test
TG, transglutaminase
TGF, transforming growth factor
Th, T helper type
TLR, toll-like receptor
TMEP, telangiectasia macularis eruptiva perstans
TMP-SMX, trimethoprim-sulfamethoxazole
TMPT, thiopurine S-methyltransferase
TNFα, tumor necrosis factor alpha
TRAPS, TNF receptor–associated periodic syndrome
T-regs, regulatory T cells
TSC, tuberous sclerosis complex
TSEBT, total skin electron beam therapy
TSH, thyroid-stimulating hormone
TSS, toxic shock syndrome
TSST-1, toxic shock syndrome toxin 1
TT, tuberculoid leprosy

TTE, transthoracic echocardiogram
TTP, thrombotic thrombocytopenic purpura
TV, tinea versicolor
T-VEC, talimogene laherparepvec
TYK2, tyrosine kinase 2

U

UA, urinalysis
UPEP, urine protein electrophoresis
URI, upper respiratory infection
US, ultrasound OR United States
UV, ultraviolet
UVA, ultraviolet A
UVB, ultraviolet B
UVR, ultraviolet radiation

V

VAC, vacuum-assisted closure
VAMP, vesicle-associated membrane protein
VCM, verrucous venucapillary malformation
VDRL, Venereal Disease Research Laboratory
VEGF, vascular endothelial growth factor
VHK, Vogt-Koyanagi-Harada
VIN, vulvar intraepithelial neoplasia
VM, venous malformation
VP, variegate porphyria
VZV, varicella-zoster virus

W

WAS, Wiskott-Aldrich syndrome
WBC, white blood cell
WHIM, warts, hypogammaglobulinemia, infections, and
    myelokathexis
WHO, World Health Organization
WILD, warts, immunodeficiency, lymphedema, and dysplasia
WLE, wide local excision

X

XLD, X-linked dominant
XLR, X-linked recessive
XO, xanthine oxidase
XP, xeroderma pigmentosum
XR, x-ray

Index

Note: Pages followed by t or f refer to tables or figures, respectively.

A

Abacavir
  drug reaction with eosinophilia and systemic symptoms (DRESS), 156
  morbilliform drug eruption, 154
Abnormal epidermis, 530
Abscess
  bacterial, 293
  chronic granulomatous disease (CGD), 294
Absolute risk increase (ARI), 41
Absolute risk reduction (ARR), 42
Absorbable sutures, 551, 555
Absorption, 36
Absorption spectrum, 22
Aβ-type fiber, 7
Acantholytic acanthoma, 370t
Acantholytic dyskeratosis, 100
Acanthoma fissuratum, 361
Acanthosis nigricans, 62
  clinicopathological features, 63
  epidemiology, 63
  evaluation, 64
  management, 64
Accelerated rheumatoid nodulosis, 137
Accessory tragus, 459, 459t, 460f
Accreditation Council for Graduate Medical Education (ACGME), 44
Acid-fast bacilli (AFB), 285
Acitretin, 498t
  for immunosuppressed patients, 53
  for pityriasis rubra pilaris (PRP), 58
  for psoriasis, 53
Acne
  seborrheic dermatitis, 68
  variants
    adults, 189t–190t
    children, 191t
Acne conglobata, 189t
Acne excoriée, 186, 189t
Acne fulminans, 189t, 192
Acneiform eruptions
  adults, 190t
  children, 191t
Acne keloidalis, 208–210, 209f
Acne mechanica, 190t
Acne vulgaris
  clinicopathological features, 188
  epidemiology, 188
  evaluation, 188
  management, 191
  pathogenesis, 189f
Acquired lipodystrophies, 149, 150t

Acquired perforating dermatosis (APD), 137, 140f, 140t
Acral blisters, epidermolysis bullosa acquisita, 107
Acral dry gangrene, arterial ulcer, 180
Acral erythematous macules, antineutrophil cytoplasmic antibody vasculitis, 174
Acral fibrokeratoma (AFK), 460, 460f
Acral lentiginous melanomas, 393
Acroangiodermatitis, stasis dermatitis, 69
Acrocyanosis, cryoglobulinemia, 173
Acrodermatitis chronica atrophicans, 304, 306t
Acrokeratosis
  paraneoplastica, 52
  verruciformis of Hopf, 100
Acropustulosis of infancy, 345
Acrospiroma, 446–447
Actinic cheilitis, 376
Actinic keratosis
  clinicopathological features, 376, 376f
  epidemiology, 376
  evaluation, 377
  management, 377
  topical antineoplastics for, 514, 522t
Actinic prurigo, polymorphous light eruption (PMLE), 353, 354
Actinomyces israelii, 298
Actinomycetoma, 333
Actinomycosis, 298, 299f
Action spectrum, 22
Acupuncture, prurigo nodularis, 183
Acute generalized exanthematous pustulosis (AGEP), 93–95
Acute hemorrhagic edema of infancy (AHEI), 171, 172t
Acute kidney injury (AKI), nephrogenic systemic fibrosis, 136
Acyclovir, 501t
  for eczema herpeticum, 272
  for herpes simplex virus (HSV), 270
  for herpes zoster, 274
  for pityriasis rosea (PR), 58
  for varicella, 273
Adams-Oliver syndrome, 431
Adapalene, 499t
Adaptive immunity, 25, 25t
Addison disease, erythema dyschromicum perstans, 85
Adenoid cystic carcinoma, 452t
Adenosine deaminase 2 (ADA2) deficiency, livedoid vasculopathy, 162
Adherens junctions, 3, 4f, 6f
Adhesives, 71t

Adipose neoplasms, 407
  Cowden syndrome, 411
  hibernoma, 409
  lipoma, 409–410
Adiposis dolorosa, 410
Adnexal disorders
  gland disorders, 595t–597t
  hair disorders, 597t–600t
  nail disorders, 600t–603t
Adnexal neoplasms and proliferations, 451t–452t
  with follicular matrical differentiation, 455, 457, 458t
  with follicular sheath differentiation, 455–456, 456t
  microcystic adnexal carcinoma, 448–450
  mucinous carcinoma, 450–452
  with primarily apocrine differentiation, 443–447
  with primarily eccrine differentiation, 446–448. 450
  with sebaceous differentiation, 439–443
  with superficial follicular differentiation, 450, 454t–455t
Adrenergic hormonal control, sebaceous gland, 9
Aδ-type fiber, 7
Adult-onset Still disease (AoSD), 137
Advancement flaps, 561, 562
Aedes mosquitoes, 284
Afamelanotide, 523
African trypanosomiasis, 339t
Age-dependent penetrance, Mendelian inheritance, 15
AGEP. *See* Acute generalized exanthematous pustulosis (AGEP)
Aggressive digital papillary adenocarcinoma, 452t
Agminated Spitz nevus, 391
Airway obstruction, cellulitis, 291
Albendazole, 343, 510
Albright hereditary osteodystrophy, 166
Alcohol dehydrogenase deficiency, rosacea, 195
Alcohol-induced flushing, rosacea, 195
Alemtuzumab, 523t
  for cutaneous T-cell lymphoma (CTCL), 471
  sarcoidosis and, 471
Alezzandrini syndrome, 84
Alkaptonuria, 245t
Alkylating agents, 512t
  toxic erythema of chemotherapy (TEC), 120
  traction alopecia, 205
Allele, 15
Allelic heterogeneity, 15
Allergen avoidance, 78

Allergic contact dermatitis (ACD), 24, 70
Allergic rhinoconjunctivitis, atopic dermatitis
    (AD), 65
Allodynia, complex regional pain syndrome
    (CPRS), 184, 184t
Allogeneic hematopoietic stem cell
    transplantation, cutaneous T-cell
    lymphoma (CTCL), 471
Allopurinol
    drug reaction with eosinophilia and systemic
        symptoms (DRESS), 156
    for gout, 245
    morbilliform drug eruption, 154
    in Stevens-Johnson syndrome/toxic epidermal
        necrolysis, 117
All-trans retinoic acid (ATRA),
    Sweet syndrome, 216
Allylamines, systemic antifungals, 507
Alopecia, 200
    epidermolysis bullosa acquisita, 107
    pressure injury, 361
Alopecia areata (AA)
    clinicopathological features, 201, 202f
    epidemiology, 200
    management, 201–202
    variants, 201
Alopecia totalis, 201
Alopecia universalis, 201
α-adrenergic agonists, 525–526
α-hydroxy acids, 86, 574
Alpha-2-macroglobulin-like 1, paraneoplastic
    pemphigus (PNP), 99
Alternative pathway, complement, 26, 27t
Aluminum chloride, for hyperhidrosis, 198
Amantadine, 501
Amblyomma americanum lone star tick, 303
Ambras syndrome, 211t
Amebiasis, 339t
Amelanosis, 83
Amelanotic melanoma, 393, 396
American trypanosomiasis, 339t
Amides, 547
Aminoglycoside, 301, 503–504, 580
Aminolevulinic acid (ALA), 530
Aminopenicillin-induced morbilliform drug
    eruption, 154
Amitriptyline, 498t
Amniotic band syndrome, 361
Amoxicillin
    for Lyme disease, 307
    for scarlet fever, 290
Amphotericin B
    for aspergillosis, 332
    for coccidioidomycosis, 327
    for cryptococcosis, 329
    for histoplasmosis, 327
    for mycosis, 326
Amyloidosis, 243, 243t–244t, 244f
Amyloid transthyretin (ATTR) amyloidosis, 243,
    244t
Amyopathic dermatomyositis (DM), 127
Anagen, 12
Anakinra, adult-onset Still disease (AoSD), 137
Anaphylatoxins, 32
Anaphylaxis, urticaria, 152
Anaplasmosis, 305t
Androgenetic alopecia, 204, 204f
Androgenetic alopecia (SAHA) syndrome, 68

Androgens, 500
    and hair follicles, 12
    for lipodermatosclerosis, 147
Anesthetics
    local anesthetics, 547
    nerve blocks, 548
    topical anesthetics, 547
Anetoderma, 400t
Angelman syndrome, 19
Angioedema
    acquired, 153
    hereditary, 153, 153t
    urticaria, 152
Angiofibroma, 401, 401f
Angioid streaks, pseudoxanthoma elasticum
    (PXE), 141
Angioinvasive fungal infection, 331–332
Angiokeratoma, 412–413, 412f, 412t
    circumscriptum, 412
    corpus diffusum, 412
    of Mibelli, 412
Angioleiomyoma, 461f
Angiolipoma, 410
Angioma serpiginosum, 412t
Angiosarcoma, 196, 428–429, 428f
Angiotensin-converting enzyme (ACE), 229
Angiotensin-converting enzyme inhibitors
    (ACEIs)
    acquired angioedema, 153
    lichenoid drug eruption, 114
    pityriasis rosea (PR), 58
    systemic sclerosis, 134
Angular cheilitis, 252, 323t
Anhidrosis, 198
Anifrolumab
    biologic and small molecule inhibitors, 493
    systemic lupus erythematosus, 122
Animal bites and stings, 347, 348t–349t
Ankle-brachial index (ABI)
    arterial ulcer, 180
    for venous ulcer, 179
Ankyloblepharon, mucous membrane
    pemphigoid, 106
Ankyloblepharon–ectodermal defects, 199t
Annular elastolytic giant cell granuloma, 231
Annular erythema annulare centrifugum, 154
Anogenital disorders, 589t–594t
Anogenital lichen sclerosus, 130
Anthralin, 53, 524t
Anthrax, 297–298
Anthropophilic fungi, 318
Antiandrogens, 191, 500
Antibacterials, 503f, 504f
    systemic, 503–507
    topical, 508t–509t
Antibiotics, 513t
    prophylaxis, 545–546
Antibodies, 29–30, 31t
Anticoagulants, 162, 545
Anticoagulation management, 545
Anti-collagen II, relapsing polychondritis, 136
Antidepressants, for prurigo nodularis, 183
Antifungals
    mechanisms, 507, 510f
    systemic antifungals, 507–510
    topical, 510–511, 511t
Antigen-binding fragment (Fab), 29
Antigen-presenting cells (APCs), 33

Antihistamines, 497, 498t
    for cutaneous small vessel vasculitis
        (CSVV), 170
    for prurigo nodularis, 183
Anti-hypertensives, lichenoid drug eruption, 114
Anti-laminin-332 mucous membrane
    pemphigoid (MMP), 106
Antimalarials, 489
    lichenoid drug eruption, 114
    morbilliform drug eruption, 154
    porphyria cutanea tarda, 248
    for sarcoidosis, 226
Anti-matrilin-1, relapsing polychondritis, 136
Antimetabolites, 513t
    azathioprine, 489–490, 490t
    methotrexate, 490–491
    mycophenolate, 491
    toxic erythema of chemotherapy (TEC), 120
    traction alopecia, 205
Antimicrobial peptides, 27
Antimicrobials
    antibacterials, 503–509
    antifungals, 507, 509–511
    antiparasitics, 510–511, 512t
    antivirals, 501–502
Antimicrotubule taxanes, 120, 513t
Antimony compounds
    for cutaneous leishmaniasis, 334
    systemic antiparasitics, 510
Antineoplastics
    for actinic keratosis, 514, 522
    for cutaneous T-cell lymphoma, 514, 523
    cytotoxic chemotherapies, 511–516
    hand-foot adverse events, 519f
    immunotherapies, 514, 520t, 521f
    mucocutaneous adverse events, 519f
    targeted, 514, 516t–517t, 518f, 519f
    topical, 514, 522
Antineutrophil cytoplasmic antibody (ANCA)
    livedoid vasculopathy, 162
    small vessel vasculitis, 169
Antineutrophil cytoplasmic antibody vasculitis,
    174–175, 175f
Antioxidants, 574
Antiparasitics
    systemic, 510–511
    topical, 512t
Antiphospholipid antibody syndrome (APLS),
    163t, 164
Antiplatelet agents
    for cholesterol emboli, 165
    for livedoid vasculopathy, 162
Antipruritic drugs, 524t
Antipsoriatic drugs, 524t
Antiretrovirals
    purine analogues, 501–502
    pyrimidine analogues, 502
    pyrophosphate analogues, 502
Antiretroviral therapy (ART), Ofuji disease, 224
Antiseptics, 548, 549t
Antivirals
    systemic, 501–502, 501t
    topical, 502t
Ants, 348t
APD. *See* Acquired perforating dermatosis
    (APD)
APECED/IPEX syndromes, 324
APECED syndrome, 324

Apert syndrome, 191t
Aphthous stomatitis, 219
    recurrent, 217, 218f
Aplasia cutis congenita (ACC), 431
Apocrine bromhidrosis, 198
Apocrine chromhidrosis, 198
Apocrine differentiation, primarily
    cylindroma and spiradenoma, 443–444
    hidradenoma, 446–447
    hidradenoma papilliferum, 444–445
    syringocystadenoma papilliferum, 444–445
Apocrine glands, 9–10
Apocrine miliaria, 200
Apoptosis, 19
Apremilast, 53, 492
Aprepitant, 183
Aquagenic palmoplantar keratodermas, 61t
Arciform erythema annulare centrifugum, 154
Areola, 14–15
Argininosuccinic aciduria, 245t
Argyll Robertson pupil, 308
Argyria, 509f
Aromatic anticonvulsants
    for cutaneous lymphoid hyperplasia (CLH), 476
    drug reaction with eosinophilia and systemic
        symptoms (DRESS), 156
    morbilliform drug eruption, 154
    for Stevens-Johnson syndrome/toxic
        epidermal necrolysis, 118
Arrector pili muscle, 12
Arrhythmia
    burns, 360
    dermatomyositis (DM), 127
Arsenical keratoses, 19, 376
Arsenic, 513t
Arsenic poisoning
    actinic keratosis, 376
    Mees lines, 212
    traction alopecia, 205
    vitiligo, 85
Arterial catheterization, cholesterol emboli, 164
Arterial insufficiency, 180
Arterial ulcer, 180
Arteriovenous malformation (AVM), 418–419,
    419f
Arteriovenous shunting, 418
Arthralgias
    cryoglobulinemic vasculitis, 173
    cutaneous small vessel vasculitis (CSVV), 169
    dengue, 284
    immunoglobulin A vasculitis, 171
    Lyme disease, 304
    serum sickness-like eruption, 170
Arthritis
    cryoglobulinemic vasculitis, 173
    immunoglobulin A vasculitis, 171
    Lyme disease, 304
    reactive, 54–55
    serum sickness-like eruption, 170
Arthroconidia, 320
Arthropod bites, 347
Asboe-Hansen sign, 117
Ascertainment bias, 42
Ascher syndrome, 153
Aspergillosis, 332, 332f
Aspirin (ASA)
    for anticoagulation management, 545
    Kawasaki disease, 158
Association, 37

Asteatotic dermatitis, 67
Atherosclerosis
    diffuse dermal angiomatosis (DDA), 180
    pseudoxanthoma elasticum (PXE), 141
Atherosclerotic disease, cholesterol emboli, 164
Atopic dermatitis (AD)
    clinicopathological features, 65–66
    epidemiology, 65
    evaluation, 66
    management, 66–67
Atopic march, 65
Atopy
    alopecia areata (AA), 200
    keratosis pilaris, 79
    periorificial dermatitis, 196
Atrioventricular block, Lyme disease, 304
Atrophia maculosa varioliformis cutis, 400t
Atrophic papulosis, malignant, 164
Atrophic scar
    acne vulgaris, 188
    epidermolysis bullosa acquisita, 107
Atrophies, 399–400, 400t
Atypical epithelioid Spitz nevus, 391
Atypical fibroxanthoma (AFX), 406, 408f
Atypical mycobacterial infections, 312t
Atypical nevi, 387, 388f, 389
Atypical Spitz nevus, 391
Auricular hematoma, 360
Auspitz sign, 49
Autoantibodies
    dermatomyositis, 129t
    lupus erythematosus (LE), 126t
    morphea, 133t
    rheumatoid arthritis, 137
Autoeczematization, stasis dermatitis, 69
Autoimmune Bullous Skin Disorder Intensity
        Score (ABSIS), 98
Autoimmune progesterone dermatitis, 76
Autoimmune thyroid disease, alopecia areata
        (AA), 200
Autoinflammatory syndromes, 137, 138t–139t
Autosensitization, stasis dermatitis, 69
Autosomal dominant hyper-immunoglobulin E
        syndrome, 343
Avelumab, for Merkel cell carcinoma, 437
Axillae
    interdigital erythrasma, 296
    morbilliform eruption, 155
    neutrophilic eccrine hidradenitis (NEH), 217
    primary focal hyperhidrosis, 198
Azathioprine
    antimetabolites, 489–490
    drug reaction with eosinophilia and systemic
        symptoms (DRESS), 156
    Sweet syndrome, 216
Azelaic acid, 508t
    for acne vulgaris, 191
    for erythema dyschromicum perstans, 86
    for papulopustular rosacea (PPR), 196
Azole cream
    for tinea, 320
    for tinea nigra, 317
    for tinea versicolor, 316

B

Babesiosis, 340t
Baboon syndrome, 120
Bacillary angiomatosis, 304

Bacille Calmette-Guérin (BCG) vaccine,
        dermatomyositis (DM), 127
Bacitracin, 289, 508t
Bacteria, 285, 286t–287t
Bacterial diseases
    abscess, 293
    actinomycosis, 298
    anthrax, 297–298
    cat scratch disease, 303
    cellulitis, 291–292
    chronic granulomatous disease, 294
    ecthyma gangrenosum, 300–301, 301f
    erysipelas, 292
    erythrasma, 296–297, 297f
    folliculitis, 294
    impetigo, 288–289
    infective endocarditis, 299–300
    leprosy, 313, 313f, 313t, 315
    Lyme disease, 304, 307
    malakoplakia, 301–303
    necrotizing fasciitis, 292–293
    paronychia, 295
    pitted keratolysis, 295–296
    Rocky Mountain spotted fever (RMSF), 303,
        305t
    scarlet fever, 290, 290t
    septic vasculitis, 299–300
    staphylococcal scalded skin syndrome (SSSS),
        289
    syphilis, 308–309
    toxic shock syndrome (TSS), 291
    tuberculosis, 309, 312
Baker's itch, 344t
Balanitis circinata, 54
Balanitis xerotica obliterans, 129
Balloon cell nevus, 387
Barbour-Stoenner-Kelly agar, 304
Bartonella hensela, 303
Bartonella infections, 304
Bart-Pumphrey syndrome, 60t
Bart syndrome, 431
Basal cell carcinoma (BCC)
    clinicopathological features, 371, 372f–373f
    epidemiology, 370–371
    evaluation, 371
    hereditary disorders, 371t
    management, 371, 373
Basal cell nevus syndrome (BCNS), 374, 374t
Basal keratinocyte hemidesmosomes, 4
Basement membrane zone (BMZ), 4–5, 5f
Basophils, 31–32
Bazex-Christol-Dupré syndrome, 371t
Bazex sign, 52
B-cell lymphoproliferative disorders/plasma cell
        dyscrasias, 153
B cells, 25, 33
Beaked nose, systemic sclerosis, 134
Bean syndrome, 415, 416
Beare-Stevenson cutis gyrata syndrome, 63
Beau lines, 211–212, 212f
Becker nevus, 211t, 462
    clinicopathological features, 463, 463f
    epidemiology, 463
    evaluation, 463
    management, 463
Beckwith-Wiedemann syndrome, 414t
Bed bug infestation, 344t
Bedside diagnostics, 620t, 624t–625t, 626f
Bees, 348t

Beetles, 349t
Behavior modification therapy
for prurigo nodularis, 183
for trichotillomania, 203
Behçet disease, 219, 219t
Belimumab, systemic lupus erythematosus, 122
Bell palsy
herpes zoster, 274
Lyme disease, 304
Benzalkonium, 549t
Benzathine penicillin, for syphilis, 309
Benzodiazepines, 118, 546
Benzophenones, photoinduced contact
dermatitis, 70
Benzyl benzoate, 512t
Benzoyl peroxide, 508t
for bacterial diseases, 294
for pitted keratolysis, 296
β-blockers
generalized pustular psoriasis (GPP), 49
for pityriasis rosea (PR), 58
systemic sclerosis, 134
telogen effluvium, 205
β-catenin, 457
β-hydroxy acids, 86
β-lactams, 504
acute generalized exanthematous pustulosis,
93
morbilliform drug eruption, 154
serum sickness-like eruption, 170
toxic erythema of chemotherapy (TEC), 120
Bevacizumab, for Kaposi sarcoma, 427
Bexarotene, 471, 498t, 499t, 523t
Bias, 42
Billing
evaluation and management codes, 637, 638t,
639t
modifiers, 640t
procedure codes, 640t
Bimatoprost, 526
Bioavailability, 36
Biologic and small molecule inhibitors, 493–496
Biopsy
calciphylaxis, 166
eosinophilic fasciitis, 135
livedoid vasculopathy, 162
morphea, 132
systemic sclerosis, 134
Biotinidase deficiencies, 245t, 252
Birt-Hogg-Dubé (BHD) syndrome, 455
Bisphosphonates, for calciphylaxis, 166
Bite fibroma/morsicatio buccarum, 361
Björnstad syndrome, 213t
Black heel and palm, 364, 365f
Black piedra, 318
Blaschkitis lichen striatus, 114
Blastic plasmacytoid dendritic cell neoplasm
(BPDCN), 478
Blastomycosis, 325–326, 326f
Blau syndrome, 230
Bleomycin, systemic sclerosis, 134
Blindness
mucous membrane pemphigoid, 106
in paraneoplastic pemphigus, 99
Blistering distal dactylitis, cellulitis, 291
Blood urea nitrogen (BUN)/creatinine
cutaneous small vessel vasculitis (CSVV), 169
drug reaction with eosinophilia and systemic
symptoms (DRESS), 156

livedoid vasculopathy, 162
prurigo nodularis, 182
systemic sclerosis, 134
Blood vessels, 7, 8f, 541
Bloom syndrome, 357t, 435t
BLOT compass, 40f
Blue lunulae, 215f
Blue nevus, 386, 386f
Blue-rubber-bleb nevus syndrome, 415
B lymphocyte stimulator (BLyS), 33
Body contouring, 582–583
Body dysmorphic disorder, 186
Body-focused repetitive behavior disorder, 186
Body surface area (BSA), psoriasis severity
measurement, 53, 54f
Bonnet-Dechaume-Blanc syndrome, 414t
Borderline fibrous neoplasms, 404t–405t
Borderline personality disorder, factitial
dermatitis, 187
Borrelia burgdorferi infection, morphea, 131
Borrelial lymphocytoma, 306t
Bortezomib
for Kaposi sarcoma, 427
Stevens-Johnson syndrome/toxic epidermal
necrolysis-like reactions, 117
Sweet syndrome and, 216
Botryomycosis, abscess, 293
Botulinum neurotoxins (BoNTs), 579t, 579f
cause, 578
clinical applications, 578–579
functional complications, 580t
safety, 579–580
Bovine collagen, 580
Bowel-associated dermatosis-arthritis syndrome
(BADAS), 222
Bowel perforation, malignant atrophic papulosis,
164
Bowel reanastamosis, 222
BP Disease Area Index (BPDAI), 104
Brachydactyly, calciphylaxis, 166
BRAF inhibitors, 517t
erythema nodosum, 144
keratosis pilaris-like reaction, 79
morbilliform drug eruption, 154
seborrheic dermatitis-like reaction, 68
Sweet syndrome, 216
BRAF mutations
melanoma, 394
nevocellular nevus, 387
Spitz nevus, 391
Brain natriuretic peptide (NT-pro-BNP),
systemic sclerosis, 134
Branchial arch syndromes and anomalies, 459t
Branchial cleft cyst, 459t, 468t
Breast adenocarcinoma, 367, 481, 481t
Brentuximab vedotin, 471, 523t
Breslow thickness, melanoma, 394
Brimonidine, for erythematotelangiectatic
rosacea (ETTR), 196
Broadband ultraviolet B (bbUVB), 529
Brocq alopecia, 206
Bromhidrosis, 198
Bronchiolitis obliterans, 99
Bronchogenic cyst, 459t, 468t
Bronze diabetes, 85
Brooke-Spiegler syndrome, 371t
Brunsting-Perry pemphigoid, 106
Buerger disease, 180
Bulb, hair, 11

Bullous arthropod bites, 347
Bullous impetigo, 288
Bullous pemphigoid, 102–105
clinicopathological features, 103, 103f
epidemiology, 103
evaluation, 103–104, 104t, 105f
management, 104
Bullous pemphigoid antigen 1 (BPAG1), 107
Bullous pyoderma gangrenosum, 220
Burning, factitial dermatitis, 187
Burning mouth syndrome, 184t
Burning pain, complex regional pain syndrome
(CPRS), 184, 184t
Burning scalp syndrome, 184t
Buruli ulcer, 312t
Butcher wart, 278t
Butenafin, 511t
Butterfly bite, 349t
Butterfly rash, 124f
Butterfly sign, 183f
Bywaters lesions, rheumatoid arthritis, 137

C

Café-au-lait macules, 435t
Calcifying and ossifying disorders, 167f
Calcifying aponeurotic fibroma, 404t
Calcineurin inhibitors
for atopic dermatitis (AD), 67
for granuloma faciale, 223
immunosuppressants and immunomodulators,
491
for prurigo nodularis, 183
for psoriasis, 53
for vitiligo, 85
Calciphylaxis, 165–166, 166t
Calcipotriene, for psoriasis, 53, 524t
Calcium channel blockers (CCBs)
acute generalized exanthematous pustulosis,
93
eczematous drug eruptions, 66
for Raynaud phenomenon, 134
Calcium intake, calciphylaxis, 166
Calluses, 361
Camphor, 524t
Camouflage
facial foundation, 86
for vitiligo, 85
Camptodactyly, 230
Candidal balanitis/vulvovaginitis, 322, 323t
Candidal folliculitis, 323t
Candidal intertrigo, 322, 323t
Candida species, 323t
Candidemia, 323t
Candidiasis, 322–325
clinicopathological features, 322, 324f
congenital, 322
epidemiology, 322
evaluation, 322
management, 322
neonatal, 322
variants, 323t
Candy cane nails, 101f
Cantharidin, 502t
Capecitabine, for pyogenic granuloma, 423
Capillaritis, pigmented purpura, 168
Capillary malformation (CM), 414t–415t, 416f
clinicopathological features, 413, 416f
epidemiology, 413–415

evaluation, 415
management, 415
Capsaicin, 524t
Caput succedaneum, 360
Carbamazepine, 117
Carcinogenesis, 19–21, 20f, 21f, 22t
Carcinoid syndrome, rosacea, 195
Cardiac troponin 1, 158
Cardiofaciocutaneous syndrome, 387
Cardiovascular syphilis, 308
Carmustine, 523t
Carney complex, 384t, 386, 433
Carotenemia, 85
Carvajal syndrome, 61t
Case-control studies, 41
Case reports, 41
Caspases, 19
Castleman disease, 99
Catagen, 12
Cataracts, varicella, 273
Catechols, hypopigmentation/depigmentation, 85
Caterpillars, 349t
Cathelicidin upregulation, rosacea, 194
Cat scratch disease, 303, 304
Causation, 37
Cavernous sinus, 541
Cavernous sinus thrombosis, cellulitis, 291
CBCL. *See* Cutaneous B-cell lymphoma (CBCL)
CCCA. *See* Central centrifugal cicatricial alopecia (CCCA)
CCR5 inhibitors, 501t
CD4/CD25+ regulatory T cells (T-regs), 33
CD8+ cytotoxic T cells, 33
CD4+ helper T cells, 33
Cefaclor, serum sickness-like eruption, 170
Cefuroxime, for perianal streptococcal infection, 292
Celiac disease, 107
Cell cycle, 19, 20f
Cell extraction, 38, 39t
Cell-mediated cytotoxicity, paraneoplastic pemphigus (PNP), 99
Cell-mediated immunity, 25
Cellular blue nevus, 386
Cellular components measurement, 38, 39t–40t
Cellulitis, 291–292
clinicopathological features, 291–292
epidemiology, 291
evaluation, 292
management, 292
Centipedes, 349t
Central centrifugal cicatricial alopecia (CCCA), 208, 208f
Cephalexin
for cellulitis, 292
for impetigo, 289
Cephalocele, 431
Cephalohematoma, 360
Ceramide, 1
Cercarial dermatitis, 342t
Cervarix vaccine, for wart, 280
Cervicofacial actinomycosis, 298
Cetirizine, 498t
Cetirizine, photoinduced contact dermatitis, 70
CGD. *See* Chronic granulomatous disease (CGD)
Chancroid, 308
Checkerboard parakeratosis, 59f

Checkpoints, cell cycle, 19
Chemical sunscreens, 25t
Chemical exposure injury, 362
Chemical peels, for erythema dyschromicum perstans, 86
Chemical resurfacing
chemical peels, 574, 575t
indications, 574
safety, 575–576
Chemokines, 29, 30
Cherry angioma, 424, 424f
Cheyletiellosis, 344t
Chigger bites, 344t
Chikungunya virus, 284
Child abuse, skin signs, 362t
Chloracne, 190t
Chloramphenicol, 303, 504
Chlorhexidine, 294, 549t
Chloroma, 478
Chlorotrichosis, 362
Chlorpheniramine, 498t
Cholestasis, 117
Cholesterol emboli, 164–165, 165f
Chondrodermatitis nodularis helicis (CNH), 365, 365f
Chorioretinitis
cytomegalovirus infection, 275
varicella, 273
Chromhidrosis, 198
Chromoblastomycosis, 326, 326f
Chromophores, 22
Chromosomal genetic disorders, 18–19
Chromosomal translocation, melanoma, 394
Chronic actinic dermatitis (CAD), 355
Chronic granulomatous disease (CGD), 30, 294
Chronic infective endocarditis, 303
Chronic kidney disease (CKD), 136
Chronic lymphocytic leukemia (CLL), 99
Chronic mucocutaneous candidiasis (CMC), 324
Chronic sun-damaged (CSD) skin, 393
Ciclopirox,511t
Cidofovir, 276
Cigarette smoking
arterial ulcer, 180
diffuse dermal angiomatosis (DDA), 180
Cimetidine, 498t
Cinacalcet, 166
C1-inhibitor (C1-inh), 27
C1-inhibitor deficiency
acquired, 153t
hereditary, 153t
Ciprofloxacin, 298
Circumcision, balanitis xerotica obliterans, 130
Circumscribed hypopigmentation/depigmentation, 83
Circumscribed vitiligo, 85
Cirrhosis, calciphylaxis, 166
Citrullinemia, 245t
c-KIT proto-oncogene mutation, 32
Classical pathway, complement, 26, 27t
Classic dermatomyositis (DM), 127
Clear cell acanthoma, 370, 370f, 370t
Clear cell sarcoma, 394
Cleft lip/palate, 459t
Cleft lip/palate syndrome, 199t
Clindamycin, 508t
for acne vulgaris, 191
for cellulitis, 292

for impetigo, 289
for pitted keratolysis, 296
Clinical studies, 41–42
Clinical tests, 42–43
Clofazimine, 504
Clomipramine, 203
Clonidine, 196
Clopidogrel/ticlopidine, 545
Clotrimazole, 511t
Clouston syndrome, 199t
CLOVES syndrome, 414t
Clutton joints, 309
Coagulopathies
cutaneous manifestations, 163t
systemic, 163t
vascular, 163t
Coal tar preparations, for psoriasis, 53, 524t
Coarse facies, hyper-immunoglobulin E syndrome, 343
Cobb syndrome, 414t
Coccidioides immitis, 327
Coccidioidomycosis, 327, 328f
erythema nodosum, 144
molluscum contagiosum, 281
Cockayne syndrome, 356t
Coffin-Siris syndrome, 214t
Cohort studies, 41
COL1A1-PDGFB fusion, 406
Colchicine, 492
for cutaneous small vessel vasculitis (CSVV), 170
for erythema nodosum, 147
for gout, 245
for recurrent mucocutaneous lesions, 219
for Sweet syndrome, 217
traction alopecia, 205
Cold injury, 360
Colicky abdominal pain, immunoglobulin A vasculitis, 171
Colitis, cytomegalovirus infection, 275
Collagen degeneration, chondrodermatitis nodularis helicis (CNH), 365
Collagen disorders, 6
Collagen III, 399
Collodion membrane, 79
Colloid milium, 244f
Colon adenocarcinoma, 367, 481t
Coma bulla, pressure injury, 361
Combined oral contraceptive pills, 500–501
Common Spitz nevus, 391
Common wart, 278t
Complement, 26–27, 27f
disorders, 28t
pathways, 26, 27f
Complementarity-determining regions (CDRs), 29
Complement receptor type 1 (CR1), 27
Complete blood count (CBC)
cutaneous small vessel vasculitis (CSVV), 169
drug reaction with eosinophilia and systemic symptoms (DRESS), 156
for erythema nodosum, 147
livedoid vasculopathy, 162
prurigo nodularis, 182
urticaria, 152
Complex aphthosis, 217
Complex regional pain syndrome (CPRS), 184–185, 184t, 185f

Compound nevi, 387
Confidence interval (CI), 37
Confluent and reticulated papillomatosis
(CARP), 64
Confounding, 42, 43f
Congenital hemidysplasia with ichthyosiform
erythroderma and limb defects (CHILD)
syndrome, 236
Congenital inclusion cyst, 465t
Congenital livedo reticularis, 161
Congenital syphilis, 308–309
Congenital toxoplasmosis infection, 334
Congenital varicella, 273
Conical teeth, 88
Conjunctival involvement, mucous membrane
pemphigoid, 106
Conjunctivitis, 54, 136
Connective tissue disorders, hereditary,
141t–143t
Connective tissue nevus, 404t
Constant fragment, 29–30
Contact allergens, 71t–74t
Contact dermatitis, 70, 71f, 71t–76t, 76–78
clinicopathological features, 71, 76
contact allergens, 71t–74t
epidemiology, 70
evaluation, 76–78, 77f
management, 78
pathogenesis, 71f
Contact irritants, 74t–75t
Contact urticaria, 76
Cooling agents/counterirritants, prurigo
nodularis, 183
Cooling and limb elevation, erythromelalgia, 181
Copper deficiency, 252, 252t
Coral bead papules, 236f
Corn/callus, 361
Cornelia de Lange syndrome, 211t
Cornification disorders, 3t
Coronary catheterization, cholesterol emboli, 164
Coronavirus disease 2019 (COVID-19), 283–284
Cortex, hair, 12
Corticosteroids
for acne fulminans, 192
for acute generalized exanthematous
pustulosis, 93
adult-onset Still disease (AoSD), 137
adverse events, 487–488
for alopecia areata (AA), 202
for atopic dermatitis (AD), 67
for Behçet disease, 219
for bullous pemphigoid, 104
for contact dermatitis, 78
for cryoglobulinemia, 173
for cutaneous small vessel vasculitis (CSVV),
170
dosing notes, 488
for drug reaction with eosinophilia and
systemic symptoms (DRESS), 157
drug selection, 487
for eosinophilic fasciitis, 135
FDA-approved dermatology indications, 487
for frontal fibrosing alopecia/lichen
planopilaris, 206
for giant cell arteritis (GCA), 177
for graft-versus-host disease (GVHD), 121
for granuloma faciale, 223
for hypereosinophilic syndrome (HES), 225

for juvenile-onset dermatomyositis (DM), 127
lichen planus (LP), 113
for lichen sclerosus, 130
mechanism, 487
monitoring parameters, 488
morbilliform eruption, 155
for mucous membrane pemphigoid (MMP),
107
for pemphigus foliaceus, 96
pemphigus vulgaris, 98
periorificial dermatitis, 196
pharmacodynamics, 488–489
pharmacokinetics, 488
for polyarteritis nodosa, 177
pregnancy risk, 488–489
for prurigo nodularis, 183
for psoriasis, 53, 524t
for pyoderma gangrenosum (PG), 220
for recurrent aphthous stomatitis, 217
for relapsing polychondritis, 136
for sarcoidosis, 226
for sebaceous gland hyperplasia, 440
for Stevens-Johnson syndrome/toxic
epidermal necrolysis, 118
for Sweet syndrome, 217
topical, 489t
for urticaria, 152
vitiligo, 85
for Wells syndrome, 224
Corynebacterial infections, 296, 297t
Cosmeceuticals, 574
Cosmetics
astringents, 573–574
body contouring, 582–583
botulinum neurotoxins, 578–580
chemical and mechanical skin resurfacing,
574–576
cleansers, 573
Glogau photoaging classification-wrinkle
scale, 573t
hair restoration, 583–584
lasers, 576–578, 576f
moisturizers, 573
safety, 574
sclerotherapy, 583, 584
soft-tissue dermal fillers, 580–582
Costochondral joint, relapsing polychondritis,
136
Cowden syndrome, 384t, 411, 411t
Cowpox, 282t
Coxsackieviruses, hand-foot-mouth disease
(HFMD), 284
CPRS. See Complex regional pain syndrome
(CPRS)
C-reactive protein (CRP)
cutaneous small vessel vasculitis (CSVV), 169
drug reaction with eosinophilia and systemic
symptoms (DRESS), 156
for erythema nodosum, 147
urticaria, 152
Cream, 37
Crisaborole, 67
Critical line of Auber, 11
Crohn disease, erythema nodosum, 144
Cromolyn sodium, 497
Cronkite-Canada syndrome, 384t
Cross-sectional surveys, 41
Crotamiton, 512t

Cryoglobulinemia, 172–173, 173, 173f, 174f
Cryoglobulinemic vasculitis, 137, 173, 174f
Cryopyrin, 28
Cryopyrin-associated periodic syndromes
(CAPS), 28
Cryosurgery, 532, 532t
Cryotherapy
actinic keratosis, 377
for basal cell carcinoma (BCC), 373
vs. electrosurgery, 535
for Kaposi sarcoma, 427
for keloid, 400
for porokeratosis, 375
seborrheic keratosis, 368
squamous cell carcinoma (SCC), 380
wart, 280
Cryptococcosis, 281, 329, 330f
CSVV. See Cutaneous small vessel vasculitis
(CSVV)
CTCL. See Cutaneous T-cell lymphoma (CTCL)
Ctenocephalides felis (cat flea), 303
C-type fiber, 8
Curly hair, 12
Current Procedural Terminology (CPT) codes,
637
Cutaneous anthrax, 298
Cutaneous B-cell lymphoma (CBCL), 476, 477f
Cutaneous ciliated cyst, 468t
Cutaneous coccidioidomycosis, 327
Cutaneous cryptococcosis, 329
Cutaneous Dermatomyositis Disease Area and
Severity Index (CDASI), 127
Cutaneous focal mucinosis, 241t
Cutaneous involvement
mucous membrane pemphigoid, 106
systemic sclerosis, 134
Cutaneous larva migrans
clinicopathological features, 336–337, 342f
epidemiology, 336
evaluation, 337, 343
management, 343
Cutaneous leishmaniasis, 334
Cutaneous lichen planus (LP), 111
Cutaneous lymphoid hyperplasia (CLH), 476,
478f
Cutaneous melanoacanthoma, 367
Cutaneous sclerosis
eosinophilic fasciitis, 135
lichen sclerosus, 129
morphea, 131
systemic sclerosis, 134
Cutaneous small vessel vasculitis (CSVV),
169–170, 170f
Cutaneous T-cell lymphoma (CTCL)
antineoplastics for, 514t, 523t
clinicopathological features, 471, 473f
clonal T cell–related dermatoses
associated, 55
epidemiology, 471
evaluation, 471, 474
management, 471
variants, 472t
Cutaneous vasculitis, 158, 161t–
Cutibacterium acnes, 530
Cutis gyrata, 63, 400t
Cutis marmorata, 161
Cutis marmorata telangiectatica congenita
(CMTC), 161

Cyclic citrullinated peptide (CCP), rheumatoid arthritis, 137
Cyclic neutropenia, recurrent aphthous stomatitis, 217
Cyclin-dependent kinase inhibitor 2A (CDKN2A), 19
Cyclobutene-pyrimidine dimers, 23, 376
Cyclophosphamide
    in dermatomyositis (DM), 127
    immunosuppressants and immunomodulators, 492
    for mucous membrane pemphigoid (MMP), 107
Cyclosporine
    for psoriasis, 53
    for pyoderma gangrenosum (PG), 220
    for sebaceous gland hyperplasia, 440
    for Stevens-Johnson syndrome/toxic epidermal necrolysis, 118
Cylindroma, 443–444, 444f
CYP3A4 interactions, 37f
Cyproheptadine, 498t
Cysticercosis, 342t
Cystic hygroma, 417
Cysts
    with nonstratified squamous epithelium, 467, 468t, 469f
    pseudocysts, 468–470
    with stratified squamous epithelium, 464–467, 465t, 466f
Cytarabine, Sweet syndrome, 216
Cytochrome p-450 (CYP) enzymes, 36, 37t
Cytokines, 29, 29t
    inhibitors, 31t
    signatures, 30t
    treatments, 30t
Cytomegalovirus infection, 275–276, 276f
Cytopenias, 117
Cytophagic histiocytic panniculitis, 148f
Cytotoxic chemotherapies, 382, 511, 512t–513t, 514, 515f
    mucocutaneous adverse events, 515f–516f
Cytotoxic keratinocyte damage, 122

D

Dactylitis, 50
Dalfopristin, 505
Damage-associated molecular patterns (DAMPs), 28
Dapsone, 508t
    for acne vulgaris, 191
    for bullous pemphigoid, 104
    for cutaneous small vessel vasculitis (CSVV), 170
    for dermatitis herpetiformis (DH), 110
    drug reaction with eosinophilia and systemic symptoms (DRESS), 156
    for granuloma faciale, 223
    for IgA pemphigus, 99
    immunosuppressants and immunomodulators, 492
    for mucous membrane pemphigoid (MMP), 107
    in Stevens-Johnson syndrome/toxic epidermal necrolysis, 117
    for Sweet syndrome, 217
    for urticarial vasculitis, 172

Daptomycin, for impetigo, 289
Darier disease, 100, 101f, 101t, 102f
Darier-Roussy syndrome, 227t
Decapitation secretion, apocrine gland, 10
Deck-chair sign, 224f
Decubitus ulcer, 292, 361
Deep burns, 360
Deep folliculitis, 294
Deep mycoses, 325–331
    blastomycosis, 325–326, 326f
    chromoblastomycosis, 326, 326f
    coccidioidomycosis, 327
    cryptococcosis, 329
    dimorphic fungi, 325, 325f
    histoplasmosis, 327, 329, 329f
    lobomycosis, 329, 331f
    paracoccidioidomycosis, 326, 326f
    sporotrichosis, 330–331, 331f
    talaromycosis, 327
Deep peroneal block, 548
Dehydroepiandrosterone sulfate (DHEA-S), for acne vulgaris, 188
Delayed-type, cell-mediated (type IV) reaction
    chronic actinic dermatitis (CAD), 355
    drug reaction with eosinophilia and systemic symptoms (DRESS), 156
    erythema nodosum, 144
    lichenoid drug eruption, 114
    morbilliform drug eruption, 154
    photoallergic/phototoxic eruption, 358
    polymorphous light eruption (PMLE), 353
    severe cutaneous adverse reaction (SCAR), 93
Delusions of parasitosis, 186
Dematiaceous onychomycosis, 321
Demodex folliculorum mites, rosacea, 194
Demodex mites, 334
Demodicosis, 344t
Dengue, 284
Denileukin diftitox, 471, 523t
De novo mutations, Mendelian inheritance, 15
Dental restorative materials, lichen planus (LP), 111
Depigmentation, 83, 85
Depositional disorders, 237, 240–255
Dercum disease, 409
Dermal melanocytosis, 385, 385f, 385t
Dermatitis herpetiformis (DH)
    clinicopathological features, 110, 110f
    differential diagnosis, 110
    epidemiology, 107, 110
    management, 110
Dermatitis neglecta, 362t
Dermatofibroma (DF)
    clinicopathological features, 403–405, 404f
    epidemiology, 403
    evaluation, 403
    management, 406
Dermatofibrosarcoma protuberans (DFSP), 406–407, 407f
Dermatologic pruritus, 181, 182t
Dermatologic signs
    internal malignancy, 605t–607t
    metabolic disorders, 609t–610t
    pregnancy, 611t–612t
Dermatomyositis (DM), 127–129, 128f
    clinicopathological features, 127, 128f
    differential diagnosis, 127
    epidemiology, 127

evaluation, 127
    malignant atrophic papulosis, 164
    skin findings, 128f
Dermatomyositis Skin Severity Index (DSSI), 127
Dermatophyte test medium (DTM), 320
Dermatosis papulosa nigra (DPN), 367
Dermis, 5, 7
Dermoid cyst/sinus, 431, 465t
Dermoscopy
    actinic keratosis, 377
    basal cell carcinoma (BCC), 371
    clear cell acnthoma, 370
    definition, 613
    eight-level criterion ladder, 613, 614t
    lichen planus (LP), 112
    melanocytic lesions, 613, 616f–618f
    melanocytic neoplasms, 382
    molluscum contagiosum, 281
    nonmelanocytic lesions, 613, 619f
    nonneoplastic disorders, 613, 620t
    pattern analysis, 613t–616t
    psoriasis, 53
    scabies, 345
    seborrheic keratosis, 367
    squamous cell carcinoma (SCC), 378
    trichoscopy, 613, 620t–621t, 623f
Desensitization, morbilliform eruption, 155
Desmocollins, paraneoplastic pemphigus (PNP), 99–100, 100f
Desmoglein, pemphigus foliaceus (PF), 96
Desmoglein compensation theory, 96, 96f, 97
Desmogleins 1 and 3, 107
Desmoid tumor, 405t
Desmoplastic/neurotropic melanoma, 393
Desmoplastic trichoepithelioma, 450t
Desmosomes, 3, 4f, 6f
Desquamative gingivitis, 97, 106
Detal hydantoin syndrome, 211t
DF. See Dermatofibroma (DF)
DFSP. See Dermatofibrosarcoma protuberans (DFSP)
DH. See Dermatitis herpetiformis (DH)
Diabetes insipidus, 233t
Diabetes mellitus
    arterial ulcer, 180
    calciphylaxis, 166
    candidiasis, 322
    erythema dyschromicum perstans, 85
    familial dysautonomia, 185
    necrobiosis lipoidica, 232
    rosacea, 195
    syringoma, 446
    zygomycosis, 332
Diabetic dermopathy, 400t
Diabetic ulcer, 292
Diaper dermatitis, 49, 62, 68, 76
    candidiasis, 322
    cellulitis, 292
    impetigo, 288
    Kawasaki disease, 158
    miliaria, 200
    and scabies, 343
    syphilis, 309
    zinc deficiency, 252
Diascopy
    lupus miliaris disseminatus faciei (LMDF), 197
    sarcoidosis, 226
Diclofenac, 522t

Dicloxacillin
  for cellulitis, 292
  for impetigo, 289
  for staphylococcal scalded skin syndrome
    (SSSS), 289
Diethylcarbamazine, 510–511
Diethyltoluamide (Deet), 284
Difelikefalin, for prurigo nodularis, 183
Diffuse alopecia areata, 201
Diffuse alveolar hemorrhage, 174
Diffuse cutaneous mastocytosis, 480t
Diffuse cutaneous systemic sclerosis, 134
Diffuse dermal angiomatosis (DDA), 180
Diffuse hereditary palmoplantar keratodermas,
    59, 60t
Diffuse hypopigmentation/depigmentation, 83
Diffuse large B-cell lymphoma, 476–477
Diffuse vitiligo, 85
Digital mucous cyst, 241t, 468–470
Digitate dermatosis, 55
Dihydroxyacetone, 25
Diltiazem, 93
Dimorphic fungi, 325, 325f
Dimple, 431
Dipeptidyl peptidase-4 (DPP-4) inhibitors,
    bullous pemphigoid, 103
Diphenhydramine, 498t, 524t
Diphtheria, 297t
Direct immunofluorescence (DIF), 93, 634t
Direct oral anticoagulants (DOACs), 545
Dispersive electrode, 533
Disseminated coccidioidomycosis, 327
Disseminated cryptococcosis, 329
Disseminated eczema, stasis dermatitis, 69
Disseminated herpes zoster, 274
Disseminated sporotrichosis, 330
Distal matrix, nail, 13
Distal subungual onychomycosis, 321
Distribution, drug, 36
Disulfiram reaction, rosacea, 195
Diuretics
  for edema blister, 177
  lichenoid drug eruption, 114
DM. *See* Dermatomyositis (DM)
Docosanol, 502t
Dominant negative effect, 15
Dorsal pterygium, 106
Dose, 22
Double-blind randomized controlled trials
    (RCTs), 41
Double-headed pseudocomedone, 193t
Doughnut sign, 240
Down syndrome, 417t
Down syndrome, keratosis pilaris, 79
Doxepin, 498t, 524t
  for excoriation disorder, 187
  for pruritus, 183
Doxycycline
  for anthrax, 298
  for bullous pemphigoid, 104
  for Lyme disease, 307
  for ocular rosacea, 196
  for periorificial dermatitis, 196
  for Rocky Mountain spotted fever (RMSF),
    303
D-penicillamine, dermatomyositis (DM), 127
Dracunculiasis, 341t
DRESS syndrome, 274

Driver mutations, 19
Drospirenone, 191
Drug excretion, 37
Drug-induced acne, 190t
Drug-induced hyperpigmentation/discoloration,
    86t–87t
Drug-induced pityriasis rosea (PR) like
    eruption, 58
Drug-induced Sweet syndrome, 216
Drug reaction with eosinophilia and systemic
    symptoms (DRESS), 155–157
Dry flush, rosacea, 195
Dupilumab
  antineutrophil cytoplasmic antibody
    vasculitis, 174
  for atopic dermatitis (AD), 67
  biologic and small molecule inhibitors, 493
  for bullous pemphigoid, 104
  psoriasis, 49
Duplex ultrasonography, for venous ulcer, 179
Dutasteride, 201, 500
Dysacusis/tinnitus, 84
Dyschezia, anogenital lichen sclerosus, 130
Dyschromatoses, pigmentary disorders, 83
Dysesthesia, 181
  regional, 184, 184t
  in sensory neuropathies, 185f
Dysesthetic anogenital pain syndromes, 184t
Dyshidrosis lamellosa sicca, 67
Dyshidrotic eczema, 67–68
Dyspareunia, 130
Dysphagia, 127
Dystrophic calcification, 165
  dermatomyositis (DM), 127
  pseudoxanthoma elasticum (PXE), 141
  systemic sclerosis, 134
Dysuria, anogenital lichen sclerosus, 130

E

EAC. *See* Erythema annulare centrifugum (EAC)
Ear, 15
Early-onset psoriasis, 49
Ear pit, 459t, 465t
EBA. *See* Epidermolysis bullosa acquisita (EBA)
Ecchymoses, 159, 159t
Eccrine angiomatous hamartoma, 451t
Eccrine bromhidrosis, 198
Eccrine chromhidrosis, 198
Eccrine differentiation, primarily
  poroma, 446–447
  syringoma, 446, 448, 450
Eccrine glands, 10–11
Echinocandins, 507
Econazole, 511t
Ecthyma, 288
Ecthyma gangrenosum, 300–301, 301f
Ectoderm, skin, 15
Ectodermal dysplasias, 198, 198t
Ectoparasite infestations, 343, 344t
Ectoparasites, 336t
Ectopic ACTH syndrome, erythema
    dyschromicum perstans, 85
Ectothrix tinea capitis, 320
Eculizumab, 164
Eczema coxsackium, 284
Eczema herpeticum, 272
Eczematous dermatitis

differential diagnosis, 66
  hyper-immunoglobulin E syndrome, 343
  stages, 65
Eczematous dermatoses
  asteatotic dermatitis, 67
  atopic dermatitis, 65–67
  contact dermatitis, 70, 71f, 71t–76t, 76–78
  dyshidrotic eczema, 67–68
  hereditary ichthyoses and
    erythrokeratodermas, 79
  ichthyosis vulgaris, 78–79
  nummular dermatitis, 68
  seborrheic dermatitis, 68–69
  stasis dermatitis, 69, 70f
Edema
  cold injury, 360
  eosinophilic fasciitis, 135
  stasis dermatitis, 69
Edema blister, 177
Edwards syndrome, 417t
Effect modification, 42
Eflornithine, 210, 526
Ehlers-Danlos syndrome (EDS), calciphylaxis,
    165
Ehrlichiosis, 305t–306t
Elastic tissue disorders, 400t
Elastofibroma dorsi, 400t
Elastoma, 400t
Elastosis perforans serpiginosa (EPS), 134, 137,
    140f
Elder self-neglect, 362t
Electrocautery, 533–535, 534f
Electrocoagulation, 533, 533t
Electrodesiccation and curettage (ED&C)
  basal cell carcinoma (BCC), 373
  squamous cell carcinoma (SCC), 380
Electrodessication, 533, 533t
Electrofulguration, 533, 533t
Electromagnetic spectrum, 23
Electrosection, 533, 533t
Electrosurgery, 533–535, 533t, 534f
Elephantiasis nostras verrucosa, lymphedema,
    178
Embryology, 15
Emollient therapy
  for atopic dermatitis (AD), 67
  for psoriasis, 53
  and seborrheic dermatitis, 69
EMPD. *See* Extramammary Paget disease
    (EMPD)
Encephalopathy, Lyme disease, 304
Endemic Burkitt lymphoma, 275
Endothelin 1, Kawasaki disease, 158
Endothrix tinea capitis, 320
End-stage renal disease (ESRD)
  calciphylaxis, 166
  ichthyosis vulgaris, 78
Enoxaparin, 545
Enteritis, 54
Enteropathy-associated T-cell lymphoma, 107
Enthesitis, 50
Entropion, 106
Environmental allergies, atopic dermatitis (AD),
    65
Envoplakin
  mucous membrane pemphigoid (MMP), 107
  paraneoplastic pemphigus, 99
Enzyme deficiencies, hereditary, 245t–247t

Enzyme-linked immunosorbent assay (ELISA)
  for bullous pemphigoid, 104
    epidermolysis bullosa acquisita, 107
    mucous membrane pemphigoid (MMP), 107
    paraneoplastic pemphigus, 99
    pemphigus foliaceus, 96
Eosinophilia-myalgia syndrome, 133t
Eosinophilic esophagitis, 65
Eosinophilic fasciitis, 135, 135f
Eosinophilic granuloma, 222
Eosinophilic granulomatosis with polyangiitis
      (EGPA), 175
Eosinophilic pustular folliculitis (EPF), 223–224,
      224f
Eosinophilic ulcer, oral mucosa, 361
Eosinophils, 30
Eotaxin, 30
EPF. *See* Eosinophilic pustular folliculitis (EPF)
Epidemiology and statistics, 41–45
Epidermal growth factor receptor (EGFR)
      inhibitors, asteatotic dermatitis and, 67
Epidermal neoplasms
    actinic keratosis, 376–377
    basal cell carcinoma (BCC), 370–374
    basal cell nevus syndrome (BCNS), 374, 374t
    benign, 370t
    clear cell acanthoma, 370, 370f, 370t
    epidermal nevus, 369, 369f
    extramammary Paget disease (EMPD), 382,
      382f
    keratoacanthoma, 381, 381f
    mammary Paget disease (MPD), 381–382, 382f
    porokeratosis, 375, 375t, 376f
    seborrheic keratosis, 367–368, 368f, 368t
    squamous cell carcinoma (SCC), 377–380
Epidermal nevus, 369, 369f
Epidermis, 1, 2f
Epidermodysplasia verruciformis (EDV), 280,
      281f
Epidermoid cyst, 464–466, 465t
Epidermolysis bullosa acquisita (EBA), 107,
      108t–109t, 109f
    variants, 108t–109t
    vs. bullous systemic lupus erythematosus, 109f
Epidermolysis bullosa (EB) simplex, 15
Epidermolytic acanthoma, 370t
Epidermolytic hyperkeratosis, 62f
Epidermolytic ichthyosis (EI), 18
Epigenetics, 15
Epithelioid blue nevus, 386
Epithelioid hemangioendothelioma, 429t
Epithelioid hemangioma, 420t
Epithelioid sarcoma, 406–407, 408f
Eponychium, 13
EPS. *See* Elastosis perforans serpiginosa (EPS)
Epstein-Barr virus (EBV) infection, dermatologic
      signs, 274, 275t
Erdheim-Chester disease, 235t
Erosio interdigitalis blastomycetica, 323t
Erosion, wound healing, 35
Eruptive syringoma, 448
Eruptive xanthoma, 236, 238t
Erysipelas, 292
Erythema, 150
    acute generalized exanthematous
      pustulosis, 93
    acute lipodermatosclerosis, 147
    asteatotic dermatitis and, 67

cellulitis, 291
  cold injury, 360
  erysipelas, 292
  erythema annulare centrifugum (EAC), 154,
      154f
  erythromelalgia, 181
  necrotizing fasciitis, 293
  staphylococcal scalded skin syndrome (SSSS),
      289
  stasis dermatitis, 69
  Stevens-Johnson syndrome/toxic epidermal
      necrolysis, 117
Erythema ab igne (EAI), 363
Erythema annulare centrifugum (EAC), 154,
      154f
Erythema dyschromicum perstans, 85–86,
      86t–87t
Erythema elevatum diutinum (EED), 172
Erythema infectiosum, 283
Erythema migrans, 307
Erythema multiforme, 116, 116f
    major, 116
    minor, 116
Erythema multiforme (EM)-like pityriasis rosea,
      57
Erythema nodosum, 116
    clinicopathological features, 144
    epidemiology, 144
    evaluation, 147
    management, 147
Erythematotelangiectatic rosacea (ETTR), 194
    clinicopathological features, 194
    evaluation, 195
    treatment, 196
Erythematous skin rash, familial dysautonomia,
      185
Erythema toxicum neonatorum, 93, 94t
Erythrasma, 296–297, 297f, 297t
Erythrocyte sedimentation rate (ESR)
    cutaneous small vessel vasculitis (CSVV), 169
    drug reaction with eosinophilia and systemic
      symptoms (DRESS), 156
    Kawasaki disease, 158
    urticaria, 152
Erythroderma, 156
    atopic dermatitis (AD), 65
    contact dermatitis, 76
    differential diagnosis, 52–53
    idiopathic, 53
    morbilliform drug eruption, 154
    pityriasis rubra pilaris (PRP), 58, 59f
    seborrheic dermatitis, 68
Erythrodermic psoriasis, 50t
Erythromelalgia, 181
Erythromelanosis follicularis faciei et colli, 79
Erythromycin, 508t
    for acne vulgaris, 191
    for erythrasma, 297
    for pitted keratolysis, 296
    for pityriasis rosea (PR), 58
Esophageal dysmotility, systemic sclerosis, 134
Esophagitis, cytomegalovirus infection, 275
Esters, 547
Estrogen, and hair follicles, 12
Etanercept, for psoriasis, 53
Etelcalcetide, for hyperparathyroidism, 166
Ethylenediamine, photoinduced contact
      dermatitis, 70

Etretinate, 498t
ETTR. *See* Erythematotelangiectatic rosacea
      (ETTR)
Eumelanin, 3
Eumycetoma, 333
European Registry of Severe Cutaneous Adverse
      (Drug) Reactions (RegiSCAR) scoring
      system, 156, 156t
Eutectic mixture of local anesthesia (EMLA), 547
Evaluation and management (E/M codes) codes,
      637, 638t, 639t
Excessive tanning behavior, 187t
Excoriation disorder, 186–187
Exon, 15
Experimental studies, 41
External carotid artery (ICA), 541
Extracellular pathogens, 25
Extracorporeal photopheresis (ECP)
    for cutaneous T-cell lymphoma (CTCL), 471
    phototherapy, 529
Extramammary Paget disease (EMPD), 382, 382f
Eyelid, 14f, 15

F

Fabry disease, 246t
Face, 14f, 15
    cosmetic subunits, 536f
    danger triangle, 541f
Facial nerve
    motor innervation, 543, 544t
    sensory innervation, 542
Factitial dermatitis, 187–188
Factor V Leiden mutation, livedoid vasculopathy,
      162
Famciclovir
    for herpes simplex virus (HSV), 270
    for herpes zoster, 274
Familial atypival multiple mole melanoma
      (FAMMM) syndrome, 398
Familial dysautonomia, 185
Familial hyperlipoproteinemia, 238t
Famotidine, 498t
Fanconi anemia, 435t
Favus, 320
Febrile ulceronecrotic Mucha-Habermann
      disease variant, PLEVA lesions, 56
Febuxostat, for gout, 245
Felty syndrome, rheumatoid arthritis, 137
Female pattern alopecia, 204
Ferguson-Smith variant, keratoacanthoma, 381,
      381f
Ferriman and Gallwey scale, 210
Fetal alcohol syndrome, 211t
Fever
    serum sickness-like eruption, 170
    Stevens-Johnson syndrome/toxic epidermal
      necrolysis, 117
    telogen effluvium, 205
Fexofenadine, 498t
FFA. *See* Frontal fibrosing alopecia (FFA)
Fiberglass, contact dermatitis, 70
Fibrodysplasia ossificans progressiva (FOP),
      165–166
Fibrofolliculoma, 454t
Fibromatosis, 400t
Fibromatosis colli, 404t
Fibrous hamartoma, infancy, 404t

Fibrous neoplasms
angiofibroma, 401
atypical fibroxanthoma (AFX), 406, 408
dermatofibroma, 403–406
dermatofibrosarcoma protuberans, 406–407
epithelioid sarcoma, 406–408
keloid, 399–401
tuberous sclerosis complex (TSC), 402–403
Filaggrin deficiency, 65, 79
Filariasis, 341t
Filgrastim, 216
Finasterid, for androgenetic alopecia, 201
Fingernails, 14
Fish tank granuloma, 312t
Fixed cutaneous sporotrichosis, 330
Fixed drug eruption (FDE), 119, 119f
Flaps
advancement, 561t, 562f
nomenclature, 561t
rotation, 561, 563t, 563f
transposition, 562, 564t, 565f
Flat wart, 278t
Flies/fleas, 349t
Florid cutaneous papillomatosis, 63
Fluconazole, for cryptococcosis, 329
Fluctuant nodule, abscess, 293
Flucytosine, 507, 509
Fludarabine, 99
Fluoroquinolone prophylaxis, 301
Fluoroscopy-induced radiation dermatitis, 531
5-Fluorouracil (5-FU)
for actinic keratosis, 377
for mammary and extramammary Paget
disease, 382
for porokeratosis, 375
FMS-like tyrosine kinase 3 (FLT3) inhibitors,
Sweet syndrome, 216
Foam, 37
Focal epithelial hyperplasia, 278t
Focal hereditary palmoplantar keratodermas,
59, 60t
Folate, recurrent aphthous stomatitis, 217
Folic acid, 490
Follicular hyperkeratosis, pachyonychia
congenita (PC), 213
Follicular hyperkeratotic spicules, 188
Follicular matrical differentiation, 455, 457–458
Follicular mucinosis, 66, 241t
Follicular occlusion tetrad, 210
Follicular sheath differentiation, 455–456
Folliculitis, bacterial, 294
Folliculitis decalvans, 208
Food allergies
atopic dermatitis (AD), 65
Forceps, 549, 550f
Forchheimer spots, 274, 290
Foreign body granulomas, 228, 229f
Foscarnet
for cytomegalovirus infection, 276
for herpes simplex virus (HSV), 271
Fournier gangrene, 293
Fox-Fordyce disease, 200
Fractionated metanephrines, rosacea, 195
Fragrances, 71t–72t
Frey syndrome, hyperhidrosis, 198
Frictional lichenoid eruption, 66
Friction bulla, 361
Friction injury, 211, 361–362

Frontal fibrosing alopecia (FFA), 206, 207f
Functional mosaicism, 18
Fungal diseases
angioinvasive fungal infection, 331–332
deep mycoses, 325–331
superficial and deep mycoses, 322–325
superficial mycoses, 315–322
Fungi
classification, 316t
forms, 315
Furocoumarins, photoinduced contact
dermatitis, 70
Furuncles, abscess, 293
Fusariosis, 332, 332f
Fusion inhibitors, 501t
Fusion proteins, 493, 493t

G

GA. *See* Granuloma annulare (GA)
Gabapentin, 183
Gain-of-function mutations, 19
Ganciclovir, for cytomegalovirus infection, 276
Ganglioneuroma, 438t
Gap junctions, 4, 6f
Gardasil 4-valent vaccine, 280
Gardasil 9-valent vaccine, 280
Gardner-Diamond syndrome, 187
Gardner syndrome, 12, 467, 467t
Gastric adenocarcinoma, 367
Gastric carcinoma, 63
Gastroesophageal reflux disease (GERD), 127
Gastrointestinal actinomycosis, 298
Gastrointestinal anthrax, 298
Gastrointestinal involvement
cutaneous small vessel vasculitis (CSVV), 169
immunoglobulin A vasculitis, 171
Gastrulation, 15
Gaucher disease, 246t
GCT. *See* Granular cell tumor (GCT)
Gel, 37
Gemcitabine, 471
Generalized eruptive histiocytoma, 235t
Generalized vitiligo, 84
Genetic disorders, 15, 17–19
Genetic modification, 40t
Genetics, 15–19
Genetic test
basal cell nevus syndrome (BCNS), 374
Cowden syndrome, 411
familial atypival multiple mole melanoma
(FAMMM) syndrome, 398
Gardner syndrome, 467
hereditary ichthyoses and
erythrokeratodermas, 79
hereditary palmoplantar keratodermas, 62
incontinentia pigmenti, 88
Genital herpes, herpes simplex virus (HSV), 269
Genital leiomyoma, 461
Genital wart, 278t
Genodermatoses, 22
Genomic mosaicism, 18
Genotype, 15
Gentamicin, 508t
Geographic tongue, 55, 55f
Geophilic fungi, 318
Gianotti-Crosti syndrome, 275t
Giant cell arteritis (GCA), 177

Giant cell fibroblastoma, 406
Gingival hyperplasia, 174
Gland disorders, 188–200, 595t–597t
chemical exposure, 362
heat injury, 360
mechanical injury, 361
Glands
apocrine glands, 9–10
eccrine glands, 10–11
sebaceous glands, 8–9
Glandular cheilitis, 376
Gliadin, 107
Glogau photoaging classification-wrinkle scale,
573
Glomeruloid hemangioma, 420t
Glomus cells, 7
Glomus tumor, 429–430, 430f
Glomuvenous malformation (GVM), 429–430,
430f
Glossopharyngeal nerve, 542
Gluten avoidance, dermatitis herpetiformis
(DH), 110
Gluten sensitivity, 107
Glycopeptides, 504
Glycopyrrolate, 526
Glycopyrronium, 198
GNA11 mutations, blue nevus, 386
GNAQ mutations, blue nevus, 386
Gnathostomiasis, 341t
Goeckerman therapy, for psoriasis, 53
Gonococcal urethritis/cervicitis, 308
Gonococcemia, 299t
Gout, 245, 247
Gouty arthritis, acute, 245
Grafts
stages of, 564–565
types, 564, 566t
Graft-*versus*-host disease (GVHD), 120–121,
121f
Graham Little-Piccardi-Lassueur syndrome, 206
Gram-negative coccus infections, 299t
Gram-negative (GN) bacteria, 285
Gram-negative rod infections, 302t
Gram-positive (GP) bacteria, 285
Gram-positive rod infections, 297t
Gram stain and bacterial culture
bacterial diseases, 294
paronychia, 295
Granular cell tumor (GCT), 436–437, 437f
Granular parakeratosis, 62, 63f
Granulocytopenia, 137
Granuloma annulare (GA)
clinicopathological features, 230, 231f
epidemiology, 230
evaluation, 231
vs. rheumatoid nodule, 231f
Granuloma faciale, 223, 223f
Granuloma gluteale infantum/adultorum, 76
Granuloma inguinale, 308
Granulomatosis with polyangiitis (GPA), 174
Granulomatous dermatoses, 137
Granulomatous rosacea, 194t
Granulosis rubra nasi, 198
Granzymes, 33
Graves disease, 156
Griseofulvin
systemic antifungals, 509
for tinea capitis, 321

Grocer's itch, 344t
Ground itch, 341t
Grover disease, 102
Gumma, 308
Gustatory hyperhidrosis, 198
Guttate hypopigmentation, 83, 85
Guttate psoriasis, 49, 50t
Guttate vitiligo, 85
GVHD. *See* Graft-*versus*-host disease (GVHD)

H

Haber syndrome, 194t
Habit-tic deformity, beau lines, 211
Haemophilus influenzae type b (Hib) vaccine, 495t
Hailey-Hailey disease, 15, 100, 101f, 101t, 102f
Haim-Munk syndrome, 61t
Hair, 11–12, 11f
    development, 15, 16f
    ectodermal dysplasia, 198
    products, 72t
HAIR-AN syndrome, 188
Hair collar sign, 211t, 431
Hair disorders, 200–211, 597t–600t
    acne keloidalis, 208–210
    alopecia areata, 200–202
    androgenetic alopecia, 204, 204f
    central centrifugal cicatricial alopecia (CCCA), 208
    chemical exposure, 362
    friction injury, 361
    heat injury, 360
    hereditary, 213t–214t
    hypertrichosis, 210, 211t, 2110t
    mechanical injury, 361
    pressure injury, 361
    telogen effluvium, 205–206
    traction alopecia, 205
    trichotillomania, 203, 203f
Hair restoration, 583–584
Hair strength, 12
Hair transplantation methods, 583, 584t
Hairy cell leukemia, 176
Half-life, 36
Halo nevus, 387, 390–391, 391f
Halo scalp ring, 361
Hamilton-Norwood system, 204
Hands and feet
    nerve blocks, 548f
    sensory nerves, 543f
Hand/finger edema, systemic sclerosis, 134
Hand-foot-mouth disease (HFMD), 284–285
    clinicopathological features, 284
    epidemiology, 284
    evaluation, 285
    management, 285
Hand-foot syndrome (HFS), 120
Hand-Schüller-Christian disease, 222
Hansen sign, 97
Haploinsufficiency, 15
Hard corns, 361
Harlequin ichthyosis, 79
Hartnup disease, 246t
Hashimoto-Pritzker disease, 222
Hashimoto thyroiditis, dermatitis herpetiformis (DH), 107
Hay-Wells syndrome, 199t

Headache, dengue, 284
Head and neck
    arteries, 541f
    motor nerves, 544f
    sensory nerves, 542f
    surgical danger zones, 454t
Hearing loss, relapsing polychondritis, 136
Heat, rosacea, 194
Heat injury, 360
Heavy metal hyperpigmentation/discoloration, 86t–87t
Heck disease, 278t
Hedgehogs, 349t
Heel sticks, 165
Heerfordt syndrome, 227t
Helminth infections, 335t, 341t–324t
Hemangioma
    clinicopathological features, 419–421, 421f
    epidemiology, 419
    evaluation, 420
    management, 420–421
    variants, 420t
Hematolymphoid neoplasms
    cutaneous B-cell lymphoma (CBCL), 476–477
    cutaneous lymphoid hyperplasia (CLH), 476, 478
    cutaneous T-cell lymphoma (CTCL), 471–474
    leukemia cutis, 478–479
    lymphomatoid papulosis (LyP), 472, 475
    mastocytosis, 480
Hematopoietic stem cell transplantation (HSCT), allogeneic, 120
Heme biosynthetic pathway, 237, 249f
Hemidesmosome, 6f
Hemizygous genotype, 15
Hemochromatosis, 85
    erythema dyschromicum perstans, 85
    porphyria cutanea tarda, 248
Hemorrhage, pseudoxanthoma elasticum (PXE), 141
Hemorrhagic disease, 245
Hemorrhagic fever, dengue, 284
Heparin, telogen effluvium, 205
Hepatic cirrhosis, edema blister, 177
Hepatitis
    cryoglobulinemic vasculitis, 173
    Stevens-Johnson syndrome/toxic epidermal necrolysis, 117
    varicella, 273
Hepatitis A vaccine, 495t
Hepatitis B vaccine, 495t
Hepatitis B virus (HBV) infection, lichen planus (LP), 111
Hepatitis C virus (HCV) infection, lichen planus (LP), 111
Hepatobiliary disease, lupus erythematosus (LE), 122
Hereditary angioedema, 153, 153t
Hereditary connective tissue disorders, 141t–143t
Hereditary disorders
    basal cell carcinoma (BCC), 371t
    café-au-lait macules, 435t
    capillary malformation, 414t
    macrocystic lymphatic malformations, 417t
Hereditary epidermolysis bullosa acquisita, 107

Hereditary hemorrhagic telangiectasia (HHT), 252
Hereditary ichthyoses and erythrokeratodermas, 79, 80t–82t
Hereditary immunodeficiency syndromes, 268t–269t
Hereditary leiomyomatosis and renal cell cancer (HLRCC), 462
Hereditary palmoplantar keratodermas, 59, 60t–61t, 62f
Herpangina, 285
Herpes simplex virus (HSV), 265, 269–271
    in adults, 269, 270t
    clinicopathological features, 269, 271f
    congenital, 269, 270t
    diagnostic tests, 270
    epidemiology, 269
    erythema multiforme, 116
    evaluation, 269–270
    management, 270–271
    neonatal, 269, 270t
Herpes zoster, 273–274
    clinicopathological features, 273–274
    epidemiology, 273
    evaluation, 274
    management, 274
Herpetiform tense blisters, 105, 106f
Heterozygous genotype, 15
Hexachlorophene, 549t
HFMD. *See* Hand-foot-mouth disease (HFMD)
Hibernoma, 409, 409f
Hidradenitis suppurativa (HS), 193, 193t
    therapeutic ladder, 193t
Hidradenoma, 446–447, 447f
Hidradenoma papilliferum (HPAP), 444–445, 445f
Hidrocystoma, 467–469, 468t
Hidrotic ectodermal dysplasia, 199t
Higoumenakis sign, 309
Hirsutism, 68, 210
Histiocytoses, 225–226
Histopathology
    direct immunofluorescence patterns, 634t
    histopathological bodies, 627t
    immunohistochemical stains, 630t–633t
    molecular tests, 633t
    special stains, 628t–629t
Histoplasma capsulatum, erythema multiforme, 116
Histoplasmosis, 281, 327, 329, 329f
History of present illness (HPI), 637
Hodgkin lymphoma, 78, 275
Holocarboxylase synthetase deficiencies, 245t, 252
Holocrine secretion, sebaceous gland, 9
Homocystinuria, 161
Homozygous genotype, 15
Homozygous protein C deficiency, 164
Hordeolum, abscess, 293
Hori nevus, 385t
Hormonal acne, 190t
Hormonal drugs
    androgens, 500
    antiandrogens, 500
    combined oral contraceptive pills, 500–501
Hornets, 348t
Hortaea werneckii, 317
Howel-Evans syndrome (TOC), 61t

HPAP. *See* Hidradenoma papilliferum (HPAP)
HRAS mutations
  nevus spilus, 390
  spitz nevus, 391
HS. *See* Hidradenitis suppurativa (HS)
HSV. *See* Herpes simplex virus (HSV)
Human herpes virus (HHV), pityriasis rosea
    (PR), 56
Human immunodeficiency virus (HIV) infection
  mucocutaneous signs, 265, 267t
  recurrent aphthous stomatitis, 217
  seborrheic dermatitis, 68
  syphilis, 308
Human leukocyte antigen (HLA), 25
  disorders, 26t
  incompatibility, 120
Human papillomavirus (HPV) vaccine, 495t
Humoral autoimmunity-mediated cytotoxicity,
    paraneoplastic pemphigus (PNP), 99
Humoral immunity, 25, 25t
Hurley staging system, 193t
Hutchinson sign, 274, 394f
Hutchinson teeth, 309
Hutchinson triad, 309
Huxley layer, inner root sheath, 11
Hyaline fibromatosis syndrome, 405t
Hyalohyphomycosis, 315
Hydroa vacciniforme (HV), 274, 354
Hydrocephalus, 334
Hydrogen peroxide, 549t
Hydrops fetalis, erythema infectiosum, 283
Hydroquinone, 86, 523, 525
Hydroxychloroquine
  for dermatomyositis (DM), 127
  for lupus erythematosus (LE), 122
  for polymorphous light eruption (PMLE), 354
Hydroxyurea
  in dermatomyositis (DM), 127
  for sickle cell disease, 364
Hydroxyzine, 498t
Hyperalgesia, complex regional pain syndrome
    (CPRS), 184, 184t
Hyperandrogenism, insulin resistance, AN
    (HAIR-AN) syndrome, 63
Hypereosinophilic syndrome (HES)
  primary, 225
  secondary, 225
Hyperhidrosis, 197–198
  pitted keratolysis, 295
  primary focal, 198
  secondary, 198
Hyper-IgE syndromes, abscess, 293
Hyper-immunoglobulin E syndromes, 343
Hyperlipoproteinemia, 238t, 239f
Hypermelanosis, pigmentary disorders, 83
Hyperpigmentation
  chronic lipodermatosclerosis, 147
  erythema ab igne (EAI), 363
  erythema dyschromicum perstans, 85–86
  lichen simplex chronicus (LSC), 183
  patterns, 515f
  prurigo nodularis, 181
Hypertension, lipodermatosclerosis, 147
Hyperthermia, ectodermal dysplasias, 198
Hyperthyroidism, erythema dyschromicum
    perstans, 85
Hypertrichosis, 200, 431
  acquired, 210t

congenital, 211t
  lanuginosa, 12
  porphyria cutanea tarda, 249
Hypertrophic scar, 399f
Hypertrophies, 399, 400t
Hypoalbuminemia
  edema blister, 177
  Muehrcke lines, 212
Hypocomplementemia, 172
Hypocomplementemic urticarial vasculitis, 137,
    172, 173t
Hypodermis, 7
Hypodontia, 88
Hypohidrosis, 198, 232
Hypohidrotic ectodermal dysplasia, 199t
Hypomelanosis, 83
Hypomethylaters, 216, 513t
Hypomyopathic dermatomyositis (DM), 127
Hyponychium, nail, 13
Hypopigmentation, 83, 114
Hypoplasia, varicella, 273
Hyporeflexia, familial dysautonomia, 185
Hypotension, urticaria, 152
Hypothyroidism, 67
  erythema dyschromicum perstans, 85
  ichthyosis vulgaris, 78

I

Iamotrigine, 476
IBD. *See* Inflammatory bowel disease (IBD)
Ibrutinib, 545
Ichthyosis vulgaris, 66, 78–79, 78f
ICIs. *See* Immune checkpoint inhibitors (ICIs)
Idiopathic palmoplantar hidradenitis, 217
Idiopathic thrombocytopenic purpura (ITP),
    273
Idiosyncratic drug reactions, 38, 38t
Illness anxiety disorder, 187t
Imatinib
  for dermatofibrosarcoma protuberans,
    406–407
  for hypereosinophilic syndrome (HES), 225
  for Kaposi sarcoma, 427
  for mastocytosis, 480
  for neurofibromatosis, 435
Imidazoles, 507
Imipramine, 498t
Imiquimod, 520t
  for actinic keratosis, 377
  and generalized pustular psoriasis (GPP), 49
  for mammary and extramammary Paget
    disease, 382
  for porokeratosis, 375
  for wart, 280
Immune checkpoint inhibitors (ICIs), 521f
  acute generalized exanthematous pustulosis,
    93
  alopecia areata (AA), 200
  bullous pemphigoid, 103
  in dermatomyositis (DM), 127
  drug reaction with eosinophilia and systemic
    symptoms (DRESS), 156
  eczematous drug eruptions, 66
  erythema nodosum, 144
  generalized pustular psoriasis (GPP), 49
  lichenoid drug eruption, 114
  morbilliform drug eruption, 154

Stevens-Johnson syndrome/toxic epidermal
    necrolysis-like reactions, 117
  Sweet syndrome, 216
Immune checkpoints, 34, 35t
Immune privilege, 12
Immunization schedule, 493, 494t–495t
Immunoglobulin, 31f
Immunoglobulin A (IgA)
  pemphigus, 98–99, 99f
  vasculitis, 171, 172t
Immunoglobulin A monoclonal
    gammopathy, 98
  pyoderma gangrenosum (PG), 219
  urticarial vasculitis, 172
Immunohistochemical stains, 630t–633t
Immunologic contact urticaria, 66
Immunologic drug reactions, 38t
Immunology, 25–34
  cellular effectors, 30–34, 32f
  molecular effectors, 26–30
Immunomodulation, 23
Immunosuppressants and immunomodulators
  antimalarials, 489
  antimetabolites, 489–491
  biologic and small molecule inhibitors,
    493–496
  calcineurin inhibitors, 491
  colchicine, 492
  corticosteroids, 487–489
  cyclophosphamide, 492
  dapsone, 492
  intravenous immunoglobulin, 497
  phosphodiesterase 4 inhibitors, 492
  potassium iodide, 492
  thalidomide, 492–493
Immunotherapies, 502t, 514, 520t, 521f–522f
Impetigo
  clinicopathological features, 288, 288f
  epemiology, 288
  evaluation, 289
  management, 289
Implantable cardioverter-defibrillators (ICDs),
    533
Imprinting, Mendelian inheritance, 15
Impulse control disorder, 203
Incision and drainage (I&D), 292, 557
Incomplete penetrance, 17
Incontinentia pigmenti, 88, 89f
Indeterminate cell histiocytosis, 235t
Indeterminate leprosy, 313
Indinavir, for pyogenic granuloma, 423
Indomethacin
  for gout, 245
  for Ofuji disease, 224
Infantile acne, 191t
Infantile digital fibroma, 405t
Infantile myofibromatosis, 405t
Infants
  candidiasis, 322
  cellulitis, 292
  contact dermatitis, 76
  impetigo, 288
  Kawasaki disease, 158
  miliaria, 200
  physiologic livedo reticularis, 161
  scabies, 335
  seborrheic dermatitis, 68
  warts, 278

Infections
and atopic dermatitis (AD), 65
cutaneous small vessel vasculitis (CSVV), 169
erythema nodosum, 144
Infectious eczematous dermatitis, 76
Infectious mononucleosis, 154, 274–275
Infectious mononucleosis-like syndrome, 275
Infective endocarditis, 299–300
Inflammasomes, 28
Inflammatory bowel disease (IBD)
alopecia areata (AA), 200
erythema nodosum, 144
pyoderma gangrenosum (PG), 219
recurrent aphthous stomatitis, 217
Inflammatory linear verrucous epidermal nevus,
369f
Inflammatory phase, wound healing, 35, 36t
Inflammatory polyarthritis, 127
Inflammatory retiform purpura, 160t
Influenza inactivated (IIV) vaccine, 494t
Influenza live attenuated (ILAV) vaccine, 494t
Influenza recombinant (RIV) vaccine, 494t
Information bias, 42
Infundibulofolliculitis, disseminate and
recurrent, 65
Infundibulum, 12
Ingenol mebutate, 522t
Ink-jet lentigo, 383
Innate immunity, 25, 25t
Insulin-dependent diabetes mellitus, 107
Insulin resistance, 63
Integrase inhibitors, 501t
Integrins, 4
Intercellular junctions, keratinocyte, 3–4, 4f
Interdigital erythrasma, 296
Interface dermatoses, 110–115
Interferon γ (IFNγ), 33
Interferon (IFN)
for cutaneous T-cell lymphoma (CTCL), 471
generalized pustular psoriasis (GPP), 49
Interferonopathies, 283
Interfollicular repigmentation, 12
Intermittent claudication, arterial ulcer, 180
Internal carotid artery (ICA), 541
Internal malignancy
monoclonal gammopathies, 607t
and paraneoplastic syndromes, 605t–607t
Interstitial granulomatous dermatitis (IGD), 137
Interstitial keratitis, 309
Interstitial lung disease (ILD), 127
Intracorneal hematoma, black heel and palm, 364
Intraepidermal neutrophilic subtype, IgA
pemphigus, 98, 99f
Intralesional avotermin, for keloid, 400
Intralesional IL-10, 400
Intralesional insulin, 400
Intralesional Kenalog, 400
Intraluminal pathology, livedo reticularis, 161
Intravascular large B-cell lymphoma, 476
Intravascular papillary endothelial hyperplasia
(IPEH), 180
Intravenous immunoglobulin (IVIG), 30, 497
dyshidrotic eczema, 67
for juvenile-onset dermatomyositis (DM), 127
for Stevens-Johnson syndrome/toxic
epidermal necrolysis, 118
urticaria, 152
Intron, 15

Iodinated radiocontrast media
drug reaction with eosinophilia and systemic
symptoms (DRESS), 156
morbilliform drug eruption, 154
toxic erythema of chemotherapy (TEC), 120
Iodoquinol, 508t
Iron deficiency, 252, 252t
Irradiance, 22
Irritants
and atopic dermatitis (AD), 65
avoidance, 78
Isavuconazole, 329
Isoniazid, 504–505
Isopropyl alcohol, 549t
Isotretinoin, 498t
for acne keloidalis, 210
for pityriasis rubra pilaris (PRP), 58
Isthmus, 12
Itraconazole
for coccidioidomycosis, 327
for cryptococcosis, 329
for histoplasmosis, 327
for mycosis, 326
for sporotrichosis, 331
Ivermectin, 511, 512t
for cutaneous larva migrans, 343
for papulopustular rosacea (PPR), 196
IVIG. See Intravenous immunoglobulin (IVIG)

J

Jacquet erosive diaper dermatitis, 76
Janeway lesions, 300
Janus kinase (JAK) enzymes, 29
Janus kinase (JAK) inhibitors
for alopecia areata (AA), 202
for sarcoidosis, 226
Jarisch-Herxheimer reaction, 309
Jellyfish, 349t
Jewish ancestry
pemphigus foliaceus, 96
pemphigus vulgaris, 97
Joint contractures
eosinophilic fasciitis, 135
morphea, 131
nephrogenic systemic fibrosis, 136
systemic sclerosis, 134
Junctional nevi, 387
Junctions
basement membrane zone (BMZ), 4–5, 5f
disorders of, 6f
intercellular, 3–4, 4f
Juvenile-onset dermatomyositis (DM), 127
Juvenile plantar dermatosis, 66
Juvenile spring eruption, polymorphous light
eruption (PMLE), 353

K

Kabuki syndrome, 84
Kaposiform hemangioendothelioma (KHE),
424–425, 425f
Kaposi sarcoma (KS)
clinicopathological features, 426, 427f
epidemiology, 426
evaluation, 426
management, 426–427
types, 426t

Kawasaki disease, 158, 158t
Keloids
clinicopathological features, 399, 399f
epidemiology, 399
evaluation, 399–400
management, 400
Keratin-degrading proteases, 295
Keratinocytes, 1, 2f, 34
immune reactions, 34
intercellular junctions, 3–4, 4f
stem cells, 12
Keratinocytic epidermal nevi, 369
Keratoacanthoma, 381, 381f
Keratoderma blennorrhagicum, 54
Keratolysis exfoliativa, 67–68
Keratosis lichenoides chronica, 111
Keratosis pilaris, 79, 83, 83f, 83t
Keratosis pilaris atrophicans, 83t
Keratosis pilaris rubra (KPR) variant, 79
Kerion, 320
Ketoconazole, 69, 511t
KHE. See Kaposiform hemangioendothelioma
(KHE)
Kindler syndrome, 109t
Klinefelter syndrome (47, XXY), 179
Klippel-Trenaunay syndrome, 414t
Koebnerization, 84, 111
Koebner phenomenon, 49
Koilonychia, 249f
Kojic acid, for erythema dyschromicum
perstans, 86
Krause end bulbs, 8
KS. See Kaposi sarcoma (KS)
Kveim-Sitzbach test, sarcoidosis, 226
Kwashiorkor, 252t

L

Laboratory techniques, 38, 39t, 40t
Lacazia loboi, 329
Lacrimation impairment, familial dysautonomia,
185
Lactation, drug interactions and, 38
Lamina densa, 4
Lamina lucida, 4, 5, 6f
Lamina lucida type linear immunoglobulin A
bullous dermatosis, 105, 106f
Laminins, 5
Lamivudine, 423
Lamotrigine
drug reaction with eosinophilia and systemic
symptoms (DRESS), 156
for Stevens-Johnson syndrome/toxic
epidermal necrolysis, 118
in Stevens-Johnson syndrome/toxic epidermal
necrolysis, 117
Langerhans cell histiocytosis (LCH), 69, 223,
223t, 224f
Langerhans cells, 1
Lanugo, 12
Large cell acanthoma, 370t
Large plaque parapsoriasis, 55
LASERs. See Light amplification by stimulated
emission of radiation (LASERs)
L-asparaginase, 195, 513t
Laugier-Hunziker syndrome, 384t
LE. See Lupus erythematosus (LE)
Lectin pathway, complement, 26, 27t

Leg elevation and compression
 for edema blister, 177
 erythema nodosum, 147
 lipodermatosclerosis, 147
 lymphedema, 178
 venous insufficiency/hypertension, 179
Legius syndrome, 435t
Leg ulcers
 cryoglobulinemia, 173
 rheumatoid arthritis, 137
Leiomyoma, 461–462
Leishmaniasis, 334, 339t
Leishmaniasis recidivans, 334
Lentigo maligna melanomas, 393
Lentigo simplex, 382–383, 384t
Lepromatous leprosy, 313, 314f
Leprosy, 313, 313f, 313t, 315
Leprosy reactions, 313, 313t
Leptospirosis, 307t
Lesch-Nyhan syndrome, 246t
Lesional skin biopsy
 dermatomyositis (DM), 127
 lupus erythematosus, 122
Letterer-Siwe disease, 222
Leukemia cutis, 478, 479f
Leukocyte chemotaxis, 27
Leukotriene inhibitors, 174, 497
Levetiracetam, 118
Levofloxacin, 298
LFTs. *See* Liver function tests (LFTs)
Lhermitte-Duclos disease, 411
Lice, 344t
 clinicopathological features, 343, 345
 epidemiology, 343
 evaluation, 345
 treatment, 347
Lichen myloidosis, 243t
Lichen myxedematosus, 241t
Lichen nitidus, 115, 115f
Lichenoid drug eruption, 114
Lichen planopilaris (LPP), 206, 207f
Lichen planus (LP)
 clinicopathological features, 111–112, 112t,
  113f
 epidemiology, 111
 evaluation, 112
 management, 113
 variants, 112t
Lichen sclerosus
 anogenital, 130
 clinicopathological features, 129–130
 epidemiology, 129
 evaluation, 130
 extragenital, 129
 management, 130
Lichen simplex chronicus (LSC), 50, 183–184
Lichen spinulosus, 83
Lichen striatus, 114–115, 115f
Lidocaine, 183, 547
Li Fraumeni syndrome, 393
Light amplification by stimulated emission of
  radiation (LASERs)
 chromophores, 576–577
 clinical applications, 577t
 hair removal, 578
 parameters, 576
 pigmented lesions, 578
 safety, 578

 scars and laser resurfacing, 578
 tattoos, 578
 vascular lesions, 578
Limb abnormalities, varicella, 273
Limb necrosis, purpura fulminans, 164
Lincomycins, 505
Lindane, 512t
Lindsay nails, 212, 212f
Linear hypopigmentation/depigmentation, 83
Linear immunoglobulin A bullous dermatosis
  (LABD), 105–106, 106f
Linear lichen striatus, 114
Linear morphea, 131
Linear vitiligo, 85
Linezolid, 289, 505
Lipodermatosclerosis, stasis dermatitis, 69
Lipodystrophy
 acquired, 149, 150t
 corticosteroids and, 487
 hereditary, 149, 149t
Lipoid proteinosis, 148f, 246t, 248
Lipoma, 409–410, 410f, 431
Liposarcoma, 410
Lip pits, 459t
Lipschutz ulcer, 275t
Liquid nitrogen, 532
Lithium, generalized pustular psoriasis (GPP), 49
Livedoid vasculopathy, 69, 162, 163f
Livedo racemosa, 161
Livedo reticularis
 cholesterol emboli, 164
 clinicopathological features, 161
 cryoglobulinemia, 173
 epidemiology, 161
 evaluation, 162
 management, 162
 physiologic, 161
 primary, 161–162
 secondary, 161
Liver function tests (LFTs)
 cutaneous small vessel vasculitis (CSVV), 169
 drug reaction with eosinophilia and systemic
  symptoms (DRESS), 156
 livedoid vasculopathy, 162
 prurigo nodularis, 182
 urticaria, 152
LMDF. *See* Lupus miliaris disseminatus faciei
  (LMDF)
Lobomycosis, 329, 331f
Lobular panniculitis, 144f
Local anesthetics
 adverse effects, 547
 chemical structure, 547
 loss of sensation, 547
 properties, 547
Localized vitiligo, 84
Locus, 15
Locus heterogeneity, 15
Löffler syndrome, 336
Löfgren syndrome, 227t
Loiasis, 341t
Longitudinal melanonychia, 387
Loose anagen hair syndrome, 213t
Loratadine, 498t
Loricrin, 1
Loricrin keratoderma, 60t
Loss of heterozygosity, 17
Lotion, 37

Louis-Bar syndrome, 357t
LP. *See* Lichen planus (LP)
LPP. *See* Lichen planopilaris (LPP)
LSC. *See* Lichen simplex chronicus (LSC)
Ludwig angina, cellulitis, 291
Ludwig system, 204
LUMBAR syndrome, 422
Lung carcinoma, 481, 482t
Lunula, 215f
Lupus band test, 122
Lupus erythematosus (LE)
 antinuclear antibody patterns, 126f
 autoantibodies, 126t
 clinicopathological features, 122, 125f
 epidemiology, 121–122
 evaluation, 122
 management, 122
 subtypes, 123t–124t
Lupus-like syndrome, chronic granulomatous
  disease (CGD), 294
Lupus miliaris disseminatus faciei (LMDF), 197,
  197f
Lyme disease, 304, 306t, 307
Lymphadenopathy
 chronic actinic dermatitis (CAD), 355
 lobomycosis, 329
 serum sickness-like eruption, 170
 Stevens-Johnson syndrome/toxic epidermal
  necrolysis, 117
 tinea capitis, 320
Lymphangioma circumscriptum, 417
Lymphatic malformation (LM), 417–418, 418f
Lymphedema
 cellulitis, 291
 primary, 178, 179t
 secondary, 178
Lymph node dissection, lymphedema, 178
Lymphocutaneous sporotrichosis, 330
Lymphoma, seborrheic keratosis, 367
Lymphomatoid granulomatosis, 275
Lymphomatoid papulosis (LyP), 472, 475, 475f
Lysosomal enzymes, 30

M

Macrocephaly, 411
Macrocystic lymphatic malformations, 417t
Macrolides, 93, 505
Macrophages, 30
Macular amyloidosis, 243t
Macular and lichen amyloidosis, 243
Macular purpura, 159t
Madarosis, 201
Mafenide, 509t
Maffucci syndrome, 415, 416
Magnetic resonance imaging (MRI)
 for dermatomyositis (DM), 127
 eosinophilic fasciitis, 135
 graft-*versus*-host disease (GVHD), 121
 necrotizing fasciitis, 293
Majocchi granuloma, 319t, 320
Major basic protein (MBP), 30
Major histocompatibility complex (MHC), 25–26
 MHC class I, 26
 MHC class II, 26
Malakoplakia, 301–303
Malar flush, rosacea, 195
Malaria, 340t

Malassezia folliculitis, 315
Malassezia furfur, 315
Malassezia globosa, 315
Malassezia species, 68
Malathion, 512t
Mal de Meleda nonepidermolytic PPK, 60t
Male pattern alopecia, 204
Malignancy-associated Sweet syndrome, 216
Malignancy risk, dermatomyositis (DM), 127, 129
Malignant atrophic papulosis, 164, 165f
Malignant peripheral nerve sheath tumor (MPNST), 432
Mammalian target of rapamycin (MTOR) inhibitors (sirolimus), 517
   for angiofibroma, 401
   for tuberous sclerosis complex, 402
Mammary Paget disease (MPD), 381–382, 382f
Marasmus, 252t
   ichthyosis vulgaris, 78
   telogen effluvium, 205
Marjolin ulcer, 360
Marshall syndrome, 217
Martorell hypertensive ischemic ulcer, 180
Mast cells, 31–32
   degranulation, 27
   mediators, 32
Mastocytosis, 480, 480f
   rosacea, 195
   variants, 480t
Matchbox sign, 186
Mat telangiectasias, 134
MCC. *See* Merkel cell carcinoma (MCC)
McCune-Albright syndrome, 435t
Mean, 41
Measles, mumps, and rubella (MMR) vaccine, 277, 494t
Mechanical injury, 360–361
Mechanical skin resurfacing
   definition, 574
   indications, 574
   safety, 575–576
Mechanoreceptors, 3
Mechlorethamine, 523t
Median, 41
Median nail dystrophy, 211, 212f
Median nerve block, 548
Median raphe cyst, 468t
Median rhomboid glossitis, 323t
Medical decision-making (MDM) types, 637, 638t
Medical treatments
   antihistamines, 497, 498t
   antimicrobials, 501–512
   antineoplastics, 511–523
   hormonal drugs, 500–501
   immunosuppressants and immunomodulators, 487–497
   miscellaneous drugs, 523–526
   retinoids, 497, 498t, 499, 499t
Mediterranean spotted fever, 305t
Mees lines, 212, 212f
Meglumine antimonate, 334
Meissner corpuscles, 8
Melan-A, 396
Melanocortin-1 receptor (MC1R), 3
Melanocytes, 1, 3, 12, 14
Melanocyte-stimulating hormone (MSH), 3

Melanocytic lesions, 613, 616f–618f
Melanocytic neoplasms, 382–398
   blue nevus, 386, 386f
   dermal melanocytosis, 385, 385f, 385t
   familial atypival multiple mole melanoma (FAMMM) syndrome, 398
   halo nevus, 390–391, 391f
   lentigo simplex, 382–383, 384t
   melanoma, 393–396
   nevocellular nevus and atypical nevus, 387, 388f, 389
   nevus spilus, 390
   spitz nevus, 391–392
Melanocytic nevi
   congenital, 389, 389f
   gene mutations, 387
Melanoma, 393–396, 481
   cancer staging, 398
   clinicopathological features, 393–394, 395f–396f
   epidemiology, 393
   evaluation, 394
   gene mutations, 393, 393t
   management, 394, 396
   TNM classification, 397t
Melanoma leukoderma, 394
Melanosomes, 3
Melasma, 85
Melkersson-Rosenthal syndrome, 226
Membrane attack complex, 27
Membranoproliferative glomerulonephritis, 173
Mendelian inheritance patterns, 17
Meningococcal A, C, W, Y (MenACWY) vaccine, 495t
Meningococcal B (MenB) vaccine, 495t
Meningococcemia, 299t
Meningoencephalitis
   for Rocky Mountain spotted fever (RMSF), 303
   varicella, 273
Menkes kinky hair disease, 213t, 252
Menthol, 524t
Merkel cell carcinoma (MCC), 437–439, 438f
Merkel cell polyomavirus (MCPyV), 437
Merkel cells, 3
Merocrine secretion, eccrine gland, 10
Mesoderm, skin, 15
Metabolic acidosis, 166
Metabolic disorders
   dermatologic signs of, 609t–610t
   erythema dyschromicum perstans, 85
Metabolic syndrome, acquired lipodystrophies, 149
Metabolism, drug, 36
Metastatic melanoma, 394
Methimazole, 431
Methotrexate
   for adult-onset Still disease (AoSD), 137
   antimetabolites, 490–491
   for cutaneous T-cell lymphoma (CTCL), 471, 523t
   for lichen sclerosus, 130
   for lymphomatoid papulosis (LyP), 475
   for psoriasis, 53
   psoriasis therapy, 53
   for rheumatoid arthritis, 137
8-Methoxsalen (8-MOP), 529
Methyl aminolevulinate (MAL), 529

Metronidazole, 505, 508t
   for papulopustular rosacea (PPR), 196
   rosacea, 195
Mevalonate kinase deficiency (MKD), 217
Mevalonate pathway, 375
MF. *See* Mycosis fungoides (MF)
Microcystic adnexal carcinoma (MAC), 448–450, 449f
Microstomia, 134
Microvenular hemangioma, 420t
Mid-borderline leprosy, 313
Midchildhood acne, 191t
Migratory poliosis, 201
Mikulicz syndrome, 227t
Milia, 107
Miliaria, 200
Miliaria crystallina, 200
Miliaria profunda, 200
Miliaria rubra, 200
Millipedes, 349t
Mineral oil preparation, for scabies, 345
Minimal erythema dose (MED), 24
Minocycline, 508t
   for acne vulgaris, 191
   for bullous pemphigoid, 104
   drug reaction with eosinophilia and systemic symptoms (DRESS), 156
   morbilliform drug eruption, 154
   pigmentation, 506f
Minoxidil, 526
   for androgenetic alopecia, 201
   telogen effluvium, 205
Misclassification bias, 42
Mites, 348t
Mitochondrial disorders, 246t
Mitochondrial inheritance, 17
Mitogen-activated protein kinase (MAPK) signaling pathway, 19–20
Mitogen-activated protein kinase (MEK) 1/2 inhibitors, 67
Mitral valve prolapse (MVP), 141
Mixed cryoglobulinemia, 173
MMP. *See* Mucous membrane pemphigoid (MMP)
Mnemonics, 17
Mode, 41
Mogamulizumab, 471, 523t
Mohs micrographic surgery (MMS)
   basal cell carcinoma (BCC), 373
   definition, 558
   indications, 558, 560f
   mammary and extramammary Paget disease, 382
   technique, 558–561
Mold, 315
Molecular signaling pathway, 19–20, 21f, 22f
   mutations, 22
Molluscum contagiosum, 280, 281, 282f, 282t
Molluscum-type central umbilicated papules, 327
   cryptococcosis, 329
   histoplasmosis, 327
Monilethrix, 214t
Monkeypox, 282t
Monoclonal antibodies, 493t
Monoclonal gammopathy, 607t
   necrobiotic xanthogranuloma, 234
   scleredema, 240
   scleromyxedema, 240

Monogenic (Mendelian) disorders, 15
Mononeuritis multiplex
  antineutrophil cytoplasmic antibody vasculitis,
    174
  cryoglobulinemic vasculitis, 173
Monosodium urate (MSU) crystal deposition,
  245
Montenegro-Leishman test, 334
Montgomery syndrome, 235t
Morbihan disease, 194t
Morbilliform drug eruption, 154–155
  dengue, 284
  serum sickness-like eruption, 170
Morgellons disease, 186
Morning stiffness, 50, 54
Morphea, 131–132, 133t
  clinicopathological features, 131, 132t
  epidemiology, 131
  evaluation, 132
  variants, 131t
Morpheaform basal cell carcinoma (BCC), 371
Mosaicism, 17, 18
Moths, 349t
Motor innervation, 543, 544
Mouth and genital ulcers with inflamed cartilage
  (MAGIC) syndrome, 136
MPD. See Mammary Paget disease (MPD)
Mucinous carcinoma, 450–452
Mucinous nevus, 241t
Mucocutaneous adverse events
  anifrolumab, 493
  antibacterials and antimicrobials, 508t–509t
  antihistamines, 498t
  antimalarials, 489
  antineoplastics, 516t–517t
  antiretrovirals, 501t
  antivirals, 502t
  azathioprine, 490
  β-lactams, 504
  calcineurin inhibitors, 491
  clofazimine, 504
  corticosteroids, 487
  cytotoxic chemotherapies, 512t–514t,
    515f–516f
  dapsone, 492
  diethylcarbamazine, 510
  dupilumab, 493
  echinocandins, 507
  glycopeptides, 504
  griseofulvin, 509
  imidazoles and triazoles, 507
  immunotherapies, 521f–522f
  intravenous immunoglobulin, 497
  isoniazid, 504
  macrolides, 505
  methotrexate, 490
  minoxidil, 526
  omalizumab, 496
  phosphodiesterase 4 inhibitors, 492
  polyenes, 509
  pyrophosphate analogues, 504
  quinolones, 505
  retinoids, 497
  rifampin, 505
  radiation therapy, 530
  saturated solution of potassium iodide, 492
  sulfonamides, 505
  tetracyclines, 506

TNFα inhibitors, 493f
  vaccines, 494t–495t
Mucocutaneous disorders, 589t–594t
Mucocutaneous end organs, 8
Mucocutaneous leishmaniasis, 334
Mucosa, 14f, 15
Mucosal disorders
  heat injury, 360
  mechanical injury, 361
  mucocutaneous and anogenital disorders,
    589t–594t
  oral cavity, 587t, 588f
Mucosal melanotic macule, 383
Mucosal ulcers, 218f
Mucous membrane pemphigoid (MMP),
  106–107, 106f
Mucous membranes, drug absorption, 37
Muehrcke lines, 212, 212f
Muir-Torre syndrome (MTS), 381, 443
Multibacillary (MB) leprosy, 315
Multikinase inhibitors, 516t
Mupirocin, 289, 508t
Muscles, 537, 540f
Mutator phenotype, 19
Myalgias, dengue, 284
Mycetoma, 333, 333t
Mycobacterium fortuitum complex infection, 312t
Mycobacterium kansasii infection, 312t
Mycophenolate, 491
Mycoplasma pneumoniae-induced rash and
  mucositis (MIRM), 116
Mycosis fungoides (MF), 471, 472t, 474t
Myelodysplastic syndrome (MDS), 136
Myeloid differentiation factor 88 (MyD88), 28
Myeloproliferative disorder
  eosinophilic fasciitis, 135
  erythromelalgia, 181
Myiasis, 344t
Myocardial infarction, pseudoxanthoma
  elasticum (PXE), 141

N

N-acetylcysteine, 186
Naftifine, 511t
Nail avulsion, 570
Nail disorders, 600t–603t
  beau lines, 211–212, 212f
  chemical exposure injury, 362
  friction injury, 361–362
  hereditary, 213t–214t
  mechanical injury, 361
  pressure injury, 361
  water exposure injury, 362
Nailfold thromboses, 137
Nail-patella syndrome (HOOD), 214t
Nail psoriasis, 49, 50t
Nails
  bed, 13
  development, 15, 16f
  ectodermal dysplasia, 198
  folds, 13
  growth, 14f
  matrix, 12–13
  plate, 13
Nail shedding, 284
Nail unit
  biopsy techniques, 570f

lentigo, 383
surgery
  anesthetic considerations, 569
  complications, 571
  instruments, 569, 570f
  techniques, 570
Naltrexone, 183
Narrowband ultraviolet B (nbUVB)
  phototherapy, 529
  for psoriasis, 53
Nasal glioma, 431, 459t
Nasolacrimal duct cyst, 431
Nasopharyngeal carcinoma, 275
Natural killer cells, 33
Naxos disease, 61t
Necrobiosis lipoidica, 232, 232f
Necrobiotic xanthogranuloma, 234, 235t–236t
Necrotizing fasciitis, 292–293
Necrotizing ulcerative gingivitis, abscess, 293
Needles and needle drivers, 549–551, 550f
Negative predictive value (NPV), 43
Neglect, 362
NEH. See Neutrophilic eccrine hidradenitis
  (NEH)
Neomycin, 508t
Neonatal acne, 191t
Neonatal purpura fulminans, 164
Neonatal varicella, 273
Neonates
  miliaria, 200
  physiologic livedo reticularis, 161
Neoplasms and cysts
  accessory tragus, 459–460
  adipose neoplasms, 407, 409–411
  adnexal neoplasms and proliferations, 439–452
  Becker nevus, 462, 463
  cutaneous small vessel vasculitis (CSVV), 169
  epidermal neoplasms, 367–382
  fibrous neoplasms, 399–408
  hair, 450, 452–458
    follicular matrical differentiation, 455,
      457–458
    follicular sheath differentiation, 455–456
    superficial follicular differentiation, 450,
      452–455
  hematolymphoid neoplasms, 470–480
  hereditary leiomyomatosis and renal cell
    cancer (HLRCC), 462
  leiomyoma, 461–462
  melanocytic, 382–398
  molecular signaling pathway mutations, 22
  nails, 458
  neural malformations, 430–439
  rudimentary supernumerary digit, 460
  solid organ metastasis, 481–482
  vascular malformations, 412–430
Nephritis
  immunoglobulin A vasculitis, 171
  Stevens-Johnson syndrome/toxic epidermal
    necrolysis, 117
Nephrogenic systemic fibrosis, 136
Nerves, 9f
  encapsulated nerve endings, 8
  motor innervation, 543, 544
  nonencapsulated nerve endings, 7–8
  sensory innervation, 541–543
Neural neoplasms
  aplasia cutis congenita, 431

granular cell tumor, 436–437
histopathological features, 438t–439t
Merkel cell carcinoma, 437–439
neurofibroma, 432
neurofibromatosis, 434–435
neuroma, 435–436
schwannoma, 432–433
Neural tube defects, 431, 431t
Neuroblastoma, 439t
Neurocutaneous disorders, 181
complex regional pain syndrome (CPRS),
184–185, 184t, 185f
familial dysautonomia, 185
lichen simplex chronicus, 183–184
prurigo nodularis, 181–183
Neurocutaneous melanosis (NCM), 389
Neurofibroma, 432, 432f
Neurofibromatosis (NF), 424t, 434–435
Neurofibromin 1 and 2 (NF-1 and 2), 434
Neurologic pruritus, 181, 182t
Neuroma, 435–436, 436f
Neuromodulators, 183
Neuropathic ulcers, 185
Neuropathy, Lyme disease, 304
Neuropeptides, 3
Neurosyphilis, 308
Neurothekeoma, 438t
Neutrophil count, Kawasaki disease, 158
Neutrophilic and eosinophilic dermatoses
aphthous stomatitis, recurrent, 217, 218f
Behçet disease, 219, 219t
bowel-associated dermatosis- arthritis
syndrome (BADAS), 222
eosinophilic pustular folliculitis, 223–224, 224f
granuloma faciale, 223, 223f
neutrophilic eccrine hidradenitis (NEH), 217,
218f
pyoderma gangrenosum (PG), 219–220, 220t,
221f, 221t
Sweet syndrome, 215–217
syndromic pyoderma gangrenosum, 222
Neutrophilic eccrine hidradenitis (NEH), 217,
218f
Neutrophils, 30
Nevirapine
drug reaction with eosinophilia and systemic
symptoms (DRESS), 156
morbilliform drug eruption, 154
Nevocellular nevus, 387, 388f, 389
Nevoid hypertrichosis, 211t
Nevus comedonicus, 452, 452f
Nevus of Ito, 385t
Nevus of Ota, 385t
Nevus sebaceous, 439, 440f
Nevus spilus, 390, 390f
New oral anticoagulants (NOACs), 545
Niacinamide, 380
Nicotinamide, 104
Nicotinic stomatitis, 360
Niemann-Pick disease, 246t
Nifedipine
for pernio, 363
for Raynaud phenomenon, 134
Nikolsky sign, 97
staphylococcal scalded skin syndrome (SSSS),
289
Stevens-Johnson syndrome/toxic epidermal
necrolysis, 117

Nitro blue tetrazolium test, 294
N, N-diethyl-3-methylbenzamide (DEET), 347
Nocardiosis, 298
Nodular amyloidosis, 243t
Nodular basal cell carcinoma (BCC), 371
Nodular fasciitis, 405t
Nodular melanomas, 393
Nodular vasculitis, 148f
Nonabsorbable sutures, 551, 555
Nonblanchable erythema, 361
Nonbullous bullous pemphigoid, 103
Nonbullous impetigo, 288
Noncaseating granulomas, 226
Nonepidermolytic PPK, 60t
Non-Hodgkin lymphoma (NHL), 99
Nonimmunologic drug reactions, 38, 38t
Noninflammatory acne vulgaris, 188
Noninflammatory retiform purpura, 159t
Noninvoluting congenital hemangioma (NICH),
420t
Non-Langerhans cell histiocytoses
in adults, 234, 235t
in childrens, 234, 235t
Nonmelanoma skin cancer (NMSC), 370
Nonneoplastic disorders, 613, 620t
calciphylaxis, 165–166, 166t
cholesterol emboli, 164–165, 165f
depositional disorders, 237, 240–255
eczematous dermatoses, 64–83
gland disorders, 188–200
hair disorders, 200–211
histiocytoses, 225–226
immunoglobulin A vasculitis, 171, 172t
livedoid vasculopathy, 162, 163f
livedo reticularis, 161–162
malignant atrophic papulosis, 164
nail disorders, 211–215
neonatal purpura fulminans, 164
neurocutaneous and psychocutaneous
disorders, 181–188
neutrophilic and eosinophilic dermatoses,
215–225
noninfectious granulomas, 225
papulosquamous disorders, 49–64
pigmentary disorders, 83–92
pigmented purpura, 168, 168t, 169f
serum sickness–like eruption, 170
small vessel vasculitis, 169–170, 170f
urticaria and erythema, 150–158
urticarial vasculitis, 171–172, 173f, 173t
vesiculobullous disorders, 93–110
xanthomas, 226
Nonnucleoside reverse transcriptase inhibitors
(NNRTIs), 501t
drug reaction with eosinophilia and systemic
symptoms (DRESS), 156
Stevens-Johnson syndrome/toxic epidermal
necrolysis, 117
Nonpitting edema, 298
Nonsteroidal anti-inflammatory drugs (NSAIDs)
acquired angioedema, 153
adult-onset Still disease (AoSD), 137
for anticoagulation management, 545
for cutaneous small vessel vasculitis (CSVV),
170
in dermatomyositis (DM), 127
erythema nodosum, 144, 147
for gout, 245

for polyarteritis nodosa, 177
reactive arthritis, 55
in Stevens-Johnson syndrome/toxic epidermal
necrolysis, 117
Nonstratified squamous epithelium, 467–469
Nonsuicidal self-injury, 187t
Nonsyndromic hereditary ichthyoses and
erythrokeratodermas, 79
Nonuremic calciphylaxis, 166
Nonvenereal sclerosing lymphangitis, 361
Noonan syndrome, 417t
Noonan syndrome with lentigines, 384t
Normocomplementemic urticarial vasculitis, 172
Nortriptyline, 498t
Nose, relapsing polychondritis, 136
NRAS mutations, nevocellular nevus, 387
Nuclear factor k-light-chain-enhancer of
activated B-cells (NF-kB), 28
Nucleoside reverse transcriptase inhibitors
(NRTIs)/nucleotide reverse transcriptase
inhibitors (NtRTIs), 501t
Nucleotide-binding domain leucine-rich repeat-
containing receptor 3 (NLRP3), 28
Nucleotide excision repair (NER) pathway, 356
Null hypothesis, 37
Nullizygous genotype, 15
Number needed to harm (NNH), 41
Number needed to treat (NNT), 42
Nummular dermatitis, 68
Nutritional deficiencies, 237
acquired, 252t–254t
Nystatin, 511t

O

Obesity, calciphylaxis, 166
Observational studies, 41
Obsessive-compulsive and related disorders, 186,
186t
Ochronosis, 525f
Occult spinal dysraphism, 431
Occupational acne, 190t
Ocular findings, atopic dermatitis (AD), 65
Ocular inflammation, 136
Ocular involvement
herpes zoster, 274
varicella, 273
Ocular mucous membrane pemphigoid, 106
Ocular rosacea, 194, 196
clinicopathological features, 194
evaluation, 195
treatment, 196
Oculocutaneous albinism (OCA), 3
Odds ratio (OR), 41
Ofuji disease, 223
Ointment, 37
Olecranon bursitis, 333
Olmstead syndrome, 61t
Omalizumab
antineutrophil cytoplasmic antibody
vasculitis, 174
biologic and small molecule inhibitors,
493, 496
for bullous pemphigoid, 104
urticaria, 152
Omphalomesenteric duct cyst, 468t
Onchocerciasis, 341t
Onychoatrophy, 107

Onychodystrophy, 213
Onychogryphosis, 362t
Onychomadesis, 284
Onychomatricoma, 458
Onychomycosis, 321–322, 321f
Open use test, contact dermatitis, 77–78
Ophiasis, 201
Ophthalmic veins, 541
Opioid antagonists/agonists, 183
Oral cavity, 587t, 588f
Oral hairy leukoplakia, 275t
Oral lichen planus (LP), 111
Ornithine decarboxylase (ODC), 12
Orolabial herpes, 269
Oropharyngeal candidiasis, 322, 323t
Oroya fever, 304
Orthopoxvirus, 282t
Osler nodes, 300
Ovarian adenocarcinoma, 481t
Oxymetazoline, 196

P

P53, 19
Pachydermoperiostosis, 214t
Pachyonychia congenita (PC), 213
Pacinian (lamellar) corpuscles, 8
Pain
  acute lipodermatosclerosis, 147
  eosinophilic fasciitis, 135
  morphea, 131
  nephrogenic systemic fibrosis, 136
  systemic sclerosis, 134
Palatal petechiae, 274
Palisaded encapsulated neuroma, 436f
Palisaded epidermal nevus (PEN), 369
Palisaded epidermal nevus with "skyline" basal
    cell layer (PENS), 369
Palisaded neutrophilic granulomatous dermatitis
    (PNGD), 137
Palmoplantar, 14f, 15
Palmoplantar wart, 278t
Palms
  neutrophilic eccrine hidradenitis (NEH), 217
  primary focal hyperhidrosis, 198
Palpable purpura, 159t
Pancreatic panniculitis, 148f
Panniculitis and lipodystrophy
  in adults, 145t
  in children, 145t–146t
  erythema nodosum, 144–147
  hereditary lipodystrophies, 149, 149t–150t
  lipodermatosclerosis, 147, 148f
  lobular, 144, 148f
  septal, 144
Panuveitis, 219
Papillary eccrine adenoma, 451t
Papillary intralymphatic angioendothelioma
    (PILA), 429t
Papillon- Lefèvre syndrome, 61t
Papular eczema, 65
Papular pruritic eruption (PPE), 224
Papular purpuric gloves and socks syndrome, 283
Papular urticaria, 347
Papulopustular rosacea (PPR), 194
  clinicopathological features, 194
  evaluation, 195
  treatment, 196

Papulosquamous disorders
  acanthosis nigricans, 62–64
  confluent and reticulated papillomatosis, 64
  geographic tongue, 55, 55f
  granular parakeratosis, 62, 63f
  hereditary palmoplantar keratodermas, 59,
      60t–61t, 62f
  parapsoriasis, 55–56
  pityriasis lichenoides, 56, 57f
  pityriasis rosea (PR), 56–58
  pityriasis rubra pilaris, 58–59, 58t, 59f
  psoriasis, 49–53
  reactive arthritis, 54–55
Paracoccidioidomycosis, 326, 326f
Paraneoplastic pemphigus (PNP), 99–100, 100f
Paraneoplastic syndromes, 605t–607t
Parapsoriasis, 55–56
Parasites, 334
  classification, 335t–336t
Parasitic diseases
  arthropod bites, 347
  cutaneous larva migrans, 336, 337, 343
  hyper-immunoglobulin E syndromes, 343
  leishmaniasis, 334
  scabies and lice, 343–347
Parathyroidectomy, 166
Parathyroid hormone (PTH), calciphylaxis, 166
Parinaud oculoglandular syndrome, 303
Parkes Weber syndrome, 414t
Parkinson disease
  bullous pemphigoid, 103
  seborrheic dermatitis, 68
Paronychia, 295
Parrot lines, 309
Partially involuting congenital hemangioma
    (PICH), 420t
Parvovirus B19, erythema infectiosum, 283
Passenger mutations, 19
Paste, 37
Patau syndrome, 417t
Patch test, contact dermatitis, 76–77
Patent safety
  issues, dermatology, 44
  sample safety program, 45t
Pathogen-associated molecular patterns
    (PAMPs), 28
Patient-centered care, 43–44
Patterned alopecia areata, 201
Paucibacillary (PB) leprosy, 315
Pauci-immune crescentic necrotizing
    glomerulonephritis, 174
Pauci-immune vasculitis, 174
Pediculosis capitis, 344t
Pediculosis corporis, 344t
Pediculosis pubis, 344t
Peliosis hepatis, 303
Pembrolizumab, 437
Pemphigoid vegetans, 103
Pemphigus Disease Area Index (PDAI), 98
Pemphigus erythematosus, 96, 122
Pemphigus foliaceus (PF), 96, 97f
Pemphigus herpetiformis, 97
Pemphigus syphiliticus, 309
Pemphigus vegetans, 97
Pemphigus vulgaris
  clinicopathological features, 97, 98f
  differential diagnosis, 97–98
  epidemiology, 97

evaluation, 97–98
  management, 98
Penicillin, 504
  for actinomycosis, 298
  for erysipelas, 292
  for perianal streptococcal infection, 292
  for scarlet fever, 290
Penicilliosis, 281
Penile lentigines, 411
Pentoxifylline, 147, 523
Perforins, 33
Performance measures, patient safety, 45
Perianal pseudoverrucous papules/nodules, 76
Perineurioma, 438t
Perioral dermatitis, 194t
Periorificial dermatitis, 66, 196
Peripheral arterial disease (PAD), 180
Peripheral hypereosinophilia, 135
  atopic dermatitis (AD), 65
  bullous pemphigoid, 103
  cholesterol emboli, 165
  eosinophilic pustular folliculitis (EPF), 224
  hypereosinophilic syndrome (HES), 225
  urticaria, 152
Peripheral neuropathy
  antineutrophil cytoplasmic antibody
      vasculitis, 174
  cryoglobulinemic vasculitis, 173
  familial dysautonomia, 185
Periplakin
  mucous membrane pemphigoid (MMP), 107
  paraneoplastic pemphigus, 99
Peristomal pyoderma gangrenosum, 220
Periungual/subungual keratotic tumors, 88
Permanent peripheral neuropathy, 362
Permethrin, 345, 512t
Pernicious anemia, 107
Pernio, 363, 363f
Pernio-like skin lesions, 283, 363
Petechiae, 69, 159t
Peutz-Jeghers syndrome, 384t
PHACE(S) syndrome, 422, 422t
Phaeohyphomycosis, 315
Phakomatosis, 414t
Phakomatosis pigmentokeratotica, 390, 439
Phakomatosis pigmentovascularis, 390
Pharmacodynamics, 36
Pharmacokinetics, 36
Pharmacology, 36–38
  drug reactions, 38, 38t
  skin absorption and penetration, 37–38
Pharyngitis, 290
Phenobarbital, 117
Phenotype, 15
Phenylketonuria, 247t
Pheochromocytoma, rosacea, 195
Pheomelanin, 3
Phimosis, 129
Phosphodiesterase 4 inhibitors, 492
Phosphoinositide 3-kinase (PI3K) signaling
    pathway, 20
Photoaging, 23
  cutaneous signs, 359, 359t
Photoallergic contact dermatitis, 24
Photoallergic/phototoxic eruption, 358, 358f
Photoallergy, 23
Photobiology, 22–25, 23f, 24t
  absorption spectrum, 22

Photocarcinogenesis, 23
Photodermatoses
    chronic actinic dermatitis (CAD), 355
    hydroa vacciniforme, 354
    photoallergic/phototoxic eruption, 358
    photopatch testing, 353
    photoprovocation testing, 353
    phototesting, 353
    poikiloderma of Civatte, 359
    polymorphous light eruption (PMLE),
        353–354–354f
    UVR exposure, 353
    xeroderma pigmentosum, 356, 356t–357t
Photodynamic therapy (PDT)
    basal cell carcinoma, 373
    phototherapy, 529–531
    porokeratosis, 375
    squamous cell carcinoma (SCC), 380
Photoinduced contact dermatitis, 70
Photoonycholysis, 358
Photopatch testing, 353, 358, 358f
Photoprotection, 24–25
    chronic actinic dermatitis (CAD), 355
    erythema dyschromicum perstans, 86
    hydroa vacciniforme, 354
    lupus erythematosus (LE), 122
    photoallergic/phototoxic eruption, 358, 358f
    polymorphous light eruption (PMLE), 354
    porphyria cutanea tarda, 249
    xeroderma pigmentosum, 356
Phototherapy
    for atopic dermatitis (AD), 67
    for cutaneous T-cell lymphoma (CTCL), 471
    for extragenital lichen sclerosus, 130
    for lymphomatoid papulosis (LyP), 475
    for parapsoriasis, 56
    photodynamic therapy, 529–531
    physical treatments, 529
    for prurigo nodularis, 183
    for psoriasis, 53
    scleredema, 240
    for vitiligo, 85
Phototoxic eruption, 531
Phototoxicity, 23
Phrynoderma, 83
Phymatous rosacea, 194, 196
    clinicopathological features, 194
    evaluation, 195
    treatment, 196
Physical agents and disorders
    black heel and palm, 364, 365f
    chondrodermatitis nodularis helicis (CNH),
        365, 365f
    cold injury, 360
    erythema ab igne (EAI), 363
    friction injury, 361–362
    heat injury, 360
    mechanical injury, 360–361
    pernio, 363, 363f
    photodermatoses, 353–359
    pressure injury, 361
    sickle cell disease, 364
    vibration injury, 362
    water exposure injury, 362
Physical sunscreens, 25t, 249
Physical therapy
    for eosinophilic fasciitis, 135
    for juvenile-onset dermatomyositis (DM), 127

    morphea, 133
    nephrogenic systemic fibrosis, 136
    systemic sclerosis, 134
Physical treatments
    cryosurgery, 532
    electrocautery and electrosurgery, 533–535
    phototherapy, 529
    radiation therapy, 531
Physiologic livedo reticularis, 161
Piedra, 318
Piezogenic pedal papules, 400t
Pigmentary changes, eczematous dermatitis, 65
Pigmentary demarcation lines, 87
Pigmentary disorders, 83–92
    erythema dyschromicum perstans, 85–86,
        86t–87t
    hereditary, 89t–92t
    hyperpigmentation, 83
    hypopigmentation, 83
    incontinentia pigmenti, 88, 89f
    pigmentary demarcation lines, 87
    prurigo pigmentosa, 88
    vitiligo, 84–85
Pigmented basal cell carcinoma (BCC), 371
Pigmented purpura, 168, 168t, 169f
Pigmented spindle cell nevus of Reed, 391, 392f
Pilar cyst, 465t
Pilar sheath acanthoma, 456t
Piloleiomyoma, 461, 461f
Pilomatricoma, 457, 457f, 458t
Pimecrolimus, for psoriasis, 53
Pimozide, 525
Pincer deformity, 213
Pinta, 307t
Pinworm infection, 341t
Piperacillin-tazobactam, 292
Pitted keratolysis, 295–296
    clinicopathological features, 295, 296f
    epidemiology, 295
    evaluation, 296f
    management, 296
Pityriasis alba, 66
Pityriasis amiantacea, 57
Pityriasis folliculorum, 194t
Pityriasis lichenoides, 56, 57f
Pityriasis lichenoides chronica (PLC), 56
Pityriasis lichenoides et varioliformis acuta
        (PLEVA), 56
Pityriasis rosea (PR)
    clinicopathological features, 56–57, 57f
    epidemiology, 56
    evaluation, 57–58
    management, 58
Pityriasis rotunda, 57, 309
Pityriasis rubra pilaris (PRP), 58–59, 58t, 59f
Pityriasis simplex capillitii, 68
Plakoglobin, 3
Plakophilin, 99
Plane xanthoma, 236, 238t
Plant allergens, 75t–76t, 77f
Plaque-type morphea, 131
Plasma cell dyscrasias, 234
Plasma cells, 29
Platelet-rich plasma, 526
Platonychia, 249f
Pleomorphic dermal sarcoma, 406, 408
Pleomorphic fibroma, 405t
Pleomorphic lipoma, 410

Plexiform fibrohistiocytic tumor, 405t
Plexiform neurofibroma, 211t
PMLE. See Polymorphous light eruption (PMLE)
Pneumococcal conjugate (PCV13) vaccine, 495t
Pneumococcal polysaccharide (PPSV23) vaccine,
        495t
Pneumonia, 136
Pneumonitis, 303
    cytomegalovirus infection, 275
    varicella, 273
PNP. See Paraneoplastic pemphigus (PNP)
Podofilox, 502t
Podophyllin, 502t
Pohl-Pinkus constriction
    alopecia areata, 201
    traction alopecia, 205
Poikiloderma of Civatte, 359
Poliosis, 84
Polyarteritis nodosa (PAN), 176–177, 176f
Polycyclic erythema annulare centrifugum, 154
Polycystic ovarian syndrome (PCOS), 188
Polyenes, 509, 510
Polygenic disorders, 18
Polymerase chain reaction (PCR)
    for leishmaniasis, 334
    onychomycosis, 322
Polymorphic eruption of pregnancy (PEP), 157,
        157f
Polymorphous light eruption (PMLE)
    clinicopathological features, 353, 354f
    epidemiology, 353
    evaluation, 353
    management, 354
    prevalence, 353
Polymyalgia rheumatica (PMR), 177
Polymyxin B, 508t
Polypodium leucotomos (Heliocare), 25
Polythelia, 15
Pomade acne, 190t
Porokeratosis, 375, 375t, 376f
Poroma, 446–447, 447f
Porphyria cutanea tarda, 248–249, 251f
Porphyrias, 237
    hereditary, 250t
Port-wine stain (PWS), 413, 415
Posaconazole, 329
Positive predictive value (PPV), 43
Posterior tibial block, 548
Postherpetic neuralgia (PHN), 274
Poststreptococcal glomerulonephritis (GAS)
    impetigo, 288
    rheumatic fever, 290
Posttransplant lymphoproliferative disorder
        (PTLD), 275
Potassium hydroxide (KOH)
    candidiasis, 322
    dimorphic fungi, 325
    onychomycosis, 322
    piedra, 318
    tinea, 320
    tinea capitis, 320
    tinea nigra, 317
    tinea versicolor, 316
Potassium iodide, 492
Povidone-iodine, 549t
Power, 41
Poxvirus infections, 281, 282t
PPR. See Papulopustular rosacea (PPR)

PR. *See* Pityriasis rosea (PR)
Prader-Willi syndrome, 19
Pramoxine, 183, 524t
Preadolescent acne, 191t
Prebiotics, 67
Precision, clinical tests, 42, 43f
Prednisone, 78
Pregabalin, 183
Pregnancy, 38
    androgenetic alopecia, 204
    dermatologic signs, 611t–612t
    drug interactions and, 38
    erythema dyschromicum perstans, 86
    polymorphic eruption, 157, 157f
    telogen effluvium, 205
    tinea versicolor, 315
Prepubertal hypertrichosis, 210t
Preservatives, 73t
Pressure injury
    chondrodermatitis nodularis helicis (CNH),
        365
    mechanical injury, 361
Pressure ulcer, 361
Prick tests, urticaria, 152
Prilocaine, 183
Primary biliary cirrhosis (PBC), 85
Primary cutaneous diffuse large B-cell
        lymphoma, leg type (PCDLBL, LT), 476
Primary cutaneous follicle center lymphoma
        (PCFCL), 476
Primary cutaneous marginal zone lymphoma
        (PCMZL), 476
Primary cutaneous mucinoses, 241t
Primary total dystrophic onychomycosis, 321
Probability value (P-value), 41
Probenecid, 37
Probiotics, atopic dermatitis (AD), 67
Prodromal pruritus, 224
Progeria, 357t
Progestins, 191
Progressive macular hypomelanosis (PMH), 85
Prolidase deficiency, 247t
Proliferative phase, wound healing, 35, 36t
Proline-serine-threonine phosphatase-
        interacting protein 1 (PSTPIP1), 28
Promethazine, 498t
Proopiomelanocortin (POMC) polypeptide, 3
Propofol, for mastocytosis, 480
Propranolol, 422
Propranolol, for hemangioma, 420
Prostate adenocarcinoma, 482t
Protease inhibitors, 501t
Protein contact dermatitis, 76
Protein-energy malnutrition, 237
Proteosome inhibitors, 517t
Proteus syndrome, 414t
Prothrombotic abnormality, livedoid
        vasculopathy, 162
Protoporphyrin IX, 529
Prototheca wickerhamii, 333
Prototheciasis, 328f, 333
Protozoa, 335t
Protozoan infections, 339t–340t
Proximal matrix, nail, 13
Proximal subungual onychomycosis, 321
PRP. *See* Pityriasis rubra pilaris (PRP)
Prurigo nodularis
    clinicopathological features, 181, 183f

epidemiology, 181
    evaluation, 182
    management, 183
Prurigo pigmentosa, 88
Pruritus, 182t
    anogenital lichen sclerosus, 130
    dyshidrotic eczema, 68
    mediators, 8
    systemic, 181, 182t
Pseudoainhum, 59
Pseudocysts, 468, 469f, 470f
Pseudodominant inheritance, 17
Pseudofolliculitis barbae, 209
Pseudogout, 245
Pseudohypoparathyroidism, 166
Pseudomembranous conjunctivitis, 99
Pseudomonal infections, 300t
Pseudopelade of Brocq, 206
Pseudoporphyria, 249, 358
Pseudo-pseudohypoparathyroidism, 166
Pseudosyndactyly, 107
Pseudoxanthoma elasticum (PXE), 141, 143f
Psoralen ultraviolet A (PUVA)
    phototherapy, 529
    for psoriasis, 53
Psoriasiform alopecia, 49
Psoriasis
    biologic and small molecule inhibitors,
        493–494, 494t
    clinicopathological correlation, 52f
    clinicopathological features, 49–50
    differential diagnosis, 52
    epidemiology, 49
    evaluation, 52–53
    management, 53
    pathogenesis, 49, 51f
    variants, 50t
Psoriasis Area and Severity Index (PASI), 53
Psoriatic arthritis, 49, 50, 51t
Psoriatic pitting, 52f
Psychiatry referral
    for delusions of parasitosis, 186
    for excoriation disorder, 187
Psychocutaneous disorders, 181, 187t
    delusions of parasitosis, 186
    excoriation disorder, 186–187
    factitial dermatitis, 187–188
Psychogenic pruritus, 181, 182t
Pterygium, 113f
Pulicosis, 344t
Pulmonary actinomycosis, 298
Pulmonary anthrax, 298
Pulmonary arterial hypertension (PAH), 134
Pulmonary coccidioidomycosis, 327
Pulmonary cryptococcosis, 329
Pulmonary edema, 303
Pulsed dye laser (PDL)
    capillary malformation, 415
    hemangioma, 421
Punctate hereditary palmoplantar keratodermas,
        59, 60t
Punctate palmoplantar keratodermas, 60t
Purified protein derivative (PPD) test, erythema
        nodosum, 147
Purine analogues, 501–502
Purpura, 158
    fulminans, 164
    macular, 159t

palpable, 159t
    pigmented, 168, 168t, 169f
    primary, 159t–160t
    retiform, 159t, 160f
Purpuric pityriasis rosea, 57
Pustular pityriasis rosea, 57
Pustular psoriasis, 49, 50t
Pustular pyoderma gangrenosum, 220
Pustulosis
    acute generalized exanthematous, 93–95
    differential diagnosis, 53
Pyoderma gangrenosum (PG)
    age-focused initial evaluation, 221t
    bullous, 220
    clinicopathological features, 220
    diagnostic criteria, 220t
    epidemiology, 219
    evaluation, 220
    management, 220
    peristomal, 220
    pustular, 220
    syndromic, 222
    ulcerative, 220, 221f
    vegetative, 220
Pyogenic granuloma (PG), 423, 423f
Pyomyositis, abscess, 293
Pyostomatitis vegetans, 220
Pyrethrins, 512t
Pyrimidine analogues, 502
Pyrin, 28
Pyrophosphate analogues, 502

Q

Q fever, 306t
Quality control checkpoints, 558, 559t
Quality improvement, 44
Quinolones, 505
Quinupristin, 505

R

Radial nerve block, 548
Radiation acne, 190t, 531
Radiation dermatitis, 531f
Radiation-induced morphea, 133t
Radiation stomatitis, 531
Radiation therapy, 531
    for basal cell carcinoma (BCC), 373
    for cutaneous T-cell lymphoma (CTCL), 471
    for Kaposi sarcoma, 427
    and keloid, 400
    and lymphedema, 178
    for mammary and extramammary Paget
        disease, 382
    and mucocutaneous adverse events, 530
    for squamous cell carcinoma (SCC), 380
    and Sweet syndrome, 216
    for tufted angioma and KHE, 425
Radioallergosorbent tests (RASTs), urticaria, 152
Ramsey-Hunt syndrome, 274
Randomized controlled trials (RCTs), 41
Rapidly involuting congenital hemangioma
        (RICH), 420t
Rapp-Hodgkin syndrome, 199t
Raynaud phenomenon
    cryoglobulinemia, 173

systemic sclerosis, 134
Reactive arthritis, 54–55
Reactive granulomatous dermatitis, 231
Reactive perforating dermatosis, 137, 140f
Red eye, 194
Red lunulae, 137, 215f
Red man syndrome, 53, 504
Regeneration, wound healing, 35
Regional dysesthesias, 184, 184t
Relapsing fever, 307t
Relapsing polychondritis, 136
Remodeling phase, wound healing, 35, 36t
Renal disease, edema blister, 177
Renal involvement
    immunoglobulin A vasculitis, 171
    systemic sclerosis, 134
Renbök phenomenon, 50
Repigmentation, vitiligo, 85
Reproduction, drug interactions, 38
Resident memory T cells, 33
Restrictive cardiomyopathy, systemic sclerosis,
        134
Retapamulin, 289, 508t
Reticular erythematous mucinosis, 241t
Reticulated hyperpigmentation, prurigo
        pigmentosa, 88
Reticulohistiocytosis, 235t
Retiform hemangioendothelioma, 429t
Retiform purpura, 159t, 160f, 283
Retinal vascular abnormalities, 88
Retinoid acid receptors (RARs), 497
Retinoids
    asteatotic dermatitis and, 67
    for hereditary ichthyoses and
        erythrokeratodermas, 79
    hereditary palmoplantar keratodermas, 62
    for pityriasis rubra pilaris (PRP), 58
    for psoriasis, 53
    for squamous cell carcinoma (SCC), 380
    systemic, 497, 498t, 499
    telogen effluvium, 205
    topical, 499, 499t
Retinoid X receptors (RXRs), 497
Retroorbital pain, dengue, 284
Revertant mosaicism, 18
Review of systems (ROS), 637
Revised Jones criteria for acute rheumatic fever,
        290, 290t
Rheumatic fever, 290
Rheumatoid arthritis (RA), 136–137
    cutaneous small vessel vasculitis (CSVV), 169
    pyoderma gangrenosum (PG), 219
    urticarial vasculitis, 172
Rheumatoid factor (RF), psoriatic arthritis, 53
Rheumatoid neutrophilic dermatosis,
        rheumatoid arthritis, 137
Rheumatoid nodules, 137, 231f
Rheumatoid vasculitis, 137
Rhinocerebral infection, zygomycosis, 332
Rhinosporidiosis, 328f, 340t
Ribonucleotide, 514t
Richner-Hanhart syndrome, 61t
Rickets, 245
Rickettsial infections, 305t–306t
Rickettsialpox, 305t
Rifampin, 505
Riga-Fede disease, 185, 361
Risperidone, 525

Rituximab
    biologic and small molecule inhibitors, 496
    for Merkel cell carcinoma, 437
    for mucous membrane pemphigoid (MMP),
        107
    in paraneoplastic pemphigus, 99
    for pemphigus vulgaris, 98
    in Stevens-Johnson syndrome/toxic epidermal
        necrolysis, 117
    systemic lupus erythematosus, 122
    urticaria, 152
Rocky Mountain spotted fever (RMSF), 303, 305t
Roflumilast, 53
Rombo syndrome, 371t
Romidepsin, 471, 523t
Rosacea
    clinicopathological features, 194, 195f
    epidemiology, 194
    evaluation, 195
    management, 196
    variants and related disorders, 194, 194t
Rosacea conglobata, 194t
Rosacea fulminans, 194t
Rosai-Dorfman disease, 235t
Roseola, 277, 277t
Rotation flaps, 561, 563
Rothmund-Thomson syndrome, 357t
Rotterdam criteria, 188
Round follicles, 12
Rowell syndrome, 116, 122
Rubber products, 73t
Rubella, 277, 277t
Rubeola, 277, 277t
Rubinstein-Taybi syndrome, 211t, 415t
Rudimentary supernumerary digit, 460, 460f
Ruffini corpuscles, 8
Russell-Silver syndrome, 435t

S

Saber shins, 309
Saddle nose, 309
Salicylic acid, 502t
Salicylic acid, for psoriasis, 53
Salmon patch, 413
Salt split-skin technique, 105f
    linear immunoglobulin A bullous
        dermatosis, 106
    mucous membrane pemphigoid, 107
    subepidermal autoimmune blistering
        disorders, 105f
Saphenous and superficial peroneal block, 548
Sarcoidosis
    epidemiology, 226
    erythema nodosum, 144
    evaluation, 226
    histopathological features, 228t
    ichthyosis vulgaris, 78
    management, 226
    variants, 227t
Sarcoptes scabiei var. hominis, 343
SARS-CoV-2 vaccine, 495t
Saturated solution of potassium
        iodide (SSKI), 492
    for erythema nodosum, 147
    for sporotrichosis, 331
    for Sweet syndrome, 217
Scabies, 344t

clinicopathological features, 343, 346f
    epidemiology, 343
    evaluation, 343, 345
    management, 345
Scalp, 14f, 15
Scalpel handles and blades, 549, 550f
Scarlet fever, 290, 290t
Scarring, wound healing, 35
Scarring alopecia, 106, 531
    necrobiosis lipoidica, 232
    tuberculosis, 309
SCC. See Squamous cell carcinoma (SCC)
Schimmelpenning syndrome, 439
Schistosomiasis, 342t
Schizophrenia spectrum, 186
Schnitzler syndrome, 152
Schöpf-Schulz-Passarge syndrome, 199t, 371t
Schwannoma, 432–433, 433f
Scleredema, 240, 241t, 242f
Sclerodactyly, 134
Scleromyxedema, 240, 241t, 242f
Sclerosing disorders, exogenous substances, 132,
        133t
Sclerotherapy
    cosmetics, 583, 584t
    for venous malformation (VM), 416
Sclerotic fibroma, 405t
Scorpions, 348t
SCORTEN, 118t
Scrotal involvement, candidiasis, 322
Scrotal sparing, 320
Scrotum, 15
    drug absorption, 37
Scurvy, 7f
Sea cucumbers, 349t
Sea lice, 349t
Sea urchins, 349t
Sebaceoma, 441–442, 441f
Sebaceous adenoma, 441–442, 441f
Sebaceous carcinoma, 442, 442f
Sebaceous differentiation
    Muir-Torre syndrome, 443
    nevus sebaceous, 439–440
    sebaceous adenoma and sebaceoma, 441–442
    sebaceous carcinoma, 442
    sebaceous gland hyperplasia, 440–441
Sebaceous gland hyperplasia (SGH), 440–441,
        440f
Sebaceous glands, 8–9
Sebopsoriasis, 50, 68
Seborrheic dermatitis, 50
    clinicopathological features, 68, 69f
    epidemiology, 68
    evaluation, 69
    management, 69
Seborrheic keratosis
    clinicopathological features, 367
    epidemiology, 367
    evaluation, 367
    management, 368
    variants, 367, 368f, 368t
Sebum, 9
Segmental vitiligo, 84, 85
Selectins, 30
Selection bias, 42
Selective serotonin reuptake inhibitors (SSRIs),
        187
Selenium deficiency, 252t

Selumetinib, 435
Semimobile papulonodules, 137
Senear-Usher syndrome, 96, 122
Senile gluteal dermatosis, 361
Senile-onset atopic dermatitis (AD), 65
Sensitivity, clinical tests, 42
Sensory innervation, 541–543
Sensory neuropathies, 184t
Sepsis, calciphylaxis, 166
Septal panniculitis, 144f
Septic vasculitis, 299–300
Seronegative inflammatory arthritis, 136
Serum sickness-like eruption, 170
Sesquiterpene lactone exposure, contact
    dermatitis, 70
Setleis syndrome, 431
Severe acute respiratory syndrome coronavirus 2
    (SARS-CoV-2), 283
Sexual abuse, 362
Sezary syndrome, 471, 472t
SGH. *See* Sebaceous gland hyperplasia (SGH)
Shar-Pei sign, 240
SHH signaling pathway, 20
Shinbone fever, 304
Shingrix, for herpes zoster, 274
Short stature, calciphylaxis, 166
Shoulder parakeratosis, 59f
Sickle cell disease, 364
Sildenafil, for Raynaud phenomenon, 134
Silver sulfadiazine, 509t, 549t
Simple aphthosis, 217
Sinecatechins, 502t
Sinusoidal hemangioma, 420t
Sirolimus
    for angiofibroma, 401
    for Kaposiform hemangioendothelioma, 425
    for neurofibromatosis, 435
    for tuberous sclerosis complex, 402
Sisaipho, 201
Sjögren syndrome
    cutaneous small vessel vasculitis (CSVV), 169
    urticarial vasculitis, 172
SJS/TEN. *See* Stevens-Johnson syndrome/toxic
    epidermal necrolysis (SJS/TEN)
Skin
    dermis, 5, 7
    development, 15, 16f
    embryology, 15
    epidermis, 1–3, 1f
    junctions, 3–5, 4f, 5f
    subcutis, 7
Skin biopsy
    for aspergillosis, 332
    ecthyma gangrenosum, 301
    epidermal nevus, 369
    herpes simplex virus (HSV), 270
    mammary and extramammary Paget disease,
      382
    molluscum contagiosum, 281
    polymorphous light eruption (PMLE), 353
    Stevens-Johnson syndrome/toxic epidermal
      necrolysis, 117
    urticaria, 152
Skin cracks, asteatotic dermatitis, 67
Skin disorders
    chemical exposure, 362
    cold injury, 360
    friction injury, 361

heat injury, 360
    mechanical injury, 360–361
    pressure injury, 361
    vibration injury, 362
    water exposure injury, 362
Skin tension lines, 539, 540f
Skin tightness
    eosinophilic fasciitis, 135
    morphea, 131
    nephrogenic systemic fibrosis, 136
    systemic sclerosis, 134
Skirt syndrome, 156
SLE. *See* Systemic lupus erythematosus (SLE)
Small fiber neuropathy, 181
Small plaque parapsoriasis, 55
Small vessel vasculitis, 169–170, 170f
SMO inhibitors
    for basal cell carcinoma (BCC), 373
    for basal cell nevus syndrome (BCNS), 374
Snake bite, 349t
Sneddon syndrome, 162
Soak and smear technique, 67
Sodium stibogluconate, for cutaneous
    leishmaniasis, 334
Sodium thiosulfate (STS), for calciphylaxis, 166
Soft corns, 361
Soft-tissue dermal fillers, 582f
    for acne vulgaris, 191
    clinical applications, 580–582, 581t
    safety, 580, 582
Solar lentigines, 367
Solar lentigo, 383
Solar urticaria, 355
Soles
    neutrophilic eccrine hidradenitis (NEH), 217
    primary focal hyperhidrosis, 198
Solid organ metastasis, 481, 481t–482t, 482f
Solitary angiokeratoma, 412
Solitary mastocytoma, 480t
Solution, 37
Somatic hypermutation, 29
Somatic symptom disorder, 187t
Sonic hedgehog (SHH), 12
Sorafenib, for Kaposi sarcoma, 427
SPAP. *See* Syringocystadenoma papilliferum
    (SPAP)
Specificity, clinical tests, 42
Spider nevus, 412t
Spiders, 348t
Spina bifida, 431
Spindle cell hemangioma, 420t
Spindle cell lipoma, 410
Spinosad, 512t
Spiradenoma, 443–444, 444f
Spirochete infections, 304, 306t–307t
Spironolactone, for acne vulgaris, 191
Spitz nevus
    clinicopathological features, 391–392, 392f
    epidemiology, 391
    evaluation, 392
    management, 392
Splenomegaly, rheumatoid arthritis, 137
Splinter hemorrhages, 300f
Spongiotic dermatitis, 76
Spontaneous abortion, pityriasis rosea (PR), 56
Sporothrix schenckii, 330
Sporotrichosis, 330–331, 331f
    clinicopathological features, 330, 331f

epidemiology, 330
    evaluation, 331
    management, 331
Squamous cell carcinoma (SCC)
    Brigham and Women's Hospital tumor staging
      system, 378, 380t
    clinicopathological features, 377, 379f–380f
    epidemiology, 377
    evaluation, 377–378
    management, 378, 380
    premalignant *vs.* verrucous carcinoma, 378t
Standard deviation (SD), 41
Standard error (SE), 37
Staphylococcal scalded skin syndrome (SSSS),
    289
Staphylococcal toxic shock syndrome (TSS), 291
Starch-iodine technique, hyperhidrosis, 198
Stasis dermatitis, 69, 70f
Statins
    asteatotic dermatitis, 67
    dermatomyositis (DM), 127
Steatocystoma, 465t
Steroid-induced rosacea, 194t
Stevens-Johnson syndrome/toxic epidermal
    necrolysis (SJS/TEN), 117–118, 117f, 118t
Stiff skin syndrome, 132
STING-associated vasculopathy with onset in
    infancy (SAVI), 161
Straight hair, 12
Stratified squamous epithelium
    epidermoid cyst, 464–466
    Gardner syndrome, 467
Stratum basale, 3
Stratum corneum, 14f, 15
Stratum lucidum, 14f, 15
Strengthening the Reporting of Observational
    studies in Epidemiology (STROBE)
    guidelines, 41
Streptococcal infections, erythema nodosum, 144
Striae, 400t
Striate palmoplantar keratodermas, 60t
Stroke, malignant atrophic papulosis, 164
Strongyloidiasis, 341t
Stucco keratosis, 367
Sturge-Weber syndrome, 415t
Stye, abscess, 293
Subacute nodular migratory panniculitis (EN
    migrans), 144
Subcorneal pustular dermatosis subtype, IgA
    pemphigus, 98, 99f
Subcutaneous fat necrosis, 148f
Subcutis, 7
Subepidermal autoimmune blistering disorders,
    103, 104t
    salt split-skin technique, 105f
Subepidermal hemorrhagic bullae, 129
Subgaleal hemorrhage, 360
Sublamina densa, 4, 6f
Sublamina densa type linear immunoglobulin A
    bullous dermatosis, 105, 106f
Substance-induced formication, 186
Substance P, 8, 32
Subungual hyperkeratosis, 213
Sucquet-Hoyer canal, 7
Suction blister, 361
Sulfacetamide, 509t
Sulfacetamide, for papulopustular
    rosacea (PPR), 196

Sulfhydryls, hypopigmentation, 85
Sulfonamides, 505–506
    drug reaction with eosinophilia and systemic symptoms (DRESS), 156
    erythema nodosum, 144
    morbilliform drug eruption, 154
    porphyria cutanea tarda, 248
    in Stevens-Johnson syndrome/toxic epidermal necrolysis, 117
    Sweet syndrome, 216
Sulfur, 196, 512t
Sun protection factor (SPF), 24
Sunscreen components, 73t–74t
Sunscreens, 25t
Superficial basal cell carcinoma (BCC), 371
Superficial follicular differentiation, 450
    Birt-Hogg-Dubé syndrome, 455
    nevus comedonicus, 452
    trichoepithelioma, 453–454
Superficial folliculitis, 294
Superficial musculoaponeurotic system (SMAS), 538
Superficial mycoses
    onychomycosis, 321–322
    piedra, 318
    tinea, 318–320
    tinea capitis, 320–321
    tinea nigra, 317, 317f
    tinea versicolor, 315–317
Superficial spreading melanoma, 393
Supportive care
    cholesterol emboli, 165
    immunoglobulin A vasculitis, 171
    small vessel vasculitis, 170
Suppurative granulomas, 294
Suprabulbar zone, hair, 12
Sural nerve block, 548
Surgery
    anesthetics, 546–548
    antibiotic prophylaxis, 545, 546f
    anticoagulation management, 545
    antiseptics, 548, 549t
    blood vessels, 541
    complications, 568t–569t
    ears, 537, 539f
    emergencies, 566, 567t
    eyelids, 537, 538f
    face, 537, 539f
    flaps, 561–564
    grafts, 564–566
    head and neck, 543, 545
    instruments, 549–552
        chalazion clamps, 551
        curettes, 551
        hemostats, 551
        needles and needle drivers, 549–551, 550f
        scissors, 551t, 552f
    for Kaposi sarcoma, 427
    lips, 537, 538f
    Mohs micrographic surgery (MMS), 558–561
    muscles, 537, 540f
    nail unit surgery, 569–571
    nerves, 541–544, 541f
    nose, 537, 538f
    procedures, 557–559
        biopsy, 557, 558t
        excision, 557–559, 558t, 559f
        incision and drainage, 557

scalp, 537, 539f
skin tension lines, 539, 540f
topical hemostasis materials, 551, 553f
wound closure materials, 551, 554, 555
wound dressings, 554, 557t
Sutures
    absorbable sutures, 551, 555t
    knots, 553
    nonabsorbable sutures, 551, 555t
    properties of, 551, 554t
    removal, 553
    techniques, 553, 556t
Sweat, 11
Sweat gland
    disorders, 198
    ectodermal dysplasia, 198
Sweet syndrome
    classic, 216
    clinicopathological features, 216, 216f
    diagnostic criteria, 216t
    epidemiology, 216
    evaluation, 216–217
    rheumatoid arthritis, 137
Swimming pool granuloma, 312t
Sycosis, 294
Symblepharon
    mucous membrane pemphigoid, 106
    Stevens-Johnson syndrome/toxic epidermal necrolysis, 117
Symmetrical drug-related intertriginous and flexural exanthema (SDRIFE), 70
Syndromic hereditary ichthyoses and erythrokeratodermas, 79
Syndromic hereditary palmoplantar keratodermas, 60–61
Syndromic pyoderma gangrenosum, 222
Syphilis, 307t, 308–309
    clinicopathological correlation, 310f
    diagnosis, 309, 311
    latent, 308–309
    stages, 308
    treatment, 309
Syringocystadenoma papilliferum (SPAP), 444–445, 445t
Syringofibroadenoma, 452t
Syringoma, 446, 448f, 450t
Systemic lupus erythematosus (SLE)
    classification criteria, 124t
    cutaneous small vessel vasculitis (CSVV), 169
    malignant atrophic papulosis, 164
    urticarial vasculitis, 172
Systemic sclerosis, 134–135

T

Tachycardia, urticaria, 152
Tacrolimus, for psoriasis, 53
Talaromyces marneffei, 327
Talaromycosis, 327
Talimogene laherparepvec (T- VEC), melanoma, 396
Tattoo reactions, 227t
Tazarotene, 53, 499t, 524t
T-cell receptor (TCR), 33
T cells, 33, 34t
Telangiectasia
    in adults, 412t
    in children, 413t

lichen sclerosus, 129
Telangiectasia macularis eruptive perstans (TMEP), 480, 480t
Telogen, 12
Telogen effluvium, 205–206
Telomeres, 19
Temporal triangular alopecia, 214t
Tendinous xanthoma, 236, 238t
Tendonitis, 50
Terbinafine, 511t
    for onychomycosis, 322
    for tinea capitis, 321
Terfenadine, 498t
Terminal hairs, 12
Terra firma-forme dermatosis, 78
Terry nails, 212, 212f
Tetanus, diphtheria, pertussis (Tdap) vaccine, 494t
Tetracyclines, 506–507
    for acne vulgaris, 191
    for bullous pemphigoid, 104
    erythema nodosum, 144
    for impetigo, 289
    porphyria cutanea tarda, 248
    for sarcoidosis, 226
    Sweet syndrome, 216
Thalidomide, 492–493
    for actinic prurigo, 354
    for prurigo nodularis, 183
Thallium poisoning
    Mees lines, 212
    traction alopecia, 205
T helper type 1 (Th1) cell, 33
T helper type 17 (Th17) cell, 33
T helper type 22 (Th22) cell, 33
T helper type 2 (Th2) cells, 33
Therapeutic phlebotomy
    for porphyria cutanea tarda, 249
Thermal burn, 362
Thermoregulation, eccrine gland, 10
Thick drop method, 334
Thrombocythemia, 181
Thrombocytopenia
    lupus erythematosus (LE), 122
    for Rocky Mountain spotted fever (RMSF), 303
    varicella, 273
Thymoma, 99
Thyroglossal duct cyst, 459t, 468t
Thyroid carcinoma, 481t
Thyroid disorder, 205
Thyrotoxicosis, rosacea, 195
Tick bites, 344t
Ticks, 348t
Tight junctions, 3, 4f
Timolol, for hemangioma, 420
Tinea
    clinicopathological features, 318, 319f
    epidemiology, 318
    evaluation, 320
    management, 320
    variants, 319t
Tinea barbae, 319t
Tinea capitis, 320–321, 320f
Tinea corporis gladiatorum, 319t
Tinea cruris, 319t
Tinea faciei, 319t
Tinea imbricata, 319t

Tinea incognita, 319t
Tinea manus, 319t
Tinea nigra, 317, 317f
Tinea pedis, 319t
Tinea profunda, 319t
Tinea versicolor, 315–317
   clinicopathological features, 315, 317f
   epidemiology, 315
   evaluation, 315–316
   management, 316–317
Tirbanibulin, 522t
Tissue adhesives, 553–554
Tocilizumab, 137
Tocopherol, 23
Toenails, 14
Tolnaftate, 511t
Toll-like receptors (TLRs), 28, 28t
Tonsillitis, scarlet fever, 290
Topical anesthetics, 547
Topoisomerase inhibitors, 205, 514t
Total skin electron beam therapy (TSEBT), 471
Toxic erythema of chemotherapy (TEC), 120, 120f
Toxic oil syndrome, 133t
Toxic shock syndrome (TSS), 291
Toxoplasmosis, 340t
Traction alopecia, 205
Transient neonatal pustular melanosis, 93, 94t
Transposition flaps, 562, 564, 565
Transverse leukonychia, 212
Transverse nail lines, 212
Traumatic neuroma, 436f
Trench fever, 304
Tretinoin, 498t, 499t
Triangular lunulae, 215f
Triazoles
   for pitted keratolysis, 296
   systemic antifungals, 507
Trichiasis, 106
Trichinosis, 341t
Trichloroacetic acid chemical reconstruction of skin scars (TCA-CROSS) technique, 191
Trichoadenoma, 454t
Trichoblastoma, 458t
Trichodiscoma, 454t
Trichodysplasia spinulosa, 188
Trichoepithelioma, 453, 453f, 454t
Trichofolliculoma, 454t
Tricholemmoma, 411, 455, 456f, 456t
Trichomycosis axillaris, 297t
Trichonodosis, mechanical injury, 361
Trichophyton rubrum, 318
Trichophyton schoenleinii, 320
Trichoptilosis, 361
Trichorrhexis nodosa, 361
Trichoschisis, 361
Trichoscopy, 613, 620t–621t
   alopecia areata (AA), 201
   androgenetic alopecia, 201
   frontal fibrosing alopecia/lichen planopilaris, 206
   hair shaft abnormalities, 622f–623f
   patterns, 623f
   telogen effluvium, 206
   tinea capitis, 320
Trichostasis spinulosa, 188
Trichotillomania, 203, 203f
Trifarotene, 499t

Trigeminal nerve
   motor innervation, 543
   sensory innervation, 542
Tripe palms syndrome, 63
Tropical acne, 190t
Tuberculids, 309
Tuberculoid leprosy, 313, 314f, 315
Tuberculosis, 309, 312
   clinicopathological correlation, 312f
   cutaneous, 309
   variants and tuberculids, 311t
Tuberous sclerosis complex (TSC), 402–403, 402t
Tuberous/tuberoeruptive xanthoma, 236, 238t
Tubular apocrine adenoma, 451t
Tufted angioma, 424–425, 425f
Tularemia, 306t
Tumor necrosis factor alpha (TNFa) inhibitors
   for adult-onset Still disease (AoSD), 137
   biologic and small molecule inhibitors, 493–495
   cutaneous small vessel vasculitis (CSVV), 169
   in dermatomyositis (DM), 127
   eczematous drug eruptions, 66
   erythema nodosum, 144
   for erythema nodosum, 147
   psoriasis, 49
   for pyoderma gangrenosum (PG), 220
   for reactive arthritis, 55
   for rheumatoid arthritis, 137
   sarcoidosis, 226
   for sarcoidosis, 226
   for Stevens-Johnson syndrome/toxic epidermal necrolysis, 118
Tungiasis, 344t
Turner syndrome, 417t
Typhus, 305t, 306t
Tyrosinase, 3

U

Ubiquitin-proteasome pathway, 20
Ulcer
   arterial, 180
   venous, 178–179
Ulceration, wound healing, 35
Ulcerative colitis
   erythema nodosum, 144
   IgA pemphigus, 98
Ulcerative pyoderma gangrenosum, 220
Ulceroglandular differential diagnosis, anthrax, 298
Ulnar nerve block, 548
Ultraviolet radiation, 23, 24t
Umbilical granuloma, 226
Uncombable hair syndrome, 214t
Undecylenic acid, 511t
Unilateral laterothoracic exanthem, 155
Universal hypertrichosis, 211t
μ-opioid receptor agonists, 8
Urachal cyst, 468t
Urea, 502t
Urethritis, 54
Uric acid nephrolithiasis, 245
Uricosuric agents, 245
Urticaria, 32
   clinicopathological features, 152
   differential diagnosis, 152
   epidemiology, 150, 152

   evaluation, 152
   inducible, 151
   management, 152
Urticaria-like follicular mucinosis, 241t
Urticarial vasculitis, 171–172, 173f, 173t
Urticaria pigmentosa, 480, 480t
Usnic acid exposure, contact dermatitis, 70
Ustekinumab, for psoriasis, 53
Uveitis, 84

V

Vaccines, 493, 494t–495t
Vaccinia, 282t
Valacyclovir
   for herpes simplex virus (HSV), 270
   for herpes zoster, 274
Valganciclovir, for cytomegalovirus infection, 276
Valproic acid
   for cutaneous lymphoid hyperplasia (CLH), 476
   for Stevens-Johnson syndrome/toxic epidermal necrolysis, 118
Vancomycin
   for impetigo, 289
   linear immunoglobulin A bullous dermatosis, 105
Varicella, 272–273
Varicosities, stasis dermatitis, 69
Variola vaccine, 495t
Vascular disorders, 158
Vascular endothelial growth factor (VEGF), 7
Vascular lasers, granuloma faciale, 223
Vascular malformations
   angiokeratoma, 412–413
   angiosarcoma, 428–429
   arteriovenous malformation (AVM), 418–419
   capillary malformation (CM), 413–416
   cherry angioma, 424
   glomus tumor, 429–430
   glomuvenous malformation, 429–430
   hemangioma, 419–421
   Kaposiform hemangioendothelioma, 424–425
   Kaposi sarcoma, 426–427
   lymphatic malformation (LM), 417–418
   PHACE(S) and LUMBAR syndrome, 422
   pyogenic granuloma, 423
   tufted angioma, 424–425
   venous malformation (VM), 415–416
Vascular occlusion, 127, 158
Vasculitis, 158
   cutaneous, 161t
   rheumatoid arthritis, 137
Vasculopathy, 158
Vasomotor dysfunction, complex regional pain syndrome (CPRS), 184, 184t
Vasospasm, livedo reticularis, 161, 162
Vectors, 337t, 338f
Vegetative pyoderma gangrenosum, 220
Vellus, 12
Vellus hair cyst, 465t
Venereal bacterial infections, 308
Venous insufficiency, 178–179
   lipodermatosclerosis, 147
   stasis dermatitis, 69
Venous malformation (VM), 415–416
Venous ulcer, 69, 178–179

Verruciform xanthoma, 236, 238t
  epidermolysis bullosa acquisita, 107
  lymphedema, 178
Verrucous lymphangioma circumscriptum, 417–418
Vesicular pityriasis rosea, 57
Vesiculobullous disorders
  acute generalized exanthematous pustulosis, 93–95
  bullous pemphigoid, 102–105
  dermatitis herpetiformis, 107, 110, 110f
  epidermolysis bullosa acquisita (EBA), 107, 108t–109t, 109f
  Grover disease, 102
  Hailey-Hailey disease and Darier disease, 100, 101f, 101t, 102f
  immunoglobulin A (IgA) pemphigus, 98–99, 99f
  immunoglobulin A pemphigus, 98–99
  interface dermatoses, 110–115
  linear immunoglobulin A bullous dermatosis (LABD), 105–106, 106f
  mucous membrane pemphigoid (MMP), 106–107, 106f
  paraneoplastic pemphigus (PNP), 99–100
  pemphigus foliaceus (PF), 96
  pemphigus vulgaris, 96–99
Vestibular dysfunction, relapsing polychondritis, 136
Vibration injury, 362
Vimentin, 7
Vinblastine, for cutaneous T-cell lymphoma (CTCL), 471, 523t
Viral classification and associations, 265, 266t–267t
Viral diseases
  coronavirus disease 2019 (COVID-19), 283–287
  cytomegalovirus infection, 275–276, 276f
  dengue, 284
  eczema herpeticum, 272
  epidermodysplasia verruciformis (EDV), 280, 281f
  erythema infectiosum, 283
  hand-foot-mouth disease (HFMD), 284–285
  herpes simplex, 265, 269–271
  herpes zoster, 273–274
  infectious mononucleosis, 274–275
  molluscum contagiosum, 280, 281, 282f
  rubella, and roseola, 277
  rubeola, 277

  varicella, 272–273
  wart, 278, 278t, 279f, 280
Viral exanthem, 155
Viral infection
  urticaria, 152
Viruses, 265
Visceral leishmaniasis, 334
Vismodegib
  for basal cell carcinoma (BCC), 373
  for basal cell nevus syndrome (BCNS), 374
Vitamin A deficiency, ichthyosis vulgaris, 78
Vitamin B12 deficiencies, 217
Vitamin C, 7f, 86
Vitamin D
  calciphylaxis, 166
  for psoriasis, 53
Vitamin K deficiency, calciphylaxis, 166
Vitiligo, 84–85
  alopecia areata (AA), 200
  clinicopathological features, 84, 84f
  differential diagnosis, 85
  epidemiology, 84
  evaluation, 85
  halo nevus, 391
  management, 85
Vitiligo ponctué, 84
Vitiligo vulgaris, 84
Vogt-Koyanagi-Harada (VHK) syndrome, 84
Vohwinkel syndrome, 60t
Von Hippel-Lindau syndrome, 415t
von Recklinghausen disease, 434
von Willebrand factor, 7
Voriconazole, for cryptococcosis, 329
Vorinostat, 471, 523t
Vörner-Unna-Thost epidermolytic PPK, 60t
Vulvar intraepithelial neoplasia (VIN), 130

W

Wallace lines, 87
Warfarin
  for anticoagulation management, 545
  calciphylaxis risk, 166
Wart, 278, 278t, 279f, 280
  clinicopathological features, 278, 279f
  epidemiology, 278
  evaluation, 280
  management, 280
  variants, 278t
Warty dyskeratoma, 370t
Wasps, 348t

Water exposure injury, 362
Water resistance, 24
Water-resistant sunscreens, 24
Waxy orange-red pityriasis rubra pilaris, 58
Weibel-Palade bodies, 7
Weil-Felix test, 303
Wells syndrome, 224, 224f
White piedra, 318
White sponge nevus, 369
White superficial onychomycosis, 321
Wickham striae, lichen planus (LP), 112
Wilson disease, 247t, 252
Wimberger sign, 309
Witkop tooth and nail syndrome, 199t
Wood's lamp, vitiligo diagnosis, 85
Woronoff ring, 49
Wound closure materials
  staples, 553
  suture, 551, 553–556
  tissue adhesives, 553–554
Wound dressings, 554, 557t
Wound healing process, 35, 36t

X

Xanthine oxidase inhibitors, for gout, 245
Xanthoma, 226, 236–237
  and hyperlipoproteinemia, 239f
  variants, 236, 238t
Xanthoma disseminatum, 235t
Xeroderma pigmentosum, 356, 356t–357t
Xerosis, 67

Y

Yaws, 307t
Yeast, 315
Yellow nail syndrome, 178, 179f

Z

Zika virus, 284
Zinc deficiency, 252, 252t, 255f
Zinsser-Engman-Cole syndrome, 357t
Zonula adherens, 3
Zonula occludens, 3
Zoon balanitis/vulvitis, 361
Zoophilic fungi, 318
Zoster live (ZVL) vaccine, 495t
Zoster recombinant (RZV) vaccine, 494t
Zygomycosis, 332, 332f